ILLUSTRATED DICTIONARY OF IMMUNOLOGY

THIRD EDITION

ILLUSTRATED DICTIONARY OF IMMUNOLOGY

THIRD EDITION

Julius M. Cruse, B.A., B.S., D. Med. Sc., M.D., Ph.D., Dr. *h.c.*,
F.A.A.M., F.R.S.H., F.R.S.M.

Guyton Distinguished Professor
Professor of Pathology
Distinguished Professor of the History of Medicine
Director of Immunopathology and Transplantation Immunology
Director of Graduate Studies in Pathology
Department of Pathology
Associate Professor of Medicine and Associate Professor of Microbiology
University of Mississippi Medical Center
Historian of the American Association of Immunologists
Historian of the American Society for Histocompatibility and Immunogenetics
Jackson, MS

Robert E. Lewis, B.S., M.S., Ph.D., F.R.S.H., F.R.S.M.

Professor of Pathology
Director of Immunopathology and Transplantation Immunology
Department of Pathology
University of Mississippi Medical Center
Jackson, MS

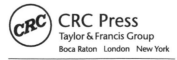

CRC Press
Taylor & Francis Group
Boca Raton   London   New York

CRC Press is an imprint of the
Taylor & Francis Group, an **informa** business

CRC Press
Taylor & Francis Group
6000 Broken Sound Parkway NW, Suite 300
Boca Raton, FL 33487-2742

© 2009 by Taylor & Francis Group, LLC
CRC Press is an imprint of Taylor & Francis Group, an Informa business

First issued in paperback 2019

No claim to original U.S. Government works

ISBN 13: 978-0-367-45245-2 (pbk)
ISBN 13: 978-0-8493-7987-1 (hbk)

Library of Congress Cataloging-in-Publication Data

Cruse, Julius M., 1937-
  Illustrated dictionary of immunology / Julius M. Cruse, Robert E. Lewis. -- 3rd ed.
    p. ; cm.
  ISBN 978-0-8493-7987-1 (hardcover : alk. paper)
  1. Immunology--Dictionaries. I. Lewis, R. E. (Robert Edwin), 1947- II. Title.
  [DNLM: 1. Allergy and Immunology--Dictionary--English. QW 513 C957i 2009]

QR180.4C78 2009
616.07'903--dc22   2008052010

Visit the Taylor & Francis Web site at
http://www.taylorandfrancis.com

and the CRC Press Web site at
http://www.crcpress.com

The Authors

Julius M. Cruse, B.A., B.S., D.Med.Sc., M.D., Ph.D., D.D.H.C. is a Guyton Distinguished Professor, Professor of Pathology, Director of Immunopathology and Transplantation Immunology, Distinguished Professor of the History of Medicine and Director of Graduate Studies in Pathology, Associate Professor of Medicine and Associate Professor of Microbiology. Dr. Cruse formerly was a Professor of Immunology and Biology at the University of Mississippi Graduate School.

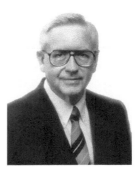

Dr. Cruse earned B.A. and B.S. degrees in chemistry in 1958 from the University of Mississippi. He was a Fulbright Fellow at the University of Graz (Austria) Medical Faculty, where he wrote a thesis on Russian tick-borne encephalitis virus and earned a D. Med. Sc. *summa cum laude* in 1960. On his return to the United States, he entered the M.D.–Ph.D. program at the University of Tennessee College of Medicine, Memphis, completing the M.D. in 1964 and the Ph.D. in pathology (immunopathology) in 1966. Dr. Cruse also trained in pathology at the University of Tennessee Center for the Health Sciences, Memphis.

He is a member of numerous professional societies including the American Association of Immunologists (Historian), the American Society for Investigative Pathology, the American Society for Histocompatibility and Immunogenetics (council member, 1997–1999; former chairman, 1987–1995, member of Publications Committee), the Societé Francaise d'Immunologie, the Transplantation Society, and the Society for Experimental Biology and Medicine, among many others. He is a Fellow of the American Academy of Microbiology, a Fellow of the Royal Society of Health (U.K.) and a Fellow of the Royal Society of Medicine (London). He was named a Doctor of Divinity, *honoris causa*, in 1999 by The General Theological Seminary of the Episcopal Church, New York City.

Dr. Cruse's research has centered on transplantation and tumor immunology, autoimmunity, MHC genetics in the pathogenesis of AIDS, neuroendocrine immune interactions, and Toll-like receptors. He has received many research grants during his career, including 12 years of support from the Wilson Research Foundation for investigation of neuroendocrine–immune system interactions in spinal cord injury patients. He is the author of more than 275 publications in scholarly journals and 45 books, and has directed dissertation and thesis research for more than 40 graduate students. He is editor-in-chief of the international *Immunologic Research, Experimental and Molecular Pathology* and *Transgenics* journals and served as chief editor of *Pathobiology* from 1982–1998 and founded the *Immunologic Research, Transgenics* and *Pathobiology* journal.

Robert E. Lewis, B.A., M.S., Ph.D. is a Professor of Pathology and Director of Immunopathology and Transplantation Immunology in the Department of Pathology at the University of Mississippi Center in Jackson. He earned a B.A. and M.S. in microbiology and a Ph.D. in pathology (immunopathology) from the University of Mississippi. Following specialty post-doctoral training at several medical institutions, Dr. Lewis rose through the academic ranks from Instructor to Professor at the University of Mississippi Medical Center.

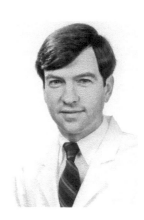

Dr. Lewis is a member of numerous professional societies including the American Association of Immunologists, the American Society for Investigative Pathology, the Society for Experimental Biology and Medicine, the American Society for Microbiology, the Canadian Society for Immunology, the American Society for Histocompatibility and Immunogenetics (member of board of directors, council member and chairman of Publications Committee), and other scientific organizations. He is a Fellow of the Royal Society of Health of Great Britain and a Fellow of the Royal Society of Medicine (U.K.). Dr. Lewis has been the recipient of a number of research grants in his career, including 12 years of support funded by the Wilson Research Foundation for his research on neuroendocrine–immune system interactions in spinal cord injury patients. His current research focuses on post-transplant monitoring and antibody identification.

Dr. Lewis has authored or co-authored more than 140 papers and 150 abstracts and has made numerous scientific presentations at national and international conferences. In addition to his work on neuroendocrine–immune interactions, his current research involves immunogenetics aspects of AIDS progression. Dr. Lewis is a founder, senior editor and deputy editor-in-chief of *Immunologic Research* and *Transgenics* and is senior editor and deputy editor-in-chief of *Experimental and Molecular Pathology*. He served as senior editor and deputy editor-in-chief of *Pathobiology* from 1982–1998.

Preface

The splendid reception of the first and second editions of this book convinced both the authors and the publisher to prepare a third edition. The 13 years since this dictionary first appeared have witnessed an exponential increase in immunological information emanating from a plethora of journals devoted to the subject. The *Journal of Immunology* is published twice monthly in an effort to accommodate an ever-increasing demand for immunological information among researchers that spans all fields of biomedicine. Besides the unprecedented advances in knowledge of cell receptors and signal transduction pathways, an avalanche of new information has been gleaned from contemporary research on immunoregulatory cytokines such as IL17 and chemokines and their receptors, with special reference to their structures and functions.

The present edition has not only been thoroughly updated but also contains multiple new entries covering immunopharmacology, newly described interleukins, comparative immunology, immunity to infectious diseases, and expansion of definitions in all of the immunological subspecialties. Thus, the reader is provided in a single volume information that would otherwise require an entire library of books on immunology to decipher. Some definitions are brief, others are more extensive; all are concise and provide thorough understandings of basic immunological concepts that often intersect the purview of other basic and clinical scientific disciplines. This book is designed to provide the most up-to-date and thorough vocabulary of immunological terms available in the complex science of immunology. It contains approximately 1200 illustrations that depict essentially every concept of importance in understanding the subject of immunology. From the beginning, immunologists developed and maintained a unique nomenclature that has often mystified and even baffled colleagues in other fields, causing them to liken immunology to a "black box." This book is designed to offer immunologists and nonimmunologists alike, including students, researchers, practitioners, and basic biomedical scientists, a resource for information about many terms encountered in contemporary immunological literature.

Simple illustrations clarify the explanations and enhance the terms and concepts described. A host of new illustrations of interleukins, cellular adhesion molecules, and other concepts is presented in a manner that facilitates better understanding of their roles in intercellular and immune reactions. Illustrated definitions that are pertinent to all of the immunological subspecialties such as transplantation, autoimmunity, immunophysiology, immunopathology, antigen presentation, and T cell and B cell receptors, to name a few, may be found in this dictionary. Individuals who need ready access to concise definitions and visual images of immunological concepts will want this book to be readily available on their bookshelves. No other book provides in one place the breadth or detail of illustrated immunological concepts as may be found in this third edition of the *Illustrated Dictionary of Immunology*. The subject matter ranges from molecular structures of recently characterized receptors and cytokines to major histocompatibility complex molecules, immunoglobulins, comparative immunology, and immunopathology, to name a few of the categories of information included.

Some of the diagrams illustrate basic concepts; others are designed for specialists interested in more detailed treatments of the subject matter of immunology. The eclectic science of immunology intersects essentially all basic biomedical and clinical sciences. If immunology becomes meaningful and demystified to readers, the effort in preparing a third edition of this book will have been well spent.

Acknowledgments

Although many individuals have offered help and suggestions in the preparation of this book, several deserve special mention. We are very grateful to Dr. Steven Bigler, Chairman of the Department of Pathology, University of Mississippi Medical Center, Jackson, for his genuine interest and generous support of our academic endeavors at this institution.

Dr. Fredrick H. Shipkey, Professor Emeritus of Pathology at the University of Mississippi Medical Center, provided valuable assistance in selecting and photographing appropriate surgical pathology specimens to illustrate immunological lesions. We express genuine appreciation to Dr. Edwin and Dr. Marsha Eigenbrodt for many photomicrographs. We thank Dr. Virginia Lockard for providing the electron micrographs that appear in the book. We also thank Dr. Robert Peace for allowing us access to a case of Job's syndrome, Dr. Ray Shenefelt for the photomicrograph of cytomegalovirus, Dr. Jonathan Fratkin for photomicrographs of eye and muscle pathology, Dr. C. J. Chen for VKH photos, Dr. Howard Shulman for GVH photos, Dr. David DeBauche for providing an illustration of the Philadelphia chromosome, and Mrs. Dorothy Whitcomb for the history photos. We also thank Dr. G. Reid Bishop of Mississippi College for his generous contributions of molecular models of cytokines and other configurations critical to immunology.

We express genuine appreciation to Ms. Julia Peteet and Mrs. Jeanann Lovell Suggs for their dedicated efforts in helping us to complete this publication in a timely manner and making valuable editorial contributions. We are very grateful for the assistance of our contributing editors Josh Goodin, Brad Suggs, and Will Singleterry, as well as our contributor Rachel Webb. We appreciate the constructive criticisms of Patsy Foley, B.S., M.T., C.H.T., C.H.S., Jay Holliday, B.S., M.T., C.H.T., John Coker, B.S., M.T., C.H.T., Josh Hammons, B.S., M.T., C.H.T., Wendy Thomson, C.H.S., Angie Bond, B.S., M.T., C.H.T., Maxine Crawford, B.S., C.H.T., and Susan Touchstone, B.S., M.T., S.B.B., C.H.T., C.H.S. We thank William Buhner for scanning selected figures. We are most grateful to Joanna Arentz, of R&D Corporation, for sharing with us a number of diagrams of immunological molecules and concepts owned by R&D. It is a pleasure to also express our genuine gratitude to INOVA Diagnostics, Inc. for permitting us to use its photomicrographs of immunological concepts. We would also like to commend the individuals at Taylor & Francis Group: Barbara Ellen Norwitz, Executive Editor; Pat Roberson, Production Coordinator; Amy Rodriguez, Project Editor; Jonathan Pennell, Art Director; Scott Hayes, Prepress Manager; and all members of their staff for their professionalism and unsparing efforts to bring this book to publication. To these individuals, we offer our grateful appreciation.

Special thanks are expressed to Dr. Daniel W. Jones, Dean of Medicine and Vice Chancellor for Health Affairs, University of Mississippi Medical Center, for his unstinting support of our research endeavors.

Illustration Credits

Figure for C1 redrawn from Arlaud GJ, Colomb MG, Gagnon J. A functional model of the human C1 complex. *Immunology Today,* 8, 107–109, 1987.

Figure for normal adult thymus reprinted from *Atlas of Tumor Pathology*, 2nd Series, Fascicle 13. Armed Forces Institute of Pathology.

Figures for the normal thymus reprinted from *Atlas of Tumor Pathology,* 3rd Series, Fascicle 21. Armed Forces Institute of Pathology.

Figures for Mac-1, CD22, CD42, subcapsular sinus lymph node, CD21, CD4, CD8, structure of CD1, structure of CD4, structure of CD8, ribbon structure of a CD8[+] T cell receptor, structure of CD5 and the structure of CD45 redrawn from *The Leukocyte Antigen Facts Book,* Academic Press, Orlando, FL, 1993.

Figures for synthetic polypeptide antigen with multichain copolymer, complement receptor, complexes on the surface of B cells, orthotopic graft, and oncofetal antigen redrawn from Bellanti JA. *Immunology II.* WB Saunders, Philadelphia, 1978.

Figure for antigen presentation, Bjorkman PJ, Saper MA, Samroui B, Bennet WS, Strominger JL, Wiley DC. Structure of the human class I histocompatibility antigen, HLA-A2. *Nature,* 329, 506–512, 1987 (Macmillan Magazines, Ltd). Reprinted courtesy of Nature Publishing Group.

Figures for mechanism of γ-globulin protection for catabolism, Brambell FWR, Hemmings WA, Morris IG. A theoretical model of gammaglobulin catabolism. *Nature*, 203, 1352–1355, 1964. (Macmillan Magazines, Ltd). Reprinted courtesy of Nature Publishing Group.

Figure for vitronectin courtesy of Mike Clark, PhD, Division of Immunology, Cambridge University, 2000.

Figure for Wu-Kabat plot, Kelvin GV, Capra JD, Edmundson AB. The antibody-combining site. *Scientific American,* 236, 50–43, 1977. Reprinted with permission from GV Kelvin.

Figure for F(ab)$_2$ fragment portions reprinted courtesy of Dr. Leon Carayannopoulos, Department of Microbiology, University of Texas Southwestern Medical School, Dallas, TX.

Figure for FcRII, Conrad DH, Keegan AD, Kalli KR, Van Dusen R, Rao M, Levine AD. Superinduction of low affinity IgE receptors on murine B lymphocytes by LPS and interleukin-4. *Journal of Immunology*, 141:1091–1097, 1988. Reprinted with permission.

Figure for Philadelphia chromosome, Cotran RS, Kumar V, Robbins SL. *Robbins Pathologic Basis of Disease.* WB Saunders, Philadelphia, 1989. Reprinted with permission.

Figure for Heymann glomerulonephritis, Cotran RS, Kumar V, Robbins SL. *Robbins Pathologic Basis of Disease.* WB Saunders, Philadelphia, 1989. Reprinted with permission.

Figures for schematic representation of CcEe and D polypeptide topology within the erythrocyte membrane; schematic representation of the biosynthetic pathways of ABH, Lewis and XY antigens; the Duffy blood group, *Human Blood Groups*, Daniels G. Blackwell Scientific, Oxford, UK, 1995. Reprinted with permission.

Figures for structure of CD3/TCR complex, Davis M. T cell receptor gene diversity and selection, *Annual Review of Biochemistry*, 59: 477, 1990. Reprinted with permission.

Figure for lymphocyte scanning electron micrograph, Deutsch M, Weinreb A. Apparatus for high-precision repetitive sequential optical measurement of lifting cells. *Cytometry*, 16: 214–226, 1994. Reprinted with permission.

Figure for preliminary three-dimensional structure of human interferon (recombinant form) redrawn from Ealick SE, Cook WJ, Vijay-Kumar S. Three-dimensional structure of recombinant human interferon. *Science*, 252: 698–702, 1991. Reprinted with permission, American Association for the Advancement of Science.

Figure for Langmuir plot redrawn from *Immunology*, Eisen H. Lippincott-Raven, New York, 1974, pp. 371, 373.

Figure for Elek plate redrawn from *Staphlococcus pyogenes and Its Relation to Disease*, Elek SD. E&S Livingstone, Edinburgh and London, 1959.

Figures for lymphocytes, small lymphocytes, plasma cell, macrophage-histiocyte inbone marrow, eosinophil, basophil, monocyte, polymorphonuclear neutrophil, lymph nodes, spleen, Peyer's patches, tonsil, Hassall's corpuscle, and renal rejection descriptions compliments of Marsha L Eigenbrodt, MD, MPH and Edwin H Eigenbrodt, MD.

Figure for abzyme (adapted), Haver E, Quartermous T, Matsueda GR, Runge MS. Innovative approaches to plasminogen activator therapy. *Science*, 243: 52–56, 1989. Reprinted with permission, American Association for the Advancement of Science.

Figure of photomicrograph of immunoglobulin light "staining" by immunoperoxidase, Harris LJ, Larson SE, Hasel KW, Day J, Greenwood, McPherson A. The three-dimensional structure of an intact monoclonal antibody for canine lymphoma, *Nature* 360: 369–372, 1992 (Macmillan Magazines, Ltd). Reprinted courtesy of Nature Publishing Group.

Figure of Paul Ehrlich, photograph courtesy of the Cruse collection; adapted from Hemmelweit F, *Collected Papers of Paul Ehrlich*, Pergamon Press, Tarrytown, NY, 1956–1960.

Figures for immunochromatography and absorption chromatography redrawn from *Practical Immunology*, Hudson L, Hay FC. Blackwell Scientific, Cambridge, MA, 1989.

Figures for CTLA-4, IL-6, IL-4, TNF-, GM-CSF, HIV-1 virus structure, LFA-1, streptococcal M protein, Fc domain of IgG, IFN-receptor, IL-1 receptor, CRP, IL-5, IL-6, cytokine receptor families, CTLA-4, IL-4 receptor, IFNs, IL-2, TGF-, Bence-Jones protein, myelin autoantibodies, TCR, CD2, VCAM-1, CD32, IL-10, IL-8, NCAM-11, B cell antigen receptor, IL-1 receptor, IL-10, and mannose receptor generated from Humphrey W, Dalke A, Schulten K. VMD: Visual Molecular Dynamics, *Journal of Molecular Graphics*, 14.1: 33–38, 1996.

Figure of the immunoglobulin superfamily redrawn from Hunkapillar T, Hood L. Diversity of the immunoglobulin gene superfamily, *Advances in Immunology,* 44, 1–63, 1989. Reprinted with permission from Elsevier.

Figure for plasma cell, immunoglobulin gene schematic, binding of Factor I to C3b adapted from Lachman PJ. *Clinical Aspects of Immunology.* Blackwell Scientific Publications, Cambridge, MA, 1993.

Figure for vitronectin courtesy of Mike Clark, PhD, Division of Immunology, Cambridge University.

Figure for HLA-DM, *Immunobiology: The Immune System in Health and Disease,* 3rd edition, Janeway CA, Jr. Travers P. pp. 4–5, 1997. Reprinted with permission from Elsevier.

The Protein Data Bank, Worldwide Protein Data Bank: Figures for CD2, ICAM-2, MIP-1, P-selectin, class I HLA molecule, CD8, Fc(IgG) receptor, FC(RI), CD4, CD4 domains 3 and 4, CD4 type I crystal form, CD8 receptor (ribbon and space-filling models), chain of TCR, human IL-1 converting enzyme, IL-1 receptor antagonist protein, human IL-4, human IL-8, IL-10, IL-13, TNF receptor, human macrophage colony-stimulating factor, IGFs, human TGF-α, leukemia inhibitory factor, IgG/gp120 complex, HIV-1 protease, HIV-1 reverse transcriptase, cyclosporine A bound to cyclophilin A, FKBP12-rapamycin, human recombinant form of FK506, rapamycin-binding protein expressed in *Escherichia coli,* HLA-0201, HLA-DR1, HLA peptide from calreticulin HLA-A 0201, HLA-DR1, HLA-B*2705 complexed with Arg-Arg-Ile-Lys-Ala-Ile-Thr-Leu-Lys (theoretical model), SV-40, Abrin-A, type 3 Sabin strain human poliovirus, hepatitis A virus 3C proteinase, influenza A subtype N2 neuraminidase, influenza B/LEE/40 neuraminidase: Abola E, Bernstein FC, Bryant SH, Koetzle TF, Weng J. *Crystallographic Databases-Information Content, Software Systems, Scientific Applications* (Allen FH, Bergerhoff G, Wievers R, Eds). Data Commission of the International Union of Crystallography, Bonn/Cambridge/Chester, 1987. Bernstein FC et al. The protein data bank: A computer-based archival file for macromolecular structures, *Journal of Molecular Biology,* 112: 535–542, 1977.

The Protein Data Bank, Worldwide Protein Data Bank: Structural image of a cytokine/receptor complex, x-ray diffraction image of IL-6 (beta sign) chain. Research Collaboratory for Structural Bioinformatics, 2003. Berman HM, Westbrook J, Feng Z, Gilliland G, Bhat TN, Weissing H, Shindyalov IN, Bourne PE. *The Protein Data Bank Nucleic Acids Research,* 2000. pp. 235–242.

Figure for Brambell receptor, Raghaven M et al. Analysis of the pH dependence of the neonatal Fc receptor/immunoglobulin G interaction using antibody and receptor variants. *Biochemistry* 34(14): 649–756, 1995 (American Chemical Society) and Junghans RP. Finally, the Brambell receptor (FcRB), *Immunologic Research* 16: 29–57, 1995.

Figure of CD16 (redrawn), Ravetch JV, Klinet JP. Fc receptors. *Annual Review of Immunology* 9: 462, 1991.

Figure of CD59 (redrawn), Rooney LA, Oblesby TJ, Atkinson JP. Complement in human reproduction: Activation and control. *Immunologic Research,* 12(3): 276–294, 1993.

Figures of schematic structures of adhesions molecules. Monoclonal Antiadhesion Molecules, presented by Seigaku Corp. November 8, 1994.

Figures for graft-vs-host disease (GVHD) and venooclusive disease (VOD) compliments of Dr Howard Shulman, Professor of Pathology, University of Washington, Member Fred Hutchinson Cancer Research Center.

Figure of *Listeria,* Tilney LG, Portnoy DA. Actin filaments and the growth, movement, and spread of the intracellular bacterial parasite, *Listeria monocytogenes. Journal of Cell Biology,* 109 (4 Pt 1): 1597–1608, 1989. With permission of the Rockefeller University Press.

Figures of type 2 "pale" and type 6 "large medullary" epithelial cells, van Wijingaert FP, Kendall MD, Schuurman HJ, Rademakers LH, Kater L. Heterogeneity of epithelial cells in the human thymus, an ultrastructural study. *Cell and Tissue Research* 237(2): 227–237, 1984.

Figures of *Psoriasis vulgaris* and relapsing polychondritis. *Immunofluorescent Patterns in Skin Diseases,* Valenquela R, Bergfeld WF, Deodhar SD. American Society of Clinical Pathologists Press, Chicago, IL, 1984.

Figures of schematic representations of membrane glycoproteins and blycosphingolipids that carry blood group antigens adapted from *Technical Manual,* 12th edition, Vengelen-Tyler V (Ed), American Association of Blood Banks, Bethesda, MD 1996, pp. 231, 282.

Figures of L Gillray cowpox cartoon, Lady Mary Wortly Montagu, Edward Jenner, Robert Koch, Svante Arrhenius, side-chain theory, Karl Landsteiner, Almorth Edward Wright, Carl Prausnitz-Giles, Elvin Abraham Kabat, Henry Hallett Dale, John Richardson Marrack, Hans Zinsser, Max Thieler, Gregory Shwartzman, Robin R.A. Coombs, Albert Hewett Coons, Ernest Witebsky, Peter Alfred Gorer, Peter Brian Medawar, Ray David Owen, Frank James Dixon, Niels Kaj Jerne, David Wilson Talmage, Frank MacFarlane Burnet, George Davis Snell, Astrid Elsa Fagraeus-Wallbom, Rosalyn Sussman Yalow, J.F.A.P. Miller, James Gowans, Rodney Robert Porter, Richard K. Gershon, Kimishige Ishizaka, Terako Ishizaka, Georges J.F. Köler, Cesar Milstein, and Susumu Tonegawa reprinted from *Immunology to 1980,* an illustrated bibliography of titles in the Middleton Health Sciences Library, which includes The Julius M Cruse Collection, Dorothy Whitcomb, editor and compiler. University of Wisconsin Center of Health Sciences, Madison, WI, 1985.

Figure of Rolf Zinkernagel and Peter Doherty courtesy of Dr Rolf Zinkernagel, Institute of Pathology, University of Zurich.

Multiple figures of caspases, apoptosis, fas, Il-23, chemokines, eph family, integrins, MCP-1, immunotoxin, SODD, VEGF and eotaxin depicted in numerous schematic representations provided through the generosity of R&D Systems; *Cytokine* bulletins, 1998–2001.

Figures for Retrovir® (zivdovudine), Epivir® (lamivudine), Ziagen® (abacavir sulfate), and Combivir® (zidovudine/lamivudine) courtesy of GlaxoWellcome.

Figure for Sustiva® (efavirenz capsules) courtesy of DuPont Pharma.

Figure for Viracept® (nelfinavir mesylate) courtesy of Agouron Pharmaceuticals.

Figure for Videx® (didanosine) courtesy of Bristol-Myers Squibb Onc/Imm.

Figure for Viramune® (nevirapine) courtesy of Roxane Laboratories.

Figure for Norvir® (ritonavir capsules) courtesy of Abbott Laboratories.

Figures for AMA, cANCA, pANCA, aANCA, centromere, crithidia, EMA, GBM, keratin, LKM, pemphigoid, and pemphigus courtesy of INOVA Diagnostics, Inc.

Special appreciation is expressed to Becton, Dickinson and Company (BD)BiosciencesPharmingen, San Diego, CA for permission to reproduce their mouse CD chart and the BD Biosciences Official Poster of the 8th International Workshop on Human Leukocyte Differentiation Antigens.

α -1 antichymotrypsin

A histiocytic marker. By immunoperoxidase staining, it is demonstrable in tumors derived from histiocytes. It may also be seen in various carcinomas.

α-1 antitrypsin (A1AT)

A glycoprotein in circulating blood that blocks trypsin, chymotrypsin, and elastase, among other enzymes. The gene on chromosome 14 encodes 25 separate allelic forms that differ according to electrophoretic mobility. The PiMM phenotype is physiologic. The PiZZ phenotype is the most frequent form of the deficiency, which is associated with emphysema, cirrhosis, hepatic failure, and cholelithiasis, with an increased incidence of hepatocellular carcinoma. It is treated with prolastin. Adenoviruses may be employed to transfer the A1AT gene to lung epithelial cells, after which A1AT mRNA and functioning A1AT become demonstrable.

abatacept

A recombinant fusion protein comprised of the extracellular domain of cytotoxic T-lymphocyte-associated antigen 4 (CTLA-4) fused with human IgG Fc. CTLA-4 is a costimulatory molecule of T cells that unites with CD80 and CD86 on antigen presenting cells. A selective costimulation modulator, abatacept blocks activation of T cells by binding to CD80 and CD86, thereby interfering with the interaction with CD28, a costimulatory signal requisite for full T lymphocyte activation, implicated in the pathogenisis of rheumatoid arthritis (RA). Activated T cells are present in the synovial of RA patients. *In vitro*, abatacept diminishes T cell proliferation and blocks the synthesis of the cytokines TNF-α, interferon-γ, and IL-2. In a rat arthritis model, abatacept diminishes inflammation, decreases anti-collagen antibody production, and reduces antigen-specific synthesis of interferon-γ. It is used for the treatment of severe rheumatoid arthritis.

A blood group

Refer to ABO blood group system.

ABO blood group antigen

Glycosphingolipid epitopes on erythrocytes and numerous other types of cells. These antigens are governed by alleles that encode enzymes needed for their synthesis. They differ among individuals and may serve as alloantigens that lead to hyperacute rejection of allografts and to blood transfusion reactions.

α chain

The immunoglobulin (Ig) class-determining heavy chain found in IgA molecules.

adalimumab

A human IgG₁ molecule used in the treatment of rheumatoid arthritis that blocks the interaction of TNF-α with TNF receptors on cell surfaces but fails to bind with TNF-β. It diminishes levels of C-reactive protein, erythrocyte sedimentation rate, IL-6 in serum, and matrix metalloproteinases MMP-1 and MMP-3. *In vitro*, it causes lysis of cells that express TNF-α when complement is present. It has a serum half-life of 2 weeks. Adalimumab binds specifically to TNF-α and inhibits its interaction with the p55 and p75 cell surface TNF receptors. It lyses surface cells *in vitro* in the presence of complement. It fails to bind or inactivate lymphotoxin (TNF-β). TNF is a naturally occurring cytokine that is involved in inflammatory and immune responses. Levels are elevated in synovial fluid in rheumatoid arthritis and psoriatic arthritis, where it plays a significant part in the inflammatory reaction and joint destruction that are hallmarks of the disease.

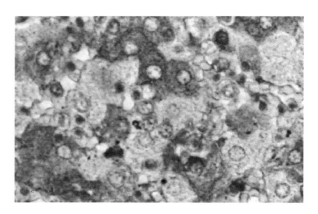

α-Fetoprotein.

α-fetoprotein

A principal plasma protein in the α globulin fraction present in the fetus. It bears considerable homology with human serum albumin. It is produced by the embryonic yolk sac and fetal liver and consists of a 590-amino acid residue polypeptide chain structure. It may be elevated in pregnant women bearing fetuses with open neural tube defects, central nervous system defects, gastrointestinal abnormalities, immunodeficiency syndromes, and various other abnormalities. After parturition, the high levels in fetal serum diminish to levels that cannot be detected. α-fetoprotein induces immunosuppression, which may facilitate neonatal tolerance. Based on *in vitro* studies, it is believed to facilitate suppressor T lymphocyte function and diminish helper T lymphocyte action. Liver cancer patients reveal significantly elevated serum levels of α-fetoprotein. In immunology, however, it is used as a marker of selected tumors such as hepatocellular carcinoma. It is detected by the avidin–biotin–peroxidase complex (ABC) immunoperoxidase technique using monoclonal antibodies.

α heavy chain disease

A rare condition in individuals of Mediterranean extraction who may develop gastrointestinal lymphoma and malabsorption with loss of weight and diarrhea. The aberrant plasma cells infiltrating the lamina propria of the intestinal mucosa and the mesenteric lymph nodes synthesize α chains alone, usually α-1, with no production of light chains. Even though the end-terminal sequences are intact, a sequence stretching from the V region through much of the Ca-1 domain is deleted. Thus, there is no cysteine residue to crosslink light chains. α heavy chain disease is more frequent than the γ type. It has been described in North Africa, in the Near East and Mediterranean areas, and in some regions of southern Europe. Rare cases have been reported in the United States. The condition may prove fatal, even though remissions may follow antibiotic therapy.

α helix

A spiral or coiled structure present in many proteins and polypeptides. It is defined by intrachain hydrogen bonds between –CO and –NH groups that hold the polypeptide chain together in a manner that results in 3.6 amino acid residues per helical turn. There is a 1.5 Å rise for each residue. The helix has a pitch of 5.4 Å. The helical backbone is formed by a peptide group and the α carbon. Hydrogen bonds link each –CO group to the –NH group of the fourth residue forward in the chain. The α helix may be left or right handed. Right-handed α helices are the ones found in proteins.

α2 macroglobulin (α₂M)

A 725-kDa plasma glycoprotein that plays a major role in inhibition of proteolytic activity generated during various extracellular processes. α_2M is synthesized in the liver and reticuloendothelial system. α_2M is produced by lymphocytes and is found associated with the surface membranes of a subpopulation of B cells. It has the unique property of binding all active endopeptidases. Other enzymes or even the inactive forms of proteinases are not bound. Complexes of α_2M with proteinase are rapidly cleared from circulation (in minutes), in contrast to the turnover of α_2M that requires several days. Some of the roles of α_2M include: (1) regulation of the extracellular proteolytic activity resulting from clotting, fibrinolysis, and proteinases of inflammation; and (2) specific activity against some proteinases of fungal or bacterial origin. It is elevated significantly in nephrotic syndrome. Increased levels have also been reported in atopic dermatitis and ataxia telangiectasia.

α1-microglobulin

A 30-kDa protein that belongs to the lipocalin family and possesses hydrophobic prosthetic groups. It is synthesized in the liver and is present in the urine and serum. α_1M may be complexed with monomeric IgA and may be increased in IgA nephropathy. Elevated serum α_1M in patients with acquired immune deficiency syndrome (AIDS) may signify renal pathology. α_1M blocks antigen stimulation and migration of granulocytes, plays a role in immunoregulation, and functions as a mitogen.

α2-plasmin inhibitor–plasmin complex (α₂PIPC)

Complex formed by the combination of α_2-PI or α_2-macroglobulin with plasmin, the active principle in fibrinolysis. These complexes are found in elevated quantities in plasma of systemic lupus erythematosus (SLE) patients with vasculitis compared to plasma of SLE patients without vasculitis.

AA amyloid

A nonimmunoglobulin amyloid fibril of the type seen following chronic inflammatory diseases such as tuberculosis and osteomyelitis or, more recently, chronic noninfectious

inflammatory disorders. Kidneys, liver, and spleen are the most significant areas of amyloid-associated (AA) deposition. The precursor for AA protein is apo-SAA (serum amyloid associated), which has a monomer mol wt of 12.5 kDa and is found in the circulation as a 220- to 235-kDa molecular complex because it is linked to high density lipoproteins. Interleukin-6 stimulates its synthesis. AA deposition is either associated with an amyloidogenic isotypical form of SAA or results from the inability to completely degrade SAA. Amyloid consists of nonbranching fibrils 7.5 to 10 nm in width and of indefinite length. Chemically, amyloid occurs in two classes. The AL (amyloid light) chain type consists of immunoglobulin light chains or parts of them. The AA type is derived from the SAA protein in the serum. SAA acts like an acute phase reactant, increasing greatly during inflammation. Thus, AA protein is the principal type of amyloid deposited in chronic inflammatory diseases. AL amyloid consists of either whole immunoglobulin light chains or their N-terminal fragments, or a combination of the two. The λ light chain especially gives rise to AL. AL amyloid protein is often deposited following or during B cell disorders. Other biochemical forms of amyloid include transthyretin, β_2 microglobulin, and β_2 amyloid protein, among others. Amyloid filaments stained with Congo red exhibit green birefringence with polarized light.

AB blood group

Refer to ABO blood group system.

ABC method

A unique immunoperoxidase procedure for localizing a variety of histologically significant antigens and other markers. The procedure employs biotinylated antibody and a preformed avidin–biotinylated enzyme complex and has been termed the "ABC" technique. Because avidin has such an extraordinarily high affinity for biotin, the binding of avidin to biotin is essentially irreversible. In addition, avidin has four binding sites for biotin, and most proteins including enzymes can be conjugated with several molecules of biotin. These properties allow macromolecular complexes (ABCs) to be formed between avidin and biotinylated enzymes.

αβ T cell receptor (αβ TCR)

The structure on both CD4+ and CD8+ T lymphocytes that recognizes peptide antigen presented in the context of a major histocompatibility complex (MHC) molecule. The variable (V) regions of both α and β chains comprise the antigen binding site. The αβ TCR also contains constant (C) regions. There is structural homology between TCR V and C regions and the corresponding regions of an immunoglobulin molecule. The αβ TCR is the most common form of T cell receptor, accounting for approximately 95% of T cells in human blood, with γδ TCR comprising the remaining 5%.

αβ T cells

T lymphocytes that express αβ chain heterodimers on their surfaces. The vast majority of T cells are of the αβ variety. Their antigen receptor is comprised of α and β polypeptide chains. This population, to which most T cells belong, includes all those that recognize peptide antigen presented by major histocompatibility complex (MHC) class I and class II molecules.

αβ TCR checkpoint

The second principal checkpoint in development of T cells. Positive selection of DP thymocytes that manifest a T cell

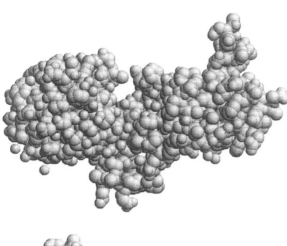

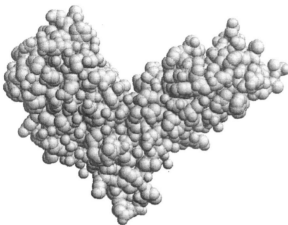

β Chain of a T cell antigen receptor of a mouse.

receptor that is totally functional facilitates the survival of thymocyte clones that identify self-MHC alleles with moderate avidity. Autoreactive thymocyte clones are deleted by negative selection.

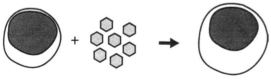

Immature B cell　Abelson murine leukemia virus (A-MuLV) bearing the v-abl oncogene　Tumor B cell clones corresponding to earlier stages in B cell development (i.e., Pre-B cells)

Abelson murine leukemia virus.

Abelson murine leukemia virus (A-MuLV)

A B cell murine leukemia-inducing retrovirus that bears the v-*abl* oncogene. The virus has been used to immortalize immature B lymphocytes to produce pre-B cells or less differentiated B cell lines in culture. These have been useful in unraveling the nature of immunoglobulin differentiation, such as heavy- and light-chain immunoglobulin gene assembly, as well as class switching of immunoglobulin.

ablastin

An antibody with the exclusive property of preventing reproduction of such agents as the rat parasite *Trypanosoma lewisi*. It does not demonstrate other antibody functions.

ABO antigens

Refer to ABO blood group substances.

ABO blood group substances

Glycopeptides with oligosaccharide side chains manifesting ABO epitopes of the same specificity as those present on red blood cells of the individual in whom they are detected. Soluble ABO blood group substances may be found in such mucous secretions of humans as saliva, gastric juice, ovarian cyst fluid, etc. Such persons are termed secretors, whereas those without the blood group substances in their secretions are nonsecretors. ABO blood group differences between donor and recipient can lead to hyperacute graft rejection as well as serious blood transfusion reactions.

ABO blood group system

The first described of the human blood groups based upon carbohydrate alloantigens present on red cell membranes. Anti-A or anti-B isoagglutinins (alloantibodies) are present only in the blood sera of individuals not possessing that specificity; that is, anti-A is found in the sera of group B individuals, and anti-B is found in the sera of group A individuals. This serves as the basis for grouping humans into phenotypes designated A, B, AB, and O. Type AB subjects possess neither anti-A nor anti-B antibodies, whereas group O persons have both anti-A and anti-B antibodies in their serum. Blood group methodology to determine the ABO blood type makes use of the agglutination reaction. The ABO system remains the most important in the transfusion of blood and is also critical in organ transplantation. Epitopes of the ABO system are found on oligosaccharide terminal sugars. The genes designated A/B, Se, H, and Le govern the formation of these epitopes and of the Lewis (Le) antigens. The two precursor substances type I and type II differ only in that the terminal galactose is joined to the penultimate *N*-acetylglucosamine in the b 1–3 linkage in type I chains, but in the b 1–4 linkage in type II chains.

aboriginal mouse

An animal that has lived apart from humans.

abortive infection

A condition in which a pathogen is able to enter the body but is unable to propagate.

abrin

A powerful toxin and lectin used in immunological research by Paul Ehrlich (*circa* 1900). It is extracted from the seeds of the jequirity plant and causes agglutination of erythrocytes.

absorption

The elimination of antibodies from a mixture by adding soluble antigens or the elimination of soluble antigens from a mixture by adding antibodies.

absorption elution test

Identification of the ABO type in semen or blood stains on clothing. ABO blood group antibodies are applied to the stain after it has been exposed to boiling water. Following washing to remove unfixed antibody, the preparation is heated to 56°C in physiological saline. An antibody that may be eluted from the stain is tested with erythrocytes of known ABO specificity to determine the ABO type. This technique is being replaced by DNA analysis of such specimens by forensics experts.

ABVD chemotherapy

A therapeutic cocktail comprised of adriamycin (doxorubicin), bleomycin, vinblastine, and dacarbazine.

A

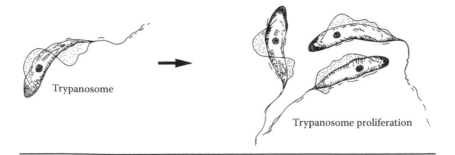

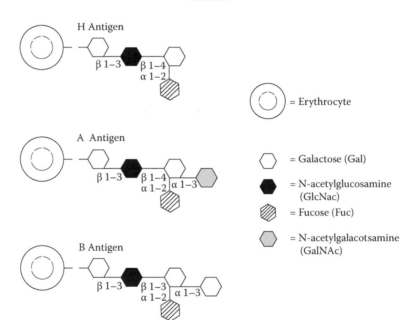

Ablastin.

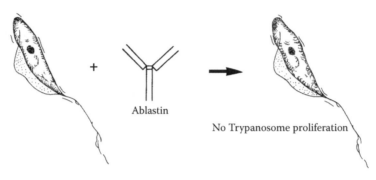

( ) = Erythrocyte

⬡ = Galactose (Gal)

⬣ = N-acetylglucosamine (GlcNac)

▨ = Fucose (Fuc)

⬡ = N-acetylgalacotsamine (GalNAc)

Chemical structures of A, B, and H antigens of the ABO blood group system.

abzyme

The union of antibody and enzyme molecules to form a hybrid catalytic molecule. Specificity for a target antigen is provided through the antibody portion and for a catalytic function through the enzyme portion. Thus, these molecules have numerous potential uses. They are capable of catalyzing various chemical reactions and show great promise as protein-clearing antibodies, as in the dissolution of fibrin clots from occluded coronary arteries in myocardial infarction.

acanthosis nigricans

A condition in which the afflicted subject develops insulin receptor autoantibodies associated with insulin-resistant diabetes mellitus, as well as thickened and pigmented skin.

accessory cell

A cell such as a dendritic or Langerhans' cell, monocyte, or macrophage that facilitates T cell responses to protein antigens. B cells may also act as antigen-presenting cells, thereby serving an accessory cell function.

accessory molecules

Molecules other than the antigen receptor and major histocompatibility complex (MHC) that participate in cognitive, activation, and effector functions of T lymphocyte responsiveness. Adhesion molecules facilitating the interaction of T lymphocytes with other cells that signal transducing molecules that participate in T cell activation or migration are classified as accessory molecules. Other examples

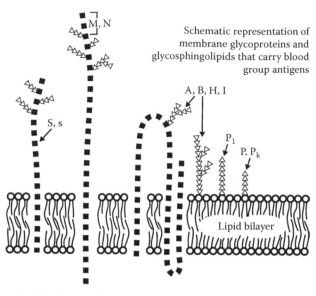

Schematic representation of membrane glycoproteins and glycosphingolipids that carry blood group antigens

△ Carbohydrate residues
■ Amino acid residues

Membrane glycoproteins and glysosphingolipids that carry blood group antigens.

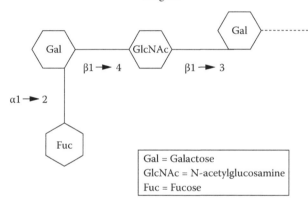

Gal = Galactose
GlcNAc = N-acetylglucosamine
Fuc = Fucose

Chemical structure of H antigen which is a specificity of the ABO blood group system.

Blood type	Red blood cell surface antigen	Antibody in serum
A	A antigen	Anti-B
B	B antigen	Anti-A
AB	AB antigens	No antibody
O	No A or B antigens	Both anti-A and anti-B

ABO blood group antigens and antibodies.

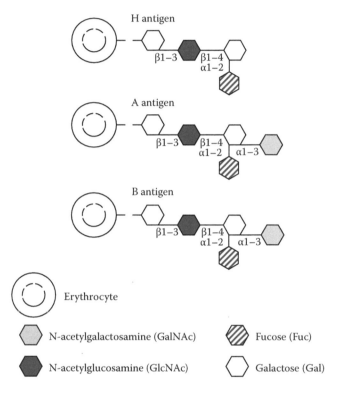

Erythrocyte

N-acetylgalactosamine (GalNAc)   Fucose (Fuc)

N-acetylglucosamine (GlcNAc)   Galactose (Gal)

Tabelle I, betreffend das Blut sechs anscheinend gesunder Männer.

Sera						
Dr. St.	−	+	+	+	+	−
Dr. Plecn.	−	−	+	+	−	−
Dr. Sturl.	−	+	−	−	+	−
Dr. Erdh.	−	+	−	−	+	−
Zar.	−	−	+	+	−	−
Landst.	−	+	+	+	+	−
Blutkörperchen von:	Dr. St.	Dr. Plecn.	Dr. Sturl.	Dr. Erdh.	Zar.	Landst.

Tabelle II, betreffend das Blut von sechs anscheinend gesunden Puerperae.

Sera						
Seil.	−	−	+	−	−	+
Linsm.	+	−	+	+	+	+
Lust.	+	−	−	+	+	−
Mittelb.	−	−	+	−	−	+
Tomsch.	−	−	+	−	−	+
Graupn.	+	−	−	+	+	−
Blutkörperchen von:	Seil.	Linsm.	Lust.	Mittelb.	Tomsch.	Graupn.

Table illustrating ABO blood groups. (From *Wien. klin. Wschr.*, 14, 1132–1134, 1901.)

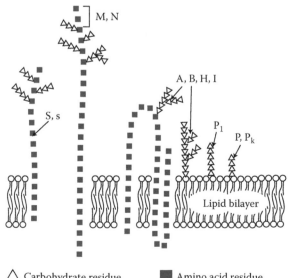

△ Carbohydrate residue   ■ Amino acid residue

Membrane glycoproteins and glycosphingolipids that carry blood group antigens.

A

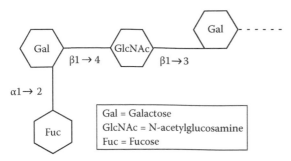

Chemical structure of H antigen which is a specificity of the ABO blood group system.

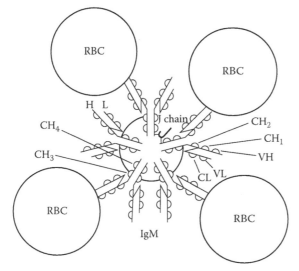

Agglutination of human red blood cells (RBCs) by natural isohemagglutinins that are antibodies of the IgM class.

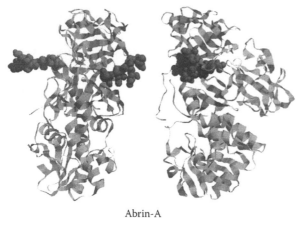

Abrin-A

Abrin.

include the CD4 and CD8 coreceptors, CD3 components of the T cell receptor, adhesion molecules, and costimulatory molecules.

acetaldehyde adduct autoantibodies

Antibodies found in approximately 73% of alcoholic and in 39% of nonalcoholic liver disease (e.g., primary biliary cirrhosis, chronic active hepatitis, acute viral and drug-induced hepatitis). The highest titers of these autoantibodies are found in advanced stages of alcoholic and nonalcoholic liver disease. Alcoholics develop acetaldehyde

adduct autoantibodies to apo B-containing lipoproteins, particularly very low density lipoproteins (VLDLs); 33% of alcoholic patients with heart muscle disease develop cardiac–protein–acetaldehyde adduct autoantibodies that could be potential markers for this heart condition.

acetylcholine receptor (AChR) antibodies

IgG autoantibodies that cause loss of function of AChRs that are critical to chemical transmission of the nerve impulse at the neuromuscular junction. This represents a type II mechanism of hypersensitivity, according to the Coombs and Gell classification. AChR antibodies are heterogeneous, with some showing specificity for antigenic determinants other than those that serve as acetylcholine or α-bungarotoxin binding sites. As many as 85 to 95% of myasthenia gravis patients may manifest AChR antibodies.

acetylcholine receptor (AChR) autoantibodies

Autoantibodies binding acetylcholine receptors react with several epitopes other than the binding site for ACh or α-bungarotoxin. They are found in 88% of patients with generalized myasthenia gravis (MG), 70% of patients with ocular myasthenia, and 80% of patients with MG in remission. They decrease in titer when weakness is reduced with immunosuppressive therapy. AChR-blocking autoantibodies react with the AChR binding site. They are found in 50% of patients with MG, in 30% of patients with ocular MG, and in 20% of patients with MG in remission. AChR-modulating autoantibodies crosslink AChRs and induce their removal from muscle membrane surfaces. They are present in more than 90% of patients with MG. AChR autoantibodies of one or more types are present in at least 80% of patients with ocular MG.

acoelomate

A lower invertebrate animal lacking a body cavity.

acquired agammaglobulinemia

Refer to common variable immunodeficiency.

acquired B antigen

The alteration of A1 erythrocyte membrane through the action of such bacteria as *Escherichia coli, Clostridium tertium,* and *Bacteroides fragilis* to make it react as if it were a group B antigen. The named microorganisms can be associated with gastrointestinal infection or carcinoma.

acquired C1 inhibitor deficiency

A condition in which the C1 inhibitor is inactivated, resulting in elevated C4 and C2 cleavage as C1 is activated. Patients experience repeated laryngeal, intestinal, and subcutaneous tissue swelling. A kinin-like peptide derived from C2b promotes vascular permeability and produces symptoms. Subjects with B lymphocyte or plasma cell monoclonal proliferation may develop acquired C1 inhibitor deficiency. These syndromes include multiple myeloma, Waldenström's macroglobulinemia, and B cell lymphoma. Subjects may develop antiidiotypic antibodies against membrane immunoglobulins or myeloma proteins. Idiotype–anti-idiotype interactions at cell membranes may result in C1 fixation and may increase utilization of C4 and C2 as well as C1 inhibitor.

acquired immune deficiency syndrome (AIDS)

A retroviral disease marked by profound immunosuppression that leads to opportunistic infections, secondary neoplasms, and neurologic manifestations. It is caused by the human immunodeficiency virus 1 (HIV-1), the causative agent for most cases worldwide, with a few cases in western

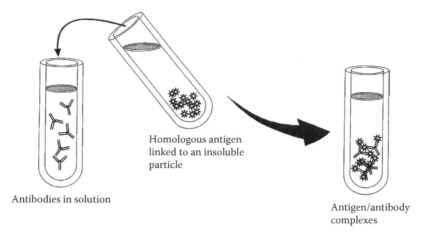

Absorption is the elimination of antibodies from the mixture by adding soluble antigens or the elimination of soluble antigen from a mixture by adding antibodies.

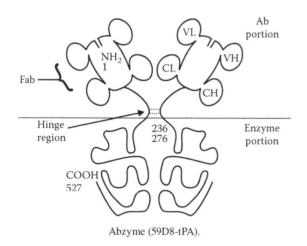

Abzyme (59D8-tPA).

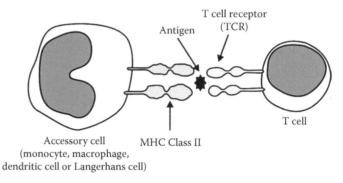

Accessory molecules.

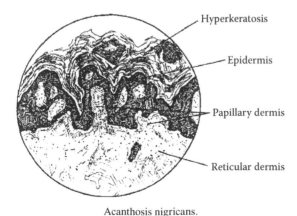

Acanthosis nigricans.

Africa attributable to HIV-2. Principal transmission routes include sexual contact, parenteral inoculation, and passage of the virus from infected mothers to their newborns. Although originally recognized in homosexual or bisexual men in the United States, AIDS is increasingly a heterosexual disease. It appears to have originated in Africa, where it is a heterosexual disease, and it has been reported in more than 193 countries. The CD4 molecules on T lymphocytes serve as high affinity receptors for HIV. HIVgp 120 must also bind to other cell surface molecules termed coreceptors for cell entry. They include CCR5 and CXCR4 receptors for β chemokines and α chemokines. Some HIV strains are macrophage tropic, whereas others are T cell tropic. Early in the disease, HIV colonizes the lymphoid organs. The striking decrease in CD4$^+$ T cells is a hallmark of AIDS that accounts for the immunodeficiency late in the course of HIV infection, but qualitative defects in T lymphocytes may be discovered in HIV-infected persons who are asymptomatic. Infection of macrophages and monocytes is very important, and the dendritic cells in lymphoid tissues are the principal sites of HIV infection and persistence. In addition to the lymphoid system, the nervous system is the major target of HIV infection. It is widely accepted that HIV is carried to the brain by infected monocytes. The microglia in the brain are the principal cell types infected in that tissue. The natural history of HIV infection is divided into three phases: (1) early acute, (2) middle chronic, and (3) final crisis. Viremia, measured as HIV-1 RNA, is the best marker of HIV disease progression and is valuable clinically in the management of HIV-infected patients. Clinically, HIV infection can range from a mild acute illness to a severe disease. The adult AIDS patient may present with fever, weight loss, diarrhea, generalized lymphadenopathy, multiple infections, neurologic disease, and in some cases secondary neoplasms. Opportunistic infections account for 80% of deaths in AIDS patients. Prominent among these is pneumonia caused by *Pneumocystis carinii* as well as other common pathogens. AIDS patients also have a high incidence of certain tumors, especially Kaposi sarcoma, non-Hodgkin lymphoma, and cervical cancer in women. No effective vaccine has yet been developed.

Opsonic—promote ingestion and killing by phagocytic cells (IgG)

Block attachment (IgA)

Neutralize toxins

Agglutinate bacteria—may aid in clearing

Render motile organisms nonmotile

Abs only rarely affect metabolism or growth of bacteria (Mycoplasma)

Abs, combining with antigens of the bacterial surface, activate the complement cascade, thus inducing an inflammatory response and bringing fresh phagocytes and serum Abs into the site

Abs, combining with antigens of the bacterial surface, activate the complement cascade, and through the final sequences the membrane attack complex (MAC) involving C5b-C9 is formed

Antimicrobial Actions of Antibodies

---

acquired immunity

Protective resistance against an infectious agent generated as a consequence of infection with a specific microorganism or as a result of deliberate immunization. Refer also to primary immune response, secondary immune response, and adaptive immunity.

acquired immunodeficiency

A decrease in the immune response to immunogenic (antigenic) challenge as a consequence of numerous diseases or conditions, including acquired immunodeficiency syndrome (AIDS), chemotherapy, immunosuppressive drugs such as corticosteroids, psychological depression, burns, nonsteroidal antiinflammatory drugs, radiation, Alzheimer's disease, celiac disease, sarcoidosis, lymphoproliferative disease, Waldenström's macroglobulinemia, multiple myeloma, aplastic anemia, sickle cell disease, malnutrition, aging, neoplasia, and diabetes mellitus, among others.

acquired tolerance

Immunologic tolerance induced by the inoculation of a neonate or fetus *in utero* with allogeneic cells prior to maturation of the recipient's immune response. The inoculated antigens are accepted as self. Immunologic tolerance to some soluble antigens may be induced in neonates by low-dose injections of the antigen or in older animals by larger doses; the so-called low dose and high dose tolerance, respectively. Refer also to immunologic tolerance.

acridine orange

A fluorescent substance that binds nonspecifically to RNA with red fluorescence and to DNA with green fluorescence. It also interacts with polysaccharides, proteins, and glycosaminoglycans. It is a nonspecific tissue stain that identifies increased mitoses and shows greater sensitivity but less specificity than the Gram stain. It is carcinogenic and of limited use in routine histology.

ACT-2

A human homolog of murine MIP-1b that chemoattracts monocytes but prefers activated CD4$^+$ cells to CD8$^+$ cells. T cells and monocytes are sources of ACT-2.

actin

In immunology, the principal muscle protein that together with myosin causes muscle contraction and is used in surgical pathology as a marker for the identification of tumors of muscle origin. Actin is identified through immunoperoxidase staining of surgical pathology tissue specimens.

activated dendritic cells

Refer to dendritic cells.

activated leukocyte cell adhesion molecule (ALCAM/CD166)

A member of the immunoglobulin (Ig) gene superfamily. It is expressed by activated leukocytes and lymphocyte antigen CD6. The extracellular region of ALCAM contains five Ig-like domains. The N terminal Ig domain binds specifically to CD6. ALCAM/CD6 interactions have been implicated in T cell development and regulation of T cell function. ALCAM may also play a role in the progression of human melanoma.

activated lymphocyte

A lymphocyte whose cell surface receptors have interacted with a specific antigen or with a mitogen such as phytohemagglutinin, concanavalin A, or staphylococcal protein A. The morphologic appearance of the activated (or stimulated) lymphocyte is characteristic, and in this form the cells are called

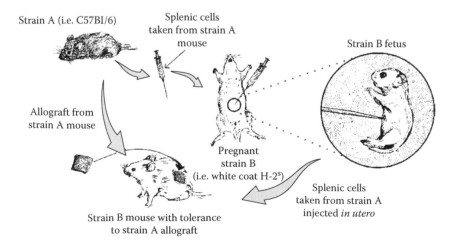

Strain A (i.e. C57Bl/6)

Splenic cells taken from strain A mouse

Strain B fetus

Allograft from strain A mouse

Pregnant strain B (i.e. white coat H-2^s)

Splenic cells taken from strain A injected *in utero*

Strain B mouse with tolerance to strain A allograft

Acquired immunologic tolerance.

immunoblasts. The cells increase in size from 15 to 30 mm in diameter, show increased cytoplasmic basophilia, and develop vacuoles, lysosomes, and ribosomal aggregates. Pinocytotic vesicles are present on the cell membrane. The nucleus contains little chromatin, which is limited to a thin marginal layer, and the nucleolus becomes conspicuous. The array of changes following stimulation is called transformation. Such cells are called transformed cells. An activated B lymphocyte may synthesize antibody molecules, whereas an activated T cell may mediate a cellular immune reaction.

activated macrophage

A macrophage that has been stimulated in some manner or by some substance to increase its functional efficiency with respect to phagocytosis, intracellular bactericidal activity, or lymphokine (i.e., IL-1) production. A lymphokine-activated mononuclear phagocyte is double the size of a resting macrophage. Major histocompatibility complex (MHC) class II antigen surface expression is elevated, and lysosomes increase. The latter changes facilitate antimicrobial defense.

activation

Stimulation of lymphocytes or macrophages to increase their functional activity or initiation of the multicomponent complement cascade in serum consisting of a series of enzyme–substrate reactions leading to the generation of functionally active effector molecules.

activation-induced cell death (AICD)

A phenomenon first observed in T hybridomas that die within 24 hours of stimulation. It was also observed *in vivo* following systemic stimulation by bacterial sAgs or peptide antigens. AICD represents a heightened sensitivity of recently stimulated cells to apoptosis induced by T cell receptor (TCR) crosslinking, linked to the cell cycle. It can also eliminate T cells immediately at the time of initial stimulation, especially in virus-infected individuals. In clonal exhaustion, AICD can lead to the complete elimination of all antigen-reactive cells and may represent the basis for high dose tolerance. Frequently mediated by the *Fas* pathway or *TNFR1* pathway.

activation-induced deaminase (AID)

A purported RNA- or DNA-editing enzyme requisite for isotype switching as well as somatic hypermutation. Germinal center B cells express it selectively.

activation phase

A stage in the adaptive immune response following recognition that is associated with lymphocyte proliferation and differentiation into effector cells.

activation protein-1 (AP-1)

DNA-binding transcription factors composed of dimers of two proteins linked to each other through a shared structural motif termed a leucine zipper. An example of an AP-1 factor is one comprised of Fos and Jun proteins. Among the many different genes of the immune system in which AP-1 exerts transcriptional regulation of cytokine genes.

activation unit

Interaction of C3b with C4b2a bound to the cell membrane.

active anaphylaxis

The anaphylactic state induced by natural or experimental sensitization in atopic subjects or experimental animals. See also anaphylaxis.

active immunity

Protection attained as a consequence of clinical or subclinical infection or deliberate immunization with an infectious agent or its products. A type of adaptive immunity in which lymphocytes are activated in response to a foreign antigen to which they have been exposed. Compare with passive immunity.

active immunization

The induction of an immune response either through exposure to an infectious agent or by deliberate immunization with products of the microorganism inducing the disease to develop protective immunity. A clinical disease or subclinical infection or vaccination may be used to induce the desired protective effect. Booster immunization injections given at intervals after primary exposure may lead to long-lasting immunity through activation of immunological memory cells. Refer also to vaccination.

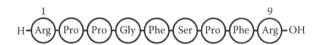

Primary structure of serum bradykinin.

active kinins

The active kinin compounds are characterized by a nonapeptide amino acid sequence whose prototype is bradykinin, the active kinin generated from plasma kininogen. Generation of the other forms depends on the enzyme and substrate used, and they differ in length and the additional residues. Tissue kallikreins are best activated by enzymes such as trypsin and hydrolyze, both low molecular weight kininogen (LMK) and high molecular weight kininogen (HMK) to yield kallidin, a tissue form of kinin. Bradykinin is formed by the action of plasma kallikrein on HMK or by the action of trypsin on both LMK and HMK. *Met-lys*-bradykinin, another kinin, results from hydrolysis by plasma kallikrein activated by acidification. Other active kinins have also been described. Besides being the precursors for the generation of kinins, kininogens also affect the coagulation system, with activation of the Hageman factor (HF) being the link between the two systems.

active site

A crevice formed by the VL and VH regions of an immunoglobulin's Fv region. It may differ in size or shape from one antibody molecule to another. Its activity is governed by the amino acid sequence in this variable region and differences in the manner in which VL and VH regions relate to one another. Antibody molecule specificity is dependent on the complementary relationship between epitopes on antigen molecules and amino acid residues in the recess comprising the antibody active site. The VL and VH regions contain hypervariable areas that permit great diversity in the antigen-binding capacity of antibody molecules.

acumentin

A neutrophil and macrophage motility protein that links to the actin molecule to control actin filament length.

acute AIDS syndrome

Within the first to sixth week following HIV-1 infection, some subjects develop the flu-like symptoms of sore throat, anorexia, nausea and vomiting, lymphadenopathy, maculopapular rash, wasting, and pain in the abdomen, among other symptoms. The total leukocyte count is slightly depressed, with possible CD4 to CD8 ratio inversion.

A

Detectable antibodies with specificity for HIV constituents gp120, gp160, p24, and p41 are not detectable until at least 6 months following infection. Approximately 33% of the infected subjects manifest acute AIDS syndrome.

acute cellular rejection

Acute graft rejection mediated by recipient cytotoxic T lymphocytes and delayed-type hypersensitivity reactions against allogeneic graft cells.

acute disseminated encephalomyelitis

Brain inflammation that may be a sequela of certain acute viral infections such as measles in children or following vaccination. It was reported in some subjects following smallpox vaccination and in early recipients of rabies vaccine containing nervous system tissues. Symptoms include neck stiffness, headache, disorientation, and coma. Elevated quantities of protein and lymphocytes appear in the cerebrospinal fluid. Histopathologically, lymphocytes, plasma cells, and polymorphonuclear leukocytes may form perivascular infiltrates. The pathological changes are probably attributable to immune reactivity against the central nervous system constituent myelin basic protein and may represent the human equivalent of experimental allergic encephalomyelitis produced in animals. Refer also to the animal model of this condition, termed experimental allergic encephalomyelitis (EAE).

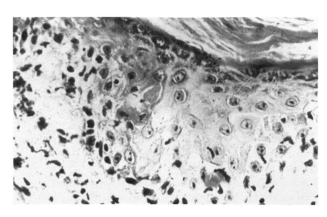

Acute graft-vs.-host reaction. Histologically, there is an intense interface dermatitis with destruction of basilar cells, particular at the tips of the rete ridges, incontinence of melanin pigment, and necrosis of individual epithelial cells, referred to as apoptosis.

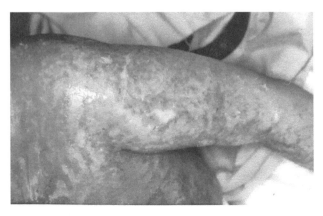

Diffuse erythematous to morbilliform rash in a child with acute graft-vs.-host disease (GVHD).

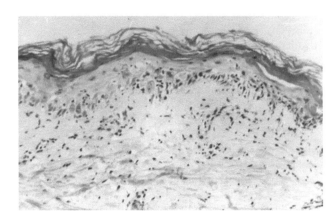

Histological appearance of the skin in graft-vs.-host disease with disruption of the basal cell layer, hyperkeratosis, and beginning sclerotic change.

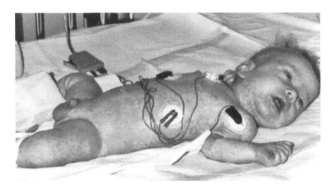

Diffuse erythematous skin rash in a patient with acute graft-vs.-host disease (GVHD).

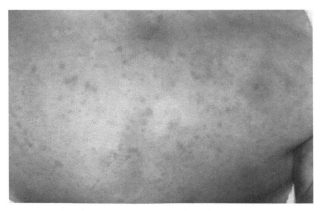

Papulosquamous rash in graft-vs.-host disease.

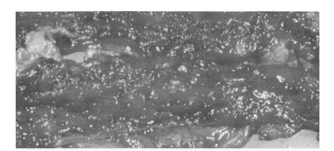

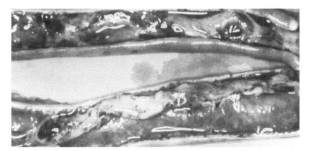

Sloughing of mucosal lining of the gut in graft-vs.-host disease.

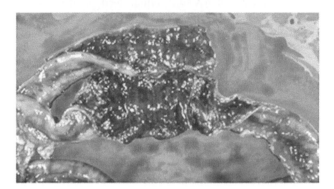

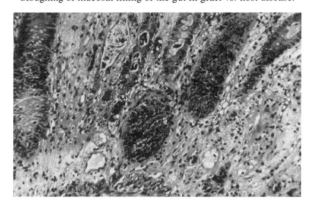

Gastrointestinal graft-vs.-host disease in which there is a diffuse process that usually involves the ileum and cecum most severely, resulting in secretory diarrhea. Grossly, diffuse erythema, granularity, and loss of folds are observed; when severe, undermining and sloughing of the entire mucosa lead to fibrinopurulent clots of necrotic material. Frank obstruction is sometimes found in patients with intractable graft-vs.-host disease.

Histologically, graft-vs.-host disease in the gut begins as a patchy destructive enteritis localized to the lower third of the crypts of Lieberkühn.

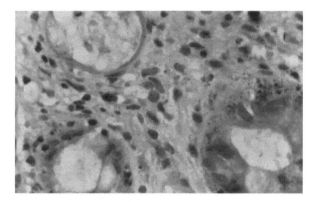

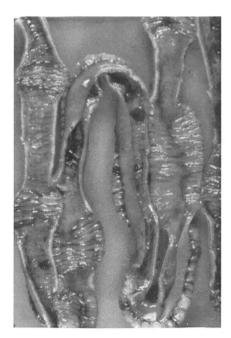

The earliest lesions are characterized by individual enterocyte necrosis with karyorrhectic nuclear debris, the so-called exploding crypt, which progresses to a completely destroyed crypt, as shown in the upper left corner.

Stenotic and fibrotic segments alternating with more normal appearing dilated segments of gut in graft-vs.-host disease.

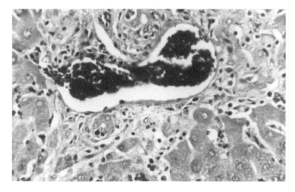

acute graft rejection

Recipient host rejection of a transplanted solid organ or tissue transplant within days or weeks following transplantation. The mechanism may be acute cellular rejection or antibody-mediated acute humoral rejection.

Hepatic graft-vs.-host disease is characterized by a cholestatic hepatitis with characteristic injury and destruction of small bile ducts that resemble changes seen in rejection. This section of early acute disease shows mile portal infiltrates with striking exocytosis into bile ducts associated with individual cell necrosis and focal destruction of the bile ducts.

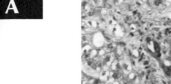

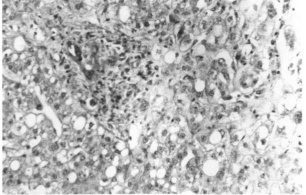

This liver section from a patient with graft-vs.-host disease demonstrates the cholestatic changes that evolve from hepatocellular ballooning to cholangiolar cholestasis with bile microliths, signifying prolonged disease.

acute graft-vs.-host reaction

The immunopathogenesis of acute graft-vs.-host disease (GVHD) consists of recognition, recruitment, and effector phases. Epithelia of the skin, gastrointestinal tract, small intrahepatic biliary ducts, and lymphoid system constitute primary targets of acute GVHD. GVHD development may differ in severity based on relative antigenic differences between donor and host and the reactivity of donor lymphocytes against non-human leukocyte antigens (HLAs) of recipient tissues. The incidence and severity of GVHD have been ascribed also to HLA-B alleles (i.e., increased GVHD incidence is associated with HLA-B8 and HLA-B35). Epithelial tissues serving as targets of GVHD include keratinocytes, erythrocytes, and bile ducts that may express Ia antigens following exposure to endogenous interferon produced by T lymphocytes. When Ia antigens are expressed on nonlymphoid cells, they may become antigen-presenting cells for autologous antigens and aid perpetuation of autoimmunity. Cytotoxic T lymphocytes mediate acute GVHD. While most immunohistological investigations have implicated CD8+ (cytotoxic/suppressor) lymphocytes, others have identified CD4+ (T helper lymphocytes) in human GVHD, whereas natural killer (NK) cells have been revealed as effectors of murine but not human GVHD. Following interaction between effector and target cells, cytotoxic granules from cytotoxic T or NK cells are distributed over the target cell membrane, leading to perforin-induced large pores across the membrane and nuclear lysis by deoxyribonuclease. Infection, rather than failure of the primary target organ (other than gastrointestinal bleeding), is the major cause of mortality in acute GVHD. Within the first few months post-transplant, all recipients demonstrate diminished immunoglobulin synthesis, decreased T helper lymphocytes, and increased T suppressor cells. Acute GVHD patients manifest an impaired ability to combat viral infections and demonstrate an increased risk of cytomegalovirus (CMV) infection, especially CMV interstitial pneumonia. GVHD may also reactivate other viral diseases such as herpes simplex. Immunodeficiency in the form of acquired B cell lymphoproliferative disorder (BCLD) represents another serious complication of bone marrow transplantation. Bone marrow transplant patients treated with pan-T cell monoclonal antibody or those in which T lymphocytes have been depleted account for most cases of BCLD, which is associated with severe GVHD. All transformed B cells in cases of BCLD have manifested the Epstein–Barr viral genome.

acute humoral rejection

A type of acute graft rejection in which antibodies are produced against allogeneic antigens in the graft, leading to vascular inflammation and neutrophil infiltration. Referred to also as delayed graft rejection or delayed vascular rejection. Characterized by C4d "staining" by immunofluorescence of peritubular capillaries in renal allotransplants undergoing acute humoral rejection.

acute inflammation

A reaction of sudden onset marked by the classic symptoms of pain, heat, redness, swelling, and loss of function. Also observed are dilation of arterioles, capillaries, and venules with increased permeability and blood flow; exudation of fluids, including plasma proteins; and migration of leukocytes into the inflammatory site. Inflammation is a localized protective response induced by injury or destruction of tissues. It is designed to destroy, dilute, or wall off both the offending agent and the injured tissue.

acute inflammatory response

An early defense mechanism to contain an infection and prevent its spread from the initial focus. When microbes multiply in host tissues, two principal defense mechanisms mounted against them are antibodies and leukocytes. The three major events in acute inflammation are (1) dilation of capillaries to increase blood flow, (2) changes in the microvasculature structure leading to escape of plasma proteins and leukocytes from the circulation, and (3) leukocyte emigration from the capillaries and accumulation at the site of injury. Widening of interendothelial cell junctions of venules or injury of endothelial cells facilitates the escape of plasma proteins from the vessels. Neutrophils attached to the endothelium through adhesion molecules escape microvasculature and are attracted to sites of injury by chemotactic agents. This process is followed by phagocytosis of microorganisms that may lead to their intracellular destruction. Activated leukocytes may produce toxic metabolites and proteases that injure endothelium and tissues when they are released. Activation of the third complement component (C3) is also a critical step in inflammation. Multiple chemical mediators of inflammation derived from plasma cells have been described. Mediators and plasma proteins such as complement are present as precursors in intracellular granules, such as histamine and mast cells. These substances are secreted following activation. Other mediators such as prostaglandins may be synthesized following stimulation. These mediators are quickly activated by enzymes or other substances such as antioxidants. A chemical mediator may also cause a target cell to release a secondary mediator with similar or opposing action. Besides histamine, other preformed chemical mediators in cells include serotonin and lysosomal enzymes. Those that are newly synthesized include prostaglandins, leukotrienes, platelet-activating factors, cytokines, and nitric oxide. Chemical mediators in plasma include complement fragments C3a, C5a, and the C5b–g sequence. Three plasma-derived factors—kinins, complement, and clotting factors—are involved in

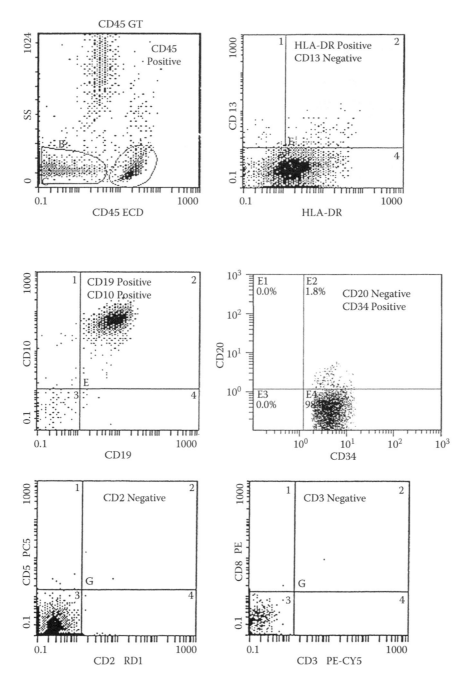

Precursor B cell acute lymphoblastic leukemia.

inflammation. Bradykinin is produced by activation of the kinin system. It induces arteriolar dilation and increased venule permeability through contraction of endothelial cells and extravascular smooth muscle. Activation of bradykinin precursors involves activated factor XII (Hageman factor) generated by its contact with injured tissues. During clotting, fibrinopeptides produced during the conversion of fibrinogen to fibrin increase vascular permeability and are chemotactic for leukocytes. The fibrinolytic system participates in inflammation through the kinin system. Products produced during arachidonic acid metabolism also affect inflammation. These include prostaglandins and leukotrienes that can mediate essentially every aspect of acute inflammation.

acute lymphoblastic leukemia (ALL)

An undifferentiated and very aggressive type of lymphoid neoplasm that results from uncontrolled growth of a progenitor cell that is believed to give rise to both B and T lymphoid cell lineages. It consists of a heterogeneous group of lymphopoietic stem cell disorders in which lymphoblasts accumulate in the bone marrow and suppress normal hemopoietic cells. Of all ALL cases, 80% are of the B cell type, whereas the remainder are T cell with rare cases of null cell origin. Ten percent (10%) of leukemias are ALL, and 60% of ALL cases occur in children. Chromosomal abnormalities have been found in most cases of ALL. B-ALL (L3) is characterized by one of three chromosomal translocations. Most B-ALL cases involve

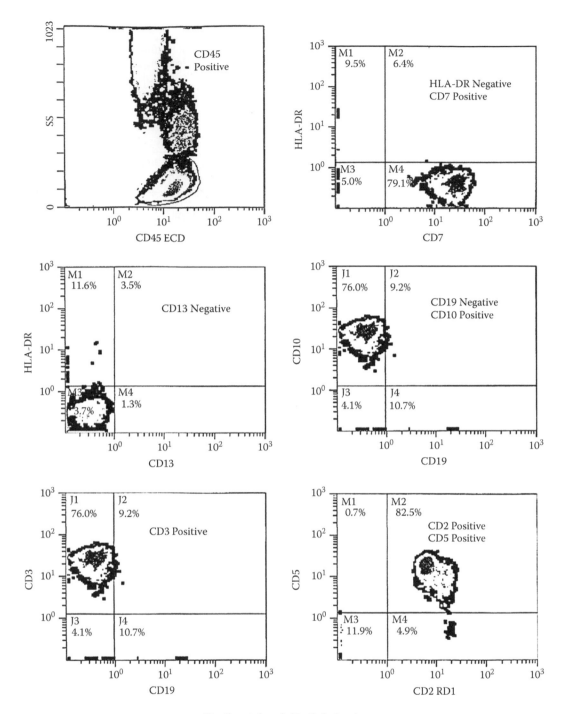

T cell acute lymphoblastic leukemia.

translocation of c-*myc* protooncogene on chromosome 8 to the immunoglobulin coding gene region on chromosome 14. Lymphoblasts that are unable to differentiate and mature continue to accumulate in the bone marrow. ALL patients develop anemia, granulocytopenia, and thrombocytopenia. L1, L2, and L3 lymphoblast cytologic subtypes are recognized. ALL is diagnosed by the demonstration of lymphoblasts in the bone marrow. The total leukocyte count is normal or decreased in half of the cases with or without lymphoblasts in the peripheral blood. An elevated leukocyte count is usually accompanied by lymphoblasts

in the peripheral blood. Patients develop a normochromic, normocytic anemia with thrombocytopenia and neutropenia. They may develop weakness, malaise, and pallor secondary to anemia. Half the individuals develop bleeding secondary to thrombocytopenia, and many develop bacterial infections secondary to neutropenia. Patients also experience bone pain. Generalized lymphadenopathy especially affects the cervical lymph nodes. Frequently, hepatosplenomegaly and leukemic meningitis are present. The age at onset and initial total blood leukocyte count are valuable prognostic features. Ninety percent (90%) of

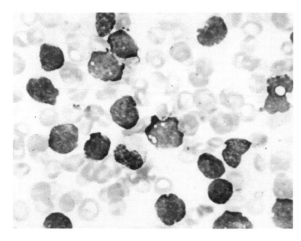

Acute lymphoblastic leukemia.

children with L1 morphology cells experience complete remission with chemotherapy. Patients may experience a profound reduction in the concentration of the serum immunoglobulins, possibly due to malignant expansion of suppressor T lymphocytes.

acute myelogenous leukemia (AML)

A heterogeneous group of disorders characterized by neoplastic transformation in a multipotential hematopoietic stem cell or in one of restricted lineage potential. Because multipotential hematopoietic stem cells are the precursors of granulocytes, monocytes, erythrocytes, and megakaryocytes, one or all of these cell types may be affected. Differentiation usually ends at the blast stage, causing myeloblasts to accumulate in the bone marrow. AML is diagnosed by the discovery of 30% myelogenous blasts in the bone marrow, whether or not they are present in the peripheral blood. The total peripheral blood leukocyte count may be normal, low, or elevated. There may be thrombocytopenia, neutropenia, and anemia. The presenting symptoms and signs are nonspecific and may be secondary to anemia. Patients may experience fatigue, weakness, and pallor. One third of AML patients are found to have hepatosplenomegaly. One third of patients may have bleeding secondary to thrombocytopenia. Gastrointestinal tract or central nervous system hemorrhage may occur when platelet counts fall below 20,000/μL. Decreased neutrophil counts may increase secondary infections. Unfavorable prognostic findings include: (1) an age at diagnosis above 60 years, (2) 5q- and 7q- chromosomal abnormalities, (3) a history of myelodysplastic syndrome, (4) a history of radiation or chemotherapy for cancer, and (5) a leukocytosis exceeding 100,000/μL. If untreated, AML leads to death in less than 2 months through hemorrhage or infection. Both chemotherapy and bone marrow transplantation are modes of therapy.

acute-phase proteins

Plasma proteins, synthesized by the liver, that increase in concentration during inflammation. They are active during early phases of host defense against infection. They include mannose-binding protein (MBP), C-reactive protein (CRPJ), fibrinogen, selected complement components, and interferons. These proteins interact with cell wall constituents of microorganisms and activate complement.

acute-phase reactants

Serum proteins that increase during acute inflammation. These proteins, which migrate in the α-1 and α-2 electrophoretic regions, include α-1 antitrypsin, α-1 glycoprotein, amyloid A&P, antithrombin III, C-reactive protein, C1 esterase inhibitor, C3 complement, ceruloplasmin, fibrinogen, haptoglobin, orosomucoid, plasminogen, and transferrin. Most of the acute-phase reactant proteins are synthesized in the liver and increase soon after infection as part of the systemic inflammatory response syndrome (SIRS). Inflammatory cytokines upregulate these molecules, including interleukin-6 (IL-6) and tumor necrosis factor (TNF). Acute-phase reactants participate in the natural or innate response to microorganisms.

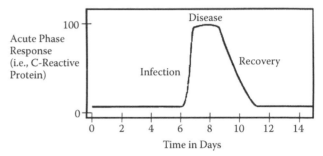

Acute-phase response.

acute-phase response (APR)

A nonspecific response by an individual stimulated by interleukin-1, interleukin-6, interferons, and tumor necrosis factor. C-reactive protein may show a striking rise within a few hours. Infection, inflammation, tissue injury, and, very infrequently, neoplasm may be associated with APR. The liver produces acute-phase proteins at an accelerated rate, and the endocrine system is affected with elevated gluconeogenesis, impaired thyroid function, and other changes. Immunologic and hematopoietic system changes include hypergammaglobulinemia and leukocytosis with a shift to the left. Diminished formation of albumin, elevated ceruloplasmin, and diminished zinc and iron are also observed. Cellular elements may also be produced in addition to the acute-phase proteins.

acute-phase serum

A serum sample drawn from an infectious disease patient in the acute phase.

acute poststreptococcal glomerulonephritis

A disease of the kidney, with a good prognosis for most patients, that follows streptococcal infection of the skin or streptococcal pharyngitis by 10 days to 3 weeks in children. The subject presents with hematuria, fever, general malaise, facial swelling, and smoky urine, as well as mild proteinuria and red blood cells in the urine. These children often have headaches, are hypertensive, and have elevated blood pressure. Serum C3 levels are decreased. The erythrocyte sedimentation rate (ESR) is elevated, and an abdominal x-ray may reveal enlarged kidneys. Renal biopsy reveals infiltration of glomeruli by polymorphonuclear leukocytes and monocytes and a diffuse proliferative process. Immunofluorescence shows granular deposits of IgG and C3 on the epithelial sides of peripheral capillary loops. Electron microscopy shows subepithelial "humps." The process usually resolves spontaneously within 1 week after onset of renal signs and symptoms, the patient becomes afebrile, and the malaise disappears. The disease is attributable to nephritogenic streptococci of types 1, 4, 12, and 49.

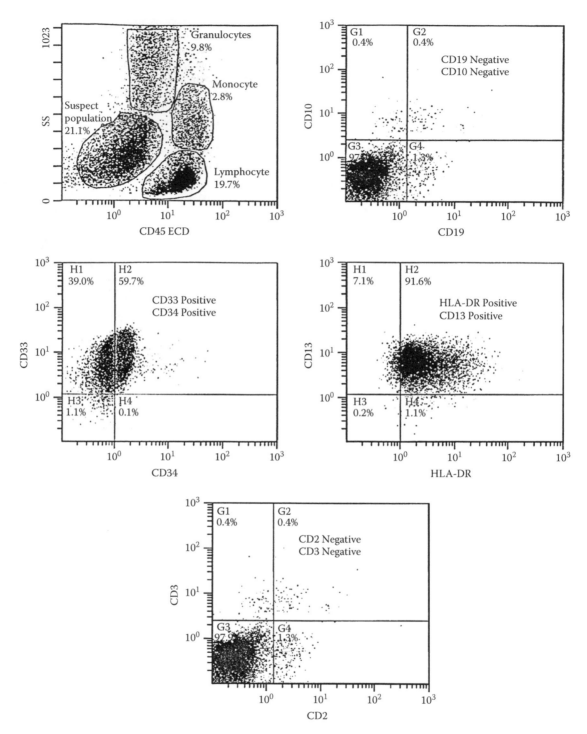

Acute myeloid leukemia.

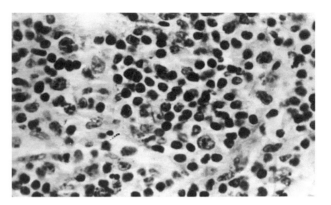

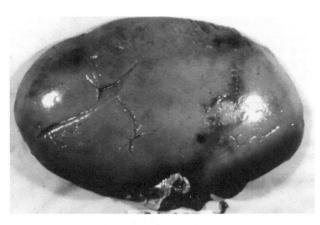

Acute rejection of a renal allograft in which the capsular surface shows several hemorrhagic areas. The kidney is tremendously swollen.

Microscopic view of the interstitium revealing predominantly cellular acute rejection. There is an infiltrate of variably sized lymphocytes and an infiltrate of eosinophils.

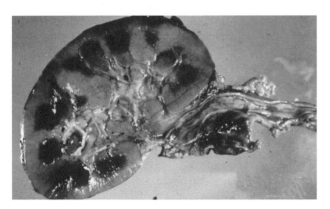

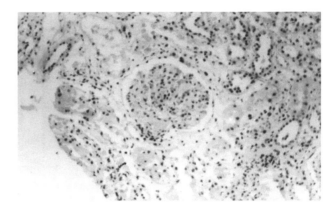

Acute rejection of bivalved kidney. The cut surface bulges, is variably hemorrhagic, and shows fatty degeneration of the cortex.

Microscopic view of acute rejection showing interstitial edema. Mild lymphocytic infiltrate. In the glomerulus, there is also evidence of predominantly vast rejection with a thrombus at the vascular pole.

acute rejection

A type of graft rejection in which T lymphocytes, macrophages, as well as antibodies may mediate tissue and vascular injury that may commence a week following transplantation. The response to the graft includes the activation of effector T lymphocytes and the formation of antibodies that may mediate the process.

acute rheumatic fever

Following a group A hemolytic streptococcal infection of the throat, inflammation of the heart, joints, and connective tissue may follow. Arthritis may affect several joints in a migratory pattern. Carditis, inflammation of the heart, may be associated with the development of high titer heart-reactive antibodies (HRAs) that have been implicated in the pathogenesis of rheumatic fever. A patient may develop HRA, rheumatic fever, or both. HRA development in rheumatic fever represents molecular mimicry. Selected anti-streptococcal cell wall M protein antibodies are crossreactive through molecular mimicry with myocardial epitopes of the human heart. These serve as sites of attachment for IgG and

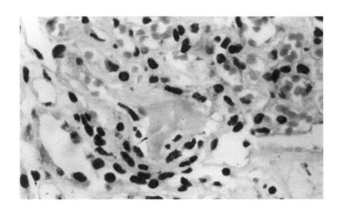

A higher magnification of the thrombus at the hilus of the glomerulus.

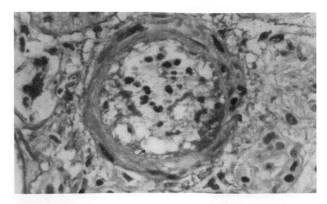

A trichrome stain of a small interlobular artery showing predominantly humoral rejection. There is tremendous swelling of the intima and endothelium with some fibrin deposition and a few polymorphonuclear leukocytes.

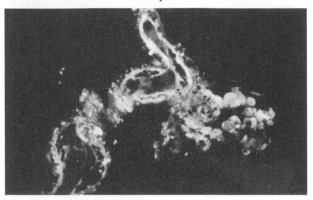

Immunofluorescence preparation showing humoral rejection with high intensity fluorescence of arteriolar walls and some glomerular capillary walls. This pattern is demonstrable in anti-immunoglobulin and anti-complement stained sections.

complement molecules that are detectable by immunofluorescence examination. The antibodies on the cardiac muscle are found at sarcolemmal and subsarcolemmal sites and in the pericardium. The crossreactivity also involves heart valve glycoproteins and the myocardial conduction system. A cell-mediated immune attack, as revealed by the accumulation of CD4 T lymphocytes in valvular tissues may occur. There appears to be a positive correlation between the development of rheumatic fever and HRA titers.

acyclic adenosine monophosphate (cAMP)

Adenosine 3′,5′-(hydrogen phosphate). A critical regulator within cells. It is produced through the action of adenylate cyclase on adenosine triphosphate; it activates protein kinase C and serves as a "second messenger" when hormones activate cells. Elevated cAMP concentrations in mast cells diminish their responses to degranulation signals.

acyclic guanosine monophosphate (cGMP)

Guanosine cyclic 3′,5′-(hydrogen phosphate). A cAMP antagonist produced by the action of guanylate cyclase on guanosine triphosphate. Elevated cGMP concentrations in mast cells accentuate their responses to degranulation signals.

acyclovir 9 (2-hydroxyethoxy-methylguanine)

An antiviral nucleoside analog that blocks herpes simplex virus type 2 (HSV-2), the causative agent of genital herpes. HSV thymidine kinase activates acyclovir through monophosphorylation, followed by triple phosphorylation with host enzymes to yield a powerful blocking action of the DNA polymerase of HSV-2. Acyclovir is prescribed for the treatment of HSV-2 genital infection.

ADA

Abbreviation for adenosine deaminase.

adaptive differentiation

Acquisition of the ability to identify major histocompatibility complex (MHC) class II antigens by thymocytes undergoing differentiation and maturation to CD4+ T helper/inducer cells in the thymus.

adaptive immune response

The response of B and T lymphocytes to a specific antigen and the development of immunological memory. The response involves clonal selection of lymphocytes that respond to a specific antigen. Also called acquired immune response.

adaptive immunity

Protection from an infectious disease agent as a consequence of clinical or subclinical infection with that agent or by deliberate immunization against that agent with products from it. This type of immunity is mediated by B and T lymphocytes following exposure to a specific antigen. It is characterized by specificity, immunological memory, and self/nonself recognition. This type of immunity is in contrast to natural or innate immunity.

adaptor proteins

Critical linkers between receptors and downstream signaling pathways that serve as bridges or scaffolds for recruitment of other signaling molecules. They are functionally heterogeneous, yet share an SH domain that permits interaction with phosphotyrosine residues formed by receptor-associated tyrosine kinases. During lymphocyte activation, they may be phosphorylated on tyrosine residues, which enables them to combine with other homology-2 (SH2) domain-containing proteins. LAT, SLP-76, and Grb-2 are examples of adaptor molecules that participate in T cell activation.

ADCC

Abbreviation for antibody-dependent cell-mediated cytotoxicity. Cell lysis induced by the interaction of the Fc region of a surface-bound antibody with an FcR expressed by effector cells such as eosinophils and NK cells. Other cells capable of mediating ADCC include macrophages, neutrophils, and monocytes.

Addison's disease

Refer to autoimmune adrenal disease.

addressin

A molecule such as a peptide or protein that serves as a homing device to direct a molecule to a specific location (an example is ELAM-1). Lymphocytes from Peyer's patches home to mucosal endothelial cells bearing ligands for the lymphocyte homing receptor. Mucosal addressin cell adhesion molecule-1 (MadCAM) is the Peyer's patch addressin in the intestinal wall that links to the integrin α4β7 on T lymphocytes that home to the intestine. Thus, endothelial cell addressins in separate anatomical locations bind to lymphocyte homing receptors, leading to organ-specific lymphocyte homing.

adenoids

Mucosa-associated secondary lymphoid tissues located in the nasal cavity. Refer also to tonsils.

adenosine

Adenosine is normally present in the plasma in concentrations of 0.03 μM in humans and 0.04 μM in dogs. In various clinical states associated with hypoxia, the α adenosine level increases five- to ten-fold, suggesting that it may play a role in the release of mediators. Experimentally, adenosine is a powerful potentiator of mast cell function. The incubation of mast cells with adenosine does not induce the release of mediators. However, by preincubation with adenosine and subsequent challenge with a mediator-releasing agent, the response is markedly enhanced.

adenosine deaminase (ADA)

A 38-kDa deaminating enzyme that prevents increased levels of adenosine, adenosine trisphosphate (ATP), deoxyadenosine, deoxy-ATP, and S-adenosyl homocysteine. It is encoded by the chromosome 20q13-ter gene. Elevated adenosine levels block DNA methylation within cells, leading to their death. Increased levels of deoxy-ATP block ribonucleoside-diphosphate reductase, which participates in the synthesis of purines. The absence of adenosine deaminase (ADA) enzyme, which participates in purine metabolism, causes toxic purine nucleosides and nucleotides to accumulate, leading to the deaths of developing thymic lymphocytes.

ADA deficiency.

adenosine deaminase (ADA) deficiency

A form of severe combined immunodeficiency (SCID) in which affected individuals lack an enzyme, adenosine deaminase (ADA), which catalyzes the deamination of adenosine as well as deoxyadenosine to produce inosine and deoxyinosine, respectively. Cells of the thymus, spleen, and lymph nodes and red blood cells contain free ADA enzyme. In contrast to the other forms of SCID, children with ADA deficiency possess Hassall's corpuscles in the thymus. The accumulation of deoxyribonucleotides in various tissues, especially thymic cells, is toxic and is believed to be a cause of immunodeficiency. As deoxyadenosine and deoxy-ATP accumulate, the latter substance inhibits ribonucleotide reductase activity, which inhibits formation of the substrate needed for synthesis of DNA. These toxic substances are especially injurious to T lymphocytes. Autosomal recessive ADA deficiency leads to death. Two fifths of SCID cases are of this type. The patient's signs and symptoms reflect defective cellular immunity with oral candidiasis, persistent diarrhea, failure to thrive, and other disorders, with death occurring prior to 2 years of age. T lymphocytes are significantly diminished. Eosinophilia and elevated serum and urine adenosine and deoxyadenosine levels are present. As bone marrow transplantation is relatively ineffective, gene therapy is the treatment of choice.

adenovirus infection and immunity

Species-specific icosahedral DNA viruses that belong to numerous serotypes. They produce multiple clinical syndromes in humans including respiratory, genitourinary, gastrointestinal, and conjunctival infections. They are resistant to most antiviral chemotherapy. An oral vaccine has been very successful in preventing acute respiratory disease in military personnel. Humans develop serotype-specific neutralizing antibodies to the structural proteins, thereby preventing reinfection with the same serotype. Early (E) nonstructural proteins produce significant immunologic effects. The virus has a double-stranded linear DNA and more than 12 structural proteins. There is no virus envelope. The viral polypeptides serve as antigens for host immune responses generated as a consequence of infection or as a result of immunization with a vaccine. The internal structural proteins are not believed to be involved in humoral or cell-mediated immunity.

ADEPT

Abbreviation for antibody-directed enzyme/pro-drug therapy. Treatment for cancer in which an immunoconjugate comprised of monoclonal antibody is united with an enzyme with the capacity to transform an inert pro-drug into an active cytotoxic drug.

adherent cell

A cell such as a macrophage (mononuclear phagocyte) that attaches to the wall of a culture flask, thereby facilitating the separation of such cells from B and T lymphocytes that are not adherent.

adhesins

Bacterial products that split proteins. They combine with human epithelial cell glycoprotein or glycolipid receptors, which may account for the increased incidence of pulmonary involvement attributable to *Pseudomonas aeruginosa* in patients who are intubated.

adhesion molecule

Molecules that mediate cell adhesion to their surroundings and to neighboring cells. In the immune system, adhesion molecules are critical to most aspects of leukocyte function, including lymphocyte recirculation through lymphoid organs, leukocyte recruitment into inflammatory sites, antigen-specific recognition, and wound healing. The five principal structural families of adhesion molecules are (1) integrins, (2) immunoglobulin superfamily (IgSF) proteins, (3) selectins, (4) mucins, and (5) cadherins.

adhesion molecule assays

Cell adhesion molecules are cell surface proteins involved in the binding of cells to each other, to endothelial cells, or to the extracellular matrix. Specific signals produced in response to wounding and infection control the expression and activation of the adhesion molecule. The interactions and responses initiated by the binding of these adhesion molecules to their receptors and ligands play important roles in the mediation of the inflammatory and immune reactions.

adhesion proteins

Extracellular matrix proteins that attract leukocytes from the circulation. For example, T and B lymphocytes possess lymph node homing receptors on their membranes that facilitate their passage through high endothelial venules. Neutrophils migrate to areas of inflammation in response to endothelial leukocyte adhesion molecule 1 (ELAM-1) stimulated by tumor necrosis factor (TNF) and interleukin-1 (IL-1) on the endothelia of vessels. B and T lymphocytes that pass

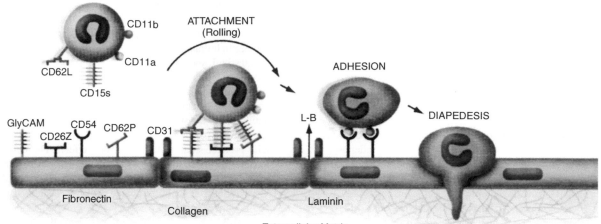

Adhesion molecule.

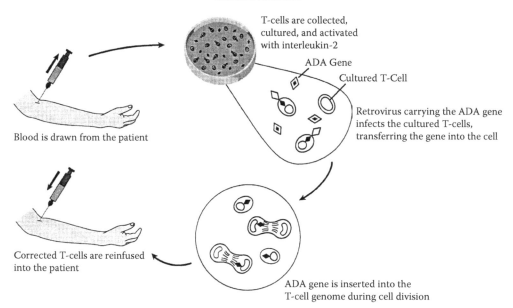

T-cells are collected, cultured, and activated with interleukin-2

ADA Gene

Cultured T-Cell

Retrovirus carrying the ADA gene infects the cultured T-cells, transferring the gene into the cell

Blood is drawn from the patient

Corrected T-cells are reinfused into the patient

ADA gene is inserted into the T-cell genome during cell division

Gene therapy for ADA deficiency.

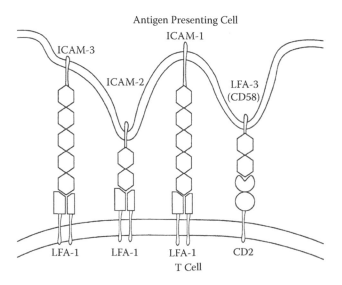

Antigen Presenting Cell

ICAM-3

ICAM-1

ICAM-2

LFA-3 (CD58)

LFA-1   LFA-1   LFA-1   CD2

T Cell

Adhesion receptors.

through high endothelial venules have lymph node homing receptors.

adhesion receptors

Proteins in cell membranes that facilitate the interaction of cells with matrix. They play a significant role in adherence and chemoattraction in cell migration. They are divided into three groups, the first of which is the immunoglobulin superfamily that contains the T cell receptor/CD3, CD4, CD8, MHC class I, MHC class II, sCD2/LFA-2, LFA-3/ CD58, ICAM-1, ICAM-2, and VCAM-2. The second group of adhesion receptors is made up of the integrin family containing LFA-1, Mac-1, p150,95, VLA-5, VLA-4/LPAM-1, LPAM-2, and LPAM-3. The third family consists of selectin molecules including Mel-14/LAM-1, ELAM-1, and CD62.

adjuvant

Substance that facilitates or enhances the immune response to an antigen with which it is combined. Various types have been described, including Freund's complete and incomplete adjuvants, aluminum compounds, and muramyl dipeptide. Some of these act by forming a depot in tissues from which an antigen is slowly released. In addition, Freund's adjuvant

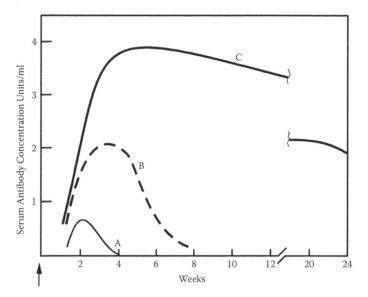

Effect of adjuvants. Schematic representation of the quantities of antibodies formed by rabbits following a single injection of a soluble protein antigen (arrow) such as a bovine gamma globulin in dilute physiologic saline solution (A), adsorbed on precipitated alum (B), or incorporated into Freund's complete adjuvant (C).

attracts a large number of cells to the area of antigen deposition to provide increased immune responsiveness to it. Modern adjuvants include such agents as muramyl dipeptide. The ideal adjuvant is biodegradable, allowing elimination from tissues once its immunoenhancing activity has been completed. An adjuvant nonspecifically facilitates an immune response to antigen. An adjuvant usually combines with the immunogen but is sometimes given prior to or following antigen administration. Adjuvants represent a heterogeneous class of compounds capable of augmenting the humoral or cell-mediated immune response to a given antigen. They are widely used in experimental work and for therapeutic purposes in vaccines. Adjuvants include compounds of a mineral nature, products of microbial origin, and synthetic compounds. The primary effect of some adjuvants is postulated to be the retention of antigen at the inoculation site so that the immunogenic stimulus persists for a longer period. However, the mechanism by which adjuvants augment the immune response is poorly understood. The macrophages may be the targets and mediators of action of some adjuvants, whereas others may require T cells for their response augmenting effects. Adjuvants such as lipopolysaccharide (LPS) may act directly on B lymphocytes. Adjuvants enhance activation of T lymphocytes by facilitating the accumulation and activation of accessory cells at a site of antigen exposure. They facilitate expression by accessory cells of T cell activating costimulators and cytokines and are believed to prolong the expression of peptide–MHC complexes on the surfaces of antigen-presenting cells (APCs).

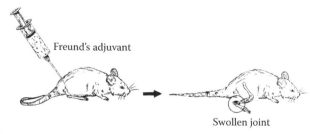

Adjuvant disease.

adjuvant disease

The injection of rats with Freund's complete adjuvant, a water-in-oil emulsion containing killed, dried mycobacteria (e.g., *Mycobacterium tuberculosis*), leads to the production of aseptic synovitis, which closely resembles rheumatoid arthritis (RA) in humans. Sterile inflammation occurs in the joints and lesions of the skin. In addition to swollen joints, inflammatory lesions of the tail may also result in animals developing adjuvant arthritis that represent animal models for RA.

adjuvant granuloma

A tissue reaction that occurs at a local site following the injection of such adjuvant materials as Freund's complete adjuvant and alum, both of which have been used extensively in immunologic research in past years.

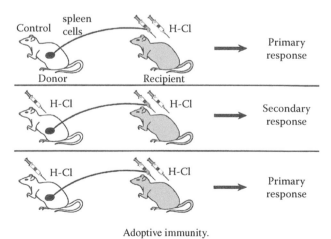

Adoptive immunity.

adoptive immunity

Term assigned by Billingham, Brent, and Medawar (1955) to transplantation immunity induced by the passive transfer of specifically immune lymph node cells from an actively immunized animal to a normal (previously nonimmune) syngeneic recipient host.

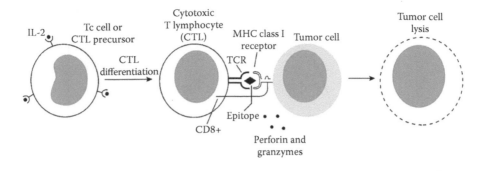

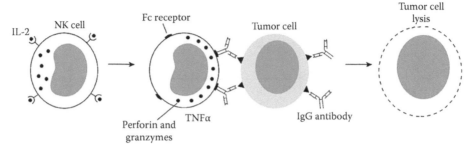

Interleukin-2 (IL-2) immunotherapy.

adoptive immunization

The passive transfer of immunity by the injection of lymphoid cells from a specifically immune individual to a previously nonimmune recipient host. The recipient is said to have adoptive immunity.

adoptive immunotherapy

The experimental treatment of terminal cancer patients who have metastatic tumors unresponsive to other modes of therapy by the inoculation of lymphokine-activated killer (LAK) cells or tumor-infiltrating lymphocytes (TILs) together with interleukin-2 (IL-2). This mode of therapy has shown some success in approximately one tenth of treated individuals who have melanoma or renal cell carcinoma.

adoptive tolerance

The passive transfer of immunologic tolerance with lymphoid cells from an animal tolerant to that antigen to a previously nontolerant and irradiated recipient host animal.

adoptive transfer

A synonym for adoptive immunization; the passive transfer of lymphocytes from an immunized individual to a nonimmune subject with immune system cells such as CD4+ T lymphocytes. Tumor-reactive T cells have been adoptively transferred for experimental cancer therapy.

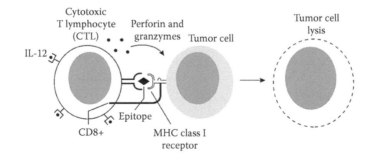

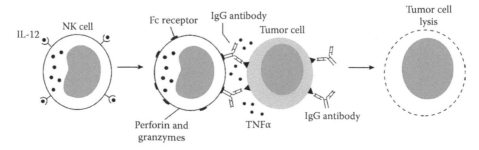

Interleukin-12 (IL-12) immunotherpy.

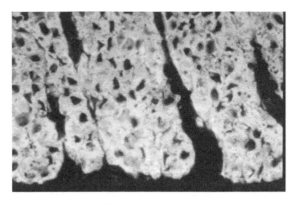

Adrenal autoantibody.

adrenal autoantibody (AA)

Autoantibody found in two thirds of idiopathic (autoimmune) patients with Addison's disease. Although once the most common cause of Addison's disease, tuberculosis is now only infrequently associated with it. Adrenal autoantibodies react with the zona glomerulosa of the adrenal cortex. The autoantigens linked to this disease are cytochrome P-450 enzyme family members that participate in steroidogenesis in the adrenal and other steroid-producing organs. The enzyme autoantigens include P-450 steroid 21 hydroxylase (21 OH), P-450 side chain cleavage enzyme (P-450 scc), and 17 α-hydroxylase (17-α-OH). Autoantibodies in adult patients with autoimmune Addison's disease may be directed against cytochrome P-450 steroid 21 OH, the only adrenal-specific enzyme. Other autoantibodies such as those against P-450 scc present in the adrenals, gonads, and placenta, and 17-α-OH present in the adrenals and gonads are found in autoimmune polyglandular syndromes (APGSs). APGS type I autoimmune polyendocrinopathy–candidiasis–ectodermal dystrophy (APECED) begins in early childhood with mucocutaneous candidiasis followed by Addison's disease and often gonadal failure in hypoparathyroidism. APS type II (Schmidt syndrome) is mostly an adult disease inherited in an autosomal-dominant manner and is marked by a variable combination of Addison's disease, insulin-dependent type I diabetes mellitus (IDDM) and autoimmune thyroid disorders. It is likened to HLA-DR3. Steroid cell antibodies have been associated with autoimmune gonadal failure. They are present in 18% of patients with Addison's disease, alone or in association with APGS. The most frequently encountered autoantigen in Addison's disease is the adrenal cytochrome P-450 enzyme 21 OH. Autoantibodies to 17-α-OH are found in 55% of APTS type I patients and in 33% of APGS type II patients. Autoantibodies against P-450 scc are found in 45% of APGS type I patients and 42% of APGS type II patients.

adrenergic receptor agonists

The β2-adrenergic receptor is expressed on Th1 but not on Th2 clones. An agonist for this receptor selectively suppresses IFN-γ synthesis *in vitro*; increases IL-4, IL-5, and IL-10 synthesis in spleen cells from treated mice; and increases IgE levels *in vivo*. Epinephrine and norepinephrine inhibit IL-12 synthesis but enhance IL-10 formation. β2-adrenergic receptor stimulation favors Th2 immune responses.

adrenergic receptors

Structures on the surfaces of various types of cells that are designated α or β and interact with adrenergic drugs.

adrenocorticotrophic hormone (ACTH) antibody

A polyclonal antibody preparation useful in immunoperoxidase procedures to stain corticotroph cells of the pituitary gland and benign and malignant tumors arising from these cells in formalin-fixed, paraffin-embedded tissue biopsies.

adsorption

The elimination of antibodies from a mixture by adding particulate antigen or the elimination of particulate antigen from a mixture by adding antibodies. The incubation of serum-containing antibodies such as agglutinins with red blood cells or other particles may allow their removal due to sticking to the particle surface.

adsorption chromatography

A method to separate molecules based on their adsorptive characteristics. Fluid is passed over a fixed solid stationary phase.

adult respiratory distress syndrome (ARDS)

Embarrassed respiratory function as a consequence of pulmonary edema caused by increased vascular permeability.

adult T cell leukemia lymphoma (ATLL)

A lymphoproliferative neoplasm of mature lymphocytes that progresses rapidly. It has been linked to the HTLV-1 retrovirus infection observed in Japan, Africa, the Caribbean, and southeastern United States. Patients develop hypercalcemia, progressive skin changes, enlarged hilar, retroperitoneal, and peripheral lymph nodes without mediastinal node enlargement. Involvement of the lungs, gastrointestinal tract, and central nervous system and opportunistic infections may also be observed. The condition occurs in five clinical forms.

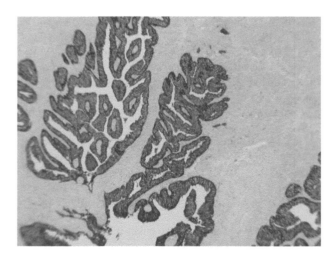

Cytokeratin cocktail—prostate.

AE1/AE3 pan-cytokeratin monoclonal antibody

An antibody that provides the broadest spectrum of keratin reactivity among the 19 catalogued human epidermal keratins and produces positive staining in virtually all epithelia.

AET rosette test (historical)

A technique used previously to enumerate human T cells based upon the formation of sheep red cell rosettes surrounding them. The use of sheep red cells treated with aminoethylthiouridium bromide renders the rosettes more stable than using sheep red cells untreated by this technique. The rosette test technique was replaced by the use of anti-CD2 monoclonal antibodies and flow cytometry.

A

afferent lymphatic vessels

The channels that transport lymph, which may contain antigens draining from connective tissue or from sites of infection in many anatomical locations, to the lymph nodes.

affinity

The strength of binding between antigen and antibody molecules. It increases along with linkage stability. The affinity constant reflects the strength of binding. The paratope of an antibody molecule views the epitope as a three-dimensional structure. Affinity (K_A) is a thermodynamic parameter that quantifies the strength of the association between antigen and antibody molecules in solution. It applies to a single species of antibody-combining sites interacting with a single species of antigen-binding sites. Affinity describes the strength of binding between a single binding site of an antibody molecule and its ligand or antigen. The dissociation constant (K_d) represents the affinity of molecule A for ligand B. This is the concentration of B required to occupy the combining sites of half the A molecules in solution. A smaller K_d signifies a stronger or higher affinity interaction, and a lower concentration of ligand is requisite to bind with the sites.

affinity chromatography

A method to isolate antigen or antibody based upon antigen–antibody binding. Antibody molecules fixed to a solid support such as plastic or agarose beads in a column, constituting the solid phase, may capture antigen molecules in solution passed over the column. Subsequent elution of the antigen is then accomplished with acetate buffer at pH 3.0 or diethylamine at pH 11.5.

affinity constant

Determination of the equilibrium constant by applying the law of mass action to the interaction of an epitope or hapten with its homologous antibody. The lack of covalent bonds between the interacting antigen and antibody permits a reversible reaction.

affinity labeling

A method to label the binding sites of proteins by virtue of a ligand analog to which a chemically reactive or photoreactive group has been attached. The latter can bind covalently with a suitably oriented amino acid in the binding site. A labeling reagent of this type is comprised of a biologically active substance that forms a reversible complex with a particular protein and a properly positioned chemically or photochemically reactive leaving group. During incubation, the affinity label reacts with its protein counterpart, leading to the production of an irreversible protein–ligand complex. The first affinity labeling studies of antibodies employed diazonium labeling reagents attached to a benzene arsonate hapten.

affinity maturation

The sustained increase in the affinity of antibodies for an antigen with time following immunization. The genes encoding the antibody variable regions undergo somatic hypermutation with the selection of B lymphocytes whose receptors express high affinity for the antigen. The immunoglobulin G (IgG) antibodies that form following the early, heterogeneous IgM response manifest greater specificity and less heterogeneity than do the IgM molecules.

African swine fever (ASF)

A very contagious acute hemorrhagic disease of pigs that is induced by a large icosahedral DNA virus that produces a broad range of clinical signs. Protective immunity has been induced *in vivo* but it is now accompanied by the development of neutralizing antibodies. No vaccine is available.

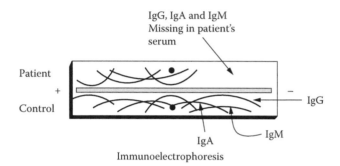

Agammaglobulinemia.

agammaglobulinemia

Refer to hypogammaglobulinemia. Agammaglobulinemia was used in earlier years before the development of methods sufficiently sensitive to detect relatively small quantities of gamma globulin in the blood. Congenital defects in B cell signaling may lead to one of several primary immunodeficiencies characterized by lack of antibodies. Primary agammaglobulinemia was attributed to defective immunoglobulin formation, whereas secondary agammaglobulinemia referred to immunoglobulin depletion, as in losses due to inflammatory bowel disease or through the skin in burn cases.

agar gel

A semisolid substance prepared from seaweed agar that was widely used in the past in bacteriology, and is used in immunology for diffusion of antigen and antibody in Ouchterlony-type techniques, electrophoresis, immunoelectrophoresis, and related methods.

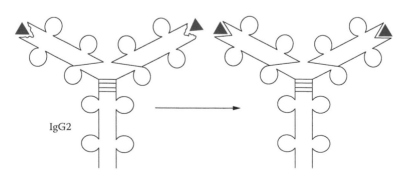

Affinity maturation.

agarose

A neutral polygalactoside consisting of alternating *d*-galactose and 3,6-anhydrogalactose linear polymer, the principal constituent of agar. Gels made from agarose are used for the hemolytic plaque assay and for leukocyte chemotaxis assays, as well as for immunodiffusion and nucleic acid/protein electrophoresis.

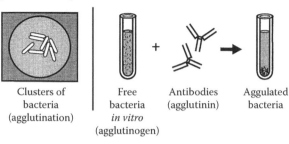

Clusters of bacteria (agglutination) | Free bacteria *in vitro* (agglutinogen) | Antibodies (agglutinin) | Aggulated bacteria

Agglutination.

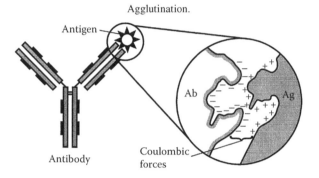

Antigen-antibody complex. Role of positive and negative charges in agglutination of antigen by antibody.

agglutination

The combination of soluble antibody with particulate antigens in an aqueous medium containing electrolyte, such as erythrocytes, latex particles bearing antigen, or bacterial cells, to form an aggregate that may be viewed microscopically or macroscopically. If antibody is linked to insoluble beads or particles, they may be agglutinated by soluble antigen through reverse agglutination. Agglutination is the basis for multiple serological reactions, including blood grouping, diagnosis of infectious diseases, rheumatoid arthritis (RA) testing, etc. To carry out an agglutination reaction, serial dilutions of antibody are prepared, and a constant quantity of particulate antigen is added to each antibody dilution. Red blood cells may serve as carriers for adsorbed antigen (e.g., the tanned red cell or *bis*-diazotized red cell technique). Like precipitation, agglutination is a secondary manifestation of antigen–antibody interaction. As specific antibody crosslinks particulate antigens, aggregates that form become macroscopically visible and settle out of suspension. Thus, the agglutination reaction has a sensitivity 10 to 500 times greater than that of the precipitin test with respect to antibody detection.

agglutination inhibition

Diminished clumping of particles bearing antigen on their surfaces by the addition of soluble antigen that interacts with and blocks the agglutinating antibody.

agglutination titer

The highest dilution of a serum that causes clumping of particles such as bacteria. Titer is an approximation of the antibody activity in each unit volume of a serum sample. The term is used in serological reactions and is determined by preparing serial dilutions of antibody to which a constant amount of antigen is added. The end point is the highest dilution of antiserum in which a visible reaction with antigen, e.g., agglutination, can be detected. The titer is expressed as the reciprocal of the serum dilution that defines the endpoint. If agglutination occurs in the tube containing a 1:240 dilution, the antibody titer is said to be 240. Thus, the serum would contain approximately 240 units of antibody per milliliter of antiserum. The titer provides only an estimate of antibody activity. For absolute amounts of antibody, quantitative precipitation or other methods must be employed.

agglutinin

An antibody that interacts with antigen on the surfaces of particles such as erythrocytes, bacteria, or latex cubes to cause their aggregation or agglutination in an aqueous environment containing electrolyte. Substances other than agglutinin antibody that cause agglutination or aggregation of certain specificities of red blood cells include hemagglutinating viruses and lectins.

agglutinogen

Antigens on the surfaces of particles such as red blood cells that react with the antibody known as agglutinin to produce aggregation or agglutination. The most widely known agglutinogens are those of the ABO and related blood group systems.

aggregate anaphylaxis

Form of anaphylaxis caused by aggregates of antigen and antibody in the fluid phase. The aggregates bind complement-liberating complement fragments C3a, C5a, and C4a, also called anaphylatoxins that induce the release of mediators. Preformed aggregates of antigen–antibody complexes in the fluid phase fix complement. Fragments of complement components, the anaphylatoxins, may induce the release of mediators from mast cells. There is no evidence that these components play a role in anaphylactic reactions *in vivo*. Aggregates of antigen–IgG antibody, however, may induce anaphylaxis, the manifestations of which are different in the various species.

aging and immunity

Aging is accompanied by many changes in the immune system. The involution of the thymus gland sets the pace for immune senescence. There are changes in the distribution and function of both T and B lymphocytes. A striking feature of immune senescence is the increased frequency of autoimmune reactions in both humans and experimental animals. There is also an increased instance of neoplasia with increasing age as immune surveillance mechanisms falter.

agonist

A molecule that combines with a receptor and enables it to function.

agonist ligand

A molecule that unites with a receptor for antigen and exerts a positive influence on downstream signaling and cellular function.

agonist peptides

Peptide antigens that activate specific lymphocytes, enabling them to synthesize cytokines and to proliferate.

agranulocytosis

A striking decrease in circulating granulocytes including neutrophils, eosinophils, and basophils as a consequence of suppressed myelopoiesis. The deficiency of polymorphonuclear leukocytes leads to decreased resistance and increased susceptibility to microbial infection. Patients may present with pharyngitis. The etiology may be unknown or follow

A

exposure to cytotoxic drugs such as nitrogen mustard or follow administration of the antibiotic chloramphenicol.

agretope

The region of a protein antigen that combines with a major histocompatibility complex (MHC) class II molecule during antigen presentation. This is then recognized by the T cell receptor MHC class II complex. Amino acid sequences differ in their reactivity with MHC class II molecules.

agrin

An aggregating protein crucial for formation of the neuromuscular junction. It is also expressed in lymphocytes and is important in reorganization of membrane lipid microdomains in setting the threshold for T cell signaling. T cell activation depends on a primary signal delivered through the T cell receptor and a secondary costimulatory signal mediated by coreceptors. Costimulation is believed to act through the specific redistribution and clustering of membrane and intracellular kinase-ridge lipid raft microdomains at the contact sites between T cells and antigen-presenting cells. This site is known as the immunological synapse. Endogenous mediators of raft clustering in lymphocytes are essential for T cell activation. Agrin induces the aggregation of signaling proteins and the creation of signaling domains in both immune and nervous systems through a common lipid raft pathway.

AH50

An assay to measure the functional activity of the alternative complement pathway. This alternative pathway (AP) hemolytic assay (AH50) employs complement-mediated lysis of rabbit red blood cells in Mg^{2+}-EGTA buffer. The EGTA chelates the Ca^{2+} needed for complement C1 macromolecular assembly, thereby blocking classical complement pathway activity. The AH50 assay is valuable to screen for homozygous deficiencies of AP constituents including C3, factor I, factor B, properdin, factor H, and factor D. Deficiencies of the fluid phase regulatory proteins of the AP, factor I, or factor H induce a secondary deficiency of C3, properdin, and factor B as a result of uncontrolled consumption of these proteins. The lack of hemolysis in both the AH50 and CH50 assays strongly suggests a deficiency in a complement terminal pathway component (C5–C9). When the AH50 values are normal and there is no lysis in CH50, a classical pathway component deficiency (C1, C2, or C4) occurs. A normal CH50 and a lack of hemolysis in AH50 firmly suggest an AP component deficiency. A lack of lysis strongly points to homozygous deficiency. Low levels of lysis in AH50 or CH50 assays suggest either heterozygous deficiency or complement activation. Hemolytic functional assays for individual complement components facilitate the detection of homozygous and some heterozygous deficiencies in addition to mutations that lead to inactive complement protein. Usually, AP deficiency is associated with recurrent bacterial infections. Homozygous factor H deficiency has been observed in patients with glomerulonephritis, recurrent pyogenic infection, hemolytic–uremic syndrome, or systemic lupus erythematosus and in healthy subjects. Factor D deficiency has been linked to recurrent upper respiratory infections with *Neisseria* species.

AICD

Abbreviation for activation-induced cell death.

AIDS (acquired immune deficiency syndrome)

A disease induced by the human immunodeficiency retrovirus (designated HIV-1). The two genetically different but antigenically similar HIV viruses are designated HIV-1 and HIV-2. HIV-1 is more common in the United States, Europe and central Africa, whereas HIV-2 produces a similar disease mainly in west Africa. Although first observed in homosexual men, the disease affects both males and females equally in central Africa and is now affecting a greater number of heterosexuals, with cases reported in both males and females in western countries, including North America and Europe. Viral entry into a cell requires CD4 and coreceptors that are chemokine receptors. This involves binding of viral gp120 and fusion with the cell via viral gp41 protein. The principal cellular targets include CD4+ helper T cells, macrophages, and dendritic cells. The provirus genome integrates into host cell DNA. Virus expression is initiated by stimuli that activate infected cells. Acute infection is associated with viremia with dissemination of the virus. There is latent infection of lymphoid tissue cells with continuing viral replication and progressive loss of CD4+ T cells. HIV is transmitted by blood and body fluids but is not transmitted through casual contact or through air, food, insect bites, or other means. Besides homosexual and bisexual males, others at high risk include intravenous drug abusers, recipients of blood transfusions, and hemophiliacs (rare since 1985), the offspring of HIV infected mothers, and sexual partners of HIV-infected individuals in the above groups. The two most important laboratory parameters in following an HIV infected patient include the absolute CD4 lymphocyte count, which gives information concerning the patient's immune status at that time, and viral load, i.e., the number of viral transcripts, which indicates disease progression. Clinically, HIV infection is marked by various opportunistic infections, neoplasms, and CNS involvement. Clinically there are three phases including: (1) early phase; (2) middle chronic phase; (3) final crisis phase. The acute phase is marked by nonspecific symptoms such as sore throat, myalgia, fever, rash and, occasionally, aseptic meningitis. There are high levels of virus production during this phase, which induces a virus-specific immune response associated with seroconversion within 3 to 17 weeks of exposure and development of virus-specific CD8+ cytotoxic T lymphocytes. During the middle chronic phase, which may last for several years, there is continued HIV replication but relative containment of the virus. Virus replication continues in the lymphoid tissues during this phase; CD4+ T cells continue to be lost; and HIV levels increase. Without treatment, most HIV infected patients develop AIDS after a chronic phase ranging from 7 to 10 years. The final crisis phase is characterized by a profound breach of host defenses characterized by increased viremia and clinical illness. Patients often present with fever, fatigue, weight loss and diarrhea, and diminished CD4 T cell counts ≤200/µl and opportunistic infections. Great strides have been made in HIV therapy including cocktails that may be altered to account for antigenic variation of the virus. Atripla™ represents a remarkable improvement in reducing the previously numerous medications required for HIV therapy to one dose of medication per day. Attempts to develop an HIV vaccine remain elusive, however.

AIDS belt

A geographic area across central Africa that describes a region where multiple cases of heterosexual AIDS related to sexual promiscuity have been reported. Nations in this belt include Burundi, Kenya, Central African Republic, Rwanda, the Congo, Malawi, Zambia, Tanzania, and Uganda.

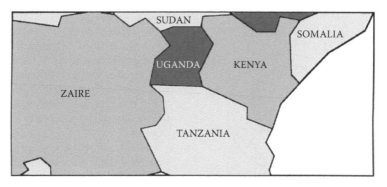

AIDS belt.

AIDS dementia complex

Up to two thirds of AIDS patients may develop central nervous system signs and symptoms, such as sustained cognitive behavior and motor impairment believed to be associated with infection of microglial cells with the HIV-1 virus. This may be due to the structural similarity of gp120 of HIV-1 to neuroleukin. Patients have memory loss, are unable to concentrate, have poor coordination of gait, and have altered psychomotor function, among other symptoms. The subcortical white matter and deep gray matter degenerate, lateral and posterior spinal cord columns show white matter vacuolization, and the gp120 of HIV serves as a calcium channel inhibitor, causing toxic levels of calcium within neurons.

AIDS embryopathy

A condition in children born to HIV-infected mothers who are intravenous drug abusers. Affected children have craniofacial region defects that include microcephaly, hypertelorism, cube-shaped head, saddle nose, widened palpebral fissures with bluish sclera, triangular philtrum, and widely spreading lips.

AIDS encephalopathy

AIDS dementia. Refer to AIDS dementia complex.

AIDS enteropathy

A condition that may be seen in patients with AIDS-related complex marked by diarrhea (especially nocturnal), wasting, possibly fever, and defective d-xylose absorption, leading to malnutrition. The small intestine may demonstrate atrophy of villi and hyperplasia of crypts. Both small and large intestines may reveal diminished plasma cells, elevated intraepithelial lymphocytes, and viral inclusions.

AIDS-related complex (ARC)

A preamble to AIDS that consists of a constellation of symptoms and signs including a temperature above 38°C, a greater than 10% loss of body weight, lymphadenopathy, diarrhea, night sweats of more than 3 months' duration, and fatigue. Laboratory findings include CD4+ T lymphocyte levels of less than 0.4×10^9, a CD4 to CD8 T lymphocyte ratio below 1.0, leukopenia, anemia, and thrombocytopenia. There may be a decreased response to PHA, principally a T cell mitogen, and anergy, manifested as failure to respond to skin tests. In contrast, a polyclonal gammopathy may be present. A diagnosis of ARC requires at least two of the clinical manifestations and two of the laboratory findings listed above.

AIDS serology

Within 3 to 6 weeks after infection with HIV-1, high levels of HIV p24 antigen are found in the plasma. One week to 3 months following infection, an HIV-specific immune response results in the formation of antibodies against

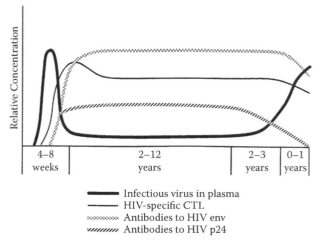

AIDS serology.

HIV envelope protein gp120 and HIV core protein p24. HIV-specific cytotoxic T lymphocytes are also formed. The result of this adaptive immune response is a dramatic decline in viremia and a clinically asymptomatic phase lasting 2 to 12 years. As CD4+ T cell numbers decrease, the patient becomes clinically symptomatic. HIV-specific antibodies and cytotoxic T lymphocytes decline, and p24 antigen increases.

AIDS treatment

Although no drug is curative, zidovudine (azidothymidine-AZT), ddC (dideoxycytidine), and ddI (dideoxyinosine) are effective in delaying progression of the disease. Many experimental preparations are under investigation, such as DAB/486 IL-2, which is cytotoxic for high-affinity IL-2 receptors expressed on HIV-infected T lymphocytes.

AIDS vaccine

Several experimental AIDS vaccines are under investigation. HIV-2 inoculation into cynomolgus monkeys apparently prevented them from developing simian AIDS following injection of the SIV virus.

AIDS virus

See human immunodeficiency virus (HIV).

AILA

Abbreviation for angioimmunoblastic lymphadenopathy.

AIRE gene

Abbreviation for the autoimmune regulator gene mapped to chromosome region 21q22.3 mutations in the autoimmune regulator gene. Responsible for autoimmune polyendocrinopathy–candidiasis–ectodermal dystrophy (APECED).

A

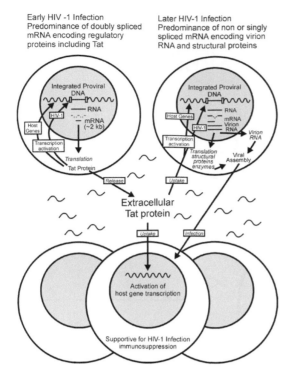

Early HIV -1 Infection
Predominance of doubly spliced mRNA encoding regulatory proteins including Tat

Later HIV-1 Infection
Predominance of non or singly spliced mRNA encoding virion RNA and structural proteins

Uninfected cells

Possible AIDS vaccine.

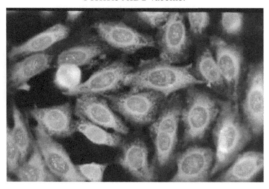

Alanyl-tRNA synthetase antibodies.

airway hyper-responsiveness

Airway narrowing induced by nonspecific stimuli in an asthmatic person.

airway remodeling

The removal of superior layers of bronchial epithelium and thickening of the submucosae as a consequence of collagen deposition beneath the basement membrane in an asthmatic patient.

alanyl-tRNA synthetase antibodies

Autoantibodies against the synthetases (histidyl-, threonyl-, alanyl-, isoleucyl-, and glycyl-tRNA synthetases) have been detected in some patients with polymyositis (PM) and dermatomyositis (DM). Histidyl-tRNA synthetase (Jo-1) antibodies are the most common (20 to 30% of patients with PM/DM).

albumin agglutinating antibody

An antibody that does not agglutinate erythrocytes in physiological saline solution but does cause their aggregation in 30% bovine serum albumin (BSA). Antibodies with this property have long been known as "incomplete antibodies" and are of interest in red blood cell typing.

albumin, serum

The principal protein of human blood serum that is soluble in water and in 50% saturated sodium sulfate. At pH 7.0, it is negatively charged and migrates toward the anode during electrophoresis. It is important in regulating osmotic pressure and in the binding of anions. Serum albumin (e.g., bovine serum albumin, BSA) is commonly used as an immunogen in experimental immunology.

alefacept

An immunosuppressive agent that interferes with lymphocyte activation by binding specifically to CD2 lymphocyte antigen and inhibiting leukocyte function-associated antigen-3 (LFA-3)/CD2 interaction. Used to treat patients with moderate to severe chronic plaque psoriasis. T lymphocyte activation involving the interaction between LFA-3 on antigen-presenting cells and CD2 on T lymphocytes is important in chronic plaque psoriasis. Most T lymphocytes in psoriatic lesions are memory effector cells with the CD45RO markers that express activation markers CD25, CD69 and release inflammatory cytokines such as interferon γ. Alefacept leads to a decrease in CD2+ T lymphocyte subsets, mainly CD45RO+. Treatment with alefacept leads to a decrease in circulating total CD4+ and CD8+ T lymphocytes.

alemtuzumab

A humanized IgG$_1$ that contains a κ light chain that binds to CD52 present on normal and malignant B and T lymphocytes, NK cells, monocytes, macrophages, and a minor population of granulocytes. It is approved for treatment of B cell chronic lymphocytic leukemia patients who have failed standard treatment. It diminishes leukemic and normal cells by direct antibody-dependent lysis, leading to lymphopenia, and sometimes neutropenia, anemia, and thrombocytopenia.

Aleutian mink disease

A parvovirus-induced disease of minks and ferrets associated with a polyclonal proliferation of B cells and a significant elevation of gamma globulin in the blood. It bears similarity both clinically and pathologically to human systemic lupus erythematosus and polyarteritis nodosa. The viscera reveal lymphocytes and plasma cells, and renal glomeruli trap immune complexes that are also present in small- and medium-sized arteries of the kidney, brain, and heart. The immune deposits lead to inflammation, resulting in glomerulonephritis, hepatitis, and arteritis, in addition to the hypergammaglobulinemia.

alexine (or alexin)

Historical synonym for complement. Hans Buchner (1850–1902) found that the bactericidal property of cell-free serum was destroyed by heat. He named the active principle alexine (which in Greek means to ward off or protect). Jules Bordet (1870–1961) studied this thermolabile and nonspecific principle in blood serum which induces the lysis of cells (e.g., bacterial cells) sensitized with specific antibody. Bordet and Gengou went on to discover the complement fixation reaction. (Bordet received the Nobel Prize for Medicine in 1919.)

ALG

Abbreviation for antilymphocyte globulin.

alkaline phosphatase (AP)

A Zn^{2+} metalloenzyme present in many living organisms. In humans, it consists of three tissue-specific isozymes encoded by three separate genes. The separate forms of AP are detectable in intestine, placenta, kidney, bone, and liver. They are glycoproteins comprised of single polypeptide chains containing 500 amino acid residues and are membrane bound. Calf intestine alkaline phosphatase is used in immunology in ELISA assays, immunoblotting, and molecular cloning. AP deletes 5′-phosphate from linear DNA terminals. It is also used in DNA recombinants to inhibit recircularization that diminishes background for DNA. It is also used to treat genomic DNA fragments to prevent two or more fragments from ligating to each other. It may be employed to prepare 5′-32P-N-labeled DNA.

ALL
Abbreviation for acute lymphoblastic leukemia.

allele
One of the alternative forms of a gene at a single locus on a chromosome that encodes the phenotypic features of a certain inherited characteristic. The presence of multiple alleles, such as at the MHC locus, leads to polymorphism.

allelic dropout
In the amplification of a DNA segment by the polymerase chain reaction, one of the alleles may not be amplified, leading to the false impression that the allele is absent. The phenomenon takes place at 82 to 90°C in the thermocycler.

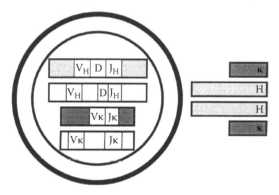

Allelic exclusion.

allelic exclusion
Only one of two genes for which the animal is heterozygous is expressed, whereas the remaining gene is not. Immunoglobulin genes manifest this phenomenon. Allelic exclusion accounts for the ability of a B cell to express only one immunoglobulin or the capacity of a T cell to express a T cell receptor of a single specificity. Investigations of allotypes in rabbits established that individual immunoglobulin molecules have identical heavy chains and light chains. Immunoglobulin-synthesizing cells produce only a single class of heavy chain and one type of light chain at a time. Thus, by allelic exclusion, a cell that is synthesizing antibody expresses only one of two alleles encoding an immunoglobulin chain at a particular locus. The synthesis of a functional μ heavy chain from the IgH locus on one chromosome blocks more V(D)J recombination and μ chain synthesis from the other IgH allele.

allelic exclusion (TCR locus)
The synthesis of a functional TCR β chain from one chromosome's TCR β locus prevents more V(D)J recombination and synthesis of TCR β chains from the other TCR β allele and V(D)J recombination in the TCR γ locus on both chromosomes.

allelic variant
It explains human leukocyte antigen (HLA) associations with rheumatoid arthritis, type I diabetes, multiple sclerosis, and

celiac disease. A minimum of 6 α and 8 β genes occur in distinct clusters, termed HLA-DR, DQ, and DP, within the HLA class II genes. DO and DN class II genes are related but map outside DR, DQ, and DP regions. The two types of dimers along the HLA cell-surface HLA-DR class II molecules are made up of either DRα-polypeptide associated with DRβ$_1$-polypeptide or DR with DRβ$_2$-polypeptide. Structural variation in class II gene products is linked to functional features of immune recognition leading to individual variations in histocompatibility, immune recognition, and susceptibility to disease. The two types of structural variations appear among DP, DQ, and DR products in primary amino acid sequence by as much as 35% and individual variations attributable to different alleleic forms of class II genes. The class II polypeptide chain possesses domains that are specific structural subunits containing variable sequences that distinguish among class II α genes or class II β genes. It has been suggested that these allelic variation sites form epitopes that represent individual structural differences in immune recognition.

allergen
An antigen that induces an allergic or hypersensitivity response in contrast to a classic immune response produced by the recipient host in response to most immunogens. Allergens include such environmental substances as pollens (i.e., their globular proteins) from trees, grasses, and ragweed, certain food substances, animal danders, and insect venom. Selected subjects are predisposed to synthesize IgE antibodies in response to allergens and are said to be atopic. The crosslinking of IgE molecules anchored to the surfaces of mast cells or basophils through their Fc regions results in the release of histamine and other pharmacological mediators of immediate hypersensitivity from mast cells or basophils.

allergen immunotherapy
Desensitization treatment. Refer to desensitization.

allergenic extracts
Substances derived individually from various biological sources containing antigens that demonstrate immunologic activity. They are classified based on standardization and dose form. Standardization systems include: (1) biological activity expressed in allergenic units (AUs); (2) weight-to-volume (w/v); and (3) protein nitrogen units (PNUs). Dose forms include aqueous, glycerinated, and alum-precipitated. The mechanism of action is ill-defined. Specific IgG appears in the serum after inoculation of allergenic extracts. IgG competes with specific IgE for a specific antigen. After binding to receptors on mast cell membranes, IgE produces an allergenic reaction by releasing histamine and other pharmacological mediators upon uniting with an antigen. Serum IgE levels diminish over time. Decreased leukocyte sensitivity to allergens and increased numbers of T-suppressor cells for IgE-producing plasma cells are also observed. Hyposensitization may diminish the release of pharmacological mediators such as histamine in the responses of basophils to a specific allergen.

allergic alveolitis
Refer to farmer's lung.

allergic asthma
Bronchial constriction that is a consequence of an allergic reaction to an inhaled antigen.

allergic conjunctivitis
A hypersensitivity reaction in the conjunctiva of the eye, often induced by airborne antigens.

A

allergic contact dermatitis

Delayed-type hypersensitivity mediated by specifically sensitized T lymphocytes (type IV hypersensitivity) in response to the covalent linkage of low molecular weight chemicals, often less than 1000 M_r, to proteins in the skin. The inflammation induced by these agents is manifested as erythema and swelling approximately 12 hours after contact and is maximal at 24 to 48 hours. Blisters form that are filled with serum, neutrophils, and mononuclear cells. There is perivascular cuffing with lymphocytes, vesiculation, and necrosis of epidermal cells. Basophils, eosinophils, and fibrin deposition appear together with edema of the epidermis and dermis. Langerhans' cells in the skin serve as antigen-processing cells where the allergen has penetrated. Sensitization lasts for many years and becomes generalized in the skin. Chemicals become conjugated to skin proteins and serve as haptens; therefore, the hapten alone can elicit the hypersensitivity once sensitization is established. After blistering, crust formation and weeping of the lesion occur. The condition is intensely pruritic and painful. Metal dermatitis, such as that caused by nickel, occurs as a patch that corresponds to the area of contact with a metal or jewelry. Dyes in clothing may produce skin lesions at points of contact with the skin. The patch test is used to detect sensitivity to contact allergens. Rhus dermatitis represents a reaction to urushiols in poison oak and ivy that elicit vesicles and bullae on affected areas. Treatment is with systemic corticosteroids or the application of topical steroid cream to localized areas. Dinitrochlorobenzene (DNCB) and dinitrofluorobenzene (DNFB) have been used to induce allergic contact dermatitis in both experimental animals and humans.

allergic disease immunotherapy

The principal immunologic, as opposed to environmental or pharmacologic, treatment of allergic diseases that include allergic rhinitis, conjunctivitis, and asthma. The allergen to which a patient exhibits immunoglobulin E (IgE)-dependent sensitivity is first identified followed by subcutaneous administration of minute quantities of natural extracts containing these allergens. The aim is to modify the immune response responsible for maintaining atopic symptoms.

allergic granulomatosis

A type of pulmonary necrotizing vasculitis with granulomas in the lung and pulmonary vessel walls. There may be infiltrates of eosinophils in the tissues and asthma. Also called Churg–Strauss syndrome.

allergic orchitis

The immunization of guinea pigs with autologous extracts of the testes incorporated into Freund's complete adjuvant leads to lymphocytic infiltrate in the testes and antisperm cytotoxic antibodies in the serum 2 to 8 weeks after inoculation. Human males who have been vasectomized may also develop allergic orchitis.

allergic reaction

A response to antigens or allergens in the environment as a consequence of either preformed antibodies or effector T cells. Allergic reactions are mediated by a number of immune mechanisms, the most common of which is type I hypersensitivity in which IgE antibody specific for an allergen is carried on the surfaces of mast cells. Combining with specific antigen leads to the release of pharmacological mediators, resulting in clinical symptoms of asthma, hay fever, and other manifestations of allergic reactions.

allergic response

A response to antigen (allergen) that leads to a state of increased reactivity or hypersensitivity rather than a protective immune response.

allergic rhinitis

A condition characterized by a pale and wet nasal mucosa with swollen nasal turbinates. When hay fever is seasonal or environmental it is allergic. One must first distinguish between infectious and noninfectious rhinitis. Both types of patients may have nasal polyps, and are often anosmic. Noninfectious rhinitis that is perennial is difficult to establish as allergic.

allergoids

Allergens that have been chemically altered to favor the induction of immunoglobulin G (IgG) rather than IgE antibodies to diminish allergic manifestations in hypersensitive individuals. These formaldehyde-modified allergens are analogous to toxoids prepared from bacterial exotoxins. Some of the physical and chemical characteristics of allergens are similar to those of other antigens; however, the molecular weights of allergens are lower.

allergy

A term coined by Clemens von Pirquet in 1906 to describe the altered reactivity of the animal body to antigen. Currently, the term refers to altered immune reactivity to a spectrum of environmental antigens including pollen, insect venom, and food. Allergy is also referred to as hypersensitivity and usually describes type I immediate hypersensitivity of the atopic/anaphylactic type. Allergy is a consequence of the interaction of antigen (or allergen) and antibody or T lymphocytes produced by previous exposure to the same antigen or allergen.

allergy, infection

Hypersensitivity, especially of the delayed T cell type, that develops in subjects infected with certain microorganisms such as *Mycobacterium tuberculosis* or certain pathogenic fungi.

alloantibody

An antibody that interacts with an alloantigen, such as the antibodies generated in the recipient of an organ allotransplant (such as kidney or heart) that then may react with the homologous alloantigen of the allograft. Alloantibodies interact with antigens that result from allelic variation at polymorphic genes. Examples include those that recognize blood group antigens and human leukocyte antigen (HLA) class I and class II molecules.

alloantigen

An antigen present in some members or strains of a species, but not in others. Alloantigens include blood group substances on erythrocytes and histocompatibility antigens present in grafted tissues that stimulate alloimmune responses in the recipient not possessing them, as well as various proteins and enzymes. Two animals of a given species are said to be allogeneic with respect to each other. Alloantigens are commonly products of polymorphic genes.

alloantiserum

An antiserum generated in one member or strain of a species not possessing the alloantigen (e.g., histocompatibility antigen) with which the strain or species has been challenged and derived from another member or strain of the same species.

allogeneic (or allogenic)

An adjective that describes genetic variations or differences among members or strains of the same species. The term refers to organ or tissue grafts between genetically dissimilar humans or unrelated members of other species.

allogeneic bone marrow transplantation

Hematopoietic cell transplants are performed in patients with hematologic malignancies, certain nonhematologic neoplasms, aplastic anemias, and certain immunodeficiency states. In allogeneic bone marrow transplantation, the recipient is irradiated with lethal doses to destroy malignant cells or create a graft bed. The problems that arise include graft-vs.-host disease (GVHD) and transplant rejection. GVHD occurs when immunologically competent cells or their precursors are transplanted into immunologically crippled recipients. Acute GVHD occurs within days to weeks after allogeneic bone marrow transplantation and primarily affects the immune system and epithelia of the skin, liver, and intestines. Rejection of allogeneic bone marrow transplants appears to be mediated by NK cells and T cells that survive in the irradiated host. Natural killer (NK) cells react against allogeneic stem cells that are lacking self major histocompatibility complex (MHC) class I molecules and therefore fail to deliver the inhibitory signals to NK cells. Host T cells react against donor MHC antigens in a manner resembling their reaction against solid tissue grafts.

allogeneic disease

Pathologic consequence of immune reactivity of bone marrow allotransplants in immunosuppressed recipient patients as a result of graft-vs.-host reactivity in genetically dissimilar members of the same species.

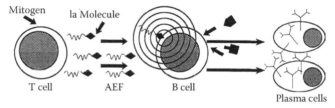

Allogeneic effect.

allogeneic effect

The synthesis of antibody by B cells against a hapten in the absence of carrier-specific T cells, provided allogeneic T lymphocytes are present. Interaction of allogeneic T cells with the major histocompatibility complex (MHC) class II molecules of B cells causes the activated T lymphocytes to produce factors that facilitate B cell differentiation into plasma cells without the requirement for helper T lymphocytes. There is allogeneic activation of T cells in the graft-vs.-host reaction.

allogeneic graft

An allograft consisting of an organ, tissue, or cell transplant from a donor individual or strain to a genetically different individual or strain within the same species.

allogeneic inhibition

Homozygous tumors grow better when transplanted to homozygous syngeneic hosts of the strain of origin than they grow when transplanted to F1 hybrids between the syngeneic (tumor) strain and an allogeneic strain. This is manifested as a higher frequency of tumor and shorter latency period in syngeneic hosts. The better growth of tumor in syngeneic than in heterozygous F1 hybrid hosts was initially termed syngeneic preference. When it became apparent that selective pressure against the cells in a mismatching environment produced the growth difference, the phenomenon was termed allogeneic inhibition.

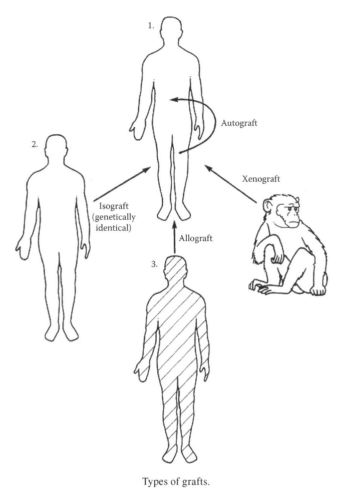

Types of grafts.

allograft

An organ, tissue, or cell transplant from one individual or strain to a genetically different individual or strain within the same species. Also called homograft.

allogroup

Several allotypes representing various immunoglobulin classes and subclasses inherited as a unit. Alleles that are closely linked encode the immunoglobulin heavy chains in an allogroup. An allogroup is a form of a haplotype.

alloimmune hemolytic anemia

Lysis of erythrocytes following exposure of an individual to allogeneic red blood cells, which leads to the formation of antibodies against foreign red blood cell antigens. Transfusion reactions attributable to mismatched ABO blood group antigens and Rh disease are examples.

alloimmune thrombocytopenia

Decreased blood platelets mediated by alloantibodies against platelet surface antigens by a type II hypersensitivity mechanism.

alloimmunization

An immune response provoked in one member or strain of a species with an alloantigen derived from a different member or strain of the same species. Examples include the immune response of a human following transplantation of a solid organ graft such as a kidney or heart. Alloimmunization with red blood cell antigens in humans may lead to pathologic sequelae such as hemolytic disease of the newborn (erythroblastosis fetalis) in a third Rh(D)+ baby born to an Rh(D)- mother.

A

allophonic mouse

A tetraparental, chimeric mouse whose genetic make-up is derived from four separate parents. It is produced by the association of two early eight-cell embryos that differ genetically. A single blastocyst forms, is placed in a pseudo-pregnant female uterus, and is permitted to develop to term. Tetraparental mice are widely used in immunological research.

alloreactive

The recognition by antibodies or T lymphocytes from one member of a species cell or tissue antigens of a genetically nonidentical member.

alloreactive T cell

A T lymphocyte from one member of a species capable of responding to an allogeneic antigen from another member of the same species.

alloreactivity

Stimulation of immune system T cells by non-self major histocompatibility complex (MHC) molecules attributable to antigenic differences between members of the same species. Alloreactivity represents the immune response to an alloantigen based on recognition of allogeneic MHC.

allorecognition

The detection of allelic differences manifested by cells of one member of the species by lymphocytes of another individual. Usually concerns identification of MHC-encoded differences.

allotope

An epitope or antigenic determinant encoded by a single allelic form of a polymorphic gene within species. An allotope often designates an antigenic determinant on an antibody molecule that is encoded by C gene alleles or framework regions of V genes. The antigenic determinant of an allotype; also called allotypic determinant.

allotransplant

An organ or tissue transplanted from one individual to another member of the same species.

allotype

A distinct antigenic form of a serum protein that results from allelic variations present on the immunoglobulin heavy chain constant region. Allotypes were originally defined by antisera that differentiated allelic variants of immunoglobulin (Ig) subclasses. The allotype is due to the existence of different alleles at the genetic locus that determines the expression of a given determinant. Immunoglobulin allotypes have been extensively investigated in inbred rabbits. Currently, allotypes are usually defined by DNA techniques. To be designated as an official allotype, the polymorphism must be present in a reasonable subset of the population (approximately 1%) and follow Mendelian genetics. Allotype examples include the IgG3 Caucasian allotypes G3m[b] and G3m[g]. These two alleles vary at positions 291, 296, and 384. Another example is the allotype at the IgA2 locus. The IgA2m(1) allele is European/Near Eastern, while IgA2m(2) is African/East Asian. The allotypic differences are in $C\alpha_1$ and $C\alpha_3$, and the IgA2m(2) allele has a shorter hinge than the IgA2m(1) allele. Allotypic differences in immunoglobulin molecules have been important in solving the genetics of antibodies.

allotype suppression

The failure to produce antibodies of a given allotype by offspring of mothers who have been immunized against the paternal immunoglobulin (Ig) allotype before mating. It

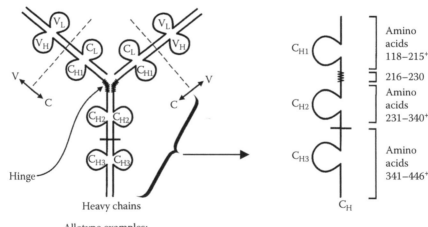

Allotype.

may also occur after administration of antibodies specific for the paternal allotype to heterozygous newborn rabbits. Animals conditioned in this way remain deficient for the suppressed allotype for months and possibly years thereafter. The animal switches to a compensatory increase in the production of the nonsuppressed allotype. In homozygotes, suppression involves heavy-chain switching from one Ig class to another.

allotypic determinant

Epitope on serum immunoglobulin (Ig) molecules present in selected members of a species. Allotypic determinants are present in addition to other markers characteristic of the molecule as a whole for the respective species. The allotypic determinants or allotopes are characteristic of a given class and subclass of immunoglobulin and have been demonstrated in several species. The inheritance of genes controlling these determinants is strictly Mendelian and is not sex linked. Both H and k L chains contain such determinants; the encoding genes are not linked and are codominant in an individual. This means that markers present both in the father and mother are expressed phenotypically in a heterozygote. However, an individual immunoglobulin-producing cell expresses only one of a pair of allelic genes, as a single cell can utilize only one parental chromosome. In an individual, some cells use the information encoded on the chromosome derived paternally and other cells use that derived from the maternal contribution. Thus, the individual is heterozygous, but a single cell secretes only the products of one allele because of allelic exclusion. The allotypic markers of human IgG are designated Gm determinants. The Km(Inv) markers are characteristic for the C region of k light chains.

allotypic marker

Refer to allotypic determinant or allotope.

allotypic specificities

Genetically different antibody classes and subclasses produced within individuals of the same species. They are detected as changes in the amino acid residues present in specific positions in various polypeptide chains. The allotypic specificities are also called genetic markers. Gm and Km(Inv) markers are examples of allotypes of human immunoglobulin G (IgG) heavy chains and k light chains, respectively.

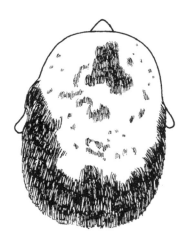

Alopecia areata.

allotypy

A term that describes the various allelic types or allotypes of immunoglobulin molecules.

alopecia areata

A partial or patchy loss of hair from the scalp or other hair site that is believed to have an autoimmune basis, even though no autoantigenic molecules in hair follicles have been identified. The inheritance is polygenic with a contribution from major histocompatibility complex (MHC) genes. Other autoimmune diseases associated with alopecia areata include the thyrogastric group, pernicious anemia, Addison's disease, and diabetes, as well as vitiligo, systemic lupus erythematosus (SLE), and others. There is supportive serological evidence for autoimmunity in alopecia areata. Organ-specific autoantibodies are increased in frequency, especially to thyroid micosomal antigen and to other tissue antigens as well. Affected hair follicles are encircled by dense lymphocytic infiltrates that consist of T cells with CD8+ T cell subset predominance.

alpha–beta T cells

T lymphocytes that express an αβ TCR. They comprise Th, Tc, and regulatory T cell populations and mediate very specific and broadly diverse adaptive immune responses.

ALPS

Abbreviation for autoimmune lymphoproliferative syndromes.

ALS (antilymphocyte serum) or ALG (anti-lymphocyte globulin)

Refer to antilymphocyte serum.

altered peptide ligand (APL)

Analog of immunogenic peptide in which the T cell receptor contact sites have been altered, usually by substitution with another amino acid. Even though these peptides fail to stimulate T cell proliferation, they activate some T cell receptor-mediated functions. Antagonist peptides specifically downmodulate the agonist-induced response. APLs can act therapeutically by modulating the cytokine patterns of T cells or they may induce a form of anergy in T cells. They stimulate partial responses from T lymphocytes specific for the agonist peptide.

altered self

The concept that the linkage of non-self peptide to major histocompatibility complex (MHC) yields a peptide–MHC structure different from any found in normal cells of the individual.

Alternaria species

Aeroallergenic fungi that can induce hypersensitivity pneumonitis (HP). These fungi cause a form of HP known as woodworker's lung disease, as well as immunoglobulin E (IgE)-mediated allergic disease.

alternative C5 convertase

A participant in the alternative pathway of complement activation, comprised of two C3b molecules linked to B ($C3b_2Bb$) and splits C5 into C5a and C5b.

alternative complement pathway

Activation of complement not by antibody but through the binding of complement protein C3b to the surface of a pathogenic microorganism. This innate immune mechanism amplifies complement activation through the classic pathway. A non-antibody-dependent pathway for

A

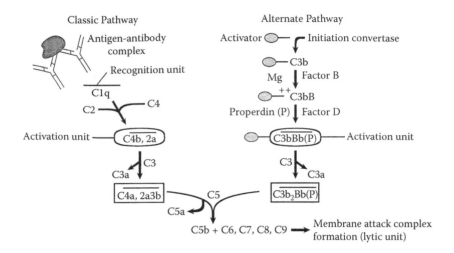

complement activation in which the early components C1, C2, and C4 are not required. It involves protein properdin factor D, properdin factor B, and C3b, leading to C3 activation and continuing to C9 in a manner identical to that which takes place in the activation of complement by the classical pathway. Substances such as endotoxin, human immunoglobulin A (IgA), microbial polysaccharides, and other agents may activate complement by the alternative pathway. The C3bB complex forms as C3b combines with factor B. Factor D splits factor B in the complex to yield the Bb active fragment that remains linked to C3b and Ba, which is inactive and is split off. C3bBb, the alternative

pathway C3 convertase, splits C3 into C3b and C3a, thereby producing more C3bBb, which represents a positive feedback loop. Factor I, when accompanied by factor H, splits the heavy chain of C3b to yield C3bi, which is unable to anchor Bb, thereby inhibiting the alternative pathway. Properdin and C3 nephritic factor stabilize C3bBb. C3 convertase stabilized by properdin activates complement's late components, resulting in opsonization, chemotaxis of leukocytes, enhanced permeability, and cytolysis. Properdin, IgA, IgG, lipopolysaccharide, and snake venom can initiate the alternative pathway. Trypsin-related enzymes can activate both pathways.

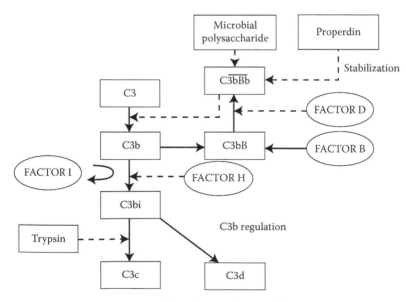

Alternative complement pathway.

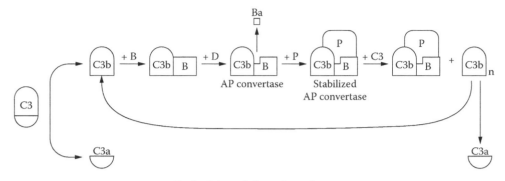

Feedback loop of alternative pathway.

alternative pathway

Activation of complement not by antibody but through the binding of complement protein C3b to the surface of a pathogenic microorganism. This innate immune mechanism amplifies complement activation through the classic pathway.

alternative pathway C3 convertase

Alternate unstable C3bB complex that splits C3 into C3a and C3b. Factor P, also known as properdin, stabilizes C3bB to yield C3bBbP. C3 nephritic factor can also stabilize C3bB.

alternative splicing

A process whereby the RNA splicing apparatus may handle primary transcripts of a selected gene at splice acceptor sites 3′ of different exons leading to mRNA populations comprising different exon subsets; exons whose splice acceptor sites are deleted from the mRNA, rendering their corresponding amino acid sequences lacking in the resulting protein. Thus, one gene can encode two or more versions of the same protein.

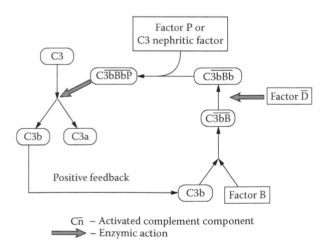

$\overline{Cn}$ – Activated complement component
⟹ – Enzymic action

Alternative pathway C3 convertase.

alum granuloma

A tissue reaction in the form of a granuloma produced at the local site of intramuscular or subcutaenous inoculation of a protein antigen precipitated from solution by an aluminum salt acting as adjuvant. Slow release of antigen from the granuloma is considered to facilitate enhanced antibody synthesis to the antigen.

alum-precipitated antigen

A soluble protein antigen such as a toxoid adsorbed to aluminum salts during precipitation from solution. The aluminum salt acts as an adjuvant that facilitates an immune response to such antigens as diphtheria and tetanus toxoids. Soluble protein antigen is combined with 1% potassium aluminum sulfate, and sodium hydroxide is added until floccules are produced.

alum-precipitated toxoid

Refer to alum-precipitated antigen.

aluminum adjuvant

Aluminum-containing substances that have a powerful capacity to adsorb and precipitate protein antigens from solution. The use of these preparations as immunogens causes depot formation in the tissues at the site of inoculation, from which the antigen is slowly released, thereby facilitating greater antibody production than if the antigen is dissipated and rapidly lost from the body. Substances used extensively in the past for this purpose include aluminum hydroxide gel, aluminum sulfate, and ammonium alum, as well as potassium alum.

aluminum hydroxide gel

Aluminum hydroxide [Al(OH)$_3$] was widely used in the past as an immunologic adjuvant by reacting antigen with 2% hydrated AL(OH)$_3$ to adsorb and precipitate the protein antigen from solution. See also aluminum adjuvant.

alums

Aluminum salts employed to adsorb and precipitate protein antigens from solution, followed by the use of the precipitated antigen as an immunogen that forms a depot in animal tissues. See also aluminum adjuvant.

A

ALVAC

An experimental AIDS vaccine developed for the first test of a human vaccine in Africa. The vaccine has undergone safety testing in the United States and France with no serious side effects reported and is being used in Uganda, where AIDS has killed nearly half a million people and left one million children orphaned.

alveolar basement membrane autoantibodies (ABM autoantibodies)

Antibodies present in the blood sera and as linear deposits on the ABMs of patients with rapidly progressive glomerulonephritis (RPGN) and pulmonary hemorrhage (Goodpasture's syndrome). The antibodies are also present in the blood sera of patients with glomerular basement membrane (GBM) nephritis. Not all patients with GBM nephritis have pulmonary involvement. This may be explained based on different reactivities with ABMs. Linear immunoglobulin staining of ABMs in ABM disease limited to the lungs is highly specific. Endothelial cell injury, such as that induced by infection, is considered significant in the pathogenesis of Goodpasture's hemorrhagic pneumonitis. Pulmonary hemorrhage has been associated with antineutrophil cytoplasmic antibodies (ANCAs) that may sometimes be immunoglobulin M (IgM) isotype-restricted. In the absence of GBM autoantibodies and ANCA, intra-alveolar hemorrhage may be associated with cardiolipin antibodies. Early diagnosis of patients with these types of clinical conditions is critical, as mortality rates exceed 75%.

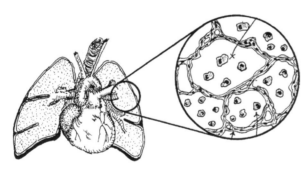

Alveolar macrophages.

alveolar macrophage

A macrophage in the lung alveoli that may remove inhaled particulate matter.

ALZ-50

A monoclonal antibody that serves as an early indicator of Alzheimer's disease by reacting with Alzheimer's brain tissue, specifically protein A-68.

Am allotypic marker

An allotypic antigenic determinant located on the heavy chain of the immunoglobulin A (IgA) molecule in humans. Of the two IgA subclasses, the IgA1 subclass has no known allotypic determinant. The IgA2 subclass has two allotypic determinants designated A2m(1) and A2m(2), based on differences in a-2 heavy chain primary structures. Allelic genes at the A2m locus encode these allotypes that are expressed on the a-2 heavy chain constant regions.

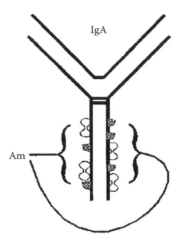

Illustration of the location of Am marker specificities on the Fc region.

amboceptor (historical)

Paul Ehrlich (*circa* 1900) considered anti-sheep red blood cell antibodies known as amboceptors to have one receptor for sheep erythrocytes and another receptor for complement. The term gained worldwide acceptance with the popularity of complement fixation tests for syphilis, such as the Wassermann reaction. The term is still used by some when discussing complement fixation.

amebocytes

Mobile phagocytic cells that mediate defense by phagocytosis in addition to digestive and excretion functions in primitive organisms lacking circulatory systems.

amino acyl tRNA synthetases

Myositis-specific autoantibodies that include antibodies against histidyl tRNA synthetase (HRS), first known as Jo-1. They are found in 20% of patients with polymyositis and dermatomyositis. Autoantibodies to analyl (PL-12), threonyl (PL-7), glycyl (EJ), and isoleucyl (OJ) tRNA synthetases have also been reported. These aminoacyl synthetases bind their corresponding amino acids to the tails of their respective tRNAs. Essentially all Jo-1-positive sera possess antibodies that react with the amino terminal (amino acids 1–44) of the protein, but most also have antibodies against epitopes positioned further toward the carboxyl end of the sequence. Anti-HRS antibodies are principally immunoglobulin G$_1$ (IgG$_1$) and persist throughout the course of the disease. Patients with autoantibodies against tRNA synthetases have several clinical features in common, including interstitial lung disease and pulmonary fibrosis (50 to 100%), arthritis (60 to 100%), Raynaud's phenomenon (60 to 93%), fever, and "mechanic's hands." In patients with antisynthetase syndrome, anti-Jo-1 antibodies are most common in polymyositis, whereas autoantibodies against other aminoacyl–tRNA synthetases are more often found in dermatomyositis. Antibodies to HRS show a strong association with HLA-DR3.

aminoethylcarbazole (AEC)

3-amino-9-ethyl carbazole is used in the ABC immunoperoxidase technique to produce a visible reaction product detectable by light microscopy when combined with hydrogen peroxide. AEC is oxidized to produce a reddish-brown pigment that is not water soluble. Peroxidase catalyzes the reaction. Because peroxidase is localized only at sites where the PAP is bound via linking antibody and primary antibody to antigen molecules, the antigen is identified by the reddish-brown pigment.

aminophylline

Refer to theophylline.

AML

Abbreviation for acute myelogenous leukemia, also called acute myeloid leukemia.

ammonium sulfate precipitation

The ammonium sulfate method is a means of measuring the primary antigen-binding capacity of antisera and detects both precipitating and nonprecipitating antibodies. It offers an advantage over equilibrium dialysis in that large, nondializable protein antigens may be used. This assay is based on the principle that certain proteins are soluble in 50% saturated ammonium sulfate, whereas antigen–antibody complexes are not. Thus, complexes may be separated from unbound antigen. Spontaneous precipitation will occur if a precipitating type of antibody is used, until a point of antigen excess at which complex aggregation no longer occurs and soluble complexes are formed is reached. Upon the addition of an equal volume of saturated ammonium sulfate (SAS) solution, these complexes become insoluble, leaving radiolabeled antigen in solution. SAS fractionation does not significantly alter the stoichiometry of the antibody–antigen reaction, and it inhibits the release or exchange of bound antigen. Thus, radioactivity of this "induced" precipitate is a measure of the antigen-binding capacity of the antisera as opposed to a measure of the amount of antigen or antibody spontaneously precipitated.

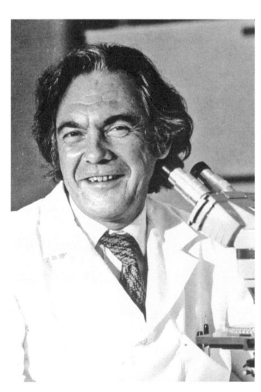

D. Bernard Amos.

Amos, D. Bernard

British immunologist trained by Peter A. Gorer, the father of modern histocompatibility testing, in the United Kingdom. He worked in the United States at Roswell Park Memorial Institute, Buffalo, New York, and spent most of his career as a professor of immunology and experimental surgery at Duke University Medical Center in Durham, North Carolina. A pioneer in human histocompatibility, having organized a number of international workshops throughout the world, he developed improved techniques to demonstrate the existence of different human tissue types. He also served as president of the American Association of Immunologists and the American Society for Histocompatibility and Immunogenetics.

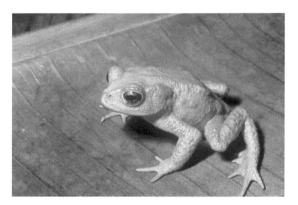

Amphibian immune system.

amphibian immune system

Amphibians serve as crucial models for developmental and comparative immunological analysis. The two species used for investigation include the axolotl and *Xenopus*. Hematopoietic precursors rapidly colonize thymus buds in *Xenopus*. The spleen consists of red and white pulp. The axolotl also has a spleen. Immunoglobulin M (IgM)-synthesizing cells are present in the digestive tract in axolotl IgM; IgX- but no IgY-synthesizing cells are found in the *Xenopus* digestive tract. Amphibian blood contains both B- and T-like cells. Monoclonal antibodies specific for different heavy and light chain immunoglobulin chain isotypes can be identified in both *Xenopus* and axolotl. A CD8 membrane glycoprotein has also been found in *Xenopus*. *Xenopus* B and T cells respond to plant mitogens in the same manner observed in mammalian T and B cells. The axolotl has B lymphocytes that proliferate in response to lipopolysaccharide (LPS). Genes that encode the α and β chains of axolotl TCR have been cloned. In *Xenopus*, IgM and IgX have high molecular weights, and IgY low molecular weight immunoglobulin classes have been identified. The *Xenopus* major histocompatibility complex (MHC) encodes both class Ia and class II molecules. This MHC region also mediates rapid rejection of grafts. Thymectomy in *Xenopus* may diminish or abolish allograft rejection.

amphipathic

An adjective describing a molecule with both hydrophobic and hydrophilic regions.

amphiphysin autoantibodies

Autoantibodies against amphiphysin, one of two known target autoantigens in stiff man syndrome (SMS), a central nervous system disease characterized by progressive muscle rigidity and painful spasms. Amphiphysin is a 125- to 128-kDa cytoplasmic, synaptic, vesicle-associated protein expressed in neurons, certain types of endocrine cells, and spermatocytes. Its biological function may involve synaptic vesicle endocytosis. Autoantibodies to glutamic acid decarboxylase (GAD) are detected in 60% of SMS. Amphiphysin autoantibodies are present in SMS patients negative for GAD autoantibody, all of whom are female breast cancer patients. The amphiphysin autoepitope is present in the C terminal region of the protein. Small-cell lung carcinoma patients who present with paraneoplastic encephalomyelitis have been reported to manifest immunoglobulin G (IgG) autoantibodies against amphiphysin.

amphiregulin

A glycoprotein member of the epidermal growth factor (EGF) family of proteins. The carboxyl terminal amino acid residues of amphiregulin positions 46 to 84 share much sequence homology with the EGF family. The actions of amphiregulin are wide ranging and include the stimulation of proliferation of certain tumor cell lines, fibroblasts, and various other normal cells. These actions are mediated by binding to EGF receptors possessing intrinsic tyrosine kinase activity.

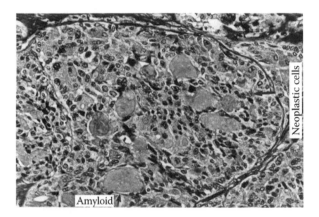

Medullary carcinoma of thyroid with amyloid deposits.

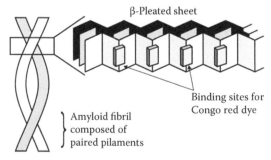

Amyloid.

amyloid

An extracellular, homogeneous eosinophilic material deposited in various tissues in disease states designated as primary and secondary amyloidosis. It is composed chiefly of protein and shows a green birefringence when stained with Congo red and observed by polarizing light microscopy. By electron microscopy, the fibrillary appearance is characteristic.

X-ray crystallography reveals a β-pleated sheet structure arranged in an antiparallel fashion that gives the protein its optical and staining properties. The amino termini of the individual chains face opposite directions, and the chains are bound by hydroxyl bonds. Amyloid consists of two principal and several minor biochemical varieties. Pathogenetic mechanisms for its deposition differ, although the deposited protein appears similar from one form to another. Amyloid is composed of nonbranching fibrils 7.5 to 10 nm wide and of indefinite length. It also has a P component that is nonfibrillary, is pentagonal in structure, and constitutes a minor component. Chemically, amyloid falls into two principal classes: AL, consisting of amyloid light chains, and AA (amyloid-associated), comprising a nonimmunoglobulin protein called AA. These molecules are antigenically different and have dissimilar deposition patterns based on the clinical situation. AL amyloid is comprised of whole immunoglobulin light chains, their N terminal fragments, or a combination of the two. Λ Light chains rather than κ are usually found in AL. Proliferating immunoglobulin-producing B cells, as in B cell dyscrasias, produce AL amyloid protein. AA amyloid fibroprotein is not an immunoglobulin and has a molecular weight of 8.5 kDa. Serum amyloid-associated (SAA) protein is the serum precursor of AA amyloid. It constitutes the protein constituent of a high density lipoprotein and acts as an acute phase reactant. Thus, its level rises remarkably within hours of an acute inflammatory response. AA protein is the principal type of amyloid deposited in the tissues during chronic inflammatory diseases. Several other distinct amyloid proteins also exist.

amyloid β fibrillosis

Every amyloid has a β-pleated sheet structure that accounts for the ability of Congo red to stain it and the ability of proteolytic enzymes to digest it. Refer also to amyloid and amyloidosis.

amyloid P component

The P component has a molecular weight of 180 kDa. It migrates in electrophoresis with the α globulin fraction, and by electron microscopy reveals a pentagonal shape, suggesting that it consists of subunits linked by hydrogen bonds. It is a minor component of all amyloid deposits and is nonfibrillar. It is a normal a_1 glycoprotein and has close structural homology with the C-reactive protein. It has an affinity for amyloid fibrils and accounts for their PAS positive staining quality.

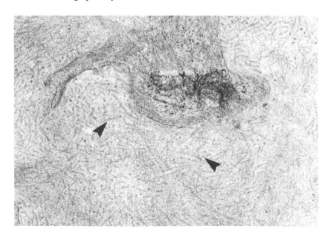

Amyloidosis: amyloid fibrils.

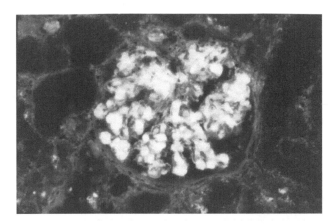

Amyloidosis: mesangial areas of glomerulus.

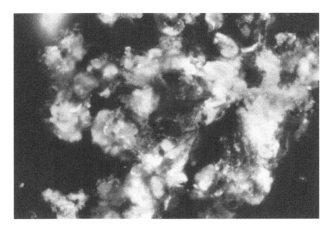

Amyloidosis: kidney.

amyloidosis

A constellation of diseases characterized by the extracellular deposition of fibrillar material that has a homogeneous and eosinophilic appearance in conventional staining methods. Amyloidosis may compromise the functions of vital organs. Diseases with which it is associated may be inflammatory, hereditary, or neoplastic. All types of amyloid link to Congo red and manifest an apple green birefrigence when viewed by polarizing light microscopy after first staining with Congo red. Under electron microscopy, amyloid has a major fibrillar component and a minor rod-like structure shaped like a pentagon with a hollow core when observed on end (the P component). All forms of amyloid share the P component in common. It is found as a soluble serum protein (SAP) in the circulation. Amyloid has a β-pleated sheet structure; it is insoluble in physiologic saline but soluble in distilled water. The classification of amyloidosis depends upon the clinical presentation, anatomic distribution, and chemical content of the amyloid. In the United States, AL amyloid is the most common type of amyloidosis and occurs in association with multiple myeloma and Waldenström's macroglobulinemia. Patients demonstrate free light chain production in association with the development of Bence–Jones proteins in myeloma. The light chain quality and degradation mechanisms are critical in determining whether Bence–Jones proteins will be deposited as amyloid. Chronic inflammation leads to increased levels of serum amyloid-associated (SAA) protein, produced by the

liver following IL-6 and IL-1 stimulation. Normally, SAA is degraded by the enzymes of monocytes. Thus, individuals with defects in the degradation process may generate insoluble AA molecules. Likewise, there may be a defect in the degradation of immunoglobulin light chains in subjects who develop AL amyloidosis. Amyloidosis secondary to chronic inflammation is severe, with kidney, liver, spleen, lymph node, adrenal, and thyroid involvement. These secondary amyloidosis deposits consist of amyloid A (AA) protein that makes up 85 to 90% of the deposits and serum amyloid P component that account for the remainder of the deposit. The AL type of amyloidosis more often involves the heart, gastrointestinal tract, respiratory tract, peripheral nerves, and tongue. Amyloidosis may also be heredofamilial or associated with aging.

ANA

Abbreviation for antinuclear antibodies.

ANAE (α-naphthyl acetate esterase)

Refer to nonspecific esterase.

anaINH

Anaphylatoxin inhibitor.

anakinra (injection)

A recombinant nonglycosylated form of human interleukin-1 receptor antagonist (IL-1Ra). It differs from native IL-1Ra in its possession of a single methionine residue at its amino terminus. Anakinra is comprised of 153 amino acids and has a molecular weight of 17.3 kDa. It is synthesized by recombinant DNA technology employing an *Escherichia coli* bacterial expression system. It blocks the biological activity of IL-1 by inhibiting IL-1 binding to the IL-1 type I receptor (IL-1RI). IL-1 is synthesized in response to inflammatory stimuli and has a wide spectrum of activities including cartilage degradation by its induction of the rapid loss of proteoglycans and stimulation of bone resorption. Levels of naturally occurring IL-1Ra in synovial fluid from RA patients are not sufficient to compete with the increased mass of locally produced IL-1.

anamnesis

Immunologic memory. Refers to the elevated immune response following secondary or tertiary administration of immunogen to a recipient previously primed or sensitized to the immunogen (i.e., the secondary response).

anamnestic

The recall response of immunologic memory that results in a rapid rise in antibody production following re-exposure to the same antigen.

anamnestic response

Accentuated immune response that occurs following exposure of immunocompetent cells to an immunogen to which they have been exposed earlier; commonly called the secondary or anamnestic response. It occurs rapidly (within hours) following secondary immunogen inoculation and does not have the lag period observed with primary immunization. Immunologic memory is involved in the production of this response that generally consists of immunoglobulin G (IgG) antibodies of high titer and high affinity. There may also be heightened T cell (cell-mediated) immune reactivity. Also called memory or booster response or secondary immune response.

anaphylactic shock

Cardiovascular collapse and suffocation attributable to tracheal swelling that results from a systemic anaphylactic

A

Schematic representation of humoral and cellular events in the primary and secondary (anamnestic) antibody responses.

(immediate hypersensitivity) reaction following an antigen that has been systemically administered. This allergic reaction is a consequence of the binding of antigen to immunoglobulin E (IgE) antibodies on mast cells in the connective tissue throughout the body, resulting in a disseminated release of inflammatory mediators.

anaphylactoid reaction

A response resembling anaphylaxis, except that it is not attributable to an allergic reaction mediated by immunoglobulin E (IgE) antibody. It is due to the nonimmunologic degranulation of mast cells such as that caused by drugs or chemical compounds such as aspirin, radiocontrast media, chymopapain, bee or snake venom, or gum acacia that cause release of the pharmacological mediators of immediate hypersensitivity including histamine and other vasoactive molecules.

anaphylatoxin inactivator

A 300-kDa globulin carboxyl peptidase in serum that destroys the anaphylatoxin activity of C5a, C3a, and C4a by cleaving their carboxyl-terminal arginine residues.

anaphylatoxin inhibitor (anaINH)

A 300-kDa globulin carboxyl peptidase that cleaves the carboxyl terminal arginine of anaphylatoxin. The enzyme acts on all three forms, including C3a, C4a, and C5a, inactivating rather than inhibiting them.

anaphylatoxins

Substances generated by the activation of complement that leads to increased vascular permeability as a consequence of the degranulation of mast cells with the release of pharmacologically active mediators of immediate hypersensitivity. These biologically active peptides of low molecular weight are derived from C3, C4, and C5. They are generated in serum during fixation of complement by antigen–antibody complexes, immunoglobulin aggregates, etc. Small blood vessels, mast cells, smooth muscles, and leukocytes in peripheral blood are targets of their action. Much is known about their primary structures. These complement fragments are designated C3a, C4a, and C5a. They cause smooth muscle contraction, mast cell degranulation with histamine release, increased vascular permeability, and the triple response in skin. They induce anaphylactic-like symptoms upon parenteral inoculation.

anaphylaxis

A shock reaction that occurs within seconds following the injection of an antigen or drug or after a bee sting to which a susceptible subject has immunoglobulin E (IgE)-specific antibodies. There is embarrassed respiration due to laryngeal

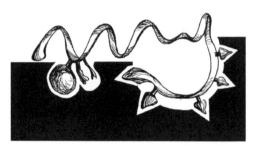

C3a/C3a57-77 –
Receptor interactions

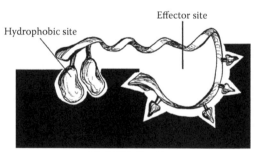

Model C3a Peptide –
Receptor interactions

Anaphylatoxin-receptor interactions.

and bronchial constriction and shock associated with decreased blood pressure. Signs and symptoms differ among species based on the primary target organs or tissues. Whereas IgE is the anaphylactic antibody in humans, IgG1 may mediate anaphylaxis in selected other species. Type I hypersensitivity occurs following the crosslinking of IgE antibodies by a specific antigen or allergen on the surfaces of basophils in the blood or mast cells in tissues. This causes the release of the pharmacological mediators of immediate hypersensitivity, with a reaction occurring within seconds of contact with the antigen or allergen. Eosinophils, chemotactic factor, heparin, histamine, and serotonin, together with selected other substances, are released during the primary response. Acute phase reactants are formed and released in the secondary response. Secondary mediators include slow-reacting substance of

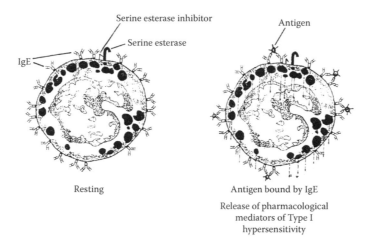

Serine esterase inhibitor
Serine esterase
IgE
Resting

Antigen
Antigen bound by IgE
Release of pharmacological
mediators of Type I
hypersensitivity

Comparison of resting basophil and mast cell in which serine esterase activity is blocked by serine esterase inhibitor with a mast cell or basophil undergoing degranulation as a consequence of antigen interaction with Fab regions of cell surface IgE molecules in which the serine esterase inhibitor activity is removed.

anaphylaxis (SRS-A), bradykinin, and platelet-activating factor. In addition to systemic anaphylaxis described above, local anaphylaxis may occur in the skin, gut, or nasal mucosa following contact with the antigen. The skin reaction, called urticaria, consists of a raised wheal surrounded by an area of erythema. Cytotoxic anaphylaxis follows the interaction of antibodies with cell surface antigens. See also aggregate anaphylaxis.

anaplastic
Tumor cells that are poorly differentiated and capable of aggressive growth.

anatoxin
Antibody specific for exotoxins produced by certain microorganisms such as the causative agents of diphtheria and tetanus. Prior to the antibiotic era, antitoxins were the treatments of choice for diseases produced by the soluble toxic products of microorganisms, such as those from *Corynebacterium diphtheriae* and *Clostridium tetani*.

anavenom
A toxoid consisting of formalin-treated snake venom that destroys the toxicity but preserves the immunogenicity of the preparation.

ancestral haplotype
An MHC haplotype that numerous families share, indicating that they probably have common ancestors. Also called HLA supratype or common extended haplotype.

anchor residues
Amino acid side chains of the peptide whose side chains fit into pockets in the peptide-binding cleft of the major histocompatibility complex (MHC) molecule. The side chains anchor the peptide in the cleft of the MHC molecule by binding two complementary amino acids in the MHC molecule.

anemia, drug-induced immune hemolytic
Acquired hemolytic anemia that develops as a consequence of immunological reactions following the administration of certain drugs. Clinically, this anemia resembles autoimmune hemolytic anemia of idiopathic origin. A particular drug may induce hemolysis in one patient, thrombocytopenia in another, neutropenia in yet another patient, and occasionally combinations of these in a single patient.
The drug-induced antibodies that produce these immune cytopenias are cell-specific. Drugs that cause hemolysis by complement-mediated lysis include quinine, quinidine, and rifampicin, as well as chlorpropamide, hydrochlorothiazide, nomifensine phenacetin, salicylazosulfapyridine, the sodium salt of *p*-aminosalicylic acid, and stibophen. Drug-dependent immune hemolytic anemia in which the mechanism is extravascular hemolysis may occur with prolonged high dose penicillin therapy or other penicillin derivatives as well as cephalosporins and tetracycline.

anergic B cell
Lymphocyte anergy, also termed clonal anergy, is the failure of B cell (or T cell) clones to react against antigen and may represent a mechanism to maintain immunologic tolerance to self. Anergic B cells express immunoglobulin D (IgD) at levels equal to that of normal B cells but they downregulate IgM 5- to 50-fold. This downregulation is associated with an inhibition in signaling, resulting in diminished phosphorylation of critical signal transduction molecules associated with surface immunoglobulin. Receptor stimulation of anergic B cells fails to release intracellular calcium, a critical step in B cell activation. Anergic B cells are unable to respond to subsequent exposure to cognate antigen. Anergy may be a means whereby the immune system silences potentially harmful B cell clones while permitting B cells to live long enough to be exported to peripheral lymphoid organs where anergic B cells may encounter a foreign antigen to which they have a higher affinity than their affinity for self antigen. If this were so, anergic B cells would be activated and contribute to a protective immune response.

anergize
Inducing anergy in a cell.

anergized
The consequence of rendering a subject anergic.

anergy
Diminished or absent delayed-type hypersensitivity (i.e., type IV hypersensitivity) as revealed by lack of responsiveness to commonly used skin test antigens including PPD, histoplasmin, candidin, etc. Decreased skin test reactivity may be associated with uncontrolled infection, tumor, Hodgkin disease, sarcoidosis, etc. There is decreased capacity of T lymphocytes to secrete lymphokines when their T cell receptors interact with a specific antigen. Anergy describes nonresponsiveness to antigen. Individuals are anergic when they cannot develop a delayed-type hypersensitivity reaction following challenge with an antigen. T and B lymphocytes are anergic when they cannot respond to their specific antigens. Often associated with lack of costimulation.

A

TCR signaling is required for T cell anergy

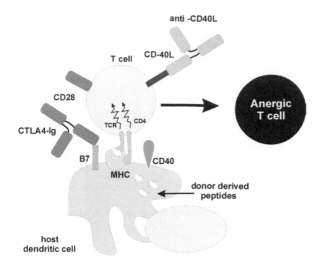

T cell anergy.

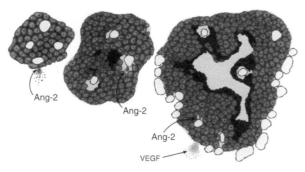

Tumor growth demonstrating progressive vessel regression correlation with expression patterns of Ang-2 and vascular endothelial growth factors 9VEGFs). (Left) A small tumor initially grows by coopting existing vessels. (Center) Ang-2 expression promotes vessel regression. (Right) Robust angiogenesis is apparent at the margin of the tumor where VEGF expression is upregulated.

aneuploidy

A condition in which the chromosome number of cells of an individual is not an exact multiple of the typical haploid set for that species.

angioedema

Significant localized swelling of tissues as a consequence of complement activation that takes place when C1 esterase inhibitor is lacking. Angioedema may also describe skin swelling following IgE-mediated allergic reactions that cause increased permeability of subcutaneous blood vessels.

angiogenesis

The formation of new blood vessels under the influence of several protein factors produced by both natural and adaptive immune system cells. It may be associated with chronic inflammation. Angiogenesis is the formation of new vessels by sprouting of new capillaries from existing vessels, a fundamental phenomenon in diseases such as atherosclerosis, cancer, and diabetes and in physiological conditions such as the menstrual cycle and pregnancy. Angiogenesis is closely related to vasculogenesis, the formation of a vascular network from stem cells in the embryo. In each case, the controlling mechanisms are the paracrine regulation of tyrosine kinase receptors, primarily on endothelial cells.

angiogenesis factor

A macrophage-derived protein that facilitates neovascularization through stimulation of vascular endothelial cell growth. Among the five angiogenesis factors known, basic fibroblast growth factor may facilitate neovascularization in type IV delayed-type hypersensitivity responses.

angiogenic factors

Fibroblast growth factors (FGFs) and vascular endothelial growth factors (VEGFs) are endothelial cell mitogens. The key factors are the five VEGFs, the VEGF receptors (VEGF-R1, -R2, and -R3), and placental growth factors (PIGFs). In addition, several newer factors, such as the angiopoietins, ephrins, leptin, and chemokines, have been shown to be important in angiogenesis.

angiogenin

A 14.4-kDa protein belonging to a family of proteins called the RNAse superfamily. Angiogenin acts as a potent inducer of blood vessel formation and is known to possess ribonuclease activity. If the ribonuclease activity is blocked, the angiogenic properties of angiogenin also appear to be inhibited. Angiogenin mRNA has been identified in a wide range of cell types.

angioimmunoblastic lymphadenopathy (AILA)

Proliferation of hyperimmune B lymphocytes. Immunoblasts, both large and small, form a pleomorphic infiltrate together

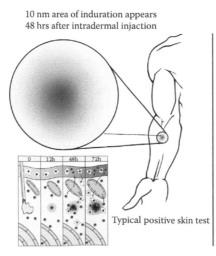

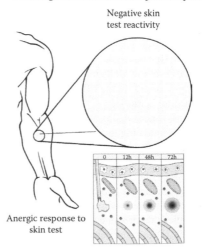

Anergy.

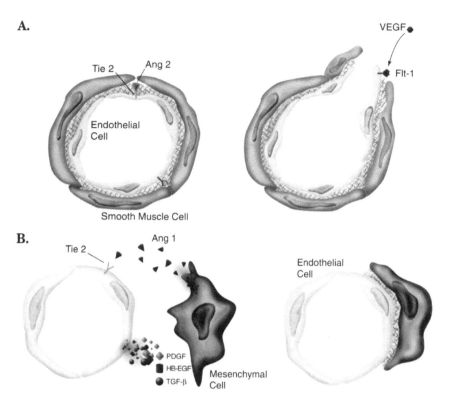

A scheme for vessel sprouting (A) and for maturation of the new vessel (B). Vessel structure is maintained by action of Ang-1 on Tie2. In (A), replacement of Ang-1 by Ang-2 destabilizes vessel integrity, facilitating vessel sprouting in response to VEGF. In (B), the new endothelial tubule interacts with surrounding mesenchymal cells, in part through Ang-1, which acts on endothelial cell Tie2 to promote association of the new tubule with periendothelial cells. The mechanism of this communication must involve other signals and is postulated to involve growth factors released from endothelial cells in response to activated Tie2.

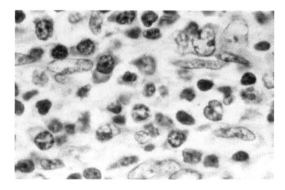

Angioimmunoblastic lymphadenopathy.

with plasma cells in lymph nodes revealing architectural efface-ment. Arborization of newly formed vessels and proliferating vessels with hyperplasia of endothelial cells is observed. In the interstitium, amorphous, eosinophilic, PAS-positive deposits, possibly representing debris from cells, are found. Fever, night sweats, hepatosplenomegaly, generalized lymphadenopathy, weight loss, hemolytic anemia, polyclonal gammopathy, and skin rashes may characterize the disease in middle-aged to older subjects. Patients live approximately 15 months, with some developing monoclonal gammopathy or immunoblastic lymphomas. AILA must be differentiated from AIDS, Hodgkin disease, immunoblastic lymphoma, histocytosis X, and a vari-ety of other conditions affecting the lymphoid tissues.

angiopoietins/Tie2

Two endothelial cell-specific tyrosine kinase receptors are Tie1 and Tie2. The ligands for Tie2 are angiopoietin-1 and angiopoietin-2 (Ang-1 and Ang-2). The ligands for Tie1 have not been identified.

angry macrophage

A term sometimes used to refer to activated macrophages.

animal reservoir

An intermediate animal host for a pathogenic microorgan-ism whose primary host is another species.

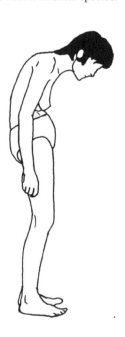

Ankylosing spondylitis

A

ankylosing spondylitis

A chronic inflammatory disease affecting the spine, sacroiliac joints, and large peripheral joints. There is a strong male predominance with onset in early adult life. The erythrocyte sedimentation rate is elevated, but subjects are negative for rheumatoid factor and antinuclear antibodies. Pathologically, there is chronic proliferative synovitis resembling that seen in rheumatoid arthritis. The sacroiliac joints and interspinous and capsular ligaments ossify when the disease advances. The disease has a major genetic predisposition, as revealed by increased incidence in selected families. Ninety percent of ankylosing spondylitis patients are positive for HLA-B27, compared to 8% among Caucasians in the United States. The HLA-B27 genes may be linked to genes that govern pathogenic autoimmunity. There may be increased susceptibility to infectious agents or molecular mimicry between HLA-B27 and an infectious agent such as *Klebsiella pneumoniae*, leading to the synthesis of a crossreacting antibody. Treatment is aimed at diminishing inflammation and pain and providing physical therapy.

ANNA

Abbreviation for antineutrophil nuclear antibodies.

annexin (lipocortin)

A protein with a highly conserved core region comprised of four or eight repeats of about 70 amino acid residues and a highly variable N terminal region. The core region mediates Ca^{2+}-dependent binding to phospholipid membranes and forms a Ca^{2+} channel-like structure. Physical and structural features of annexin proteins suggest that they regulate many aspects of cell membrane function, including membrane trafficking signal transduction, and cell–matrix interactions. Their actions resemble some of those of glucocorticoids, including anti-inflammatory, anti-edema, and immunosuppressive effects.

annexin V binding

In normal, nonapoptotic cells, phosphatidylserine (PS) is segregated to the inner leaflet of the plasma membrane. During early stages of apoptosis, this asymmetry collapses and PS becomes exposed on the outer surface cells. Annexin V is a protein that preferentially binds PS in a calcium-dependent manner. Binding of annexin V, in conjunction with dye exclusion (e.g., propidium iodide) to establish membrane integrity, can be used to identify apoptotic cells.

antagonist

Peptide with a sequence closely related to that of an agonist peptide that inhibits the responses of a cloned T cell line specific for the agonist peptide; a molecule that interferes with the function of a receptor as a consequence of binding to it.

antagonist ligand

A molecule, which when bound to a specific receptor, inhibits the action of a separate ligand for the same receptor.

antiagglutinin

A specific antibody that interferes with the action of an agglutinin.

anti-allotypic antibodies

Antibodies specific for allotopes of an immunoglobulin molecule derived from a member of the same species.

antianaphylaxis

Inhibition of anaphylaxis through desensitization. This is accomplished by repeated injections of the sensitizing agent too minute to produce an anaphylactic reaction.

antiantibody

In addition to their antibody function, immunoglobulin molecules serve as excellent protein immunogens when inoculated into another species, or they may become autoantigenic even in their own hosts. The Gm antigenic determinants in the Fc region of an immunoglobulin G (IgG) molecule may elicit autoantibodies, principally of the IgM class, known as rheumatoid factor in individuals with rheumatoid arthritis. Anti-idiotypic antibodies directed against the antigen-binding N terminal variable regions of antibody molecules represent another type of antiantibody. Rabbit anti-human IgG (Coombs' test reagent) is an antiantibody used extensively in clinical immunology to reveal autoantibodies on erythrocytes.

anti-B and T cell receptor idiotype antibodies

Antibodies that interact with antigenic determinants (idiotopes) at the variable N termini of the heavy and light chains comprising the paratope region of an antibody molecule in which the antigen-binding site is located. The idiotope antigenic determinants may be situated within the cleft of the antigen-binding region or located on the periphery or outer edge of the variable region of heavy and light chain components. Anti-idiotypic antibodies also block T cell receptors from antigens for which they are specific.

anti-bcl-2 primary antibody

A mouse monoclonal antibody. The bcl-2 oncoprotein expression is inhibited in germinal centers where apoptosis forms a part of the B cell production pathway. In 90% of follicular lymphomas, a translocation juxtaposes the *bcl-2* gene at 19q21 to an immunoglobulin gene, with subsequent deregulation of protein synthesis and cell proliferation. The bcl-2 product is considered to act as an inhibitor of apoptosis. This observation has clinical implications. Distinction of follicular hyperplasia from follicular lymphoma is a common problem in histopathology. Reactive follicles show no staining for bcl-2, whereas the cells in neoplastic follicles exhibit membrane staining.

anti-BCL-6 (PG-B6p) mouse monoclonal antibody

A monoclonal antibody against *bcl-6*, a transcriptional regulator gene that encodes a 706-amino-acid nuclear zinc finger protein. Antibodies to this protein stain the germinal center cells in lymphoid follicles, follicular cells and interfollicular cells in follicular lymphoma, diffuse large B-cell lymphomas, and Burkitt's lymphoma, and the majority of the Reed–Sternberg cells in nodular lymphocyte-predominant Hodgkin disease. In contrast, anti-BCL-6 rarely stains mantle cell lymphoma, and MALT lymphoma bcl-6 expression is seen in approximately 45% of CD30+ anaplastic large cell lymphomas but is consistently absent in other peripheral T cell lymphomas.

antibodies

Glycoprotein substances synthesized and secreted by B lymphoid lineage cells, termed plasma cells, in response to stimulation with an immunogen. They possess the ability to react *in vitro* and *in vivo* specifically and selectively with the antigenic determinants or epitopes eliciting their production or with an antigenic determinant closely related to the homologous antigen. Antibody molecules are immunoglobulins found in the blood and body fluids. Thus, all antibodies are immunoglobulins formed in response to immunogens. Antibodies may be produced by hybridoma technology in which antibody-secreting cells are fused by polyethylene glycol (PEG) treatment with a mutant myeloma cell line. Monoclonal antibodies are widely used in research and diagnostic medicine and have

A

potential in therapy. Antibodies in the blood serum of any given animal species may be grouped according to their physicochemical properties and antigenic characteristics. Immunoglobulins are not restricted to the plasma but may be found in other body fluids or tissues such as urine, spinal fluid, lymph nodes, spleen, etc. Immunoglobulins do not include the components of the complement system. Immunoglobulins (antibodies) constitute approximately 1 to 2% of the total serum proteins in health. Gamma globulins comprise 11.2 to 20.1% of the total serum content in humans. Antibodies are in the gamma globulin fraction of serum. Electrophoretically, they are the slowest migrating fraction.

antibodies to histidyl t-RNA synthetase (anti-HRS)

Antibodies with a formation closely associated with DR3 in Caucasians. DR6 may be increased in African-American patients with this autoantibody. The supertypic DR specificity DR52 is found among essentially all individuals with anti-HRS. This specificity is encoded by the DRB3 gene, which is present on haplotypes bearing DR3, DR5, or DR6 and is also represented on the DR8 molecule. Essentially all patients with anti-HRS have one or two of these DR alleles. All are DR52-positive. The first hypervariable regions of the DRB1 genes encoding DR3, DR5, DR6, and DR8 have homologous sequences. This homology is believed to predispose to the development of immune reactivity against HRS.

antibodies to Mi-1 and Mi-2

Antibodies to Mi-1 and Mi-2 have been found exclusively in diabetes mellitus (DM) patients (15 to 35%). Anti-Mi-1 has been found in a small percentage of DM patients but also in 5% of patients with systemic lupus erythematosus (SLE), including 7% of those with anti-RNP and 9% of those with anti-Sm. It has also been shown to bind bovine IgG and is not helpful in diagnosis.

antibody absorption test

A serological assay based upon the ability of a crossreactive antigen to diminish a serum sample's titer of antibodies against its homologous antigen (i.e., the antigen that stimulated its production). Crossreactive antibodies and crossreactive antigens may be detected in this way.

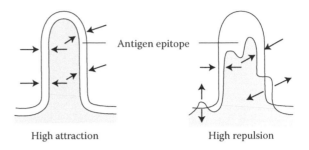

High attraction   High repulsion

Antibody affinity.

antibody affinity

The force of binding of one antibody molecule's paratope with its homologous epitope on the antigen molecule. It is a consequence of positive and negative portions affecting these molecular interactions.

antibody–antigen intermolecular forces

The various types of bonds that participate in the specific interaction between antibody and antigen molecules are relatively weak physical forces. They fall into three classes: (1) van der Waals or electrodynamic forces, (2) hydrogen bonding or polar forces, and (3) electrostatic forces. Covalent bonds are not involved in antibody–antigen interactions.

antibody-binding site

The antigen-binding site of an antibody molecule, known as a paratope and comprised of heavy chain and light chain variable regions. The paratope represents the site of attachment of an epitope to the antibody molecule. The complementarity-determining hypervariable regions play a significant role in dictating the combining site structure together with the participation of framework region residues. The T cell receptor also has antigen-binding sites in the variable regions of its α and β (or γ and δ) chains.

antibody deficiency syndrome

A few patients have been observed in which normal immunoglobulin levels are present, but the ability to mount an immune response to immunogenic challenge is impaired. This condition is associated with several separate disease states and might more properly be considered a syndrome.

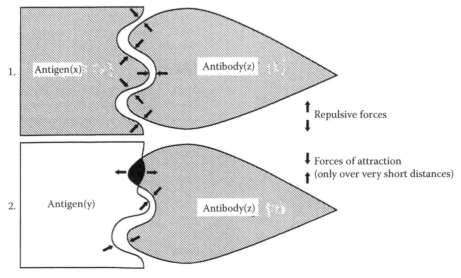

1. Antigen(x)   Antibody(z)

↕ Repulsive forces

↓
↑ Forces of attraction (only over very short distances)

2. Antigen(y)   Antibody(z)

Antibody affinity.

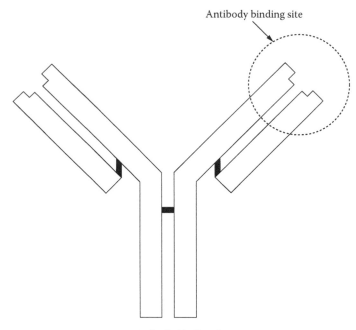

Antibody-binding site.

Some may present clinically as severe combined immunodeficiency with diminished cell-mediated immunity, lymphopenia, and infection by microorganisms of low pathogenicity. There are normal or even elevated numbers of plasma cells, and there may be no demonstrable T cell deficiency. Both findings are in contrast to the usual clinical picture of severe combined immunodeficiency (SCID). These individuals may develop autoimmune reactions and show reduced numbers of lymphoid cells with surface immunoglobulin in the circulating blood. One possible explanation for normal immunoglobulin levels and an inadequate humoral immune response to antigenic challenge may be a defect in clonal diversity resulting in an antibody response to only a limited number of antigens. Some investigators have associated the defect with T cell clonal diversity. This combined B and T cell system disorder resembles SCID, but is less pronounced. Some patients with this defect develop paraproteins with subsequent agammaglobulinemia and clinical manifestations closely resembling SCID.

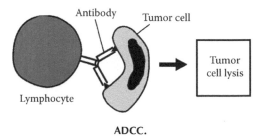

ADCC.

antibody-dependent cell-mediated cyotoxicity (ADCC)
A reaction in which T lymphocytes, natural killer (NK) cells (including large granular lymphocytes), neutrophils, and macrophages may lyse tumor cells, infectious agents, and allogeneic cells by combining through their Fc receptors with the Fc regions of immunoglobulin G (IgG) antibodies bound through their Fab regions to target cell surface antigens. Following linkage of Fc receptors with Fc regions, destruction of the target is accomplished through released cytokines, representing an example of participation between antibody molecules and immune system cells to produce an effector function. NK cells mediate most ADCC through the Fc receptor FcγRIII or CD 16 on their surfaces.

antibody detection
Techniques employed to detect antibodies include immunoprecipitation, agglutination, complement-dependent assays, labeled anti-immunoglobulin reagents, blotting techniques, and immunohistochemistry. Enzyme-based immunoassays, blotting methods, and immunohistochemistry are routine procedures to detect antibodies and characterize their specificity.

antibody-directed enzyme pro-drug therapy (ADEPT)
A type of treatment in which an antibody is used to target an enzyme to a tumor and unbound reagent is allowed to clear. A nontoxic prodrug is then given and is activated by the enzyme to form a cytotoxic drug at the tumor site. An important part of ADEPT is bystander killing. Because the drugs are activated extracellularly by the antibody–enzyme complex, neighboring cells may also be killed by a mechanism that does not require translocation across intracellular membranes. By contrast, immunotoxins kill only the cells to which they bind.

antibody-excess immune complexes (ABICs)
These complexes may result from alterations of the immunoglobulin molecules such as those seen in rheumatoid arthritis or may be produced locally as in type B hepatitis. ABICs have a short intravascular life and, in contrast to antigen-excess immune complexes, adhere to platelets and cause platelet aggregation that is due not to crosslinking of ABIC to platelets, but to changes in the adhesive properties of the latter. ABICs also bind to neutrophils and induce the release of lysosomal enzymes without prior phagocytic activity.

antibody feedback
The negative feedback system whereby antigen-specific antibodies downregulate further immune responses to

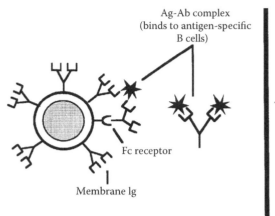

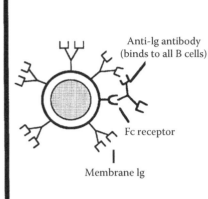

Antibody feedback.

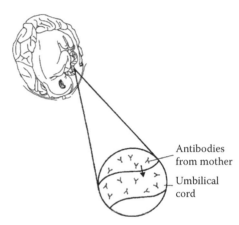

Passive immunization.

that antigen. Several mechanisms may be responsible for this including (1) removal of the initiating stimulus by the antibody, (2) binding of antigen–IgG antibody immune complexes to the Fcγ receptors of B cells, and (3) inhibition of T cell responses by antigen–antibody complexes. The use of Rh immune globulin to prevent erythroblastosis fetalis in the infants of Rh– mothers is an example of antibody feedback. Secreted IgG antibodies may downregulate antibody production when antigen–antibody complexes simultaneously engage B cell membrane immunoglobulin and Fcγ receptors (FcγRII). The cytoplasmic tails of Fcγ receptors transduce inhibitory signals inside the B cells.

antibody fragment

A product of enzymatic treatment of an antibody immunoglobulin molecule with an enzyme such as papain or pepsin. For example, papain treatment leads to the production of two Fab and one Fc fragments, whereas the use of pepsin yields the F (ab′)$_2$ fragment. Refer to the individual fragments for further information.

antibody half-life

The mean survival time of a particular antibody molecule after its formation. Half-life is the time required to rid an animal body of one half of a known amount of antibody. Thus, antibody half-life differs according to the immunoglobulin class to which the antibody belongs.

antibody humanization

The transference of the antigen-binding part of a murine monoclonal antibody to a human antibody.

antibody-mediated suppression

The feedback inhibition that antibody molecules exert on their own further synthesis.

antibody repertoire

All of the antibody specificities that an individual can synthesize.

antibody screening

Candidates for organ transplants, especially renal allografts, are monitored with relative frequency for changes in their percent reactive antibody (PRA) levels. Obviously, those with relatively high PRA values are considered less favorable candidates for renal allotransplants than those whose PRA values are low. PRA determinations may vary according to the composition of the cell panel. If the size of the panel is inadequate, it may affect the relative frequency of common histocompatibility antigens found in the population.

antibody-secreting cells

Differentiated B lymphocytes that synthesize the secretory form of immunoglobulin. Antibody-secreting cells result from antigen stimulation. They may be found in the lymph nodes, spleen, and bone marrow.

antibody specificity

A property of antibodies determined by their relative binding affinities, intrinsic capacities of the antibody-combining sites expressed as equilibrium dissociation (K_d) or association (K_a) for their interactions with different antigens.

antibody synthesis

The 10^{12} B lymphocytes that comprise the human immune system synthesize 10^{20} antibody (immunoglobulin) molecules present inside and on the surfaces of these cells and most of all in the serum. Other species have B cell and immunoglobulin molecule numbers relative to their body weights. B cells and immunoglobulin molecules are formed and degraded throughout the human lifespan.

antibody titer

The amount or level of circulating antibody in a patient with an infectious disease. For example, the reciprocal of the highest dilution of serum (containing antibodies) that reacts with antigen (e.g., agglutination) is the titer. Two separate

A

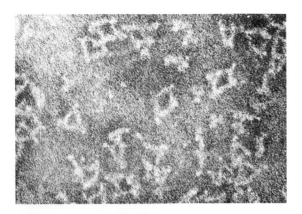

Antibody structure.

titer determinations are required to reflect an individual's exposure to an infectious agent.

antibody unit

Refer to titer.

anti-broad spectrum cytokeratin antibody

A mouse monoclonal antibody that may be used to identify cells of normal and abnormal epithelial lineage and as an aid in the diagnosis of anaplastic tumors. The cytokeratins comprise a group of intermediate filament proteins that occur in normal and neoplastic cells of epithelial origin. The 19 known human cytokeratins are divided into acidic and basic subfamilies, and they occur in pairs in epithelial tissues, with the composition of pairs varying according to the epithelial cell type, stage differentiation, cellular growth, environment, and disease state. The pankeratin cocktail recognizes most of the acidic and all of the basic cytokeratins, making it a useful general stain for nearly all epithelial tissues and their tumors. This antibody binds specifically to antigens located in the cytoplasmic regions of normal simple and complex epithelial cells. The antibody is used to qualitatively stain cytokeratins in sections of formalin-fixed paraffin-embedded tissue. Anti-pankeratin primary antibody contains a mouse monoclonal antibody raised against an epitope found on human epidermal keratins. It reacts with 56.5-, 50-, 48-, and 40-kDa cytokeratins of the acidic subfamily and 67- to 65-, 64-, 59-, 58-, 56-, and 52-kDa cytokeratins of the basic subfamily. In anaplastic tumors, the percentage of tumor cells showing cytokeratin reactivity may be small (under 5%). Unexpected antigen expression or loss of expression may occur, especially in neoplasms. Occasionally, stromal elements surrounding heavily stained tissue and/or cells will show immunoreactivity. The clinical interpretation of any staining or its absence must be complemented by morphological studies and evaluation of proper controls.

anti-BRST-2 (GCDFP-15) monoclonal antibody

An antibody specific for BRST-2 antigen expressed by apocrine sweat glands, eccrine glands (variable), minor salivary glands, bronchial glands, metaplastic epithelium of the breast, benign sweat gland tumors of the skin, and the serous cells of the submandibular gland. Breast carcinomas (primary and metastatic lesions) with apocrine features express the BRST-2 antigen. BRST-2 is positive in extra-mammary Paget's disease. Other tumors are negative.

anti-BRST-3 (B72.3) monoclonal antibody

A monoclonal antibody that recognizes TAG-72, a tumor-associated oncofetal antigen expressed by a wide variety of

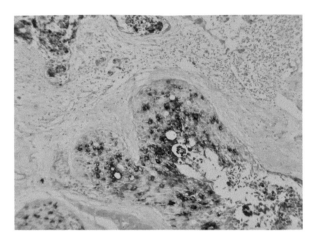

Tag 72—carcinoma of the breast.

human adenocarcinomas. This antigen is expressed by 84% of invasive ductal breast carcinoma and 85 to 90% of colon, pancreatic, gastric, esophageal, lung (non-small cell), ovarian, and endometrial adenocarcinomas. It is not expressed by leukemias, lymphomas, sarcomas, mesotheliomas, melanomas, or benign tumors. TAG-72 is also expressed on normal secretory endometrium but not on other normal tissues.

anticardiolipin antibody syndrome

Circulating lupus anticoagulant syndrome (CLAS). A clinical situation in which circulating anticardiolipin antibodies may occur in patients with lupus erythematosus in conjunction with thromboembolic events linked to repeated abortions caused by placenta vasculothrombosis, repeated myocardial infarction, pulmonary hypertension, and possibly renal and cerebral infarction. There is neurologic dysfunction, including a variety of manifestations such as myelopathy, transient ischemic attacks, chorea, epilepsy, etc. There may be hemolytic anemia, thrombocytopenia, and Coombs' positive reactivity. Immunoglobulin G (IgG) anticardiolipin antibodies manifest 80% specificity for the anticardiolipin antibody syndrome. Anticardiolipin antibodies and DNA show crossreactivity.

anti-CD1a antibody

A murine monoclonal antibody that reacts with CD1a, a nonpolymorphic major histocompatibility complex (MHC) class-I-related cell surface glycoprotein expressed in association with β_2 microglobulin. In normal tissues, the antibody reacts with cortical thymocytes, Langerhans' cells, and interdigitating reticulum cells. It also reacts with thymomas, Langerhans' histiocytosis cells (histiocytosis X), some T cell lymphomas, and leukemias. The staining is localized on the membrane.

anti-CD5 monoclonal antibody

This antibody detects CD5 antigen expressed in 95% of thymocytes and 72% of peripheral blood lymphocytes. In lymph nodes, the main reactivity is observed in T cells. CD5 antigen is expressed by many T cell leukemias, lymphomas, and activated T cells. It is also expressed on a subset of B cells. CD5 is recommended for the identification of mantle cell lymphomas. Antibodies to CD5 may prove of particular use in the detection of T cell acute lymphocytic leukemias (T-ALLs), some B cell chronic lymphocytic leukemias (B-CLLs), and B and T cell lymphomas. CD5 does not react with granulocytes or monocytes.

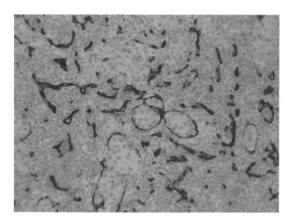

CD34—highly vascular tumor.

anti-CD34 antibody

A murine monoclonal antibody raised by immunization with human placental endothelial cells that has a specificity for the CD34 glycoprotein, which is considered the earliest known CD marker and is expressed on virtually all human hematopoietic progenitor cells.

anti-CD43 antibody

A murine monoclonal antibody directed against an epitope present on human monocytes, granulocytes, and lymphocytes. This reagent may be used to aid in the identification of cells of lymphoid lineage. It is intended for qualitative staining in sections of formalin-fixed, paraffin-embedded tissue. Anti-CD43 antibody specifically binds to antigen located in the plasma membrane and cytoplasmic regions of normal granulocytes and T lymphocytes.

anti-CD45R (leukocyte common antigen) antibody

A mouse monoclonal antibody specific for an epitope present on the majority of human leukocytes. This reagent may be used to aid in the identification of cells of lymphocytic lineage and is intended for qualitative staining in sections of formalin-fixed, paraffin-embedded tissue. It specifically binds to antigens located predominantly in plasma membranes and to a lesser degree in the cytoplasma of lymphocytes, with variable reactivity to monocytes/histiocytes, and polymorphonuclear leukocytes. Unexpected antigen expression or loss of expression may occur, especially in neoplasms. Occasional stromal elements surrounding heavily stained tissues or cells show immunoreactivity. The clinical interpretation of any staining or its absence must be complemented by morphological features and evaluation of proper controls.

anti-CD68 (human macrophage marker) antibody

A murine monoclonal antibody that stains macrophages and a wide variety of human tissues, including Kupffer's cells and macrophages in the red pulp of the spleen, in the lamina propria of the gut, in lung alveoli, and in bone marrow. Antigen-presenting cells (e.g., Langerhans' cells) are either negative or show weak and/or restricted areas of reactivity (e.g., interdigitating reticulum cells). Resting microglia in the normal white matter of the cerebrum and microglia in areas of infarction react with the antibody. Peripheral blood monocytes are also positive, with a granular staining pattern. The antibody reacts with myeloid precursors and peripheral blood granulocytes. It also reacts with the population known as "plasmacytoid T cells" present in many reactive lymph nodes and believed

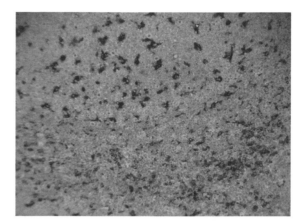

CD68—tonsil.

to be of monocyte/macrophage origin. The antibody stains cases of chronic and acute myeloid leukemia, giving strong granular staining of the cytoplasm of many cells and also reacts with rare cases of true histiocytic neoplasia. The positive staining of normal and neoplastic mast cells is seen with the antibody as well as staining of a variable number of cells in malignant melanomas. Neoplasms of lymphoid origin are usually negative, although some B cell neoplasms, most frequently small lymphocytic lymphomas and hairy cell leukemias, show weak staining of the cytoplasm, usually in the form of a few scattered granules.

anticentriole antibody

An antibody that may occur in serum specific for the mitotic spindle apparatus (MSA). These antibodies are rarely found in the sera of subjects developing connective tissue diseases such as scleroderma.

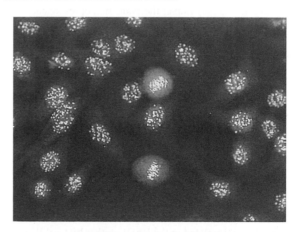

Anticentromere antibody.

anticentromere antibody

Antibody against the centromere antigens CENP-A and CENP-B present in approximately 95% of CREST syndrome patients. They are much less frequent in cases of diffuse scleroderma and are considered significant diagnostic markers for scleroderma with limited skin involvement and also have prognostic significance. Indirect immunofluorescence and immunoblotting are the suggested methods for assay. Twelve percent of primary biliary cirrhosis patients, half of whom also have manifestations of systemic sclerosis, have anticentromere

A

antibodies. The antibodies do not affect survival and pulmonary hypertension in patients with limited scleroderma; however, survival is much longer in anticentromere-positive patients with limited scleroderma than in anti-Scl-70-positive diffuse scleroderma patients.

anti-Clq antibody

Present in the majority of patients with hypocomplementemic urticarial vasculitis syndrome (HUVS) and in 30 to 60% of systemic lupus erythematosus (SLE) patients. Clq is strikingly decreased in the blood sera of HUVS patients, even though their Clr and Cls levels are within normal limits and C5 to C9 are slightly activated.

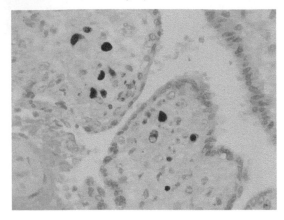

Cytomegalovirus (CMV)—placenta.

anticomplementary

The action of any agent or treatment that interferes with complement fixation through removal or inactivation of complement components or cascade reactants. Multiple substances may exhibit anticomplementary activity. These are especially significant in complement fixation serology, as anticomplementary agents may impair the evaluation of test results.

anticytomegalovirus (CMV) antibody

A mouse monoclonal antibody that reacts with CMV-infected cells giving a nuclear staining pattern with early antigen and a nuclear and cytoplasmic reaction with the late viral antigen. The antibody shows no crossreactivity with other herpesviruses or adenoviruses.

anticytoplasmic antibody

Antineutrophil cytoplasmic antibody occurring in 84 to 100% of active generalized Wegener's granulomatosis patients. This antibody is assayed by flow cytometry and indirect fluorescence microscopy. HIV-1 infected patients may be biologically false-positive for neutrophil cytoplasmic antibody.

anti-D antibody

Antibody against the Rh blood group D antigen. This antibody is stimulated in the RhD⁻ mother by fetal RhD⁺ red blood cells that enter her circulation at parturition. Anti-D antibodies become a problem usually with the third pregnancy, resulting from the booster immune response against the D antigen to which the mother was previously exposed. IgG antibodies pass across the placenta, leading to hemolytic disease of the newborn (erythroblastosis fetalis). Anti-D antibody (Rhogam®) administered up to 72 hours following parturition may combine with the RhD⁺ red blood cells in the mother's circulation, thereby facilitating their removal by the reticuloendothelial system. This prevents maternal immunization against the RhD antigen.

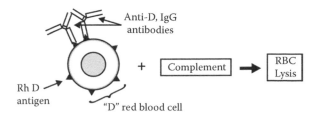

Complement-mediated lysis of RhD antigen-positive red blood cells through doublets of anti-D, IgG antibodies on the red cell surface.

antidesmin antibody

A mouse monoclonal antibody (clone DE-R-11) raised against purified porcine desmin that reacts with the 53-kDa intermediate filament desmin protein. This reagent may be used to aid in the identification of cells of myocyte lineage. The antibody is intended for qualitative staining in sections of formalin-fixed, paraffin-embedded tissue. Antidesmin primary antibody specifically binds to antigens located in the cytoplasm of myocytic cells. The clinical interpretation of any staining or its absence must be complemented by morphological studies and evaluation of proper controls.

anti-DEX antibodies

Murine α1–3 dextran specific antibodies.

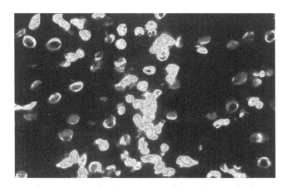

Anti-dsDNA (rim pattern).

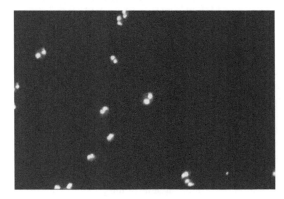

Anti-dsDNA.

anti-double-stranded DNA (anti-dsDNA)

Antibodies present in the blood sera of systemic lupus erythemastosus (SLE) patients. Among the detection methods is an immunofluorescence (IFT) technique using *Crithidia luciliae* as the substrate. Fluorescence of the kinetoplast containing mitochondrial DNA signals the presence of anti-dsDNA antibodies. This technique is useful for assaying SLE serum, which is usually positive in patients with active disease. A rim or peripheral pattern of nuclear staining of cells interacting with antinuclear antibody represents morphologic expression of anti-double-stranded DNA antibody.

anti-endothelial cell autoantibody

An antibody that may cause vasculitis as part of an autoimmune response.

anti-epithelial membrane antigen (EMA) antibody

A mouse monoclonal antibody directed against a mucin epitope present on most human epithelial cells. This antibody reacts with epithelial mucin, a heavily glycosylated molecule with a molecular weight of about 400 kDa. Epithelial membrane antigen is widely distributed in epithelial tissues and tumors arising from them. Normal glandular epithelium and tissue from non-neoplastic diseases stain in lumen membranes and cytoplasm. Malignant neoplasms of glandular epithelium frequently show a change in pattern with the appearance of adjacent cell membrane staining. EMA is of value in distinguishing both large cell anaplastic carcinoma from diffuse histiocytic lymphoma and small cell anaplastic carcinoma from well and poorly differentiated lymphocytic lymphomas.

anti-estrogen receptor antibodies

A mouse monoclonal antibody specific for estrogen receptors (ERs). The ER content of breast cancer tissue is an important parameter in the prediction of prognosis and response to endocrine therapy. Monoclonal antibodies to ER allow determination of the receptor status of breast tumors in routine histopathology laboratories. Although monoclonal antibodies that recognize ER were effective initially only on frozen sections, currently available monoclonal antibodies are effective on formalin-fixed, paraffin-embedded tissues for determining ER in routinely processed and archival material.

anti-Ewing's sarcoma marker

A mouse monoclonal anti-human MIC2 gene product (Ewing's sarcoma marker) antibody reacts only with glioblastoma and ependymoma of the central nervous system and certain islet cell tumors of the pancreas. Because the MIC2 gene products are most strongly expressed on the cell membranes of Ewing's sarcoma (ES) and primitive peripheral neuroectodermal tumors (pPNET), demonstration of the gene products allows for the differentiation of these tumors from other round cell tumors of childhood and adolescence.

anti-factor VIII antibody

A mouse monoclonal antibody that gives positive staining in the cytoplasm of normal vascular endothelial cells of arteries, veins, capillaries, and endocardial cells. Factor-VIII-related antigen is also present in megakaryocytes and platelets.

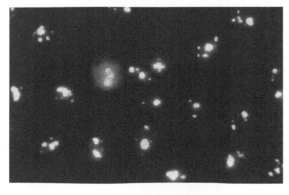

Antifibrillarin antibodies.

antifibrillarin antibodies

Antibodies to this 34-kDa protein constituent of U3 ribonucleoproteins (RNPs) are detectable in the sera of about 8% of patients with diffuse and limited scleroderma. Also called anti-U3-RNP antibodies.

antigen

A substance that reacts with the products of an immune response stimulated by a specific immunogen, including both antibodies and/or T lymphocyte receptors. Currently considered to be one of many kinds of substances with which an antibody molecule or T cell receptor may bind. These include sugars, lipids, intermediary metabolites, autocoids, hormones, complex carbohydrates, phospholipids, nucleic acids, and proteins. By contrast, the "traditional" definition of antigen is a substance that may stimulate B and/or T cell limbs of the immune response and react with the products of that response, including immunoglobulin antibodies and/or specific receptors on T cells. See immunogen definition. The "traditional" definition of antigen more correctly refers to an immunogen. A complete antigen is one that induces an immune response and also reacts with the products of the response, whereas an incomplete antigen or hapten is unable to induce an immune response alone but is able to react with the products (e.g., antibodies). Haptens may be rendered immunogenic by covalently linking them to a carrier molecule. Following the administration of an antigen (immunogen) to a host animal, antibody synthesis and/or cell-mediated immunity or immunologic tolerance may result. To be immunogenic, a substance usually needs to be foreign, although some autoantigens represent exceptions. An immunogen should usually have a molecular weight of at least 1000 and should be either a protein or a polysaccharide. Nevertheless, immunogenicity depends also upon the genetic capacity of the host to respond to, rather than merely upon, the antigenic properties of an injected immunogen. The term also alludes to any molecule capable of producing peptides that unite specifically with T cell receptors. Refer also to epitope.

antigen–antibody complex

The union of antibody with soluble antigen in solution containing electrolyte. When the interaction takes place *in vitro*, it is called the precipitin reaction, but it may also take place *in vivo*. The relative proportion in which antigen and antibody combine varies according to their molar ratio. Excess antigen may lead to soluble complexes, whereas excess antibody may lead to insoluble complexes. *In vivo*, soluble complexes are more likely to produce tissue injury, whereas larger insoluble complexes are often removed by reticuloendothelial system cells. Also called immune complex.

antigen-binding capacity

Assay of the total capacity of antibody of all immunoglobulin classes to bind antigen. This refers to primary as opposed to secondary or tertiary manifestations of the antigen–antibody interaction. Equilibrium dialysis measures the antigen-binding capacity of antibodies with the homologous hapten, and the Farr test measures primary binding of protein antigens with the homologous antibody.

antigen-binding cell (ABC) assays

The principle of this assay is the binding of cells bearing receptors for antigen to a gelatin dish in which antigen is incorporated. After incubation for a specified time and

A

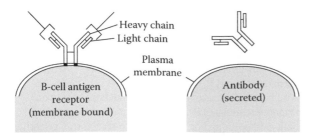

Antigen-binding site.

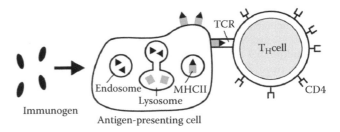

Capture, processing, and presentation of antigen by an antigen-presenting cell.

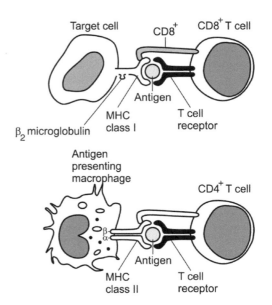

Antigen presentation.

temperature, the unbound cells are washed out, and the bound cells are collected following melting of the gelatin layer at 37°C. The harvested cells are washed, counted, and used for various other assays.

antigen-binding site

The location on an antibody molecule where an antigenic determinant or epitope combines with it. The antigen-binding site is located in a cleft bordered by the N terminal variable regions of heavy and light chain parts of the Fab region. Also called paratope. The term also refers to that part of a T cell receptor that binds antigen specifically.

antigen capture assay

A method to identify minute quantities of antigen in blood sera or supernatants. Antibodies of high titer are linked to an insoluble solid support, and the specimen containing the antigen to be evaluated is passed over the solid phase. This will bind or capture the antigen, making it available for reaction with a separate enzyme-labeled antibody that reacts with and reveals the captured antigen.

antigen clearance

Exogenous clearance is a principal immune system function. Antigen removal is by phagocytosis, cytolysis, or complement-mediated elimination. Fixed mononuclear phagocytic system cells are the principal mechanisms for eliminating antigen. The mechanism of removal depends on the biological and physical chemical properties of the antigen, its mode of presentation, and its capacity to induce a specific humoral or cellular immune response.

antigen excess

The interaction of soluble antigen and antibody in the precipitin reaction leads to occupation of all of the binding sites of the antibody molecules and leaves additional antigenic determinants free to combine with more antibody molecules if excess antigen is added to the mixture. This leads to the formation of soluble antigen–antibody complexes *in vitro* (i.e., the postzone in the precipitin reaction). A similar phenomenon may take place *in vivo* when immune complexes form in the presence of excess antigen. These are of clinical significance in that soluble immune complexes may induce tissue injury, leading to immunopathologic sequelae.

antigen masking

The ability of some parasites (e.g., *Schistosoma mansoni*) to become coated with host proteins, theoretically rendering them "invisible" to the host's immune system.

antigen presentation

The display of peptide antigens on the cell surface together with either MHC class I or class II molecules that permits T cells to recognize antigen on a target cell or antigen-

presenting cell surface. T lymphocytes recognize antigens only in the context of self-MHC molecules on the surfaces of antigen-presenting cells. During processing, intact protein antigens are degraded into peptide fragments. Most epitopes that T cells recognize are peptide chain fragments. B cells and T cells often recognize different epitopes of an antigen leading to both antibody and cell-mediated immune responses. Before antigen can bind to MHC molecules, it must be processed into peptides in the intracellular organelles. CD4+ helper T lymphocytes recognize antigens in the context of class II MHC molecules, a process known as class II MHC restriction. By contrast, CD8+ cytotoxic T lymphocytes recognize antigens in the context of class I molecules; this is known as class I MHC restriction. Following the generation of peptides by proteolytic degradation in antigen-presenting cells, peptide–MHC complexes are presented on the surface of antigen-presenting cells where they may be recognized by T lymphocytes. Antigens derived from either intracellular or extracellular proteins may be processed to produce peptides from either self or foreign proteins that are presented by surface MHC molecules to T cells. In the class II MHC processing pathway, professional antigen-presenting cells, such as macrophages, dendritic cells, or B lymphocytes incorporate extracellular proteins into endosomes where they are processed. Enzymes within the vesicles of the endosomal pathway cleave proteins in the acidic environment.

Class II MHC heterodimeric molecules united with invariant chains are shifted to endosomal vesicles from the

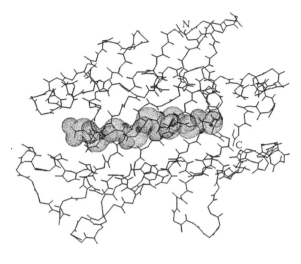

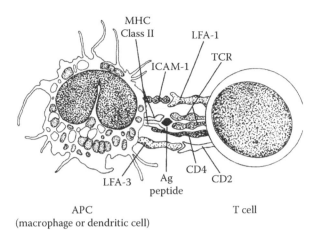

Antigen presentation.

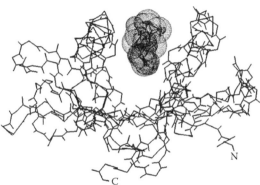

Presentation of MHC histocompatibility antigen HLA-B270S complexes with nonapeptide ARG-ARG-ILE-LYS-ALA-ILE-THR-LEU-LYS. The C terminal amino acid of the antigen-binding domain is protected by an N-methyl group. Three water molecules bridge the binding of the peptide to the histocompatibility protein.

endoplasmic reticulum. Following cleavage of the invariant chain, DM molecules remove a tiny piece of invariant chain from the MHC molecules' peptide-binding grooves. Following complexing of extracellular-derived peptide with

the class II MHC molecule, the MHC–peptide complex is transported to the cell surface where presentation to CD4+ cells occurs. Proteins in the cytosol, such as those derived from viruses, may be processed through the class I MHC route of antigen presentation. The multiprotein complex in the cytoplasm, known as the proteasome, leads to proteolytic degradation of proteins in the cytoplasm to yield many of the peptides that are presented by class I MHC molecules. TAP molecules transport peptides from the cytoplasm to the endoplasmic reticulum where they interact and bind to class I MHC dimeric molecules. Once the class I MHC molecules have become stabilized through peptide binding, the complex leaves the endoplasmic reticulum, entering the Golgi apparatus en route to the surface of the cell. Thus, mechanisms are provided through MHC-restricted antigen presentation to guarantee that peptides derived from extracellular microbial proteins can be presented by class II MHC molecules to CD4+ helper T cells and that peptides derived from intracellular microbes can be presented by class I MHC molecules to CD8+ cytotoxic T lymphocytes. The generation of microbial peptides produced through antigen processing to combine with self

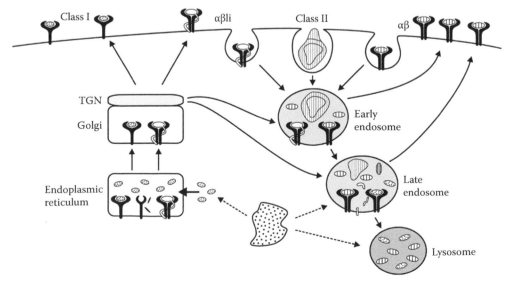

Processing pathways for class II-restricted antigen presentation.

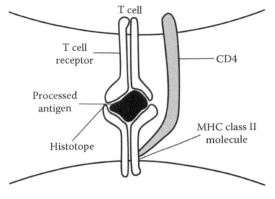

Antigen-presenting cell.

MHC molecules is critical to the development of an appropriate immune response.

antigen-presenting cell (APC)

A cell that can process a protein antigen, break it into peptides, and present it in conjunction with major histocompatibility complex (MHC) antigens on the cell surface where it may interact with appropriate T cell receptors. Professional antigen-presenting cells include dendritic cells, macrophages, and B cells that are capable of initiating T lymphocyte responsiveness to antigen. These cells display antigenic peptide fragments in association with the proper class of MHC molecules and also bear costimulatory surface molecules. Dendritic cells are the most important professional antigen-presenting cells for initiating primary T lymphocyte responses. This process is facilitated in part by their continuous high level expression of costimulatory B7 molecules. Dendritic reticulum cells, macrophages, Langerhans cells, and B cells process and present antigen to immunoreactive lymphocytes such as CD4+ T helper/ inducer cells. An MHC transporter-gene-encoded peptide supply factor may mediate peptide antigen presentation. In addition to the three types of professional APCs mentioned above, follicular dendritic cells are the main antigen-presenting cells for B cells. Non-professional antigen-presenting cells include keratinocytes and selected epithelial, endothelial, and mesenchymal cells and can act as antigen-presenting cells when activated during inflammation. Antigen-presenting cells include those that present exogenous antigen processed in their endosomal compartments and are presented together with MHC class II molecules. Other antigen-presenting cells present antigen that has been endogenously produced by the body's own cells with processing in an intracellular compartment and presentation together with MHC class I molecules. A third group of APCs present exogenous antigen that is taken into cells and processed followed by presentation together with MHC class I molecules. In addition to processing and presenting antigenic peptides in association with MHC class II molecules, an antigen-presenting cell must also deliver a costimulatory signal that is necessary for T cell activation. Nonprofessional APCs that function in antigen presentation for only brief periods include thymic epithelial cells and vascular endothelial cells.

antigen processing

The degradation of proteins into peptides capable of binding in the peptide binding groove of MHC class I or MHC class II molecules for presentation to T lymphocytes. For presentation by MHC molecules, antigens must be processed into peptides.

antigen receptor

Cell surface immunoglobulin for B cells and T cell receptor for T cells. A single antigen specificity is expressed on the surface of each lymphocyte.

antigen recognition activation motif

A conserved sequence of 17 amino acid residues that contains two tyrosine-X-X-leucine regions. This motif is found in the cytoplasmic tails of the FceRI-b and -a chains, the z and h chains of the TCR complex, the IgG and IgA proteins of membrane IgD and IgM, and the α, δ, and ε chains of CD3. The antigen recognition activation motif is thought to be involved in signal transduction.

antigen retrieval

A novel method for the rescue of antigens from formalin-fixed, paraffin-embedded tissue. It consists of heating sections in a microwave oven or pressure cooker in the presence of an antigen retrieval solution. It is designed for use in immunohistochemical staining with certain antibodies. This technique increases staining intensity and reduces background staining of many important markers in formalin-fixed tissue. Its use helps overcome false-negative staining of overfixed tissue, expands the range of antibodies useful

Cell type	Class II	Costimulators	Principal functions
Dendritic cells (Langerhans cells, lymphoid dendritic cells)	Constitutive	Constitutive	Inflammation of CD4* T cell response; allograft rejection
Macrophages	Inducible by IFN	Inducible by LPS	Development of CD4* effector T cells
B lymphocytes	Constitutive	Constitutive	Stimulation by CD4* helper T cells in humoral immune responses
Vascular endothelial cells	Inducible by IFN	Constitutive	Recruitment of antigen-specific T cells to site of antigen exposure or inflammation

Properties and functions of antigen-presenting cells.

for routinely processed tissue, and increases the usefulness of archival materials for retrospective studies. In addition to microwave heating, the pH of the antigen retrieval solution is an important cofactor for some antigens. Three antigen retrieval solutions covering a wide pH range are used. These include a citrate-based neutral pH solution, a Tris-based high pH solution, and a glycine-based low pH solution.

antigen-specific cells

Antigen-binding cells such as B lymphocytes that recognize antigen with a unique antigen receptor comprising surface immunoglobulin. Monoclonal antibodies recognizing a single clonotype of T cell receptor can be used to identify antigen-specific cells and responses using this clone. Fluorescence-activated cell sorting can also be used to identify antigen-specific cells.

antigen-specific suppressor cells

Antigen-specific Ts cells can be demonstrated both in humoral and cell-mediated immunity. The Ts cells active in the humoral response can be generated after priming with the carrier to be used in subsequent experiments with hapten–carrier conjugates. These Ts cells can suppress the hapten-specific immunoglobulin M (IgM) and IgG antibody response if recipient animals are immunized with the hapten coupled to the homologous carrier. This type of suppression may have a differential effect on IgM and IgG antibody responses according to the time frame in which the Ts cells are administered to the recipient animal. The early IgG response is relatively independent of T cell function and accordingly less susceptible to Ts cell effects. The late IgM and IgG responses are more T cell-dependent and, accordingly, more susceptible to Ts cell inhibition.

antigen, supertypic

An inclusive term describing an antigenic mosaic that can be separated into smaller but related parts called inclusions, splits, and subtypic antigens. Bw4 and Bw6 are classic examples of supertypic antigens. This implies that an antibody that detects Bw4 will also react with all antigens associated with Bw4, and an antibody that detects Bw6 will also react with all antigens associated with Bw6.

antigen, T-dependent

Refer to thymus-dependent antigen.

antigen, T-independent

Refer to thymus-independent antigen.

antigen unmasking

Exposure of tissue antigens using an antigen unmasking solution based on a citric acid formula is highly effective at revealing antigens in formalin-fixed, paraffin-embedded tissue sections when used in combination with a high temperature treatment procedure.

antigenic

An adjective that refers to the ability of a substance to induce an immune response and react with its products, which include antibodies and T lymphocyte receptors. The term *antigenic* has been largely replaced by *immunogenic*.

antigenic competition

The simultaneous injection of two closely related antigens may lead to suppression or a decrease of the immune response to one of them compared to the ability of the antigen to elicit an immune response if injected alone. Proteins that are thymus-dependent antigens are the ones with which antigenic competition occurs. The phenomenon has been claimed to be due in part to the competition by antigenic peptides for one binding site on

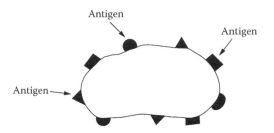

Antigenic determinants.

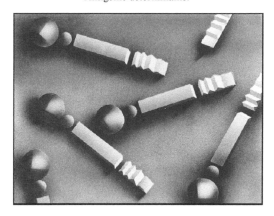

Schematic of antigenic determinants (epitopes).

major histocompatibility complex (MHC) class II molecules. Antigenic competition was observed in the early days of vaccination when it was found that the immune response of a host to the individual components of a vaccine might be less than if they had been injected individually.

antigenic deletion

Antigenic deletion describes antigenic determinants that have been lost or masked in the progeny of cells that usually contain them. Antigenic deletion may take place as a consequence of neoplastic transformation or mutation of parent cells, resulting in the disappearance or repression of the parent cell genes.

antigenic determinant

The site on an antigen molecule that is termed an epitope and interacts with the specific antigen-binding site in the variable region of an antibody molecule known as a paratope. The excellent fit between epitope and paratope is based on their three-dimensional interaction and noncovalent union. An antigenic determinant or epitope may also react with a T cell receptor for which it is specific. A lone antigen molecule may have several different epitopes available for reaction with antibody or T cell receptors.

antigenic diversion

The replacement of a cell's antigenic profile by the antigens of a different normal tissue cell. Used in tumor immunology.

antigenic drift

Spontaneous variation in pathogen surface antigens, usually through point mutations in genes, as in influenza virus, expressed as relatively minor differences exemplified by slow antigenic changes from one year to the next. Antigenic drift is believed to be due to mutation of the genes encoding the hemagglutinin or the neuraminidase components. Antigenic variants represent those viruses that have survived exposure to the host's neutralizing antibodies. Minor alterations in a viral genome may occur every few years,

A

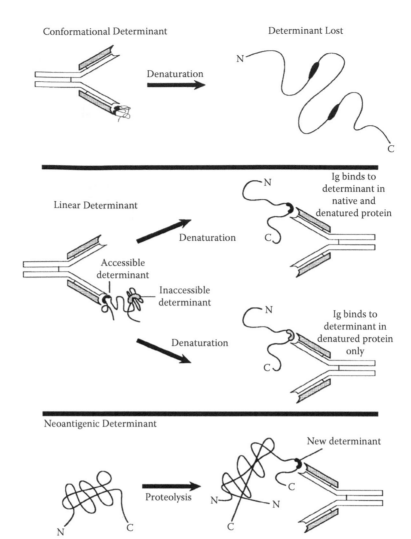

Conformational Determinant

Determinant Lost

Denaturation

Linear Determinant

Denaturation

Ig binds to determinant in native and denatured protein

Accessible determinant

Inaccessible determinant

Denaturation

Ig binds to determinant in denatured protein only

Neoantigenic Determinant

New determinant

Proteolysis

Antigenic determinant.

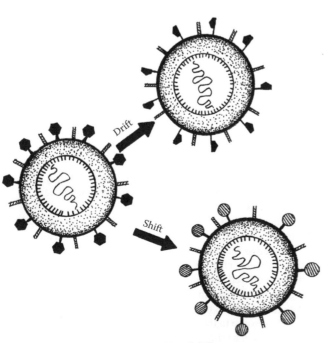

Antigenic drift and shift.

especially in influenza A subtypes that are made up of H1, H2, and H3 hemagglutinins and N1 and N2 neuraminidases. Antigenic shifts follow point mutations of DNA encoding these hemagglutinins and neuraminidases.

antigenic gain

Nondistinctive normal tissue components that are added or increased without simultaneous deletion of other normal tissue constituents.

antigenic modulation

The loss of epitopes or antigenic determinants from a cell surface following combination with an antibody. The antibodies cause the epitope to disappear or become camouflaged by covering it.

antigenic mosaicism

Antigenic variation first discovered in pathogenic *Neisseria*. It is the result of genetic transformation between gonococcal strains. It is also observed in penicillin resistance of several bacterial species when the resistant organism contains DNA from a host commensal organism.

antigenic peptide

A peptide that is able to induce an immune response and one that complexes with major histocompatibility complex (MHC), thereby permitting its recognition by a T cell receptor.

antigenic profile

The total antigenic content, structure, or distribution of epitopes of a cell or tissue.

antigenic reversion

The change in antigenic profile characteristic of an adult cell to an antigenic mosaic that previously existed in the immature or fetal cell stage of the species. Antigenic reversion may accompany neoplastic transformation.

antigenic shift

A remarkable alteration of viral surface antigens attributable to reassortment of their segmented genomes. The progeny virions generated possess new combinations of genome segments and therefore new proteins. A major antigenic change in which a strain with distinctive new antigens may appear, such as Asian or A2 influenza in 1957. Antigenic variants of type A influenza virus are known as subtypes. Influenza virus antigenic shift is attributable mainly to alterations in the hemagglutinin antigens, with less frequent alterations in the neuraminidase antigens. The appearance of a new type A influenza virus signals the addition of a new epitope, even though several original antigenic determinants are still present. In contrast to antigenic drift, antigenic shift involves a principal alteration in a genome attributable to gene rearrangement between two related microorganisms. Because antigenic shift involves the acquisition of totally new antigens against which the host population is not immune, this alteration may lead to an epidemic of significant proportions.

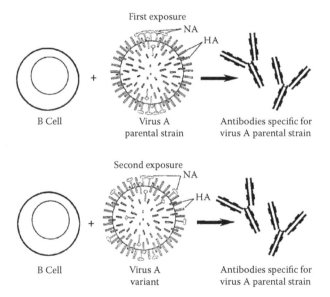

Doctrine of original antigenic sin.

antigenic sin, doctrine of original

When the immune response against a virus, such as a parental strain, to which an individual was previously exposed is greater than it is against the immunizing agent, such as type A influenza virus variant, the concept is referred to as the doctrine of original antigenic sin.

antigenic transformation

Changes in a cell's antigenic profile as a consequence of antigenic gain, deletion, reversion, or other process.

antigenic variation

A mechanism whereby selected viruses, bacteria, and animal parasites may evade the host antibody or T cell immune response, thereby permitting antigenically altered etiologic agents of disease to produce a renewed infection. The variability among infectious disease agents is of critical significance in the development of effective vaccines. Antigenic variation affects the surface antigens of the virus, bacteria, or animal parasite in which it occurs. By the time the host has developed a protective immune response against the antigens originally present, the latter have been replaced in a few surviving microorganisms by new antigens to which the host is not immune, thereby permitting survival of the microorganism or animal parasite and its evasion of the host immune response. Thus, from these few surviving viruses, bacteria, or animal parasites, a new population of infectious agents is produced. This cycle may be repeated, thereby obfuscating the protective effects of the immune response.

antigenicity

A property of a substance that renders it immunogenic or capable of stimulating an immune response. Antigenicity was more commonly used in the past to refer to what is now known as immunogenicity, although the two terms are still used interchangably by some investigators. An antigen is considered by many to be a substance that reacts with the products of immunogenic stimulation. It combines specifically with antibodies formed or with receptors of T cells stimulated during an immune response.

antigliadin antibodies (AGAs)

Antibodies specific for gliadin, a protein present in wheat and rye grain gluten. Antigliadins are requisite for the development of celiac disease with associated jejunal mucosal flattening in genetically prone subjects. Thus, antibodies against gliadin may be used for population screening for gluten-sensitive enteropathies such as celiac disease and dermatitis herpetiformis. An environmental agent such as an adenovirus in the intestine may induce an aberrant immune response to gluten in genetically susceptible subjects such as in HLA-DR3-DQw2 or HLA-B8 individuals.

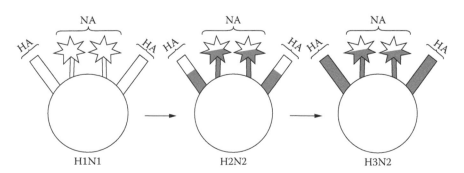

Antigenic variation.

A

antiglial fibrillary acidic protein (GFAP) antibody

A rabbit polyclonal antibody directed against glial fibrillary acidic protein present in the cytoplasm of most human astrocytes and ependymal cells. This reagent may be used to aid in the identification of cells of glial lineage. The antibody is intended for qualitative staining in sections of formalin-fixed, paraffin-embedded tissue. Anti-GFAP antibody specifically binds to the glial fibrillary acidic protein located in the cytoplasm of normal and neoplastic glial cells. Unexpected antigen expression or loss of expression may occur, especially in neoplasms. Occasionally, stromal elements surrounding heavily stained tissue and/or cells will show immunoreactivity. The clinical interpretation of any staining or its absence must be complemented by morphological studies and evaluation of proper controls.

antiglobulin

An antibody raised by immunization of one species, such as a rabbit, with immunoglobulin from another species, such as a human. Rabbit anti-human globulin has been used for many years in an antiglobulin test to detect incomplete antibodies coating red blood cells, as in erythroblastosis fetalis or autoimmune hemolytic anemia. Antiglobulin antibodies are specific for epitopes in the Fc regions of immunoglobulin molecules used as immunogens, rendering them capable of agglutinating cells whose surface antigens are combined with the Fab regions of IgG molecules whose Fc regions are exposed.

antiglobulin consumption test

An assay to test for the presence of an antibody in serum which is incubated with antigen-containing cells or antigen-containing particles. After washing, the cells or particles are treated with antiglobulin reagents and incubated further. If any antibody has complexed with the cells or particles, antiglobulin will be taken up. Antiglobulin depletion from the mixture is evaluated by assaying the free antiglobulin in the supernatant through combination with incomplete antibody-coated erythrocytes. No hemagglutination reveals that the antiglobulin reagent was consumed in the first step of the reaction and shows that the patient's original serum contained the antibody in question.

antiglobulin inhibition test

An assay based upon interference with the antiglobulin test through reaction of the antiglobulin reagent with antibody against it prior to combination with incomplete antibody-coated erythrocytes. This is the basis for the so-called antiglobulin consumption test.

antiglobulin test

When red blood cells are coated with antibodies that are not agglutinable in saline, such as those from an infant with erythroblastosis fetalis, a special anti-human immunoglobulin (Ig) prepared by immunizing rabbits with human IgG may be employed to crosslink the antibody-coated red cells to produce agglutination. Although previously considered to be incomplete antibodies, they are known to be bivalent but may be of a smaller size than saline agglutinable-type antibodies. R.R.A. Coombs developed this test in England in the 1940s. In addition to its usefulness in hemolytic disease of the newborn, the Coombs' test detects incomplete antibody-coated erythrocytes from patients with autoimmune hemolytic anemia. In the direct Coombs' test, red blood cells linked to saline nonagglutinable antibody are first washed, combined with rabbit anti-human immunoglobulin serum, and then observed for agglutination. In the indirect Coombs'

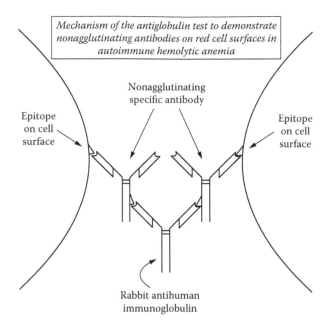

Mechanism of the antiglobulin test to demonstrate nonagglutinating antibodies on red cell surfaces in autoimmune hemolytic anemia

Nonagglutinating specific antibody

Epitope on cell surface

Epitope on cell surface

Rabbit antihuman immunoglobulin

Antiglobulin test.

test, serum containing the saline nonagglutinable antibodies is combined with red blood cells that are coated but not agglutinated. The rabbit anti-human immunoglobulin is then added to these antibody-coated red cells, and agglutination is observed as in the direct Coombs' reaction. A third assay termed the non-gamma test requires the incubation of erythrocytes with anti-C3 or anti-C4 antibodies. Agglutination reflects the presence of these complement components on red blood cell surfaces. This is an indirect technique to identify IgM antibodies that have fixed complement, such as those that are specific for Rh blood groups.

antiglutinin

Mammalian seminal plasma substance that prevents washed spermatozoa from spontaneously agglutinating (*i.e.*, autoagglutinating).

anti-GM1 antibodies

Antibodies found in 2 to 40% of Guillain–Barré syndrome (GBS) patients. They are mainly IgG_1, IgG_1, or IgA rather than IgM, even though IgM anti-GM_1 antibodies have been found in a few GBS cases. Anti-GM_1 antibodies are more frequent in GBS patients who experienced *Campylobacter jejuni* infection (up to 50% of cases). Titers are highest initially and fall as the disease progresses. These antibodies are present in spinal fluid, apparently due to disruption of the blood–nerve barrier. Anti-GM_1 antibodies recognize surface epitopes on *Campylobacter* bacteria, stains, and possibly a saccharide identical to the terminal tetrasaccharide of GM_1 that has been found in *Campylobacter* lipopolysaccharide. IgG anti-GM_1 has been postulated to selectively injure motor nerves in GBS.

antigranulocyte antibodies

Antigranulocyte antibodies play a significant role in the pathogenesis of febrile transfusion reactions, drug-induced neutropenia, isoimmune neonatal neutropenia, autoimmune neutropenia (including Felty's syndrome), Graves' disease, Evans syndrome, systemic lupus erythematosus (SLE), and primary autoimmune neutropenia of children. Antigranulocyte antibodies are best detected and quantitated by flow cytometry.

A

antigrowth hormone (GH) antibody

A rabbit polyclonal antibody against human growth hormone that positively stains the growth hormone-producing cells and somatotrophs of the pituitary gland and malignant and benign neoplasms arising from these cells.

antiheat shock protein antibodies

Heat shock proteins (hsps) have a broad phylogenetic distribution and share sequence similarities in molecules derived from bacteria, humans, or other animals. They play a significant role in inflammation. Heat shock proteins of mycobacteria are important in the induction of adjuvant arthritis by these microorganisms. Forty percent of SLE patients and 10 to 20% of RA patients have antibodies of IgM, IgG, and IgA classes to a 73-kDa protein of the hsp70 group. RA synovial fluid contains T lymphocytes that react with a 65-kDa mycobacterial heat shock protein. The significance of these observations of immune reactivity to heat shock proteins remains to be determined.

antihepatitis B virus core antigen (HBcAg) antibody

HBcAg is expressed predominantly in the nuclei of infected liver cells, although variable staining may also be seen in the perinuclear cytoplasm. This antibody labels the nuclei and occasionally cytoplasm of virus-infected cells.

antihigh molecular weight human cytokeratin antibodies

Mouse monoclonal antibodies that identify keratins of approximately 66 and 57 kDa in extracts of the stratum corneum. The antibody labels squamous, ductal, and other complex epithelia. It is reactive with both squamous and ductal neoplasms and variably with those derived from simple epithelium. Consistently positive are squamous cell carcinomas, ductal carcinomas (most notably those of the breast, pancreas, bile duct, and salivary gland), transitional cell carcinomas of the bladder and nasopharynx, thymomas, and epithelioid mesotheliomas. Adenocarcinomas are variably positive. The antibodies are largely unreactive with adenomas of endocrine organs, carcinomas of the liver (hepatocellular carcinoma), endometrium, and kidney. Mesnchymal tumors, lymphomas, melanomas, neural tumors, and neuroendocrine tumors are unreactive.

antihistamine

A substance that links to histamine receptors, thereby inhibiting histamine action. Antihistamine drugs derived from ethylamine block H1 histamine receptors, whereas those derived from thiourea block the H2 variety.

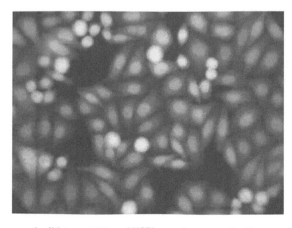

Antihistone (H2A and H2B) complex autoantibodies.

antihistone antibodies

Antibodies associated with several autoimmune diseases that include systemic lupus erythematosus (SLE), drug-induced lupus, juvenile rheumatoid arthritis, and rheumatoid arthritis. H-1 antibodies are the most common in SLE followed by anti-H2B, anti-H2A, anti-H3, and anti-H4, respectively. Antihistone antibodies are usually assayed by the ELISA technique.

anti-Hu antibodies

Autoantibodies associated with paraneoplastic encephalomyeloneuronitis (PEMN). They react with neuronal nuclei, recognizing 35- to 40-kDa antigens present in neuronal nuclei and also detectable in the nuclei of cells from small cell carcinoma of the lung. The antibody may be responsible for the death of neurons.

anti-human α-smooth muscle actin

A mouse monoclonal antibody that reacts with the α-smooth muscle isoform of actin. It reacts with smooth muscle cells of vessels and different parenchyma without exception, but with different intensity, according to the amount of α-smooth muscle actin present in smooth muscle cells, myoepithelial cells, pericytes, and some stromal cells in the intestine, testes, breast, and ovary. The antibody also reacts with myofibroblasts in benign and reactive fibroblastic lesions and perisinusoidal cells of normal and diseased human livers.

anti-human chorionic gonadotropin (HCG) antibody

An antibody that reacts with the β chain of human chorionic gonadotropin (HCG). HCG is a polypeptide hormone synthesized in the syncytiotrophoblastic cells of the placenta and in certain trophoblastic tumors. HCG is a marker for the biochemical differentiation of trophoblastic cells that often precedes their morphological differentiation. The antibody aids in the detection of HCG in trophoblastic elements of germ cell tumors of the ovaries, testes, and extragonadal sites. It crossreacts with luteinizing hormone.

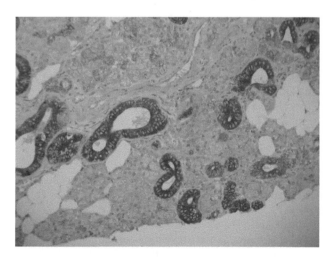

Cytokeratin 18—salivary gland.

anti-human cytokeratin (CAM 5.2) antibody

Monoclonal antibody against cytokeratins, which are polypeptide chains that form structural proteins within the epithelial cell cytoskeleton. Nineteen different molecular forms of cytokeratins have been identified in both normal

A

and malignant epithelial cell lines. Because specific combinations of cytokeratin peptides are associated with different epithelial cells, these peptides are clinically important markers for classifying carcinomas (tumors of epithelial origin) and for distinguishing carcinomas from malignant tumors of nonepithelial origin such as lymphomas, melanomas, and sarcomas. The identification of cytokeratin has gained increasing importance in immunopathology.

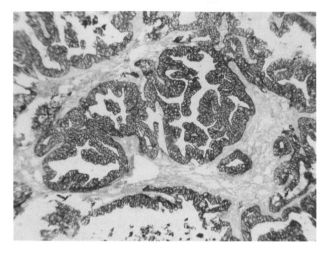

Cytokeratin 7—adenocarcinoma of the lung.

anti-human cytokeratin 7 antibody

A mouse monoclonal antibody directed against the 54-kDa cytokeratin intermediate filament protein identified as cytokeratin 7, a basic cytokeratin found in most glandular epithelia and in transitional epithelia. The antibody reacts with a large number of epithelial cell types including many ductal and glandular epithelia. In general, the antibody does not react with stratified squamous epithelia but is reactive with transitional epithelium of the urinary tract. The antibody reacts with many benign and malignant epithelial lesions. Keratin 7 is expressed in specific subtypes of adenocarcinomas from ovary, breast, and lung, whereas carcinomas from the gastrointestinal tract remain negative. Transitional cell carcinomas express keratin 7, whereas prostate cancer is generally negative. The antibody does not react with squamous cell carcinomas, rendering it a rather specific marker for adenocarcinoma and transitional cell carcinoma. In cytological specimens, the antibody permits ovarian carcinoma to be distinguished from colon carcinoma.

anti-human cytokeratin 20 antibody

A mouse monoclonal antibody that reacts with the 46-kDa cytokeratin intermediate filament protein. It reacts with intestinal epithelium, gastric foveolar epithelium, and a number of endocrine cells of the upper portions of the pyloric glands, as well as with the urothelium and Merkel's cells in the epidermis. The antibody has been tested on a series of carcinomas, including primary and metastatic lesions. There is a marked difference in expression of cytokeratin 20 among various carcinoma types. Neoplasia expressing cytokeratin 20 are derived from normal epithelia expressing cytokeratin 20. Colorectal carcinomas consistently express cytokeratin 20, whereas adenocarcinomas of the stomach express cytokeratin

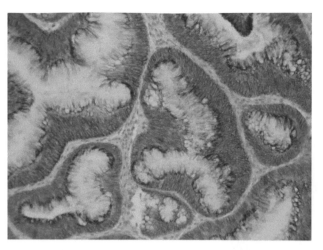

Cytokeratin 20—adenoma of the colon.

20 to a lesser degree. Adenocarcinomas of the gall bladder and bile ducts, ductal cell adenocarcinomas of the pancreas, mucinous ovarian tumors, and transitional cell carcinomas have been found to stain positively with the antibody. Most of the carcinomas from other sites are not positive using the antibody to cytokeratin 20 (e.g., adenocarcinomas of the breast, lung, and endometrium and nonmucinous tumors of the ovary). Merkel cell carcinomas of the skin stain normally with the anti-cytokeratin 20 antibody. There is a lack of positivity in small-cell lung carcinomas and in intestinal and pancreatic neuroendocrine tumor cells.

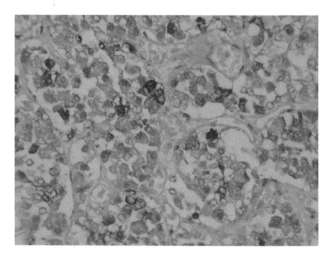

Follicle-stimulating hormone (FSH)—pituitary.

anti-human follicle-stimulating hormone (FSH) antibody

A rabbit antibody that labels gonadotropic cells in the pituitary. Positive staining for adenohypophyseal hormones assists in the classification of pituitary tumors. FSH is an adenohypophyseal glycoprotein hormone found in gonadotropic cells of the anterior pituitary glands of most mammals. Gonadotropic cells average about 10% of anterior pituitary cells. This antibody can be used for immunohistochemical staining.

anti-human gastrin antibody

A rabbit antibody that labels G cells of antropyloric mucosa of the stomach. It permits immunohistochemical detection of gastrin-secreting tumors and G cell hyperplasia.

anti-human glucagon antibody

A rabbit antibody that labels A cells of the endocrine mammalian pancreas.

anti-human hemoglobin

A rabbit antibody against hemoglobin A isolated from erythrocytes of normal adults that reacts with hemoglobin A and, due to a common α chain, also with hemoglobin A_2 and hemoglobin F.

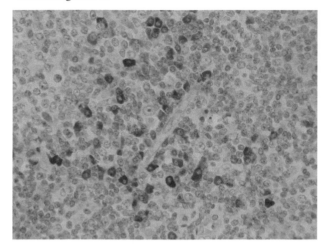

κ light chain—tonsil.

anti-human κ light chain antibody

A rabbit antibody that reacts with free κ light chains as well as κ chains in intact immunoglobulin molecules. It may be used for typing of free and bound monoclonal light chains by immunoelectrophoresis and immunofixation and for immunohistochemistry.

anti-human Ki-1 antigen (CD30) antibody

A mouse monoclonal antibody that reacts with a 595-amino acid transmembrane 121-kDa glycoprotein. It contains six cysteine-rich motifs in the extracellular domain and is homologous to members of the nerve growth factor receptor superfamily. The CD30 gene was assigned to the short arm of chromosome 1 at position 36. The CD30 antigen was initially designated Ki-1. The antibody detects a formalin-resistant epitope on the 90-kDa precursor molecule. This molecule is processed in the Golgi system into the membrane-bound, phosphorylated, mature, 120-kDa glycoprotein and into the soluble 85-kDa form of CD30, which is released from the supernatant and appears in serum at detectable levels in conditions such as infectious mononucleosis or neoplastically amplified CD30-positive blasts. The CD30 antigen is expressed by Hodgkin and Reed–Sternberg cells in Hodgkin disease, by the tumor cells of a majority of anaplastic large cell lymphomas and by a varying proportion of activated T and B cells. It is also expressed on embryonal carcinomas.

anti-human Ki-67 antibody

A mouse monoclonal antibody directed against the Ki-67 nuclear antigen that may be used to aid in the identification of proliferating cells in normal and neoplastic cell populations. It is intended for qualitative staining in sections of formalin-fixed, paraffin-embedded tissue (some form of antigen enhancement is required for paraffin-embedded samples), frozen tissue, and cytologic preparations. Ki-67 antibody specifically binds to

nuclear antigen(s) associated with cell proliferation and present throughout the active cell cycle (G_1, S, G_2, and M phases) but absent in resting (G_0) cells. Unexpected antigen expression or loss of expression may occur, especially in neoplasms. Occasionally stromal elements surrounding heavily stained tissues and or cells will show immunoreactivity. The clinical interpretation of any staining or its absence must be complemented by morphological studies and evaluation of proper controls.

anti-human λ light chain

A rabbit antibody that reacts with free λ light chains as well as the λ light chains in intact immunoglobulin molecules.

anti-human luteinizing hormone (LH)

A rabbit antibody that labels gonadotropic cells of the pituitary. Positive staining for adenohypophyseal hormones assists in classification of pituitary tumors. Luteinizing hormone (LH) is an adenohypophyseal glycoprotein hormone found in gonadotropic cells of the anterior pituitary glands of most mammals. Gonadotropic cells average about 10% of anterior pituitary cells.

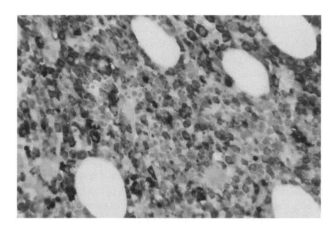

Myeloperoxidase—bone marrow.

anti-human myeloperoxidase antibody

An antibody used to discriminate between lymphoid leukemias and myeloid leukemias in formalin-fixed, paraffin-embedded tissues.

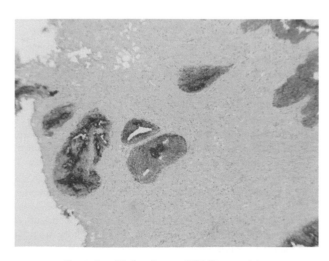

Prostatic acid phosphatase (PSAP)—prostate.

anti-human prostatic acid phosphatase (PSAP)

A rabbit antibody that reacts with prostatic ductal epithelial cells—normal, benign hypertrophic, and neoplastic. It labels the cytoplasm of prostatic epithelium, secretions, and concretions.

anti-human synaptophysin antibody

A rabbit antibody that reacts with a wide spectrum of neuroendocrine neoplasms of neural type including neuroblastomas, ganglioneuroblastomas, ganglioneuromas, pheochromocytomas, and chromaffin and nonchromaffin paragangliomas. The antibody also labels neuroendocrine neoplasms of epithelial type including pituitary adenomas, islet cell neoplasms, medullary thyroid carcinomas, parathyroid adenomas, carcinoids of the bronchopulmonary and gastrointestinal tracts, neuroendocrine carcinomas of the bronchopulmonary and gastrointestinal tracts, and neuroendocrine carcinomas of the skin.

anti-human thyroglobulin antibody

A rabbit antibody that reacts with human thyroglobulin. It labels the cytoplasm of normal and neoplastic thyroid follicle cells. Some staining of colloid may also be observed.

anti-human thyroid-stimulating hormone (TSH)

A rabbit antibody used for the immunochemical detection of thyroid-stimulating hormone (TSH) in thyrotrophic cells and in certain pituitary tumors.

anti-I antibodies

Antibodies against the I blood group antigen that is present in the majority of adult red blood cells in humans. The I/i antigens are present in the subterminal portions of oligosaccharides that are ultimately converted to H and A or B antigens. I and i configurations are present on membrane-associated glycoproteins and glycosphingolipids. The heterogeneity observed with different anti-I antisera may reflect the recognition of different parts of the branched oligosaccharide chain. Fetal erythrocytes contain abundant i antigen but few branched oligosaccharides and little I antigen. The I antigen develops during the first 2 years of life, with simultaneous loss of i. Anti-I is a common autoantibody, frequently present as a cold-reacting agglutinin. Anti-I is of pathologic significance in many cases of coronary heart disease (CHD) when it acts as a complement-binding monoclonal antibody. Auto-anti-I is of less significance in cold hemagglutinin disease than is anti-I. Thus, anti-I acting as a cold agglutinin may be detected as an autoantibody in a number of cases of cold antibody-type hemolytic anemia and in patients with *Mycoplasma pneumoniae* infection.

anti-idiotypic antibody

An antibody that interacts with antigenic determinants (idiotopes) at the variable N termini of the heavy and light chains comprising the paratope region of an antibody molecule where the antigen-binding site is located. The idiotope antigenic determinants may be situated either within the cleft of the antigen-binding region or on the periphery or outer edge of the variable regions of heavy and light chain components.

anti-idiotypic vaccine

An immunizing preparation of anti-idiotypic antibodies that are internal images of certain exogenous antigens. To develop an effective anti-idiotypic vaccine, epitopes of an infectious agent that induce protective immunity must be identified. Antibodies must be identified that confer passive immunity to this agent. An anti-idiotypic antibody prepared using these protective antibodies as the immunogen can in some instances be used as an effective vaccine. Anti-idiotypic vaccines have effectively induced protective immunity against such viruses as rabies, coronavirus, cytomegalovirus, and hepatitis B; such bacteria as *Listeria monocytogenes, Escherichia coli,* and *Streptococcus pneumoniae*; and such parasites as *Schistosoma mansoni* infections. Anti-idiotypic vaccination is especially desirable when a recombinant vaccine is not feasible. Monoclonal anti-idiotypic vaccines represent uniform and reproducible sources for immunizing preparations.

anti-immunoglobulin antibodies

Antibodies specific for immunoglobulin constant domains, which renders them useful for detection of bound antibody molecules in immunoassays. Anti-isotype antibodies are synthesized in different species; anti-allotype antibodies are made in the same species against allotypic variants; and anti-idiotype antibodies are induced against a single antibody molecule's unique determinants.

anti-intrinsic factor autoantibodies

Antibodies against the intrinsic factor glycoprotein, with a molecular weight of 44 kDa. Intrinsic factor binds vitamin B_{12}. Radioimmunoassay can detect two separate antibodies: one that reacts with the binding site for vitamin B_{12}, thereby blocking the subsequent binding of intrinsic factor with the vitamin, and another that reacts with an antigenic determinant remote from this site.

anti-isotypic antibodies

Antibodies generated in one species specific for antigenic determinants found only on one immunoglobulin isotype of a different species, e.g., goat anti-human IgM antibodies.

anti-Jo-1

Antibodies against tRNA synthetases occur frequently in polymyositis patients. Anti-Jo-1, the best known of this group, is present in 35% of adult polymyositis patients. The antibody is specific for the 54-kDa histidyl– tRNA synthetase.

anti-Ki-67 (MIB)

A mouse monoclonal antibody directed against the Ki-67 nuclear antigen. It may be used to aid in the identification of proliferating cells in normal and neoplastic cell populations. It is intended for qualitative staining in sections of formalin-fixed, paraffin-embedded tissue (some form of antigen enhancement is required for paraffin-embedded samples), frozen tissue and cytologic preparations. Ki-67 antibody specifically binds to nuclear antigen(s) associated with cell proliferation which is present throughout the active cell cycle (G_1, S, G_2, and M phases) but absent in resting (G_0) cells. Unexpected antigen expression or loss of expression may occur, especially in neoplasms. Occasionally stromal elements surrounding heavily stained tissues and or cells will show immunoreactivity. The clinical interpretation of any staining or its absence must be complemented by morphological studies and evaluation of proper controls.

anti-Ku autoantibodies

A myositis-associated autoantibody that occurs in a few (5 to 12%) Japanese patients with overlap syndrome. These antibodies are specific for 70- and 80-kDa DNA-binding proteins that represent the Ku antigen. They have also been found in patients with systemic lupus erythematosus (SLE), pure dermatomyositis, pure scleroderma, thyroid disease, and Sjögren's syndrome.

anti-La-SS-B autoantibodies

Autoantibodies found in Sjögren's syndrome and systemic lupus erythematosus (SLE). The La-SS-B antigen is a 47-kDa ribonucleic protein associated with a spectrum of small RNAs. Ls-SS-B is readily susceptible to proteolysis, resulting in many smaller (42-, 32-, and 27-kDa) but still immunoreactive polypeptides. The La-SS-B antigen primarily resides in the nucleus and is associated with RNA polymerase III transcripts. It shows strong conservation across species. The presence of autoantibodies against the La-SS-B antigen has been advocated as a diagnostic aid in patients with Sjögren's syndrome. Autoantibodies against La-SS-B are also commonly found in SLE and subacute cutaneous lupus. There is a correlation between anti-La-SS-B and the absence of nephritis in SLE patients. SLE patients with precipitating anti-Ro-SS-A antibodies have a high incidence of serious nephritis (53%), while those with both anti-Ro-SS-A and anti-La/SS-B have a low (9%) frequency of nephritis.

anti-LN1 antibody

A mouse monoclonal antibody against a sialoglycan antigen (CDw75) on cell membranes. In lymphoid tissues, the antibody reacts strongly with the B lymphocytes in the germinal centers but only faintly with B lymphocytes of the mantle zone. No reaction is observed with T lymphocytes. LN1 also reacts with certain epithelial cells, including cells of the distal renal tubules, breast, bronchus, and prostate.

anti-low molecular weight cytokeratin

A mouse monoclonal antibody directed against an epitope found on human cytokeratins. It may be used to aid in the identification of cells of epithelial lineage. The antibodies are intended for qualitative staining in sections of formalin-fixed, paraffin-embedded tissue. Antikeratin primary antibody specifically binds to antigens located in the cytoplasmic regions of normal epithelial cells. Unexpected antigen expression or loss of expression may occur, especially in neoplasm. Occasionally, stromal elements surrounding heavily stained tissue and/or cells will show apparent immunoreactivity. The clinical interpretation of any staining or its absence must be complemented by morphological studies and evaluation of proper controls.

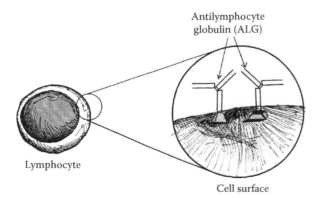

Antilymphocyte globulin (ALG)

Lymphocyte

Cell surface

Antilymphocyte globulin.

antilymphocyte serum (ALS) or antilymphocyte globulin (ALG)

An antiserum prepared by immunizing one species such as a rabbit or horse with lymphocytes or thymocytes from a different species such as a human. Antibodies present in this antiserum combine with T cells and other lymphocytes in the circulation to induce immunosuppression. ALS is used in organ transplant recipients to suppress graft rejection. The globulin fraction known as ALG rather than whole antiserum produces the same immunosuppressive effect.

antimalignin antibodies

Antibodies specific for the 10-kDa protein malignin comprised of 89 amino acids. These antibodies are claimed to be increased in cancer patients without respect to tumor cell type. It has been further claimed that antibody levels are related to survival. These claims require additional confirmation and proof to be accepted as facts.

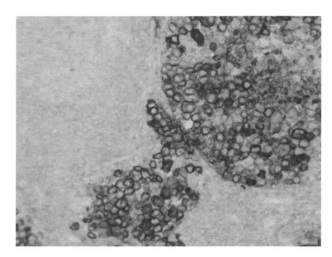

HMB-45. Melanoma in lymph node.

antimelanoma primary antibody

A mouse monoclonal antibody (clone HMB-45) raised against an extract of pigmented melanoma metastases from lymph nodes directed against a glycoconjugate present in immature melanosomes. This antibody may be used to aid in the identification of cells of melanocytic lineage. It is used for qualitative staining in sections of formalin-fixed, paraffin-embedded tissue and binds specifically to antigens located on immature melanosomes. Unexpected antigen expression or loss of expression may occur, especially in neoplasms. Clinical interpretation must be complemented by morphological studies and evaluation of proper controls.

antimetabolite

A drug that interrupts the normal intracellular processes of metabolism, such as those essential to mitosis. Antimetabolite drugs such as azathioprine, mercaptopurine, and methotrexate induce immunosuppression in organ transplant recipients and diminish autoimmune reactivity in patients with selected autoimmune diseases.

antimicrobial peptides

Small peptides that injure bacteria or fungi by rendering their cell walls permeable. Mammalian keratinocytes, or intestinal epithelial cells under pathogen attack, produce these peptides and some can be identified in neutrophil granules. These peptides include defensins and cathelicidins. Magainins, attacins, agglutinins, cecropins, and drosomycin represent microbial peptides in lower and

A

primitive animals. Antimicrobial peptides in plants include defensins, thionins, and phytoalexins.

antimuscle actin primary antibody

A mouse monoclonal antibody (clone HUC1-1) directed against an actin epitope found on muscle actin isoforms. It may be used to aid in the identification of cells of myocytic lineage and is intended for qualitative staining in sections of formalin-fixed, paraffin-embedded tissue. Antimuscle actin antibody specifically binds to antigens located in the cytoplasmic regions of normal muscle cells. Unexpected antigen expression or loss of expression may occur, especially in neoplasm. Occasionally, stromal elements surrounding heavily stained tissue and/or cells will show immunoreactivity. Clinical interpretation must be complemented by morphological studies and the evaluation of appropriate controls.

antimyelin-associated glycoprotein (MAG) antibodies

Antibodies associated with demyelinating neuropathy, which is a slowly progressive distal and symmetrical sensory or sensorimotor neuropathy involving both arms and legs; intention tremor may be present. Spinal fluid protein is often increased but cells are absent. There is demyelination and occasional axonal degeneration. Monoclonal anti-MAG and complement deposits have been found on the myelin sheaths. Selected nerves may show widening of the myelin lamellae. Most patients have a monoclonal gammopathy of the immunoglobulin M (IgM) type. The monoclonal IgM causes the neuropathy.

antimyocardial antibodies (AmyAs)

These antibodies occur in elevated titers in two thirds of coronary artery bypass patients and do not have to be related to postcardiotomy syndrome. They are also found in a majority of acute rheumatic fever patients.

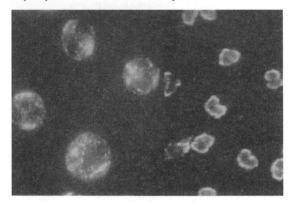

ANCA.

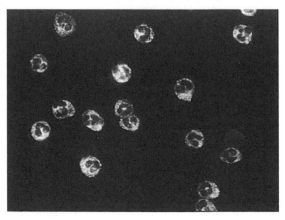

Neutrophil cytoplasmic antibody (cANCA). Formalin fixation.

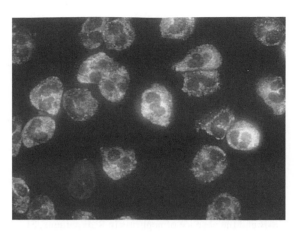

ANCA.

antineutrophil cytoplasmic antibodies (ANCAs)

A heterogeneous group of autoantibodies specific for constituents of neutrophilic granulocytes. They are valuable serological markers for the diagnostic and therapeutic management of patients with systemic vasculitides such as Wegener's granulomatosis and microscopic polyangiitis, in which they recognize well defined cytoplasmic antigens such as proteinase III and myeloperoxidase. Two well established ANCA staining patterns can be distinguished on ethanol-fixed neutrophils: a diffuse cytoplasmic fluorescent pattern (cANCA) and a fine homogeneous labeling of the perinuclear cytoplasm (pANCA). cANCA and classic pANCA in systemic vasculitides are autoantibodies specific for cytoplasmic antigens present in azurophils and specific granules of neutrophils. By contrast, atypical pANCAs in inflammatory bowel disease and hepatobiliary disorders do not react with cytoplasmic structures. Their fluorescence pattern, revealed by indirect immunofluorescence microscopy, is characterized by a broad inhomogeneous labeling of the nuclear periphery together with multiple intranuclear fluorescent foci. This antibody is assayed by flow cytometry and indirect fluorescence microscopy. HIV-1 infected patients may be biologically false-positive for neutrophil cytoplasmic antibody.

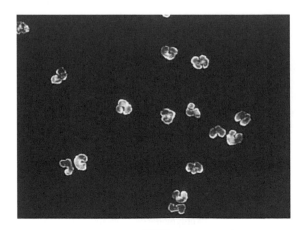

pANCA.

antineutrophil cytoplasmic autoantibodies (pANCAs)

Autoantibodies that recognize neutrophil myeloperoxidase; 50 to 80% of patients with ulcerative colitis express

A

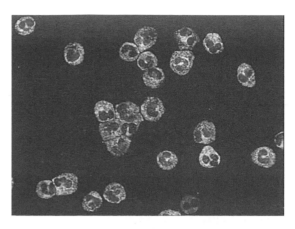

pANCA.

pANCAs. It is unlikely that ANCAs play a pathogenic role in inflammatory bowel disease since their presence does not correlate with disease activity or extent. There is no defect in neutrophil function in the presence of ANCAs.

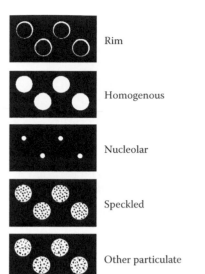

Antinuclear antibodies.

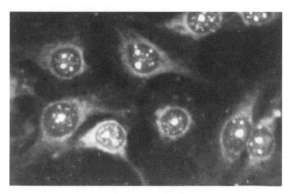

Antinuclear antibodies.

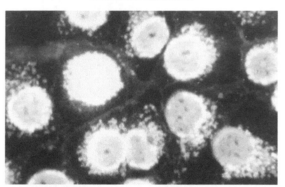

ANA/AMA mixed pattern.

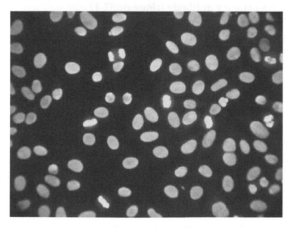

Antinuclear antibodies.

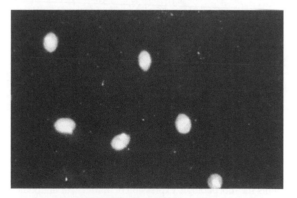

nDNA antibody; positive reaction.

anti-nRNP antibody
     Antibodies that recognize a set of proteins uniquely associated with U1-snRNP (U1-k, U1-A, and U1-C).

antinuclear antibodies (ANAs)
     Antibodies found in the circulations of patients with various connective tissue disorders. They may show specificity for various nuclear antigens including single- and double-stranded DNA, histones, and ribonucleoprotein. To detect antinuclear

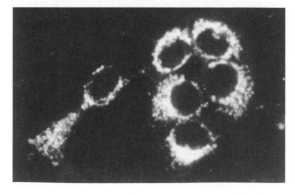

AMA positive pattern.

A

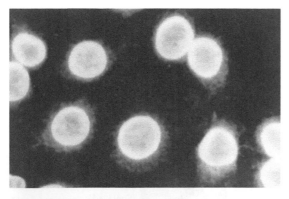

ANA peripheral pattern.

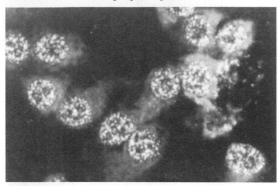

ANA speckled pattern.

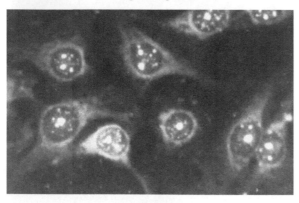

ANA nucleolar pattern.

antibodies, the patient's serum is incubated with Hep-2 cells and the pattern of nuclear staining is determined by fluorescence microscopy. The homogeneous pattern of staining represents the morphologic expression of antinuclear antibodies specific for ribonucleoprotein, which is positive in more than 95% of cases of systemic lupus erythematosus (SLE) and drug-induced lupus erythematosus and 70 to 90% of cases of diffuse systemic sclerosis and limited scleroderma (CREST) cases. It is also positive in 50 to 80% of Sjögren's syndrome and in 40 to 60% of inflammatory myopathies. The test is also positive in progressive systemic sclerosis, rheumatoid arthritis, and other connective tissue disorders. Peripheral nuclear staining represents the morphologic expression of DNA antibodies associated with SLE. Nucleolar fluorescence signifies anti-RNA antibodies of the type that occurs in progressive systemic sclerosis (scleroderma). The speckled pattern of staining is seen in several connective tissue diseases. When antinuclear antibodies (ANAs) reach elevated titers significantly above the normal serum level, ANA tests are considered positive. The indirect

immunofluorescence technique (IFT) is used as a screening technique before more specific methods are used. Most ANAs are specific for nucleic acids or proteins associated with nucleic acids. Only nucleoli in centromeres of chromosomes can be distinguished by IFT as separate antigens. Nucleosomes are irrelevant autoantigens for the formation of antibodies against nucleosomes, histones, and DNA. Antibodies against specific nuclear antigens are listed individually.

antinucleosome antibodies

Antibodies specific for nucleosomes or subnucleosomal structures that consist of DNA plus core histones. These autoantibodies were the first to be associated with systemic lupus erythematosus (SLE) and were formerly referred to as LE factors responsible for the so-called LE cell phenomenon.

antioxidants and immunity

Immune function depends on a balance between the free radical and antioxidant status of the body. Exposure of healthy adults to high levels of oxidants leads to diminished immune responses. Exposure to low levels of dietary antioxidants also decreases immune responses such as delayed-type hypersensitivity. Increased oxidative stress and immune dysfunction result from rheumatoid arthritis, aging, and cigarette smoking, leading to damage to lipids and other cellular components by free radicals. Antioxidant status is reduced in arthritic patients and smokers compared with controls. Thus, supplemental antioxidants are useful for diminishing oxidative stress and improving immune function. Increased levels of antioxidants may be needed for elderly individuals to maintain delayed-type hypersensitivity responses.

anti-p24 antibodies

Antibodies against the viral core protein p24 appear within weeks of acute human immunodeficiency virus (HIV) infection and may have a role in the decrease in plasma viremia associated with primary infection. The decline in anti-p24 antibodies is linked to HIV disease progression.

anti-p53 primary antibody (clone Bp53-11)

A mouse monoclonal antibody directed against both the mutant and wild-type of the p53 nuclear phosphoprotein. Normal cells very rarely express *p53*, but alterations in the p53 suppressor gene result in an overproduction of this protein in malignancies. This reagent may be used to aid in the identification of abnormally proliferating cells in neoplastic cell populations. It is intended for qualitative staining in sections of formalin-fixed, paraffin-embedded tissue on a Ventana automated slide staining device. Some form of antigen enhancement is required for paraffin-embedded samples. The p53 antibody specifically binds to nuclear antigen(s) associated with the normal downregulation of cell division. Increased expression of p53 in actively dividing cells is an indication of loss of function due to mutation of the p53 gene.

antipancreatic polypeptide (PP) antibody

A polyclonal antibody that detects pancreatic polypeptide in routinely fixed, paraffin-embedded or frozen tissue sections. Hyperplasia of pancreatic polypeptide-containing cells (PP cells) is often seen in patients with juvenile diabetes, chronic pancreatitis, and islet cell tumors. Hyperplasia of PP cells (greater than 10% of the islet cell population) in the nontumoral pancreas has been observed in nearly 50% of islet cell tumors. Demonstration of increased numbers of cells secreting PP found both within the islets and between the islets is characteristic of type II hyperplasia of pancreatic islets.

antipapillomavirus antibody

A rabbit antibody against papillomavirus. The structural antigens on this virus can be detected in a variety of proliferative squamous lesions. Only 50 to 60% of lesions caused by papillomavirus will express the structural antigens. This antibody staining is predominantly intranuclear in a focal or diffuse pattern, although perinuclear cytoplasmic staining of koilocytotic cells may also be seen.

antiparathyroid hormone (PTH) antibody

A polyclonal antibody against parathyroid hormone (PTH). PTH controls the concentration of calcium and phosphate ions in the blood. A decrease in blood calcium stimulates the parathyroid gland to secrete PTH, which acts on cells of bone, increasing the number of osteoclasts and leading to absorption of the calcified bone matrix and the release of calcium into the blood. Hyperparathyroidism may be caused by adenomas, rarely by carcinomas, and by ectopic PTH production. PTH is released by renal adenocarcinomas and by squamous cell cancers of the bronchi.

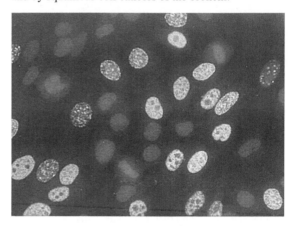

Anti-PCNA antibodies.

anti-PCNAs

Antibodies present in the sera of 3% of systemic lupus erythematosus (SLE) patients. Epitope mapping reveals that the antibodies bind conformational epitopes of this antigen.

antiphospholipid antibodies

A heterogeneous group of immunoglobulins directed against negatively charged phospholipids, protein–phospholipid complexes, and plasma proteins. Antiphospholipid antibodies occur in autoimmune disease; bacterial, fungal, and viral infections; and malignant tumors, or they may result from use of specific medications or appear in normal, healthy people. They are associated with both venous and arterial thrombosis. They occur in systemic lupus erythematosus (SLE), rheumatoid arthritis, Sjögren's syndrome, Reiter's syndrome, and possibly scleroderma and polyarteritis. They may appear as a result of HIV, Lyme disease, ornithosis, adenovirus, rubella and chicken pox, smallpox vaccination, or syphilis. Refer also to anticardiolipin antibody syndrome and to lupus anticoagulant.

antiphospholipid syndrome (APS)

An autoimmune disorder characterized by autoantibodies against constituents of the prothrombin activator complex requisite for the blood coagulation cascade. A condition with four common clinical features: venous thrombosis, arterial thrombosis, pregnancy loss, or thrombocytopenia. Fifty percent of patients present with primary APS (not associated with systemic disease), and the remaining 50% have secondary APS associated with such diseases as systemic lupus erythematosus (SLE), other connective tissue diseases, HIV or other infections, malignancy, and drug use. APS is a leading cause of hypercoagulability and thrombosis. Thrombosis is the most common presentation of APS. Anticardiolipin (ACA)-positive APS and lupus anticoagulant (LA)-positive APS are the two syndromes. ACA-APS is more common than LA-APS, with a relative prevalence of 5 to 2. Both are associated with thrombosis, fetal wastage, and thrombocytopenia. ACA-APC is associated with both arterial and venous thrombosis including deep vein thrombosis and pulmonary embolism, premature coronary artery disease, and premature cerebrovascular disease. By contrast, LA-APS is more commonly associated with venous thrombosis involving mesenteric, renal, hepatic, and portal veins and vena cava. Antiphospholipid antibodies (aPL) are demonstrated by either prolongation of a phospholipid-dependent coagulation test (lupus) or by their reactivity to anticoagulant (LA anionic phospholipids [PL]) in a solid-phase immunoassay. To diagnose APS, at least one of the above clinical features and a positive test are required.

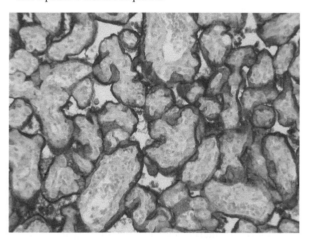

Placental alkaline phosphatase (PLAP)—placenta.

antiplacental alkaline phosphatase antibody

Placental alkaline phosphatase (PLAP) is normally produced by syncytiotrophoblasts after the 12th week of pregnancy. Human placental alkaline phosphatase is a member of a family of membrane-bound alkaline phosphatase enzymes and isoenzymes. It is expressed by both malignant somatic and germ-cell tumors. PLAP immunoreactivity can be used in conjunction with epithelial membrane antigen (EMA) and keratin to differentiate between germ cell and somatic tumor metastases. Germ cell tumors appear to be universally reactive for PLAP, whereas somatic tumors show only 15 to 20% reactivity.

antiplatelet antibodies

Autoantibodies that may be induced by drugs such as amphotericin B, cephalothin, methicillin, pentamidine, trimethoprim-sulfamethoxizole, and vancomycin.

anti-PM/Scl autoantibodies

Myositis-associated autoantibodies specific for the nucleolar antigen PM/Scl found among many patients with overlap syndrome with features such as scleroderma and polymyositis/dermatomyositis (25%). This autoantibody is found in a few patients with pure polymyositis or scleroderma. It is

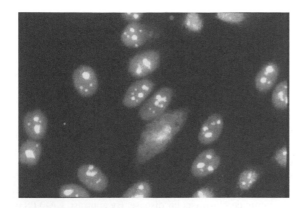

Anti-PM/Scl autoantibodies.

specific for a complex of nucleolar proteins, the principal antigen having a mass of 100 kDa, and is found mainly in Caucasian patients with overlap syndrome.

antiprogesterone receptor antibody

A mouse monoclonal antibody against human progesterone receptor; a mouse monoclonal anti-human progesterone receptor antibody that specifically recognizes the A and B forms of the receptor in Western blot purified recombinant receptor, normal endometrium, and cell lysates of the progesterone receptor-rich T47D human breast carcinoma cell line. No reactivity was observed with lysate of the progesterone receptor-negative MDA-MB-231 breast carcinoma cells. No crossreactivity was found with androgen receptor, estrogen receptor, or glucocorticoid receptor. The antibody binds an epitope found between amino acids 165 and 534, in the N terminal transactivation domain of the progesterone receptor molecule. Various tumors of the female reproductive tract have been shown to express progesterone receptor. Immunoreactivity has been demonstrated in breast carcinoma, uterine papillary serous carcinoma, endometrial carcinoma, ovarian serous borderline tumor, endometrial stromal sarcoma, uterine adenomatoid tumor, and ovarian thecoma. Other tumors shown to stain positively include medullary carcinoma of the thyroid and meningioma.

antiprolactin antibody

A rabbit antibody that gives positive staining of the prolactin cells of the anterior pituitary and benign and malignant neoplasms derived from these cells.

antiprostate-specific antigen antibody

A rabbit antibody that reacts with prostatic ductal epithelial cells: normal, benign hypertrophic, and neoplastic. It labels the cytoplasm of prostatic epithelium, secretions, and concretions.

anti-Purkinje cell antibody

An antibody detected in the circulation of patients with subacute cerebellar degeneration and in those with ovarian neoplasms and other gynecologic malignancies.

anti-RA-33 antibodies

Antibodies considered specific for rheumatoid arthritis (RA) have now been found in other autoimmune diseases and are detected by immunoblotting.

antiretroviral drugs

Therapeutic agents employed to inhibit replication and spread of HIV. They include protease inhibitors, nucleoside and non-nucleoside reverse transcriptase inhibitors, and fusion inhibitors that block fusion of the HIV viral envelope to the host cell membrane.

anti-Ri antibody

An antibody found in sera and spinal fluids of patients with opsoclonus without myoclonus that occurs in conjunction with gait ataxia in women with breast cancer. The anti-Ri antibody reacts with 55- and 80-kDa proteins present in the nuclei of central nervous system neurons and breast tumor cells. The condition may remit, manifest exacerbations and remissions, and occasionally respond to steroids or other immune interventions.

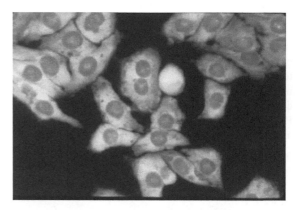

Antiribosomal RNP autoantibodies.

antiribosomal rRNP antibodies

Antibodies that react with ribosomal phosphoproteins P1 and P2. Anti-P is present in 10% of systemic lupus erythematosus (SLE) patients.

anti-scRNP (Ro-SS-A, La-SS-B)

Anti-La-SS-B antibodies are found mainly in patients with Sjögren's syndrome but also in those with systemic lupus erythematosus (SLE) and rheumatoid arthritis (RA). These antibodies are usually found together with anti-Ro-SS-A. Anti-Ro-SS-A frequently occurs alone in SLE and systemic sclerosis. There is no correlation between anti-Ro-SS-A and anti-La-SS-B antibody in patients with SLE and disease activity. Maternal anti-Ro-SS-A is the greatest single risk factor for the development of intrauterine or neonatal complete heart block in a child.

antisense oligonucleotide

An oligonucleotide created to interfere with the synthesis of a human protein by binding specifically to a complementary sequence, the "sense strand" in a primary RNA transcript or mRNA that encodes the protein concerned. The resulting duplex mRNA may inhibit the splicing of the primary transcript, stop mRNA translation, interfere with ribosomal assembly, or lead to cleavage of mRNA by RNase H activation.

antiseptic paint

A colloquial designation for the coating effect of secretory immunoglobulin A (IgA), such as that produced locally in the gut, on mucosal surfaces, thereby barring antigen access.

antiserum

A preparation of serum containing antibodies specific for a particular antigen (i.e., immunogen). A therapeutic antiserum may contain antitoxin, antilymphocyte antibodies, etc. An antiserum contains a heterogeneous collection of antibodies that bind the antigen used for immunization. Each antibody has a specific structure, antigenic specificity, and crossreactivity contributing to the heterogeneity that renders an antiserum unique.

anti-Sm autoantibodies

Autoantibodies found in the sera of patients with systemic lupus erythematosus (SLE). The antibodies are usually accompanied by antinuclear ribonucleoprotein (nRNP) antibodies. The U1RNP particle has both Sm and RNP binding specificities. The difference is that the RNP particles bound by U2, U4/6, and U5 are bound by anti-Sm autoantibodies but not by anti-nRNP autoantibodies. Sm antigen is a nonhistone nucleoprotein composed of several polypeptides of differing molecular weights. Autoantibodies against Sm antigen precipitate the U1, U2, U4/6, and U5 small nuclear RNAs. The Sm antigen is involved in normal post-transcriptional, pre-messenger RNA processing to excise introns. Autoantibodies to Sm antigen have been observed in 15 to 30% of SLE sera as diagnostic markers. It is believed that IgG anti-Sm correlates with lupus disease activity and is a useful variable in predicting exacerbation and prognosis of SLE. IgG anti-Sm is specifically detected in patients with SLE. ELISA methodology is used to quantitate this antibody.

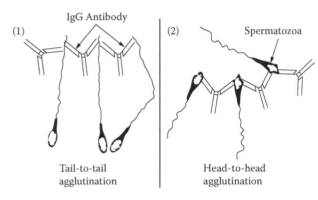

Antisperm antibody.

anti-snRNP (Sm, U1-RNP, U2-RNP)

Sm antibodies are specific for the D proteins and the BB′ doublets of Usn-RNPs. Sm-specific antibodies precipitate U1-, U2-, U4-, U5-, and U6-smRNPs. Anti-Sm autoantibodies are found exclusively in systemic lupus erythematosus (SLE) patients and are considered disease-specific. Antibodies to U1-RNP are markers for mixed connective tissue disease (MCTD).

antisomatostatin antibody

A rabbit antibody that can be used for the immunohistochemical staining of somatostatin in tumors and hyperplasias of pancreatic islets.

antisperm antibody

An antibody specific for any one of several sperm constituents. Antisperm agglutinating antibodies are detected in blood serum by the Kibrick sperm agglutination test that uses donor sperm. Sperm-immobilizing antibodies are detected by the Isojima test. The subject's serum is incubated with donor sperm and motility is examined. Testing for antibodies is of interest to couples with infertility problems. Treatment with relatively small doses of prednisone is sometimes useful in improving the situation by diminishing antisperm antibody titers. One half of infertile females manifest immunoglobulin G (IgG) or IgA sperm-immobilizing antibodies that affect the tails of spermatozoa. By contrast, IgM antisperm head-agglutinating antibodies may occur in homosexual males.

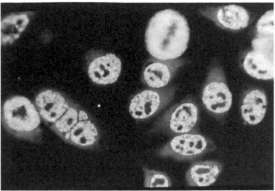

Anti-SM/RNP autoantibodies.

anti-SS-A

An anti-RNA antibody that occurs in Sjögren's syndrome patients. The antibody may pass across the placenta in pregnant females and be associated with heart block in their infants.

anti-SS-B

An anti-RNA antibody detectable in patients with Sjögren's syndrome and other connective tissue (rheumatic) diseases.

antitarget antigen antibodies

Antibodies used to block MHC class II molecules to prolong allograft survival or to remove Rh(D)+ cells to prevent sensitization of Rh(D)– mothers.

anti-T cell (CD45RO) antibody

An antibody that reacts with the CD45RO determinant of leukocyte common antigen. It reacts with most T lymphocytes, macrophages, and Langerhans' cells of normal tissues. It also reacts with peripheral T cell lymphomas, T cell leukemia, histiocytosis, and monocytic leukemia with mature phenotype. It reacts very rarely with B cell lymphoma and leukemia.

anti-T cell receptor idiotype antibodies

Antibodies that interact with antigenic determinants (idiotypes) at the variable N termini of the heavy and light chains comprising the paratope region of an antibody molecule where the antigen-binding site is located. The idiotope antigenic determinants may be situated within the cleft of the antigen-binding region or located on the periphery or outer edge of the variable regions of heavy and light chain components. Anti-idiotypic antibodies also block T cell receptors for the antigens for which they are specific.

anti-τ antibodies

Rabbit antibodies against τ, one of the microtubule-associated proteins (MAPs) in the central nervous system. In the phosphorylated form, τ is a major component of the paired helical filaments of the neurofibrillary tangles developed in Alzheimer's disease. One of its functions is to stabilize microtubules. Phosphorylation of τ reduces the stabilizing effect. The C terminal part of the τ protein shows a high degree of homology with other MAPs such as MAP2, and has been suggested to serve as a microtubule-binding domain. The antibody reacts on immunoblots with τ protein and with τ from Alzheimer's paired helical filaments. Brain tissue from patients with Alzheimer's disease is characterized by several histopathological lesions such as neurofibrillary tangles and senile plaques. For the study of lesions associated with Alzheimer's disease, the

A

anti-τ antibody may be used in combination with mouse monoclonal anti-β-amyloid and rabbit anti-ubiquitin. Neurofibrillary tangles are labeled by anti-τ, whereas the senile plaques are labeled by the β amyloid and ubiquitin antibodies.

antithymocyte globulin (ATG)

The globulin fraction of serum containing antibodies generated through immunization of animals such as rabbits or horses with human thymocytes. The fraction has been used clinically to treat rejection episodes in organ transplant recipients.

antithymocyte serum (ATS)

Antibody raised by immunizing one species such as a rabbit or horse with thymocytes derived from another such as a human. The resulting antiserum has been used to induce immunosuppression in organ transplant recipients. It acts by combining with the surface antigens of T lymphocytes and suppressing their action.

anti-topoisomerase I (Scl 70)

Anti-Scl 70 antibodies are associated with diffuse cutaneous systemic sclerosis and are specific to this disease. This renders Scl 70 as an important marker for systemic sclerosis.

antitoxin

Antibody specific for exotoxins produced by certain microorganisms such as the causative agents of diphtheria and tetanus. Prior to the antibiotic era, antitoxins were the treatments of choice for diseases produced by the soluble toxic products of microorganisms, such as those from *Corynebacterium diphtheriae* and *Clostridium tetani*.

antitoxin assay (historical)

Antitoxins are assayed biologically by their capacity to neutralize homologous toxins as demonstrated by the lack of toxic manifestations following inoculations of the mixture into experimental animals (e.g., guinea pigs). They may be tested serologically by their ability to flocculate (precipitate) toxin *in vitro*.

antitoxin unit

A unit is the amount of antitoxin present in 1/6000 g of a certain dried unconcentrated horse serum antitoxin that has been maintained since 1905 at the National Institutes of Health in Bethesda, Maryland. The standard antitoxin unit contained sufficient antitoxin to neutralize 100 MLD of the special toxin prepared and used by Ehrlich in the titration of a standard antitoxin. The American and international units of antitoxin are the same.

anti-*Toxoplasma gondii* antibody

An antibody that reacts with an epitope of *Toxoplasma gondii* that is resistant to formalin fixation and paraffin embedding. When tested by indirect immunofluorescence on infected glioma cells, anti-*T. gondii* stains the outer surfaces of tachyzoites of two different strains of *T. gondii* (RH and T626). Using an immunoperoxidase technique, both tachyzoites and encysted bradyzoites have been labeled in infected lung.

anti-U1-RNP autoantibodies

Antibodies to ribonucleoprotein (U1-RNP) have been used to partially define mixed connective tissue disease (MCTD). High titer anti-RNP occurs also in inflammatory muscle disease. Autoantibodies against nuclear ribonucleoprotein (U1-RNP) in Caucasians with or without MCTD are associated with DR4 anti-U1Sn-RNP. Autoantibodies in the Japanese demonstrate an increased frequency of DQ3,

with only a few subjects having MCTD. Further studies demonstrated an association of DRB1*0401, DRB4*0101, DQA1*03, DQB1*0301, and MCTD.

antivenin (Crotalidae) polyvalent (equine origin) injection

An antivenin raised in horses for the treatment of envenomation of crotalids (pit vipers) found in North, South, and Central America, including rattlesnakes (*Crotalus*, *Sistrurus*); copperhead and cotton mouth (*Agkistrodon*) snakes including *A. halys* of Korea and Japan; the fer-delance and other species of *Bothrops*; the tropical rattler (*C. durissus* and similar species); the cantil (*A. bilineatus*); and bushmaster (*Lachesis mutus*) of South and Central America. The antivenin consists of concentrated serum globulins from horses immunized with the venoms of *C. adamanteus* (Eastern diamond rattlesnake), *C. atrox* (Western diamond rattlesnake), *C. durissus terrificus* (tropical rattlesnake, Cascabel), and *Bothrops atrox* (fer-de-lance).

antivenin, black widow spider (*Latrodectus mactans*) (equine origin) injection

An antivenin raised in horses for passive transient protection against the toxic effects of black widow (*Latrodectus mactans*) bites and those of related spiders. The antivenin is most effective when administered within 4 hours after envenomation. It is moderately effective in the relief of pain and can be life-saving. Symptoms begin to ameliorate 1 to 3 hours after injection.

antivenin, North American coral snake (*Micrurus fulvius*) (equine origin)

An antivenin raised in horses for passive transient protection from the toxic effects of venoms of *Micrurus fulvius fulvius* (Eastern coral snake). It is also effective in neuetralizing venom of *M. fulvius tenere* (Texas coral snake). It is most effective when administered within 4 hours following envenomation. It is a refined, concentrated, lyophilized preparation of serum globulins derived from sera of horses immunized against Eastern coral snake venom.

antivenom

Antitoxin prepared specifically for the treatment of bite or sting victims of poisonous snakes or arthropods. Antibodies in this immune serum preparation neutralize the snake or arthropod venom. Also called antivenin or antivenene.

antivimentin antibody

A mouse monoclonal antibody raised against purified bovine eye. It reacts with the 57-kDa intermediate vimentin filament protein and may be used to aid in the identification of cells of mesenchymal origin. The antibody is intended for qualitative staining in sections of formalin-fixed, paraffin-embedded tissue. It binds specifically to antigens located in the cytoplasm of mesenchymal cells. The clinical interpretation of any staining or its absence must be complemented by morphological studies and evaluation of proper controls.

antiviral state

A metabolic condition in which a cell becomes resistant to virus by exposure to type I IFN derived from nearby virus-infected cells. Relies on viral RNA degradation by IFN and blocking of viral transcription and translation.

antrypol

Alternative name for suramin.

AP-1

A transcription factor that binds the IL-2 promoter, thereby regulating induction of the IL-2 gene. Some transcription factors have roles in lymphocyte activation. Immediately following T cell stimulation, c-*fos* mRNA is increased, and the c-*fos* gene product combines with the c-*jun* gene product to form AP-1. A similar series of events occurs following B cell stimulation; however, the genes regulated by B cell AP-1 are not known.

APC

Abbreviation for antigen-presenting cell.

APC licensing

The postulate that total activation of a cytotoxic T cell stimulated by antigen is enabled through costimulation by a dendritic cell whose costimulatory molecules have been upregulated following previous CD40–CD40L-mediated interaction with an antigen-activated Th lymphocyte.

APECED (autoimmune polyendocrinopathy–candidiasis–ectodermal dystrophy)

An autosomal-recessive disorder characterized by hypoparathyroidism, adrenal cortical failure, gonadal failure, candidiasis, and malabsorption. Antithymocyte globulin (ATG) immunoglobulin G (IgG) isolated from the sera of rabbits or horses hyperimmunized with human thymocytes is used to treat aplastic anemia patients and combat rejection in organ transplant recipients. Equine ATG contains 50 mg/ml of immunoglobulin and has yielded 50% recovery of bone marrow and treated aplastic anemia patients.

APD

Alternative abbreviation for autoimmune polyendocrinopathy–candidiasis–ectodermal dystrophy.

apheresis

Technique whereby blood is removed from the body, its components are separated, and some are retained for therapeutic or other use; the remaining elements are recombined and returned to the donor. Also called hemapharesis.

apical

The surface of an epithelial cell that faces the lumen rather than the tissue.

aplasia

The disappearance of a particular population of cells because of their failure to develop.

aplastic anemia

Bone marrow stem cell failure that leads to cessation of formation of cellular blood components. Bone marrow transplantation is the recommended treatment.

APO-1

Synonym for *fas* gene. Fas membrane protein ligation has been shown to initiate apoptosis. This is the reverse action of bcl-2 protein, which blocks apoptosis.

apolarity

An aqueous environment is of considerable importance to the antigen–antibody complex and it may contribute greatly to its stabilization. A net attractive force results from a decrease in energy arising from the preference of apolar or hydrophobic regions of the interacting molecules to associate with themselves rather than with solvent molecules (H_2O). The reaction is endothermic ($\Delta H > 0$); in order for it to be spontaneous ($\Delta H < 0$), it must occur through a concomitant increase in entropy through an entropy-driven reaction. This can be understood from the following thermodynamic relationship: $\Delta G = \Delta H - T\Delta S$ where ΔG is the free energy change, ΔH is the enthalpy change, T is the absolute temperature, and ΔS is the entropy change. When $\Delta H > 0$ (endothermic reaction), a positive ΔS is needed for

the overall energy decrease ($\Delta G < 0$), resulting in the attractive force. The binding of this attractive force increases (ΔG becomes more negative) as ΔH decreases and as the temperature T increases.

apolipoprotein (APO-E)

A plasma protein involved in many functions including lipid transport, tissue repair, and regulation of cellular growth and proliferation. There are three major isoforms of APO-E encoded by the ε 2, 3, or 4 alleles (APO-E2, APO-E3, APO-E4). APO-E3 is the most common variant. There is much interest in the APO-E4 variant, as it may be implicated in Alzheimer's disease. Other APO-E polymorphisms have been implicated in lipid metabolism disorders and heart disease. APO-E is a 33-kDa protein produced by nonactivated macrophages but not monocytes. It binds low-density lipids and high density cholesterol esters.

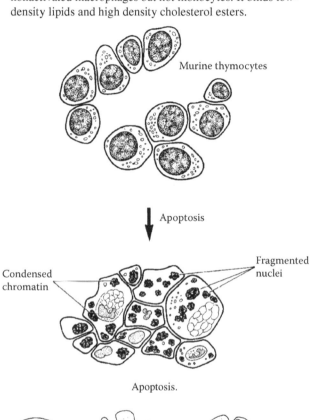

Apoptosis.

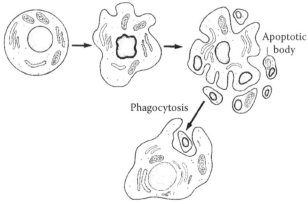

Apoptosis.

apoptosis

Programmed cell death in which the chromatin becomes condensed and the DNA is degraded. The immune

A

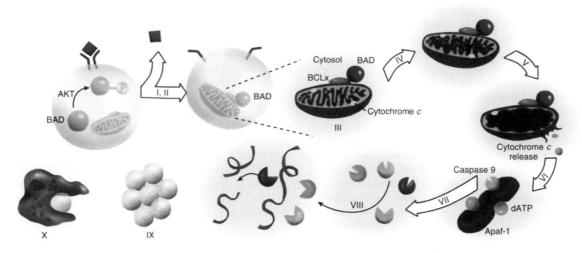

Apoptosis signaling.

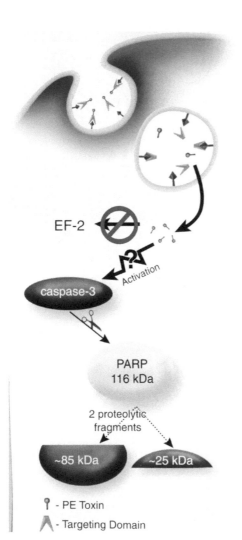

EF-2

caspase-3

Activation

PARP
116 kDa

2 proteolytic
fragments

~85 kDa   ~25 kDa

♀ - PE Toxin

Λ - Targeting Domain

Four caspase pathways involved in apoptosis.

system employs apoptosis for clonal deletion of cortical thymocytes by antigen in immunologic tolerance. A
healthy organism is an exquisitely integrated collection of
differentiated cells that maintain a balance between life
and death. Some cells are irreplaceable; some complete

their functions and are then sacrificed; and some cells
live finite lifetimes to be replaced by subsequent generations. A failure of cells to fulfill their destiny has cata-
strophic consequences for an organism. Apoptosis is the
last phase of cell destiny. It is the controlled disassembly
of a cell. When apoptosis occurs on schedule, neighboring cells and, more importantly, the total organism are
not adversely affected. Apoptosis gone awry, however,
produces dire effects. When apoptosis occurs in irreplaceable cells, as in some neurodegenerative disorders,
functions critical to the organism are lost. When cells
fail to undergo apoptosis after serving their purpose, as
in autoimmune disorders, escaped cells adversely affect
the organism. When cells become renegade and resist
apoptosis, as in cancer, the outlaw cells create a dire situation for the organism. Mistiming of or errors in apoptosis can exert devastating consequences on development.
Apoptotic fidelity is, therefore, critical to the well-being
of an organism. Mitochondrial cytochrome c is released in
the intrinsic apoptotic pathway, whereas death receptors
such as *Fas* and TNFR are activated in the extrinsic apoptotic pathway. The process of apoptosis (programmed cell
death) is regulated by signals generated when cytokines
bind to their receptors. One of the two types of cytokine-
induced signals initiates apoptosis. Cytokines producing
inductive signals include TNF-α, FAS/APO-1 ligand, and
TRAIL/APO-2 ligand. The second is an inhibitory signal
that suppresses apoptosis. Cytokines producing inhibitory
signals include those required for cell survival. Apoptosis
proceeds through cleavage of vital intracellular proteins.
Caspases are inactive until a signal initiates activation of
one, starting a cascade in which a series of other caspases
are proteolytically activated. Although both signaling processes affect caspase activation, the mechanism
differs. Apoptosis is characterized by degradation of
nuclear DNA, degeneration and condensation of nuclei,
and phagocytosis of cell residue. Proliferating cells often
undergo apoptosis as a natural process and proliferating
lymphocytes manifest rapid apoptosis during development
and during immune responses. In contrast to the internal
death program of apoptosis, necrosis describes death from
without.

A. Caspase 9- and Caspase 3-dependent apoptosis in embryonic stem cells

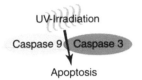

B. Caspase 9- and Caspase 3-independent apoptosis in thymocytes and splenocytes

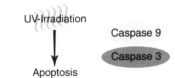

C. Caspase 9-dependent and Caspase 3-independent apoptosis in thymocytes

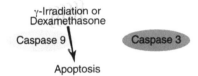

D. Caspase 9-independent and Caspase 3-dependent apoptosis in embryonic stem cells

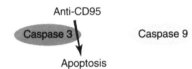

Table 1. Cell Type-specific Effect of Apoptosis-inducing Agents on Caspase 9 or Caspase 3 Deficient Mice.

| | Caspase 9 -/- | | Caspase 3 -/- | |
	resistant to	sensitive to	resistant to	sensitive to
Embryonic Stem Cells	adriamycin cisplatinum anisomycin etoposide osmotic shock γ irradiation UV irradiation		adriamycin cisplatinum anisomycin etoposide osmotic shock γ irradiation UV irradiation	
Embryonic Fibroblasts	adriamycin etoposide γ irradiation UV irradiation	CTL* killing	adriamycin etoposide γ irradiation UV irradiation	CTL killing
Thymocytes	dexamethasone γ irradiation etoposide	UV irradiation heat shock anti-CD95 TNF-α		dexamethasone γ irradiation UV irradiation
Splenocytes	γ irradiation dexamethasone	UV irradiation adriamycin cisplatinum etoposide osmotic shock	γ irradiation	UV irradiation
Activated Splenocytes		anti-CD95	anti-CD95	

* Cytotoxic T-lymphocytes

Removal of a cytokine required for cellular viability leads to the following sequential events: (1) loss of kinase (AKT) activity; (2) dephosphorylation of Bad (or some other regulator of Bcl-2/Bcl-x activity); (3) Bad binding to Bcl-2; (4) loss of normal mitochondrial physiology; (5) release of cytochrome c; (6) binding of cytochrome *c* by Apaf-1 with concomitant activation of caspase 9; (7) amplification by the caspase cascade; (8) cleavage of vital cellular proteins; (9) fission of cells into apoptotic bodies; and finally (10) disappearance of any trace of the cell when the apoptotic bodies are engulfed by either neighboring or phagocytic cells.

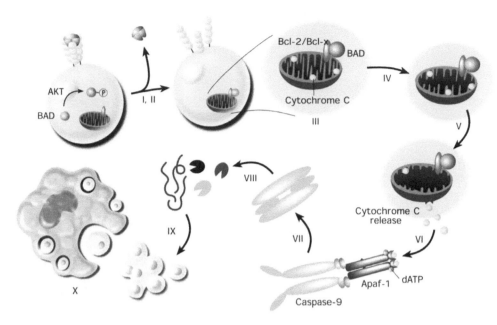

Removal of a cytokine required for cellular viability leads to the following sequential events: (1) loss of kinase (AKT) activity; (2) dephosphorylation of Bad (or some other regulator of Bcl-2/Bcl-x activity); (3) Bad binding to Bcl-2; (4) loss of normal mitochondrial physiology; (5) release of cytochrome c; (6) binding of cytochrome c by Apaf-1 with concomitant activation of caspase 9; (7) amplification by the caspase cascade; (8) cleavage of vital cellular proteins; (9) fission of cells into apoptotic bodies; and finally (10) disappearance of any trace of the cell when the apoptotic bodies are engulfed by either neighboring or phagocytic cells.

apoptosis, caspase pathway

A group of intracellular proteases called caspases are responsible for the deliberate disassembly of cells into apoptotic bodies during apoptosis. Caspases are present as inactive proenzymes activated by proteolytic cleavage. Caspases 8, 9, and 3 are situated at pivotal junctions in apoptosis pathways. Caspase 8 initiates disassembly in response to extracellular apoptosis-inducing ligands and is activated in a complex associated with the cytoplasmic death domains of many cell surface receptors for the ligands. Caspase 9 activates disassembly in response to agents or insults that trigger the release of cytochrome c from mitochondria and is activated when complexed with apoptotic protease activating factor 1 (APAF-1) and extramitochondrial cytochrome c. Caspase 3 appears to amplify caspase 8 and caspase 9 initiation signals into full-fledged commitments to disassembly. Caspase 8 and caspase 9 activate caspase 3 by proteolytic cleavage, and caspase 3 then cleaves vital cellular proteins or other caspases.

apoptosis, immunotoxin-induced

Immunotoxins are cytotoxic agents usually assembled as recombinant fusion proteins composed of targeting domains and toxins. The targeting domain controls the specificity of action and is usually derived from an antibody Fv fragment, a growth factor, or a soluble receptor. The protein toxins are obtained from bacteria (e.g., *Pseudomonas* endotoxin [PE] or diphtheria toxin [DT]) or from plants (e.g., ricin). Immunotoxins have been studied as treatments for cancer, graft-vs.-host disease, autoimmune disease, and AIDS. The PE and DT bacterial toxins act via the ADP ribosylation of elongation factor 2, thereby inactivating it. This results in the arrest of protein synthesis and subsequent cell death. These toxins can also induce apoptosis, although the mechanism is unknown. Two common features of apoptotic cell death are the activation of a group of cysteine proteases called caspases and the caspase-catalyzed cleavage

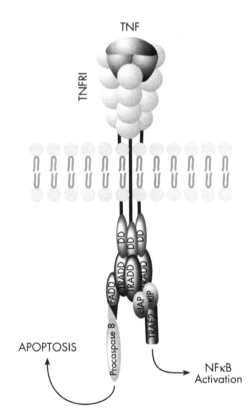

TNF-induced receptor trimerization aggregates the death domains (DD) of tumor necrosis factor (TNF) RI and recruits the adaptor protein TRADD. This in turn promotes the recruitment of the DD-containing cytoplasmic proteins FADD, TRAF2, and RIP to form an active TNF RI signaling complex. The active TNF RI signaling complex can then recruit procaspase 8. Following activation, caspase 8 can initiate caspase-mediated cell death.

of so-called "death substrates" such as the nuclear repair enzyme poly (ADP-ribose) polymerase (PARP).

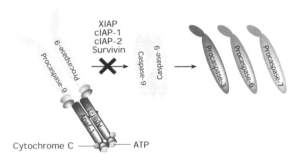

The inhibitor of apoptosis proteins XIAP, cIAP-1, and Survivin can prevent proteolytic processing of procaspases 3, 6, and 7 by blocking cytochrome-*c*-induced activation of procaspase 9.

apoptosis, necrosis and

Apoptosis and necrosis are two major processes by which cells die. Apoptosis is the ordered disassembly of cells from within. Disassembly creates changes in the phospholipid content of the plasma membrane outer leaflet. Phosphatidylserine (PS) is exposed on the outer leaflet, and phagocytic cells that recognize this change may engulf the apoptotic cell or cell-derived, membrane-limited apoptotic bodies. Necrosis normally results from a severe cellular insult. Both internal organelle and plasma membrane integrities are lost, resulting in spilling of cytosolic and organellar contents into the surrounding environment. Immune cells are attached to the area and begin producing cytokines that generate an inflammatory response. Thus, cell death in the absence of an inflammatory response may be the best way to distinguish apoptosis from necrosis. Other techniques that have been used to distinguish apoptosis from necrosis in cultured cells and in tissue sections include detecting PS at the cell surface with annexin V binding, DNA laddering, and staining cleaved DNA fragments that contain characteristic ends. At the extremes, apoptosis and necrosis clearly involve different molecular mechanisms. It is not clear whether there is cellular death involving the molecular mechanisms of both apoptosis and necrosis. Cell death induced by free radicals, however, may have characteristics of apoptosis and necrosis.

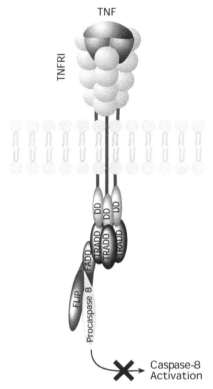

The inhibitor of apoptosis protein FLIP interacts with FADD and procaspase 8, blocking activation of caspase 8 and thereby suppressing death-receptor-induced apoptosis.

apoptosis, negative induction

Negative induction of apoptosis by loss of a suppressor activity involves the mitochondria. Release of cytochrome *c* from the mitochondria into the cytosol serves as a trigger to activate caspases. Permeability of the mitochondrial outer membrane is essential to initiation of apoptosis through this pathway. Proteins belonging to the Bcl-2 family appear to regulate the membrane permeability to ions and possibly to cytochrome *c* as well. Although these proteins can form channels in membranes, the molecular mechanisms by which they regulate mitochondrial permeability and the solutes released are less clear. The Bcl-2 family is composed of a

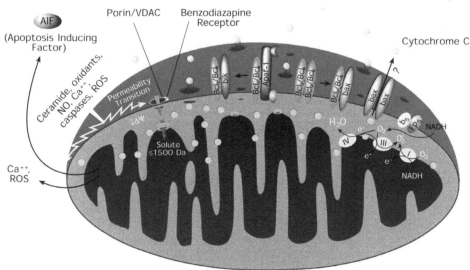

Apoptotic cell death resulting from free-radical exposure involves mitochondria. In cells undergoing apoptosis, mitochondria release AIF (apoptosis-inducing factor) and cytochrome *c*. The anti-apoptotic mitochondrial protein Bcl-2 inhibits free-radical-induced apoptosis.

A

large group of anti-apoptosis members that, when overexpressed, prevent apoptosis and a large group of pro-apoptosis members that, when overexpressed, induce apoptosis. The balance between the anti-apoptotic and pro-apoptotic Bcl-2 family members may be critical in determining whether a cell undergoes apoptosis. Thus, the suppressor activity of the anti-apoptotic Bcl-2 family appears to be negated by the pro-apoptotic members. Many members of the pro-apoptotic Bcl-2 family are present in cells at levels sufficient to induce apoptosis; however, these members do not induce apoptosis because their activity is maintained in a latent form. Bax is present in the cytosols of live cells. After an appropriate signal, Bax undergoes a conformational change and moves to the mitochondrial membranes, where it causes release of mitochondrial cytochrome c into the cytosols. BID is also present in the cytosols of live cells. After cleavage by caspase 8, it moves to the mitochondria, where it causes release of cytochrome c, possibly by altering the conformation of Bax. Similarly, BAK appears to undergo a conformational change that converts it from an inactive to an active state. Thus, understanding the molecular mechanisms responsible for regulating the Bcl-2 family activities creates the potential for pharmaceutical intervention to control apoptosis. The viability of many cells is dependent on a constant or intermittent supply of cytokines or growth factors. In the absence of an apoptosis-suppressing cytokine, cells may undergo apoptosis. Bad is a pro-apoptotic member of the Bcl-2 family and is sequestered in the cytosol when cytokines are present. Cytokine binding can activate PI3 kinase, which phosphorylates Akt/PKB, which in turn phosphorylates Bad. Phosphorylated Bad is sequestered in the cytosol by the 14-3-3 protein. Removal of the cytokine turns the kinase pathway off, the phosphorylation state of Bad shifts to the dephosphorylated form, and dephosphorylated Bad causes release of cytochrome c from the mitochondria.

apoptosis, positive induction

Two central pathways lead to apoptosis: (1) positive induction by ligand binding to plasma membrane receptor, and (2) negative induction by loss of suppressor activity. Each pathway leads to activation of cysteine proteases with homology to IL-1β-converting enzyme (ICE) (i.e., caspases). Positive induction involves ligands related to tumor necrosis factor (TNF). Ligands are typically trimeric and bind to cell surface receptors, causing aggregation (trimerization) of the receptors. Receptor oligomerization orients their cytosolic death domains into a configuration that recruits adaptor proteins. The adaptor complex recruits caspase 8. Caspase 8 is activated, and the cascade of caspase-mediated disassembly proceeds.

apoptosis, suppressors

The induction of apoptosis or progression through the process of apoptosis is inhibited by a group of proteins known as inhibitors of apoptosis (IAPs). These proteins contain baculovirus IAP repeat (BIR) domains near their amino termini. The BIR domain can bind some caspases. Many members of the IAP family of proteins block proteolytic activation of caspase 3 and 7. XIAP, cIAP-1, and cIAP-2 appear to block cytochrome-c-induced activation of caspase 9, thereby preventing initiation of the caspase cascade. Because cIAP-1 and cIAP-2 were first identified as components in the cytosolic death domain-induced complex associated with the tumor necrosis factor (TNF) family of receptors, they may inhibit apoptosis by additional mechanisms.

appendix, vermiform

A gut-associated secondary lymphoid tissue situated at the ileocecal junction of the gastrointestinal tract.

APR (acute phase response)

A nonspecific response by an individual stimulated by interleukin-1, interleukin-6, tumor necrosis factor, and interferons. C-reactive protein may show a striking rise within a few hours. Infection, inflammation, tissue injury, and very infrequently neoplasm may be associated with APR. The liver produces acute phase proteins at an accelerated rate, and the endocrine system is affected with elevated gluconeogenesis, impaired thyroid function, and other changes. Immunologic and hematopoietic system changes include hypergammaglobulinemia and leukocytosis with a shift to left. Diminished formation of albumin, elevated ceruloplasmin, and diminished zinc and iron are observed.

APT (alum-precipitated toxoid)

Refer to alum-precipitated antigen.

Aquaphor®

An emulsifying preparation of lanolin used extensively in the past to prepare the water-in-oil emulsion immunologic adjuvants of the Freund type.

aqueous adjuvants

Freund's adjuvants are not used in humans because of the ease with which hypersensitivity is induced and the unpredictability of local reactions. A number of water-soluble synthetic components comprising active moieties of mycobacterial cell walls have been synthesized in search of more adequate adjuvants. One of them is muramyl dipeptide (MDP), which is active when administered by the oral route. MDP in water is extremely active as an adjuvant and is not generally toxic when administered at high doses. It is not mitogenic, immunogenic, or antigenic and is rapidly eliminated from the animal body. The simplicity of its chemical structure allows the study of the targets of its action in the immune system. Other synthetic adjuvant compounds are polynucleotides such as poly-inosine-poly-cytidine (poly I:C), the structure of which is similar to those of native nucleotides. The mechanism of action involves signals that are rapidly received by the immune system, as such compounds are destroyed in 5 to 10 minutes by the nucleases of the serum. The prevalent concept is that adjuvants have a number of other regulatory activities on the immune response, and the term *adjuvant* may be replaced by *immunoregulatory molecule.*

arachidonic acid (AA) and leukotrienes

Critical constituents of mammalian cell membranes. AA is released from membrane phospholipids as a consequence of membrane alterations or receptor-mediated signaling that leads to activation of phospholipase A_2 (PLA_2). Oxidative metabolism of AA through cyclooxygenase leads to the formation of various prostaglandins through the cytochrome P-450 system or through one of the lipoxygenases. Molecules derived from the lipoxygenase pathway of arachidonic acid are termed leukotrienes (LTs). They are derived from the combined actions of 5-lipoxygenase (5-LOX) and 5-LOX-activating protein (FLAP). Initially 5-hydroperoxyeicosatetraenoic (5-HPETE) acid is formed followed by LTA_4. LTB_4 is an enzymatic, hydrolytic product of LTA_4. It differs from the LTC_4, LTD_4, and LTE_4 leukotrienes in that it does not have a peptide component. LTB_4 has powerful leukocytotropic effects. It is a powerful chemokinetic and chemotactic agent with the ability to induce neutrophil aggregation, degranulation, hexose uptake, and enhanced binding to endothelial cells. It can cause cation fluxes, augment cytoplasmic calcium concentrations, form intracellular pools, and activate phosphatidylinositol hydrolysis. LTB_4 can act synergistically with prostaglandins E_1 (PGE_1) and PGE_2 to induce macromolecule leakage in the skin through increased vascular permeability. When injected into the skin of a guinea pig, it can induce leukocytoclastic vasculitis. Human polymorphonuclear neutrophils have two sets of plasma membrane receptors. A high affinity receptor set mediates aggregation, chemokinesis, and increased surface adherence, whereas the low affinity receptor set mediates degranulation and increased oxidative metabolism. A fraction of $CD4^+$ and $CD8^+$ T lymphocytes bind LTB_4, but LTB_4 receptors on lymphocytes remain to be characterized.

arcitumomab

A murine $F(ab')_2$ fragment of an anti-carcinoembryonic antigen (CEA) antibody labeled with technetium 99m (^{99m}Tc) used for imaging patients with metastatic colorectal cancer by immunoscintigraphy to evaluate spread of the disease. Use of the $F(ab')_2$ fragment diminishes the immunogenicity, permitting it to be used more than once.

arenavirus immunity

Even though arenaviruses may not cause ill effects in carrier rodents, when transmitted to primates they may induce severe encephalitis, hepatitis, or hemorrhagic syndrome. LCMV is a classic member of this group and has been used to investigate virus-induced, cell-mediated immunity. Infection of mice may be either acute (inducing strong cell-mediated immunity) or persistent (associated with little cell-mediated immunity). The immune response to the acute infection either kills the mouse by causing meningitis or subsides and renders the mouse LCMV-immune. CD8+ T cells clear the virus infection and may also mediate pathological changes of choriomeningitis when injected intracerebrally. LCMV infection induces interferon γ (IFN-γ) and tumor necrosis factor α, which affect host immune responses. IFN-γ induces natural killer (NK) cell proliferation, which eliminates pathogen-infected cells and selected tumors. Arenaviruses persist in long-term carriers through antigenic variation that evades the host immune response. Mice may be protected from lethal LCMV challenge by peptide vaccination or by vaccinia vectors that express viral epitopes.

arginine and immunity

Arginine, a dibasic nitrogen-rich amino acid, has a marked immunomodulatory function. It is critical for the maintenance of nitrogen balance and physiologic functions in humans. Supplemental administration of arginine in experimental animals led to increased thymic size, lymphocyte count, and lymphocyte mitogenic response to mitogens and antigens. IL-2 synthesis is enhanced. Arginine protects against post-traumatic thymic involution and the impairment of T cell function. It enhances delayed-type hypersensitivity reactions in animal studies and also promotes host antitumor responses. Arginine is essential for the functions of various immunoregulatory proteins including thymosin, thymopentin, and tuftsin. Arginine exerts powerful effects on numerous cells and molecules of the immune system and may have potential as a pharmacologic agent in the treatment of immunocompromised patients.

Arlacel A®

A mannide monooleate used as an emulsifier to stabilize water-in-oil emulsions employed as adjuvants (e.g., Freund's adjuvant) in experimental immunology.

armed cytotoxic T lymphocyte (armed CTL)

A mature effector cytotoxic T lymphocyte that forms chemical mediators prior to contact with antigen that will be employed to fatally injure target cells with which they come into contact.

armed effector T cells

Activated effector T cells induced to mediate their effector functions as soon as they contact cells expressing the peptide–major histocompatability complex (MHC) for which they are specific. By contrast, memory T lymphocytes require activation by antigen-presenting cells to empower them to carry out effector functions.

armed macrophages

Macrophages bearing surface immunoglobulin G (IgG) or IgM cytophilic antibodies or T cell lymphokines that render them capable of inducing antigen-specific cytotoxicity.

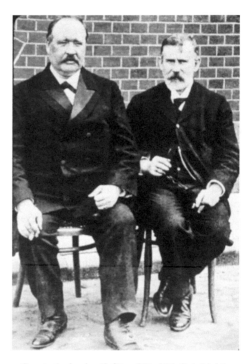

Svante Arrhenius (left) and Paul Ehrlich (right).

armed mast cell

A mast cell whose Fcε receptors have bound IgE molecules specific for antigen prior to interaction with that same allergen.

Arrhenius, Svante (1859–1927)

Arrhenius coined the *immunochemistry* term and hypothesized that antigen–antibody complexes are reversible. He was awarded the Nobel Prize for chemistry in 1903. (See Arrhenius, S., *Immunochemistry,* Macmillan Publishers, New York, 1907).

Artemis SCID

A form of severe combined immunodeficiency attributable to mutations of the Artemis gene that codes for a factor significant in both V(D)J recombination and DNA repair.

arthritis

Joint inflammation.

Arthus, Nicolas Maurice (1862–1945)

Paris physician who studied venoms and their physiological effects; first to describe local anaphylaxis or the Arthus reaction (1903). Author of *De l'Anaphylaxie a l'Immunite*, 1921.

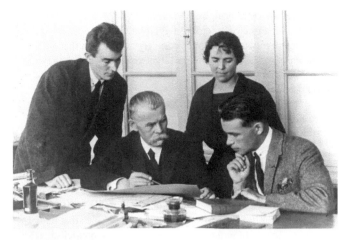

Maurice Arthus with students.

Arthus reaction

A reaction induced by repeated intradermal injections of antigen into the same skin site. It is dependent upon the development of humoral antibodies of the precipitin type that react *in vivo* with specific antigen at a local site. The reaction may also be induced by the inoculation of antigen into a local skin site of an animal possessing preformed immunoglobulin G (IgG) antibodies specific for the antigen. Immune complexes are composed of antigen, antibody, and complement formed in vessels. The chemotactic complement fragment C5a and other chemotactic peptides produced attract neutrophils to antigen–antibody–complement complexes followed by lysosomal enzyme release, which induces injury to vessel walls with the development of thrombi, hemorrhage, edema, and necrosis. Events leading to vascular necrosis include blood stasis, thrombosis, capillary compression in vascular injury which causes extravasation, venule rupture, hemorrhage, and local ischemia. There is extensive infiltration of polymorphonuclear cells, especially neutrophils, into the connective tissue. Grossly, edema, erythema, central blanching, induration, and petechiae appear. Petechiae develop within 2 hours, reach a maximum between 4 and 6 hours, and then may diminish or persist for 24 hours or longer with associated central necrosis, depending on the severity of the reaction. If the reaction is more prolonged, macrophages replace neutrophils; histiocytes and plasma cells may also be demonstrated. The Arthus reaction is considered a form of immediate-type hypersensitivity, but it does not occur as rapidly as does anaphylaxis. It takes place during a 4-hour period and diminishes after 12 hours. Thereafter, the area is cleared by mononuclear phagocytes. The passive cutaneous Arthus reaction consists of the inoculation of antibodies intravenously into a nonimmune host, followed by local cutaneous injection of antigen. The reverse passive cutaneous Arthus reaction requires the intracutaneous injection of antibodies, followed by the intravenous or incutaneous (at same site) administration of antigen. The Arthus reaction is a form of type III hypersensitivity, as it is based upon the formation of immune complexes with complement fixation. Clinical situations for which it serves as an animal model include serum sickness, glomerulonephritis, and farmer's lung.

artificial antigen

An antigen prepared by chemical modification of a natural antigen. Compare with synthetic antigen.

artificial passive immunity

The transfer of immunoglobulins from an immune individual to a nonimmune, susceptible recipient.

artificially acquired immunity

The use of deliberate active or passive immunization or vaccination to elicit protective immunity as opposed to immunity that results from unplanned and coincidental exposure to antigenic materials including microorganisms in the environment.

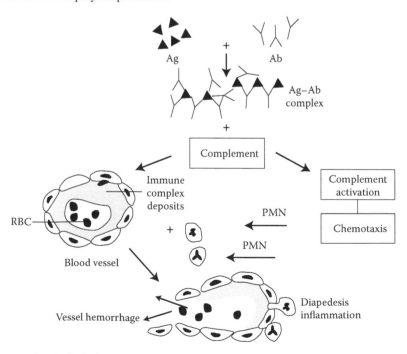

Molecular, cellular, and tissue interactions in the Arthus reaction. RBC = red blood cell. PMN = polymorphonuclear neutrophil. Ag–Ab = antigen–antibody complex.

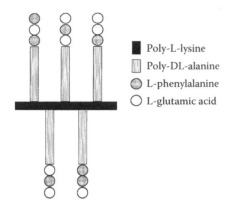

Synthetic polypeptide antigen with multichain copolymer (Phe, G)-A-L.

Poly-L-lysine
Poly-DL-alanine
L-phenylalanine
L-glutamic acid

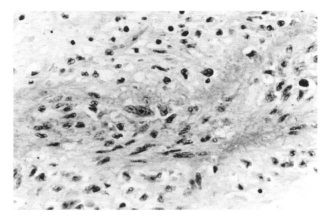

Aschoff bodies.

artificially acquired passive immunity

The transfer of immunoglobulins from an immune individual to a nonimmune, susceptible recipient. Passive immunity of this type is more often used for prophylaxis than for therapy. It provides immediate protection of the recipient for relatively short periods (few weeks). Human sera are preferred for passive immunization to avoid serum sickness induced by foreign serum proteins.

Ascaris immunity

The *Ascaris lumbricoides* roundworm infects 1.3 billion people. Infected subjects mount strong immunoglobulin G (IgG) antibody responses specific for the parasite, but most individuals respond to only a subset of parasite constituents. Only 20% of individuals respond to the ABA-1 antigen/allergen. Laboratory studies have shown that immune responses to *Ascaris* antigens in laboratory rodents is restricted by the major histocompatibility complex (MHC) class II region. Human hypersensitivity reactions to *Ascaris lumbricoides* may vary in specificity. The IgE response appears to be protective in ascariasis and is believed to be a protective mechanism in other helminth infections. Mouse experiments show that the immune response to *Ascaris* infection is dominated by T_H2 cells, which helps to explain the elevated IgE levels, eosinophilia, and mastocytosis observed in these infections. The T_H2 response is critical for immune elimination of the parasites. Although the parasite is able to alter its surface and secreted antigens, it remains to be proven that this serves as an effective mechanism to evade the host immune system. No vaccine is available.

ascertainment artifact

A reference to data that appear to show a specific finding but fail to do so because they have been derived from a population selected in a biased manner.

Aschoff bodies

Areas of fibrinoid necrosis encircled first by lymphocytes and macrophages with rare plasma cells. The mature Aschoff body reveals prominent modified histiocytes termed Anitschkow cells or Aschoff cells in the inflammatory infiltrate. These cells have round to oval nuclei with wavy ribbon-like chromatin and amphophilic cytoplasm. Aschoff bodies are pathognomonic of rheumatic fever. They may be found in any of the three layers of the heart (i.e., pericardium, myocardium, or endocardium).

ascites fluid

Fluid in the peritoneal cavity.

Ascoli's test

A ring precipitin assay used in the past to identify anthrax antigen in tissues, skins, and hides of animals infected with *Bacillus anthracis*. The simple test was considered useful in that it could identify anthrax antigen in decaying material from which anthrax bacilli could no longer be cultured.

asialoglycoprotein receptor (ASGP R) autoantibodies

Autoantibodies against this liver-specific membrane receptor occur at high frequency in autoimmune liver diseases, especially autoimmune hepatitis, and may occur also in primary biliary cirrhosis (PBC), viral hepatitis, and other liver diseases but at a lower frequency. Anti-ASGP R antibodies correlate with disease activity. Anti-ASGP R antibodies against human-specific epitopes are closely linked to autoimmune hepatitis. T lymphocytes specific for the ASGP R have been isolated from the livers of autoimmune hepatitis type I patients. Tissue expression of ASGP R is most prominent in periportal areas where piecemeal necrosis is observed as a marker of severe inflammatory activity. ASGP R antibodies may be used as diagnostic markers for autoimmune hepatitis if other markers are negative and autoimmune liver disease is suspected.

ASLT

Abbreviation for the antistreptolysin O test.

ASO (antistreptolysin O)

A laboratory technique that serves as an indicator of infection by group A β-hemolytic streptococci. Immunoglobulin M (IgM) antibody titers expressed in Todd units (TU) increase fourfold within 3 weeks after infection in untreated subjects. Penicillin treatment decreases the ASO titer. Normal level is below 166 TU; levels above 333 TU in children and above 250 TU in adults suggest recent infection. The ASO assay depends upon hemolysis inhibition. The greatest dilution of a patient's blood combined with 1 U streptolysin O that prevents the lysis of erythrocytes determines TU, the reciprocal of endpoint dilution.

Aspergillus species

Aeroallergenic fungi that may induce hypersensitivity pneumonitis (HP). *Aspergillus* species together with the thermophilic actinomyces are the most common causes of the hypersensitivity pneumonitis known as farmer's lung disease.

aspirin (acetylsalicylic acid, ASA)

An anti-inflammatory, analgesic, and antipyretic drug that blocks the synthesis of prostaglandin. It may induce atopic reactions such as asthma and rhinitis due to intolerance and idiosyncratic reactivity against the drug.

aspirin sensitivity reaction

A hypersensitivity response to aspirin (acetylsalicylic acid, ASA) as a manifestation of allergy and asthma. This allergic reaction may be manifested as either urticaria and angioedema or rhinoconjunctivitis with bronchospasm. Aspirin sensitivity is sometimes termed a pseudoallergic reaction. Possible mechanisms include cyclooxygenase blockade resulting in an altered ratio of PGE_2 (bronchodilator) to PHF_2 (bronchoconstrictor), a shunting of arachidonate from the cyclooxygenase to the 5-lipoxygenase pathway with eosinophilia, and viral infection in which altered prostaglandin regulation of cytotoxic lymphocytes is postulated. Mast cells and eosinophils in the nasal mucosa and periphery point to a possible role of these cells in aspirin hypersensitivity. Patients with this type of allergic reaction present clinically with such features as rhinitis, nasal polyps, eosinophilia in nasal smears, abnormal sinus, radiographs, and chronic asthma. ASA sensitivity is associated with various nonsteroidal anti-inflammatory drugs (NSAIDs).

association constant (KA)

A mathematical measurement of the reversible interaction between two molecular forms at equilibrium. The AB complex, free A and B concentrations at equilibrium, are expressed in K_A liters per mole by [AB], [A], and [B]. The s (molecules of substance A) interact reversibly with the t (molecules of substance B); i.e., $sA + tB1\ A_sB_t$, the association constant is $[A_sB_t]/[A]^s[B]^t$. Molar concentrations at equilibrium are indicated by the symbols in brackets.

asthma

Inflammation of the bronchi in the lungs characterized by reversible airway obstruction (in most cases). Inflammation of the airway is characterized by prominent eosinophil participation, and there is increased responsiveness by the airway to various stimuli. Bronchospasm is associated with recurrent paroxysmal dyspnea and wheezing. Some cases of asthma are allergic (i.e., bronchial allergy), mediated by immunoglobulin E (IgE) antibody to environmental allergens. Other cases are provoked by nonallergic factors that are not discussed here.

ataxia telangiectasia

A disorder characterized by cerebellar ataxia, oculocutaneous telangiectasis, variable immunodeficiency that affects both T and B cell limbs of the immune response, the development of lymphoid malignancies, and recurrent sinopulmonary infections. A consequence of a mutation of the tumor suppressor gene *ATM* associated with the nonhomologous end joining (NHEJ) pathway of DNA repair. Clinical features may appear by 2 years of age. Forty percent of patients have selective immunoglobulin A (IgA) deficiency. The disease has an autosomal recessive mode of inheritance. There may be lymphopenia, normal or decreased T lymphocyte numbers, and normal or diminished lymphocyte responses to PHA and allogeneic cells. The delayed-type hypersensitivity skin test may not stimulate any response. Some individuals may have an IgG_2, IgG_4, or IgA_2 subclass deficiency. Other patients may reveal no IgE antibody levels. Antibody responsiveness to selected antigens is diminished. B cell numbers are usually normal, and natural killer (NK) cell function is within physiologic limits. The level of T cell deficiency varies. Defects in DNA repair mechanisms lead to multiple breaks, inversions, and translocations within chromosomes, rendering them highly susceptible to the injurious actions of ionizing radiation and radiomimetic chemicals. The chromosomal breaks are especially apparent on chromosomes 7 and 14 in the regions that encode immunoglobulin genes and T cell receptor genes. The multiple chromosomal breaks are believed to be linked to the high incidence of lymphomas in these patients. α-Fetoprotein is also elevated. Endocrine abnormalities associated with the disease include glucose intolerance associated with anti-insulin-receptor antibodies and hypogonadism in males. Patients may experience retarded growth and hepatic dysfunction. Death may occur in many of the patients related to recurrent respiratory tract infections or lymphoid malignancies.

ATG

Abbreviation for antithymocyte globulin.

atherosclerosis, MCP-1 in

Chemokines are involved in the pathogenesis of atherosclerosis by promoting directed migration of inflammatory cells. Monocyte chemoattractant protein-1 (MCP-1), a CC chemokine, has been detected in atherosclerotic lesions by anti-MCP-1 antibody detection and *in situ* hybridization. MCP-1 mRNA expression has been detected in endothelial cells, macrophages, and vascular smooth muscle cells in atherosclerotic arteries of patients undergoing bypass revascularization. MCP-1 functions in the development of atherosclerosis by recruiting monocytes into the subendothelial cell layer. MCP-1 is critical for the initiation and development of atherosclerotic lesions. During the progression of atherosclerosis, there is an accumulation of low density lipoprotein (LDL) within macrophages and monocytes present in the intimal layer. Deposition of lipids within these cells leads to the formation and eventual enlargement of atherosclerotic lesions. Studies suggest a noncholesterol-mediated effect of MCP-1 in the development of atherosclerotic lesions. MCP-1 plays a crucial role in initiating atherosclerosis by recruiting macrophages and monocytes to the vessel wall.

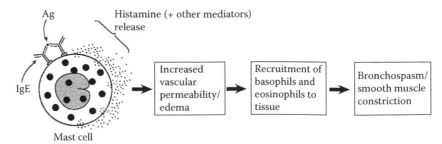

Asthma.

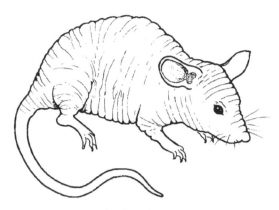

Athymic nude mouse.

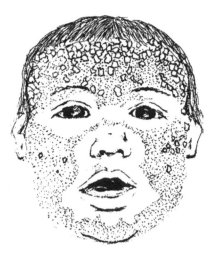

Atopic dermatitis.

athymic nude mouse

A mouse strain with no thymus and no hair. T lymphocytes are absent; therefore, no manifestations of T cell immunity are present; that is, the mice do not produce antibodies against thymus-dependent antigens and fail to reject allografts. They possess normal complements of B and natural killer (NK) cells. These nude or nu nu mice are homozygous for a mutation (v on chromosome 11) inherited as an autosomal-recessive trait. These features make the strain useful in studies evaluating thymic-independent immune responses.

atopic

Adjective referring to clinical manifestations of type I (IgE-mediating) types of hypersensitivity to environmental antigens such as pollen or house dust resulting in allergic rhinitis (hay fever), asthma, eczema, or food allergies. Individuals with such allergies are described as atopic.

atopic allergy or atopy

A genetically determined increased tendency of some members of the population to develop immediate hypersensitivity reactions, often mediated by immunoglobulin E (IgE) antibodies, against innocuous substances.

atopic dermatitis

Chronic eczematous skin reaction marked by hyperkeratosis and spongiosis, especially in children with genetic predispositions to allergy. The dermatitis is often accompanied by elevated serum immunoglobulin (IgE) levels that are not proved to produce the skin lesions. A type I hypersensitivity.

atopic hypersensitivity

Refer to atopy.

atopic rhinitis

An inflammatory reaction in the nasal mucous membranes attributable to type I hypersensitivity to an inhaled allergen. Clinical features include nasal secretions, itchy and tearing eyes. Also called hay fever.

atopy

A type of immediate (type I) hypersensitivity to common environmental allergens in humans mediated by humoral antibodies of the immunoglobulin (IgE) class, formerly termed reagins, that are able to passively transfer the effect. Atopic hypersensitivity states include hay fever, asthma, eczema, urticaria, and certain gastrointestinal disorders. There is a genetic predisposition to atopic hypersensitivities that affect more than 10% of the human population. Antigens that sensitize atopic individuals are termed allergens and include (1) grass and tree pollens; (2) dander, feathers, and hair; (3) eggs, milk, and chocolate; and (4) house dust,

bacteria, and fungi. IgE antibody is a skin-sensitizing homocytotropic antibody that occurs spontaneously in the sera of human subjects with atopic hypersensitivity. IgE antibodies are nonprecipitating (*in vitro*), heat-sensitive (destroyed by heating to 60°C for 30 to 60 minutes), unable to pass across the placenta, remain attached to local skin sites for weeks after injection, and fail to induce passive cutaneous anaphylaxis (PCA) in guinea pigs.

ATRA

Abbreviation for all trans-retinoic acid. A therapeutic agent administered orally that blocks the action of the chimeric protein in acute promyelocytic leukemia and restores hematopoietic cell maturation.

attenuate

To diminish the virulence of a pathogenic microorganism, rendering it incapable of causing disease. Attenuated bacteria or viruses may be used in vaccines to induce better protective immunity than would have been induced with a killed vaccine.

attenuated

Diminished virulence of a microorganism.

attenuated pathogen

A pathogen that has been altered to the point that it will grow in a host and induce immunity without causing clinical illness.

attenuation

Decrease of a particular effect, such as by exposing a pathogenic microorganism to suboptimal culture conditions or chemical or genetic alterations that diminish or negate its virulence but leave its antigenicity or immunogenicity intact.

AtxBm

Abbreviation for a so-called B cell mouse—a thymectomized irradiated adult mouse that has received a bone marrow transplant.

atypical pANCA

Atypical antineutrophil cytoplasmic antibodies (ANCAs) are present in patients with ulcerative colitis (UC), primary sclerosing cholangitis (PSC), and autoimmune hepatitis (AIH). Atypical pANCA reacts with nuclear envelope proteins and neutrophils. Immunoblotting has revealed reactivity to a myeloid-specific 50-kDa nuclear protein with an isoelectric point of pH 6.0 found in 92% of patients with inflammatory bowel or hepatobiliary disease and atypical pANAC. Antibodies against the 50-kDa protein reveal a nuclear rim-like fluorescence on myeloid cells observed by immunofluorescence microscopy. Thus, the atypical pANCAs in UC, PSC, or AIH recognize a 50-kDa myeloid-specific nuclear envelope protein.

Auer rods

Finely granular flat structures found in myeloid lineage leukemic cell cytoplasm.

Auer's colitis

An Arthus reaction in the intestine produced by the inoculation of albumin serving as an antigen into the colons of rabbits that have developed antialbumin antibodies. An inflammatory lesion is produced in the colon and is marked by hemorrhage and necrosis.

Australia antigen (AA)

Hepatitis B viral antigen. The name is derived from detection in an Australian aborigine. Australia antigen is demonstrable in the cytoplasm of an infected hepatocyte. In early hepatitis B, there is sublobular cell involvement, but later in the disease only some hepatocytes are antigen-positive. There is a positive correlation between the presence of hepatitis B antigen in the livers of a group of people and the group's incidence of hepatocellular carcinoma.

autoagglutination

The spontaneous aggregation of erythrocytes, microorganisms, or other particulate antigens in a saline suspension, thereby confusing interpretation of bacterial agglutination assays. The term also refers to the aggregation of an individual's cells by his own antibody.

autoallergy

Tissue injury or disease induced by immune reactivity against self antigens.

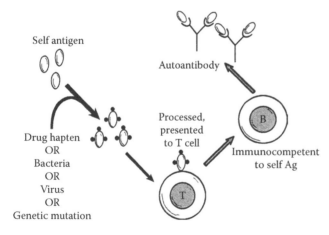

Autoantibody formation.

autoantibodies

An antibody that recognizes and interacts with an antigen present as a natural component of the individual synthesizing the autoantibody. The ability of these autoantibodies to crossreact with corresponding antigens from other members of the same species provides a method for *in vitro* detection of such autoantibodies. Autoantibodies are specific for self antigen and can lead to cell and tissue injury.

autoantibodies against lamin

Autoantibodies against lamin, a nuclear antigen, are present in the sera of chronic autoimmune disease patients manifesting hepatitis, leukocytoclastic angiitis or brain

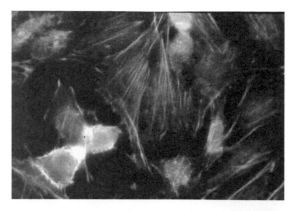

Antiactin autoantibody.

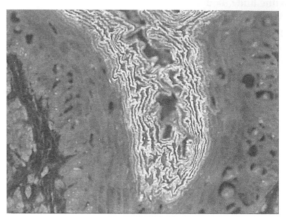

Antikeratin autoantibody.

vasculitis, cytopenia, and circulating anticoagulant or cardiolipin antibodies. They form a rim-type antinuclear staining pattern in immunofluorescence assays. A minority of systemic lupus erythematosus patients develop antibodies to lamin. The autoantibodies are found in selected patients with autoimmune and inflammatory diseases. IFA is the method of choice for their detection. Lamin autoantibodies occur in selected patients with chronic autoimmune disease marked by hepatitis, cytopenia with circulating anticoagulants or cardiolipin antibodies, cutaneous leukocytoclastic angitis, and possibly brain vasculitis. They may occur naturally, be crossreacting, or may form in response to antigen. They have no known clinical significance.

autoantibodies against pepsinogen

Autoantibodies that develop in autoimmune atrophic gastritis patients with pernicious anemia. Three fourths of peptic ulcer patients have pepsinogen antibodies.

autoantibodies to gastric parietal cells

Autoantibodies specific for both the catalytic 100-kDa (α) and the 60- to 90-kDa glycoprotein (β) subunits of gastric H+/K+ ATPase, the enzyme that acidifies gastric juice. Detection is by immunofluorescence.

autoantibodies, virus infection-associated

Viral infections may stimulate the production of autoantibodies in three ways: (1) by complexing with cell surface histocompatibility antigens to form new immunogenic units; (2) by nonspecifically stimulating the proliferation of lymphocytes (e.g., after infection with

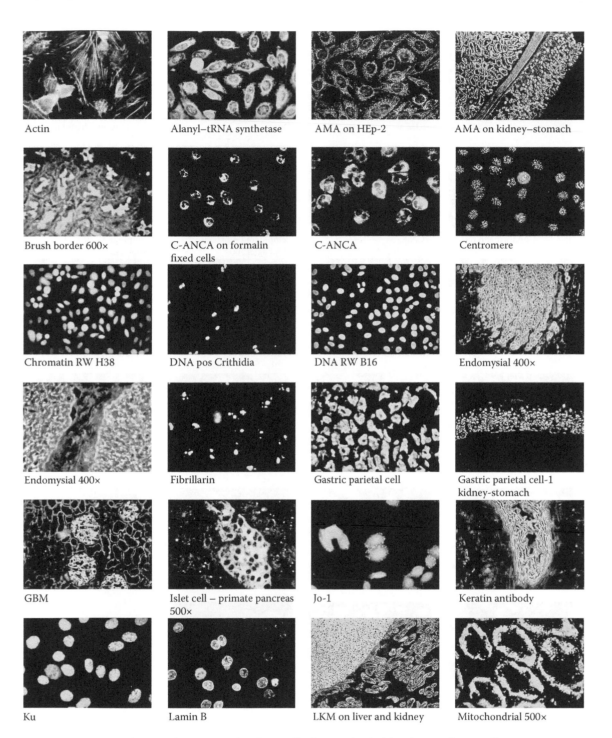

Actin | Alanyl–tRNA synthetase | AMA on HEp-2 | AMA on kidney–stomach

Brush border 600× | C-ANCA on formalin fixed cells | C-ANCA | Centromere

Chromatin RW H38 | DNA pos Crithidia | DNA RW B16 | Endomysial 400×

Endomysial 400× | Fibrillarin | Gastric parietal cell | Gastric parietal cell-1 kidney-stomach

GBM | Islet cell – primate pancreas 500× | Jo-1 | Keratin antibody

Ku | Lamin B | LKM on liver and kidney | Mitochondrial 500×

Examples of immunofluorescent stains of autoantibodies associated with various autoimmune diseases.

Epstein–Barr virus), for which the nonspecific response includes clones of cells specific for autoantigens; and (3) by inducing the expression of antigens normally repressed in host cells.

autoantibody assays

Tests for autoantibodies that can bind to self antigens include a broad spectrum of techniques such as agglutination (e.g., latex agglutination), indirect immunofluorescence, indirect immunoperoxidase, radioimmunoassay, ELISA, hemagglutination, bioassay, binding assay, and immobilization, among others.

autoantigens

Normal body constituents recognized by autoantibodies specific for them. T cell receptors may also identify autoantigens (self antigens) when the immune reactivity has induced a cell-mediated T lymphocyte response.

autobody

An antibody that exhibits the internal image of an antigen as well as a binding site for an antigen. It manifests dual binding to both idiotope and epitope. It bears an idiotope that is complementary to its own antigen-binding site or paratope. Thus, it has self-binding potential. This type of

A

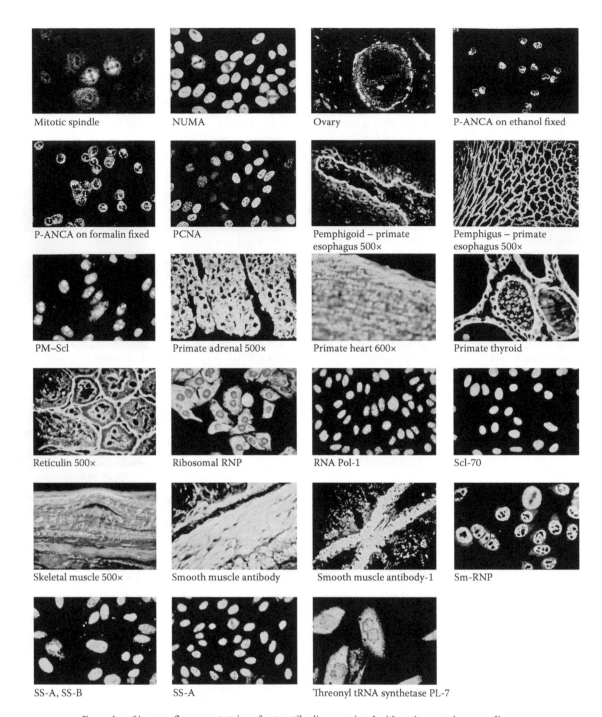

Mitotic spindle	NUMA	Ovary	P-ANCA on ethanol fixed
P-ANCA on formalin fixed	PCNA	Pemphigoid – primate esophagus 500×	Pemphigus – primate esophagus 500×
PM–Scl	Primate adrenal 500×	Primate heart 600×	Primate thyroid
Reticulin 500×	Ribosomal RNP	RNA Pol-1	Scl-70
Skeletal muscle 500×	Smooth muscle antibody	Smooth muscle antibody-1	Sm-RNP
SS-A, SS-B	SS-A	Threonyl tRNA synthetase PL-7	

Examples of immunofluorescent stains of autoantibodies associated with various autoimmune diseases.

anti-idiotypic antibody has features of Ab1 and Ab2 on the same molecule, causing it to be designated Ab1–2, or "autobody." The name points to the potential for self aggregation of the molecules and the potential participation of autobodies in autoimmune phenomena. Antibodies to phosphorylcholine (PC) epitope raised in Balb/c mice expressing the T15 idiotype self aggregate (i.e., bind to one another).

autochthonous

Pertaining to self; occurring in the same subject. Also called autologous.

autocrine

The action of a hormone, cytokine, or other secreted molecule on the same cell that synthesized it.

autocrine factor

A molecule that acts on the same cell that synthesized it, such as interleukin-2 (IL-2) stimulating the T lymphocyte that produced it to undergo mitosis.

autofluorescence

Natural fluorescence.

autogenous vaccine

The isolation and culture of microorganisms from an infected subject. The microorganisms in culture are killed and used as an immunogen (i.e., a vaccine) to induce protective immunity in the same subject from which they were derived. In earlier years, this was a popular method to treat *Staphylococcus aureus*-induced skin infections.

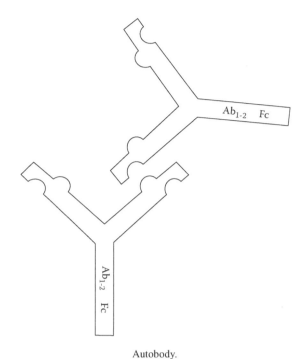

Autobody.

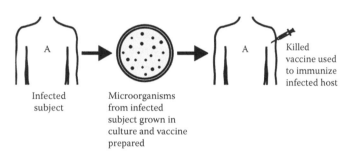

Autogenous vaccine.

autograft

A graft of tissue taken from one area of the body and placed in a different site on the body of the same individual, such as grafts of skin transferred from unaffected areas to burned areas.

autoimmune adrenal failure

Autoimmune destruction of the adrenal gland or idiopathic adrenal atrophy is the principal cause of primary adrenal failure in North America. The eponym for this condition is Addison's disease. It typically presents in females 20 to 30 years old. It may be part of a polyglandular endocrine disorder, but in half of the cases it is an isolated autoimmune endocrine disorder. One study recorded 93 cases per 1,000,000 population, with 40% manifesting autoimmune disease and 27% remaining unclassified. Autoimmune adrenal disease is believed to comprise approximately two thirds of the cases of primary adrenal disease in North America. The pathologic findings in the adrenal gland consist of inflammation with lymphocyte and plasma cell infiltration. By the time of diagnosis, fibrosis is present. Germinal centers are rare and antibody binding to cortical cells can be detected by immunohistochemistry. In the advanced stages of the disease, the adrenal cortex is completely destroyed. Autoantibodies are present in 60 to 75% of patients with autoimmune adrenal disease and are more

common with polyglandular syndrome. These antibodies are directed against specific cytochrome P-450 enzymes involved in steroidogenesis. Antibodies to 17 α-hydroxylase (P-450 C17), 21 α-hydroxylase (P-450 C21), and the side chain cleavage enzyme (P-450 scc) have all been identified. The major symptom of acute insufficiency is postural hypotension.

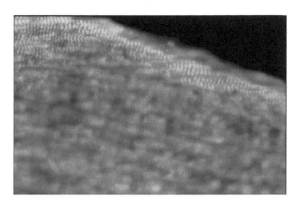

Autoimmune cardiac disease.

autoimmune cardiac disease

Rheumatic fever is a classic example of microbial-induced autoimmune heart disease. The immune response against the M protein of group A streptococci crossreact with cardiac proteins such as tropomyosin and myosin. The M protein contains numerous epitopes that participate in these crossreactions. A second crossreactive protein in the streptococcal membrane has been purified to a series of four peptides ranging in molecular weight from 23 to 22kD. Patients with rheumatic fever may develop antibodies that bind to the cytoplasm of cells of the caudate nucleus with specificity for its cells. Autoantibodies against microorganisms crossreact with cardiac tissue. A monoclonal antibody termed D8/17 identifies all rheumatics. It is not related to the MHC system and serves as a B cell marker associated with rheumatic fever, although no specific role for the antigen in the disease has been demonstrated. Numerous microbes and viruses can induce acute myocarditis. These cases are characterized by the presence of lymphocytic infiltrates and increased titers of heart-reactive antibodies. Important causative agents include group B coxsackieviruses that cause acute cardiac inflammation in humans. Rose et al., using an experimental mouse model, showed that only those mice with heart-reactive antibodies in their sera went on to develop chronic cardiomyopathy with antibodies primarily against the cardiac isoform of myosin in their model of acute myocarditis. Postpericardiotomy syndrome occurs in both adults and children 10 to 14 days after surgery and is characterized by fever, chest pain, and pericardial and pleural effusions. This condition is associated with the presence of high titer, heart reactive antibodies in the sera. The heart-specific antibodies are believed to play a role in disease pathogenesis. Since many microbes share epitopes with human tissues, crossreactions between antibodies against the microbe and human tissues may be harmless or may lead to serious autoimmune consequences in genetically susceptible hosts. Although much attention has been given to antibodies, cell-mediated immunity may play a larger role than previously thought in both rheumatic fever and Chagas' disease in which T cells are specifically cytotoxic for the target organ. Cytotoxic T cells specific for cardiac myofibers appear in both rheumatic fever and Chagas' disease. Only selected individuals with cardiomyopathy develop progressive autoimmune disease after active infection.

autoimmune complement fixation reaction

The ability of sera from patients with certain autoimmune diseases such as systemic lupus erythematosus, chronic active hepatitis, etc., to fix complement when combined with kidney, liver, or other tissue suspensions in saline.

autoimmune disease

Pathogenic consequences, including tissue injury, produced by autoantibodies or autoreactive T lymphocytes interacting with self epitopes (i.e., autoantigens). The mere presence of autoantibodies or autoreactive T lymphocytes does not prove a cause-and-effect relationship between these components and a patient's disease. To show that autoimmune phenomena are involved in the etiology and pathogenesis of human disease, Witebsky suggested that certain criteria be fulfilled (see Witebsky's criteria). In addition to autoimmune reactivity against self constituents, tissue injury in the presence of immunocompetent cells corresponding to the tissue distribution of the autoantigen, duplication of the disease features in experimental animals injected with the appropriate autoantigen, and passive transfer with either autoantibody or autoreactive T lymphocytes to normal animals offer evidence in support of autoimmune pathogenesis. Individual autoimmune diseases are discussed under their own headings, such as systemic lupus erythematosus (SLE), autoimmune thyroiditis, etc. Autoimmune diseases may be either organ-specific (thyroiditis, diabetes) or systemic (SLE).

autoimmune disease animal models

Studies of human autoimmune disease have always been confronted with the question of whether immune phenomena, including the production of autoantibodies, represent a cause or a consequence of the disease. The use of animal models (rats, mice, guinea pigs, rabbits, monkeys, chickens, and dogs, among other species) has helped answer many of these questions. A broad spectrum of human autoimmune diseases has been clarified through the use of animal models that differ in detail but nevertheless provided insight into pathogenic mechanisms, converging pathways, and disturbances of normal regulatory function related to the development of autoimmunity.

autoimmune disease spontaneous animal models

Animal strains based on years of selective breeding develop certain organ-specific or systemic autoimmune diseases spontaneously without experimental manipulation. These models resemble the human condition to a remarkable degree in many cases and serve as valuable models to investigate pathogenetic mechanisms underlying disease development. Spontaneous animal models for organ-specific autoimmune diseases include the obese strains of chickens that serve as animal models for Hashimoto's thyroiditis. Animal strains with spontaneous insulin-dependent diabetes mellitus (IDDM) include NOD mice and DP-BB rats, both of which develop humoral and cellular autoimmune responses against islet β cells of the pancreas. Spontaneous animal models of systemic autoimmune diseases include the University of California at Davis (UCD) 200 strain as an animal model for progressive systemic sclerosis

(SSc)–scleroderma. Several mouse strains develop systemic lupus erythematosus-like autoimmunity. These include the New Zealand black (NZB), (NZB × New Zealand White [NZW])F1, (NZB × SWR)F1, BXSB, and MRL mice. These animal models have contributed greatly to knowledge of the etiopathogenesis, genetics, and molecular defects responsible for autoimmunity. Mechanisms include defects in lymphoid lineage, endocrine alterations, target organ defects, endogenous viruses, and/or mutations in immunologically relevant molecules such as major histocompatibility complex (MHC) and cell receptor genes. Many of these have been implicated in animal autoimmune diseases and in some cases of human disease.

autoimmune gastritis

An organ-specific autoimmune disease in which autoantibodies are formed against gastric antigens and mononuclear cells infiltrate through target organs with destruction. The disease is associated with a regenerative response of the affected tissue to corticosteroid and immunosuppressive drugs, familial predisposition, and other autoimmune diseases. The molecular target of parietal cell autoantibodies is the gastric H^+/K^+ ATPase located on secretory membranes of gastric parietal cells. Refer also to pernicious anemia.

autoimmune hemolytic anemia

Although both warm antibody and cold antibody types are known, the warm type is the most common and is characterized by a positive direct antiglobulin (Coombs' test) associated with lymphoreticular cancer or autoimmune disease and splenomegaly. Patients may have anemia, hemolysis, lymphadenopathy, hepatosplenomegaly, or features of autoimmune disease. They commonly exhibit normochromic, normocytic anemia with spherocytosis and nucleated red blood cells in the peripheral blood. Leukocytosis and thrombocytosis may also occur, along with a significant reticulocytosis and an elevated serum indirect (unconjugated) bilirubin. Immunoglobulin G (IgG) and complement adhere to red blood cells. Antibodies are directed principally against Rh antigens. The indirect antiglobulin test is positive in 50% of cases, and agglutination of enzyme-treated red blood cells is positive in 90% of cases. In the cold agglutinin syndrome, IgM antibodies with an anti-I specificity are involved. Warm autoantibody autoimmune hemolytic anemia has a fairly good prognosis.

autoimmune hemophilia

An acquired disorder that resembles the inborn disease of coagulation due to a deficiency or dysfunction of Factor VIII. Patients develop an autoantibody that can inactivate Factor VIII. This auto-anti-Factor VIII antibody leads to an acquired hemophilia that resembles inherited hemophilia. This is a rare disorder that presents with spontaneous bleeding that can be life threatening. It may occur spontaneously or may be associated with other autoimmune disorders. It may result from the treatment of inherited hemophilia with preparations of Factor VIII. Soft tissues and muscles, the gut, the postpartum uterus, and retroperitoneum all represent sites of hemorrhage. Bleeding may also occur following surgery. The acquired antibody to Factor VIII is usually immunoglobulin G (IgG), of the IgG_4 subclass. Anti-idiotypic antibodies may also be formed against anti-Factor VIII antibodies.

autoimmune hepatitis

Approximately 10 to 20% of chronic hepatitis cases are attributable to autoimmune hepatitis. The diagnosis of autoimmune hepatitis is based on clinical and laboratory criteria defined by the International Autoimmune Hepatitis Group (IAHG). Circulating autoantibodies are hallmarks of this syndrome. Whereas immune defects occur during the chronic course of viral hepatitis, loss of tolerance to autologous liver tissue is the principal pathogenic mechanism in autoimmune hepatitis. It is important to distinguish between autoimmune and viral hepatitis because interferons administered for viral hepatitis are contraindicated in autoimmune liver disease. Immunosuppression prolongs survival in autoimmune hepatitis but favors viral replication. Drug-induced liver injury may also be immune mediated.

autoimmune lymphoproliferative syndromes (ALPS)

A group of rare primary immunodeficiency disorders in children characterized by lymphocytosis, hypergammaglobulinemia, hepatosplenomegaly, prominent lymphadenopathy, antinuclear and anti-red blood cell antibodies and accumulation of CD4⁻CD8⁻ T cells. It is believed to be associated with a defect in the Fas–Fas L apoptosis signaling system. Some children with the disorder have autoimmune hemolytic anemia, neutropenia, and thrombocytopenia. ALPS is associated with inherited genes that encode defective versions of the Fas protein. *Fas* alleles in children with ALPS have been shown to be heterozygous and manifest interference with T cell apoptosis. *Fas* mutations in these children include single- or multiple-based lesions, substitutions, or duplications leading to premature termination of transcription or aberrant *Fas* mRNA splicing. These alterations produce truncated or elongated forms of *Fas* and are not detected in normal persons. Murine *lpr* and *gld* disease models are being used to investigate how *Fas* molecule mutations may interfere at the molecular level with cell death signaling and contribute to human lymphoproliferative and autoimmune disorders. Like *lpr* and *gld* mice, children develop double negative T cells and hypergammaglobulinemia. Unlike the mouse mutations, affected patients rarely develop antinuclear antibodies or lupus-like renal pathology. There may be increased susceptibility, based on long-term observations of a few patients.

autoimmune myocarditis

Inflammation associated with an autoimmune response to myocardial tissues of the heart. Cardiac myosin has been postulated to be the target autoantigen. May result in chronic heart disease or dilated cardiomyopathy.

autoimmune neutropenia

This can be an isolated condition or appear secondary to autoimmune disease. Patients may exhibit recurrent infections or remain asymptomatic. Antigranulocyte antibodies may be demonstrated. Bone marrow function is normal, with myeloid hyperplasia and a shift to the left as a result of increased granulocyte destruction. The autoantibody may suppress myeloid cell growth. The condition is treated by immunosuppressive drugs, corticosteroids, or splenectomy. Patients with systemic lupus erythematosus (SLE), Felty's syndrome (rheumatoid arthritis, splenomegaly, and severe neutropenia), and other autoimmune diseases may manifest autoimmune neutropenia.

autoimmune polyendocrinopathy–candidiasis–ectodermal dystrophy (APECED)

An autoimmune disease associated with a mutation in *AIRE*, a transcriptional co-activator requisite for thymic epithelial cells to express peripheral self-antigens. A deficiency in *AIRE* leads to a defect in central tolerance. The disorder is marked by chronic mucosal yeast infection and autoimmune assaults on several endocrine glands, including thyroid, pancreas, and adrenal. Also called autoimmune polyglandular disease (APD). Refer also to autoimmune polyglandular syndrome (APS).

autoimmune polyglandular syndrome (APS)

A designation for Addison's disease and associated diseases based on classification into type I, II, and III APSs. Type I APS patients have chronic mucocutaneous candidiasis, adrenal insufficiency, and hypoparathyroidism and may also have gonadal failure, alopecia, malabsorption, pernicious anemia, and chronic active hepatitis. Candidiasis and malabsorption may also be present. Type II APS consists of three primary disorders: Addison's disease, insulin-dependent diabetes mellitus, and autoimmune thyroid disease. Type III APS consists of a subgroup of type II without Addison's disease but with thyroid autoimmunity and pernicious anemia, as well as vitiligo.

autoimmune response

An antibody or T cell immune response to self antigens.

autoimmune skin diseases

Autoimmune diseases of the skin include pemphigus, pemphigoid, epidermolysis bullosa acquisita, linear bullous IgA disease, herpes gestationes, and cutaneous lupus erythematosus. Probable autoimmune skin diseases may also include psoriasis, lichen ruber planus, alopecia areata, actinic reticuloid, morphea, and scleroderma. Possible autoimmune diseases include pyoderma gangrenosum, parapsoriasis, and sarcoidosis.

autoimmune thrombocytopenia

Decreased blood platelets attributable to interaction with platelet-specific autoantibodies that mediate thrombocyte destruction through phagocytosis. This may be an acute or chronic condition that has a type II hypersensitivity mechanism. May be manifested in immune thrombocytopenic purpura (ITP) and thrombotic thrombocytopenic purpura (TTP).

autoimmune thrombocytopenic purpura

A disease in which patients synthesize antibodies specific for their own blood platelets. The antibody–platelet reactants become bound to cells bearing Fc receptors and complement receptors, leading to decreased blood platelets followed by purpura or bleeding.

autoimmune thyroiditis

Refer to thyroiditis, autoimmune.

autoimmune tubulointerstitial nephritis

A renal disease believed to be mediated by anti-tubular basement membrane (TBM) antibody. It is characterized by linear deposition of immunoglobulin G (IgG) and occasionally complement along tubular basement membranes. Occurs with serum anti-TBM antibodies in 10 to 20% of cases. Symptoms include tubular dysfunction with polyuria, proteinuria, aminoaciduria, and glucosuria. TBM antigens that have been identified include a 58-kDa TIN-antigen. Other nephritogenic tubular interstitial antigens have also been identified in both animal models of the disease and in humans.

A

autoimmune uveoretinitis

An ocular inflammation and the leading cause of visual impairment in a significant segment of the population. T cell autoimmunity is postulated to play a significant role in the pathogenesis of at least some of these conditions. An organ-specific inflammatory autoimmune disease of the neural retina of the eye with Th1 lymphocyte and monocyte infiltration across the blood–retina barrier. Autoantibodies against retinal antigens may also be detected.

autoimmunity

Immune reactivity involving either antibody-mediated (humoral) or cell-mediated limbs of the immune response against the body's own (self) constituents (i.e., autoantigens). May induce autoimmune disease if there has been a breach in peripheral tolerance mechanisms. When autoantibodies or autoreactive T lymphocytes interact with self epitopes, tissue injury may occur; for example, in rheumatic fever, the autoimmune reactivity against heart muscle sarcolemmal membranes occurs as a result of crossreactivity with antibodies against streptococcal antigens (molecular mimicry). Thus, the immune response can be a two-edged sword, producing beneficial (protective) effects while also leading to severe injury to host tissues. Reactions of this deleterious nature are referred to as hypersensitivity reactions that are subgrouped into four types.

autoinflammatory syndromes

Primary immunodeficiencies marked by episodes of severe local inflammation and extended periods of fever without any clear pathogenic etiology.

autologous

Derived from self. The adjective describes grafts or antigens taken from and returned to the same subject from which they were derived.

autologous bone marrow transplantation (ABMT)

A bone marrow transplant by a donor who may later become the recipient of the same transplant. Leukemia patients in remission may donate marrow that can be readministered to them after a relapse. Leukemic cells are removed from the bone marrow, which is cryopreserved until needed. Prior to reinfusion of the bone marrow, the patient receives supralethal chemoradiotherapy. This therapy has improved considerably the survival rates of some leukemia patients.

autologous graft

The donation of tissue such as skin or bone marrow by an individual who will subsequently receive it either at a different anatomical site, as in skin autografts for burns, or at a later date, as in autologous bone marrow transplants.

autologous graft-vs.-host disease

A condition that may occur following autologous bone marrow transplantation in cyclosporine-A-treated patients. Autologous graft-vs.-host disease is associated with the emergence of autoreactive T cells recognizing self major histocompatibility complex (MHC) class II antigens and the elimination of a T cell-dependent peripheral autoregulatory mechanism. The induction of autograft-vs.-host disease may be of benefit to autologous bone marrow transplant patients by providing a graft-vs.-tumor effect.

autolymphocyte therapy (ALT)

An unconfirmed immunotherapeutic treatment for metastatic renal carcinoma. Leukocytes from a patient are isolated and activated with monoclonal antibodies to induce the leukocytes to synthesize and secrete cytokines. Cytokines produced in the supernatant are combined with a sample of the patient's own lymphocytes and reinjected. Preliminary reports claim success, but these have not been confirmed.

autoradiography

A method employed to localize radioisotopes in tissues or cells from experimental animals injected with radiolabeled substances. The radioisotopes serve as probes bound to specific DNA or RNA segments. Radioactivity is detected by placing the x-ray or photographic emulsion into contact with the tissue sections or nylon/nitrocellulose membranes in which they are localized to record sites of radioactivity. The technique permits the detection of radioactive substances by analytical methods involving electrophoresis, Southern blotting, and Northern blot hybridization.

autoreactive T lymphocytes

Autoreactive T cells in selected diseases may represent a failure of normal regulation; when present in a normal healthy individual, they may be necessary aspects of the immune system. Autoreactive T cells develop from mature antigen-dependent precursor cells that have changed physiologically in a manner that restores their thymic-selected ability to respond to self. Any mechanism that returns T cells to a resting state would halt autoreactive expansion until stimulation is induced once again by a specific foreign antigen. Chronic stimulation in the presence of continuous expression of high levels of major histocompatibility complex (MHC) class II molecules together with abnormal immune regulation can lead to severe and persistent inflammation.

autoreactivity

An immune response against self antigens.

autosensitization

Reactivity against one's own antigens (i.e., autoantigens) that occurs in autoimmunity and autoimmune disease.

autosomal, autosomes

Nonsex (nonX and nonY) chromosomes.

Avery, Oswald T.

Investigator at the Rockefeller Institute for Medical Research, New York in the 1940s. Together with MacLeod and McCarty, he identified DNA as the transforming principle in a landmark paper in the *Journal of Experimental Medicine* titled "Studies on the chemical nature of the substance inducing transformation of pneumococcal types."

avian immunity

Although turkeys, ducks, pigeons, and Japanese quail have been investigated, the domestic chicken is the principal representative of this biological group. There is much similarity between the avian and the mammalian immune systems, especially with respect to lymphoid organ structure, the generation of antibody variability, and the arrangements of immunoglobulin and major histocompatibility complex (MHC) genes. More than a dozen highly inbred chicken strains have been used in research. Chickens are usually excellent antibody producers. Their immune responses develop early. They form immunoglobulin M (IgM) prior to IgG and develop poor affinity maturation, reflecting the lack of extensive generation of antibody variability in peripheral tissues. Monoclonal antibodies are difficult to prepare from chicken cells. B lymphoid cell development takes place in a distinct primary lymphoid organ, the bursa of Fabricius.

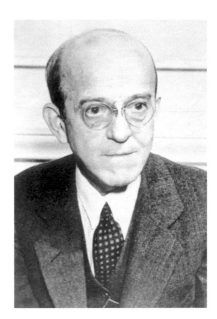

Oswald T. Avery.

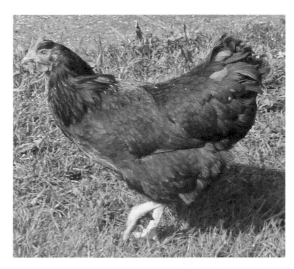

Avian immunity.

Another difference from the mammalian immune system is the multilobed thymus comprised of six to seven distinct lobes on one side of the neck. Chicken T cells develop from precursors that enter the thymus during development. Avian nonlymphoid hematopoietic cells are well defined as are the chicken immunoglobulin classes IgM and IgA and an IgG-like class termed IgY. Chicken β_2-microglobulin and MHC class I α (BF) and class II (BL) molecules are homologous to their mammalian counterparts both structurally and functionally. Chicken T cell surface constituents are similar to mammalian T cell receptors (TCRs), in addition to CD3, CD4, CD5, CD6, CD8, CD28, and CD45 antigens and the interleukin-2 (IL-2) receptor α chain (CD25). Whereas λ and γ chain genes are linked closely, light and heavy chain gene complexes are not linked. Chicken TCR $\alpha\beta\gamma$ and δ genes have been cloned and sequenced. The chicken MHC (B complex) is situated on microchromosome 16, which bears the nucleolar organizer region (NOR). The avian immune system is especially susceptible to the avian leukoses, Marek's disease, and infectious bursal disease

(IBD). Vaccines against IBD and other diseases of chicks are available.

avidin

A 68-kDa tetrameric egg-white glycoprotein that has a very high affinity for and binds biotin, a water-soluble vitamin. Four identical 128-amino-acid-residue subunits that bind a single biotin molecule each comprise the avidin molecule. It also has an *N*-linked oligosaccharide and one disulfide bridge. Avidin's strong affinity for biotin has made it useful as an indicator molecule in a number of methods. An enzyme can be linked to avidin, and the complex can be bound to an antibody linked to biotin. The avidin–biotin–peroxidase complex (ABC) method is an immunoperoxidase reaction used extensively in antigen identification in histopathological specimens, especially in surgical pathological diagnosis. See also streptavidin.

avidin–biotin–peroxidase complex (ABC) technique

A method useful for the localization of peptide hormones or other antigens in formalin-fixed tissues. After incubating the tissue section with primary antibody specific for the antigen sought, biotin-labeled secondary antibody is applied. This is followed by avidin-biotinylated horseradish peroxidase complex that then binds to the biotinylated secondary antibody. The specific antigenic markers may be visualized in tissue sections by conventional light microscopy following incubation in a solution of peroxidase substrate. The technique makes use of the very high affinity of the 68-kDa avidin glycoprotein from egg white for biotin. The ease with which biotin may be covalently linked to antibody makes the ABC staining system feasible. In addition to the widespread use of the technique in surgical pathologic diagnosis, the principle can be applied to *in situ* hybridization, gene mapping, double labeling, immuno-electron microscopy, Southern blotting, radioimmunoassay, solid-phase ELISA, hybridoma screening, etc.

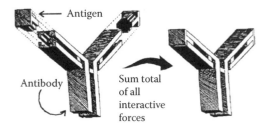

Avidity.

avidity

The strength of binding of an antibody and its specific antigen. The stability of this union is a reflection of the number of binding sites they share. Avidity is the binding force or intensity between a multivalent antigen and a multivalent antibody. Multiple binding sites on both the antigen and the antibody (e.g., IgM or multiple antibodies interacting with various epitopes on the antigen) and reactions of high affinity between each of the antigens and its homologous antibody all increase the avidity. Nonspecific factors such as ionic and hydrophobic interactions also increase avidity. Whereas affinity is described in thermodynamic terms, avidity is not; it is described according to the assay procedure employed. The sum of the forces contributing to the avidity of an antigen and antibody interaction may

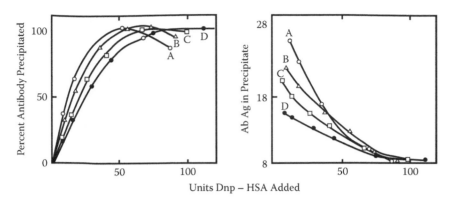

Precipitation curves showing differences in avidity of four antisera for the same antigen. The order of avidity of the sera is A > B > C > D.

be greater than the strength of binding of the individual antibody–antigen combinations contributing to the overall avidity of a particular interaction. K_A, the association constant for the Ab + Ag = AbAg interaction, is frequently used to indicate avidity. Avidity may also describe the strength of cell-to-cell interactions mediated by numerous binding interactions between cell surface molecules. Avidity is distinct from affinity, which describes the strength of binding between a single molecular site and its ligand.

avidity hypothesis

Previously known as the affinity hypothesis of T cell selection in the thymus, the avidity hypothesis is based on the concept that T cells must have a measurable affinity for self major histocompatibility complex (MHC) molecules to mature but not an affinity sufficient to cause activation of the cell when it matures, as this would necessitate deletion of the cell to maintain self tolerance.

Avionics®

Interferon-β-1a preparation approved for the treatment of multiple sclerosis.

avr-R system

Plant immune response mechanism in which the disease resistance (R) plant genes and microbial avirulent (*avr*) interact. For a plant to be able to isolate or wall off and degrade a pathogen, its R product and the *avr* product of the invading pathogen must match.

axenic

Free from association with or contamination by other organisms, e.g., germ-free mice raised in isolation; also refers to pure cultures of microorganisms. Also referred to as gnotobiotic and germ-free.

azathioprine

A slow-acting immunosuppressive agent that suppresses delayed hypersensitivity and cellular cytotoxicity to a greater degree than antibody responses. Immunosuppressive and therapeutic effects in animal models are dose-related. A nitroimidazole derivative of 6-mercaptopurine, a purine antagonist. Following administration, it is converted to 6-mercaptopurine *in vivo*. Its principal action is to interfere with DNA synthesis. It interferes with purine nucleic acid metabolism at stages requisite for lymphoid cell proliferation following antigenic stimulation. The purine analogs act as cytotoxic agents that fatally injure stimulated lymphoid cells. These

(6-[(1-methyl-4-nitro-1H-imidazol-5-yl)thio]-1H-purine)

Structure of azathioprine.

analogs have less effect on messenger RNA synthesis needed for sustained antibody formation by plasma cells than on nucleic acid in proliferating cells. The cytotoxic agents can depress cellular immunity as well as primary and secondary serum antibody responses. Of less significance is the ability to impair RNA synthesis. Azathioprine has a greater inhibitory effect on T cell than on B cell responses, even though it suppresses both cell-mediated and humoral immunity. It diminishes circulating natural killer (NK) and killer cell numbers. It has been used successfully to maintain renal allografts and treat various autoimmune disorders including rheumatoid arthritis, other connective tissue diseases, autoimmune blood diseases, and immunologically mediated neurological disorders. It is active chiefly against reproducing cells. The drug has little effect on immunoglobulin levels or antibody titers, but it does diminish neutrophil and monocyte numbers in the circulation. The major toxic effect is bone marrow suppression, often manifested as leukopenia.

azidothymidine

Synonym for zidovudine.

azoprotein

The joining of a substance to a protein through a diazo linkage –N=N–. Karl Landsteiner (in the early 1900s) made extensive use of diazotization to prepare hapten–protein conjugates to define immunochemical specificity. See also diazo reaction.

AZT

3′-azido-3′-deoxythymidine. Refer to zidovudine.

B

4-1BB:

A TNF receptor family molecule that binds specifically to 4-1BB ligand.

4-1BB ligand (4-1BBL)

A TNF family molecule that binds to 4-1BB.

β selection

The initial principal checkpoint in T cell development. It is the pathway in which the T cell receptor β chain receptor expressed by a DN3 thymocyte interacts in a pre-TCR that enables the thymocyte to receive a survival/proliferation signal (pre-TCR activation) and become committed to the αβ T cell lineage.

B-1 cells

B lymphocytes that express the CD5 glycoprotein and synthesize antibodies of broad specificities. They comprise a minor population of B cells. Also called CD5 B cells.

B-1a B cells (CD5)

A small population of B cells that express CD5, but to a lesser degree than CD5 expression on T cells. CD5 is a negative regulator of T cell receptor signaling. It participates in apoptosis of B-1a cells induced by B cell receptors.

B-2 cells

B lymphocytes that fail to express the CD5 glycoprotein and synthesize antibodies of narrow specificities. They comprise most of the B cell population.

b4, b5, b6, and b9

The four alleles whose κ chains vary in multiple constant region amino acid residues.

B7

A homodimeric immunoglobulin superfamily protein whose expression is restricted to the surfaces of cells that stimulate growth of T lymphocytes. The ligand for B7 is CD28. B7 is expressed on the surfaces of professional antigen-presenting cells (APCs) and is important in costimulatory mechanisms. Some APCs may upregulate expression of B7 following activation by various stimuli, including IFN-α, endotoxin, and major histocompatibility complex (MHC) class II binding. B7 is also referred to as BB1, B7.1, or CD80.

B7.1 costimulatory molecule

A 60-kDa protein that serves as a costimulatory ligand for CD28 but as an inhibitory ligand upon interacting with CTLA-4 molecules. Also called CD80.

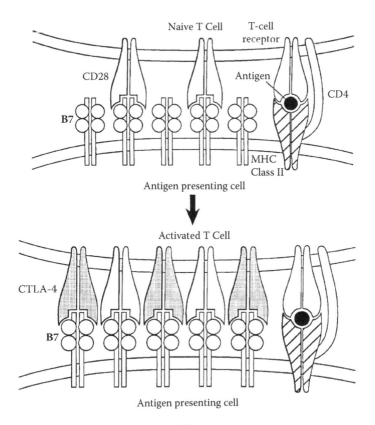

B7.

B

B7.2 costimulatory molecule

A costimulatory molecule whose sequence resembles that of B7. Dendritic cells, monocytes, activated T cells, and activated B lymphocytes may express B7.2, which is an 80-kDa protein that serves as a costimulatory ligand for CD28 but as an inhibitory ligand upon interacting with CTLA-4 molecules. Also called CD86.

B220

A form of CD45, a protein tyrosine phosphatase.

b allotype

A rabbit immunoglobulin κ light chain allotype encoded by alleles at the *K*1 locus.

B antigen, acquired

The alteration of A1 erythrocyte membrane through the action of such bacteria as *Escherichia coli, Clostridium tertium,* and *Bacteroides fragilis* to make it react as if it were a group B antigen. The named microorganisms may be associated with gastrointestinal infection or carcinoma.

B blood group

Refer to ABO blood group system.

B cell activation

B cell response to antigen, whether T-independent or T-dependent, results in the conversion of small resting B cells to large lymphoblasts and then into either plasma cells that form specific antibody or long-lasting memory B cells. Thymic-independent antigens such as bacterial polysaccharides can activate B cells independently of T cells by crosslinking of the B cell receptor. By contrast, protein antigens usually require the intimate interaction of B cells with helper T cells. Antigen stimulation of the B cell receptor leads to endocytosis and degradation of the antigen captured by the B cell receptor. Peptides that result from degraded antigen are bound to major histocompatibility complex (MHC) class II molecules and transported to the cell surface for presentation to T lymphocytes. T

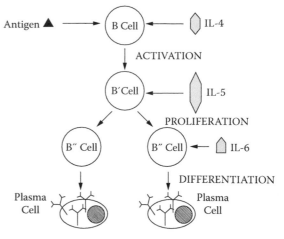

B cell activation.

cells bearing a specific T cell receptor that recognizes the peptide–MHC complex presented on the B cell surface are activated. Activated T cells help B cells either via soluble mediators such as cytokines (i.e., IL-4, IL-5, and IL-6) or membrane-bound stimulatory molecules such as the CD40 ligand. In germinal centers, B cells are converted to large replicating centroblasts and then to nonreplicating centroblasts. In germinal centers, frequent immunoglobulin (Ig) region mutations and the switch from IgM to IgG, IgA, or IgE production occur. Mutation increases the diversity of antigen-binding sites. Mutations that lead to loss of antigen binding cause the cells to die by apoptosis. The few cells for which mutation gives an immunoglobulin product that has high affinity for antigen are selected for survival. These antigen-selected cells differentiate into plasma cells that produce antibody or into small long-lived memory B cells that enter the blood and lymphoid tissues.

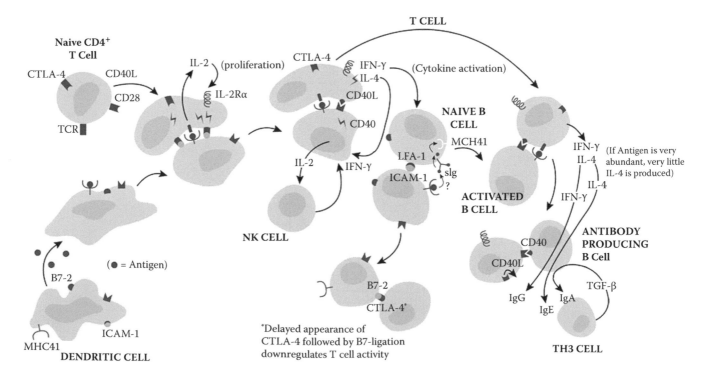

Hypothetical B7/CD40 pathway for B cell activation.

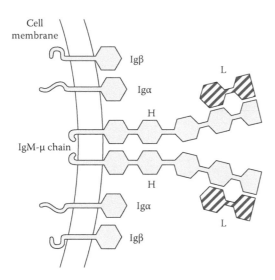

B cell antigen receptor.

B cell antigen receptor (or) B cell receptor

An antibody expressed on antigen reactive B cells that is similar to secreted antibody but is membrane-bound due to an extra domain at the Fc portion of the molecule. Upon antigen recognition by the membrane-bound immunoglobulin, noncovalently associated accessory molecules mediate transmembrane signaling to the B cell nucleus. The immunoglobulin and accessory molecule complex is similar in structure to the antigen receptor–CD3 complex of the T lymphocyte. The cell-surface, membrane-bound immunoglobulin molecule serves as a receptor for antigen together with two associated signal-transducing Iα/Igβ molecules.

B cell chronic lymphocytic leukemia/small lymphocytic lymphoma (B-CLL/SLL)

The most common leukemia in the Western world. The malignant cell is a small, fragile B lymphocyte with a immunophenotype resembling that of lymphocytes in the mantle zones (MZs) of secondary lymphoid follicles. The most distinctive feature is the coexpression of CD5 with CD19 and CD20 with very faint amounts of monoclonal surface immunoglobulin. The finding of somatic mutation in half the cases indicates that a memory B cell has been exposed to antigen in germinal centers of secondary follicles. The remaining cases that show no mutations originate from naïve B cells that have not responded to antigen. The prognosis of cases arising from naïve B cells is worse than the prognosis for cases arising from memory B cells. The disease has an insidious onset and is not curable. Patients are predisposed to repeated infections and have abdominal discomfort and bleeding from mucosal surfaces. They may have general localized or generalized lymphadenopathy, splenomegaly, hepatomegaly, petechiae, and pallor and develop an absolute lymphocytosis with small lymphocytes expressing modest amounts of pale basophilic cytoplasm and nuclei with round contours and mature or "blocky" chromatin clumping with or without a small nucleolus. By immunophenotyping, the CD5+/CD10−/CD23+ profile in a mature monoclonal B lymphocytosis is virtually diagnostic of B-CLL/SLL. Eighty percent of cases show clonal aberrations. The most common involve deletions at 13q. This is a lymphoproliferative disorder characterized by sustained lymphocytosis of

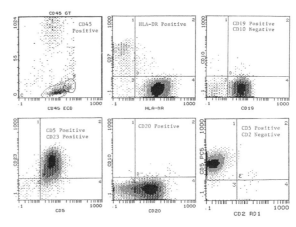

Immunoreceptor tyrosine-based activation motif (ITAM) signaling region of B cell antigen receptor.

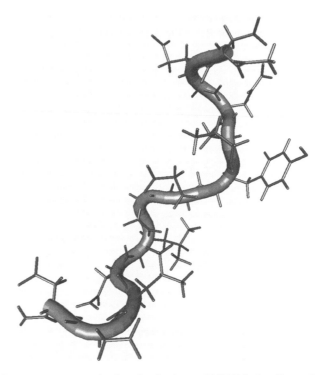

B cell chronic lymphocytic leukemia (B-CLL).

lymphocytes that are light chain restricted. Splenomegaly, lymphadenopathy, and hepatomegaly occur, with lymphocytosis ranging from 4×10^9/L to lymphocyte counts exceeding 400×10^9/L. The lymphocytes are relatively small with condensed nuclear chromatin and sparse cytoplasm. They have a uniform appearance, and injured cells are often present. Nucleoli are usually not visible. The mixed cell type may reveal both large and small lymphocytes. The more diffuse the pattern of involvement, the more aggressive the disease. B-CLL lymphocytes express pan-B cell antigens and meager quantities of light chain-restricted immunoglobulins on cell surfaces. The lymphocytes usually express CD5, a pan-T cell antigen, and rosette spontaneously with mouse red blood cells. One half to three fourths of B-CLL patients are hypogammaglobulinemic. Autoimmune hemolytic anemia, neutropenia, or thrombocytopenia develop in 15 to 30% of cases. B-CLL cases that become aggressive with pyrexia, weight loss, fatigue, and large cell lymphoma are referred to as having undergone Richter transformation, usually leading to death.

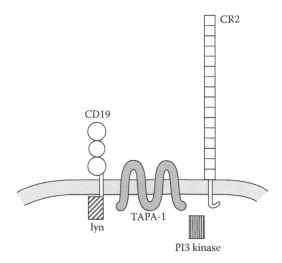

B cell coreceptor.

B cell coreceptor

A three-protein complex that consists of CR2, TAPA-1, and CD19 that associates with the B cell receptor and facilitates its response to specific antigen. CR2 unites not only with an activated component of complement but also with CD23. TAPA-1 is a serpentine membrane protein. The cytoplasmic tail of CD19 is the mechanism through which the complex interacts with lyn, a tyrosine kinase. Activation of the coreceptor by ligand binding leads to the union of phosphatidyl inositol–3′ kinase with CD19, resulting in activation. This produces intracellular signals that facilitate B cell receptor signal transduction.

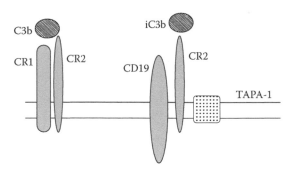

Complement receptor complexes on the surfaces of B cells include CR1, C3b, CR2, CR19, iC3B, CR2 (CD21), and TAPA-1. B cell markers used routinely for immunophenotyping by flow cytometry include CD19, CD20, and CD21.

B cell corona

The zone of splenic white pulp comprised mainly of B cells.

B cell differentiation and growth factors

T-lymphocyte-derived substances that promote differentiation of B lymphocytes into antibody-producing cells. They can facilitate the growth and differentiation of B cells *in vitro*. Interleukins 4, 5, and 6 belong in this category of factors.

B cell growth factor (BCGF)

See interleukins 4, 5, and 6.

B cell growth factor I (BCGF-1)

An earlier term for interleukin-4.

B cell growth factor II (BCGF-2)

An earlier term for interleukin-5.

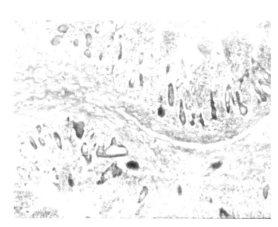

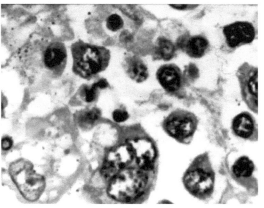

B cell lymphoma in the gut.

B cell leukemias

These leukemias may be classified as pre-B cell, B cell, or plasma cell neoplasms. They include Burkitt's lymphoma, Hodgkin disease, and chronic lymphocytic leukemia (CLL). Neoplasms of plasma cells are associated with multiple myeloma and Waldenström's macroglobulinemia. Many of these conditions are associated with hypogammaglobulinemia and a diminished capacity to form antibodies in response to the administration of an immunogen. In CLL, more than 95% of individuals have malignant leukemic cells that are identifiable as B lymphocytes expressing surface immunoglobulin. These patients frequently develop infections and have autoimmune manifestations such as autoimmune hemolytic anemia. Chronic lymphocytic leukemia/small lymphocytic lymphoma patients may have secondary immunodeficiency that affects both B and T limbs of the immune response. Diminished immunoglobulin levels are due primarily to diminished synthesis.

B cell lymphoproliferative syndrome (BLS)

A rare complication of immunosuppression in bone marrow or organ transplant recipients. Epstein–Barr virus appears to be the etiologic agent. The syndrome occurs in fewer than 1% of human leukocyte antigen (HLA)-identical bone marrow recipients and is more likely in those whose anti-CD3 monoclonal antibodies have been used to treat graft-vs.-host disease. Clinically, it may be either a relatively mild infectious mononucleosis or a proliferating and relentless lymphoma that produces high mortality. Monoclonal antibodies to the B cell antigens, CD21 and CD24, have proven effective in controlling the B cell proliferation, but further studies are needed.

B cell mitogen
Substance that induces B cell division and proliferation.

B cell receptor (BCR) complex
The antigen receptors of B cells, each of which makes a single type of immunoglobulin. The form of this immunoglobulin on the cell surface is the B cell receptor for the antigen of interest in addition to the membrane-bound immunoglobulin monomers of the intracellular signaling molecules that comprise the accessory Igα/Igβ complex.

B cell-specific activator protein (BSAP)
A transcription factor that has an essential role in early and later stages of B cell development. It is encoded by the gene *Pax-5*.

B cell-stimulating factor 1 (BSF-1)
An earlier term for interleukin-4.

B cell-stimulating factor 2 (BSF-2)
An earlier term for interleukin-6.

B cell tolerance
B cell tolerance is manifested as a decreased number of antibody-secreting cells following antigenic stimulation, compared to a normal response. Hapten-specific tolerance can be induced by inoculation of deaggregated haptenated γ-globulins (Ig). Induction of tolerance requires membrane Ig cross-linking. Tolerance may have a duration of 2 months in B cells of the bone marrow and 6 to 8 months in T cells. Whereas prostaglandin E (PGE) enhances tolerance induction, interleukin-1 (IL-1), lipopolysaccharide (LPS), and 8-bromoguanosine block tolerance instead of an immunogenic signal. Tolerant mice carry a normal complement of hapten-specific B cells. Tolerance is not attributable to a diminished number or isotype of antigen receptors. It has also been shown that the six normal activation events related to membrane Ig turnover and expression do not occur in tolerant B cells. Although tolerant B cells possess a limited capacity to proliferate, they fail to do so in response to antigen. Antigenic challenge of tolerant B cells induces them to enlarge and increase expression, yet they are apparently deficient in a physiologic signal requisite for progression into a proliferative stage.

B cell tyrosine kinase (Btk)
Src family tyrosine kinase that plays a critical role in the maturation of B lymphocytes. *Btk* gene mutations lead to X-linked agammaglobulinemia in which B cell maturation is halted at the pre-B stage.

B cells
The B lymphocytes that derive from the fetal liver in the early embryonal stages of development and from the bone marrow thereafter. In birds, maturation takes place in the bursa of Fabricius, a lymphoid structure derived from an outpouching of the hindgut near the cloaca. In mammals, maturation is in the bone marrow. Plasma cells that synthesize antibody develop from precursor B cells.

B complex
The major histocompatibility complex (MHC) in chickens. Genes at these loci determine MHC class I and II antigens and erythrocyte antigens.

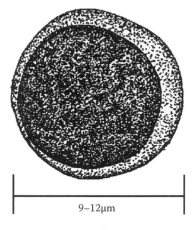

9–12μm

B cell.

B genes
Situated within the major histocompatibility complex (MHC) locus on the short arm of chromosome 6, they are called MHC class III genes. TNF-α and TNF-β genes are situated between the C2 and HLA-B genes. Another gene designated FD lies between the *Bf* and *C4a* genes. C2 and B complete primary structures have been deduced from cDNA and protein sequences. C2 is comprised of 732 residues and is an 81-kDa molecule, whereas B contains 739 residues and is a 83-kDa molecule. Both proteins have three domains. Certain HLA alleles occur at a higher frequency in individuals with particular diseases than in the general population. This type of data permits estimation of the relative risk (RR) of developing a disease for every known HLA allele. For example, there is a strong association between ankylosing spondylitis, an autoimmune disorder involving the vertebral joints, and the major histocompatibility complex (MHC) class I allele, HLA-B27. There is a strong association between products of the polymorphic class II alleles HLA-DR and DQ and certain autoimmune diseases, as MHC class II molecules are of great importance in the selection and activation of CD4[+] T lymphocytes that regulate immune responses against protein antigens. For example, 95% of Caucasians with insulin-dependent (type I) diabetes mellitus have HLA-DR3, HLA-DR4, or both. There is also a strong association of HLA-DR4 with rheumatoid arthritis. Numerous other examples exist and are the targets of current investigations, especially in extended studies employing DNA probes. Methods of calculating the RR and absolute risk (AR) can be found under definitions for those terms.

B locus
The major histocompatibility locus in the chicken.

B lymphocyte
Lymphocytes of the B cell lineage that mature under the influence of the bursa of Fabricius in birds and in the bursa equivalent (bone marrow) in mammals. B cells occupy follicular areas in lymphoid tissues and account for 5 to 25% of all human blood lymphocytes that number 1000 to 2000 cells per mm[3]. They comprise most of the bone marrow lymphocytes, one third to one half of the lymph node and spleen lymphocytes sites, but less than 1% of those in the thymus. Nonactivated B cells circulate through the lymph nodes and the spleen. They are concentrated in follicles and marginal zones around the follicles. Circulating B cells may interact

B

and be activated by T cells at extrafollicular sites where the T cells are present in association with antigen-presenting dendritic cells. Activated B cells enter the follicles, proliferate, and displace resting cells. They form germinal centers and differentiate into both plasma cells that form antibody and long-lived memory B cells. Those B cells synthesizing antibodies provide defense against microorganisms including bacteria and viruses. Surface and cytoplasmic markers reveal the stage of development and function of lymphocytes in the B cell lineage. Pre-B cells contain cytoplasmic immunoglobulins, whereas mature B cells express surface immunoglobulin and complement receptors. B lymphocyte markers include CD9, CD19, CD20, CD24, Fc receptors, B1, BA-1, B4, and Ia. Refer also to B cells.

B lymphocyte antigen receptor (BCR) complex

A B lymphocyte surface multiprotein complex that identifies antigen and transduces activating signals into cells. The BCR comprises membrane immunoglobulin that binds antigen and Igα and Igβ proteins that initiate signals.

B lymphocyte chemokine (BLC)

A CXC chemokine that induces B lymphocytes and activated T cells to enter peripheral lymphoid tissue follicles by binding to the CXCR5 receptor.

B lymphocyte hybridoma

A clone formed by the fusion of a B lymphocyte with a myeloma cell. Activated splenic B lymphocytes from a specifically immune mouse are fused with myeloma cells by polyethylene glycol. Thereafter, the cells are plated in HAT medium in tissue culture plates containing multiple wells. The only surviving cells are the hybrids, as the myeloma cells employed are deficient in HAT medium and fail to grow in HAT medium. Wells with hybridomas are screened for antibody synthesis. This is followed by cloning carried out by limiting the dilution or in soft agar. The hybridomas are maintained either in tissue culture or through inoculation into the peritoneal cavity of a mouse that corresponds genetically to the cell strain. The antibody-producing B lymphocyte confers specificity and the myeloma cell confers immortality upon the hybridoma. B lymphocyte hybridomas produce monoclonal antibodies.

B lymphocyte receptor

Immunoglobulin anchored to the B lymphocyte surface. Its combination with antigen leads to B lymphocyte division and differentiation into memory cells, lymphoblasts, and plasma cells. The original antigen specificity of the immunoglobulin is maintained in the antibody molecules subsequently produced. B lymphocyte receptor immunoglobulins

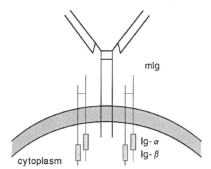

Schematic representation of immunoglobulin (Ig) on a cell membrane.

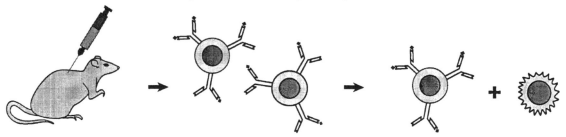

Immunize mouse with antigen   Isolate antibody-producing spleen cells   Mix spleen cells producing desired antibody with myeloma cells and fusing agent

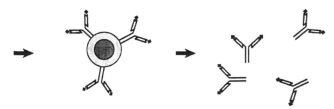

Select and culture immortalized fused spleen/myeloma cells producing desired antibody   Purify antibody from hybridoma culture medium

Making of a hybridoma for monoclonal antibody production.

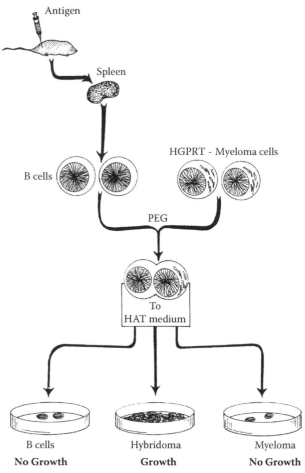

B lymphocyte hybridoma.

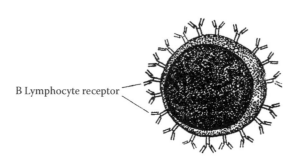

B lymphocyte receptor.

are to be distinguished from those in the surrounding medium that adhere to the B cell surface through Fc receptors. Refer to membrane immunoglobulin.

B lymphocyte stimulator (BlyS)

A naturally occurring protein that stimulates the immune system to produce antibodies. It is being tested as a potential drug for the treatment of immunodeficiency that occurs in higher than normal levels in rheumatoid arthritis and lupus patients and could account for their immune systems becoming overactive and attacking joints in rheumatoid arthritis (RA) or connective tissues in systemic lupus erythematosus (SLE).

B lymphocyte stimulatory factors

See interleukins 4, 5, and 6.

B lymphocyte tolerance

Immunologic nonreactivity of B lymphocytes induced by relatively large doses of antigen. It is of relatively short duration. By contrast, T cell tolerance requires less antigen and has a longer duration. Exclusive B cell tolerance leaves T cells immunoreactive and unaffected.

B-type virus (*Aspergillus macaques*)

An Old World monkey virus that resembles herpes simplex. Clinical features include intermittent shedding and reactivation in the presence of stress and immunosuppression. Humans who tend these monkeys may become infected with fatal consequences. B-type viruses possess eccentric nuclear cores.

babesiosis immunity

The host immune response to babesiosis, a malaria-like disease transmitted by parasitized *Ixodes* ticks, depends in part on the spleen, which has a central role in immune defense. Patients in whom the spleen has been removed are more susceptible to infection by *Babesia* and manifest elevated parasitemia. Complement activation by *Babesia* may lead to formation of TNF-α and IL-1, promoting local defense. Complement levels decrease in babesiosis. Patients develop increased circulating C1q binding activity and decreased C4, C3, and CH50 levels. The formation of TNF-α and IL-1 may account for many of the clinical features of the disease. Besides macrophages, other cellular immune functions are critical parts of the response to *Babesia*. T cell-deficient mice manifest significantly increased parasitemia. Cellular immunity is diminished by the disease, which is also associated with increased CD8+ T lymphocytes, diminished monocyte mitogen responsiveness, and polyclonal hypergammaglobulinemia.

bacille Calmette-Guérin

An attenuated strain of *Mycobacterium bovis* that has been employed as a vaccine against tuberculosis. Refer to BCG.

Bacillus anthracis immunity

Protective immunity against anthrax is induced only by the antigen designated PA. The *B. anthracis* polypeptide capsule is only weakly immunogenic and is not believed to contribute to naturally acquired immunity or induce protection against anthrax. The Ca⁻/tx⁺ strains of *B. anthracis* are protective. One of these strains is used to prepare a very successful live-spore animal vaccine. It is considered unsuitable in the West for use in humans because it retains some residual virulence. Human vaccine developed half a century ago consists of aluminum hydroxide-adsorbed, cell-free filtrates of cultures of a noncapsulating, nonproteolytic derivative of strain V770. Several doses are required. An immune response to PA but not to LF or EF is critical for protection. Immunization with strains synthesizing either PA and EF or PA and LF resulted in higher antibody responses to EF or LF, respectively. There is a synergistic relationship between PA and LF or EF in immunoprotection. Some cellular immune mechanisms are believed to be significant in the induction of protective immunity. PA has been shown with monoclonal antibodies to have at least three non-overlapping antigenic regions. It is anticipated that the elucidation of protective motifs on PA may lead to the development of a subunit-based vaccine. Passive immunity in the treatment of anthrax has been unsuccessful.

B

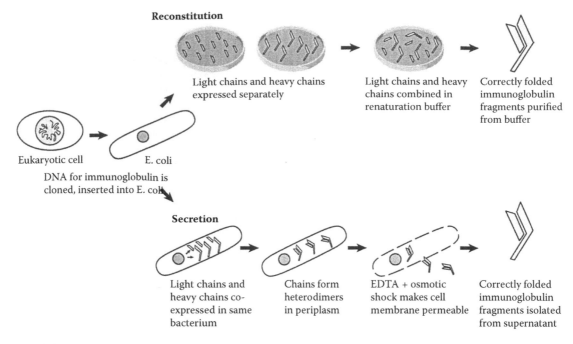

Reconstitution

Light chains and heavy chains expressed separately

Light chains and heavy chains combined in renaturation buffer

Correctly folded immunoglobulin fragments purified from buffer

Eukaryotic cell   E. coli

DNA for immunoglobulin is cloned, inserted into E. coli

Secretion

Light chains and heavy chains co-expressed in same bacterium

Chains form heterodimers in periplasm

EDTA + osmotic shock makes cell membrane permeable

Correctly folded immunoglobulin fragments isolated from supernatant

Beyond hybridoma technology, immunoglobulin subunits and fragments have been produced using cloned DNA expressed in bacteria.

backcross

The crossing of a heterozygous organism and a homozygote. Commonly refers to the transfer of a particular gene from one background strain or stock to an inbred strain via multigenerational matings to the desired strain. Breeding an F_1 hybrid with either one of the strains that produced it.

back typing

The interaction of antibodies in an individual's serum with known antigens of an erythrocyte panel; used to ascertain whether serum contains antierythrocyte antibodies. Also called reversed typing.

bacteremia

The presence of bacteria in the blood.

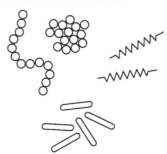

Morphology of bacteria.

bacteria

Prokaryotic microorganisms found throughout nature; they are responsible for many infectious diseases of humans and other animals.

bacterial agglutination

Antibody-mediated aggregation of bacteria. This technique has been used for a century in the diagnosis of bacterial diseases through the detection of an antibody specific for a particular microorganism or for the identification of a microorganism isolated from a patient.

bacterial allergy

Delayed-type hypersensitivity of infection such as in tuberculosis.

bacterial hypersensitivity

Refer to delayed-type hypersensitivity (type IV).

bacterial immunity

Bacteria produce disease by toxicity, invasiveness, or immunopathology or combinations of these three mechanisms. Immune mechanisms may require the development of a neutralizing antitoxin or mechanisms to destroy the microorganism. The animal body provides both nonspecific and specific defenses. Nonspecific defenses include natural barriers such as the skin, acidity in the gut and vagina, mucosal coverings, etc. Those microorganisms not excluded may be recognized by acute phase proteins, formol peptide receptors, receptors for bacterial cell wall components, complement, and receptors that promote cytokine release. Other factors influence the T_H1/T_H2 balance of the T cell response. Cytokines play a protective role during nonspecific recognition and early defense. Bacteria may interact with complement, leading to three types of protective function. Antibodies are important in neutralizing bacterial toxins. Secretory IgA can inhibit the binding of bacteria to epithelial cells. This antibody may also sensitize bacterial cells and render them susceptible to injury by complement. Phagocytic cells are important antibacterial defenses. Monocytes and polymorphonuclear cells have both oxygen-dependent and oxygen-independent antimicrobial mechanisms. Oxygen-independent killing may be accomplished by exposure to lysozyme and neutroproteases. Cell-mediated immunity mediated by T lymphocytes is another important antibacterial mechanism. T lymphocytes function through the release of lymphokines that have various types of consequences. Cytotoxic T cells and natural killer (NK) cells also play an important role in antimicrobial immunity. Mechanisms of immunopathology include septisemic shock

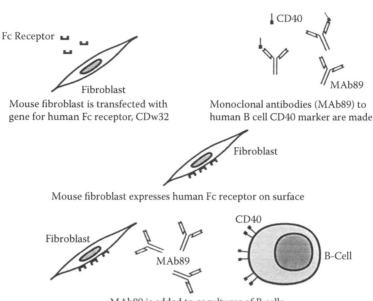

Fc Receptor

Fibroblast

Mouse fibroblast is transfected with gene for human Fc receptor, CDw32

Monoclonal antibodies (MAb89) to human B cell CD40 marker are made

Fibroblast

Mouse fibroblast expresses human Fc receptor on surface

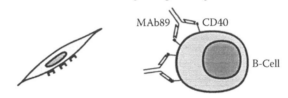

Fibroblast   CD40

MAb89   B-Cell

MAb89 is added to cocultures of B cells and fibroblasts expressing Fc receptor

MAb89   CD40

B-Cell

MAb89 binds to CD40 expressed on B-cells. The bound antibodies then bind, through their Fc fragments, to the fibroblasts expressing Fc receptors.

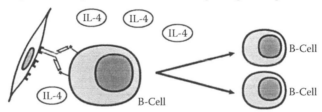

IL-4   IL-4

IL-4

IL-4

B-Cell

B-Cell

B-Cell

The cross-linking of CD40 glycoproteins on B-cell surface triggers B-cell proliferation, which is sustained in the presence of interleukin-4

System for producing factor-dependent B cell lines.

in adult respiratory distress syndrome, the Shwartzman reaction, the Koch phenomenon, necrotizing T cell-dependent granulomas, heat shock proteins, and the possible development of autoimmunity. Thus, the immune response to bacteria is varied and complex but effective in the animal organism with an intact immune response.

bacterial immunoglobulin-binding proteins

Molecules expressed by selected microorganisms that interact with immunoglobulin at sites other than their antigen-combining regions. Thus, the ability of an antibody to bind its homologous antigen is not impaired. Gram-positive bacteria express six types of IgG-binding protein, including protein A (type I) which is expressed on *Staphylococcus aureus*. Most human group A streptococci express type II receptors and exhibit great variability in immunoglobulin-binding capacity. Protein G, the type III IgG binding protein, is expressed by most human group C and G streptococcal isolates. Types IV, V, and VI immunoglobulin-binding proteins require further investigation.

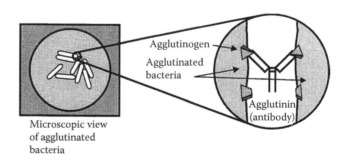

Agglutinogen

Agglutinated bacteria

Agglutinin (antibody)

Microscopic view of agglutinated bacteria

Bacterial agglutination.

bacterial vaccine

A suspension of killed or attenuated bacteria prepared for injection to generate active immunity to the same microorganism.

bacteriicidin

An agent such as an antibody or nonantibody substance in blood plasma that destroys bacteria.

bacterin

A vaccine comprised of killed bacterial cells in suspension. Inactivation is by either chemical or physical treatment.

bacteriolysin

An agent such as an antibody or other substance that lyses bacteria.

bacteriolysis

The disruption of bacterial cells by such agents as antibody and complement or lysozyme, causing the cells to release their contents.

bacteriophage λ

λ bacteriophage.

bacteriophage neutralization test

Refer to phage neutralization assay.

***Bacteroides* immunity**

Bacteroides fragilis has a capsular polysaccharide that serves as a virulence factor that led to use of the polysaccharide as a vaccine in rats. The vaccine produced excellent antibody levels but did not prevent abscess formation. In the rat model, the findings strongly point to the role of T cells in the immune response to *B. fragilis* in abscess prevention. Murine studies confirmed the rat findings and demonstrated that immune T cells are antigen-specific. Abscess formation and prevention in response to *B. fragilis* are mediated by T cell mechanisms. Abscess formation requires a precursor-type T cell. Prevention of abscess requires T cells belonging to the suppressor phenotype that communicate via a small polypeptide factor. These cells are antigen-specific but not major histocompatibility complex (MHC)-restricted.

BAFF

B lymphocyte activating factor that is a member of the TNF family. A survival factor needed for the maturation of splenic transitional T1 B cells into transitional T2 B cells. BAFF is necessary for the appearance of mature B cells in the periphery. BAFF signaling is believed to activate NF-κB and induces Bcl-2 expression. Autoimmunity develops in mice when BAFF is overexpressed, and elevated serum levels of BAFF have been described in human autoimmune diseases. It is produced mainly by monocytes, macrophages, and dendritic cells, but not by B cells. Proinflammatory stimuli stimulate its expression by macrophages. It occurs as both a homotrimeric transmembrane molecule and in a soluble homotrimeric form. It binds to three receptors, BAFF-R, TACI, and BCMA.

bagassosis

Hypersensitivity among sugar cane workers to the *Thermoactinomyces saccharic fungus* that thrives in the pressings from sugar cane. The condition is expressed as a hypersensitivity pneumonitis. Subjects develop type III (Arthus reaction) hypersensitivity following inhalation of dust from molding hot sugar cane bagasse.

Bak^a

A normal human platelet (thrombocyte) antigen. Anti-Bak^a IgG antibody synthesized by a Bak^a-negative pregnant female may be passively transferred across the placenta to induce immune thrombocytopenia in the neonate.

balancing selection

A form of evolutionary selection that maintains various phenotypes such as MHC isoforms in a population.

BALB/c mice

An inbred white mouse strain that responds to an intraperitoneal inoculation of mineral oil and Freund's complete adjuvant with a myeloproliferative reaction.

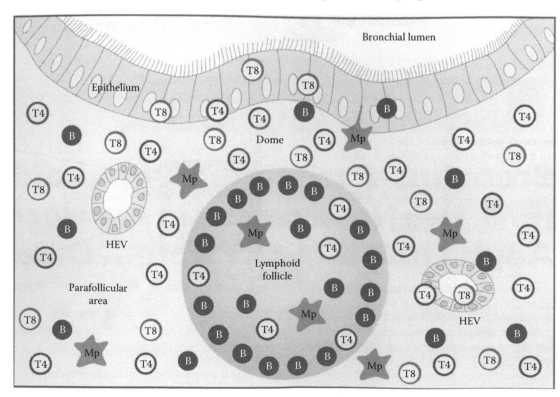

BALT.

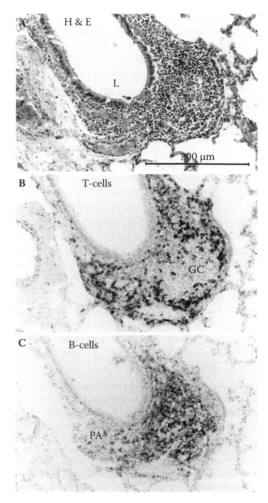

BALT.

BALT
See bronchial-associated lymphoid tissue and MALT.

band test
Antigen–antibody deposits at the dermal–epidermal junctions in patients with lupus erythematosus. They may consist of IgG, IgM, IgA, and C3. Deposits are not found in uninvolved areas of the dermal–epidermal junctions in discoid lupus erythematosus (DLE) but are present in both involved and uninvolved areas of the junctions in systemic lupus erythematosus (SLE). Immune complexes at the dermal–epidermal junction appear in 90 to 95% of SLE patients. Ninety percent reveal them in skin exposed to sunlight, and 50% have deposits in skin not exposed to the sun. Also called lupus band test. Immunofluorescence bands also occur in some cases of anaphylactoid purpura, atopic dermatitis, contact dermatitis, autoimmune thyroiditis, bullous pemphigoid, cold agglutinin syndrome, dermatomyositis, hypocomplementemic vasculitis, polymorphous light eruption, rheumatoid arthritis, scleroderma, and a number of other conditions.

bare lymphocyte syndrome (BLS)
Rare autosomal-recessive disorders in which individuals manifest little or no expression of human leukocyte antigen (HLA) major histocompatibility proteins. BLS has been classified into three types that are of varying severity with respect to phenotypic HLA expression and loss of immune function. BLS type I patients have little or no expression of HLA class I molecules on peripheral blood cells. They may have a broad range of immunodeficiency, with some individuals even revealing normal immunity. Type II BLS is characterized by a reduction or complete loss of HLA class II protein expression on all cells. This disorder is usually expressed as a severe combined immunodeficiency. In BLS type III, there is decreased expression of both HLA class I and class II antigen expression. These patients have severe immunodeficiency. HLA class I deficiency is sometimes referred to as type I BLS. It is believed that low expression of class I molecules may be sufficient for immune responses against pathogens, whereas complete deficiency would be lethal. Contrary to type II and III BLS, characterized by early onset of severe combined immunodeficiency (SCID), class I antigen deficiencies are not accompanied by specific pathologic features during the first years of life, although chronic lung disease develops in late childhood. In contrast to type II or III BLS, pathology of the gastrointestinal tract (diarrhea) is not observed. The lack of MHC molecule expression on the cells is due to a deficiency of the RFX or CIITA components of the SXY-CITTA regulatory system. Thus, the syndrome may be attributable to various different regulatory gene defects leading to severe immune deficiency.

barrier filter
A device in the eyepiece of an ultraviolet light source microscope employed for fluorescent antibody techniques to protect the viewer's eyes from injury by ultraviolet radiation. It also facilitates observation of the fluorescence by blocking light of the wavelength that produces fluorochrome excitation.

bas
Mutation in an mRNA splicing acceptor site in the rabbit that leads to diminished expression of the principal type of immunoglobulin κ light chain (MO-κ-1). Rabbits with the bas mutation have λ light chains, although a few have the κ-2 isotype of light chains.

basement membrane
A structure comprised of collagen, laminin, heparan sulfate, and glycosaminoglycan beneath an overlying epithelial or endothelial cell layer.

basement membrane antibody
Antibody specific for the basement membranes of various tissues such as lung basement membranes, glomerular basement membranes, etc. This antibody is usually observed by immunofluorescence and less often by immunoperoxidase technology.

basiliximab (injection)
An immunosuppressive agent that acts as an IL-2 receptor antagonist by binding with high affinity to the α chain of the high affinity IL-2 receptor complex and inhibiting IL-2 binding. It is specific for IL-2Rα, which is expressed on activated T cell surfaces. High affinity binding of basiliximab to IL-2Rα inhibits IL-2 mediated activation of lymphocytes, which is critical in cellular immune responsiveness in allograft rejection. It blocks responses of the immune system to antigenic challenges when in the circulation.

basolateral
The epithelial cell surface that faces the tissue instead of the lumen.

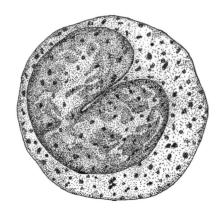

A peripheral blood basophil showing a bilobed nucleus and cytoplasmic granules that represent storage sites of pharmacological mediators of immediate type I hypersensitivity.

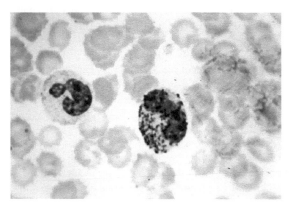

Neutrophil and basophil in peripheral blood.

basophil

A polymorphonuclear leukocyte of myeloid lineage with distinctive basophilic secondary granules in the cytoplasm that frequently overlie the nucleus. These granules are storage depots for heparin, histamine, platelet-activating factor, and other pharmacological mediators of immediate hypersensitivity. Degranulation of the cells with release of these pharmacological mediators takes place following crosslinking by allergens or antigens of Fab regions of IgE receptor molecules bound through Fc receptors to cell surfaces. They comprise less than 0.5% of peripheral blood leukocytes. Following crosslinking of surface-bound IgE molecules by specific allergen or antigen, granules are released by exocytosis. Substances liberated from the granules are pharmacological mediators of immediate (type I) anaphylactic hypersensitivity.

basophil-derived kallikrein (BK-A)

BK-A represents the only known instance in which an activator of the kinin system is generated directly from a primary immune reaction. The molecule is a high molecular weight enzyme with arginine esterase activity. It is stored in the producing cells in a preformed state. Its release depends on basophil–IgE interactions with antigen and parallels the release of histamine.

basophilic

An affinity of cells or tissues for basic stains leading to a bluish tint.

BCDF

Abbreviation for B cell differentiation factor.

BCG (*bacille* Calmette–Guérin)

A *Mycobacterium bovis* strain maintained for more than 75 years on potato, bile, glycerine agar that preserves the immunogenicity but dissipates the virulence of the microorganism. It has long been used in Europe as a vaccine against tuberculosis, although it never gained popularity in the United States. It has also been used in tumor immunotherapy to nonspecifically activate immune responses in selected tumor-bearing patients, such as those with melanoma or bladder cancer. It has been suggested as a possible vector for genes that determine human immunodeficiency virus (HIV) proteins such as *gag, pol, env,* gp20, gp40, reverse transcriptase, and tetanus toxin. In certain countries with high incidences of tuberculosis, BCG provides effective immunity against the disease, diminishing the risk of infection by approximately 75%. The vaccine has the disadvantage of rendering skin testing for tuberculosis inaccurate, especially in the first 5 years after inoculation, because it induces hypersensitivity to tuberculin. Intended for protection against tuberculosis in individuals not previously infected with *Mycobacterium tuberculosis* who are at high risk for exposure. Designed for percutaneous use as an attenuated live culture preparation of the Bacillus of Calmette and Guerin (BCG) strain of *M. bovis*. The TICE strain was developed at the University of Illinois from a strain originated at the Institut Pasteur in Paris.

BCGF (B cell growth factor)

See interleukins 4, 5, and 6.

BCG vaccine

Refer to BCG (*bacille* Calmette-Guérin).

Bcl-2

A 25-kDa human oncoprotein that is believed to play a regulatory role in tissue development and maintenance in higher organisms by preventing the apoptosis of specific cell types. The inhibitory effect of Bcl-2 is influenced by the expression of other gene products such as *bax, bcl-xs, bak,* and *bad* that promote apoptosis. Bcl-2 is situated at the outer membranes of mitochondria, the endoplasmic reticulum, and the nuclear membrane and may prevent apoptosis either by acting at these locations or as an antioxidant that neutralizes the effects of reactive oxygen species that promote apoptosis or by obstructing mitochondrial channel openings, thereby preventing the release of factors that promote apoptosis. Bcl-2 is involved in the development of the adult immune system as demonstrated by studies with Bcl-2 knockout mice. Failure to induce normal levels of apoptosis due to overexpression of Bcl-2 may contribute to the development of lymphoproliferative disorders and acceleration of autoimmunity under the appropriate genetic background. The role of Bcl-2 in human systemic lupus erythematosus (SLE) and PSS has not yet been fully defined.

Bcl-2 family

The Bcl-2 family consists of proteins that share homology to Bcl-2 in one or more of the Bcl-2 homology regions designated BH1, BH2, BH3, and BH4. Many of the family members have carboxyl-terminal mitochondrial membrane targeting sequences. All have two central membrane-spanning helices surrounded by additional amphipathic helices. X-ray crystallographic studies have shown that Bcl-x$_L$ has structural similarity to diphtheria toxin and colicins. Diphtheria toxin is endocytosed by cells. Acidification of the endosome induces a conformational change in diphtheria toxin that triggers membrane insertion of the membrane-spanning domains. Pore formation by dimerization is thought to occur, and the toxic subunit diphtheria toxin is translocated from the endosomal lumen into the cytosol. It is clear from reconstitution assays that many members of the Bcl-2 family can form a pore that allows passage of ions or elicits the release of cytochrome *c* from isolated mitochondria. Passage of ions is more dramatic at low pH. The carboxyl mitochondria targeting sequence is not required for *in vitro* pore formation.

Bcl-2 proteins

Proteins that regulate the rate at which apoptotic signaling events initiate or amplify caspase activity. Bcl-2 alters the apoptotic threshold of a cell rather than inhibiting a specific step in programmed cell death. Cells that overexpress Bcl-2 still carry out programmed cell death in response to a wide spectrum of apoptotic initiators. The dose of the initiator is greater than in the absence of Bcl-2. Several Bcl-2-related proteins have been identified. Whereas some Bcl-2 family members promote cell survival, others enhance the sensitivity of a cell to programmed death. Five homologs of Bcl-2 with antiapoptotic properties include Bcl-x_L, Bcl-w, Mcl-1, NR-13, and A-1. By contrast, two proapoptotic members of the Bcl-2 family include Bax and Bak. Bcl-2-related proteins are present in the intracellular membranes, including the endoplasmic reticulum, outer mitocondrial membrane, and outer nuclear membrane. Bcl-2 proteins are hypothesized to regulate membrane permeability.

Bcl-X_L

A Bcl-2-related protein that is upregulated through the action of the costimulatory molecules CD28 and CD40. Bcl-X_L expression is claimed to prevent cell death in response to growth factor limitation or Fas signal transduction. Signal transduction through CD28 or CD40 induces Bcl-X_L expression only in antigen-activated cells. Without antigen–receptor engagement, CD40 engagement promotes cell death. Bcl-x_L induction by either CD28 or CD40 is transient, persisting only 3 to 4 days. Protection of cells from death lasts only as long as Bcl-x_L is expressed.

BCR/cABL

Fusion gene that can be detected by either chromosomal analysis or polymerase chain reaction (PCR)-based molecular assays. There is also a total lack of leukocyte alkaline phosphatase.

BDB

Refer to *bis*-diazotized benzidine.

Behçet's disease

Oral and genital ulcers, vasculitis, and arthritis that recur as a chronic disease in young men. It is postulated to have an immunologic basis and possibly to be immune complex-mediated. Perivascular infiltrates of lymphocytes may occur. The serum contains immune complexes, and immunofluorescence may reveal autoantibodies against the oral mucous membrane. It is associated with HLA-1 in ethnic groups, but not Caucasians. The principal immunologic dysfunction in Behçet's disease is neutrophil hyperfunction, shown by augmented chemotactic responsiveness and superoxide production. Behçet's disease is an inflammatory condition of uncertain cause. No autoimmune mechanism has been proven.

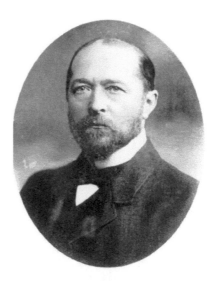

Emil Adolph von Behring (1854–1917).

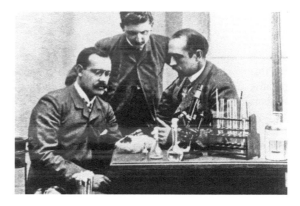

Emil Adolph von Behring with colleagues in the laboratory.

Behring, Emil Adolph von (1854–1917)

German bacteriologist who, with Kitasato, demonstrated that circulating antitoxins against diphtheria and tetanus conferred immunity. Received the first Nobel Prize for Medicine in 1901 for this work. (Related works include *Die Blutserumtherapie,* 1902; *Gesammelte Abhandlungen,* 1915; *Behring, Gestalt und Werk,* 1940; *Emil von Behring zum Gedachtnis,* 1942.)

beige mice

A mutant strain of mice that develops abnormalities in pigment, defects in natural killer cell function, and heightened tumor incidence, serving as a model for the Chediak–Higashi disease in humans. There is a defect in granule function. The strain has also been used as an NK cell-deficient murine model.

Benacerraf, Baruj (1920–)

American immunologist born in Caracas, Venezuela. His multiple contributions include the carrier effect in delayed-type hypersensitivity, lymphocyte subsets, major histocompatibility complex (MHC), and Ir immunogenetics, for which he received the Nobel Prize in 1980. (Benacerraf, B. and Unanue, E., *Textbook of Immunology,* Williams & Wilkins, Baltimore, Maryland, 1979.)

Bence–Jones (B–J) proteins

Represent the light chains of either the κ or λ variant excreted in the urine of patients with a paraproteinemia as

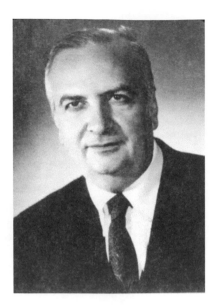

Baruj Benacerraf.

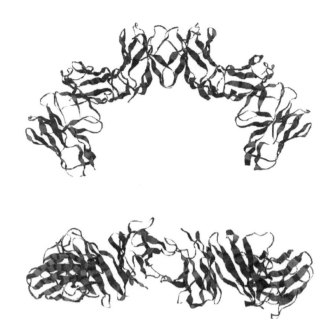

Bence–Jones protein.

a result of excess synthesis of such chains or from mutant cells that make only such chains. Both mechanisms appear operative, and more than 50% of patients with multiple myeloma, a plasma cell neoplasm, have B–J proteinuria. The highest frequency of B–J excretion is seen in IgD myeloma; the lowest is seen in IgG myeloma. The daily amount excreted parallels the severity of the disease. These proteins are secreted mostly as dimers and show unusual heat solubility properties. They precipitate at temperatures between 40 and 60°C and redissolve again near 100°C. With proper pH control and salt concentration, precipitation may detect levels as low as 30 mg/100 mL of urine. Better identification is by protein electrophoresis.

benign
A nonmalignant neoplasm or a mild clinical illness.

benign lymphadenopathy
Lymph node enlargement that is not associated with malignant neoplasms. Histologic types of benign lymphadenopathy include nodular, granulomatous, sinusoidal, paracortical, diffuse or obliterative, mixed,

and depleted; clinical states are associated with each histologic pattern.

benign lymphoepithelial lesion
Autoimmune lesion in lacrimal and salivary glands associated with Sjögren's syndrome. Myoepithelial cell aggregates together with extensive lymphocyte infiltration are present.

benign monoclonal gammopathy
A paraproteinemia that occurs in normal healthy subjects who develop the serum changes characteristic of myeloma (i.e., a myeloma protein-type immunoglobulin spike on electrophoresis). They have none of the clinical signs and symptoms of multiple myeloma and their prognosis is excellent.

benign tumor
An abnormal proliferation of cells that leads to a growth that is localized and contained within epithelial barriers. It does not usually lead to death, in contrast to a malignant tumor.

bentonite (Al$_2$O$_3$·4SiO$_2$·H$_2$O)
Aluminum silicate that is hydrated and colloidal. This insoluble particulate substance has been used to adsorb

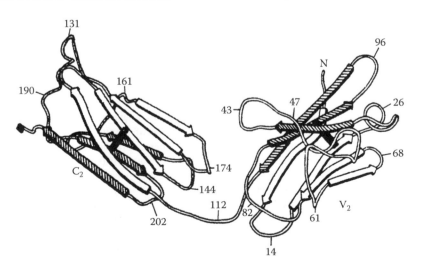

Bence–Jones protein.

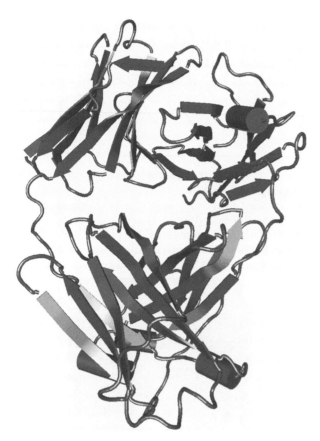

Bence-Jones (B-J) protein.

proteins, including antigens. It was used in the past in the bentonite flocculation test.

bentonite flocculation test

An assay in which bentonite particles are used as carriers to adsorb antigens. These antigen-coated bentonite particles are then agglutinated by the addition of a specific antibody.

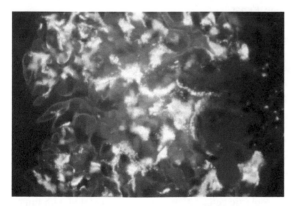

Berger's IgA nephropathy.

Berger's disease

A type of glomerulonephritis in which prominent IgA-containing immune deposits are present in mesangial areas. Patients usually present with gross or microscopic hematuria and often mild proteinuria. Under light microscopy, mesangial widening or proliferation may be observed. However, immunofluorescence microscopy demonstrating IgA and C3, fixed by the alternative pathway, is requisite for diagnosis. Electron microscopy confirms the presence of

electron-dense deposits in mesangial areas. Half of the cases progress to chronic renal failure over a 20-year course.

berylliosis

A disease induced by the inhalation of beryllium in dust. Subjects may develop a delayed-type hypersensitivity (type IV) reaction to beryllium–macromolecular complexes. An acute chemical pneumonia or chronic pulmonary granulomatous disease that resembles sarcoidosis may develop. Granulomas may form and lead to pulmonary fibrosis. The skin, lymph nodes, or other anatomical sites may be affected. Subjects who develop chronic progressive granulomatous pulmonary disease appear to be sensitized by beryllium.

Besredka, Alexandre (1870–1940)

Born in Odessa, Besredka was a Parisian immunologist who worked with Metchnikoff at the Pasteur Institute. He contributed to studies of local immunity, anaphylaxis, and anti-anaphylaxis. (See *Anaphylaxie et Antianaphylaxie,* 1918; *Histoire d'une Idee: L'Oeuvre de Metchnikoff,* 1921; *Etudes sur l'Immunite dans les Maladies Infectieuses,* 1928.)

β barrel

Refer to β sheet.

β cells

Insulin-secreting cells in the islets of Langerhans of the pancreas.

β lysin

A thrombocyte-derived antibacterial protein that is effective mainly against Gram-positive bacteria. It is released when blood platelets are disrupted, as occurs during clotting. β lysin acts as a nonantibody humoral substance that contributes to nonspecific immunity.

β-pleated sheet

A protein configuration in which the β sheet polypeptide chains are extended and have a 35-nm axial distance. Hydrogen bonding between NH and CO groups of separate polypeptide chains stabilizes the molecules. Adjacent molecules may be either parallel or antiparallel. The β-pleated sheet configuration is characteristic of amyloidosis and is revealed by Congo red staining followed by polarizing light microscopy, which yields an apple-green birefringence. Ultrastructurally, it consists of nonbranching fibrils.

β propiolactone

A substance employed to inactivate the nucleic acid cores of pathogenic viruses without injuring the capsids. This permits the development of an inactivated vaccine, as the immunizing antigens that induce protective immunity are left intact.

β₁A globulin

A breakdown product of β₁C globulin. It has a molecular weight less than that of β₁C globulin, and its electrophoretic mobility is more rapid than that of β₁C globulin. β₁A degradation is linked to the disappearance of C3 activity.

β₁C globulin

The globulin fraction of serum that contains complement component C3. On storage of serum, β₁C dissociates into β₁A globulin, which is inactive.

β₁E globulin

The globulin fraction of serum that contains complement component C4 activity.

β₁F globulin

The globulin fraction of serum that contains complement component C5 activity.

B

β₁H
Refer to factor H.

β-2 glycoprotein-I autoantibodies
Autoantibodies against β-2 glycoprotein-1 (β-2-GP1), a natural serum coagulation inhibitor. These autoantibodies represent one of the interactions of antiphospholipid antibodies with components of the clotting system. Antiphospholipid autoantibodies occur in antiphospholipid syndrome (APS), which is associated with recurrent thrombotic events, repeated fetal loss, and/or thrombocytopenia, usually associated with systemic lupus erythematosus (SLE), as well as in patients without autoimmune disease. β-2-GP1, a 50-kDa plasma protein binds to phospholipids (PLs) and lipoproteins. Binding to PLs inhibits the intrinsic blood coagulation pathway, prothrombinase activity, and ADP-dependent platelet aggregation and induces a conformational change in β-2-GP1, causing β-2-GPI autoantibodies to bind only to β-2-GP1 when it is complexed to PLs.

β₂ microglobulin (β₂M)
A thymic epithelium-derived polypeptide that is 11.8 kDa and makes up part of the major histocompatibility complex (MHC) class I molecules that appear on the surfaces of nucleated cells. It is noncovalently linked to the MHC class I polypeptide chain. It promotes maturation of T lymphocytes and serves as a chemotactic factor. β₂M makes up part of the peptide–antigen class I–β₂M complex involved in antigen presentation to cytotoxic T lymphocytes. Nascent β₂M facilitates the formation of antigenic complexes that can stimulate T lymphocytes. This monomorphic polypeptide accumulates in the serum in renal dialysis patients and may lead to β₂ microglobulin (β₂M)₂-induced amyloidosis. The extracellular protein β₂M is encoded by a nonpolymorphic gene outside the MHC. It is homologous structurally to an immunoglobulin domain and is invariant among all class I molecules.

β-adrenergic receptor autoantibodies
Autoantibodies against β1-adrenoreceptors are detected in a significant proportion of individuals with dilated cardiomyopathy. The human heart contains both β1-adrenoreceptors and a substantial number of β2-adrenoreceptors. Both types are diminished in chronic heart failure. β1-adrenoreceptors are decreased in all types of heart failure, whereas β2-adrenoreceptors are diminished in mitral valve disease, tetralogy of Fallot, and end-stage ischemic cardiomyopathy; 30 to 40% of dilated cardiomyopathy, 22% of ischemic cardiomyopathy, and 25% of alcoholic cardiomyopathy patients develop autoantibodies against β-adrenoreceptors. In familial, idiopathic, dilated cardiomyopathy, 62% of affected family members manifest the β-adrenoreceptor autoantibodies, compared to 29% in unaffected members. Dilated cardiomyopathy patients have increased frequency of HLA-DR4 antigen compared to normal persons, and 60 to 80% of patients with HLA-DR4 and dilated cardiomyopathy develop β-adrenoreceptor antibodies.

beta-gamma bridge
Patients with chronic liver disease such as that caused by alcohol, chronic infection, or connective tissue disease may synthesize sufficient polyclonal proteins whose electrophoretic mobilities are in the β–γ range to cause obliteration of the β and γ peaks, forming a "bridge" from one to the other.

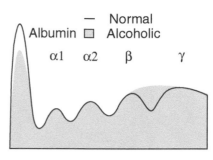

Beta-gamma bridge.

β thromboglobulin (βTG)
A chemokine generated through successive proteolysis of platelet basic protein (PBP), a 94-amino-acid protein present in the α granules of platelets. The plasma concentrations of both βTG and PF4 granule constituents are assayed for platelet activation in allergic states and asthma.

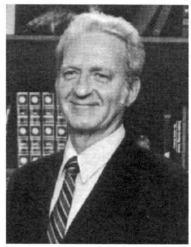

Ernst Beutner.

Beutner, Ernst
A member of the Buffalo Immunology Group.

bevacizumab
A humanized IgG₁ monoclonal antibody that unites with vascular endothelial growth factor (VEGF) and blocks VEGF binding to its receptor, mainly on endothelial cells. It has an antiangiogenic effect, inhibiting blood vessel growth in tumors. It is used to treat patients with metastatic colorectal cancer.

BFPR
Abbreviation for biological false-positive reaction.

biclonality
In contrast to uncontrolled proliferation of a single clone of neoplastic cells which is usually associated with tumors, rarely two neoplastic cell clones may proliferate simultaneously, leading to a biclonality. For example, either neoplastic B or T lymphocytes may demonstrate this effect.

bifunctional antibodies
Artificially formed immunoglobulins that manifest double, well-defined antigen specificity. They are used to focus the activity of an effector cell on a target cell by their ability to bind with one combining site on the effector cell and with another on the target cell. Antibodies to helper and cytotoxic effector T cell receptors can mimic antigen and activate the T cells to proliferate, release lymphokines, or become cytotoxic.

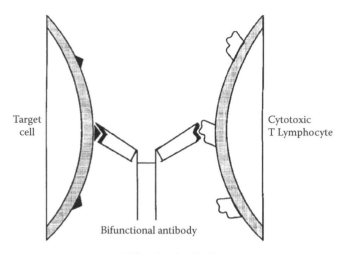

Bifunctional antibody.

Bispecific antibodies that bind to both effector and target cells can activate the effector cell and guarantee intimate contact between effector and target cells. The three basic techniques to prepare bispecific molecules are (1) heteroconjugate bispecific antibodies produced by chemical linkage of two immunoglobulin molecules with different binding specificities; (2) hybridoma-specific antibodies formed by hybridomas produced by fusing two lymphocytes that synthesize antibodies of different specificities; and (3) bispecific molecules produced by genetic engineering which permits the insertion, within or adjacent to the genes encoding an immunoglobulin molecule, of oligonucleotides encoding another immunoglobulin, a desired immunogenic epitope, or an epitope responsible for interaction with a viral antigen. Bispecific antibodies were developed to redirect or enhance immune effector responses toward tumors and induce killing of target cells in a non-MHC-restricted manner. One limb of the bispecific antibody recognizes a cell-surface antigen on the cytotoxic effector cell, while the other limb is specific for a tumor antigen. Recombinant DNA technology has permitted the generation of bispecific scFv, minibodies, diabodies, and multivalent bispecific antibodies. Single-chain bispecific antibodies are composed of linked variable domains fused to human Fc domains. Miniantibodies comprise an scFv joined by a linker to a dimerization domain while diabodies exploit the intrinsic nature of VH and VL within an Fv to pair.

Billingham, Rupert (1921–2002)

Together with P.B. Medawar proved that the rejection of grafts between unrelated individuals, i.e., allografts or homografts, has an immunological basis. Pioneer of acquired immunological tolerance reported in classic paper in *Nature* 1953.

binding constant

Refer to association constant.

binding protein

Also called immunoglobulin heavy chain-binding protein.

binding site

The paratope area of an antibody molecule that binds antigen or the part of a T cell receptor that is antigen binding.

biochemical sequestration

Antigenic determinants that are hidden in a molecule may be unable to act as immunogens or react with antibody. Structural alterations in the molecule may render them identifiable and capable of serving as immunogens.

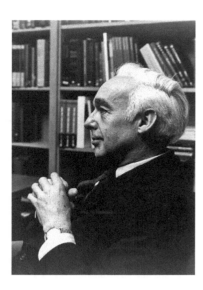

Rupert Billingham, colleague of P.B. Medawar, who was also a pioneer in immunologic tolerance.

biogenic amines

Nonlipid substances of low molecular weight, such as histamine, that have an amine group in common. Biogenic amines are stored in the cytoplasmic granules of mast cells, from which they may be released to mediate the biological consequences of immediate hypersensitivity reactions. Also called vasoactive amines.

biolistics

The coating of small particles such as colloidal gold with an agent such as a drug, nucleic acid, or other substance to be conveyed into a cell. A helium-powered gun is employed to fire particles into the recipient's dermis.

biological false-positive reaction

A positive serological test for syphilis, such as the VDRL (Venereal Disease Research Laboratory) serological test produced by the serum of an individual who is not infected with *Treponema pallidum*. The reaction is attributable to antibodies reactive with antigens of tissues such as the heart, from which cardiolipin antigen used in the test is derived. The sera of patients with selected autoimmune diseases, including systemic lupus erythematosus (SLE), may contain antibodies that give biological false-positive results for syphilis.

biological response modifiers (BRMs)

A wide spectrum of molecules such as cytokines that alter immune responses. They include substances such as interleukins, interferons, hematopoietic colony-stimulating factors, tumor necrosis factor, B lymphocyte growth and differentiating factors, lymphotoxins, and macrophage-activating and chemotactic factors, as well as macrophage inhibitory factor, eosinophil chemotactic factor, osteoclast activating factor, etc. BRMs may modulate the immune system of a host to augment antitumor defense mechanisms. Some have been produced by recombinant DNA technology and are available commercially. An example is α interferon used in the therapy of hairy cell leukemia.

biologicals

Natural or engineered proteins employed to activate or interefere with the proliferation, metabolism, or functioning of normal or neoplastic cells. Substances used for therapy that include antitoxins, vaccines, products prepared from pooled blood plasma, and biological response modifiers

B

(BRMs). BRMs are prepared by recombinant DNA technology and include lymphokines such as interferons, interleukins, tumor necrosis factor, etc. Monoclonal antibodies for therapeutic purposes also belong in this category. Biologicals have always presented problems related to chemical and physical standardization to which drugs are subjected. Biologicals are regulated by the Food and Drug Administration within the United States.

biotin–avidin system

Avidin is an egg-white-derived glycoprotein with an extraordinarily high affinity (affinity constant $> 10^{15}\,M^{-1}$) for biotin. Streptavidin is similar in properties to avidin but has a lower affinity for biotin. Many biotin molecules can be coupled to a protein, enabling the biotinylated protein to bind more than one molecule of avidin. If biotinylation is performed under gentle conditions, the biological activity of the protein can be preserved. By covalently linking avidin to different ligands such as fluorochromes, enzymes, or EM markers, the biotin–avidin system can be employed to study a wide variety of biological structures and processes. This system has proven particularly useful in the detection and localization of antigens, glycoconjugates, and nucleic acids by employing biotinylated antibodies, lectins, or nucleic acid probes.

biovin antigens

Salmonella O antigens. These carbohydrate–lipid–protein complexes withstand trichloroacetic acid treatment.

Biozzi mice

Murine lines that are genetically selected for high (H) or low (L) antibody responsiveness. Selections I, II, III, IV, and V have been carried out. The character selected was the maximal or minimal antibody response at a given time following an optimal dose of the various antigens used in the different selections.

BiP

A chaperonin that binds unassembled heavy and light chains after they are synthesized in the endoplasmic reticulum. Chains that are malformed are not allowed to leave the ER and thus are not used in immunoglobulin assembly.

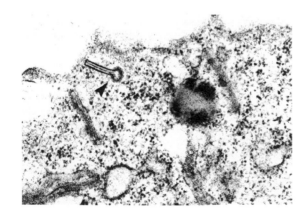

Birbeck granule.

Birbeck granule

A round, 10- to 30-nm-diameter cytoplasmic vesicle present in the cytoplasm of Langerhans' cells in the epidermis.

bird fancier's lung

Respiratory distress in a subject who is hypersensitive to plasma protein antigens of birds following exposure to bird

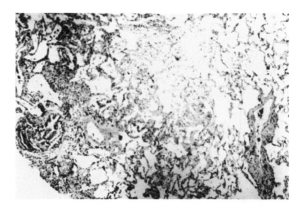

Bird fancier's lung. Lung biopsy shows an interstitial granulomatous pneumonitis consistent with bird fancier's lung.

feces or skin and feather dust. Hypersensitive subjects have an Arthus type of reactivity or type III hypersensitivity to the plasma albumin and globulin components. Precipitates may be demonstrated in the blood sera of hypersensitivity subjects.

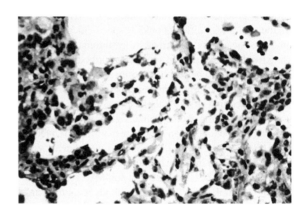

Bird fancier's lung. Lung biopsy shows an interstitial granulomatous pneumonitis consistent with bird fancier's lung.

BI-RG-587

A powerful inhibitor of reverse transcriptase in humans. This dipyridodiazepinone can prevent the replication of HIV-1 *in vitro*. It can be used in conjunction with such nucleoside analogs as zidovudine, ddI, and ddC, and in subjects whose HIV-1 infections no longer respond to these drugs.

$$Cl^-\ \overset{+}{N}N\!\!\bigcirc\!\!\bigcirc\!\!N\overset{+}{N}\ Cl^-$$

bis-diazotized benzidine.

***bis*-diazotized benzidine**

A chemical substance that serves as a bivalent coupling agent that can link to protein molecules. It was used in the past to conjugate erythrocytes with antigens for use in the passive agglutination test.

bispecific antibodies

Molecules that have two separate antigen-binding specificities. They may be produced by either cell fusion or chemical techniques. An immunoglobulin molecule in which one of two antigen-binding sites is specific for one antigen-binding specificity, whereas the other antigen-binding site is specific for a different antigen specificity. This never occurs in nature, but can be produced *in vitro* by treating two separate antibody specificities with mild reducing agents, converting the central disulfide bonds of both antibody molecules to sulfhydryl groups, mixing the two specificities of half molecules together, and allowing them to reoxidize to form whole molecules, some of which will be bispecific. They also may be produced by fusing hybridomas that synthesize different monoclonal antibodies. Bispecific antibodies were developed to redirect or enhance immune effector responses toward tumors and induce killing of target cells in a non-MHC-restricted manner. One limb of the bispecific antibody recognizes a cell-surface antigen on the cytotoxic effector cell, while the other limb is specific for a tumor antigen. Recombinant DNA technology permitted the generation of bispecific scFv, minibodies, diabodies, and multivalent bispecific antibodies. Single-chain bispecific antibodies are composed of linked variable domains fused to human Fc domains. Miniantibodies comprise a scFv joined by a linker to a dimerization domain, while diabodies exploit the intrinsic nature of VH and VL within a Fv to pair.

BLA-36
An antigen demonstrable by immunoperoxidase staining in Reed–Sternberg cells of all types of Hodgkin disease and in activated B lymphocytes and B cell lymphomas.

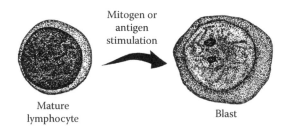

Blastogenesis.

blast cell
A relatively large cell (greater than 8 μm in diameter) with abundant RNA in the cytoplasm, a nucleus with loosely arranged chromatin, and a prominent nucleolus. Blast cells are active in synthesizing DNA and contain numerous polyribosomes in the cytoplasm.

blast crisis (in chronic myelogenous leukemia)
Chronic myelogenous leukemia, late phase, characterized by blast-like leukemia cells that comprise more than 30% of the patient's blood or bone marrow cells. There may be extramedullary tissue infiltration.

blast transformation
The activation of small lymphocytes to form blast cells.

blastocyst
Stage in early animal development (typically the 16-cell stage in mice) characterized by the formation of a multicellular spherical shell enclosing a fluid-filled cavity (the blastocoele).

blastogenesis
The activation of small lymphocytes to form blast cells.

blastoma
Highly undifferentiated malignant tumors of children. The cells appear similar to those of a blastocyst.

blocking
Prevention of nonspecific interaction of an antibody with a certain antigenic determinant (the identification of which is sought) by washing with mammalian serum other than that used in the test system. For example, the enzyme-linked immunosorbent assay (ELISA) employs blocking.

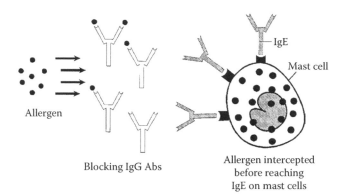

Blocking antibody.

blocking antibody
(1) An incomplete immunoglobulin G (IgG) antibody that, when diluted, may combine with red blood cell surface antigens and inhibit agglutination reactions used for erythrocyte antigen identification. This can lead to errors in blood grouping for Rh, K, and k blood types. Pretreatment of red cells with enzymes may correct the problem. (2) An IgG antibody specifically induced by exposure of allergic subjects to specific allergens to which they are sensitive in a form that favors IgG rather than IgE production. The IgG specific for the allergens to which the subjects are sensitized competes within IgE molecules bound to mast cell surfaces, thereby preventing their degranulation and inhibiting a type I hypersensitivity response. (3) A specific immunoglobulin molecule that may inhibit the combination of a competing antibody molecule with a particular epitope. Blocking antibodies may also interfere with the union of T cell receptors with an epitope for which they are specific, as occurs in some tumor-bearing patients with blocking antibodies that may inhibit the tumoricidal action of cytotoxic T lymphocytes.

blocking factor
Agents such as immune complexes in the sera of tumor-bearing hosts that interfere with the capacity of immune lymphoid cells to mediate cytotoxicity of tumor target cells.

blocking test
An assay in which the interaction between an antigen and its homologous antibody is inhibited by the previous exposure of the antigen to a different antibody that has the same specificity as the first one but does not have the same biological function. In a different situation, a hapten may be used to prevent the reaction of an antibody with its intended antigen. This is referred to as the hapten inhibition test. An example would be blood group substance-soluble molecules equivalent to erythrocyte surface isoantigen epitopes found in body fluids. Refer to ABO blood group substances.

blood group
The classification of erythrocytes based on their surface isoantigens. Among the well known human blood groups are the ABO, Rh, and MNS systems.

B

blood group antigens

Erythrocyte surface molecules that may be detected with antibodies from other individuals such as ABO blood group antigens. Various blood group antigen systems including Rh (Rhesus) may be typed in routine blood banking procedures. Other blood group antigen systems may be revealed through cross matching.

blood grouping

The classification of erythrocytes based on their surface isoantigens. Among the well-known human blood groups are the ABO, Rh, and MNS systems.

TABELLE I

betreffend das blut sechs anscheinend gesunder männer

	Sera					
Dr. St.	−	+	+	+	+	−
Dr. Plecn.	−	−	+	+	−	−
Dr. Sturl.	−	+	−	−	+	−
Dr. Erdh.	−	+	−	−	+	−
Zar.	−	−	+	+	−	−
Landst.	−	+	+	+	+	−
Blutköperchen von:	Dr. St.	Dr. Plecn.	Dr. Sturl.	Dr. Erdb.	Zar.	Landst.

Table illustrating ABO blood groups. (*From Wien. klin. Wschr., 14, 1132–1134, 1901.*)

TABELLE II

betreffend das blut von sechs anscheinend gesunder puerperae

	Sera					
Seil	−	−	+	−	−	+
Linsm.	+	−	+	+	+	+
Lust.	+	−	−	+	+	−
Mittelb.	−	−	+	−	−	+
Tomsch.	−	−	+	−	−	+
Graupn.	+	−	−	+	+	−
Blutköperchen von:	Seil.	Linsm.	Lust.	Mittelb.	Tomsch.	Graupn.

ABO blood group antigens and antibodies.

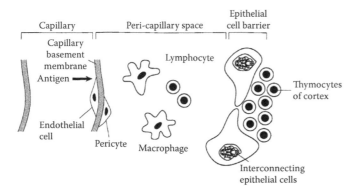

Three levels of lymphocyte protection that form the blood–thymus barrier: capillary wall, macrophages in pericapillary space, and a wall of epithelial cells.

blood–thymus barrier

Protects thymocytes from contact with antigen. Lymphocytes reaching the thymus are prevented from contact with antigen by a physical barrier. The first level is represented by the capillary wall endothelial cells inside the pericytes outside of the lumen. Potential antigenic molecules that escape the first level of control are taken over by macrophages present in the pericapillary space. Further protection is provided by a third level, represented by the mesh of interconnecting epithelial cells that enclose the thymocyte population. The effects of thymus and thymic hormones on the differentiation of T cells is demonstrable in animals congenitally lacking thymus glands (nu/nu animals), in neonatal or adult thymectomized animals, and in subjects with immunodeficiencies involving T cell function. Differentiation is associated with surface markers whose presence or disappearance characterizes the different stages of cell differentiation. Extensive proliferation of the subcapsular thymocytes occurs. The largest proportion of these cells die, but remaining cells continue to differentiate. The differentiating cells become smaller in size and move through interstices in the thymic medulla. The fully developed thymocytes pass through the walls of the postcapillary venules to reach the systemic circulation and seed in the peripheral lymphoid organs. Some of them recirculate but do not return to the thymus.

Bloom syndrome (BS)

A very rare clinical entity characterized by a strikingly small but well-proportioned body size. It is the consequence of either homozygosity or compound heterozygosity of a mutation of *BLM*, a gene that encodes a phylogenetically, highly conserved nuclear protein. It has been suggested that this condition should be grouped with the genetically determined immunodeficiencies. Respiratory tract infections occur much more commonly in patients with BS than in the general population; if not treated promptly, these infections become life threatening, yet 37% of BS patients manifest no increased tendency to infection of any kind. The disease is characterized by diminished numbers of T lymphocytes, decreased antibody levels, and increased susceptibility to respiratory infections, tumors, and radiation injury. Mutations in a DNA helicase cause the disorder. Genomic instability is a characteristic of this rare autosomal recessive primary immunodeficiency that is attributable to mutation of the *BLM* gene associated with the homologous recombination pathway of DNA repair.

blot

The transfer of DNA, RNA, or protein molecules from an electrophoretic gel to a nitrocellulose or nylon membrane by osmosis or vacuum, followed by immersion of the membrane in a solution containing a complementary (i.e., mirror-image) molecule corresponding to the one on the membrane. This is known as a hybridization blot.

BLR-1/MDR-15

Burkitt's lymphoma receptor-1/monocyte-derived receptor-15 (BLR-1/MDR-15) is a member of the G protein-coupled receptor family, the chemokine receptor branch of the rhodopsin family. It is expressed on B cells and memory T cells, chronic B lymphoid leukemia and non-Hodgkin lymphoma cells, peripheral blood monocytes, and lymphocytes. It is expressed in tonsils and secondary lymphoid organs and in selected other tissues. Most Burkitt's lymphoma cell lines express the receptor. Interleukin-4 (IL-4) and IL-6 downregulate BLR-1. The receptor is also downregulated by monoclonal antibodies against CD40 and CD3. Jurkat cells expressing BLR-1 do not bind known chemokines. Also called BLR-1 and MDR-15.

BlyS

A tumor necrosis factor (TNF) cytokine family molecule that is secreted by T lymphocytes and is critical in the formation of germinal centers and plasma cells and may be significant in maturation of dendritic cells.

***bm* mutants**

Mouse H-2 *bm* mutants have served as elegant genetic tools for performing detailed analyses of the H-2 gene structure and its relationship to functions of the gene products. The mutants are especially useful when intact animals are needed to investigate a particular process. These mutants have aided in the assignment of diverse biological and immunologic functions to single H-2 genes. They also influence mating preferences, as evidenced by the ability of mice to use urine odor to distinguish parental animals from those carrying *bm* mutations.

BMT

Abbreviation for bone marrow transplantation.

Bombay phenotype

The O_h phenotype is an ABO blood group antigen variant on human erythrocytes in rare subjects. These red blood cells do not possess A, B, or H antigens on their surfaces, even though the subject's serum contains anti-A, anti-B, and anti-H antibodies. The Bombay phenotype may cause difficulties in crossmatching for transfusion.

bombesin

A neuropeptide of 14 residues analogous to a gastrin-releasing peptide that is synthesized in the gastrointestinal (GI) tract and induces GI smooth muscle contraction and the release of stomach acid and the majority of GI hormones, with the exception of secretin. Bombesin injection into the brain may induce hyperglucagonemia, hyperglycemia, analgesia, and hypothermia. Bombesin facilitates bronchial epithelial cell proliferation and pancreas and small cell carcinoma. Antibombesin antibodies may prove useful in the future for the treatment of small cell lung carcinoma, the cells of which bear bombesin receptors.

bone marrow

Soft tissue within bone cavities that contains hematopoietic precursor cells and hematopoietic cells that are maturing into erythrocytes, the five types of leukocytes, and thrombocytes. Whereas red marrow is hematopoietic and is present in developing bone, ribs, vertebrae, and long bones, some of the red marrow may be replaced by fat and become yellow marrow. In mammals, the bone marrow is the site of B cell development and the source of stem cells from which T lymphocytes develop following migration to the thymus, where they mature. A stromal framework comprised of fibroblasts, fat cells, endothelial cells and fibers supports the developing hematopoietic cells. Bone marrow transplantation may supply all of the cellular elements of the blood, including those needed for adaptive immunity.

bone marrow cell

Stem cells from which the formed elements of the blood, including erythrocytes, leukocytes, and platelets, are derived. B lymphocyte and T lymphocyte precursors are abundant. The B lymphocytes and pluripotent stem cells in bone marrow are important for reconstitution of an

irradiated host. Bone marrow transplants are useful in the treatment of aplastic anemias, leukemias, and immunodeficiencies. Patients may donate their own marrow for subsequent bone marrow autotransplantation if they are to receive intensive doses of irradiation.

bone marrow chimera

The inoculation of an irradiated recipient mouse with bone marrow from an unirradiated donor mouse which ensures that lymphocytes and other cellular elements of the blood will be of donor genetic origin. The technique has been useful in demonstrating lymphocyte and other blood cell development.

bone marrow transplantation

The inoculation of a recipient with donor bone marrow including stem cells that serve as precursors for all mature cellular elements of the blood including lymphocytes; a procedure used to treat both nonneoplastic and neoplastic conditions not amenable to other forms of therapy. It has been especially used in cases of aplastic anemia, acute lymphoblastic leukemia, and acute nonlymphoblastic leukemia. A high degree of histocompatibility between donor and recipient is required. Using an HLA-matched donor, 750 mL of bone marrow are removed from the iliac crest. Following appropriate treatment of the marrow to remove bone spicules, the cell suspension is infused intravenously into an appropriately immunosuppressed recipient who has received whole-body irradiation and immunosuppressive drug therapy. Bone marrow cells derived from a patient during disease remission may be held frozen in liquid nitrogen for a future autologous bone marrow transplant that will permit the subject to receive his or her own cells. Graft-vs.-host episodes, acute graft-vs.-host disease, or chronic graft-vs.-host disease may follow bone marrow transplantation in selected subjects. The immunosuppressed patients are highly susceptible to opportunistic infections. See graft-vs.-host disease.

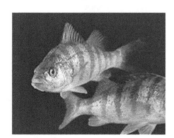

Bony fish (teleosts)

T and B lymphocyte functions become separate and distinctive, NK cells appear, and important cytokines such as IL-2 and IFN appear in bony fish. A polymorphic major histocompatibility complex (MHC) system resembling mammalian MHC is demonstrable in zebrafish.

booster

A second administration of immunogen to an individual primed months or years previously by a primary injection of the same immunogen. The purpose is to deliberately induce a secondary or anamnestic or memory immune response to facilitate protection against an infectious disease agent.

booster injection

The administration of a second inoculation of an immunizing preparation, such as a vaccine, to which an individual has been previously exposed. The booster inoculation elicits

B

a recall or anamnestic response through stimulation of memory cells that encountered the same antigen previously. Booster injections are given after a passage of time sufficient for a primary immune response specific for the immunogen to have developed. Booster injections are frequently given to render the subject immune prior to the onset of a particular disease or protect the individual when exposed to subjects infected with the infectious disease agent against which immunity is desired.

booster phenomenon
An expansion in the diameter of a tuberculin reaction following the administration of a subsequent PPD skin test for tuberculosis. The reaction is usually larger than 6 mm and shows an increase in size from below 10 mm to more than 10 mm in diameter following the secondary challenge. A positive test suggests an increased immunologic recall as a consequence of either previous infection with *Mycobacterium tuberculosis* or other mycobacteria. It is seen in older subjects with previous *M. tuberculosis* infections who fail to convert to active disease.

booster response
The secondary antibody response produced during immunization of subjects primed by earlier exposure to the same antigen. Also called anamnestic response and secondary response.

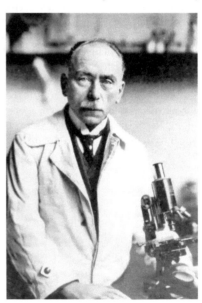

Jules Jean Baptiste Vincent Bordet.

Bordet, Jules Jean Baptiste Vincent (1870–1961)
Belgian physician who graduated from the University of Brussels as a doctor of medicine. He served as a preparateur in Metchnikoff's laboratory at the Institut Pasteur from 1894 to 1901 where he discovered immune hemolysis and elucidated the mechanisms of complement-mediated bacterial lysis. He and Gengou described complement fixation and pointed to its use in the diagnosis of infectious diseases. Their technique was subsequently used by von Wassermann to develop a complement fixation test for syphilis that enjoyed worldwide popularity. Bordet's debates with Paul Ehrlich on the nature of antigen–antibody–complement interactions stimulated much useful research. He was awarded the 1919 Nobel Prize in Medicine or Physiology

for his studies on immunity. (Refer to *Traite de l'Immunite dans les Maladies Infectieuses,* 1920.)

Bordetella immunity
Bordetella pertussis produces the respiratory disease known as whooping cough or pertussis. Both humoral and cell-mediated immune responses follow infection. The neutralizing antibodies believed to be the principal protective mechanism against infection with *B. pertussis* are formed against the *B. pertussis* antigens PT, FHA, PRN, and fimbriae associated with protection against pertussis. Pertussis infection can lead to long-lasting immunity against subsequent pertussis. Patients recovering from the infection develop anti-*B. pertussis* immunoglobulin A (IgA) in serum and saliva, pointing to the role of mucosal antibodies. Cell-mediated immunity is also believed to be significant, as T_H1 cells specific for the microorganism occur in persons following either infection or vaccination. High-titer IgG antibodies may clear bacteria in respiratory infections, as revealed by animal studies, but cell-mediated immunity is necessary to completely eliminate the microorganism from mouse lungs. In humans, immunity that follows infection may prevent respiratory colonization, whereas immunity that follows vaccination may protect against toxin-mediated disease. *B. pertussis* antigens suppress the host response to pertussis both *in vitro* and *in vivo*. The whole-cell vaccine comprised of killed, whole, virulent *B. pertussis* has been replaced with an acellular preparation combined with diphtheria and tetanus toxoid in the currently used DTaP vaccine. It provides fewer and milder side effects than the whole-cell vaccine preparation and is more effective in inducing serum antibody responses and protection from pertussis.

Bordetella pertussis
The etiologic agent of whooping cough in children. Killed *Bordetella pertussis* microorganisms are administered in a vaccine together with diphtheria toxoid and tetanus toxoid as DPT. The endotoxin of *B. pertussis* has an adjuvant effect that can facilitate antibody synthesis.

Borrelia immunity
Relapsing fever and Lyme disease are produced by members of this genus. *Borrelia burgdorferi* sensu lato spirochetes are the causative agents of Lyme disease. These microorganisms are covered by a slime layer comprised of self molecules that block immune recognition. The slime layer acting as a capsule prevents phagocytosis, but the microbe is killed when it is incubated with specific antibody in complement. The principal surface proteins in the exterior cell membrane include A, B, C, D, E, and F, which are designated as outer surface proteins (Osps). The proteins are heterogeneous, but their function remains to be determined. Spirochetes that cause Lyme disease upregulate or downregulate Osp A and Osp C during the course of human infection. Other antigens in the outer membrane of *Borrelia burgdorferi* sensu lato include 16-, 27-, 55-, 60-, 66-, and 83-kDa proteins. Osp A is the principal candidate for a Lyme disease vaccine. Soon after infection with *Borrelia burgdorferi* sensu lato, the microorganisms become refractory to the action of bactericidal antibodies.

botulinum toxin
A toxin formed by *Clostridium botulinum*. The 150-kDa, type A toxin is available in purified form and is employed to treat neuromuscular junction diseases such as dystonias. It acts by combining with the presynaptic cholinergic nerve terminals where it is internalized and prevents exocytosis of

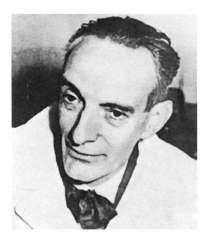

Daniel Bovet.

acetylcholine. Subsequently, sprouting takes place, and new terminals are formed that reinnervate the muscle.

Botulism immune globulin IV (human) (BIG-IV)

Indicated for the treatment of patients under 1 year of age who have infant botulism caused by toxin type A or B.

Bovet, Daniel (1907– 1992)

Primarily a pharmacologist and physiologist, Bovet received the Nobel Prize in 1957 for his contributions to the understanding of the role histamine plays in allergic reactions and the development of antihistamines. (Refer to *Structure chimique et Activite Pharmacodynamique des Medicaments du Systems Nerveux Vegetatif,* 1948; *Curare and Curare-Like Agents,* 1959.)

bovine serum albumin (BSA)

Albumin in the sera of cows that is used extensively as an antigen in experimental immunologic research.

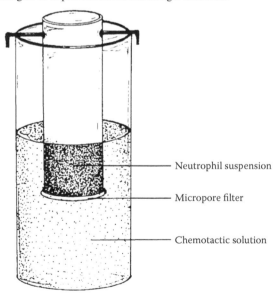

- Neutrophil suspension
- Micropore filter
- Chemotactic solution

Boyden chamber.

Boyden chamber

A two-compartment structure used to assay chemotaxis. The two chambers in the apparatus are separated by a micropore filter. The cells to be tested are placed in the upper chamber and a chemotactic agent such as f–met–leu–phe is placed in the lower chamber. As cells in the upper chamber settle to the filter surface, they migrate through the pores if the agent below chemoattracts them. On staining of the filter, cell migration can be evaluated.

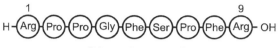

Primary Structure of
Serum Bradykinin

Active Kinins.

bradykinin

A 9-amino-acid peptide split by plasma kallikrein from plasma kininogens. It produces slow, sustained, smooth muscle contraction; its action is slower than that of histamine. It is produced in experimental anaphylaxis in animal tissues, and its sequence is Arg–Pro–Pro–Gly–Phe–Ser–Pro–Phe–Arg. Bradykinin is also increased in endotoxin shock. Lysyl-bradykinin (kallidin), which is split from kininogens by tissue kallikreins, also has a lysine residue at the amino terminus.

brain death

Irreversible loss of brain function without trauma to other body systems. Artificial maintenance of the subject's respiration can be employed to preserve organs for transplantation.

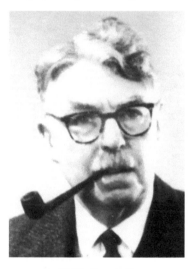

F.W.R. Brambell.

Brambell, F.W.R. (1901–1970)

A pioneer in transmission of immunity from mother to fetus who described a receptor that conserves IgG by binding to its Fc region and protects it from catabolism by lysosomes. It is an Fc receptor that transports IgG across epithelial surfaces and is named the Brambell receptor.

Brambell receptor (FcRB)

An Fc receptor that transports immunoglobulin G (IgG) across epithelial surfaces. Its structure resembles that of a major histocompatibility complex (MHC) class I molecule. It conserves IgG by binding to its Fc region and protects it from catabolism by lysosomes. The mechanism of binding is pH-dependent. In the low pH of the endosomes, the receptor FcRB binds to IgG. IgG is then transported to the luminal surface of the catabolic cell, where the neutral pH mediates release of the bound IgG. Refer to FcRn.

BrdU labeling

A technique to assay cellular proliferation. Based on the incorporation of bromo-deoxyuridine into the DNA of dividing cells.

B

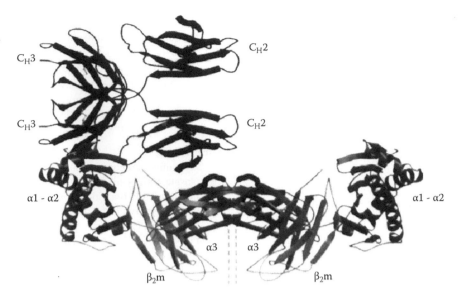

Brambell receptor.

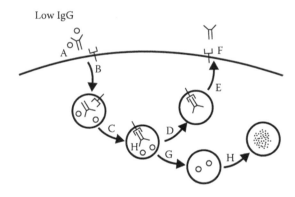

Structure of brequinar sodium (BQR).

Low IgG

High IgG

Mechanism of γ-globulin protection from catabolism. IgG (Y) and plasma proteins (°) (A) are internalized into endosomes of endothelium (B) without prior binding. In the low pH (H⁺) of the endosome (C), binding of IgG is promoted. (D), (E), (F) IgG retained by receptor recycles to the cell surface and dissociates in the neutral pH of the extracellular fluid, returning to circulation. (G), (H) Unbound proteins are shunted to the lysosomes for degradation. With low IgG, receptor efficiently rescues IgG from catabolism. With high IgG, receptor is saturated and excess IgG passes to catabolism for a net acceleration of IgG catabolism.

brequinar sodium (BQR)

An antineoplastic and immunosuppressive agent. Its major activity is inhibition of the *de novo* biosynthesis of pyrimidine nucleosidases, resulting in inhibition of both DNA and RNA synthesis. BQR has also been shown to interfere with immunoglobulin M (IgM) production by interleukin-6 (IL-6)-stimulated SKW6.4 cells, although in a manner independent of DNA synthesis. In transplantation studies, BQR has been shown to inhibit both humoral and cellular immune responses of the host, thereby significantly suppressing acute and antibody-mediated graft rejection.

Bretscher–Cohn theory

A theory that allows self/not-self discrimination to occur at any stage of lymphoreticular development. The concept is based on three principles: (1) engagement of the lymphocyte receptor by antigen, providing signal 1; signal 1 alone is a tolerogenic signal for the lymphocyte; (2) provision of signal 1 in conjunction with signal 2, a costimulatory signal, results in lymphocyte induction; and (3) delivery of signal 2 requires associative recognition of two distinct epitopes on the antigen molecule. The requirement for associative recognition blocks the development of autoimmunity in an immune system where diversity is generated randomly throughout an individual's lifetime.

bright

An adjective used in flow cytometry to indicate the relative fluorescence intensity of cells being analyzed, with *bright* designating the greatest intensity and *dim* representing the lowest intensity of fluorescence.

BRM

Abbreviation for biological response modifier.

bromelin

An enzyme used to render erythrocyte surfaces capable of being agglutinated by incomplete antibody.

bronchial-associated lymphoid tissue (BALT)

BALT is present in birds and mammals, including humans. In many areas it appears as a collar containing nodules located deep around the bronchus and connected with the epithelium by patches of loosely arranged lymphoid cells. Germinal centers are absent (except in chickens), although cells in the centers of nodules stain lighter than do those at the periphery. Plasma cells are occasionally present beneath the epithelium. The cells in BALT have a high turnover rate and apparently do not produce immunoglobulin G (IgG). BALT development is independent of that of the peripheral lymphoid tissues or antigen exposure. The cells of BALT apparently migrate there from other lymphoid areas. This tissue plays an important role in mounting an immune response to inhaled antigens in respiratory infectious agents. Refer also to MALT.

bronchial asthma

Intermittent and reversible airway obstruction that results from repeated hypersensitivity reactions leading to inflammatory disease in the lung. Chronic inflammation of the bronchi with eosinophils, hypertrophy, and hyperreactivity of bronchial smooth muscle cells occur.

bronchiectasis

Chronic dilatation of the bronchi of the lungs associated with expectoration of mucopurulent material.

bronchodilator

Quick acting aerosolized β adrenergic drug that inhibits mast cell degranulation and relieves bronchoconstriction during acute asthma attacks.

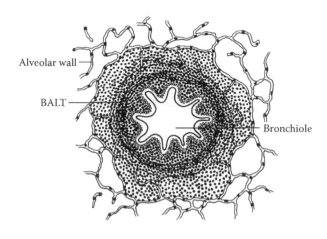

Bronchial-associated lymphoid tissue (BALT).

BRST-2 (GCDFP-15), monoclonal antibody (murine)

Detects BRST-2 antigen expressed by apocrine sweat glands, eccrine glands (variable), minor salivary glands, bronchial glands, metaplastic epithelium of the breast, benign sweat gland tumors of the skin, and the serous cells of the submandibular gland. Breast carcinomas (primary and metastatic lesions) with apocrine features express the BRST-2 antigen. BRST-2 is positive in extramammary Paget's disease. Other tumors tested are negative.

***Brucella* immunity**

The immune response to *Brucella* infection is marked by early immunoglobulin M (IgM) synthesis followed by a switch to IgG and IgA. IgE is also detected. IgM persists for an unusually long time, possibly responding to the T cell-independent antigen lipopolysaccharide (LPS). Antibodies are important for the serodiagnosis of *Brucella* infection. The only protective role of the antibody is probably as a pre-existing mucosal antibody that decreases

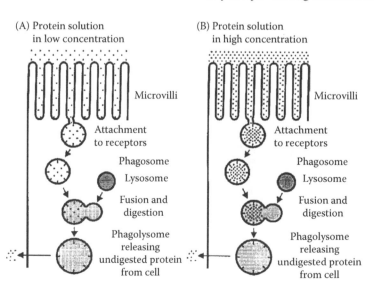

Mechanism of γ-globulin transmission by the cell. (A) Concentration of γ-globulin is only a little more than sufficient to saturate the receptors and the proportion degraded is less than 40%. (B) Concentration is about four times that in (A); hence over 80% is degraded. The amount released from the cell remains constant, regardless of concentration.

initial infection. Cell-mediated immune responses confer protective immunity. *Brucella* is a facultative, intracellular bacteria controlled by macrophage activation and granuloma formation to isolate the infectious agents. Both CD4⁺ and CD8⁺ T lymphocytes participate in the experimental infection in mice. The CD4⁺ T cells synthesize interferon-γ (IFN-γ) and the CD8⁺ T cells lyse ineffective macrophages. Interleukin-12 (IL-12) is important in controlling the differentiation of T cells and natural killer (NK) cells to produce IFN-γ, which facilitates cell-mediated immunity. IL-1, TNF-α, IL-6, M-CSF, and G-CSF are all produced during experimental infection. Minute granulomata comprised of epithelioid cells, neutrophils, mononuclear leukocytes, and giant cells are produced in the tissues of humans infected with *Brucella* species. Hepatosplenomegaly is a common clinical feature. Delayed-type hypersensitivity, which is a correlate of cell-mediated immunity, induces immuno-pathological changes. The granulomata is accompanied by development of a severe, generalized, delayed-type hypersensitivity response that mimics many features of the infection. Diagnosis depends on testing for antibodies in the serum. Most of the antibodies are directed against LPS. The agglutination test is the one most widely used but is being replaced by ELISA. Whereas *B. abortus* strain 19 is employed to immunize cattle and *B. melitensis* stain Rev 1 is used to immunize sheep and goats, human vaccination has been employed essentially only in Russia. Other preventive measures include pasteurization of milk products.

Brucella vaccine
A preparation used for the prophylactic immunization of cattle. It contains live, attenuated *Brucella abortus* microorganisms. A second vaccine comprised of McEwen strain 45/20 killed microorganisms in a water-in-oil emulsion (adjuvant) has also been used.

brucellin
A substance similar to tuberculin but derived from a culture filtrate of *Brucella abortus* that is used to test for the presence of delayed-type hypersensitivity to *Brucella* antigens. The test is of questionable value in diagnosis.

brush border
Dense microvilli on the apical surfaces of intestinal epithelial cells that significantly increase their surface area.

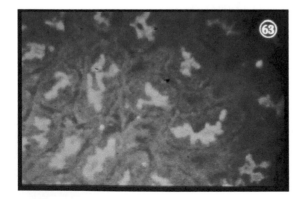

brush-border autoantibodies
Antibodies associated with Heymann nephritis in rats as well as in half of patients with ulcerative proctocolitis, in

20% of patients with antibodies to *Yersinia enterocolitica* 0:3, and in patients who are extensively burned.

Bruton's agammaglobulinemia
Synonym for X-linked agammaglobulinemia.

Bruton's X-linked agammaglobulinemia
One of the more common immunodeficiencies. There is a failure of B cell precursors, i.e., pro-B cells and pre-B cells, to mature into B cells. The defect is in rearrangement of immunoglobulin heavy chain genes. B cell maturation ceases after the heavy chain genes are rearranged. Light chains are not produced, which prevents assembly of the complete immunoglobulin molecule. The block in differentiation is attributable to mutations in cytoplasmic B cell tyrosine kinase (*Btk*). It occurs almost entirely in males and is apparent after 6 months of age following disappearance of the passively transferred maternal immunoglobulins. Patients have recurrent sinopulmonary infections caused by *Haemophilus influenzae, Streptococcus pyogenes, Staphylococcus aureus, and Streptococcus pneumoniae*. These patients have absent or decreased B cells and decreased serum levels of all immunoglobulin classes. The T cell system and cell-mediated immunity appear normal.

BSA
Abbreviation for bovine serum albumin.

BSF (B lymphocyte stimulatory factor)
Refer to interleukins 4, 5, and 6.

B symptoms
Inexplicable rapid weight loss, fatigue, fever, and night sweats often associated with chest pain that occur in lymphoma patients.

Btk
A protein tyrosine kinase coded for by the defective gene in X-linked agammaglobulinemia (XLA). B lymphocytes and polymorphonuclear neutrophils express the Btk protein. In patients with XLA (Bruton's disease), only the B lymphocytes manifest the defect, and the maturation of B lymphocytes stops at the pre-B cell stage. Rearrangement of heavy chain but not light chain genes occurs. The Btk protein may have a role in linking the pre-B cell receptor to nuclear changes that result in growth and differentiation of pre-B cells.

bubble boy
A 12-year-old male child maintained in a germ-free (gnotobiotic) environment in a plastic bubble from birth because of his severe combined immunodeficiency (SCID). A bone marrow transplant from a histocompatible sister was treated with monoclonal antibodies and complement to diminish alloreactive T lymphocytes. The boy died of a B cell lymphoma as a consequence of Epstein–Barr virus-induced polyclonal gammopathy that transformed into monoclonal proliferation, leading to lymphoma.

Buchner, Hans (1850–1902)
German bacteriologist who was a professor of hygiene in Munich in 1894 and discovered complement. Through his studies of normal serum and its bactericidal effects, he became an advocate of the humoral theory of immunity.

buffy coat
The white cell layer that forms between the red cells and plasma when anticoagulated blood is centrifuged.

bullous pemphigoid
A blistering skin disease with fluid-filled bullae developing at flexor surfaces of extremities, groin, axillae, and inferior abdomen. Immunoglobulin G (IgG) is deposited in a linear

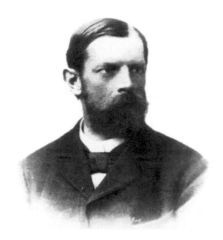

Hans Buchner (1850–1902).

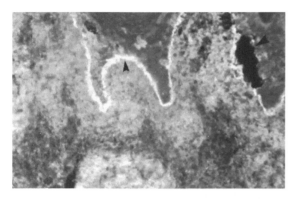

▲ Bulla formation
▲ Linear IgG and C3
   at dermal-epidermal junction

Bullous pemphigoid.

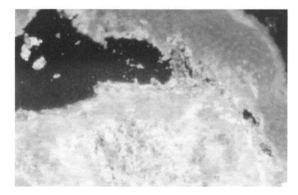

Bullous pemphigoid.

pattern at the lamina lucida of the dermal–epidermal junction in most patients (50 to 90%) and at linear C3 in nearly all cases. The blisters are subepidermal bullae filled with fluid containing fibrin, neutrophils, eosinophils, and lymphocytes. Antigen–antibody–complement interaction and mast cell degranulation release mediators that attract inflammatory cells and facilitate dermal–epidermal separation.

bullous pemphigoid antigen

The principal antigen is a 230-kDa basic glycoprotein produced by keratinocytes in the epidermis. Autoantibody and complement react with this antigen to produce bullous pemphigoid skin lesions.

bungarotoxin

An anticholinergic neurotoxin extracted from the venom of Australian snakes belonging to the genus *Bungarus*. It binds to acetylcholine receptors of the nicotinic type and inhibits depolarization of the neuromuscular junction's postsynaptic membrane, leading to muscular weakness.

Bunyaviridae immunity

Bunyaviridae are very immunogenic, stimulating the formation of neutralizing antibodies that are type-specific and reveal limited crossreactivity within the genus. Solid immunity that follows infection protects against reinfection. The immune responses in some individuals may be too late to prevent central nervous system or liver invasion. For example, Rift Valley fever virus may lead to liver necrosis and high mortality. Some American hantaviruses produce the greatest effect on the lungs rather than the liver, kidneys, or central nervous system, leading to hantavirus pulmonary syndrome. G1 glycoprotein antibodies neutralize viral infectivity and prevent hemagglutination. The dominant antigen is nucleocapsid protein in complement-fixation assays. Little is known regarding the role of cell-mediated immunity in resistance. Formalin-inactivated veterinary vaccines against Rift Valley fever and Nairobi sheep disease are available.

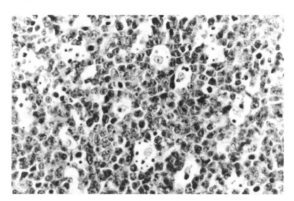

Burkitt's lymphoma.

Burkitt's lymphoma

An Epstein–Barr virus-induced neoplasm of B lymphocytes that affects the jaws and abdominal viscera. It is seen especially in African children. The Epstein–Barr virus is present in tumor cells that may reveal rearrangement between the c-*myc*-bearing chromosome and the immunoglobulin-heavy chain gene-bearing chromosome. Burkitt's lymphoma patients have antibodies to the Epstein–Barr virus in their blood sera. The disease occurs in geographic regions that are hot and humid and where malaria is endemic. It occurs in subjects with acquired immunodeficiency and in other immunosuppressed individuals. There is an effective immune response against the lymphoma that may lead to remission.

Burnet, Frank Macfarlane (1899–1985)

Australian virologist and immunologist who shared the Nobel Prize in Medicine or Physiology with Peter B. Medawar in 1960 for the discovery of acquired immunological tolerance. Burnet was a theoretician who made major contributions to the developing theories of self tolerance and clonal selection in antibody formation. Burnet and

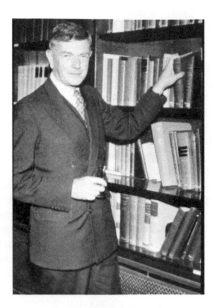

Frank Macfarlane Burnet.

Fenner's suggested explanation of immunologic tolerance was tested by Medawar et al., who confirmed the hypothesis in 1953 using inbred strains of mice. (Refer to *Production of Antibodies* [with Fenner], 1949; *Natural History of Infectious Diseases,* 1953; *Clonal Selection Theory of Antibody Formation,* 1959; *Autoimmune Diseases* [with Mackay], 1962; *Cellular Immunology,* 1969; *Changing Patterns* [autobiography], 1969.)

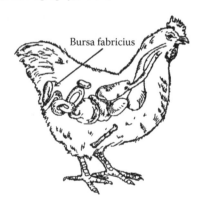

Bursa fabricius

Bursa of Fabricius.

bursa of Fabricius

An outpouching of the hindgut located near the cloaca in avian species that governs B cell ontogeny. This specific lymphoid organ is the site of migration and maturation of B lymphocytes. The bursa is located near the terminal portion of the cloaca and, like the thymus, is a lymphoepithelial organ. The bursa begins to develop after the 5th day of incubation and becomes functional around the 10th to 12th day. It has an asymmetric sac-like shape and a star-like lumen, which is continuous with the cloacal cavity. The epithelium of the intestine covers the bursal lumen but lacks mucous cells. The bursa contains abundant lymphoid tissue, forming nodules beneath the epithelium. The nodules show a central medullary region containing epithelial cells and project into the epithelial coating. The center of the medullary region is less structured and also

contains macrophages, large lymphocytes, plasma cells, and granulocytes. A basement membrane separates the medulla from the cortex; the latter is composed mostly of small lymphocytes and plasma cells. The bursa is well developed at birth but begins to involute around the fourth month; it is vestigial at the end of the first year. There is a direct relationship between the hormonal status of the bird and involution of the bursa. Injections of testosterone may lead to premature regression or even lack of development, depending on the time of hormone administration. The lymphocytes in the bursa originate from the yolk sac and migrate there via the bloodstream. They are composed of B cells that undergo maturation to immunocompetent cells capable of antibody synthesis. Bursectomy at the 17th day of incubation induces agammaglobulinemia, with the absence of germinal centers and plasma cells in peripheral lymphoid organs.

bursacyte

A lymphocyte that undergoes maturation and differentiation under the influence of the bursa of Fabricius in avian species. This cell synthesizes the antibody that provides humoral immunity in this species. A bursacyte is a B lymphocyte.

bursal equivalent

The anatomical site in mammals and other nonavian species that resembles the bursa of Fabricius in controlling B cell ontogeny. Mammals do not have a specialized lymphoid organ for maturation of B lymphocytes. Although lymphoid nodules are present along the gut, forming distinct structures called Peyer's patches, their role in B cell maturation is no different from that of lymphoid structures in other organs. After commitment to B cell lineage, the B cells of mammals leave the bone marrow in a relatively immature stage; likewise, after education in the thymus, T cells migrate from the thymus, also in a relatively immature stage. Both populations continue their maturation process away from the site of origin and are subject to influences originating in the environment in which they reside.

$$H_3C-\overset{\overset{\displaystyle O}{\|}}{\underset{\underset{\displaystyle O}{\|}}{S}}-O-CH_2-CH_2-CH_2-CH_2-O-\overset{\overset{\displaystyle O}{\|}}{\underset{\underset{\displaystyle O}{\|}}{S}}-CH_3$$

1,4–butanediol dimethanesulfonate

Structure of busulfan.

bursectomy

The surgical removal or ablation of the bursa of Fabricius, an outpouching of the hindgut near the cloaca in birds. Surgical removal of the bursa prior to hatching or shortly thereafter followed by treatment with testosterone *in vivo* leads to failure of the B cell limb of the immune response responsible for antibody production.

busulfan (1,4-butanediol dimethanesulfonate)

An alkylating drug that is toxic to bone marrow cells and is used to condition bone marrow transplant recipients.

butterfly rash

A facial rash in the form of a butterfly across the bridge of the nose seen especially in patients with lupus erythematosus. These areas are photosensitive and consist of

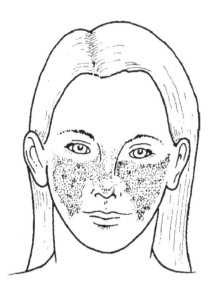

Butterfly rash.

erythematous and scaly patches that may become bulbous or secondarily infected. The rash is not specific for lupus erythematosus; it may appear in various other conditions including AIDS, dermatomyositis, ataxia–telangiectasia, erysipelas, pemphigus erythematosus, pemphigus foliaceus, etc.

BXSB mice

A mouse strain genetically prone to developing lupus erythematosus-like disease spontaneously. The strain manifests serologic aberrations and immune complex glomerulonephritis but demonstrates a distinct and significant acceleration of the disease in males. Among other features, BXSB strains develop moderate lymphadenopathy 10 to 20 times greater than normal. The B cell content of these proliferating male lymph nodes may reach 70%. The B cell content also develops significant levels of antinuclear antibodies, including anti-DNA, diminished complement, and immune complex-mediated renal injury. Acceleration of this autoimmune disease in the male rather than in the female has been shown not to be hormone-mediated.

byssinosis

A disease of cotton, flax, jute, and hemp employees, probably attributable to hypersensitivity to vegetable fiber dust. These patients develop tightness in the chest upon returning to work after several days' absence.

bystander activation

B cell stimulation with T cell help provided by a T helper cell responding to an unrelated antigen.

bystander B cells

Non-antigen-specific B cells in the area of B cells specific for antigen. Released cytokines activate bystander B cells that synthesize nonspecific antibody following immunogenic challenge.

bystander effects

Indirect, non-antigen-specific phenomena that result in polyclonal responses. In contrast to antigen-specific interactions, bystander effects are the results of cellular interactions that take place without antigen recognition or under conditions in which antigen and receptors for antigen are not involved. Bystander effects are phenomena linked to the specific immune response in that they do not happen on their own but only in connection with a specific response. Cells not directly involved in the antigen-specific response are trans-stimulated or "carried along" in the response.

bystander lysis

Tissue cell lysis that is nonspecific. The tissue cells are not the specific targets during an immune response but are killed as innocent bystanders because of their proximity to the site where nonspecific factors are released near the actual target of the immune response. Bystander lysis may occur by the Fas/FasL pathway, depending on the polarity and kinetics of FasL surface expression and downregulation after T cell receptor (TCR) engagement. This cytotoxicity pathway may give rise to bystander lysis of Fas$^+$ target cells.

C

c allotype

A rabbit immunoglobulin λ light chain allotype 100 designated as c7 and c21.

C domain

Refer to constant domain.

C gene

DNA encoding the constant region of immunoglobulin heavy and light polypeptide chains. The heavy chain *C* gene is comprised of exons that encode the different homology regions of the heavy chain.

C gene segment

DNA coding for a T cell receptor or an immunoglobulin polypeptide chain constant region. One or more exons may be involved. Constant region gene segments comprise immunoglobulin and T cell receptor gene loci DNA sequences that encode TCR α and β chains and nonvariable regions of immunoglobulin heavy and light polypeptide chains.

C region

Refer to constant region.

C region (constant region)

Abbreviation for the constant region carboxyl terminal portion of immunoglobulin heavy or light polypeptide chain that is identical in a particular class or subclass of immunoglobulin molecules. C_H designates the constant region of the heavy chain of immunoglobulin, and C_L designates the constant region of the light chain.

C segment

An exon that encodes an immunoglobulin molecule's constant region domain.

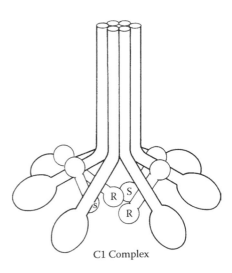

C1 Complex.

C1

A 750-kDa multimeric molecule comprised of one C1q, two C1r, and two C1s subcomponents. The classical pathway of complement activation begins with the binding of C1q to immunoglobulin M (IgM) or IgG molecules. C1q, C1r, and C1s form a macromolecular complex in a Ca^{2+}-dependent manner. The 400-kDa C1q molecule possesses three separate polypeptide chains that unite into a heterotrimeric structure resembling a stem that contains an amino terminal in triple helix and a globular structure at the carboxyl terminus resembling a tulip. Six of these tulip-like structures with globular heads and stems form a circular and symmetric molecular complex in the C1q molecule that has a central core. The serine esterase molecules designated $C\overline{1}r$ and C1s are needed for the complement cascade to progress. These single chain 85-kDa proteins unite in the presence of calcium to produce a tetramer comprised of two C1r and two C1s subcomponents to form a structure that is flexible and has a C1s–C1r–C1r–C1s sequence. When at least two C1q globular regions bind to IgM or IgG molecules, the $C\overline{1}r$ in a tetramer associated with the C1q molecule becomes activated, leading to splitting of the C1r molecules in the tetramer with the formation of 57- and a 28-kDa chains. The latter, termed C1r, functions as a serine esterase, splitting the $C\overline{1}s$ molecules into 57- and 28-kDa chains. The 28-kDa chain derived from the cleavage of C1s molecules, designated C1s, also functions as a serine esterase, cleaving C4 and C2 and causing progression of the classical complement pathway cascade.

C1 deficiencies

Only a few cases of C1q, C1r, or C1r and C1s deficiencies have been reported. The deficiencies have an autosomal-recessive mode of inheritance. Patients with these defects may manifest systemic lupus erythematosus (SLE), glomerulonephritis, or pyogenic infections. They exhibit increased incidence of type III (immune complex) hypersensitivity diseases. Half of C1q-deficient persons may contain physiologic levels of mutant C1q that are not functional.

C1 esterase inhibitor

A serum protein that counteracts activated C1. This diminishes the generation of C2b which facilitates development of edema.

C1 inhibitor (C1 INH)

A 478-amino acid residue, single polypeptide chain protein in the serum. It blocks C1r activation, prevents $C\overline{1}r$ cleavage of $C\overline{1}s$, and inhibits $C\overline{1}s$ splitting of C4 and C2. The molecule is highly glycosylated, with carbohydrates making up approximately one half of its content. It contains seven O-linked oligosaccharides linked to serine and six N-linked oligosaccharides tethered to an asparagine residue. Besides its effects on the complement system, C1 INH blocks factors in the blood clotting system, including kallikrein, plasmin, factor XIa, and factor XIIa. C1 INH is an α_2 globulin and is a normal serum constituent that inhibits serine protease. The 104-kDa C1 INH interacts with activated C1r or C1s to produce a stable complex that prevents these serine protease molecules from splitting their usual substrates. Either C̄1s or C̄1r can split C1 INH to uncover an active site in the inhibitor that becomes bound to the proteases through a covalent ester bond. By binding to most of the C1 in the blood, C1 INH blocks the spontaneous activation of C1. C1 INH binding blocks conformational alterations that would lead to spontaneous activation of C1. When an antigen–antibody complex binds C1, the inhibitory influence of C1 INH on C1 is relinquished. Genes on chromosome 11 in humans encode C1 INH. C1r and C1s subcomponents disengage from C1q following their interaction with C1 INH. In hereditary angioneurotic edema, C1 INH formation is defective. In acquired C1 INH deficiency, catabolism of C1 INH is elevated.

C1 inhibitor (C1 INH) deficiency

The absence of C1 INH is the most frequently found deficiency of the classic complement pathway and may be seen in patients with hereditary angioneurotic edema. This syndrome may be expressed as either a lack of the inhibitor substance or a functionally inactive C1 INH. The patient develops edema of the face; of the respiratory tract, including the glottis and bronchi; and of the extremities. Severe abdominal pain may occur with intestinal involvement. Because C1 INH can block Hagemann factor (factor XII) in the blood clotting mechanism, its absence can lead to the liberation of kinin and fibrinolysis resulting from the activation of plasmin. The disease is inherited as an autosomal-dominant trait. When edema of the larynx occurs, the patient may die of asphyxiation. When abdominal attacks occur, watery diarrhea and vomiting may occur. These bouts usually span 48 hours and are followed by a rapid recovery. During an attack of angioedema, C1r is activated to produce C̄1s, which depletes its substrates C4 and C2. The action of activated C1s on C4 and C2 leads to the production of a substance that increases vascular permeability, especially that of postcapillary venules. C1 and C4 cooperate with plasmin to split this active peptide from C2. Of the families of patients with hereditary angioneurotic edema, 85% do not have C1 INH. Treatment is by preventive maintenance. Patients are given inhibitors of plasmin such as ε-aminocaproic acid and tranexamic acid. Methyl testosterone, which causes synthesis of normal C1 INH in angioneurotic edema patients, is effective by an unknown mechanism.

C1q

An 18-polypeptide-chain subcomponent of C1, the first component of complement. It commences the classical complement pathway. The three types of polypeptide chains are designated A, B, and C. Disulfide bonds link these chains. The triple helix structures of the C1q molecule are parallel and resemble the stems of six tulips in the amino terminal half of the structure. They then separate into six globular regions that resemble the heads of a tulip. The molecule is arranged in a heterotrimeric rod-like configuration, bearing a collagen-like triple helix at its amino terminus and a tulip-like globular region at its carboxyl terminus. The combination of six of the rod-shaped structures leads to a symmetric molecular arrangement comprised of three helices at one terminus and the globular (tulip-like) heads at the

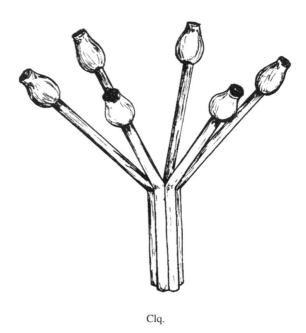

C1q.

other terminus. The binding of antibody to C1q initiates the classic complement pathway. It is the globular C-terminal region of the molecule that binds to either immunoglobulin M (IgM) or IgG molecules. A tetramer comprised of two molecules of C1r and two molecules of C1s bind by Ca^{2+} to the collagen-like part of the stem. The C1q A chain and C1q B chain are coded for by genes on chromosome 1p in humans. The interaction of C1q with antigen–antibody complexes represents the basis for assays for immune complexes in patients' serum. IgM, IgG_1, IgG_2, and IgG_3 bind C1q, whereas IgG_4, IgE, IgA, and IgD do not.

C1q autoantibodies

Autoantibodies are detectable in 14 to 52% of patients with systemic lupus erythematosus (SLE), in 100% of patients with hypocomplementemic urticarial vasculitis syndrome (HUVS), in patients with rheumatoid arthritis (RA) (5% of patients with uncomplicated RA and 77% of RA patients with Felty's syndrome), in 73% of patients with membranoproliferative glomerulonephritis type I, in 45% of patients with membranoproliferative glomerulonephritis types II and III, in 94% of patients of mixed connective tissue disease, and in 42% of patients with polyarteritis nodosa. Lupus nephritis patients usually reveal the immunoglobulin G (IgG) isotype. Rising levels of C1q autoantibodies portend renal flares in patients with SLE. The rare HUVS condition can occur together with SLE and is marked by diminished serum C1q and recurrent idiopathic urticaria with leukocytoclastic vasculitis.

C1q binding assay for circulating immune complexes (CICs)

There are two categories of methods to assay circulating immune complexes: (1) the specific binding of CICs to complement components, such as C1q, or the binding of complement activation fragments within the CICs to complement receptors, as in the Raji cell assay; and (2) precipitation of large and small CICs by polyethylene glycol. The C1q binding assay measures those CICs capable of binding C1q, a subcomponent of the C1 component of complement, and capable of activating the classical complement pathway.

C1q deficiency

Deficiency of C1q may be found in association with lupus-like syndromes. C1r deficiency, which is inherited as an autosomal-recessive trait, may be associated with respiratory tract infections, glomerulonephritis, and skin manifestations that resemble a systemic lupus erythematosus (SLE)-like disease. C1s deficiency is transmitted as an autosomal-dominant trait, and patients may again show SLE-like signs and symptoms. Their antigen–antibody complexes can persist without resolution.

C1q receptor (C1q-R)

A receptor that binds the collagen segments of C1q fixed to antigen–antibody complexes. The C1q globular head is the site of binding of the Fc region of immunoglobulin. Thus, the C1q-R can facilitate the attachment of antigen–antibody complexes to cells expressing C1q-R and Fc receptors. Neutrophils, B cells, monocytes, macrophages, natural killer (NK) cells, endothelial cells, platelets, and fibroblasts all express C1q-R. C1q-R stimulation on neutrophils may lead to a respiratory burst.

C1r

A subcomponent of C1, the first component of complement in the classical activation pathway. It is a serine esterase. Ca^{2+} binds C1r molecules to the stem of a C1q molecule. Following binding of at least two globular regions of C1q with immunoglobulin M (IgM) or IgG, C1r is split into a 463-amino acid residue α chain, the N terminal fragment, and a 243-amino acid residue carboxyl-terminal β chain fragment where the active site is situated. C1s becomes activated when C1r splits its arginine–isoleucine bond. Refer also to C1.

C1s

A serine esterase that is a subcomponent of C1, the first component of complement in the classical activation pathway. Ca^{2+} binds two C1s molecules to the C1q stalk. Following activation, C1r splits the single-chain, 85-kDa C1s molecule into a 431-amino acid residue A chain and a 243-amino acid residue B chain where the active site is located. C̄1s splits a C4 arginine–alanine bond and a C2 arginine–lysine bond.

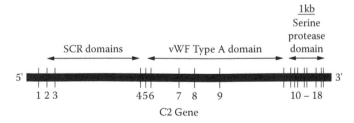

Schematic representation of the exon/intron organization of the human *C2* gene. Exons, represented by vertical bars, are numbered.

C2 (complement component 2)

The third complement protein to participate in the classical complement pathway activation. C2 is a 110-kDa single polypeptide chain that unites with C4b molecules on cell surfaces in the presence of Mg^{2+}. C1s splits C2 following its combination with C4b at the cell surface. This yields a 35-kDa C2b molecule and a 75-kDa C2a fragment. Whereas C2b may leave the cell surface, C2a continues to be associated with surface C4b. The complex of C4b2a constitutes classical pathway C3 convertase. This enzyme is able to bind and split C3. C4b facilitates combination with C3. C2b catalyzes the enzymatic cleavage. C2a contains the active site of classical pathway C3 convertase (C4̄b2̄a). C2 is encoded by genes on the short arm of chromosome 6 in humans. *C2A*, *C2B*, and *C2C* alleles encode human C2. Murine C2 is encoded by genes at the S region of chromosome 17.

C2a

The principal substance produced by C̄1s* cleavage of C2. N-linked oligosaccharides may combine with C2a at six sites. The 509 carboxyl terminal amino acid residues of C2 constitute C2a. The catalytic site for C3 and C5 cleavage is located in the 287-residue carboxyl terminal sequence. The association of C2a with C4b yields the C3 convertase (C4̄b2̄a)* of the classical pathway.

C2b

A 223-amino acid terminal residue of C2 that represents a lesser product of C̄1s cleavage of C2. Three abbreviated 68-amino acid residue homologous repeats in C2b are present in C3- or C4-binding proteins. N-linked oligosaccharides combine with C2b at two sites. A peptide split from the carboxyl terminus of C2b by plasmin has been implicated in the formation of edema in hereditary angioneurotic edema patients.

C2 and *B* genes

The *C2* and *B* genes are situated within the major histocompatibility complex (MHC) locus on the short arm of chromosome 6. They are termed MHC class III genes. TNFα and TNFβ genes are situated between the *C2* and *HLA-B* genes. Another gene designated *FD* lies between the *Bf* and *C4a* genes. C2 and B complete primary structures have been deduced from cDNA and protein sequences. C2 is comprised of 732 residues and is an 81-kDa molecule, whereas B contains 739 residues and is an 83-kDa molecule. Both proteins have a three-domain globular structure. During C3 convertase formation, the amino terminal domains, C2b or Ba, are split off. They contain consensus repeats that are present in CR1, CR2, H, DAF, and C4bp, which all combine with C3 and/or C4 fragments and regulate C3 convertases. The amino acid sequences of the C2 and B consensus repeats are known. C2b contains site(s) significant for C2 binding to C4b. Ba, resembling C2b, manifests binding site(s) significant in C3 convertase

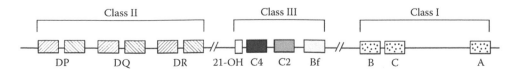

C2 and *B* genes are situated within the major histocompatibility complex (MHC) locus on the short arm of chromosome 6.

C

assembly. Available evidence indicates that C2b possesses a C4b-binding site and that Ba contains a corresponding C3b-binding site. In considering assembly and decay of C3 convertases, initial binding of the three-domain structures C2 or B to activator-bound C4b or C3b, respectively, requires one affinity site on the C2b/Ba domain and another on one of the remaining two domains. A transient change in C2a and Bb conformation results from C2 or B cleavage by $\overline{C1s}$ or D. This leads to greater binding affinity, Mg^{2+} sequestration, and acquisition of proteolytic activity for C3. C2a or Bb dissociation leads to C3 convertase decay. Numerous serum-soluble and membrane-associated regulatory proteins control the rate of formation and association of C3 convertases.

C2 deficiency

Rare individuals may demonstrate a failure to express C2. Although no symptoms are normally associated with this trait, which has an autosomal-recessive mode of inheritance, autoimmune-like manifestations that resemble features of certain collagen-vascular diseases, such as systemic lupus erythematosus (SLE), may appear. Thus, many genetically determined complement deficiencies are not associated with signs and symptoms of disease. When they do occur, it is usually manifested as an increased incidence of infectious diseases that affect the kidneys, respiratory tract, skin, and joints.

C3 (complement component 3)

A 195-kDa glycoprotein heterodimer that is linked by disulfide bonds. It is the fourth complement component to react in the classical pathway, and it is also a reactant in the alternative complement pathway. C3 contains α and β polypeptide chains and has an internal thioester bond that permits it to link covalently with surfaces of cells and proteins. Much of the C3 gene structure has now been elucidated. It is believed to contain approximately 41 exons. Eighteen of 36 introns have now been sequenced. The human C3 gene is located on chromosome 19. Hepatocytes, monocytes, fibroblasts, and endothelial cells can synthesize C3. More than 90% of serum C3 is synthesized in the liver. The concentration of C3 in serum exceeds that of any other complement component. Human C3 is generated as a single chain precursor which is cleaved into the two-chain mature state. C3 molecules are identical antigenically, structurally, and functionally, regardless of cell source. Hepatocytes and monocytes synthesize greater quantities of C3 than do epithelial and endothelial cells. C3 convertases split a 9-kDa C3a

fragment from the α chain of C3. The other product of the reaction is C3b, which is referred to as metastable C3b and has an exposed thioester bond. Approximately 90% of the metastable C3b thioester bonds interact with H_2O to form inactive C3b byproducts that have no role in the complement sequence. Ten percent of C3b molecules may bind to cell substances through covalent bonds or with the immunoglobulin bound to $\overline{C4b2a}$. This interaction leads to the formation of $\overline{C4b2a3b}$, which is classical pathway C5 convertase, and serves as a catalyst in the enzymatic splitting of C5, which initiates membrane attack complex (MAC) formation. When C3b, in the classical complement pathway, interacts with E (erythocyte), A (antibody), C1 (complement 1), and 4b2a, EAC14b2a3b is produced. As many as 500 C3b molecules may be deposited at a single EAC14b2a complex on an erythrocyte surface. *C3S* (slow electrophoretic mobility) and *C3F* (fast electrophoretic mobility) alleles on chromosome 19 in humans encode 99% of C3, with rare alleles accounting for the remainder. C3 has the highest concentration in serum of any complement system protein with a range of 0.552 to 1.2 mg/ mL. Following splitting of the internal thioester bond, it can form a covalent link to amino or hydroxyl groups on erythrocytes, microorganisms, or other substances. C3 is an excellent opsonin. It was known in the past as $\beta_1 C$ globulin.

C3 convertase

An enzyme that splits C3 into C3b and C3a. There are two types: one in the classical pathway designated $\overline{C4b2a}$ and one in the alternative pathway of complement activation termed $\overline{C3bBb}$. An amplification loop with a positive feedback is stimulated by alternative pathway C3 convertase. Each of the two types of C3 convertase lacks stability, leading to the ready disassociation of their constituents. However, C3 nephritic factor can stabilize both classical and alternative pathway C3 convertases. Properdin may stabilize alternative pathway C3 convertase. C2a and Bb contain the catalytic sites.

C3 deficiency

An extremely uncommon genetic disorder that may be associated with repeated serious pyogenic bacterial infections and may lead to death. C3-deficient individuals are deprived of appropriate opsonization, prompt phagocytosis, and the ability to kill infecting microorganisms. Classical and alternative pathway activation is defective. Besides infections, these individuals may also develop an immune complex disease such as glomerulonephritis. C3 levels that

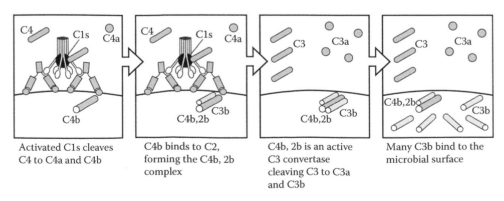

Activated C1s cleaves C4 to C4a and C4b

C4b binds to C2, forming the C4b, 2b complex

C4b, 2b is an active C3 convertase cleaving C3 to C3a and C3b

Many C3b bind to the microbial surface

Classical pathway of complement activation generates a C3 convertase.

are one half normal in heterozygotes are apparently sufficient to avoid the clinical consequences induced by a lack of C3 in the serum.

C3 nephritic factor (C3NeF)

An immunoglobulin G (IgG) autoantibody to the alternate complement pathway C3 convertase that mimics the action of properdin. C3NeF is present in the sera of patients with membranoproliferative glomerulonephritis type II (dense deposit disease). It stabilizes the alternate pathway C3 convertase, thereby enhancing the breakdown of C3, and produces hypocomplementemia. Rarely, C3NeF may be IgG autoantibodies to C3 convertase ($\overline{C4b2a}$) of the classical pathway. Patients with systemic lupus erythematosus (SLE) may contain antibodies against $\overline{C4b2a}$ which stabilize the classical pathway C3 convertase, leading to increased *in vivo* cleavage of C3.

C3 PA (C3 proactivator)

An earlier designation for factor B.

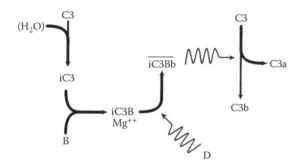

C3 tickover mechanism.

C3 tickover

Alternative pathway C3 convertase perpetually generates C3b. C3 internal thioester bond hydrolysis is the initiating event.

C3a

A low molecular weight (9-kDa) peptide fragment of complement component C3. It is comprised of the 77 N terminal end residues of the C3 α chain. This biologically active anaphylatoxin that induces histamine release from mast cells and causes smooth muscle contraction is produced by the cleavage of C3 by either classical pathway C3 convertase (i.e., $\overline{C4b2a}$) or alternative complement pathway C3 convertase (i.e., $\overline{C3bBb}$). Anaphylatoxin inactivator, a carboxyl peptidase N, can inactivate C3a by digesting the C terminal arginine of C3a.

C3a receptor (C3a-R)

A protein on the surface membranesof mast cells and basophils. It serves as a C3a anaphylatoxin receptor.

C3a/C4a receptor (C3a/C4a-R)

C3a and C4a share a common receptor on mast cells. When a C terminal arginine is removed from C3a and C4a by serum carboxyl peptidase N (SCPN), these anaphylatoxins lose their ability to activate cellular responses. Thus, $C3a_{des\,Arg}$ and $C4a_{des\,Arg}$ lose their ability to induce spasmogenic responses. C3a-R has been demonstrated on guinea pig platelets. Eosinophils have been found to bind C3a.

C3b

The principal fragment produced when complement component C3 is split by either classical or alternative pathway convertases (*i.e.,* $\overline{C4b2a}$ or $\overline{C3bBb}$, respectively). It results

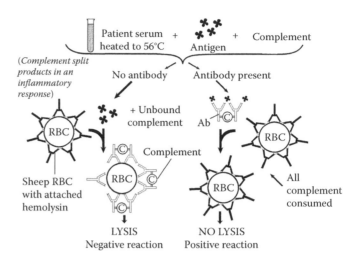

Complement fixation.

from C3 convertase digestion of the α chain of C3. It is an active fragment, as revealed by its combination with factor B to produce $\overline{C3bBb}$, the alternative pathway C3 convertase. Classical complement pathway C5 convertase is produced when C3b combines with $\overline{C4b2a}$ to yield $\overline{C4b2a3b}$. Factor I splits the arginine–serine bonds in C3b, if factor H is present, to yield C3bi. This produces the C3f peptide. Particle-bound C3b interacts with complement receptor 1. C3b interacts with C3b receptors on macrophages, B lymphocytes, polymorphonuclear neutrophils (PMNs), and possibly T cells. It promotes phagocytosis and immune adherence and may function as an opsonin.

C3b inactivator

Refer to factor I.

C3b receptor

Refer to complement receptor 1 (CR1).

C3bi (iC3b)

The principal molecular product when factor I cleaves C3b. If complement receptor 1 or factor H is present, factor I can split the arginine–glutamic acid bond of C3bi at position 954–955 to yield C3c and C3dg. C3bi attached to particles promotes phagocytosis when combined with complement receptor 3 on the surfaces of polymorphonuclear neutrophils (PMNs) and monocytes. It also promotes phagocytosis by binding to conglutinin in the sera of cows.

C3c

The principal molecule that results from factor I cleavage of C3bi when factor H or complement receptor 1 is present. C3c is comprised of 27- and 43-kDa α chain fragments linked through disulfide bonds to a whole β chain.

C3d

A 33-kDa B cell growth factor formed by proteolytic enzyme splitting of a lysine–histidine bond in C3dg at position 1001–1002. C3d is comprised of the carboxyl terminal 301-amino acid residues of C3dg. It interacts with complement receptor 2 on the surfaces of B cells. C3d contains the C3 α chain thioester.

C3dg

A 41-kDa, 349-amino acid residue molecule formed by the cleavage of C3bi, with factor H or complement receptor 1 present. Polymorphonuclear neutrophil leukocytes express complement receptor 4, which is reactive with C3dg. Complement receptor 2 on B cells is also a C3dg receptor.

C

C3e

A C3c α chain nonapeptide that causes leukocytosis. The peptide is comprised of Thr–Leu–Asp–Pro–Glu–Arg– Leu–Gly–Arg.

C3f

A 17-amino acid residue peptide split from the α chain of C3b by factor I, with factor H or complement receptor 1 present.

C3g

An 8-kDa molecule comprised of the amino terminal, 47-amino acid residues of C3dg. Trypsin digestion of C3dg yields C3g, whose function is unknown.

C3H/HeJ mouse

A mutant substrain of C3H mice that manifests a suppressed response by macrophages and B cells to challenge with lipopolysaccharide. Their macrophages do not produce interleukin-1 (IL1) and tumor necrosis factor (TNF) following the lipopolysaccharide challenge. This mutation has an autosomal-dominant mode of inheritance and is encoded by genes on chromosome 4. This immunosuppression leads to an increased incidence of microbial infections in these mice.

C4 allotype

Complement component 4 (C4) is encoded by two genes designated C4A and C4B, located within the major histocompatibility complex (MHC) class III region on the short arm of chromosome 6 in humans. Each locus has numerous allelic forms, including nonexpressed or null alleles. C4A is usually Rodgers-negative and Chido-negative, whereas C4B is usually Rodgers-negative and Chido-positive. C4 protein is highly polymorphic with more than 40 variants that include null alleles (C4Q0) at both loci. Null alleles are defined by the absence of C4 protein in plasma and exist in normal populations at frequencies of 0.1 to 0.3%. The presence and number of null alleles determine the expected reference range of serum C4.

C4 (complement component 4)

A 210-kDa molecule comprised of α, β, and γ chains. The α chain has an internal thioester bond linking a cysteine residue and adjacent glutamate residue. C4 reacts immediately following C1 in the classical pathway of complement activation. $\overline{C1s}$ splits the α chain of C4 at position 76–77, where an arginine–alanine bond is located. This yields a 8.6-kDa C4a fragment, an anaphylatoxin, and C4b, which is a larger molecule. C4b remains linked to C1. Many C4b molecules can be formed through the action of a single $\overline{C1s}$ molecule. Enzymatic cleavage renders the α chain thioester bond of the C4b fragment very unstable. The chemically active form of the molecule is termed metastable C4b. C4bi intermediates form when C4b thioester bonds and water molecules react. C4b molecules may become bound covalently to cell surfaces when selected C4b thioester bonds undergo trans-esterification, producing covalent amide or ester bonds with proteins or carbohydrates on the cell surface. This enables complement activation to take place on the surfaces of cells where antibodies bind. C4b may also link covalently with antibody. C4 is first formed as a 1700-amino acid residue chain that contains α, β, and γ chain components joined through connecting peptides. C4A and C4B genes located at the major histocompatibility complex on the short arm of chromosome 6 in humans encode C4. Slp and Ss genes located on chromosome 17 in the mouse encode murine C4.

C4 deficiency

An uncommon genetic defect with an autosomal-recessive mode of inheritance. Affected individuals have defective classical complement pathway activation. Those who manifest clinical consequences of the defect may develop systemic lupus erythematosus (SLE) or glomeruloneophritis. Half of the patients with C4 and C2 deficiencies develop SLE, but deficiencies in these two complement components are not usually linked to increased infections.

C4a

A 76-amino acid terminal residue peptide produced by $\overline{C1s}$ cleavage of C4. Together with C3a and C5a, C4a is an anaphylatoxin that induces degranulation of mast cells and basophils associated with histamine release and the features of anaphylaxis. However, the anaphylatoxin activity of C4a is 100 times weaker than those of the other two anaphylatoxin molecules.

C4A

A very polymorphic molecule expressing the Rodgers epitope encoded by the C4A gene. The equivalent murine gene encodes a sex-limited protein (SLP). It has less hemolytic activity than does C4B. C4A and C4B differ in only four amino acid residues in the C4d region of the α chain. C4A is Pro–Cys–Pro–Bal–Leu–Asp, whereas C4B is Leu–Ser–Pro–Bal–Ile–His.

C4b

The principal molecule produced when $\overline{C1s}$ splits C4. C4b is that part of the C4 molecule that remains after C4a has been split off by enzymatic digestion. C4b unites with C2a to produce $C\overline{4b2a}$, an enzyme known as the classical pathway C3 convertase. Factor I splits the arginine– asparagine bond of C4b at position 1318–1319 to yield C4bi, if C4b binding protein is present. C4b linked to particulate substances reacts with complement receptor 1.

C4B

A polymorphic molecule that usually expresses the Chido epitope and is encoded by the C4B gene. The murine equivalent gene encodes an Ss protein. It shows greater hemolytic activity than does C4A.

C4b-binding protein (C4bp)

A 600-kDa protein in serum capable of binding six C4b molecules at once by means of seven spokes extending from a core at the center. C4b halts progression of complement activation. Factor I splits C4b molecules captured by C4bp. C4bp belongs to the regulators of complement activity molecules. C4bp interferes with C2a association with C4b. It also promotes C4b2a dissociation into C4b and C2a and is necessary for the action of factor I in splitting C4b to C4bi and of C4bi into C4c and C4d. The C4bp gene is located on chromosome 1q3.2.

C4b inactivator

Refer to factor I.

C4bi (iC4b)

When factor I splits C4b, C4bi is the principal product of the reaction. When C4b-binding protein is present, C4bi splits an α chain arginine–threonine bond to yield C4c and C4d.

C4c

The principal product of factor I cleavage of C4bi when C4b-binding protein is present. This 145-kDa molecule of unknown function is comprised of β and γ chains of C4 and two α chain fragments.

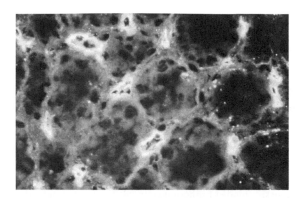

Immunofluorescence staining of C4d in peritubular capillaries.

C4d

A 45-kDa molecule produced by factor I cleavage of C4bi when C4b-binding protein is present. C4d is the molecule in which Chido and Rodgers epitopes are located. It is also the location of the C4 α chain's internal thioester bond. C4d staining of peritubular capillaries, demonstrable by immunofluorescence, in renal allotransplants suggests a humoral antibody component of renal allograft rejection.

C5 (complement component 5)

A component comprised of α and β polypeptide chains linked by disulfide bonds that react in the complement cascade following C1, C4b, C2a, and C3b fixation to complexes of antibody and antigen. The 190-kDa dimeric C5 molecule shares homology with C3 and C4 but does not possess an internal thioester bond. C5 combines with C3b of C5 convertase of either the classical or the alternative pathway. C5 convertases split the α chain at an arginine–leucine bond at position 74–75, producing an 11-kDa C5a fragment that has both chemotactic action for neutrophils and anaphylatoxin activity. It also produces a 180-kDa C5b fragment that remains anchored to the cell surface. C5b maintains a structure that is able to bind with C6. C5 is a $\beta_1 F$ globulin in humans. C5b complexes with C6, C7, C8, and C9 to form the membrane attack complex (MAC), which mediates immune lysis of cells. Murine C5 is encoded by genes on chromosome 2.

C5 convertase

A molecular complex that splits C5 into C5a and C5b in both the classical and the alternative pathways of complement activation. Classical pathway C5 convertase is comprised of $\overline{C4b2a3b}$, whereas alternative pathway C5 convertase is comprised of $\overline{C3bBb3b}$. C2a and Bb contain the catalytic sites.

C5 deficiency

A very uncommon genetic disorder that has an autosomal recessive mode of inheritance. Affected individuals have only trace amounts of C5 in their plasma and have a defective ability to form the membrane attack complex (MAC) necessary for the efficient lysis of invading microorganisms. They have increased susceptibility to disseminated infections by *Neisseria* microorganisms such as *N. meningitidis* and *N. gonorrhoeae*. Heterozygotes may manifest 13 to 65% of C5 activity in their plasma and usually show no clinical effects of their partial deficiency. C5-deficient mice have also been described.

C5a

A peptide split from C5 through the action of C5 convertases, $\overline{C4b2a3b}$ or $\overline{C3bBb3b}$. It is comprised of the 74 amino terminal residues of the C5 α chain. It is a powerful chemotactic factor and an anaphylatoxin, inducing mast cells and basophils to release histamine. It also causes smooth muscle contraction, promotes the production of superoxide in polymorphonuclear neutrophils (PMNs), and accentuates CR3 and Tp150,95 expression in their membranes. In addition to chemotaxis, it may facilitate PMN degranulation. Human serum contains anaphylatoxin inactivator that has carboxyl peptidase N properties. It deletes the C terminal arginine of C5a which yields $C5a_{des\ Arg}$. Although deprived of anaphylatoxin properties, $C5a_{des\ Arg}$ demonstrates limited chemotactic properties.

C5a receptor (C5a-R)

A receptor found on phagocytes and mast cells that binds the anaphylatoxin C5a, which plays an important role in inflammation. Serum carboxyl peptidase N (SCPN) controls C5a function by eliminating the C-terminal arginine. This produces $C5a_{des\ Arg}$. Neutrophils are sites of C5a catabolism. C5a-R is a 150- to 200-kDa oligomer comprised of multiple 40- to 47-kDa C5a-binding components. C5a-R mediates chemotaxis and other leukocyte reactions.

$C5a_{74des\ Arg}$

That part of C5a that remains following deletion of the carboxyl terminal arginine through the action of anaphylatoxin inactivator. Although deprived of the anaphylatoxin function of C5a, $C5a_{74des\ Arg}$ demonstrates limited chemotactic properties. This very uncommon deficiency of C2 protein in the serum has an autosomal-recessive mode of inheritance. Affected persons show increased likelihood of developing type III hypersensitivity disorders mediated by immune complexes, such as systemic lupus erythematosus (SLE). Whereas affected individuals possess the C2 gene, mRNA for C2 is apparently absent. Individuals who are heterozygous possess 50% of the normal serum levels of C2 and manifest no associated clinical illness.

C5aR

This C5 anaphylatoxin receptor belongs to the G-protein-coupled receptor family, the chemokine receptor branch of the rhodopsin family. COS-7 cells and HEK 293 cells expressing C5aR bind C5a with high affinity. C5aR mRNA is present in peripheral blood monocytes, granulocytes, and the myeloid fraction of bone marrow. C5aR message is present in the KG-1 monocytic cell line.

C5b

The principal molecular product that remains after C5a has been split off by the action of C5 convertase on C5. It has a binding site for C6 and complexes with it to begin generation of the membrane attack complex (MAC) of complement that leads to cell membrane injury and lysis.

C6 (complement component 6)

A 128-kDa single polypeptide chain that participates in the membrane attack complex (MAC). It is encoded by *C6A* and *C6B* alleles. It is a β_2 globulin.

C6 deficiency

A highly uncommon genetic defect with an autosomal recessive mode of inheritance in which affected individuals have only trace amounts of C6 in their plasma. They are defective in the ability to form a membrane attack complex (MAC)

C

and have increased susceptibility to disseminated infections by *Neisseria* microorganisms, including gonococci and meningococci. C6-deficient rabbits have been described.

C7 (complement component 7)

An 843-amino acid residue polypeptide chain that is a β_2 globulin. C5b67 is formed when C7 binds to C5b and C6. The complex has the appearance of a stalk with a leaf type of structure. C5b constitutes the leaf, and the stalk consists of C6 and C7. The stalk facilitates introduction of the C5b67 complex into the cell membrane, although no transmembrane perforation is produced. C5b67 anchored to the cell membrane provides a binding site for C8 and C9 in formation of the membrane attack complex (MAC). N-linked oligosaccharides bind to asparagine at positions 180 and 732 in C7.

C7 deficiency

A highly uncommon genetic disorder with an autosomal-recessive mode of inheritance in which the sera of affected persons contain only trace amounts of C7 in the plasma. Patients have a defective ability to form a membrane attack complex (MAC) and show an increased incidence of disseminated infections caused by *Neisseria* microorganisms. Some may manifest an increased propensity to develop immune complex (type III hypersensitivity) diseases such as glomerulonephritis or systemic lupus erythematosus (SLE).

C8 (complement component 8)

A 155-kDa molecule comprised of a 64-kDa α chain, a 64-kDa β chain, and a 22-kDa γ chain. Disulfide bonds join the α and γ chains. Noncovalent bonds link α and γ chains to the β chain. The C5b678 complex becomes anchored to the cell surface when the γ chain inserts into the membrane's lipid bilayer. When the C8 β chain combines with C5b in C5b67 complexes, the α chain regions change in conformation from β-pleated sheets to α helixes. The

C5b678 complex has a limited capacity to lyse the cell to which it is anchored because the complex can produce a transmembrane channel. The α chain of C8 combines with a single molecule of C9, thereby inducing C9 polymerization in the membrane attack complex (MAC). Genes at three different loci encode C8 α, β, and γ chains. One third of the amino acid sequences are identical between C8 α and β chains. These chains share the identity of one fourth of their amino acid sequences with C7 and C9. C8 is a β_1 globulin. In humans, the C8 concentration is 10 to 20 μ/mL.

C8 deficiency

A highly uncommon genetic disorder with an autosomal-recessive mode of inheritance in which affected individuals are missing C8 α, β, or γ chains. The disorder is associated with a defective ability to form a membrane attack complex (MAC). Individuals may have an increased propensity to develop disseminated infections caused by *Neisseria* microorganisms such as meningococci.

C9 (complement component 9)

A 535-amino acid residue single chain protein that binds to the C5b678 complex on the cell surface. It links to this complex through the α chain of C8, changes in conformation, significantly increases its length, and reveals hydrophobic regions that can react with the cell membrane lipid bilayer. With Zn^{2+} present, a dozen C9 molecules polymerize to produce 100-nm diameter hollow tubes positioned in the cell membrane to produce transmembrane channels. The interaction of 12 to 15 C9 molecules with one C5b678 complex produces the membrane attack complex (MAC). When viewed by an electron microscope, the pores in the plasma membrane produced by the poly-C9 have a 110-Å internal diameter, a 115-Å stalk anchored in the membrane's lipid bilayer, and a 100-Å structure above the membrane that gives an appearance of a doughnut when viewed from

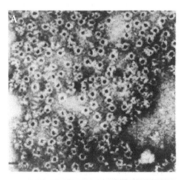

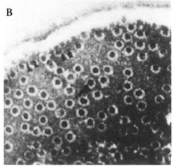

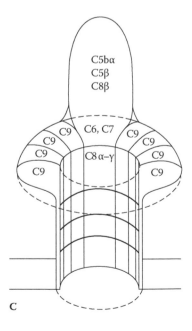

A: Electron micrograph of complement lesions (approximately 100 C) in erythrocyte membranes formed by poly C9 tubular complexes. B: Electron micrograph of complement lesions (approximately 160 C) induced on a target cell by a cloned cytolytic T lymphocyte (CTL) line. CTL- and natural killer (NK)-induced membrane lesions are formed by tubular complexes of perforin which is homologous to C9. Therefore, except for the larger internal diameter, the morphology of the lesions is similar to that of complement-mediated lesions. C: Model of MAC subunit arrangement.

above. Similar pores are produced by proteins released from cytotoxic T lymphocytes and natural killer (NK) cells called perforins or cytolysins. Sodium and water quickly enter the cells through these pores, leading to cell swelling and lysis. C9 shares one fourth of the amino acid sequence identity with the α and β chains of C7 and C8. It resembles perforin structurally. No polymorphism is found in C9, which is encoded by genes on chromosome 5 in humans.

C9 deficiency

A highly uncommon genetic disorder with an autosomal-recessive mode of inheritance in which only trace amounts of C9 are present in the plasma of affected persons. There is a defective ability to form the membrane attack complex (MAC). The sera of C9-deficient subjects retain lytic and bactericidal activities, even though the rate of lysis is decreased compared to that induced in the presence of C9. There are usually no clinical consequences associated with this condition. The disorder is more common in the Japanese than in most other populations.

C10

A chemokine of the β (CC) family that has been found in mice but not humans. Its biological significance is unknown. It is expressed on bone marrow cells, myeloid cell lines, macrophages, and T lymphocytes.

CA-15-3

An antibody specific for an antigen frequently present in the sera of metastatic breast carcinoma patients.

CA-19-9

A tumor-associated antigen found on the Lewis A blood group antigen that is sialylated or in mucin-containing tissues. In individuals whose serum levels exceed 37 U/mL, 72% have carcinoma of the pancreas. In individuals whose levels exceed 1000 U/mL, 95% have pancreatic cancer. Anti-CA-19-9 monoclonal antibody is useful to detect the recurrence of pancreatic cancer following surgery and to distinguish between neoplastic and benign conditions of the pancreas; however, it is not useful for pancreatic cancer screening.

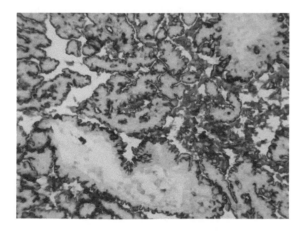

CA-125 papillary carcinoma of the ovary.

CA-125

A mucinous ovarian carcinoma cell-surface glycoprotein detectable in blood serum. Increasing serum concentrations portend a grave prognosis. It may also be found in the sera of patients with other adenocarcinomas, such as breast, gastrointestinal tract, uterine cervix, and endometrium.

CA-125 antibody

A mouse monoclonal antibody that reacts with malignant ovarian epithelial cells. The antigen is formalin-resistant, permitting the detection of ovarian cancer by immunohistochemistry, although serum assays for this protein are widely used to monitor ovarian cancer. CA-125 also reacts with antigens in seminal vesicle carcinoma and anaplastic lymphoma.

cachectin

An earlier name for tumor necrosis factor α found in the blood serum and associated with wasting. See tumor necrosis factor α (TNFα).

cachexia

Body wasting attributable to unregulated cellular catabolism. Elevated levels of tumor necrosis factor cause cachexia in patients with malignant tumors.

cadaveric organ

A solid organ secured from a recently deceased donor, i.e., a cadaver, for the purpose of transplantation.

cadherins

One of four specific families of cell adhesion molecules that enable cells to interact with their environment. Cadherins help cells communicate with other cells in immune surveillance, extravasation, trafficking, tumor metastasis, wound healing, and tissue localization. Cadherins are calcium-dependent. The five different cadherins include N-cadherin, P-cadherin, T-cadherin, V-cadherin, and E-cadherin. Cytoplasmic domains of cadherins may interact with proteins of the cytoskeleton. They may bind to other receptors based on homophilic specificity, but they still depend on intracellular interactions linked to the cytoskeleton.

caecal tonsils

Lymphoid aggregates containing germinal centers found in the gut wall in birds, specifically in the wall of the cecum.

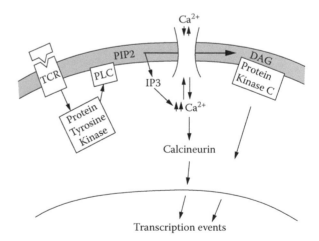

Schematic representation of cellular events upon binding of an activated T cell.

calcineurin

A protein phosphatase that is serine- and threonine-specific. Activation of T cells apparently requires deletion of phosphates from serine or threonine residues. Its action is inhibited by the immunosuppressive drugs cyclosporin-A and FK506 (tacrolimus). Cyclosporin-A and FK506 combine with immunophilin intracellular molecules to form a complex that combines with calcineurin and inhibits its activity.

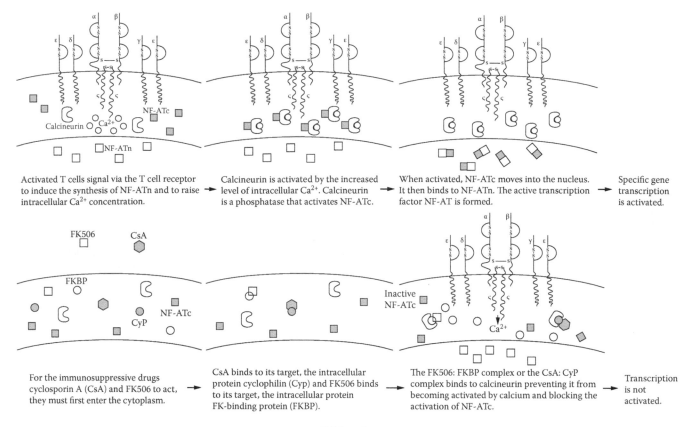

Activated T cells signal via the T cell receptor to induce the synthesis of NF-ATn and to raise intracellular Ca²⁺ concentration. → Calcineurin is activated by the increased level of intracellular Ca²⁺. Calcineurin is a phosphatase that activates NF-ATc. → When activated, NF-ATc moves into the nucleus. It then binds to NF-ATn. The active transcription factor NF-AT is formed. → Specific gene transcription is activated.

For the immunosuppressive drugs cyclosporin A (CsA) and FK506 to act, they must first enter the cytoplasm. → CsA binds to its target, the intracellular protein cyclophilin (Cyp) and FK506 binds to its target, the intracellular protein FK-binding protein (FKBP). → The FK506: FKBP complex or the CsA: CyP complex binds to calcineurin preventing it from becoming activated by calcium and blocking the activation of NF-ATc. → Transcription is not activated.

Calcineurin.

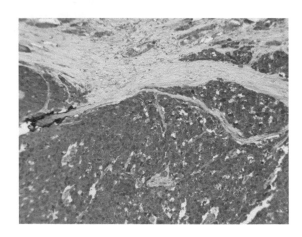

Calcitonin—medullary carcinoma of the thyroid.

calcitonin

A hormone that influences calcium ion transport. Immunoperoxidase staining demonstrates calcitonin in thyroid parafollicular or C cells. It serves as a marker characteristic of medullary thyroid carcinoma and APUD (amine precursor uptake and decarboxylation) neoplasms. Lung and gastrointestinal tumors may also form calcitonin.

calcivirus immunity

Human calciviruses (HuCVs) have been shown to cause gastric distress. Antibodies against members of this group such as small, round, structured viruses (SRSV) that include Norwalk virus (NV) may crossreact with other viruses of this same form; thus a rise in antibody titer is insufficient for diagnosis. Immunoglobulin A (IgA) antibody responses appear more specific. Reinfection by NV is common as preformed antibody correlates with susceptibility to the illness. Thus, people who recover often become susceptible again on rechallenge. High titers attained after several infections are protective in some studies, although this has not been confirmed. Antibody to HuCV is protective and mainly type-specific. Vaccines are available for FCV and RHDV.

CALLA

Common acute lymphoblastic leukemia antigen; also known as CD10.

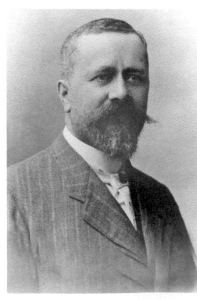

Albert Calmette (1863–1933).

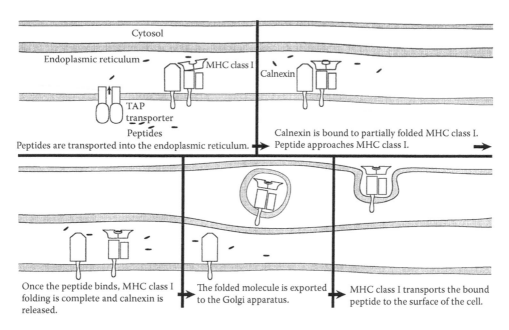

Calnexin.

Calmette, Albert (1863–1933)

French physician who was subdirector of the Institut Pasteur in Paris. In a popular book published in 1920 titled *Bacillary Infection and Tuberculosis*, he emphasized the necessity of separating tuberculin reactivity from anaphylaxis. With Guérin, he perfected the BCG (bacille Calmette–Guérin) vaccine and also investigated snake venom and plague serum.

calnexin

An 88-kDa membrane molecule that combines with newly formed α chains that also interact with nascent β$_2$-microglobulin. Calnexin maintains partial folding of major histocompatibility complex (MHC) class I molecules in the endoplasmic reticulum. It also interacts with MHC class II molecules, T cell receptors, and immunoglobulins that are partially folded.

calreticulin

A calnexin structurally-related soluble protein present in the endoplasmic reticulum that facilitates proper folding of major histocompatibility complex (MHC) molecules and other glycoproteins; a molecular chaperone that binds to MHC class I and class II, as well as other immunoglobulin-like domains containing proteins, including antigen receptors for both T and B cells. Calreticulin resembles calnexin structurally and functionally.

CAM (cell adhesion molecule)

Cell-selective proteins that promote adhesion of cells to one another and are calcium-independent. They are believed to help direct migration of cells during embryogenesis. The majority of lymphocytes and monocytes express this antigen, which is not found on other cells. The "humanized" antibodies specific for this epitope are termed Campath-1H. Refer to CD52.

campath-1 (CD52) CAMPATH-1M

A rat immunoglobulin M (IgM) monoclonal antibody against the CD52 antigen. It is able to lyse cells using human complement, making no other manipulation necessary to deplete T cells other than to add donor serum. This antibody has been used to deplete T cells to prevent graft-vs.-host disease. It is a lipid-anchored glycoprotein with a very small peptide constituent. Anti-CD52 antibodies are potent lytic agents, killing cells *in vitro* with human complement as well as *in vivo*. These antibodies have been used for therapy of leukemia, bone marrow transplantation, organ transplantation, rheumatoid arthritis, vasculitis, and multiple sclerosis. Campath-1H (human IgG$_1$) was the first monoclonal antibody to be humanized. It was formed by transplanting complementarity-determining regions of campath-1G into human heavy and light chain genes. Even though initial binding affinity was decreased, this was corrected by modifying framework residues. Patients receiving this humanized antibody developed very low antiglobulin responses compared with the original rat antibodies. The CD52 antigen is a glycoprotein with only 12 amino acids. It is a complex carbohydrate consisting of sialylated polylactosamine units with fucosylated mannose cores. It is attached to Asn3 at the C terminus as a glycosylphosphatidylinositol (GPI) anchor. The campath-1 epitope is comprised of the C terminal amino acids and part of the GPI anchor, which means that the antibodies bind near the cell membrane, facilitating cell lysis. The antigen is expressed abundantly on all lymphocytes except plasma cells and also on monocytes, macrophages, and eosinophils. It is not found on any other tissues except the male reproductive tract, where it is strongly expressed on epithelial cells lining the epididymis, vas deferens, and seminal vesicle. The CD52 antigen is a principal membrane protein of sperm.

Campylobacter immunity

Circulating antibodies develop rapidly in patients with *Campylobacter enteritis*. These antibodies fix complement, are bactericidal, and agglutinate. Following an initial but short-lived immunoglobulin M (IgM) response, a rapid IgA response peaks 14 days after onset of symptoms but declines by the fifth week. IgG antibodies appear by the tenth day after infection and are present for several months. Antibodies are believed to limit the infection. Serologic tests for diagnosis depend on an acid-extractable surface antigen that consists mainly of flagellin, which is the immunodominant surface antigen. Antiflagellin antibodies appear early during an infection and are believed to be protective. MOMP is also immunogenic. All of these antibodies have specificity for homologous and heterologous strains. Lipopolysaccharides (LPSs) induce variable antibody responses. Half of the cases of *C. enteritis* develop during Guillain-Barré syndrome. These patients develop increased circulating IgG and IgM that bind to GM1 and GD1 ganglioside epitopes and crossreact with the LPSs of certain serotypes of *C. jejuni*. Definitive studies of T cell responses to *Campylobacter* remain to be performed.

Canale–Smith syndrome

A rare autoimmune and lymphoproliferative syndrome (ALPS) that leads to lymphoid enlargement and immune cytopenia. It is a consequence of a dominant, nonfunctional Fas molecule. Children develop "double-negative" T lymphocytes and hypergammaglobulinemia. Unlike *lpr* and *gld* mice, human patients rarely develop antinuclear antibodies or lupus-like renal pathology; however, in the few cases studied, they showed increased susceptibility to malignancy.

cancer

An invasive, metastatic, and highly anaplastic cellular tumor that leads to death. Neoplasms are often divided into the two broad categories of carcinoma and sarcoma.

cancer–testis antigens

Proteins normally present only on spermatogonia and spermatocytes that become tumor-associated antigens when they appear on other types of cells as a consequence of transformation.

Candida immunity

Resistance against *Candida* begins with the nonspecific barriers such as intact skin and mucosal epithelium in addition to the indigenous bacterial flora that compete for binding sites. Once these protective barriers have been breached, the major cellular defense is neutrophils, which phagocytose the *Candida* microorganisms with intracellular killing through oxidative mechanisms. Monocytes and eosinophils also participate in this process. Microabscesses may form in infected tissues. Mononuclear cells constitute the main inflammatory response in more chronic infections. Immunoglobulin G (IgG), IgM, and IgA classes of *Candida*-specific antibodies have been found in infected patients. Local mucosal immunity, such as in the vagina, is associated with the development of IgA antibodies in secretions. Even though antibody titers are elevated in infected patients, the humoral immune response does not have a principal role in host defense against *Candida*. Patients with defects in cell-mediated immunity, such as AIDS patients and those with chronic mucocutaneous candidiasis, have increased susceptibility to *Candida* infections. Vaccination has been determined to be ineffective in preventing *Candida* infections.

canine distemper virus

A virus that induces disease in dogs and is associated with demyelination, probably induced by myelin-sensitive lymphocytes.

canine immunity

The canine immune system, using the dog as the classic example, is structurally and functionally very similar to its mouse and human counterparts. As in humans, dogs have numerous natural resistance mechanisms that prevent disease-causing agents by nonimmunologic means, including,

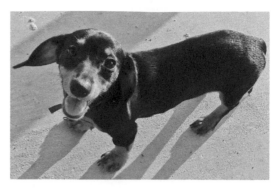

Canine immunity.

for example, the skin and mucous membranes. Dogs have the same immunoglobulin classes as described in humans. Canine cell-mediated immunity is essentially no different from the murine and human equivalents. The major histocompatibility complex (MHC) in the dog is known as DLA, which encodes the DLA class I and class II histocompatibility antigens. Natural killer (NK) cells, killer (K) cells, and T suppressor cells have also been described in dogs. There are also multiple inherited canine immunodeficiencies. Acquired immune deficiencies may also be associated with vitamin and mineral deficiencies, and various autoimmune conditions have been described including systemic lupus erythematosus (SLE), which is associated with MHC DLA-A7.

canine parvovirus vaccine

Initially, a live and attenuated feline enteritis vaccine was used, based on its crossreactivity with canine parvovirus. Canine parvovirus may have originated from the feline enteritis organism by mutation. This vaccine was later replaced with attenuated canine parvovirus vaccine.

canonical structure

A frequently encountered molecular sequence or molecular arrangement.

capillary leak syndrome

The therapeutic administration of GM-CSF (granulocyte–macrophage colony-stimulating factor) may lead to progressive dyspnea and pericarditis in the treatment of patients bearing metatastic solid tumors. Interleukin-2 (IL2) may likewise induce the effect when used to treat tumor patients. IL2 treatment may lead to the accumulation of 10 to 20 L of fluid in peripheral tissues with resultant disorientation, confusion, and pronounced fever.

Caplin's syndrome

Rheumatoid nodules in the lungs of subjects such as hard coal miners in contact with silica.

capping

The migration of antigens on the cell surface to a cell pole following crosslinking of antigens by a specific antibody. These antigen–antibody complexes coalesce or aggregate into a "cap" produced by the interaction of antigen with cell-surface immunoglobulin M (IgM) and IgD molecules at sites distant from each other, as revealed by immunofluorescence. Capping is followed by internalization of the antigen after which the cell surface is left bereft of immunoglobulin receptors until they are re-expressed.

capping phenomenon

The migration of surface membrane proteins toward one pole of a cell following crosslinking by a specific antibody, antigen, or mitogen. Bivalent or polyvalent ligands cause the surface

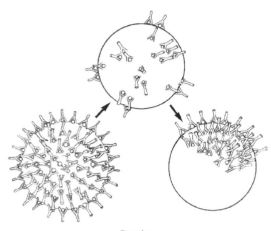

Capping.

molecules to aggregate into patches. This passive process is referred to as patching. The ligand–surface molecule aggregates move in patches to a pole of the cell, where they form a cap. If a cell with patches becomes motile, the patches move to the rear, forming a cluster of surface molecule–ligand aggregates that constitutes a cap. The process of capping requires energy and may involve interaction with microfilaments of the cytoskeleton. In addition to capping in lymphocytes, the process occurs in numerous other cells.

caprinized vaccine

A preparation containing microorganisms attenuated by passage through goats and used for therapeutic immunization.

capromab pendetide

A murine monoclonal antibody specific for prostate-specific membrane antigen. When labeled with isotopic indium (^{111}In), it is useful for immunoscintigraphy in prostate cancer patients.

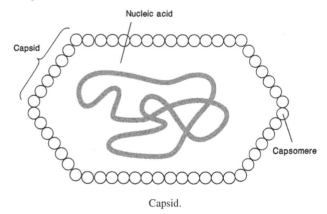

Capsid.

capsid

A virus protein envelope comprised of subunits that are called capsomers.

capsular polysaccharide

A constituent of the protective coating around a number of bacteria such as pneumococcus (*Streptococcus pneumoniae*). Chemically, is a polysaccharide and stimulates the production of antibodies specific for its epitopes. In addition to pneumococcus, other microorganisms such as *Streptococci* and certain *Bacillus* species have polysaccharide capsules.

capsule

Refer to capsular polysaccharide.

capsule swelling reaction

Pneumococcus swelling reaction. Refer to Quellung reaction.

capture assay

Technique to measure antigens or antibodies in which antibodies bound to plastic capture antigens or antigens bound to plastic capture antibodies. Labeled antigens or antiimmunoglobulins may be used to measure antibody binding to a plate-bound antigen. Antigen binding to an antibody bound to a plate can be assayed with an antibody that binds to a different antigenic determinant or epitope on the antigen.

carbohydrate antigen

The best known carbohydrate antigen is the specific soluble substance of the capsule of *Streptococcus pneumoniae* that is immunogenic in humans. Heidelberger developed the first effective vaccines against purified pneumococcal polysaccharide in the early 1940s; the vaccines were effective in the treatment of pneumonia caused by these microorganisms, yet interest in the vaccine waned as antibiotics were developed for treatment. With increased resistance of bacteria to antibiotics, however, there is a renewed interest in immunization with polysaccharide-based vaccines. Polysaccharides alone are relatively poor immunogens, especially for infants and immunocompromised hosts. Pneumococci have 84 distinct serotypes, further complicating the matter. Polysaccharides are classified as T cell-independent immunogens. They fail to induce the immunologic memory needed for booster responses in an immunization protocol. Only a few B cell clones are activated, leading to restricted yet polyclonal heterogeneity. The majority of polysaccharides can induce tolerance or unresponsiveness and fail to induce delayed-type hypersensitivity. Polysaccharide immunogenicity increases with molecular weight. Polysaccharides below 50 kDa are nonimmunogenic. Thus, immunization with purified polysaccharides has not been as effective as desired. The covalent linkage of a polysaccharide or of its epitopes to a protein carrier to form a conjugate vaccine has facilitated enhancement of immunogenicity in both humans and other animals and induces immunologic memory. Antibodies formed against the conjugate vaccine are protective and bind the capsular polysaccharide from which they were derived. An example of this type of immunogen is HIV polysaccharide linked to tetanous toxoid, which has been successful in infant immunization.

carbohydrates, immunogenic

Carbohydrates are important in various immunological processes that include opsinization and phagocytosis of microorganisms and cell activation and differentiation. They exert their effects through interactions with carbohydrate-binding proteins or lectins that have a widespread distribution in mammalian tissues including the immune system. Immunogenic carbohydrates are usually large polymers of glucose (glucans and lentinans), mannose (mannans), xylose, (hemicelluloses), fructose (levans), or mixtures of these sugars. Complex carbohydrates may stimulate the immune system by activating macrophages with fungal glycans or stimulating T cells with lentinan. Acemannin activates microphages and T cells, thereby influencing both cellular and humoral immunity. Glucans stimulate immunity against bacterial diseases by activating macrophages and stimulating their lysosomal and phagocytic activity. Complex carbohydrates may activate the immune systems of patients or experimental animals with neoplastic diseases. Some mannans and glucans are powerful anticancer agents. Lentinin derived from an edible mushroom has an antineoplastic effect against several different allogeneic and syngeneic tumors without mediating cytotoxicity of the tumor cells. Mannans derived from yeast also exert significant antitumor effects, as do levans that activate not only macrophages but B and T cells as well. Pectin is a galactose-containing carbohydrate concentrated in citrus and has an antitumor effect.

carbon clearance test

An assay to judge mononuclear phagocyte system activity *in vivo*. Blood samples are collected at designated intervals following the intravenous inoculation of a colloidal carbon particle suspension. Following dissolution of the erythrocytes in blood samples, their carbon particle content is determined colorimetrically. This permits determination of the rate at which blood phagocytes remove carbon. The logarithms of the readings in the colorimetry are plotted against time to yield the desired slope.

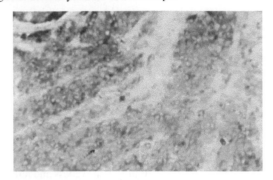

Carcinoembryonic antigen (CEA).

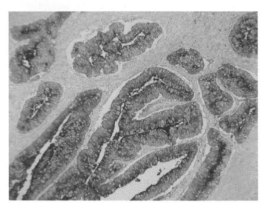

Carcinoembryonic antigen (CEA)—carcinoma of the colon.

carcinoembryonic antigen (CEA)

A 200-kDa membrane glycoprotein epitope present in the fetal gastrointestinal tract under normal conditions. However, tumor cells, such as those in colon carcinoma, may re-express it. CEA was first described as a screen for identifying carcinoma by detecting nanogram quantities of the antigen in serum. It was later shown to be present in certain other conditions. CEA levels are elevated in almost one third of patients with colorectal, liver, pancreatic, lung, breast, head and neck, cervical, bladder, medullarythyroid, and prostatic carcinoma. However, the level may also be elevated in patients with malignant melanoma or lymphoproliferative disease and in smokers. Regrettably, CEA levels also increase in a variety of non-neoplastic disorders including inflammatory bowel disease, pancreatitis, and cirrhosis of the liver. Nevertheless, determination of CEA levels in the serum is valuable for monitoring the recurrence of tumors in patients whose primary neoplasm has been removed. A CEA

level elevated 35% compared to the level immediately following surgery may signify metastases. This oncofetal antigen is comprised of one polypeptide chain with one variable region at the amino terminus and six constant region domains. CEA belongs to the immunoglobulin superfamily. It lacks specificity for cancer, thereby limiting its diagnostic usefulness. It is detected with a mouse monoclonal antibody directed against a complex glycoprotein antigen present on many human epithelial-derived tumors. This reagent may be used to aid in the identification of cells of epithelial lineage. The antibody is intended for qualitative staining in sections of formalin-fixed, paraffin-embedded tissue. Anti-CEA antibodies specifically bind to antigens located in the plasma membrane and cytoplasmic regions of normal epithelial cells. Unexpected antigen expression or loss of expression may occur, especially in neoplasms. Occasionally, stromal elements surround heavily stained tissue and/or cells that show immunoreactivity. Clinical interpretation of any staining or its absence must be complemented by morphological studies and evaluation of proper controls.

carcinogen

Any chemical or physical agent that produces cancer through mutation or deregulating oncogenes, tumor-suppressor genes, or DNA repair genes. Carcinogens are of two types: (1) the epigenetic type that does not damage DNA but causes other physiological alterations that predispose to cancer, and (2) the genotoxic type that reacts directly with DNA or with micromolecules that then react with DNA.

carcinogenesis

A multistep sequence consisting of initiation, promotion, progression, and malignant conversion through which a cell may progress to deregulation of cell growth resulting in malignant transformation.

carcinoma

A malignant tumor comprised of epithelial cells that infiltrate surrounding tissues and lead to metastases.

carcinoma-associated antigens

Self antigens whose epitopes have been changed due to effects produced by certain tumors. Self antigens are transformed into a molecular structure for which the host is immunologically intolerant. Examples include the T antigen, which is an MN blood group precursor molecule exposed by the action of bacterial enzymes, and the Tn antigen, which is a consequence of somatic mutation in hematopoietic stem cells caused by inhibition of galactose transfer to *N*-acetyl-d-galactosamine.

carcinomatous neuropathy

Neurological findings in tumor-bearing patients who have no nervous system metastasis. Sensory carcinomatous neuropathy, in which patients develop autoantibodies specific for neurone cytoplasm RNA-protein, is an example of a carcinomatous neuropathy.

cardiac disease, autoimmune

Rheumatic fever is a classic example of microbial-induced autoimmune heart disease. The immune response against the M protein of group A *Streptococci* crossreacts with cardiac proteins such as tropomyosin and myosin. The M protein contains numerous epitopes that participate in these crossreactions. A second crossreactive protein in the streptococcal membrane has been purified to a series of four peptides ranging in molecular weight from 22 to 23 kDa. Patients with rheumatic fever may develop antibody that binds to the cytoplasm of cells of the caudate nuclei with specificity for its cells. Autoantibodies against microorganisms crossreact with cardiac tissue. A monoclonal antibody termed D8/17 identifies all rheumatics. This antibody is not related to the major histocompatibility complex (MHC) system and serves as a B cell marker associated with rheumatic fever, although no specific role for the antigen in the disease has been demonstrated. Numerous microbes and viruses can induce acute myocarditis. These cases are characterized by the presence of lymphocytic infiltrates and increased titers of heart-reactive antibodies. Important causative agents include group B coxsackieviruses that cause acute cardiac inflammation in humans. Rose et al., using an experimental mouse model, showed that only those mice with heart-reactive antibodies in their sera went on to develop chronic cardiomyopathy with antibodies primarily against the cardiac isoform of myosin in their model of acute myocarditis. Postpericardiotomy syndrome occurs in both adults and children 10 to 14 days after surgery and is characterized by fever, chest pain, and pericardial and pleural effusions. This condition is associated with the presence of high-titer, heart-reactive antibodies in the blood sera. The heart-specific antibodies are believed to play a role in the disease pathogenesis. Because many microbes share epitopes with human tissues, crossreactions between antibodies against the microbe and human tissues may be harmless or may lead to serious autoimmune consequences in genetically susceptible hosts. Despite the attention given to antibodies, cell-mediated immunity may play a larger role than previously thought in both rheumatic fever and Chagas' disease in which T cells are specifically cytotoxic for the target organ. Cytotoxic T cells specific for cardiac myofibers appear in both rheumatic fever and Chagas' disease. Only selected individuals with cardiomyopathy develop progressive autoimmune disease after active infection.

cardiolipin

Diphosphatidyl glycerol, a phospholipid extracted from beef heart as the principal antigen in the Wassermann complement fixation test for syphilis used earlier in the century.

cardiolipin antibodies

Anticardiolipin antibodies (ACAs) may be linked to thrombocytopenia, thrombotic events, and repeated fetal loss in patients with systemic lupus erythematosus (SLE). Caucasian but not Chinese patients with SLE may have a relatively high incidence of valve defects associated with the presence of these antibodies. Other conditions associated with ACA include adrenal hemorrhage and Addison's disease, livedo reticularis (LR), and livedo reticularis with cardiovascular disease (Sneddon syndrome), as well as possibly polymyalgia rheumatica/giant cell arteritis and focal central nervous system lupus.

cardiolipin autoantibodies

Immunoglobulin G (IgG), IgM, and IgA cardiolipin autoantibodies are assayed by enzyme immunoassay (EIA) for the detection of antiphospholipid antibodies (aPLs) in patients believed to have antiphospholipid syndrome (APS). Combined testing for phosphatidylserine autoantibodies and lupus anticoagulant in addition to anticardiolipin autoantibodies improves the sensitivity for the detection of antiphospholipid antibodies. High anticardiolipin autoantibody concentrations are associated with an increased risk of venous and arterial thrombosis, recurrent pregnancy loss, and thrombocytopenia.

Carrel, Alexis (1873–1944)

French surgeon working at the Rockefeller Institute for Medical Research in New York City, who first successfully

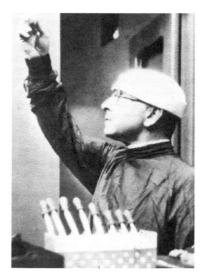

Alexis Carrel.

sewed blood vessels together after approximating their ends by triangulation suture. The technique earned him a Nobel Prize in Medicine and made organ and tissue grafts surgically possible.

carriage (HIV)

The expeditious transmission of HIV through a bicellular conjugate (an infectious synapse) from an infected antigen-presenting cell to T cells in lymph nodes. The transport of infected T cells to additional secondary lymphoid tissues creates numerous reservoirs for virus dissemination throughout the body.

carrier (person)

An individual with a latent infection who can serve unknowingly as a source of infection to other persons.

carrier (protein)

An immunogenic macromolecular protein such as ovalbumin to which an incomplete antigen termed a hapten may be conjugated either *in vitro* or *in vivo*. Whereas the hapten alone is not immunogenic, conjugation to the carrier molecule renders it immunogenic. When self proteins are appropriately modified by the hapten, they may serve as carriers *in vivo*, a mechanism operative in allergy to drugs. The carrier protein supplies T cell epitopes that are requisite for B cell–T cell cooperation.

carrier effect

To achieve a secondary immune response to a hapten, both the hapten and the carrier used in the initial immunization must be employed.

carrier specificity

That part of an immune response, either humoral antibody or cell-mediated immunity, that is specific for the carrier portion of a hapten–carrier complex used as an immunogen. The carrier-specific part of the immune response does not react with the hapten either alone or when conjugated to a different carrier.

cartilaginous fish immunity

Major milestones in the evolution of immunity included the development by cartilaginous fishes, including sharks, of the thymus, the anamnestic (secondary or memory) antibody response, plasma cells for antibody synthesis, and the spleen. Cartilaginous vertebrates have both 7S and 18S disulfide-linked IgM immunoglobulins. The low and high

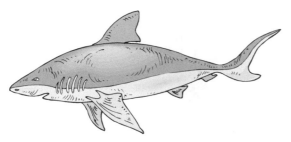

Cartilaginous fishes.

molecular weights are probably attributable to polymerization rather than differences in heavy chain class. The classic complement pathway components also make their debut.

cartwheel nucleus

The arrangement of chromatin in the nucleus of a typical plasma cell based on the more and less electron-dense areas observed by electron microscopy. Euchromatin makes up the less electron-dense spokes of the wheel, whereas heterochromatin makes up the more electron-dense areas.

cascade reaction

A sequential event in such enzymatic reactions as complement fixation and blood coagulation in which each stage of the reaction triggers the next appropriate step.

caseation necrosis

A type of necrosis present at the centers of large granulomas such as those formed in tuberculosis. The white cheesy appearance of the central necrotic area is the basis for the term.

caseous necrosis

Tissue destruction that occurs in tuberculosis and has the appearance of cottage cheese.

Casoni test

A diagnostic skin test for hydatid disease in humans induced by *Echinococcus granulosus* infection. In sensitive individuals, a wheal and flare response develops within 30 minutes following intradermal inoculation of a tapeworm or hydatid cyst fluid extract. This is followed within 24 hours by an area of induration produced by this cell-mediated, delayed-hypersensitivity reaction.

caspase substrates

The specificity of caspases translates into an order disassembly of cells by proteolytic cleavage of specific cellular protein. The paradigm substrate for caspase cleavage is PARP (polyADP-ribose polymerase). During apoptosis, intact 121-kDa PARP is cleaved by caspases into fragments of approximately 84 and 23 kDa. Generation of these fragments tends to be an inductor of apoptosis. Cleavage inactivates the enzymatic activity of PARP.

caspases

Closely related cysteine proteases that cleave protein substrates at the C terminal sides of aspartic acid residues and represent components of enzymatic cascades that lead to apoptotic cell death. There are two pathways of activation of caspases in lymphocyte. One involves mitochondrial permeability changes in growth factor-deprived cells, and the other involves signals from death receptors in plasma membranes. Cytosolic aspartate-specific proteases, called caspases, are responsible for the deliberate disassembly of cells into apoptotic bodies. Caspases are present as inactive proenzymes, most of which are activated by proteolytic cleavage. Caspase 8, caspase 9, and caspase 3 are situated at the pivotal junctions in apoptotic pathways. Caspase 8 initiates disassembly in response to extracellular apoptosis-inducing ligands and is activated in a complex associated

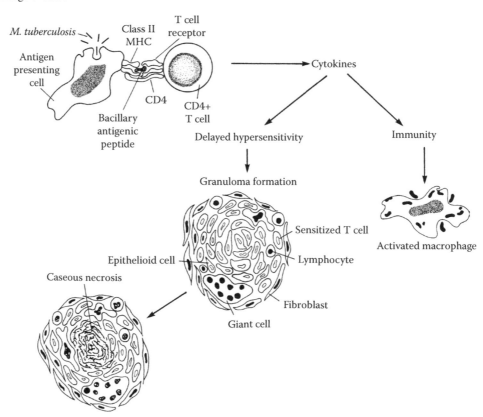

Caseation necrosis.

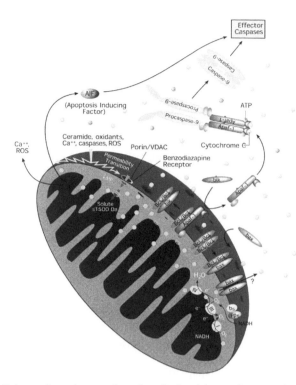

Release of cytochrome c from the mitochondria can trigger a series of events leading to the activation of effector caspases. For example, procaspase 9 is activated when complexed with dATP, APAF-1, and extramitochondrial cytochrome *c*. Following activation, caspase 9 can inhibit apoptosis by cleaving additional caspases.

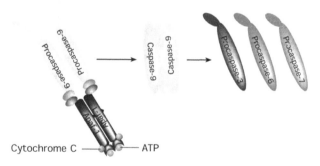

Activation of procaspase 9 can occur upon formation of a complex with Apaf-1 and cytochrome *c*. Caspase 9 may then activate additional caspases through proteolytic cleavage (*e.g.* procaspases-3, -6, and -7).

with the cytoplasmic death domains of the receptor. Caspase 9 activates disassembly in response to agents or insults that trigger release of cytochrome *c* from the mitochondria and is activated when complexed with dATP, APAF-1, and extramitochondrial cytochrome *c*. Caspase 3 appears to amplify caspase 8, and caspase 9 signals into a full-fledged commitment to disassembly. Both caspase 8 and caspase 9 can activate caspase 3 by proteolytic cleavage, and caspase 3 may then cleave vital cellular proteins or activate additional caspase by proteolytic cleavage. Many other caspases have been described. Caspases proteolytically disassemble cells. They are present in healthy cells as inactive proforms. During apoptosis, most caspases are activated by proteolytic cleavage. Caspase 9, however, may be active without being proteolytically cleaved. Activation is through autoproteolysis or cleavage by other caspases. Cleavage of caspases generates a pro-domain fragment and subunits of approximately 20 and 10 kDa. Active caspases appear to be tetramers consisting of two identical 20-kDa subunits and two identical 10-kDa subunits. Detection of either the 20- or 10-kDa subunit by immunoblotting may imply activation of the caspase. Colorimetric and fluorometric assays using fluorogenic peptide substrates can be used to measure caspase activity in apoptotic cells. Caspases cleave substrate proteins at the carboxyl termini of specific aspartates. Tetrameric peptides with fluorometric or colorimetric groups at the carboxyl terminal have been used to determine the Km values of caspases. Although there is preference for peptides with certain amino acid (aa) sequences, the aa sequence may have some variance. Caspases also have overlapping preferences for the tetrameric aa sequence (*i.e.*, the same substrates can be cleaved by multiple caspases although one caspase may have a lower Km). Peptides containing groups that form covalent bonds with the cysteine residing at the active site of the caspase are often used to inhibit caspase activities.

Castleman's disease

Also called giant lymph node hyperplasia. A disease of unknown etiology that involves both lymph nodes and extranodal tissues. Two histopathologic subtypes have been described. The first, termed hyaline-vascular angiofollicular lymph node hyperplasia, accounts for 90% of the cases. It usually affects young men who present with an asymptomatic mass in the mediastinum. Histopathologically, it reveals numerous small, follicle-like structures, frequently with radially penetrating, thick-walled, hyalinized vessels, concentrically arranged small lymphocytes around the follicular structures, called "onion skinning," and extensive proliferation of capillaries in the interfollicular areas. The second type of Castleman's disease is plasma cell angiofollicular lymph node hyperplasia, which comprises 10% of the cases. It is either a localized mass or a multicentered systemic disorder. The mass may consist of multiple matted lymph nodes with histopathologic features that include large hyperplastic follicles with fewer permanent penetrating vessels than in the hyaline-vascular type, with pronounced interfollicular plasma cytosis and permanent vascularity. A multicentric type of the plasma cell variant of angiofollicular lymph node hyperplasia is more aggressive. Affected patients may have increased risk for developing Kaposi's sarcoma or immunoblastic lymphoma. Clinical features of plasma cell angiofollicular hyperplasia include fever, polyclonal hypergammaglobulinanemia, elevated sedimentation rate, and anemia.

cat scratch disease

Regional lymphadenitis, common in children following a cat scratch. The condition is induced by a small Gram-negative bacillus. Erythematous papules may appear on the hands or forearms at the site of the injury. Patients may develop fever, malaise, swelling of the parotid gland, lymphadenopathy that is regional or generalized, maculopapular rash, anorexia, splenic enlargement, and encephalopathy. Hyperplasia of lymphoid tissues, formation of granulomas, and abscesses may occur. A positive skin test, together with history, establishes the diagnosis. Gentamycin and ciprofloxacin have been used in treatment.

catalase

An enzyme present in activated phagocytes that causes degradation of hydrogen peroxide and superoxide dismutase.

catalytic antibodies

Antibodies that are exclusively specific for a particular ligand and are also catalytic. Approximately 100 reactions have been catalyzed by antibodies. Among these are pericyclic processes,

C

elimination reactions, bond-forming reactions, and redox processes. Most antibody-catalyzed reactions are highly stereospecific. For efficient catalysis, it is necessary to introduce catalytic functions within the antibody-combining site properly juxtaposed to the substrate. Catalytic antibodies resemble enzymes in processing their substrates through a Michaelis M complex, in which the chemical transformation takes place followed by a product dissociation. Refer also to abzyme.

catalytic antibody

A monoclonal antibody into whose antigen-binding site the catalytic activity of a specific biological enzyme has been introduced. This permits enzymatic catalysis of previously arranged specificity to take place. Site-directed mutagenesis, in which a catalytic residue is added to a combining site by amino acid substitution, is used to attain the specificity. Specific catalysts can be generated by other mechanisms, such as alternation of enzyme sites genetically or chemical alternation of receptors with catalytic properties.

catch-up vaccine

The immunization of unvaccinated children at a convenient time, such as the first day of school, rather than at the optimal time for antibody synthesis. This procedure provides a second opportunity for disease prevention and control for many children who miss vaccines at regularly scheduled intervals.

cathepsins

Thiol and aspartyl proteases that have broad substrate specificities. Cathepsins represent the most abundant proteases of endosomes in antigen-presenting cells. They are believed to serve an important function in the generation of peptide fragments from exogenous protein antigens that bind to major histocompatibility complex (MHC) class II molecules. Significant for *Ii* chain degradation into diminutive fragments, leading to CLIP formation. Critical components of exogenous antigen processing and presentation.

cationic proteins

Phagocytic cell granule constituents that have antimicrobial properties.

CBA mouse

A strain of inbred mice from which many substrains have been developed, such as CBA/H-T6.

CBA/N mouse

A CBA murine mutant that is incapable of responding immunologically to linear polysaccharides and selected other thymus-independent immunogens. The B cells of this mutant strain are either defective or immature. The Lyb3, Lyb5, and Lyb7 B lymphocyte subsets are not present in these mice. This mutation is designated *xid* and has an X-linked recessive mode of inheritance. The serum immunoglobulin G (IgG) concentrations for these mice are diminished. They mount only weak immune responses to thymus-dependent immunogens.

CC CKR-1

CC chemokine receptor 1 belongs to the G protein-coupled receptor family, the chemokine receptor branch of the rhodopsin family. It is expressed on neutrophils, monocytes, eosinophils, B cells, and T cells. Tissue sources include the placenta, lung, and liver. CC CKR-1 RNA is present in peripheral blood and synovial fluid of patients with rheumatoid arthritis (RA) but not in patients with osteoarthritis. Also termed MIP-1α receptor, RANTES receptor, and CCR-1.

CC CKR-2

CC chemokine receptor 2 belongs to the G protein-coupled receptor family, the chemokine receptor branch of the rhodopsin family. Ligands include MCP-1 and MCP-3. It is expressed on monocytes. Tissue sources include kidney, heart, bone marrow, lung, liver, and pancreas. Also called MCP-1 receptor and CCR2 A and B.

CC CKR-3

CC chemokine receptor 3 belongs to the G-protein-coupled receptor family, the chemokine receptor branch of the rhodopsin family. Tissue sources include the human monocyte cDNA library. Also termed eosinophil chemokine receptor, RANTES receptor, CCR3, and eotaxin receptor.

CC CKR-4

CC chemokine receptor 4 mRNA is present in leukocyte-rich tissue. It is found in interleukin-5 (IL5)-treated basophils. Ligands include MIP-1α, RANTES, and MCP-1. Tissue sources include the immature basophilic cell line KU-812. Also termed CCR4.

CCL2

A chemokine generated from activated T cells that directs macrophages to an area of infection. Known previously as macrophage chemotactic protein (MCP).

CCL21

A vascular endothelial cell-derived chemokine associated with leukocyte extravasation. Known previously as SLC.

CC subgroup

A chemokine subgroup in which adjacent cysteines are linked by disulfide bonds.

CD antigen

A molecule of the cell membrane that is employed to differentiate human leukocyte subpopulations based upon their interactions with monoclonal antibodies. The monoclonal antibodies that interact with the same membrane molecule are grouped into a common cluster of differentiation (CD).

CD antigens

Cluster of differentiation antigen identified by monoclonal antibodies. The CD designation refers to a cluster of monoclonal antibodies, all of which have identical cellular reaction patterns and identify the same molecular species. Anti-CD refers to anti-idiotype and should not be employed to name CD monoclonal antibodies. The CD designation was subsequently used to describe the recognized molecule but it had to be clarified by using the term antigen or molecule. CD nomenclature is used by most investigators to designate leukocyte surface molecules. Provisional clusters are designated as CDw.

CD (cluster of differentiation)

Refer to cluster of differentiation. Molecular weights for the CD designations that follow are given for reduced conditions.

CD molecules

Cell-surface molecules found on immune system cells that are designated a cluster of differentiation (CD) followed by a number, such as CD33. **For a complete listing of CD markers, refer to Appendix V.**

CD1

An antigen that is a cortical thymocyte marker that disappears at later stages of T cell maturation. The antigen is also found on interdigitating cells, fetal B cells, and Langerhans' cells. These chains are associated with β_2-microglobulin, so the antigen is thus analogous to classical histocompatibility antigens but is coded for by a different chromosome. More recent studies have

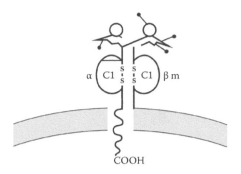

Structure of CD1.

shown that the molecule is coded for by at least five genes on chromosome 1, of which three produce recognized polypeptide products. CD1 may participate in antigen presentation.

CD1a

An antigen (molecular weight of 49,12 kDa) that is a membrane glycoprotein. It is expressed strongly on cortical thymocytes.

CD1b

An antigen (molecular weight of 45,12 kDa) that is a membrane glycoprotein. It is expressed moderately on thymocytes.

CD1c

An antigen (molecular weight of 43,12 kDa) that is a membrane glycoprotein. It is expressed weakly on cortical thymocytes.

CD2

A T cell adhesion molecule that binds to the LFA-3 adhesion molecule of antigen-presenting cells. Also called LFA-2.

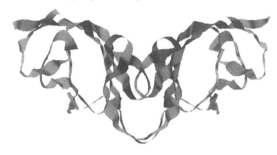

CD2. Ribbon diagram. Resolution = 2.0 Å.

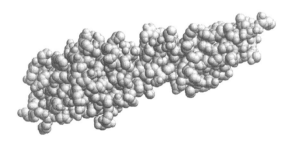

CD2. Space fill. Resolution = 2.0 Å.

CD2R

A molecule (molecular weight of 50 kDa) that is restricted to activated T cells and some natural killer (NK) cells. The CD2R epitope is unrelated to LFA-3 sites. The antigen is of importance in T cell maturation, as certain CD2 antibodies in combination with CD2R antibodies or LFA-3 may induce T cell proliferation. CD2R is a conformational form of CD2 that is activation-dependent.

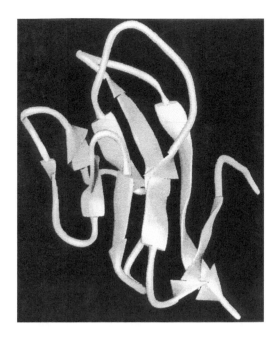

CD2. Ribbon structure.

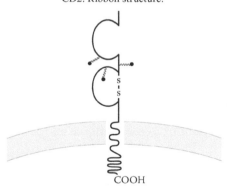

Structure of CD2.

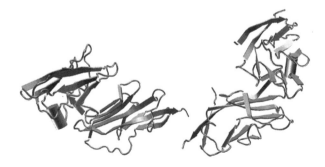

Heterophilic adhesion complex between CD2 and LFA-3..

CD3

A molecule, also referred to as the T3 antigen, that consists of five different polypeptide chains with molecular weights ranging from 16 to 28 kDa. The five chains are designated γ, δ, ε, ζ, and ή, with most CD3 antibodies being against the 20-kDa ε chain. They are closely associated physically and also with the T cell antigen receptor in the T cell membrane. Incubation of T cells with CD3 antibodies induces calcium flux and proliferation. This group of molecules may therefore transmit a signal to the cell interior following binding of the antigen to the antigen receptor.

C

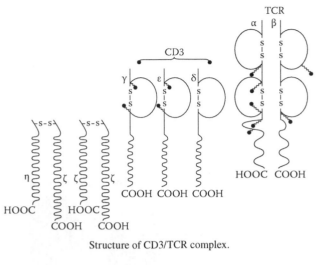

Structure of CD3/TCR complex.

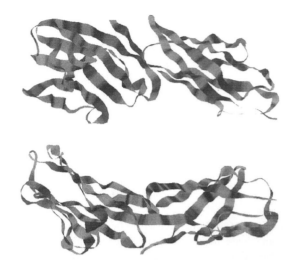

Ribbon structure of T cell surface glycoprotein CD4.

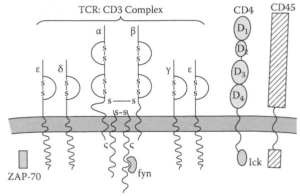

Structure of TCR/CD3 complex showing the lck, fyn, and ZAP phospho-tyrosine kinases.

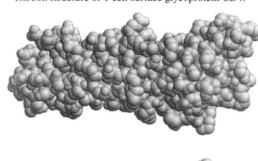

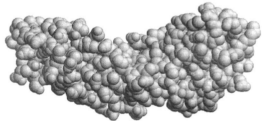

Space-filling model of CD4 type 1 crystal form. Human recombinant form expressed in Chinese hamster ovary cells.

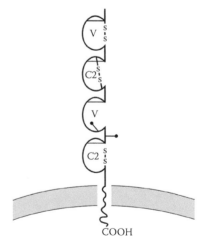

Structure of CD4.

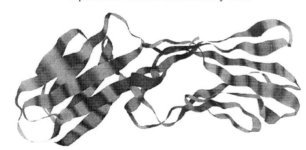

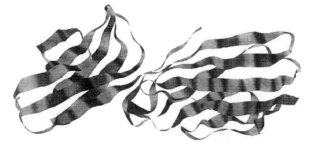

Ribbon structures of CD4 domains 3 and 4. Rat recombinant form expressed in Chinese hamster ovary cells.

CD3 complex

A combination of α:β or γ:δ T cell receptor chains with the invariant subunits CD3γ, δ, and ε and the dimeric ζ chains.

CD4

A cell-surface glycoprotein on T cells that recognizes antigens presented by major histocompatibility complex (MHC) class II molecules. CD4 binds to the MHC class II molecules on the antigen-presenting cell and serves as a coreceptor binding to the lateral faces of the MHC class II molecules.

C

CD4 molecule

Exists as a monomer and contains four immunogloblin-like domains. The first domains form a rigid rod-like structure linked to the two carboxyl terminal domains by a flexible link. The binding site for major histocompatibility complex (MHC) class II molecules is believed to involve the D_1 and D_2 domains of CD4.

CD4 T cells

The T cell subset that expresses the CD4 coreceptor and recognizes peptide antigens presented by major histocompatibility complex (MHC) class II molecules.

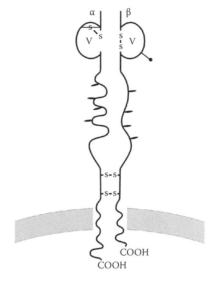

Structure of CD8.

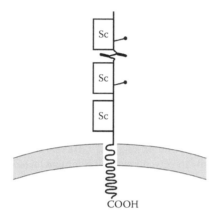

Structure of CD5.

CD5

Initially described as an alloantigen termed Ly-1 on murine T cells. Subsequently, a pan T cell marker of similar molecular mass was found on human lymphocytes using monoclonal antibodies and named CD5. Thus, CD5 is homologous at the DNA level with Ly-1. It is a 67-kDa type I transmembrane glycoprotein comprised of a single polypeptide of approximately 470 amino acids. The signal peptide is formed by the first 25 amino acids. CD5 is expressed on the surfaces of all $\alpha\beta$ T cells but is absent or of low density on $\gamma\delta$ T cells. It has been discovered on many murine B cell lymphomas and on endothelial cells of blood vessels in the pregnant sheep uterus. CD72 on B cells is one of its three ligands. CD5 is present on thymocytes and most peripheral T cells. It is believed to be significant for the activation of T cells and possibly B1 cells. CD5 is also present on a subpopulation of B cells (B1 cells) that synthesize polyreactive and autoreactive antibodies as well as the "natural antibodies" present in normal serum. Human chronic lymphocytic leukemia cells express CD5 which points to their derivation from this particular B cell subpopulation.

CD5 B cells

An atypical, self-renewing class of B lymphocytes that reside mainly in the peritoneal and pleural cavities in adults and have far less diverse receptor repertoires than do conventional B cells.

CD6

A molecule, sometimes referred to as the T12 antigen. It is a single chain glycopolypeptide with a molecular weight of 105 kDa and is present on the majority of human T cells (similar in distribution to CD3). It stains some B cells weakly.

CD7

An antigen (molecular weight of 40 kDa) that is present on the majority of T cells and is useful as a marker for T cell

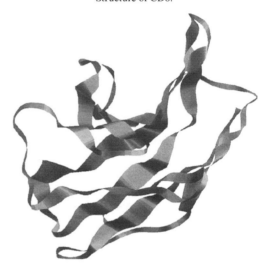

Ribbon structure of a human CD8 T cell receptor.

neoplasms when other T cell antigens are absent. The CD7 antigen is probably an Fc receptor for immunoglobulin M (IgM).

CD8

A cell surface glycoprotein on T cells that recognizes antigens presented by major histocompatibility complex (MHC) class I molecules. It binds to MHC class I molecules on antigen-presenting cells and serves as a coreceptor to facilitate the T cell response to antigen.

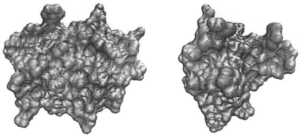

This structure consists of the N terminal 114 residues of CD8. These residues make up a single immunoglobulin axis which coincides with a crystallographic two-fold axis.

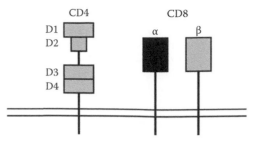

Outline structure of CD4 and CD8 coreceptor molecules.

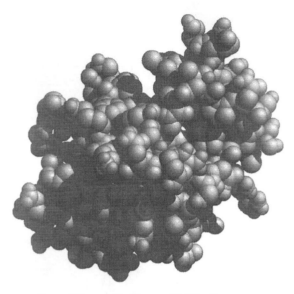

Space-filling model of human CD8 T cell receptor.

CD8 molecule

A heterodimer of an α and β chain that are covalently associated by disulfide bond. The two chains of a dimer have similar structures, each having a single domain resembling an immunoglobulin variable domain and a stretch of peptide believed to be in a relatively extended confirmation.

CD8 T cells

The T cell subset that expresses CD8 coreceptor and recognizes peptide antigens presented by major histocompatibility complex (MHC) class I molecules.

CD9

A single chain protein (molecular weight of 24 kDa) that is present on pre-B cells, monocytes, granulocytes, and platelets. Antibodies against the molecule can cause platelet aggregation. The CD9 antigen has protein kinase activity. It may be significant in aggregation and activation of platelets.

CD10

An antigen, also referred to as common acute lymphoblastic leukemia antigen (CALLA), that has a molecular weight of 100 kDa. CD10 is now known to be a neutral endopeptidase (enkephalinase). It is present on many cell types, including stem cells, lymphoid progenitors of B and T cells, renal epithelium, fibroblasts, and bile canaliculi.

CD11

A family of three leukocyte-associated, single chain molecules identified in recent years (sometimes referred to as the leukocyte function-associated antigen [LFA]/Mac-1 family). They all consist of two polypeptide chains; the larger of these chains (α) is different for each member of the family; the smaller chain (β) is common to all three molecules (see CD11a, CD11b, CD11c).

CD11a

The α chain of the leukocyte function associated-1 antigen (LFA-1) molecule. It has a molecular weight of 180 kDa and is present on leukocytes, monocytes, macrophages, and granulocytes but not on platelets. LFA-1 binds the intercellular adhesion molecules ICAM-1 (CD54), ICAM-2, and ICAM-3.

CD11b

The α chain of Mac-1 (C3bi receptor). It has a molecular weight of 170 kDa and is present on granulocytes, monocytes, and natural killer (NK) cells.

CD11c

The α chain of the p150,95 molecule. It has a molecular weight of 150 kDa and is present on granulocytes, monocytes, and natural killer (NK) cells. It reacts very strongly with hairy cell leukemia. The antigen is weakly expressed on B and T cell subsets.

CD12

Little is known about this antigen, which has a molecular weight of 90 to 120 kDa. It is present on some monocytes, granulocytes, and platelets.

CD13

An antigen (molecular weight of 130 kDa) that is a single chain membrane glycoprotein. It is present on monocytes, granulocytes, some macrophages, and connective tissue. CD13 has recently been shown to be aminopeptidase-N. It functions as a zinc metalloproteinase.

CD14

An antigen (molecular weight of 55 kDa) that is a single chain membrane glycoprotein. It is found principally on monocytes but also on granulocytes, dendritic reticulum cells, and some tissue macrophages. It serves as a receptor for lipopolysaccharide (LPS) and for lipopolysaccharide-binding protein (LBP).

CD15

A carbohydrate antigen that is often referred to as hapten X and consists of galactose, fucose, and N-acetyl-glucosamine linked in a specific sequence. The antigen appears to be particularly immunogenic in mice and numerous monoclonal antibodies of this oligosaccharide specificity have been produced. CD15 is present in neutrophil secondary granules of granulocytic cells that express the antigen strongly late in their maturation. It is also present on eosinophils, monocytes, and Reed–Sternberg and Hodgkin cells but can also be found on non-Hodgkin cells. CD15 is also termed Lewis-x (Le^x).

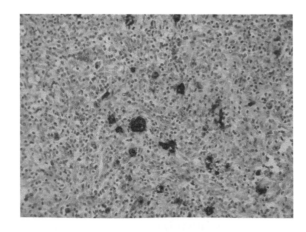

Leu M1 in Hodgkin disease.

CD15 (Leu M1)

A monoclonal antibody that recognizes the human myelo-monocytic antigen lacto-N fucopentose III. It is present on more than 95% of mature peripheral blood eosinophils and neutrophils and is present at low density on circulating monocytes. In lymphoid tissue, CD15 reacts with Reed–Sternberg cells of Hodgkin disease and with granulocytes. It also reacts with few tissue macrophages and does not react with dendritic cells.

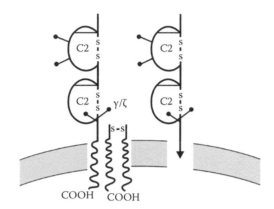

Structure of CD16.

CD16

An antigen that is also known as the low-affinity Fc receptor for complexed IgG–FcγRIII. It is expressed on natural killer (NK) cells, granulocytes, neutrophils, and macrophages. Structural differences in the CD16 antigen from granulocytes and NK cells have been reported. This apparent polymorphism suggests two different genes for the FcγRIII molecule in polymorphonuclear leukocytes (PMNs) and in NK cells. The CD16 molecule in NK cells has a transmembrane form, whereas it is phosphatidylinositol (PI)-linked in granulocytes. CD16 mediates phagocytosis. It is the functional receptor structure for performing antibody-dependent, cell-mediated cytotoxicity (ADCC). CD16 is also termed FcγRIII.

CDw17

An antigen that is a cell surface glycosphingolipid moiety, lactosylceramide, and is present principally on granulocytes but also on monocytes and platelets.

CD18

An antigen (molecular weight of 95 kDa) that is an integral membrane glycoprotein. This integrin β_2 subunit is noncovalently linked to CD11a, CD11b, and CD11c molecules and is expressed on leukocytes. It is important for cell adhesion. The immunodeficiency known as leukocyte adhesion deficiency (LAD) has been shown to be caused by a genetic defect of the CD18 gene.

CD19

A constituent of the B cell coreceptor.

CD20

A B cell marker (molecular weight of 33, 35, and 37 kDa) that appears relatively late in B cell maturation (after the pro-B cell stage) and persists for some time before the plasma cell stage. Its molecular structure resembles that of a transmembrane ion channel. The gene is on chromosome 11 at band q12–q13. It may be involved in regulating B cell activation.

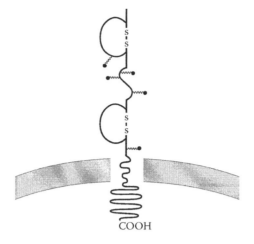

Structure of CD19.

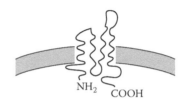

Structure of CD20—tonsil.

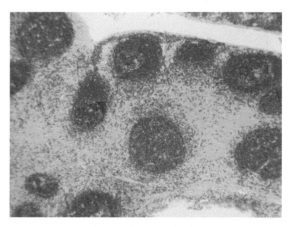

CD20 primary antibody.

CD20 primary antibody

A mouse monoclonal antibody (clone L26) directed against an intracellular epitope of the CD20 antigen present on human B lymphocytes. It may be used to aid in the identification of cells of B lymphocytic lineage and is intended for qualitative staining in sections of formalin-fixed, paraffin-embedded tissue. Anti-CD20 antibodies specifically bind to antigens located in the plasma membrane and cytoplasmic regions of normal B lymphocytes that may also be expressed in Reed–Sternberg cells. Unexpected antigen expression or loss of expression may occur, especially in neoplasms. Occasional stromal elements surrounding heavily stained tissue and/or cells may show immunoreactivity. The clinical interpretation of any staining, or its absence, must be complemented by morphological studies and evaluation of proper controls.

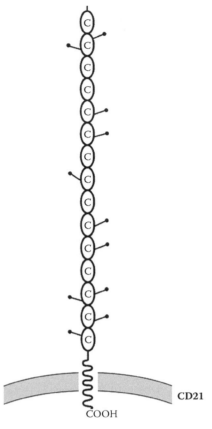

Structure of CD21.

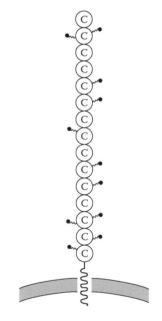

Structure of CD21.

CD21

A 145-kDa glycoprotein that is a component of the B cell receptor. CD21 is a membrane molecule that participates in transmitting growth-promoting signals to the interiors of B cells. It is the receptor for the C3d fragment of the third component of complement, CR2. The CD21 antigen is a restricted B cell antigen expressed on mature B cells. It is present at high

density on follicular dendritic cells (FDCs), the accessory cells of the B zones. Also called complement receptor 2 (CR2).

CD21 antigen

A restricted B cell antigen expressed on mature B cells. The antigen is present at high denisty on follicular dendritic cells (FDCs), the accessory cells of the B zones. It shows moderate labeling of B cells and a strong labeling of FDC in cryostat sections, whereas the staining of B cells is reduced or abolished in paraffin sections. However, the labeling of FDC in paraffin sections is as strong as on cryostat sections.

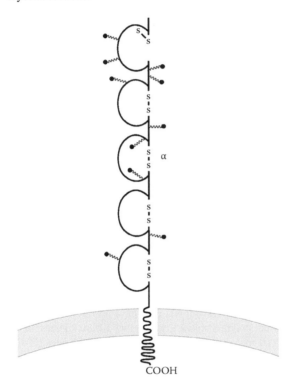

Structure of CD22.

CD22

A molecule (molecular weight of α130 and β140 kDa) expressed in the cytoplasm of B cells of the pro-B and pre-B cell stages and on the cell surfaces of mature B cells with surface immunoglobulin (Ig). The antigen is lost shortly before the terminal plasma cell phase. The molecule has five extracellular immunoglobulin domains and shows homology with myelin adhesion glycoprotein and with N-CAM (CD56). It participates in B cell adhesion to monocytes and T cells. Also called BL-CAM.

CD23

An antigen (molecular weight of 45 to 50 kDa) that is an integral membrane glycoprotein. The CD23 antigen has been identified as the low affinity Fc-IgE receptor (FceRII). Two species of FceRII/CD23 have been found. FceRIIa and FceRIIb differ only in the N terminal cytoplasmic region and share the same C terminal extracellular region. FceRIIa is strongly expressed on IL4-activated B cells and weakly on mature B cells. FceIIa is not found on circulating B cells and bone marrow B cells positive for surface IgM, IgD. FceRIIb is expressed weakly on monocytes, eosinophils, and T cell lines. However, IL4-treated monocytes show a

C

stronger staining. The CD23 molecule may also be a receptor for B cell growth factor (BCGF).

CD23(1B12)

Anti-CD23 mouse monoclonal antibody. A B-cell antibody that is useful to differentiate between B-CLL and B-SLLs that are CD23-positive from mantle cell lymphomas and small cleaved lymphomas that are CD23-negative. This antibody reacts with the antigen that is found on a subpopulation of peripheral blood cells, B lymphocytes, and on EBV transformed B lymphoblastoid cell lines.

CD24

An antigen that is a glycoprotein found on B cells, granulocytes, interdigitating cells, and epithelial cells. The CD24 antigen, with a molecular weight of 41/38 kDa, is expressed on B cells from the late pro-B cell stage and is lost before the plasma cell stage. It may be a homolog in humans of murine heat-stable antigen (HSA) or J11d.

CD25

A single chain glycoprotein, often referred to as the α chain of the interleukin-2 receptor (IL2R) or the Tac antigen, that has a molecular weight of 55 kDa and is present on activated T and B cells and activated macrophages. It functions as a receptor for IL2. Together with the β chain of the IL2R (p75, molecular weight of 75 kDa), the CD25 antigen forms a high affinity receptor complex for IL2. The gene for IL2R has been located as a single gene on chromosome 10. It associates with CD122 and complexes with the IL2R$\beta\gamma$ high-affinity receptor. It facilitates T cell growth.

CD26

An antigen (molecular weight of 110 kDa) that is a single chain glycoprotein. It is present on activated T and B cells and also on macrophages, bile canaliculi, and splenic sinusoidal lining cells. It has recently been shown to be a dipeptidyl peptidase IV (DPP-IV), which is a serine-type protease, and may play a role in cell proliferation together with the CD25 antigen. Although the CD4 molecule is requisite for binding HIV particles, it is not sufficient for efficient entry of the virus and infection. The cofactor is dipeptidyl peptidase IV (DPP-IV), also termed CD26.

CD27

A T cell antigen (molecular weight of 110 kDa) that is a disulfide-linked homodimer of two polypeptide chains, each with a molecular weight of 55 kDa. It is found on a subpopulation of thymocytes, on the majority of mature T cells, and on transformed B lymphocytes. CD27 antigen expression is unregulated on activated cells.

CD28

A T cell low affinity receptor that interacts with B7 costimulatory molecules to facilitate T lymphocyte activation. More specifically, B7-1 and B7-2 ligands are expressed on the surfaces of activated antigen-presenting cells (APCs). Signals from CD28 to the T cell elevate expression of high affinity interleukin-2 (IL2) receptor and increase the synthesis of numerous cytokines, including IL2. CD28 regulates the responsiveness of T cells to antigen when they are in contact with APCs. It serves as a costimulatory receptor because its signals are synergistic with those provided by the T cell antigen receptor (TCR-CD3) in promoting T cell activation and proliferation. Without the signal from TCR-CD3, the signal of CD28 is only able to stimulate minimal T cell proliferation and may even lead to T cell unresponsiveness.

CD29

An antigen (molecular weight of 130 kDa) that is very widely distributed on human tissues (e.g., nerve, connective tissue, endothelium), as well as on many white cell populations. The structure recognized is now known to be the platelet gpIIa, the integrin β-1 chain, the common β subunit of very late antigens (VLA) 1 to 6, and the fibronectin receptor. The CD29 antigen is termed gpIIa in contrast to CD31, which is called gpIIa'. Together with α^1 chain (CDw49), it forms a heterodimeric complex. CD29 associates with CD49a in VLA-1 integrin. Antibodies against CD29 appear to define a subset of cells among CD4-positive T cells which provide help for antibody production. Like the antibody belonging to CD45RO (UCHL1), CD29 antibodies appear to be reciprocal (when T4 positive cells are analyzed) to those of CD45RA antibodies against the B-cell-restricted form of leukocyte common antigen (LCA). This form recognizes a T cell subset of CD4-positive cells suppressing antibody production. The molecule is involved in the mediation of cell adhesion to cells or matrix, especially in conjunction with CD49.

CD30

A molecule (molecular weight of 105 kDa) that is a single chain glycoprotein, also referred to as the Ki-1 antigen, present on activated T and B cells, embryonal carcinoma cells, and Hodgkin and Reed–Sternberg cells. It is also found on a minority of non-Hodgkin lymphomas (referred to as anaplastic large-cell lymphomas), with a characteristic anaplastic morphology.

CD31

An antigen (molecular weight of 140 kDa) that is a single chain membrane glycoprotein. It is found on granulocytes, monocytes, macrophages, B cells, platelets, and endothelial cells. Although it is termed gpIIa', it is different from the CD29 antigen. At present, its function is unknown. It may be an adhesion molecule. Also called PECAM-1 (platelet endothelial cell adhesion molecule-1).

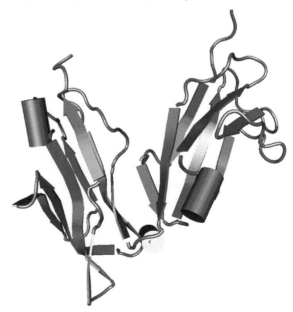

CD32 receptor.

CD32

An antigen (molecular weight of 40 kDa) also known as FcγRII receptor, which is a low affinity Fc receptor for IgG,

C

aggregated immunoglobulin/immune complexes. Several different isoforms that are coded for by closely related genes exist. D32 is found on granulocytes, B cells, monocytes, platelets, and endothelial cells. FcγRII functions as the receptor for aggregated IgG and is involved in cell activation.

CD33

An antigen (molecular weight of 67 kDa) that is a single chain transmembrane glycoprotein. It is restricted to myeloid cells and is found on early progenitor cells, monocytes, myeloid leukemias, and weakly on some granulocytes.

CD34

A single chain transmembrane glycoprotein (molecular weight of 105 to 120 kDa) present on immature haematopoietic cells and endothelial cells as well as bone marrow stromal cells. Three classes of CD34 epitopes have been defined by differential sensitivity to enzymatic cleavage with neuraminidase and with glycoprotease from *Pasteurella haemolytica*. Its gene is on chromosome 1. It is the ligand for L-selectin (CD62L).

CD35

An antigen that is known as CR1 that binds C3b and C4b. The CD35 antigen includes four different allotypes, C, A, B, and D, with molecular weights of 160, 190, 220, and 250 kDa, respectively. The antigen is widely distributed on various cell types, including erythrocytes, B cells, monocytes, granulocytes (negative on basophils), some natural killer (NK) cells, and follicular dendritic cells. The functions of CR1 are the processing of immune complexes and promotion of binding and phagocytosis of C3b-coated particles/cells.

CD36

An antigen (molecular weight of 88 kDa) that is a single chain membrane glycoprotein found on monocytes, macrophages, platelets, some endothelial cells, and weakly on B cells. The CD36 antigen is also referred to as gpIV or gpIIIb. The antigen acts as a receptor for thrombospondin and collagen. Furthermore, it is the endothelial cell receptor for erythrocytes infected with *Plasmodium falciparum*.

CD37

A B cell antigen (molecular weight of 40 to 52 kDa) that is an integral glycoprotein that appears at the late pre-B cell stage and then persists throughout B cell maturation until shortly before the terminal plasma cell stage. The antigen is also weakly expressed on macrophages, on neutrophils and monocytes, and on resting and activated T cells. The function of CD37 antigen is unknown.

CD38

A molecule that is an integral glycoprotein and is also referred to as the T10 antigen. It has a molecular weight of 45 kDa and is found on plasma cells, pre-B cells, immature T cells, and activated T cells.

CD39

An antigen (molecular weight of 100 to 70 kDa) that is present on a number of cell types, including B cells (mantle zone), most mature B cells with surface-bound immunoglobulin G (IgG), monocytes, some macrophages, and vascular endothelial cells. Its function is yet to be determined, but it may mediate B cell adhesion. Also called gp80.

CD40

An integral membrane glycoprotein (molecular weight of 48/44 kDa) that is also referred to as gp50. The antigen shares similarities with many nerve growth factor receptors. The CD40 antigen is expressed on peripheral blood and tonsillar B cells from the pre-B cell stage until the plasma cell stage, where it is lost. It is also expressed on B cell leukemias and lymphomas, on some carcinomas, weakly on monocytes, and on interdigitating cells. The CD40 antigen is active in B cell proliferation. The CD40 ligand is gp39. CD40 binds CD40-L, the CD40 ligand. It is the receptor for the costimulatory signal for B cells. Its interaction with CD40 ligand on T cells induces B cell proliferation. CD40 belongs to the TNF receptor family of molecules.

CD40-L

A 39-kDa antigen present on activated CD4+ T cells. It is the ligand for CD40. It is also called T-BAM or gp39.

CD40 ligand

A molecule on T cells that interacts with CD40 on B cell proliferation.

CD41

An antigen, equivalent to glycoprotein IIb/IIIa, that is found on platelets and megakaryocytes. This structure is a Ca²⁺-dependent complex between the 110-kDa gpIIIa (CD61) and the 135-kDa gpIIb molecules. The gpIIb molecule consists of two chains: an α chain of 120 kDa and a β chain of 23 kDa. The gpIIIa (CD61) is a single chain protein, but both gpIIIa (CD61) and gpIIb contain transmembrane domains. The molecule is a receptor for fibrinogen, but it also binds von Willebrand factor, thrombospondin, and fibronectin. It is absent or reduced in Glanzmann's thrombasthenia (hereditary gpIIb/IIIa deficiency). It has a role in platelet aggregation and activation.

CD42a

An antigen, equivalent to glycoprotein IX, that is a single chain membrane glycoprotein with a molecular weight of 23 kD. It is found on megakaryocytes and platelets. CD42a forms a noncovalent complex with CD4b (gpIb) which acts as a receptor for von Willebrand factor. It is absent or reduced in the Bernard–Soulier syndrome.

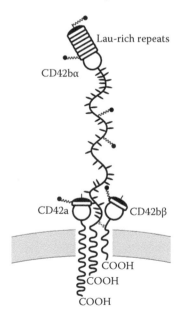

Structure of CD42.

CD42b

An antigen, equivalent to glycoprotein Ib, that is a two-chain membrane glycoprotein with a molecular weight of

170 kDa. CD42b has an α chain of 135 kDa and a β chain of 23 kDa. It is found on platelets and megakaryocytes. It forms a noncovalent complex with CD42a (gpIX) which acts as a receptor for von Willebrand factor. The antigen is absent or reduced in the Bernard–Soulier syndrome.

CD42c

A 22-kDa antigen found on platelets and megakaryocytes. It is also referred to as GPIB-β.

CD42d

An 85-kDa antigen present mainly on platelets and mega-karyocytes. It is also referred to as GPV.

CD43

A 90- to 100-kDa sialylated glycoprotein found on leu-kocytes, including T cells, granulocytes, erythrocytes, epithelial cell lines, and brain cells. The CD43 antigen is not present on peripheral B cells. The molecule is involved in activation of T cells, B cells, natural killer (NK) cells, and monocytes. It binds CD54 (ICAM-1).

CD44

A ubiquitous multistructural and multifunctional cell sur-face glycoprotein that participates in adhesive cell-to-cell and cell-to-matrix interactions. It also plays a role in cell migration and cell homing. Its main ligand is hyaluronic acid (HA), hyaluronate, and hyaluronan. It is expressed by numerous cell types of lymphohematopoietic origin, including erythrocytes, T and B lymphocytes, natural killer (NK) cells, macrophages, Kupffer cells, dendritic cells, and granulocytes. It is also expressed in other types of cells such as fibroblasts and central nervous system cells. In addition to hyaluronic acid, CD44 also interacts with other ECM ligands such as collagen, fibronectin, and laminin. In addition to these functions, CD44 facilitates lymph node homing via binding to high endothelial venules, presenta-tion of chemokines or growth factors to migrating cells, and growth signal transmission. CD44 concentration may be observed in areas of intensive cell migration and prolifera-tion, as in wound healing, inflammation, and carcinogen-esis. Many cancer cells and their metastases express high levels of CD44. It may be used as a diagnostic or prognostic marker for selected human malignant diseases.

CD45

An antigen that is a single chain glycoprotein referred to as the leukocyte common antigen (or T200). It consists of at least five high molecular weight glycoproteins present on the surfaces of the majority of human leukocytes (molecu-lar weights of 180, 190, 205, and 220 kDa). The different isoforms arise from a single gene via alternative mRNA splicing. The variation among the isoforms is all in the extracellular region. The larger (700-amino acid) intracel-lular portion is identical in all isoforms and has protein tyrosine phosphatase activity. It can potentially interact with intracellular protein kinases such as p56[lck], which may be involved in triggering cell activation. By dephosphory-lating proteins, CD45 would act in a fashion opposite that of a protein kinase. It facilitates signaling through B and T cell antigen receptors. Leukocyte common antigen (LCA) is present on all leukocyte surfaces. It is a transmembrane tyrosine phosphatase that is expressed in various isoforms on different types of cells, including the different subtypes of T cells. The isoforms are designated by CD45R fol-lowed by the exon whose presence gives rise to distinctive antibody-binding patterns.

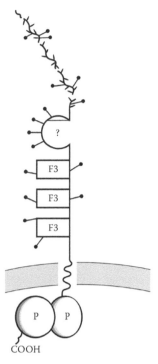

Structure of CD45, also known as leukocyte common antigen.

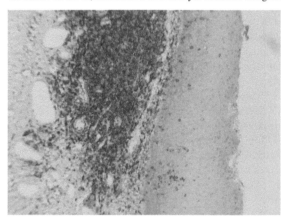

CD45—tonsil.

CD45R

A subfamily that is now divided into three isoforms: CD45RO, CD45RA, and CD45RB. The designation CD45R has been maintained for those antibodies that have not been tested on appropriate transfectants.

CD45RA

A 220/205-kDa isoform of CD45 (sequence encoded by exon A) that is found on B cells, monocytes, and a subtype of T cells. T cells expressing this isotype are naïve or virgin T cells and nonprimed CD4 and CD8 cells.

CD45RB

A molecule consisting of four isoforms of CD45 (sequence encoded by exon B), with molecular weights of 220, 205, and 190 kDa, that is found on B cells, subset of T cells, monocytes, macrophages, and granulocytes.

CD45RO

A 180-kDa isoform of CD45 (sequence not encoded by exons A, B, or C) found on T cells, a subset of B cells, monocytes, and macrophages. T cells expressing this anti-gen are T memory cells or primed T cells.

CD46

An antigen that is a dimeric protein with a molecular weight of 66/56 kDa. It has a broad tissue distribution. It is present on hematopoietic and nonhematopoietic nucleated cells. The CD46 antigen shows sequence homology to complement-associated molecules such as decay-accelerating factor (DAF, CD55) and the complement receptors CR1 (CD35) and CR2 (CD21). It is a membrane cofactor protein that binds C3b and C4b, allowing their degradation by factor I.

CD47

A single chain glycoprotein (molecular weight of 47 to 52 kDa) that is widely distributed and may be associated with the Rhesus blood group.

CD47R

Formerly CDw149. Mabs actually recognized with low affinity the CD47 glycoprotein.

CD48

An antigen (molecular weight of 43 kDa) that is a phosphatidylinositol (PI)-linked glycoprotein and is widely distributed on white blood cells.

CD49a

A 210-kDa antigen present on activated T cells and monocytes. It associates with CD29 and binds collagen and laminin. It is also referred to as VLA-1 and α^1 integrin.

CD49b

A 165-kDa antigen present on B cells, platelets, and monocytes. It associates with CD29 and binds collagen and laminin. It is also referred to as VLA-2 and α^2 integrin.

CD49c

A 125-kDa antigen present on B cells. It associates with CD29 and binds laminin and fibronectin. It is also referred to as VLA-3 and α^3 integrin.

CD49d

A 150-kDa antigen present on B cells and thymocytes. It associates with CD29 and binds fibronectin, Peyer's patch HEV, and VCAM-1. It is also referred to as VLA-4 and α^4 integrin.

CD49e

A 135,25-dimer antigen present on memory T cells, platelets, and monocytes. It associates with CD29 and binds fibronectin. It is also referred to as VLA-5 and α^5 integrin.

CD49f

A 120,25-dimer antigen present on memory T cells, monocytes, and thymocytes. It associates with CD29 and binds laminin. It is also referred to as VLA-6 and as α^6 integrin.

CD50

A molecule (molecular weight of 124 kDa) that is broadly distributed on leukocytes including thymocytes, T cells, B cells (not plasma cells), monocytes, and granulocytes. However, it is not present on platelets and erythrocytes. CD50 is also called ICAM-3.

CD51

A molecule (molecular weight of 140 kDa) that is the α chain of the vitronectin receptor (VNR). The CD51 antigen consists of a disulfide-linked large subunit of 125 kDa and a smaller one of 25 kDa. The VNR α chain is noncovalently associated with the VNR β_3 chain, also termed gpIIIa or CD61. The α chain is weakly expressed on platelets. The VNR mediates cell adhesion to arg–gly–arp-containing sequences in vitronectin, von Willebrand factor, fibrinogen, and thrombospondin.

CD51/61 complex

An antigen found on platelets and on endothelial cells. It is also referred to as vitronectin receptor or as integrin $\alpha V\beta_3$.

CD52

A cluster that corresponds to the leukocyte antigen (molecular weight of 21 to 28 kDa) recognized by antibody campath-1. Anti-CD52 antibodies have been used to deplete T lymphocytes therapeutically.

CD53

A single chain glycoprotein (molecular weight of 32 to 42 kDa) that is widely distributed, for example, in monocytes, T cells, B cells, and natural killer (NK) cells.

CD54

An intercellular adhesion molecule (ICAM-1) found on phytohemagglutinin (PHA) blasts, endothelial cells, and follicular dendritic cells. The molecular weight of the antigen is 90 kDa. ICAM-1 is a lymphokine-inducible molecule and has been shown to be a ligand for LFA-1 or the CD11/CD18 complex. It is also the receptor for rhinovirus. CD54 binds CD11a/CD18 integrin (LFA-1) and CD11b/CD18 integrin (Mac-1).

CD55

A 75-kDa molecule that is a phosphatidylinositol (PI)-linked, single chain glycoprotein, also known as the decay-accelerating factor (DAF). The antigen is involved in complement degradation on the cell surface. It is broadly distributed on hematopoietic and many nonhematopoietic cells. CD55 binds C3b and disassembles C3/C5 convertase.

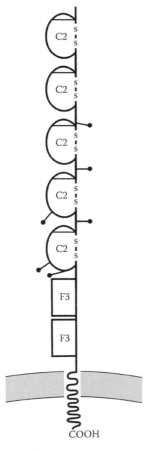

Structure of CD56.

CD56

A 220/135-kDa molecule that is an isoform of the neural adhesion molecule (N-CAM). It is used as a marker of natural killer (NK) cells, but it is also present on neuroectodermal cells.

CD57

A 110-kDa, myeloid-associated glycoprotein that is recognized by the antibody HNK1. It is a marker for natural killer (NK) cells, but it is also found on some T and B cells. It is an oligosaccharide present on multiple cell surface glycoproteins.

CD58

A 65- to 70-kDa molecule that is a single chain glycoprotein also known as LFA-3 (leukocyte function associated-3 antigen) and is the ligand to which CD2 binds. The CD58 antigen is expressed on many hematopoietic and nonhematopoietic cells.

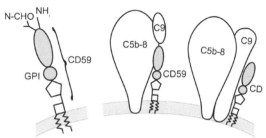

Structure of CD59.

CD59

An 18-kDa membrane glycoprotein that regulates the activity of the complement membrane attack complex (MAC). A glycosylphosphatidylinositol anchor attaches CD59 to the outer layer of the membrane. It is shed from cell surfaces into body fluid. There is no evidence for a secreted form. CD59 inhibits MAC formation by binding to sites on C8 and C9, blocking the uptake and incorporation of multiple C9 molecules into the complex. CD59 can interact with C8 and C9 from heterologous species but works best with homologous proteins, which is the basis for homologous restriction (of lysis). Paroxysmal nocturnal hemoglobinuria (PNH)-affected cells deficient in C59 and other complement regulatory proteins are very sensitive to lysis. Also called protective membrane inhibitor of reactive lysis (MIRL), homologous restriction factor 20 (HRF 20) and membrane attack complex inhibitory factor (MACIF).

CDw60

An oligosaccharide found on gangliosides. It is present on a subpopulation of lymphocytes, platelets, and monocytes.

CD61

An antigen that is also termed gpIIIa, the integrin β_3 chain, or the β chain of the vitronectin receptor (VNR β_3 chain). GpIIIa can associate with either gpIIb to form the gpIIb/IIIa complex (CD41) or with the VNR α chain (CD51). The CD61 molecule has a molecular weight of 110 kDa and is expressed on platelets and megakaryocytes.

CD62E

A 140-kDa antigen present on endothelium. CD62E is endothelium leuckocyte adhesion molecule (ELAM). It mediates neutrophil rolling on the endothelium. It also binds sialyl–Lewis-x.

CD62L

A 150-kDa antigen present on B and T cells, monocytes, and natural killer (NK) cells. CD62L is a leukocyte β_3 adhesion molecule (LAM). It mediates cell rolling on the endothelium and binds CD34 and GlyCAM. It is also referred to as L-selectin, LECAM-1, or LAM-1.

CD62P

A 75- to 80-kDa antigen present on endothelial cells, platelets, and megakaryocytes. CD62P is an adhesion molecule that binds sialyl–Lewis-x. It is a mediator of platelet interaction with monocytes and neutrophils and also mediates neutrophil rolling on the endothelium. It is also referred to as P-selectin, GMP-140, PADGEM, or LECAM-3.

CD63

A 53-kDa antigen that is a platelet-activation antigen associated with lysosomes. The CD63 molecule is also present on monocytes, on macrophages, and weakly on granulocytes, T cells, and B cells. Following activation, the CD63 lysosomal membrane protein is translocated to the cell surface.

CD64

A 75-kDa receptor that is a single chain glycoprotein. It is a high-affinity receptor IgG, also known as FcγR1, present on monocytes and some tissue macrophages.

CDw65

A 180- to 200-kDa fucoganglioside (NeuAc–Gal–GlcNac–Gal–GlcNac[Fuc]–Gal–GlcNac–Gal–GlcNac–Gal–Glc–Cer) that is present on granulocytes and monocytes.

CD66a

A 160- to 180-kDa antigen present on cells of neutrophil lineage. It is also referred to as BGP (biliary glycoprotein).

CD66b

A 95- to 100-kDa antigen present on granulocytes. It is also referred to as CGM6 (CEA gene member 6), p100. It was previously called CD67.

CD66c

A 90-kDa antigen present on neutrophils and colon β_3 carcinoma cells. It is also referred to as NCA (nonspecific crossreacting antigen).

CD66d

A 30-kDa antigen present on neutrophils. It was formerly called CGM1 (CEA gene member 1).

CD66e

A 180- to 200-kDa antigen present on adult colon epithelial cells and colon carcinoma cells. It was previously referred to as CEA (carcinoembryonic antigen).

CD67

Refer to CD66b.

CD68

A 110-kDa macrophage/myeloid marker that is principally intracellular but has weak expression under some conditions. Macrophages, monocytes, neutrophils, basophils, and large lymphocytes express it. Also called macrosialin.

CD69

A 60-kDa phosphorylated glycoprotein that is a homodimer of 34/28 kDa. CD69 is also known as AIM (activation inducer molecule) and is found on activated B and T cells, activated macrophages, and natural killer (NK) cells.

CD70

A 75-, 95-, 170-kDa antigen present on activated T and B cells and on Reed–Sternberg cells and weakly expressed on macrophages. It has also been referred to as Ki-24 antigen and CD27 ligand.

CD71

A molecule (molecular weight of 95 kDa) that is otherwise known as transferrin receptor. The antigen is a homodimeric glycoprotein present on activated T and B cells, on macrophages, and in proliferating cells. The main function of this receptor is the binding of transferrin. By internalization of the receptor and its ligand within cells, iron is delivered for cellular metabolism. Also called T9.

CD72

An antigen (molecular weight of 43 and 39 kDa) that is a heterodimeric glycoprotein. The CD72 antigen is a pan-B cell marker that occurs like the CD19 antigen at the earliest stages of B cell differentiation. The antigen is expressed from the pro-B cell stage until the plasma cell stage. It is the ligand for CD5.

CD73

A 69-kDa molecule that is an ecto-5′ nucleotidase found on B and T cell subsets, dendritic reticulium cells, epithelial cells, and endothelial cells. It is expressed weakly on pre-B cells until the final plasma cell stage, where it is lost. CD73 dephosphorylates nucleotides to permit uptake of nucleoside.

CD74

An antigen, also known as Ii, that is invariant chain of HLA-class II. It is found on B cells, macrophages, and some epithelial cells. The expression of CD74 begins during the pre-B cell stage and is lost before the plasma cell stage. Several forms (molecular weights of 41, 35, and 33 kDa) are recognized as arising via alternative splicing.

CD75

A marker of mature B cells expressing surface immunoglobulin and of a T cell subset but which is also detectable on epithelial cells. The antigen is lost before the plasma cell stage. It may be an oligosaccharide.

CD75s

An antigen (molecular weight of 85/67 kDa) that is a marker of mature B cells expressing surface immunoglobulin and a T cell subset. The CD76 antigen is lost before the plasma cell stage. Mantle zone B cells are positive, and germinal centers are negative. It may be an oligosaccharide.

CD77

A molecule that corresponds to a sugar moiety of globotriaosylceramide (Gb3) with the formula Galα1-4Galβ1-4Glc1-1 ceramide and is also recognized as the p^k blood group antigen. The CD77 antigen is only expressed on activated B cells. It is present on follicular center B cells, follicular dendritic cells, endothelium, and a variety of epithelial cell types. Also called BLA.

CDw78 (deleted by VIIth International Workshop)

A pan-B cell and macrophage subset marker that increases its expression on peripheral B cells after activation. The CDw78 antigen is expressed on pre-B cells and is lost before the plasma cell stage. Also called Ba.

CD79a

A 33,40-kDa antigen present on mature B cells. It is part of the B cell antigen receptor. It is analogous to CD3 in T cells and is needed for cell-surface expression and signal transduction. Also called MB1 or Igα.

CD79b

A 33,40-kDa antigen present on mature B cells. It is part of the B cell antigen receptor and is analogous to CD3 in T cells. It is needed for cell-surface expression and signal transduction. Also called B29 or Igβ.

CD80

A 60-kDa antigen present on a B cell subset *in vivo* and most activated B cells *in vitro*. It may also be found on dendritic cells and macrophages. It serves as a costimulator for T cell activation. It is a ligand for CTLA-4 and for CD28. Also called B7 (B7.1) or BB1.

CD81

A 22-kDa antigen present on B cells. It has broad expression including lymphocytes. It associates with CD19 and CD21 to produce the B cell coreceptor. This B cell receptor component also serves as a cell receptor for hepatitis C virus. Also termed TAPA-1.

CD82

A 50- to 53-kDa antigen. It has broad expression on leukocytes (weak) but not on erythrocytes. Also called R2, IA4, or 4F9. Its function is unknown.

CD83

A 43-kDa antigen that serves as a specific marker for circulating dendritic cells, activated B and T cells, and germinal center cells. Its function is unknown. Also called HB15.

CDw84

A 73-kDa antigen present on platelets and monocytes (strong) and circulating B cells (weak). Its function is unknown. Also called GR6.

CD85

A 120,83-kDa antigen present on circulating B cells (weak) and monocytes (strong). Its function is unknown. Also called VMP-55, GH1/75, or GR4.

CD86

An 80-kDa antigen present on circulation monocytes, germinal center cells, and activated B cells. Its function is unknown. Also called FUN-1, GR65, or BU63.

CD87

A 50- to 65-kDa antigen present on monocytes, macrophages, granulocytes, and activated T cells. It is a urokinase plasminogen activator receptor. Also called UPA-R (urokinase plasminogen activator receptor).

CD88

A 42-kDa antigen present on polymorphonuclear leukocytes, mast cells, macrophages, and smooth muscle cells. It is a receptor for complement component C5a. Also called C5a receptor or GR10.

CD89

A 55- to 70-kDa antigen present on neutrophils, monocytes, macrophages, and T and B cell subpopulations. It is the receptor for immunoglobulin A (IgA). Also called FcαR, IgA receptor.

CDw90

A 25- to 35-kDa molecule present on human CD34 prothymocytes, murine thymocytes, and T cells. It is also expressed on bone marrow, cord blood, and fetal liver. Also called Thy-1.

CD91

A 600-kD antigen present on monocytes and some nonhematopoietic cell lines. It is the α$_2$ macroglobulin receptor and is also called α$_2$M-R (α$_2$ macroglobulin receptor).

CD92

A 70-kDa antigen present on neutrophils, monocytes, endothelial cells, and platelets. Its function is unknown. Also called GR9.

CD93

A 120-kDa antigen present on neutrophils, monocytes, and endothelial cells. Its function is unknown. Also called GR11.

CD94

A 43-kDa antigen present on natural killer (NK) cells and α/β, γ/δ, and T cell subsets. Its function is unknown. Also called KP43.

CD94-NKG2 receptor

A heterodimeric inhibitory receptor that regulates natural killer (NK) cell activation. It interacts with the nonclassical human leukocyte antigen (HLA) class I molecule, HLA-E.

CD95

A 42-kDa antigen present on myeloid and T lymphoblastoid cell lines as well as various other cell lines. It binds the TNF-like ligand and causes apoptosis. Also called APO-1 or Fas.

CD96

A 160-kDa antigen present on activated T cells. Its function is unknown. Also called TACTILE (T cell activation incresed late expression).

CD97

A 74,80 89-kDa antigen present on activated cells. Its function is unknown. Also called GR1, GL-KDD/F12.

CD98

An 80,94-kDa heterodimeric antigen present on T cells and B cells (weak), monocytes (strong), natural killer (NK) cells, granulocytes, and most human cell lines. Its function is unknown. Also called 4F2 or 2F3.

CD99

A 32-kDa antigen present on peripheral blood lymphocytes and thymocytes. Also called MIC2 or E2.

CD99 (HO36-1.1)

Anti-CD99 mouse monoclonal antibody reacts with MIC-2 antigen present on the cell membranes of Ewing's sarcoma and primitive peripheral neuroectodermal tumors (PNETs). It is also present on some bone marrow, lymph nodes, spleen, cortical thymocytes, granulosa cells of the ovary, most β cells, CNS ependymal cells, Sertoli's cells of the testis, and a few endothelial cells. MIC-2 has also been identified in lymphoblastic lymphoma, rhabdomyosarcoma, mesenchymal chondrosarcoma, and thymoma.

CD99R

A 32-kDa antigen present on B and T lymphocytes and some leukemias. Also called CD99 mAb restricted.

CD100

A 150-kDa antigen that has broad expression on hematopoietic cells. Its function is unknown. Also called BB18, A8, GR3.

CDw101

A 140-kDa antigen present on granulocytes and macrophages. Its function is unknown. Also called BB27, BA27, GR14.

CD102

A 60-kDa antigen present on resting lymphocytes, monocytes, and vascular endothelial cells (strongest). It binds CD11/CD18 (LFA-1) but not CD11β/CD18 (Mac-1). Also called ICAM-2.

CD103

A 150/25-kDa antigen present on hairy cell leukemia cells, intraepithelial lymphocytes (2 to 6%), and peripheral blood lymphocytes. It is the αE integrin. Also called HML-1, αE integrin, or α6.

CD104

A 220-kDa antigen present on epithelia, Schwann cells, and some tumor cells. It functions as a β_4 integrin. Also called β_4 integrin chain or β_4.

CD105

A 95-kDa homodimeric antigen present on endothelial cells, bone marrow cell subset, and *in vitro* activated macrophages. Its function is unknown although it may be a ligand for an integrin. Also called Endoglin, TGF B$_1$ and β_3 receptor, and GR7.

CD106

A 100,110-kDa antigen present on endothelial cells that functions as an adhesion molecule. It is a ligand for VLA-4. Also called VCAM-1 or INCAM-110.

CD107a

A 110-kDa antigen present on activated platelets. Its function is unknown, but it is a lysosomal membrane protein translocated to the cell surface following activation. Also called LAMP-1 (lysosomal associated membrane protein-1).

CD107b

A 120-kDa antigen present on activated platelets. Its function is unknown, but it is a lysosomal membrane protein translocated to the cell surface following activation. Also called LAMP-2.

CD108

An 80-kDa antigen present on activated T cells in spleen and some stromal cells. Its function is unknown. Also called GR2.

CDw109

A 170/150-kDa antigen present on activated T cells, platelets, and endothelial cells. Its function is unknown. Also called platelet activation factor, 8A3, 7D1, GR56.

CD110

An 82- to 84-kDa antigen present on stem cell subsets, megakaryocytes, and platelets (very weak). Also called thrompoetin receptor or Mpl.

CD111

A 64- to 72-kDa antigen present on stem cell subsets, macrophages, and neutrophils. Commonly referred to as PRR/Nectin-1.

CD112

A 64- to 72-kDa antigen present on monocytes, neutrophils, and stem cell subsets. Also called PRR2/nectin-2.

CD113

Nothing yet assigned to this number.

CD114

A 95/139-kDa antigen present on granulocytes and monocytes. Also called G-CSF receptor.

CD115

A 150-kDa antigen present on monocytes, macrophages, and placenta. It is a macrophage colony-stimulating factor (M-CSF) receptor. Also called M-CSFR (macrophage colony-stimulating factor receptor), CSF-1R, or cFMS.

CDw116

A 75- to 85-kDa antigen present on monocytes, neutrophils, eosinophils, fibroblasts, and endothelial cells. It is a granulocyte–macrophage colony-stimulating factor (GM-CSF) receptor α chain. Also called GM-CSF R (granulocyte–macrophage colony-stimulating factor receptor) or HGM-CSFR.

C

C

CD117

A 145-kDa antigen present on bone marrow progenitor cells. It is a stem cell factor (SCF) receptor. Also called c-*kit* or stem cell factor receptor (SCF-R).

CD118

An antigen with broad cellular expression that serves as the interferon α,β receptor. Also called IFN-α,βR.

CD119

A 90-kDa antigen present on macrophages, monocytes, B cells, and epithelial cells. It is the interferon-γ receptor. Also called IFN-γR.

CD120a

A 55-kDa antigen present on most cell types, at higher levels on epithelial cell lines. It is the TNF receptor. It binds both TNFα and TNFβ. Also called TNFR-1.

CD120b

A 75-kDa antigen present on most cell types, at higher levels on myeloid cell lines. It is the TNFβ receptor, binding both TNFα and TNFβ. Also called TNFR-II.

CDw121a

An 80-kDa antigen present on T cells, thymocytes, fibroblasts, and endothelial cells. It is the type I interleukin-1 receptor and binds IL1α and IL1β. Also called IL1R (interleukin-1 receptor) type I.

CDw121b

A 68-kDa antigen present on B cells, macrophages, and monocytes. It is a type II interleukin-1 receptor, binding IL1α and IL1β. Also called IL1R type II.

CD122

A 75-kDa antigen present on natural killer (NK) cells, the resting T cell subpopulation, and some B cell lines. It is the IL2 receptor β chain. Also called IL2Rβ.

CDw123

A 70-kDa antigen present on bone marrow stem cells, granulocytes, monocytes, and megakaryocytes. It is the IL3 receptor α chain. Also called IL3Rα.

CD124

A 140-kDa antigen present on mature B and T cells, and hematopoietic precursor cells. It is the IL4 receptor. Also called IL4R.

CDw125

A 55- to 60-kDa antigen present on eosinophils and basophils. It is the IL5 receptor α chain. Also called IL5Rα.

CD126

An 80 (α subunit)-kDa antigen present on activated B cells and plasma cells (strong) and most leukocytes (weak). It is the IL6 receptor α subunit. Also called IL6Rα.

CDw127

A 75-kDa antigen present on bone marrow lymphoid presursors, pro-B cells, mature T cells, and monocytes. It serves as the IL7 receptor. Also called IL7R.

CDw128

A 58- to 67-kDa antigen present on neutrophils, basophils, and a T cell subset. It is the IL8 receptor. Also called IL8R.

CD129

Nothing yet assigned to this number.

CDw130

A 130-kDa antigen present on activated B cells and plasma cells (strong), most leukocytes (weak), and endothelial cells. It is a common subunit of IL6, IL11, oncostatin M (OSM), and leukemia inhibitory factor (LIF)

receptors. Also called IL6Rβ, IL11Rβ, OSMRβ, LIFRβ, or IL6R-gp 130SIG.

CDw131

A 130-kDa antigen present on myeloid cells. It is also referred to as common β chain for IL3, IL5, and GM-CSF receptor.

CD132

A 64-kDa molecule with broad antigenic expression that is often referred to as common γ chain for IL2, IL4, IL7, IL9, and IL15 receptors.

CD133

A 120-kDa antigen expressed on stem cell subsets. It is also called AC-133.

CD134

A 48- to 50-kDa antigen present on activated T cell subsets. It is also called OX40.

CD135

A 130- to 150-kDa antigen expressed on progenitor stem cell subsets. It is often called Flt3/Flk2.

CDw136

A 180-kDa molecule with broad antigenic expression, commonly referred to as macrophage-stimulating protein receptor.

CDw137

A 30-kDa antigen present on T cell subsets. It is also called 4-1BB.

CD138

A 20-kDa antigen expressed on plasma cells and epithelial cells. It is also called SYNDECAN-1.

CD139

A 209,228-kDa antigen present on germinal center B cells.

CD140a

A 180-kDa antigen that is undetectable on most normal cells. It is commonly called PDGF receptor α.

CD140b

A 180-kDa antigen that is present on stromal cells and endothelial cell subsets. Also called PDGF β.

CD141

A 100-kDa antigen that is expressed on endothelial cells. Also called thrombomodulin.

CD142

A 45-kDa antigen that is present on activated monocytes and endothelial cells. It is also called tissue factor.

CD143

A 170-kDa antigen that is present on endothelial cell subsets. It is commonly referred to as angiotensin converting enzyme.

CD144

A 135-kDa antigen that is present on endothelial cells. It is also called VE-cadherin.

CDw145

A 25, 90, 110 antigen expressed on endothelial cells and some stromal cells.

CD146

A 118-kDa antigen that is present on endothelial cells and activated T cells. It is also called MUC18/S-endo.

CD147

A 50- to 60-kDa antigen expressed on endothelial cells, monocytes, T cell subsets, platelets, and erythrocytes. Also called neurothelin/basigin.

CD148

A molecule present on hematopoetic cells that is commonly referred to as HPTP-ETA/DEP-1.

C

CDw149 (redesignated CD47R)

A molecule expressed on lymphocytes, monocytes, granulocytes (weak), and platelets (weak). Also called MEM-133.

CD150

A 70-kDa antigen present on T cell subsets, B cell subsets, and thymocytes. Also referred to as SLAM.

CD151

A 27-kDa antigen expressed on platelets and endothelial cells. Also called PETA-3.

CD152

A 44-kDa antigen present on activated T cells. Also referred to as CTLA-4.

CD153

A 40-kDa antigen present on activated T cells. Also called CD30 ligand.

CD154

A 330-kDa antigen present on activated T cells, mast cells, and basophils. Also called CD40 ligand.

CD155

An 80- to 90-kDa antigen present on monocytes, macrophages, and thymocytes. Also called poliovirus receptor.

CD156a

A 60-kDa antigen expressed on monocytes, macrophages, and granulocytes. Also called ADAM8.

CD156b

An 85-kDa molecule with broad antigenic expression; commonly called TACE/ADAM17.

CD157

A 42- to 45-kDa antigen present on monocytes, neutrophils, and endothelial cells. Also referred to as BST-1.

CD158

A molecule present on T cell and natural killer (NK) cell subsets. It is considered part of the KIR family.

CD158a

A 50,58-kDa antigen that is present on natural killer (NK) cells and T cell subsets. Also called p58.1 and P50.1.

CD158b

A 50,58-kDa antigen that is present on NK cells and T cell subsets. Also called p58.2 and p50-2.

CD159

Nothing yet assigned to this number.

CD159a

A 43-kDa antigen present on natural killer (NK) cells. Also called NKG2a.

CD160

A 26-kDa antigen expressed on natural killer (NK) cell and T cell subsets. Also called By55.

CD161

A 60-kDa antigen present on natural killer (NK) cells and T cell subsets. Also referred to as NKR-P1.

CD162

A 110-kDa antigen present on T cells, monocytes, granulocytes, and B cell subsets. Also called PSGL-1.

CD162R

A carbohydrate antigen present on natural killer (NK) cell subsets. Also referred to as PEN5.

CD163

A 130-kDa molecule expressed on monocytes. Also called KiM4.

CD164

An 80-kDa antigen present on T cells, monocytes, granulocytes, B cell subsets, and progenitor cells. Also called MGC-24.

CD165

A 37-kDa antigen expressed on thymocytes and thymic epithelial cells. Also called AD2/gp37.

CD166

A 100-kDa antigen present on activated lymphocytes, endothelial cells, and fibroblasts. Also called ALCAM and CD6 ligand.

CD167a

A 120-kDa antigen expressed on epithelial cells and myoblasts. Also referred to as discoidin domain receptor and DDR1.

CD168

An 84-to 88-kDa molecule present on monocytes, thymocyte subsets, and T cell subsets. Also called RHAMM.

CD169

A 185-kDa antigen expressed on macrophage subsets. Also called sialoadhesin.

CD170

A 140-kDa molecule present on macrophage subsets and neutrophils. Commonly referred to as siglec-5.

CD171

A 200-kDa antigen present on monocytes, T cell subsets, and B cells. Also called L1.

CD172a

A 110-kDa molecule expressed on monocytes, T cell subsets, and stem cells. Also called SIRPα.

CD173

A carbohydrate antigen present on red cells, stem cell subsets, and platelets. Also called blood group H type 2.

CD174

A carbohydrate antigen expressed on stem cell subsets and epithelial cells. Also called Lewis-Y.

CD175

A carbohydrate antigen present on stem cell subsets. Also called TN.

CD175s

A carbohydrate antigen present on erythroblasts. Also referred to as sialyl-Tn.

CD176

A carbohydrate antigen expressed on stem cell subsets. Also called Thomson–Friedrenreich antigen.

CD177

A 56-to 62-kDa antigen present on neutrophil subsets. Also called NB1.

CD178

A 38- to 42-kDa molecule present on activated T cells. Also referred to as Fas ligand.

CD179a

A 16-kDa antigen expressed on pro-B cells and pre-B cells. Also called V pre-β.

CD179b

A 22-kDa antigen present on pro-B cells and pre-B cells. Also called λ5.

CD180

A 95- to 105-kDa molecule present on B cell subsets, monocytes, and dendritic cells. Also called Rp105/Bgp95.

CD183

A 40-kDa antigen expressed on activated T cells and activated natural killer (NK) cells. Also called CXCR3.

CD184

A 45-kDa antigen present on T cell subsets, B cells, monocytes, dendritic cells, and endothelial cells. Commonly called CXCR4.

CD195

A 45-kDa molecule present on monocytes and T cell subsets. Also called CCR5.

CDw197

A 45-kDa antigen present on T cell subsets. Also called CCR7.

CD200

A 45- to 50-kDa antigen expressed on thymocytes, B cells, endothelium, and activated T cells. Also called OX-2.

CD201

A 50-kDa molecule present on endothelial cell subsets. Also called endothelial cell protein C receptor (EPCR).

CD202b

A 150-kDa antigen present on endothelial cells and stem cells. Also called Tie/Tek.

CD203c

A 130- to 150-kDa antigen present on basophils and megakaryocytes. Also referred to as NPP3.

CD204

A 220-kDa molecule expressed on macrophages. Also called the macrophage scavenger receptor.

CD205

A 205-kDa antigen present on dendritic cells and thymic epithelium. Also called DEC-205.

CD206

A 180-kDa antigen expressed on dendritic cell subsets, monocytes, and macrophages. Also called macrophage mannose receptor.

CD207

A 40-kDa molecule expressed on immature Langerhans' cells. Also called langerin.

CD208

A 70- to 90-kDa antigen present on interdigitating dendritic cells. Also called DC-LAMP.

CD209

A 44-kDa antigen present on dendritic cell subsets. Also called DC-SIGN.

CDw210

A 90- to 110-kDa molecule expressed on T cells, B cells, natural killer (NK) cells, monocytes, and macrophages. Also called IL10R.

CD212

A 100-kDa antigen present on activated T cells and activated natural killer (NK) cells. Also called IL12Rβ1.

CD213a1

A 65-kDa antigen present on B cells, monocytes, fibroblasts, and endothelial cells. Also called IL13Rα1.

CD213a2

A 65-kDa antigen present on B cells and monocytes. Also called IL13Rα2.

CDw217

A 120-kDa molecule with broad antigenic expression. Commonly called IL17R.

CD220

A (140 + 70)-kDa molecule with broad antigenic expression. Also called insulin receptor.

CD221

A (140 + 70)-kDa molecule with broad antigenic expression. Also called IGF-1 receptor.

CD222

A 250-kDa molecule with broad antigenic specificity. Also called IGF-2 receptor/mannose-6 phosphate receptor.

CD223

A 70-kDa antigen present on activated T cells and activated natural killer (NK) cells. Also called LAG-3.

CD224

A 27,68-kDa antigen present on leukocytes and stem cells. Commonly referred to as γ-glutamyl transferase (GGT).

CD225

A 17-kDa molecule with broad antigenic expression. Also called Leu-13.

CD226

A 65-kDa antigen present on T cells, natural killer (NK) cells, monocytes, and platelets. Also called DNAM-1.

CD227

A 300-kDa molecule present on stem cell subsets and epithelial cells. Also called MUC-1.

CD228

A 80- to 95-kDa antigen present on stem cells and melanoma cells. Also called melanotransferrin.

CD229

A 95,110-kD antigen expressed on T cells and B cells. Also called Ly-9.

CD230

A 35-kDa molecule with broad antigenic expression. A large membrane prion protein that occurs normally in neurons of the human brain and is thought to be involved in synaptic transmission. In prion diseases, such as Creutzfeldt–Jakob disease (CJD) and bovine spongiform encephalopathy (BSE), altered forms of the normal cellular protein (PrPc) can occur upon contact with an infectious prion protein (PrPsc) from another host. The altered PrPsc form differs from the host encoded PrPc in its conformational structure, but the sequence of both forms is reported to be the same. The altered PrPsc form is resistant to proteolytic degradation and accumulates in cytoplasmic vesicles of diseased individuals, forming lesions, vacuoles, and amyloid deposits. Also referred to as a prion protein.

CD231

A 30- to 45-kDa antigen expressed in conjunction with T cell leukemia and neuroblastoma. Commonly referred to as TALLA-1.

CD232

A 200-kDa molecule with broad antigenic expression. Also called VESPR (plexin C1).

CD233

A 90-kDa antigen expressed on red blood cells. Also called band 3.

CD234

A 35- to 45-kDa antigen present on red blood cells. Also called Duffy antigen.

CD235a

A 36-kDa antigen present on red blood cells. Also called glycophorin A.

CD235b

A 20-kDa antigen present on red blood cells. Also called glycophorin B.

CD236

A 32/23-kDa antigen presented on red blood cells and stem cell subsets. Also called glycophorin C/D.

CD236R

A 32-kDa antigen present on red blood cells and stem cell subsets. Also called glycophorin C.

CD238

A 93-kDa antigen present on red blood cells and stem cell subsets. Commonly called Kell antigen.

CD239

A 78- to 85-kDa antigen expressed on red blood cells and stem cell subsets. Also called B-CAM and Lutheran antigen.

CD240CE

A 30- to 320-kDa antigen present on red blood cells. Also called Rhesus 30 CE.

CD240D

A 30- to 32-kDa antigen present on red blood cells. Also called Rhesus 30 D.

CD241

A 50-kDa antigen expressed on red blood cells. Also called Rhesus 50 glycoprotein.

CD242

A 42-kDa molecule present on red blood cells. Commonly referred to as ICAM-4.

CD243

A 180-kDa antigen present on stem cells. Also called MDR-1.

CD244

A 70-kDa antigen present on natural killer (NK) cells and T cell subsets. Also called 2B4.

CD245

A 220- to 240-kDa antigen present on T cell subsets. Also called p220/240.

CD246

A 80-kDa antigen expressed in conjunction with anaplastic T cell leukemia. Also called anaplastic lymphoma kinase.

CD247

A 16-kDa antigen present on T cells and natural killer (NK) cells. Also called TCR ζ chain.

CD248

A 175-kDa antigen present on endothelial cells that functions in angiogenesis. Also called endosialin.

CD249

A 160-kDa antigen present on endothelial and epithelial cells. Also called aminopeptidase A. Converts angiotensin II to angiotensin III.

CD252

A 34-kDa antigen present on dendritic cells, activated B cells, endothelial and mast cells that has a costimulatory function.

CD253

A 40-kDa antigen present on activated T cells and NK cells; participates in apoptosis.

CD254

A 40-kDa antigen present on activated T cells, stromal cells and osteoclasts that functions in interaction between T and B cells and T cells and dendritic cells and in bone development.

CD256

A 38-kDa antigen present on leukocytes, pancreatic, and colon cells and functions in T and B cell proliferation.

CD257

A 34-kDa antigen present on activated monocytes and dendritic cells and functions in T and B cell growth and development.

CD258

A 29-kDa antigen present on activated T cells and activated monocytes. It has a costimulatory function related to T cells and induces apoptosis.

CD261

A 56-kDa antigen present on activated T cells and selected tumor cells; induces apoptosis.

CD262

A 55-kDa antigen present on leukocytes, heart, placenta, liver, and tumor cells; induces apoptosis.

CD263

A 55-kDa antigen present in low levels in most tissues. It is negative in most tumor tissues and inhibits TRAIL-induced apoptosis.

CD264

A 35-kDa antigen present in low levels in most tissues but is negative in most tumors. Inhibits TRAIL-induced apoptosis.

CD265

A 97-kDa antigen present on dendritic cells and activated monocytes. Its ligand is TRANCE (CD254).

CD266

A 14-kDa antigen present on endothelial cells. It regulates apoptosis.

CD267

A 32-kDa antigen present on B cells, whose ligand is BAFF that inhibits B cell proliferation.

CD268

A 25-kDa antigen present on B cells and a T cell subset. Its ligand is BAFF. It functions in B cell survival and maturation and in T cell activation.

CD269

A 27-kDa antigen present on B cells, whose ligand is BAFF. It has a role in plasma cell survival.

CD271

A 75-kDa antigen present on dendritic cells, B cells, monocytes and keratinocytes. Its ligand is NGF. It inhibits T cell function.

CD272

An antigen present on T cells, whose ligand is B7H4.

CD273

A 25-kDa antigen present on dendritic cells and activated monocytes, whose functions are costimulation and inhibition.

CD274

A 40-kDa antigen present on T cells, B cells, NK cells, dendritic, macrophages and epithelial cells, whose functions are costimulation and inhibition.

CD275

A 40-kDa antigen present on activated monocytes, macrophages and dendritic cells, whose function is costimulation.

CD276

A 45- to 110-kDa antigen present on dendritic cells, activated macrophages, activated T cells, activated B cells, activated NK cells, and epithelial cells that may have a role in costimulation or inhibition.

CD277

An antigen present on T cells, B cells, NK cells, monocytes, dendritic cells and endothelial cells, whose role is in T cell activation.

CD278

A 47- to 57-kDa antigen present on activated T cells whose function is T cell costimulation.

CD279

A 50- to 55-kDa antigen present on activated T cells and activated B cells that has a role in T cell tolerance, negative regulation.

CD280

A 180-kDa antigen present on fibroblasts, endothelial cells, macrophages, osteoclasts, osteocytes, and chondrocytes that has a role in remodeling uptake and degradation of collagen.

CD281

A 90-kDa antigen present on monocytes, macrophages, dendritic cells, and keratinocytes. It regulates TLR2 function. Also called TLR1.

CD282

An 86-kDa antigen present on monocytes, granulocytes, macrophages, dendritic cells, keratinocytes, and epithelial cells. It has a role in innate immune responses to some bacteria and mycoplasma pathogens. Also called TLR2.

CD283

A 120-kDa antigen present on dendritic cells, fibroblasts, and epithelial cells. It has a role in innate immune responses to viral pathogens. Also called TLR3.

CD284

A 110-kDa antigen present on monocytes, macrophages, endothelial cells, and epithelial cells that has a role in innate immune responses to gram-negative bacteria. Also called TLR4.

CD286

A 90-kDa antigen present on monocytes, macrophages, granulocytes, dendritic cells, and epithelial cells that has a role in innate immune responses to some bacteria and mycoplasma pathogens. Also called TLR6.

CD288

A 110-kDa antigen present on monocytes, macrophages, dendritic cells, neurons, and axons that has a role in antiviral immune responses, brain development, and hematopoiesis. Also called TLR8.

CD289

A 110-kDa antigen present on dendritic cells, B cells, and monocytes that has a role in innate immune responses to bacteria or viruses. Also called TLR9.

CD290

A 90-kDa antigen present on B cells and dendritic cells that functions as a coreceptor with TLR2. Also called TLR10.

CD292

A 55, 80-kDa antigen present on mesenchymal cells, epithelial cells, bone progenitors, neurons, chrondrocytes, skeletal muscles, and cardiac myocytes. It participates in kinase functions, anti-apoptosis, and embryogenesis.

CDw293

A 55, 80-kDa antigen present on mysenchymal cells, bone progenitors, chrondrocytes, epithelial cells, heart and kidney cells. It is a kinase regulating cartilage formation.

CD294

A 55- to 70-kDa antigen present on Th2 cells, basophils, and eosinophils. It regulates immune and inflammatory responses, induces Th2 cells, eosinophil and basophil migration.

CD295

A 132-kDa antigen present on hematopoietic cells, heart, placenta, liver, kidney, and pancreatic cells. It regulates fat metabolism, proliferative/anti-apoptotic T cells, and hematopoietic precursors.

CD296

A 36-kDa antigen present on neutrophils, heart cells and skeletal muscle. It transfers ADP-ribose to target proteins and regulates cellular metabolism.

CD297

A 36-kDa antigen expressed on Dombrock red blood cells, monocytes, macrophages, basophils, endothelial cells, intestinal cells, and ovarian cells. It functions in metabolism of Dombrock blood group antigen.

CD298

A 32-kDa antigen that is broadly expressed in the central nervous system and testis. A noncatalytic component of ATPase coupling exchange of Na$^+$, K$^+$.

CD299

A 45-kDa antigen present on endothelia of the liver and lymph nodes. Its ligands are ICAM-3 and HIV gp120, as well as hepatitis C virus and Ebola virus. It functions in T cell trafficking, HCV, EBOV, and HIV infection.

CD300a

A 34-kDa antigen present on monocytes and macrophages, neutrophils, dendritic cells, NK cells, mast cells, T cells, and B cells. Functions as inhibitory R.

CD300c

A 35-kDa antigen present on monocytes, macrophages, neutrophils, dendritic cells, NK cells, T cells, and B cells.

CD300e

An antigen present on monocytes, macrophages, and selected dendritic cells.

CD301

A 42-kDa antigen present on macrophages and immature dendritic cells. It functions in cell adhesion, macrophage migration, and cellular recognition.

CD302

A 30-kDa antigen present on monocytes, macrophages, and dendritic cells.

CD303

A 39-kDa antigen present on plasmacytoid dendritic cells that functions in antigen capture and inhibition of interferon α/β production.

CD304

A 103-kDa antigen present on dendritic cells, T cells, neurons, and endothelial cells that functions in angiogenesis, dendritic cell–T cell interaction, and neuritogenesis.

CD305

A 31-kDa antigen present on T cells, B cells, NK cells, dendritic cells, monocytes, and macrophages. It inhibits cellular activation and inflammation.

CD306

A 16-kDa antigen present on T cells and monocytes that inhibits cellular activation and inflammation.

CD307

An 83- to 107-kDa antigen present on B cells, germinal centers, and light zone B cells. It functions in IgR and may play a role in B cell activation and neoplasia.

CD309

A 195/235-kDa antigen present on endothelial cells, primitive stem cells, and some tumor cells that functions in angiogenesis.

CD312

A 90-kDa antigen present on macrophages, activated monocytes, dendritic, liver, and lung cells. It is involved in immune and inflammatory responses.

CD314

A 42-kDa antigen present on NK cells, CD8+ T cells, γδ T cells, and macrophages. It functions in NK cell activation.

CD315

A 135-kDa antigen present on megakaryocytes, hepatocytes, epithelial cells, and endothelial cells and is weakly expressed on B cells and monocytes. Its ligands are w/CD9 and CD81.

CD316

A 62- to 78-kDa antigen present on T cells, B cells, NK cells, and hepatocytes. It inhibits tumor cell metastasis.

CD317

A 30- to 36-kDa antigen present on plasma cells, lymphoplasmacytoid cells, stromal cells, fibroblasts, and selected dendritic cells. It may play a role in pre-B cell growth.

CD318

An 80/140-kDa antigen present on hematopoietic stem cells, epithelial cells, and selected tumor cells. Its function is in adhesion.

CD319

A 66-kDa antigen present on NK cells, most T cells, activated B cells, and mature dendritic cells. It activates NK cytotoxicity and functions in adhesion.

CD320

An antigen present on follicular dendritic cells that stimulates B cell growth.

CD321

A 35- to 40-kDa antigen present on epithelial cells, endothelial cells, leukocytes, platelets, erythrocytes, lung, placenta, and kidney. It functions in cell adhesion, leukocyte migration, and epithelial barrier maintenance.

CD322

A 48-kDa antigen present on endothelial cells, high endothelial venules in tonsils and heart cells. It functions in cell adhesion and lymphocyte homing.

CD324

A 120-kDa antigen present on epithelial cells, keratinocytes, and trophoblasts. It functions in cell-to-cell and cell-to-matrix adhesion, tumor suppression, cell growth, and differentiation.

CD325

A 130-kDa antigen present on neurons, skeletal and cardiac myocytes, fibroblasts, epithelial cells, and pancreatic and liver cells. It functions in cell-to-cell and cell-to-matrix adhesion, cell growth, and differentiation.

CD326

A 40-kDa antigen present on epithelial cells, in low concentration on thy-c and T, and tumor cells. It inhibits cellular activation and inflammation.

CD327

An antigen present on B cells, placenta trophoblastic cells, and granulocytes that functions in adhesion.

CD328

A 65- to 75-kDa antigen present on NK cells, selected T cells, monocytes, and granulocytes that inhibits NK and T cell activity.

CD329

An antigen present on monocytes, selected NK cells, B and T cells, neutrophils, hepatocytes, and myeloid leukemic cells. It inhibits immune responses.

CD331

A 60, 110- to 160-kDa antigen broadly expressed on epithelial cells, endothelial cells, fibroblasts, mesenchymal cells, cardiac myocytes, and fetal tissues. It functions in cell growth and limb development.

CD332

A 135-kDa antigen present on brain, liver, prostate, kidney, lung, spinal cord, and fetal tissues. It functions in limb induction and craniofacial development.

CD333

A 115- to 135-kDa antigen present on brain, kidney, adult testis, and fetal small intestine cells. It functions in limb induction and craniofacial development.

CD334

An 88- to 110-kDa antigen present on kidney, liver, lung and pancreatic cells, lymphocytes, and macrophages. It functions in bone and muscle development and cancer progression and metastasis.

CD335

A 46-kDa antigen present on NK cells. It functions in NK cell activation.

CD336

A 44-kDa antigen present on activated NK cells that functions in NK cell activation.

CD337

A 30-kDa antigen present on NK cells that functions in NK cell activation.

CD338

A 72-kDa antigen present on liver, kidney, intestine, lung, endothelial cells, melanoma, placenta, selected stem cells, and selected drug-resistant tumors. It functions in absorption and excretion of certain xenobiotics.

CD339

A 134-kDa antigen present on bone marrow stromal cells, thymic epithelium, endothelial cells, Schwann cells, keratinocytes, ovarian, prostate, pancreatic, placenta and heart cells. It functions in cell fate decisions in hematopoiesis and cardiovascular development.

CD340

A 185-kDa antigen present on epithelial and endothelial cells, keratinocytes, hematopoietic stem cell subsets, fetal mesodermal cells, and extraembryonic tissues. It is overexpressed on many malignant cells. It functions in cell growth and differentiation, and tumor cell metastasis.

CD344

A 48- to 53-kDa antigen present on epithelial, endothelial and mesenchymal cells, myeloid progenitors, neuronal progenitors, and intestinal neurons. It functions in cell proliferation and differentiation, embryonic development, and retinal angiogenesis.

CD349

A 64-kDa antigen present on mesenchymal stem cells, neural precursors, mammary epithelial and brain cells, fetal testis, kidney, eye, and pancreas, and selected tumors. It functions in B cell development, hippocampal development, and tissue morphogenesis.

CD350

A 65-kDa antigen present on brain, embryo, kidney, liver, pancreas, placenta, mammary and lung epithelium, and selected tumors. It functions in development of limbs and the nervous system.

CDR

Abbreviation for complementarity-determining regions.

CEA

Abbreviation for carcinoembryonic antigen.

cecropin

An antibacterial protein derived from immunized cecropia moth pupae and also found in butterflies. Cecropin is a basic protein that induces prompt lysis of selected Gram-negative and Gram-positive bacteria.

celiac disease

An inflammatory immunological disease of the intestinal mucosa attributable to an immune response against gluten proteins found in selected cereals, including wheat. Refer to gluten-sensitive enteropathy.

celiac sprue (gluten-sensitive enteropathy)

Gluten-sensitive enteropathy resulting from hypersensitivity to cereal grain storage proteins, including gluten or its product gliadin, present in oats, wheat, and barley. It is characterized by villous atrophy and malabsorption in the small intestine. It occurs mostly in Caucasians and occasionally in African-Americans, but not in Asians. Individual patients may have the disease limited to the intestines or associated with dermatitis herpetiformis, a vesicular eruption of the skin. The mucosa of the small intestine shows the greatest reactivity in areas in contact with gluten-containing food. Antigliadin antibodies are formed, and lymphocytes and plasma cells appear in the lamina propria in association with villous atrophy. Gluten-sensitive enteropathy is associated with HLA-DR3, -DR7, and -DQ2, as well as with HLA-B8. Diagnosis is made by showing villous atrophy in a biopsy of the small intestine. Administering a gluten-free diet leads to resolution of the disease. Antigliadin antibodies are of the immunoglobulin A (IgA) class. Both T and B cell limbs

of the immune response participate in the pathogenesis of this disease. Patients may also develop IgA or IgG reticulin antibodies. An α gliadin amino acid sequence shares homology with adenovirus 12Elb early protein. Patients with celiac disease develop immune reactivity for both gliadin and this viral peptide sequence. The disease occurs more frequently in individuals exposed earlier to adenovirus 12. Patients develop weight loss, diarrhea, anemia, petechiae, edema, and dermatitis herpetiformis, among other signs and symptoms. Lymphomas such as immunoblastic lymphoma may develop in 10 to 15% of untreated patients.

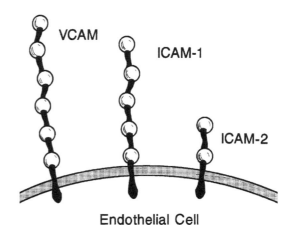

VCAM-1 bound to an endothelial cell.

cell adhesion molecules (CAMs)

Molecules on cell surfaces that facilitate the binding of cells to each other in tissues and in cell-to-cell interactions. They also facilitate cell-to-matrix adhesion and extravasation.

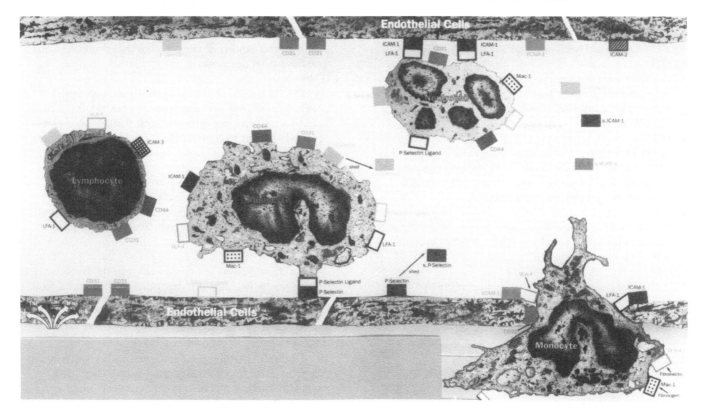

Cellular Adhesion Molecules (CAMS).

Most are grouped into protein families that include the integrins, selectins, mucin-like proteins, and the immunoglobulin superfamily.

cell-bound antibody (cell-fixed antibody)

An antibody anchored to the cell surface either through its paratopes binding to cell epitopes or attachment of its Fc region to Fc receptors. An example is cytophilic antibody or IgE which may then react with antigens as their Fab regions are available.

cell cooperation

T lymphocyte and B lymphocyte cooperation.

cell line

Cultured neoplastic cells or normal cells that have been transformed by chemicals or viruses. Transformed cell lines may be immortal, enabling them to be propagated indefinitely in culture.

cell-mediated hypersensitivity

Refer to delayed-type hypersensitivity and to type IV cell-mediated hypersensitivity.

cell-mediated immune response

Host defense mediated by antigen-specific T lymphocytes together with nonspecific cells of the immune system. The response offers protection against intracellular bacteria, viruses, and neoplasms and mediates graft rejection. It may be transferred passively with primed T lymphocytes.

cell-mediated immunity (CMI)

The limb of the immune response mediated by antigen-specific effector T cells that produce their effect through direct reaction, in contrast to the indirect effect mediated by antibodies of the humoral limb produced by B lymphocytes. CMI also includes the effector functions of natural killer (NK) and NKT cells. The development of cell-mediated immunity to an exogenous antigen first involves processing of the antigen by an antigen-presenting cell such as a macrophage. Processed antigen is presented in the context of major histocompatibility complex (MHC) class II molecules to a CD4+ T lymphocyte. IL1β is also released from the macrophage to induce IL2 synthesis in CD4+ lymphocytes. The IL2 has an autocrine effect on the cells producing it, causing their proliferation and also causing proliferation of other lymphocyte subsets including CD8+ suppressor/cytotoxic T cells, B lymphocytes that form antibodies, and NK cells. Cell-mediated immunity is critical in defenses against mycobacterial and fungal infections and resistance to tumors, and it has a role in allograft rejection.

cell-mediated immunodeficiency syndrome

Condition in which cell-mediated immunity is defective. It may be manifested as negative skin test results following the application of tuberculin, histoplasmin, or other common skin test antigens; failure to develop contact hypersensitivity following application of sensitizing substances such as dinitrochlorobenzene (DNCB) to the skin; or failure to reject an allograft, such as a skin graft. Severe combined immunodeficiency (SCID) is characterized by defective T lymphocyte and B lymphocyte limbs of the immune response. DiGeorge syndrome is characterized by failure of development of the T-cell-mediated limb of the immune response.

cell-mediated lympholysis (CML) test

Responder (effector) lymphocytes are cytotoxic for donor (target) lymphocytes after the two are combined in culture. Target cells are labeled by incubation with 51Cr at 37°C for 60 minutes. Following combination of effector and target cells in tissue culture, the release of 51Cr from target cells injured by cytotoxicity represents a measure of cell-mediated lympholysis (CML). The CML assay gives uniform results, is relatively simple to perform, and is rather easily controlled. The effector cells can result from *in vivo* sensitization following organ grafting or can be induced *in vitro*. Variations in the ratio of effector to target cell can be employed for quantification.

cell separation methods

Early cell separation techniques were based in the early 1960s on differences such as cell size and density. Subsequently, membrane receptors or surface antigens were found to be differently expressed by lymphocyte subsets. Currently, the most popular lymphocyte separation techniques include immunoselection procedures that employ monoclonal antibodies. The two methods used for lymphocyte separation based on physical differences include sedimentation separation and density gradient separation. Other methods are based on functional properties of cells such as adhesive or phagocytic properties. Selected mononuclear cell types can adhere to plastic surfaces or to nylon wool. Other techniques employ selective depletion of cells such as lymphocytes undergoing proliferation. Mitogens in culture can be employed to select given lymphocyte populations based on their ability to respond to these stimulants. Rosetting techniques permit the detection or purification of cells expressing a certain surface receptor for antigen. Immunoselection techniques employ either monoclonal or polyclonal antibodies

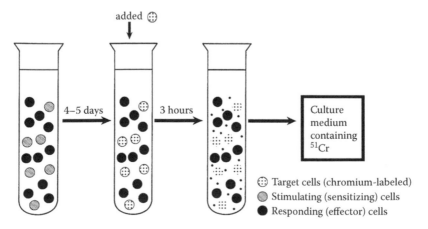

added ⊙

4–5 days   3 hours

Culture medium containing 51Cr

⊙ Target cells (chromium-labeled)
◉ Stimulating (sensitizing) cells
● Responding (effector) cells

Cell-mediated lympholysis test.

C

specific for surface antigens on lymphocyte subsets. Immunotoxicity procedures can be used to induce selective cytolysis of cells expressing a certain antigen at the cell surface by reacting the cell with antibodies. Immunoadhesion procedures make use of antibodies against cell-surface antigens bound to a solid support, permitting the capture of cells by adherence to the support. Immunomagnetic beads to which antibodies have been attached may also be used. Magnetic cell sorting is based on the use of monoclonal antibodies or lectins that bind specifically to surface antigen/receptor expressed by a certain cell subset. Flow cytometry is a precise and objective method to quantify the number of cells expressing a given surface marker and the extent to which the marker is expressed.

cell surface immunoglobulin

The B cell receptor for antigen.

cell surface molecule immunoprecipitation

A technique to analyze cell surface molecules with monoclonal antibodies and antisera. Immunoprecipitation is based on solubilization of membrane proteins by the use of nonionic detergents, subsequent interaction of specific antibody with solubilized membrane antigen, and recovery of antibody–antigen complexes by binding to an insoluble support that permits washing procedures to remove unbound molecules. Analysis of immunoprecipitates can be accomplished by sodium dodecyl sulfate (SDS)–polyacrylamide gel electrophoresis (SDS-PAGE) or isoelectric focusing (IEF).

cell surface receptors and ligands

Activation of caspases via ligand binding to cell surface receptors involves the tumor necrosis factor (TNF) family of receptors and ligands. These receptors contain an 80-amino acid death domain (DD) that, through homophilic interactions, recruits adaptor proteins to form a signaling complex on the cytosolic surface of the receptor. The signaling induced by the ligand binding to the receptor appears to involve trimerization. Based on x-ray crystallography, the trimeric ligand has three equal faces, and a receptor monomer interacts at each of the three junctions formed by the three faces. Thus, each receptor polypeptide contacts two ligands. The bringing together of three receptors, thereby orienting the intracellular DDs, appears to be the critical feature for signaling by these receptors. The adaptor proteins recruited to the aligned receptor DDs recruit either caspases or other signaling protiens. The exact mechanism by which recruitment of caspase 8 to the DD-induced complex causes activation of caspase 8 is not clear.

cell tray panel

Used to detect and identify human leukocyte antigen (HLA) antibodies. Patient serum is tested against a panel of known cells. The panel (or percent) reactive antibody (PRA) is the percent of panel cells reacting with a patient's serum. It is expressed as a percentage of the total reactivity: % PRA = (number of positive reactions/ number of cells in panel) × 100. This percentage is a useful indicator of the proportion of HLA antibodies.

cellular allergy

Refer to delayed-type hypersensitivity, type IV cell-mediated hypersensitivity, and cell-mediated immunity.

cellular and humoral metal hypersensitivity

Metal ions interact with proteins in several ways. Mercury and gold form metal–protein complexes by binding with high affinity to thiol groups of cysteine. These complexes are able to activate T lymphocytes with or without antigen or by superantigen stimulation. Mercury is used as a preservative and as a dental amalgam, but mercury compounds can induce contact sensitivity and glomerulonephritis in humans. Gold salts are used as antirheumatic drugs but can cause contact dermatitis, stomatitis, pneumonitis, glomerulonephritis, increased levels of serum immunoglobulins, antinuclear autoantibodies, thrombocytopenia, and asthma in goldminers. Cadmium chloride can induce renal tubular damage in mice via interaction with T cells with specific Hsp70 on tubular cells. Occupational exposure to beryllium salts may lead to chronic interstitial granulomatous lung disease. CD4+ T lymphocytes from patients with berylliosis react to beryllium salts in a major histocompatibility complex (MHC) class II restricted manner. Silica, silicone, and sodium silicate activate CD4+ memory T lymphocytes

TRAY POS	#CENTRL	TEST	CELL ID	RACE	A		B		C		BW	
1A		8	10571T	H	1	2	8	35	7			6
1B		8	9891T	C	1	2	44	51	1	5	4	
1C		8	9884T	B	1	2	57	82	3	6	4	6
1D		8	9898T	B	1	23	45	49	6	7	4	6
1E		8	10356T	B	1	23	58	72	6		4	6
1F		8	10990T	O	1	24	27	37	2	6	4	
2F		8	10367T	C	1	32	8	51	7		4	6
2E		8	7109T	H	1		13	64	6	8	4	6
2D		1	6606T	C	2	11	18	38	7		4	6
2C		1	10567T	C	2	11	37	60	3	6	4	6
2B		8	10988T	C	2	24	51	55	3		4	6
2A		1	10359T	C	2	25	57	62	5	6	4	6
3A		1	10549T	O	2	26	39	61	1	7		6
3B		1	10361T	O	2	26	54	62	1	3		6
3C		1	10570T	O	2	26	60	65	4	8		6
3D		1	9899T	B	2	30	8	58	7		4	6
3E		1	10352T	O	2	30	13	46	1	6	4	6
3F		1	10547T	C	2	31	35	47	4		4	6
4F		1	6688T	C	2	31	50	60	3	6		6
4E		1	10568T	H	2	32	41	61	2	7		6

Cell tray panel showing positive reactions (8s) for HLA-A1 at tray positions 1A, 1B, 1C, 1D, 1E, 1F, 2F, and 2E and a positive reaction for HLA-A24 at position 2B.

in women with silicone breast implants. Silicone hypersensitivity results in high levels of interleukin-1 (IL1) and IL1ra in the circulation. The silicone immune disease reaction is associated with the synthesis of autoantibodies to multiple endocrine organs and is compatible with an immune-mediated endocrinopathy. Nickel sulfate, potassium dichromate, cobalt chloride, palladium chloride, and gold sodium thiosulfate represent metal allergy in patients with symptoms resulting from dental restoration. Lead and cadmium can lead to suppression of cell-mediated immunity. Laboratory methods of assessment include enzyme immunoassay (EIA), memory lymphocyte immunostimulation assay (MELISA), and lymphocyte proliferation tests.

cellular hypersensitivity

Refer to delayed-type hypersensitivity, type IV cell-mediated hypersensitivity, and cell-mediated immunity.

cellular immunity

Refer to cell-mediated immunity.

cellular immunology

The study of cells involved in immune phenomena.

cellular interstitial pneumonia

Inflammation of the lung in which the alveolar walls are infiltrated by mononuclear cells.

cellular oncogene

Refer to protooncogene.

CEM-15

An RNA/DNA editing enzyme of the host that unites with HIV polyproteins and is incorporated into virions. It induces hypermutation of replicating HIV DNA, inhibiting incorporation into the host cell genome.

centiMorgan (cM)

A chromosomal unit of physical distance that corresponds to a 1% recombination frequency between two genes that are closely linked. Also termed a map unit.

central lymphoid organs

Lymphoid organs that are requisite for the development of the lymphoid and therefore of the immune system. These include the thymus, bone marrow, and bursa of Fabricius. Also termed primary lymphoid organs. Sites of lymphocyte development. Human T lymphocytes mature in the thymus, whereas B lymphocytes develop in the bone marrow.

central MHC

The location of the MHC's class III region, between the class I and class II regions.

central tolerance

The mechanism involved in the functional inactivation of cells requisite for the initiation of an immune response. Central tolerance affects the afferent limb of the immune response, which is concerned with sensitization and cell proliferation. It is established in lymphocytes developing in central lymphoid organs and prevents the emergence of lymphocytes with high affinity receptors for self antigens present in bone marrow or thymus. Induced by negative selection in the thymus and bone marrow. Peripheral tolerance protects self cells from attack by autoreactive cells that evade central tolerance.

centriole antibodies

Antibodies sometimes detected in blood sera also containing antibodies against mitotic spindle apparatus (MSA). They are only rarely found in patients developing connective tissue disease of the scleroderma category. Selected centriole antibodies may be directed against the glycolytic enzyme enolase.

centroblasts

Large, rapidly dividing cells in germinal centers. These cells, in which somatic hypermutation is thought to take place, give rise to memory and antibody-secreting B cells.

centrocyte

Germinal center B cells that are small and nonproliferating. They are derived from centroblasts and mature into plasma cells that secrete antibody or memory B cells or may undergo apoptosis, depending on the interactions between their receptors and antigen. They undergo affinity maturation, isotype switching, and somatic hypermutation.

centromere antibodies

Antibodies specific for centromeres/kinetochores are detectable in 22% of systemic sclerosis patients, most of whom have CREST syndrome rather than diffuse scleroderma. Approximately 12% of primary biliary cirrhosis patients, half of whom also manifest scleroderma, have centromere antibodies.

centromere antigen complex

Consists of the antigenic proteins CENP-A (18 kDa), CENP-B (80 kDa), and CDNP-C (140 kDa).

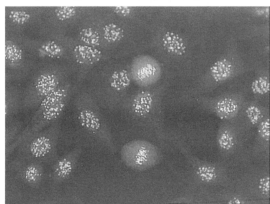

Centromere autoantibodies

centromere autoantibodies

Autoantibodies against centromeres (CENAs) occur in 22% of systemic sclerosis patients and in 12% of primary biliary cirrhosis (PBC) cases, half of whom develop scleroderma. Limited scleroderma known as CREST occurs in 4 to 18% of primary biliary cirrhosis cases. CENA-positive patients with limited scleroderma are more likely to have calcinosis and telangiectasia and less often pulmonary interstitial fibrosis compared with CENA-negative patients with limited scleroderma. When patients with Raynaud's syndrome become CENA-positive, they may be developing limited scleroderma. CENAs in patients with silicone breast implants lead to symptoms associated with connective tissue types of diseases. Antinuclear antibodies developed in 58% (470/813) of patients studied; antibody levels and clinical symptoms diminished when the implants were removed.

***c-erb*-B2 monoclonal antibody**

A murine monoclonal antibody against *c-erb*-B2 oncoprotein that is expressed by tumor cell membranes at a level detectable by immunohistochemistry in up to 20% of adenocarcinomas from various sites, including ovary, gastrointestinal tract, and breast. Immunohistochemical staining correlates with gene amplification. In the case of breast cancer, *c-erb*-B2 expression has been shown to be associated with poor prognosis. Between 15 and 30% of invasive ductal cancers are positive for c-*erb*-B2. Almost all cases of Paget's disease and approximately 70% of cases of *in situ* ductal carcinoma are positive.

cerebrospinal fluid (CSF) immunoglobulins

In normal individuals, CSF immunoglobulins are derived from plasma by diffusion across the blood–brain barrier. The amount present is dependent on the immunoglobulin concentration in the serum, the molecular size of the immunoglobulin, and the permeability of the blood–brain barrier. Immunoglobulin M (IgM) is normally excluded by virtue of its relatively large molecular size and low plasma concentration. However, in certain disease states, such as demyelinating diseases and infections of the central nervous system, immunoglobulins may be produced locally. The permeability of the blood–brain barrier is accurately reflected by the CSF total protein or albumin levels relative to those in the serum. By comparing these data, it is possible to derive information about deviation from normal. The comparative method is called Ig quotient and is calculated in various ways:

1. CSF – IgG/albumin (normal 13.9 + 14%)
2. CSF – IgG/total protein
3. CSF – IgA/albumin
4. CSF – κ/λ (ratio)

To correct for variations in the blood–brain barrier, the calculation can be modified to yield a more sensitive quotient represented as: $[(CSF\ IgG)/(serum\ IgG)]\ \Pi\ [(CSF\ albumin)/(serum\ albumin)]$. The ratio of κ to λ light chains in CSF in comparison with that of these light chains in serum is significant in that some patients with local immunoglobulin production show a change in the ratio. An increase in the IgA present in CSF appears in some viral infections of the CNS in which antiviral antibodies are also detectable.

cetuximab

A human–mouse chimeric monoclonal antibody that combines with epidermal growth factor receptor (EGFR), which blocks tumor cell growth. It has a decreasing kinase activity, matrix metalloproteinase activity, and growth factor synthesis, as well as elevated apoptosis. It is used in metastatic colorectal cancer where there is overexpression of EGRF.

CFA

Abbreviation for complete Freund's adjuvant.

CFT

Abbreviation for complement fixation test.

CFU

Abbreviation for colony-forming unit.

CFU-GEMM

A colony-stimulating factor that acts on multiple cell lines, including granulocytes, erythroid cells, megakaryocytes, and macrophages. The pancytopenia observed in myelodysplasia and Fanconi's disease has been attributable to a total lack of CFU-GEMM.

CFU-S (colony-forming units, spleen)

A mixed cell population considered to contain the ideal stem cell that is pluripotent and capable of proliferating and renewing itself.

Cγ

Immunoglobulin γ chain constant region that is subdivided into four isotypes in humans that are indicated as Cγ_1, Cγ_2, Cγ_3, and Cγ_4. The corresponding exons are shown by the same designations in italics.

CGD

Abbreviation for chronic granulomatous disease.

CH

Immunoglobulin heavy chain constant region encoded by the *CH* gene.

C$_H$1

An immunoglobulin heavy chain's first constant domain encoded by the *CH1* exon.

C$_H$2

An immunoglobulin heavy chain's second constant domain encoded by the *CH2* exon.

C$_H$3

An immunoglobulin heavy chain's third constant domain encoded by the *CH3* exon.

C$_H$4

An immunoglobulin heavy chain's fourth constant domain encoded by the *CH4* exon. Of the five immunoglobulin classes in humans, only the μ heavy chain of immunoglobulin M (IgM) and the ε heavy chain of IgE possess a fourth domain.

CH$_{50}$ unit

The amount of complement (serum dilution) that induces lysis of 50% of erythrocytes sensitized (coated) with specific antibody. More specifically, the 50% lysis should be of 5×10^8 sheep erythrocytes sensitized with specific antibody during 60 minutes of incubation at 37°C. To obtain the complement titer (i.e., the CH$_{50}$ present in 1 mL of serum that has not been diluted), the log $y/(1 - y)$, where $y = \%$ lysis, is plotted against the log of the quantity of serum. At 50% lysis, the plot approaches linearity near $y/(1 - y)$.

CHAD

Abbreviation for cold hemagglutinin disease.

challenge

Antigen deliberately administered to induce an immune reaction in an individual previously exposed to that antigen to determine the state of immunity.

challenge stock

An antigen dose that has been precisely measured and administered to an individual following earlier exposure to an infectious microorganism.

chancre immunity

Resistance to reinfection with *Treponema pallidum* that develops 3 months following a syphilis infection that is untreated.

Chagas' disease

The immune response effectively controls the high number of parasites in the acute phase, leading to essentially undetectable parasitemia in the chronic phase yet sterile immunity and complete parasite clearance and cure have not been achieved in humans or in experimental animals infected with *Trypanosoma cruzi*. The immune response does not achieve a cure but maintains a host–parasite balance that lasts for the lifetime of the infected person. Various antigens have been used in vaccine trials but most only reduce the parasitemia during the acute phase of the disease and transform lethal to non-lethal infections. No vaccination has produced complete protection; the vaccinated animals still become infected. Decreased parasitemia may diminish the incidence and severity of the chronic phase.

chaperones

A group of proteins that includes BiP, a protein that binds the immunoglobulin heavy chain. Chaperones aid the proper folding of oligomeric protein complexes. They prevent incorrect conformations or enhance correct ones. Chaperones are believed to combine with the surfaces of proteins exposed during intermediate folding and to restrict further folding to the correct conformations. They take part in transmembrane targeting of selected proteins. Chaperones hold some proteins that are to be inserted into membranes in intermediate conformation in the cytoplasm until they interact with the target membrane. Besides BiP, they include heat shock proteins 70 and 90 and nucleoplasmins.

Charcot–Leyden crystals

Crystals present in asthmatic patients' sputum that are hexagonal and bipyramidal. They contain a 13-kDa lysophospholipase derived from the eosinophil cell membrane.

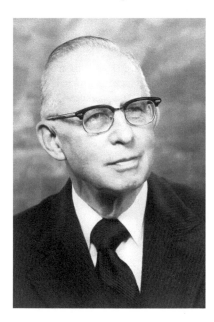

Merrill Chase.

Chase, Merrill (1905– 2004)

American immunologist who worked with Karl Landsteiner at the Rockefeller Institute for Medical Research, New York. He investigated hypersensitivity, including delayed-type hypersensitivity and contact dermatitis. He was the first to demonstrate the passive transfer of tuberculin and contact hypersensitivity and also made contributions in the fields of adjuvants and quantitative methods.

Chase–Sulzberger phenomenon

Refer to Sulzberger–Chase phenomenon.

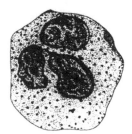
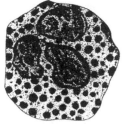

Normal   Chediak-Higashi Syndrome
PMN   PMN

Chediak–Higashi syndrome.

Chediak–Higashi syndrome

A childhood disorder with an autosomal-recessive mode of inheritance, identified by the presence of large lysosomal granules in leukocytes that are very stable and undergo slow degranulation. Induced by mutations in the CHS1 gene associated with intracellular fusion/fission activity. Multiple systems may be involved. Repeated bacterial infections with various microorganisms, partial albinism, central nervous system disorders, hepatosplenomegaly, and an inordinate incidence of malignancies of the lymphoreticular tissues may occur. The large cytoplasmic granular inclusions that appear in white blood cells may also be observed in blood platelets and can be seen by regular light microscopy in peripheral blood smears. Defective neutrophil chemotaxis and an altered ability of the cells to kill ingested microorganisms are observed. The killing time is delayed, even though hydrogen peroxide formation, oxygen consumption, and hexose monophosphate shunt are all within normal limits. Defective microtubule function leads to defective phagolysosome formation. Cyclic AMP levels may increase which causes decreased neutrophil degranulation and mobility. High doses of ascorbic acid have been shown to restore normal chemotaxis, bactericidal activity, and degranulation. Natural killer (NK) cell numbers and function are decreased. The incidence of lymphomas in patients with Chediak–Higashi syndrome is increased. There is no effective therapy other than the administration of antibiotics for the infecting microorganisms. The disease carries a poor prognosis because of the infections and neurological complications. The majority of affected individuals die during childhood, although occasionally subjects may live longer.

chemical adjuvants

Chemicals used for immunopotentiation that include the polynucleotide poly-I:C and poly-A:U, vitamin D_3, dextrand sulphate, inulin, dimethyl, dioctadecyl ammonium bromide (DDA), avridine, carbohydrate polymers similar to mannan, and trehalose dimycolate, among others. Two of the newer chemical adjuvants include polyphosphazines (initially introduced as slow release-promoting agents) and a *Leishmania* protein LeIF.

chemical "splenectomy"

Deliberate suppression of the immune system by the administration of high dose corticosteroids (1 mg/kg/day) or intravenous immunoglobulin (0.4 g/kg/day). This prevents endocytosis of cells or microorganisms opsonized by a coating of immunoglobulin or complement which blocks Fc receptors. Although the opsonized particles are bound, they are not endocytosed. This procedure has been used in the management of hypersplenism associated with certain immune disorders such as autoimmune hemolytic anemia, Felty's syndrome, or autoimmune neutropenia.

chemiluminescence

The conversion of chemical energy into light by an oxidation reaction. A high energy peroxide intermediate such as luminol is produced by the reaction of a precursor substance exposed to peroxide and alkali. The emission of light energy by a chemical reaction may occur during reduction of an unstable intermediate to a stable form. Chemiluminescence measures the oxidative formation of free radicals such as superoxide anion by polymorphonuclear neutrophils and mononuclear phagocytes. Light is released from these cells after they have taken up luminol

(5-amino-2,3-dihydro-1,4-phthalazinedione). This is a mechanism to measure the respiratory burst in phagocytes. The oxidation of luminol increases intracellular luminescence. Chronic granulomatous disease may be diagnosed by this technique.

chemoattractant

A substance that attracts leukocytes and may induce significant physiologic alterations in cells that express receptors for them.

chemokine autoantibodies

Autoantibodies against members of the chemokine family that include macrophage inflammatory proteins (MIPs) MIP-1-α (stem-cell inhibitor), MIP-1-β, MIP-2-α (GRO-β), GRO-α, MIP-2-α (GRO-γ); platelet factor-4 (PF-4); interleukin-8 (IL8); macrophage chemotactic and activating factor, IP-10; monocyte chemoattractant protein-1 (MCP-1); and RANTES. MCP-1, MIP-1, and RANTES are the mononuclear cell chemoattractant equivalent of IL8. All these molecules are able to stimulate leukocyte movement (chemokinesis) and directed movement (chemotaxis). IL8, the best known member of this subfamily, is a proinflammatory cytokine synthesized by various cells that act as neutrophil activators and chemotactic factors. It is believed to be responsible for the induction and maintenance of localized inflammation. Monoclonal antibodies against IL8 and MCP-1 receptors can distinguish between MCP-1- and IL8-responsive T lymphocyte subsets. The enzyme immunoassay (EIA) technique is the preferred method for assaying chemokines and chemokine autoantibodies.

chemokine β receptor-like 1

A member of the G protein-coupled receptor family, the chemokine receptor branch of the rhodopsin family. It is expressed on neutrophils and monocytes but not on eosinophils. It may be found in brain, placenta, lung, liver and pancreas.

chemokine receptor

Cell surface molecules that transduce signals stimulating leukocyte migration following the binding of the homologous chemokine. These receptors belong to the seven-transmembrane and α-helical, G protein-linked family. Examples include Th1 cells that manifest CCR1, CCR5, and CXCR3, which usher cells to sites of tissue inflammation; Th2 cells bearing CCR4, CCR3, and CCR8, which direct cells to mucosae; and naïve lymphocytes that bear CR7, which guides cells to lymph nodes.

chemokines

Molecules that recruit and activate leukocytes and other cells at sites of inflammation. They exhibit both chemoattractant and cytokine properties. There are two groups. Those that mainly activate neutrophils are the α chemokines (CXC chemokines). By contrast, those that activate monocytes, lymphocytes, basophils, and eosinophils are designated β chemokines (CC chemokines). Blocking chemokine function can exert a major effect on inflammatory responses.

chemokinesis

Determination of the rate of movement or random motion of cells by chemical substances in the environment. The direction of cellular migration is determined by chemotaxis, not chemokinesis.

chemotactic assays

The chemotactic properties of various substances can be determined by various methods. The most popular is the Boyden technique, which consists of a chamber separated into two compartments by a Millipore™ filter of appropriate porosity through which cells can migrate actively but not drop passively. The cell preparation is placed in the upper compartment of the chamber, and the assay solution is placed in the lower compartment. The chamber is incubated in air at 37°C for 3 hours, after which the filter is removed and the number of cells migrating to the opposite surface of the filter are counted.

chemotactic deactivation

The reduced chemotactic responsiveness to a chemotactic agent caused by prior incubation of leukocytes with the same agent, but in the absence of a concentration gradient. It can be tested by adding first the chemotactic factor to the upper chamber, washing, and then testing the response to the chemotactic factor placed in the lower chamber (no gradient being present). The mechanism of deactivation has been postulated as obstruction of the membrane channels involved in cation fluxes. Deactivation phenomena are used to discriminate between chemokinetic factors that enhance random migration and true chemotactic factors that cause directed migration. Only true chemotactic factors are able to induce deactivation.

chemotactic disorder

Condition attributable to abnormalities of the complex molecular and cellular interactions involved in mobilizing an appropriate phagocytic cell response to injuries or inflammation. It can involve defects in either the humoral or cellular components of chemotaxis that usually lead to recurrent infections. The process begins with the generation of chemoattractants. Among these chemoattractants that act *in vivo* are the anaphylatoxins (C3a, C4a, and C5a), leukotriene B$_4$ (LTB$_4$), interleukin-8 (IL8), granulocyte–macrophage colony-stimulating factor (GM-CSF), and platelet-activating factors (PAFs). Once exposed to the chemoattractant, circulating neutrophils embark upon a four-stage mechanism of emigration through the endothelial layer to a site of tissue injury where phagocytosis takes place. The four stages include: (1) rolling or initial margination by the selectins (L-, P-, E-); (2) stopping on the endothelium by CD18 integrins and ICAM-1; (3) neutrophil–neutrophil adhesion by CD11b/CD18; and (4) transendothelial migration by CD11b/CD18, CD11a/CD18, and ICAM-1. Chemotactic defects can be either acquired or inherited. Specific disorders are listed separately.

chemotactic factor

Directed migration of cells, known as chemotaxis, is mediated principally by the complement components C5a and C5a–des Arg. Neutrophil chemoattractants also include bacterial products such as *N*-formyl methionyl peptides, fibrinolysis products, oxidized lipids such as leukotriene B$_4$, and stimulated leukocyte products. Interleukin-8 (IL8) is chemotactic for polymorphonuclear neutrophils (PMNs). Chemokines that are chemotactic for PMNs include epithelial-cell-derived neutrophil-activating peptide (ENA-78), neutrophil-activating peptide 2 (NAP-2), growth-related oncogene (GRO-α, β, and γ), and macrophage inflammatory proteins 2α and β (MIP-2α and MIP-2β). Polypeptides with chemotactic activity mainly for mononuclear cells (β chemokines) include monocyte chemoattractant proteins 1, 2, and 3 (MCP-1, MCP-2, and MCP-3), macrophage inflammatory proteins 1α and β (MIP-1α and MIP-1β), and RANTES.

These chemotactic factors are derived from both inflammatory and noninflammatory cells including neutrophils, macrophages, smooth muscle cells, fibroblasts, epithelial cells, and endothelial cells. MCP-1 participates in the recruitment of monocytes in various pathologic or physiologic conditions. Neutrophil chemotaxis assays are performed using the microchamber technique. Chemotactic assays are also useful to reveal the presence of chemotaxis inhibitors in serum.

chemotactic peptide

A peptide that attracts cell migration, such as formyl-methionyl-leucyl-phenylalanine.

chemotactic receptor

Cellular receptor for chemotactic factor. In bacteria, such receptors are designated sensors and signalers and are associated with various transport mechanisms. The cellular receptors for chemotactic factors have not been isolated and characterized. In leukocytes, the chemotactic receptor appears to activate a serine proesterase enzyme, which sets in motion the sequence of events related to cell locomotion. The receptors appear specific for the chemotactic factors under consideration, and apparently the same receptors mediate all types of cellular responses inducible by a given chemotactic factor. However, these responses can be dissociated from each other, suggesting that binding to the putative receptor initiates a series of parallel, interdependent, and coordinated biochemical events leading to one or another type of response. Using a synthetic peptide, N-formyl-methionyl-leucyl-phenylalanine, about 2000 binding sites have been demonstrated for each polymorphonuclear neutrophil (PMN) leukocyte. The binding sites are specific, have a high affinity for the ligand, and are saturable. Competition for the binding sites is shown only by the parent or related compounds; the potency of the latter varies. Positional isomers may inhibit binding. Full occupancy of the receptors is not required for a maximal response, and occupancy of only 10 to 20% of them is sufficient. The presence of spare receptors may enhance the sensitivity in the presence of small concentrations of chemotactic factors and may contribute to the detection of a gradient. There also remains the possibility that some substances with chemotactic activity do not require specific binding sites on cell membranes.

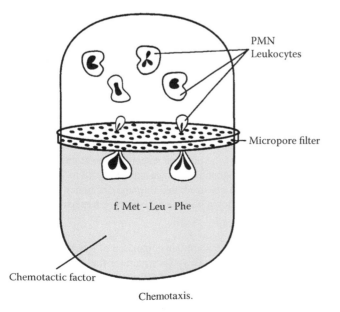

Chemotaxis.

chemotaxis

The process whereby chemical substances direct cell movement and orientation. The orientation and movement of cells in the direction of a concentration gradient constitute positive chemotaxis, whereas movement away from the concentration gradient is termed negative chemotaxis. Substances that induce chemotaxis are referred to as chemotaxins and are often small molecules, such as C5a, formyl peptides, lymphokines, bacterial products, leukotriene B_4, etc., that induce positive chemotaxis of polymorphonuclear neutrophils, eosinophils, and monocytes. These cells move into inflammatory agents by chemotaxis. Chemotaxis is measured by using a dual-chamber device called a Boyden chamber, in which phagocytic cells in culture are separated from a chemotactic substance by a membrane. The number of cells on the filter separating the cell chamber from the chemotaxis chamber reflect the chemotactic influence of the chemical substance for the cells.

chemotherapy

Treatment of neoplasia with chemical drugs that destroy tumor cells that grow more rapidly than do normal cells or have a metabolic disorder.

chickenpox (varicella)

Human herpesvirus type 3 (HHV-3) induced in acute infection that usually occurs in children below 10 years of age. There is anorexia, malaise, low fever, and a prodromal rash following a 2-week incubation period. Erythematous papules appear in crops and intensify for 3 to 4 days. They are very pruritic. Complications include viral pneumonia, secondary bacterial infection, thrombocytopenia, glomerulonephritis, myocarditis, and other conditions. HHV-3 may become latent when chickenpox resolves. Its DNA may become integrated into the dorsal route ganglion cells that may be associated with the development of herpes zoster or shingles later in life.

Phenotype	C4d Component Present	Frequency (%) Whites
Ch(a+), Rg(a+)	C4dS, C4df	95
Ch(a−), Rg(a+)	C4df	2
Ch(a+), Rg(a−)	C4dS	3
Ch(a−), Rg(a−)	None	Very rare

Chido (Ch) and Rodgers (Rg) Antigens

Chido (Ch) and Rodgers (Rg) antigens

Epitopes of C4d fragments of human complement component C4. They are not intrinsic to the erythrocyte membrane. The Chido epitope is found on C4d from C4B, whereas the Rodgers epitope is found on C4A derived from C4d. The Rodgers epitope is Val–Asp–Leu–Leu, and the Chido epitope is Ala–Asp–Leu–Arg. They are situated at residue positions 1188 and 1191 in the C4d region of the C4 α chain. Antibodies against Ch and Rg antigenic determinants agglutinate saline suspensions of red blood cells coated with C4d. Because C4 is found in human serum, anti-Ch and anti-Rg are neutralized by sera of most individuals having the relevant antigens. Ficin and papain destroy these antigens.

C

chief cell autoantibodies

Antibodies reactive with chief cells that are principal sources of PG1 (the main form of serum pepsinogen). They are significantly diminished in atrophic gastritis type A, which is associated with pernicious anemia. Autoantibodies against pepsinogen, a 41-Kda antigen, are more frequent in pernicious anemia than are intrinsic factor antibodies. Pepsinogen autoantibodies are also present in approximately 50% of active duodenal ulcer patients, a quarter of whom may have autoantibodies against H^+/K^+ ATPase.

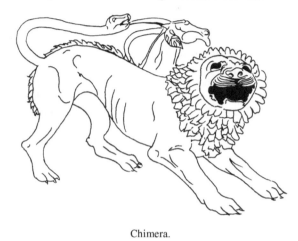

Chimera.

chimera

The presence in an individual of cells of more than one genotype. This can occur rarely under natural circumstances in dizygotic twins (such as in cattle) that share a placenta in which the blood circulation has become fused, causing the blood cells of each twin to circulate in the other. More commonly, it refers to a human or other animal that received a bone marrow transplant that provides a cell population consisting of donor and self cells. Tetraparental chimeras can be produced by experimental manipulation. The name *chimera* derives from a monster of Greek mythology that had the body of a goat, the head of a lion, and the tail of a serpent.

chimeric antibodies

Antibodies that have, for example, mouse Fv fragments for the Ag-binding portion of the molecule but Fc regions of human immunoglobulin (Ig) that convey effector functions.

chimeric protein

A molecular structure comprised of segments of at least two, or possibly more, different proteins.

chimerism

The presence of two genetically different cell populations within an animal at the same time.

Chlamydia immunity

Chlamydiae infect many animal species and various anatomical sites. No single pattern of host response can be described, but similarities in effector mechanisms may exist. The strain or serovar of the infecting microorganism is also significant. *In vitro* studies and genital respiratory and ocular animal models have provided most of the information about both protective and pathologic host responses. Acute inflammation is the initial response, with participation by polymorphonuclear leukocytes (PMNs) that may counteract the microorganisms but also cause pathologic changes. When chlamydiae infect epithelial cells, interleukin- (IL1) is released, as well as IL8, a potent PMN chemoattractant. When these microorganisms infect macrophages, lipopolysaccharide (LPS) triggers the synthesis of TNFα, IL1, and IL6. They may also activate the alternative pathway of complement. IL8, TNFα, and complement may induce chemotaxis of PMNs to the local site. ICAM-1, VCAM-1, and MAdCAM-1 are all detectable early in the infection and may be addressins responsible for PMN extravasation at sites of infection. Natural killer (NK) cells may appear early after infection of the genital tract. Chlamydial infection produces both humoral and cell-mediated immune responses. Cell-mediated immunity has been found important in both mouse and guinea pig models. The $CD4^+$ T cells are the main subset responsible for protective cell-mediated immunity. In genital infections, the T_H1 subset of CD4 T cells is the principal cell type leading to the formation of high levels of IFN-γ, which is believed to have a protective role. In some models, antibody appears to be important in the resolution of infection. Antibody may neutralize chlamydial elementary bodies *in vitro*. Immunity to chlamydial infections is short lived. No effective vaccine for chlamydia infections in humans currently exists, but a veterinary vaccine is available.

$$HOOC-CH_2-CH_2-CH_2-\!\!\!\bigcirc\!\!\!-N\Big\langle{CH_2-CH_2-Cl \atop CH_2-CH_2-Cl}$$

Structure of chlorambucil (4-[*bis* (2-chloroethyl)] amino-phenylbutyric acid).

chlorambucil (4-[*bis*(2-chloroethyl)]amino-phenylbutyric acid)

An alkylating and cytotoxic drug. Chlorambucil is not as toxic as is cyclophosphamide and has served as an effective therapy for selected immunological diseases such as rheumatoid arthritis, systemic lupus erythematosus (SLE), Wegener's granulomatosis, essential cryoglobulinemia, and cold agglutinin hemolytic anemia. Although it produces bone marrow suppression, it has not produced hemorrhagic cystitis and is less irritating to the gastrointestinal tract than cyclophosphamide. Chlorambucil increases the likelihood of opportunistic infections and the incidence of some tumors.

chlorodinitrobenzene (1-chlor-2,4-dinitrobenzene)

More often termed dinitrochlorobenzene (DNCB). A chemical substance used to test for a patient's ability to develop the type of delayed-type hypersensitivity referred to as contact hypersensitivity. This is a type IV hypersensitivity reaction. The chemical is applied to a patient's forearm. Following sufficient time for sensitization to develop, the patient's other forearm is exposed to a second (test) dose of the same chemical. In an individual with an intact cell-mediated limb of the immune response, a positive reaction develops at the second challenge site within 48 to 72 hours. Individuals with cell-mediated immune deficiency disorders fail to develop a positive delayed-type hypersensitivity reaction.

cholera toxin

A *Vibro cholerae* enterotoxin comprised of five B subunits that are cell-binding, 11.6-kDa structures that encircle a 27-kDa catalase that conveys ADP-ribose to G protein, leading to continual adenyl cyclase activation. Other toxins

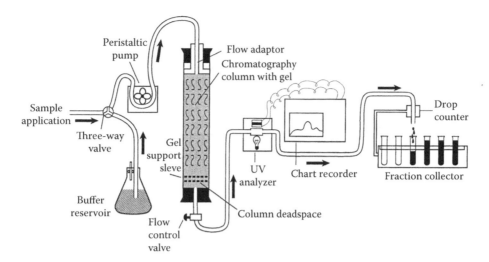

Column chromatography. Arrows indicate direction of flow. Chromatography refers to a group of methods employed for the separation of proteins.

that resemble cholera toxin in function include diphtheria toxin, exotoxin A, and pertussis toxin.

cholera vaccine

An immunizing preparation comprised of *Vibrio cholerae* smooth strains Inaba and Ogawa in addition to El Tor vibrio that have been killed by heat or formalin treatment. The vaccine is designed to induce protective active immunity against cholera in regions where it is endemic as well as in travelers to those locations. The immunity induced is effective for only about 12 weeks.

cholinergic urticaria

Skin edema induced by an aberrant response to acetylcholine that occurs following diminished cholinesterase activity.

CHOP therapy

A combination of chemotherapeutic antineoplastic substances including cyclophosphamide, [H]-doxorubicin, [O]-vincristine, and prednisolone.

chorea

Involuntary muscle twitching that occurs in cases of acute rheumatic fever and is commonly known as St. Vitus' dance.

choriocarcinoma

An unusual malignant neoplasm of the placenta trophoblast cells in which the fetal neoplastic cells are allogeneic in the host. On rare occasions, these neoplasms are "rejected" spontaneously by the host. Antimetabolites have been used in the treatment of choriocarcinoma.

chromium release assay

The release of chromium (^{51}Cr) from labeled target cells following their interaction with cytotoxic T lymphocytes or antibody and K cells (ADCC) or natural killer (NK) cells. The test measures cell death, which is reflected by the amount of radiolabel released according to the number of cells killed.

chromogenic substrate

A colorless substance transformed into a colored product by an enzymatic reaction.

chromogranin monoclonal antibody

An antibody that recognizes chromogranin A (68 kDa) and other related chromogranin polypeptides from humans, monkeys, and pigs. It is designed for the specific and quantitative localization of human chromogranin in

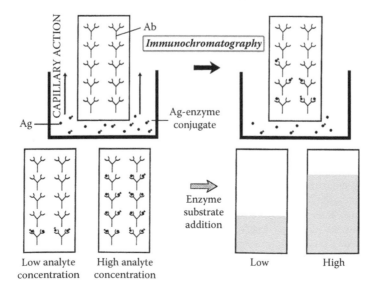

Immunochromatography.

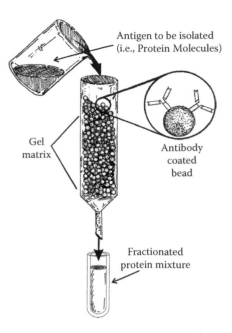

Absorption chromatography separates molecules based on their absorptive characteristics. Fluid is passed over a fixed solid stationary phase.

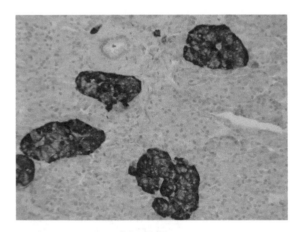

Chromogranin—pancreas.

paraffin-embedded and frozen tissue sections. It aids the localization of secretory storage granules in endocrine cells. Chromogranin A is a large, acidic protein present in catecholamine-containing granules of bovine adrenal medulla. It may be widely distributed in endocrine cells and tissues that share some common characteristics and are known as APUD (amine precursor uptake and decarboxylation) cells. Dispersed throughout the body, they are also referred to as the diffuse neuroendocrine system (DNES). Chromogranin has been demonstrated in several elements of the DNES, including anterior pituitary, thyroid parafollicular C cells, parathyroid chief cells, pancreatic islet cells, intestinal enteroendocrine cells, and tumors derived from these cells. Chromogranin immunoreactivity has also been observed in the thymus, spleen, lymph nodes, fetal liver, neurons, inner segments of rods and cones, the submandibular gland, and the central nervous system. Chromogranin is a widespread histological marker for polypeptide-producing cells (APUDs) and the tumors derived from them.

chromogranins

Acidic glycoproteins (molecular weights of 20 to 100 kDa) of neurosecretory granules in multiple tissue sites that are used as general endocrine indicators of neuroendocrine tumors using the immunoperoxidase reaction. The chromogranins are designated as A, B, and C. B and C are also termed secretogranin I and II.

chromatin remodeling

Changing a gene's chromatin structure to increase or diminish its availability for transcription.

chromatin remodeling complex

An enzymatic complex that is large, variable, and comprised of multiple components. These complexes are able to reorganize and flex DNA to either enhance or repress its transcription.

chromatography

A group of methods employed for the separation of proteins.

chromosomal translocations

DNA sequence rearrangement between two different chromosomes or two separate regions on the same chromosome, which is frequently associated with neoplasia. Lymphocyte malignancies may be associated with chromosomal translocations involving an immunoglobulin or T cell receptor locus and a chromosomal segment containing a cellular oncogene.

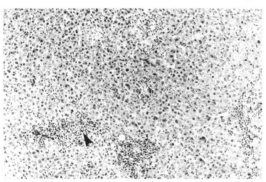

Chronic active hepatitis.

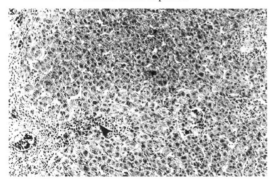

Chronic active hepatitis piecemeal necrosis.

chronic active hepatitis, autoimmune

A disease that occurs in young females who may develop fever, arthralgias, and skin rashes. They may be of the HLA-B8 and DR3 haplotype and suffer other autoimmune disorders. Most develop antibodies to smooth muscle, principally against actin, and autoantibodies to liver membranes. They also have other organ- and nonorgan-specific autoantibodies. A polyclonal hypergammaglobulinemia may be present. Lymphocytes infiltrating portal areas destroy hepatocytes. Injury to liver cells produced by these infiltrating lymphocytes produces piecemeal necrosis. The inflammation and necrosis are followed by fibrosis and cirrhosis. The T cells infiltrating the liver are CD4+. Plasma cells are also present, and immunoglobulins may be deposited on hepatocytes. The autoantibodies against liver cells do not play a pathogenetic role in liver injury. No serologic findings are diagnostic. Corticosteroids are useful in treatment. The immunopathogenesis of autoimmune chronic active hepatitis involves antibody, K cell cytotoxicity, and T cell reactivity against liver membrane antigens. Antibodies and specific T suppressor cells reactive with LSP are found in chronic active hepatitis patients, all of whom develop T cell sensitization against asialo-glycoprotein (AGR) antigen. Chronic active hepatitis has a familial predisposition.

chronic and cyclic neutropenia

A syndrome characterized by recurrent fever, mouth ulcers, headache, sore throat, and furunculosis occurring every 3 weeks in affected individuals. This chronic agranulocytosis leads to premature death from infection by pyogenic microorganisms in affected children who may have associated pancreatic insufficiency, dysostosis, and dwarfism. Antibodies can be transmitted from the maternal to fetal circulation to induce an isoimmune neutropenia that may consist of a transitory type in which the antibodies are against neutrophil antigens determined by the father or a type produced by autoantibodies against granulocytes.

chronic asthma

A clinical condition in which the airways are chronically inflamed, leading to difficulty in breathing. Whereas exposure to an allergen may initiate the condition, chronic asthma may progress in its absence.

chronic disease

A malady, such as a persistent infection, characterized by persistent or recurring symptoms.

chronic fatigue syndrome (CFS)

A disabling fatigue that persists for at least 6 months. Although the etiology is idiopathic, laboratory studies on patients reveal a consistent observation of immune system dysfunction primarily affecting the cellular immune response. CD4+ T helper cells and CD8+ suppressor/cytotoxic cells may be normal, increased, or decreased, but the CD4/DC8 ratio is usually elevated. This has been attributed to a diminished number of suppressor cells with a concomitant increase in cytotoxic T cell (CD8+, CD28+, CD11b–) numbers. The increased cytotoxic T cells express HLA–DR and/or CD38 activation markers. Manifestations of altered T cell functions also include decreased delayed-type hypersensitivity, diminished responsiveness in mitogen-stimulation assays *in vitro*, increased suppression of immunoglobulin synthesis by T cells, and elevated spontaneous suppressor activity. Natural killer (NK) cells may be normal, increased, or decreased, but there may be qualitative alterations in NK cell function. Elevated immunoglobulin G (IgG) antibody titers to Epstein–Barr virus (EBV) early antigen and capsid antigen are demonstrable in many CFS patients. Occasionally, increased antibodies against cytomegalovirus (CMV), herpes simplex, human herpesvirus type 6 (HHV-6), coxsackie B, or measles may be observed. Some CFS patients have abnormal levels of IgG, IgM, IgA, or IgD. Approximately one third of CFS patients have antibodies against smooth muscle or thyroid. Laboratory test results from CFS patients should be interpreted as one battery and not as individual tests.

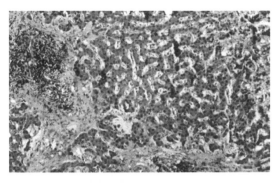

Chronic graft-vs.-host disease (GVHD) of the liver with pronounced inflammation and portal fibrosis with disappearance of bile ducts.

chronic graft rejection (CGR)

An anti-allograft immune response with features of fibrosis, collagen deposition and chronic graft vasculopathy that appear several months following transplantation and lead to cessation of allograft function.

chronic graft-vs.-host disease (GVHD)

Chronic GVHD may occur in as many as 45% of long-term bone marrow transplant recipients. It differs both clinically and histologically from acute GVHD and resembles autoimmune connective tissue diseases. For example, chronic GVHD patients may manifest skin lesions resembling scleroderma; sicca syndrome in the eyes and mouth; inflammation of the oral, esophageal, and vaginal mucosa; bronchiolitis obliterans; occasionally myasthenia gravis; polymyositis; and autoantibody synthesis. Histopathologic alterations in chronic GVHD, such as chronic inflammation and fibrotic changes in involved organs, resemble changes associated with naturally occurring autoimmune disease. The skin may reveal early inflammation with subsequent fibrotic changes. Infiltration of lacrimal, salivary, and submucosal glands by lymphoplasmacytic cells leads ultimately to fibrosis. The resulting sicca syndrome that resembles Sjögren's syndrome occurs in 80% of chronic GVHD patients. Drying of mucous membranes in the sicca syndrome affects the mouth, esophagus, conjunctiva, urethra, and vagina. The pathogenesis of chronic GVHD involves the interaction of alloimmunity, immune dysregulation, and resulting immunodeficiency and autoimmunity. The increased incidence of infection among chronic GVHD patients suggests immunodeficiency. The dermal fibrosis is associated with increased numbers of activated fibroblasts in the papillary dermis. T lymphocyte or mast cell cytokines may activate this fibroplasia, which leads to dermal fibrosis in chronic GVHD.

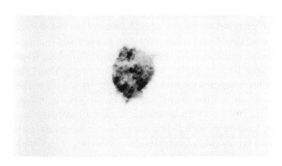

Nitroblue tetrazolium test (NBT) for diagnosis in CGD.

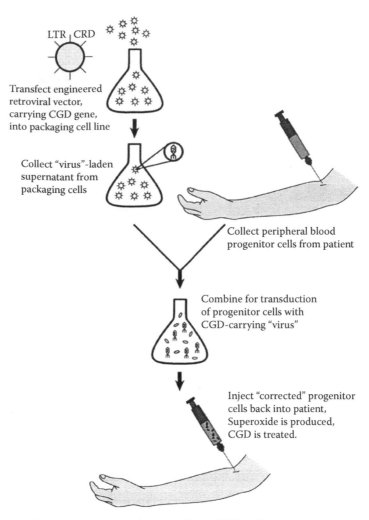

LTR   CRD

Transfect engineered retroviral vector, carrying CGD gene, into packaging cell line

Collect "virus"-laden supernatant from packaging cells

Collect peripheral blood progenitor cells from patient

Combine for transduction of progenitor cells with CGD-carrying "virus"

Inject "corrected" progenitor cells back into patient, Superoxide is produced, CGD is treated.

Strategy for gene therapy in chronic granulomatous disease (CGD) with peripheral blood progenitor cells.

chronic graft vasculopathy

Smooth muscle cell proliferation in arteries or arterioles of a graft induced by growth factors and cytokines released from recipient T cells activated by allorecognition that stimulate monocytes/macrophages in the graft and endothelial cells in blood vessel walls to release these substances. Narrowing of the graft vasculature leads to ischemia.

chronic granulomatous disease (CGD)

An immunodeficiency disorder that is inherited as an X-linked trait in two thirds of the cases and as an autosomal-recessive trait in the remaining third. Clinical features are usually apparent before the end of the second year of life. An enzyme defect is associated with NADPH oxidase. This enzyme deficiency causes neutrophils and monocytes to have decreased consumption of oxygen and diminished glucose utilization by the hexose monophosphate shunt. Although neutrophils phagocytize microorganisms, they do not form superoxide and other oxygen intermediates that usually constitute the respiratory burst. Neutrophils and monocytes also form a smaller amount of hydrogen peroxide, have decreased iodination of bacteria, and have diminished production of superoxide anions. All of this leads to decreased intracellular killing of bacteria and fungi. Thus, these individuals have increased susceptibility to infection

with microorganisms that normally are of relatively low virulence. These include *Aspergillus* spp., *Serratia marcescens,* and *Staphylococcus epidermidis.* Patients may have hepatosplenomegaly, pneumonia, osteomyelitis, abscesses, and draining lymph nodes. The quantitative nitroblue tetrazolium (NBT) test and the quantitative killing curve are both employed to confirm the diagnosis. Most microorganisms that cause difficulty in CGD individuals are catalase-positive. Therapy includes interferon-γ, antibiotics, and surgical drainage of abscesses.

chronic lymphocytic leukemia (CLL)

A peripheral B cell neoplasm in which the peripheral blood is flooded with small lymphocytes exhibiting condensed chromatin and scant cytoplasm. Disrupted tumor cells termed smudge cells represent a characteristic finding. Most patients have absolute lymphocyte counts above 4000/mm³ of blood. CLL is the most common leukemia of adults in the Western world. The tumor cells resemble a small subset of circulating B cells that express the surface marker CD45. The tumor cells express CD5, as well as the pan-B cell markers CD19 and CD20. However, they fail to express CD10. There is dim surface expression of immunoglobulin D heavy chain, and either κ or λ light chain chromosomal anomalies include trisomy 12 deletions of 13q 12–14 and deletions of 11q. CLL may be asymptomatic and may disrupt normal immune function through unknown mechanics. A prolonged disease course.

chronic lymphocytic leukemia/small lymphocytic lymphoma

Patients may have secondary immunodeficiency that affects both B and T limbs of the immune response. Diminished immunoglobulin levels are due primarily to diminished synthesis.

chronic lymphocytic thyroiditis

Profound infiltration of the thyroid by lymphocytes, leading to the extensive injury of thyroid follicular structure. Even though the gland becomes enlarged, its function diminishes, leading to hypothyroidism. Women are affected much more commonly than men. Antibodies detectable in the serum are specific for the 107-kDa thyroid microsomal peroxidase, the thyrotropin receptor, and thyroglobulin. Also called Hashimoto's thyroiditis. Thyroid hormone replacement therapy is the usual approach to treatment.

chronic mucocutaneous candidiasis

Infection of the skin, mucous membranes, and nails by *Candida albicans* associated with defective T-cell-mediated immunity specific to *Candida*. Skin tests for delayed hypersensitivity to the *Candida* antigen are negative. There may also be associated endocrinopathy. The selective deficiency in T lymphocyte immunity leads to increased susceptibility to chronic *Candida* infection. T cell immunity to non-*Candida* antigens is intact. B cell immunity is normal, which leads to an intact antibody response to *Candida* antigens. T lymphocytes form migration inhibitor factor (MIF) to most of the antigens, except for those of *Candida* microorganisms. The most common endocrinopathy is hypoparathyroidism. Clinical forms of the disease may be either granulomatous or nongranulomatous. *Candida* infection of the skin may be associated with the production of granulomatous lesions. The second most frequent endocrinopathy associated with this condition is Addison's disease. The disease is difficult to treat. The antifungal drug ketoconazole has proven effective. Intravenous amphotericin B has led to improvement. Transfer factor has been administered with variable success in selected cases.

chronic myelogenous leukemia (CML)

A disease affecting adults between the ages of 25 and 60 years that has a distinctive molecular abnormality consisting of a translocation involving the *Bcr* gene on chromosome 9 and the *Abl* gene on chromosome 22. The *Bcr/Abl* fusion gene that results controls the synthesis of a 210-kDa fusion protein that has tyrosine kinase activity; 90% of cases have the Ph1 karyotype. There is a striking increase in neoplastic granulocytic precursors in the bone marrow. The target of transformation is a pluripotent stem cell. The *Bcr/cAbl* fusion gene can be detected by either chromosomal analysis or polymerase chain reaction (PCR)-based molecular assays. There is also nearly total lack of leukocyte alkaline phosphatase. Most frequently encountered myeloproliferative disease. Marked by elevated numbers of mature and immature granulocytes. Clinically may be manifested as a chronic phase, accelerated phase, or blast crisis.

chronic myeloid leukemia

Leukemia characterized by cell types in the circulation that are in the late stages of granulocyte maturation. These include mature granulocytes, myelocytes, and metamyelocytes.

chronic progressive vaccinia (vaccinia gangrenosa) (historical)

An unusual sequela of smallpox vaccination in which the lesions produced by vaccinia on the skin became gangrenous and spread from the vaccination site to other areas of the skin. This occurred in children with cell-mediated immunodeficiency.

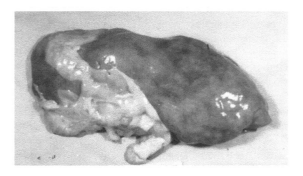

Renal allotransplant showing chronic rejection. The kidney is shrunken and malformed.

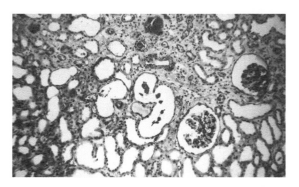

Microscopic view of chronic rejection showing tubular epithelial atrophy with interstitial fibrosis and shrinkage of glomerular capillary tufts.

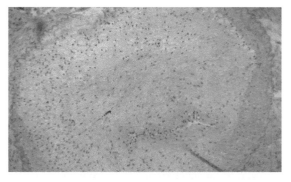

Wall of an artery seen in chronic rejection. Note obliteration of the vascular lumen with fibrous tissue; only a slit-like lumen remains.

chronic rejection

A type of allograft rejection that occurs during a prolonged period following transplantation and is characterized by structural changes such as fibrosis with loss of normal organ architecture. The principal pathologic change is degeneration and occlusion of arteries linking the graft to the host. This results from intimal smooth muscle cell proliferation and has been referred to as graft arteriosclerosis. Induced by antibodies against graft HLA class I alloantigens.

chronic thyroiditis

An autoimmune disease that leads to progressive destruction of the thyroid gland as in Hashimoto's thyroiditis. An inflammatory disease of the thyroid found most frequently in middle-age to older women. There is extensive infiltration of the thyroid by lymphocytes that completely replace the normal glandular structure of the organ. The numerous plasma cells, macrophages, and germinal centers give the appearance of a node structure within the thyroid gland. Both B cells and CD4+ T lymphocytes comprise the principal infiltrating lymphocytes. Thyroid function is first increased as inflammatory reaction injures thyroid follicles, causing them to release thyroid hormones. However, this increase is soon replaced by hypothyroidism in the later stages of Hashimoto's thyroiditis. Patients with this disease have enlarged thyroid glands. There are circulating autoantibodies against thyroglobulin, and thyroid microsomal antigens may be present (thyroid peroxidase). Cellular sensitization to thyroid antigens may also be detected. Thyroid hormone replacement therapy is given for the hypothyroidism that develops.

chronic xenograft rejection

Xenograft failure that occurs within weeks following transplantation as a consequence of cytotoxic T lymphocytes, NK cells reacting against donor endothelium. Also called cellular xenograft rejection.

chrysotherapy

Refer to gold therapy.

Churg–Strauss syndrome (allergic granulomatosis)

A combination of asthma associated with necrotizing vasculitis, eosinophilic tissue infiltrates, and extravascular granulomas.

CIA

Abbreviation for collagen-induced arthritis.

CIC

Abbreviation for circulating immune complexes.

cicatricial ocular pemphigoid

A rare blistering disorder of the conjunctival mucous membrane that may lead to scarring and result in blindness if untreated with corticosteroids. Histopathologically, the subepithelial unilocular bulla is accompanied by a mild inflammatory reaction. Direct immunofluorescence reveals a diffuse, linear deposition of immunoglobulins and components, mainly IgG and C3 at the epithelial–subepithelial junction.

CID

Abbreviation for (1) cytomegalic (CMV) inclusion disease and (2) combined immunodeficiency.

CIE

Abbreviation for counterimmunoelectrophoresis or crossed immunoelectrophoresis.

CIIV

Abbreviation for class II vesicle. Refer to MIICs.

cilia

Hair-like projections on respiratory and gastrointestinal tract epithelial cells. Cilia propel microorganisms out of the tract.

ciliary neurotrophic factor (CNTF)

A protein hormone related to the IL6 family. It performs several functions in the nervous system which are similar to those of leukemia inhibitory factor.

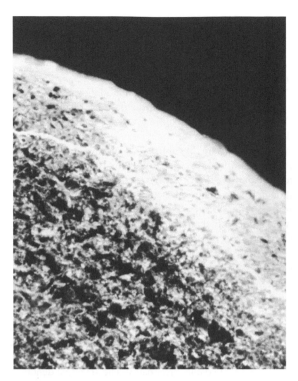

Cicatricial ocular pemphigoid stained with anti-IgG antibody.

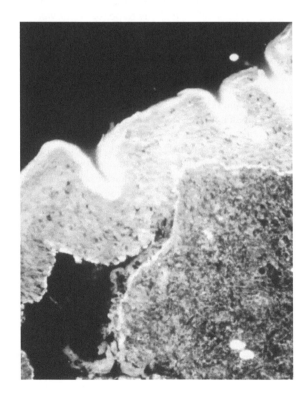

Cicatricial ocular pemphigoid stained with anti-IgG antibody.

cimetidine

An H$_2$-receptor antagonist capable of more than 90% reduction in food-stimulated and nocturnal secretion of gastric acid after a single dose. A well known treatment for peptic ulcers. This histamine H$_2$-receptor antagonist is of interest to immunologists because of its efficacy in treating common variable immunodeficiency, possibly through suppressor T lymphocyte inhibition. It also has an immunomodulating effect by reducing the activity of suppressor lymphocytes. Other drug immunomodulators, including low-dose cyclophosphamide given prior to immunization with a tumor vaccine, can augment the immune responses in animals and humans. Indomethacin can nullify the effects of suppressor macrophages.

circulating anticoagulant

Antibodies specific for one of the blood coagulation factors. They may be detected in the sera of patients treated with penicillin, streptomycin, or isoniazid; in patients with systemic lupus erythematosus (SLE); or following treatment with factor VIII or factor IX in patients with hemophilia A or B. These are often IgG4 antibodies.

circulating dendritic cell

A dendritic cell that has taken up antigen and is migrating to secondary lymphoid tissue such as a lymph node.

circulating lupus anticoagulant syndrome (CLAS)

The occurrence in lupus patients, who are often antinuclear antibody (ANA)-negative, of recurrent thromboses, kidney disease, and repeated spontaneous abortions. Immunoglobulin M (IgM) gammopathy and fetal wastage occur repeatedly.

circulating lymphocytes

The lymphocytes present in the systemic circulation represent a mixture of cells derived from different sources: (1) B and T cells exiting from bone marrow and thymus on their way to seed peripheral lymphoid organs; (2) lymphocytes exiting the lymph nodes via lymphatics, collected by the thoracic duct and discharged into the superior vena cava; and (3) lymphocytes derived from direct discharge into the vascular sinuses of the spleen. About 70% of cells in the circulating pool are recirculating; that is, they undergo a cycle during which they exit the systemic circulation to return back to lymphoid follicles, lymph nodes, and spleen and start the cycle again. The cells in this recirculating pool are mostly long-lived mature T cells. About 30% of the lymphocytes of the intravascular pool do not recirculate. They comprise mostly short-lived immature T cells that live their life spans intravascularly or are activated and exit the intravascular space. The exit of lymphocytes into the spleen occurs by direct discharge from the blood vessels. In the lymph nodes and lymphoid follicles, the exit of lymphocytes occurs through specialized structures, the postcapillary venules that differ from other venules in that they have tall endothelial coverings. The exiting lymphocytes percolate through the endothelial cells, a mechanism whose real significance is not known. A number of agents such as cortisone or *Bordetella pertussis* bacteria increase the extravascular exit of lymphocytes and prevent their return to circulation. The lymphocytes travel back and forth between the blood and lymph nodes or the marginal sinuses of the spleen. Within 24 to 48 hours they return via the lymphatics to the thoracic duct, where they then re-enter the blood.

circulatory system infection

The principal infection involving the circulatory system with immunologic sequelae is infective endocarditis. In acute endocarditis attributable to *Staphylococcus aureus*, high fever and, if untreated, fatal rapid destruction of the heart valves occur. A more indolent course is found in subacute endocarditis, and immunologic complications follow. Emboli break off from the infected heart valve. The principal causative microorganisms are streptococci including *S. veridans* and the more antibiotic-resistant entrococci. Antibody levels measured by immunoblotting are greatly increased in enterococcal or streptococcal endocarditis and are species-specific.

***cis* pairing**

Association of two genes on a single chromosome encoding the protein.

cisterna chyli

Refer to thoracic duct.

cisternal space

The endoplasmic reticulum lumens of plasma cells that contain immunoglobulin molecules prior to secretion.

Cκ

An immunoglobulin κ light chain constant region. The corresponding exon is designated $C\kappa$.

c-kit ligand

A cytokine, also termed stem cell factor, that interacts with a tyrosine–kinase membrane receptor of pluripotent stem cells. The receptor, which contains a five-immunoglobulin domain extracellular structure, is encoded by the *c-kit cellular oncogene*. Bone marrow stromal cells such as fibroblasts, endothelial cells, and adipocytes produce a 27-kDa transmembrane form and a 24-kDa secreted form of a c-kit ligand. This cytokine alone apparently does not induce colony formation but is postulated to render stem cells reactive with other colony-stimulating factors.

CL

An immunoglobulin light chain constant domain. The corresponding exon is designated C_L.

clade

HIV subtype based on sequence diversity. There is less than 10% difference among members of the same clade. Different clades varied in sequence are at least 15%.

***Cladosporium* species**

Aeroallergenic fungi that can induce hypersensitivity pneumonitis (HP) of the type known as hot tub lung disease, as well as immunoglobulin E (IgE)-mediated allergic disease that is frequent in persons with atopic disease. Symptoms of asthma that follow seasonal variations in *Cladosporium* spore counts and the demonstration of IgE reactivity aid diagnosis of allergy attributable to this microorganism.

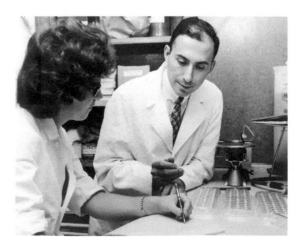

Henry Claman.

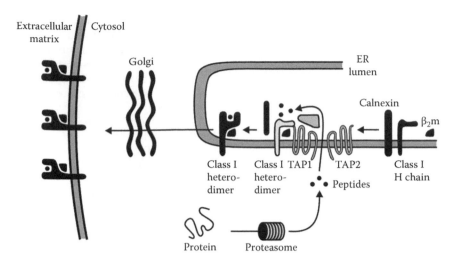

Major histocompatibility complex (MHC) class I assembly.

Claman, Henry

He conducted studies with lethally irradiated mice and proved that both bursa-derived and thymus-derived lymphocytes were needed to produce an immune response (T and B cell cooperation).

Cλ

An immunoglobulin λ light chain constant region. The corresponding exon is designated *Cλ*. There is more than one isotype in mice and humans.

class I antigen

A major histocompatibility complex (MHC) antigen found on nucleated cells on multiple tissues. In humans, class I antigens are encoded by genes at A, B, and C loci and in mice by genes at D and K loci.

class I region

The segment of the major histocompatibility complex that comprises the MHC class I heavy chain genes.

class IB genes

Genes linked to the major histocompatibility complex (MHC) class I region that code for class I-like α chains. These genes that encode molecules on cell surfaces that associate with β_2 microglobulin vary in their cell surface expression and tissue distribution from one species to another. An individual animal may have multiple class IB molecules. One such molecule has a role in presentation of peptides bearing *N*-formylated amino termini. Other class IB molecules may also be active in antigen presentation.

class I MHC molecules

Glycoproteins that play an important role in the interactions of cells of the immune system. Major histocompatibility complex (MHC) class I molecules occur on essentially all nucleated cells of the body but are absent from trophoblast cells and sperm. The cell membrane of T lymphocytes is rich in class I molecules that are composed of two distinct polypeptide chains: a 44-kDa α (heavy) chain and a 12-kDa β chain (β_2 microglobulin). There is a 40-kDa core polypeptide in the human α chain that has one N-linked oligosaccharide. Approximately 75% of the α chain is extracellular, including the amino terminus and the oligosaccharide group. The membrane portion is an abbreviated hydrophobic segment. The cytoplasm contains the 30-amino acid residue that comprises the carboxyl terminus. The β_2 microglobulin component is

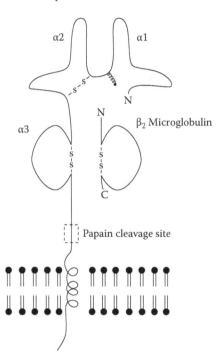

Major histocompatibility complex (MHC) class I molecules are glycoproteins that play an important role in interactions among cells of the immune system.

linked to neither the cell surface nor the α chain by covalent bonds. Its association with the α chain is noncovalent. Class I molecules consist of four parts: an extracellular amino terminal peptide-binding site, an immunoglobulin (Ig)-like region, a transmembrane segment, and a cytoplasmic portion. The main function of MHC molecules is to bind foreign peptides to form a complex that T cells can recognize. The class I molecular site that binds protein antigens is a 180-amino acid residue segment at the amino terminus of the class I α chain. The α-3 segment of the heavy chain contains approximately 90 amino acid residues between the carboxyl terminal end of the α-2 segment and the point of entrance into the plasma membrane. The α-3 segment joins the plasma membrane through a short connecting region and spans the membrane as a segment of 25 hydrophobic amino acid residues. This stabilizes the α

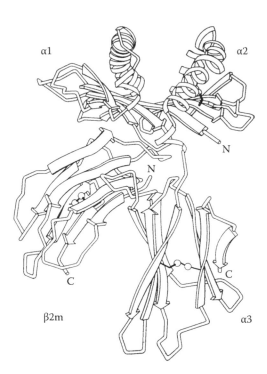

Three-dimensional structure of the external domains of a human class I HLA molecule based on x-ray crystallographic analysis. The β strands are depicted as thick arrows and the α helices as spiral ribbons. Disulfide bonds are shown as two interconnected spheres. The α_1 and α_2 domains interact to form the peptide-binding cleft. Note the immunoglobulin fold structure of the α_3 and β_2 microglobulin.

chain of MHC class I in the membrane. The carboxyl terminal region emerges as a 30-amino acid stretch in the cytoplasm. Class I histocompatibility antigens are products of the MHC locus. HLA-A, -B, and -C genes located in the MHC region on the short arm of chromosome 6 in humans encode these molecules. K, D, and L genes located on chromosome 17 in the H-2 complex in mice encode murine MHC class I antigens. The Tla complex situated near H-2 encodes additional class I molecules in mice. In T-cell-mediated cytotoxicity, CD8+ T lymphocytes kill antigen-bearing target cells. The cytotoxic T lymphocytes play a significant role in resistance to viral infection. MHC class I molecules present viral antigens to CD8+ T lymphocytes as a viral peptide class I molecular complex that is transported to the infected cell surface. Cytotoxic CD8+ T cells recognize this and lyse the target before the virus can replicate, thereby stopping the infection.

class I region

That part of the major histocompatibility complex (MHC) that contains the MHC class I heavy chain genes.

class II antigens

Major histocompatibility complex (MHC) antigens with limited distribution on such cells as B lymphocytes and macrophages. In humans, these antigens are encoded by genes at the DR, DP, and DQ loci.

class-II-associated invariant chain peptide (CLIP)

A peptide of variable length cleaved from the class II variant chain by proteases. It resides in the major histocompatibility complex (MHC) class II peptide-binding cleft and remains associated with the MHC class II molecules in an unstable form until removed by the HLA-DM protein.

class II MHC molecules

Glycoprotein histocompatibility antigens that play a critical role in immune system cellular interactions. Each major histocompatibility complex (MHC) class II molecule is comprised of a 32- to 34-kDa α chain and a 29- to 32-kDa β chain, each of which possesses N-linked oligosaccharide groups, amino termini that are extracellular, and carboxyl termini that are intracellular. Approximately 70% of both α and β chains are extracellular. Separate MHC genes encode the class II molecule α and β chains that are polymorphic. Class II molecules resemble class I molecules structurally as revealed by class II molecule nucleotide and amino acid sequences. MHC class II molecules consist of a peptide-binding region, a transmembrane segment, and an intracytoplasmic portion. The extracellular portions of α and β chains consist of α-1 and α-2 and β-1 and β-2 segments, respectively. The α-1 and α-2 segments constitute the peptide-binding region and consist of approximately 90 amino acid residues each. The immunoglobulin-like region is comprised of α-2 and β-2 segments folded into immunoglobulin domains in the class II molecule. The transmembrane region consists of approximately 25 hydrophobic amino acid residues. The transmembrane portion ends with a group of basic amino acid residues immediately followed by hydrophilic tails that extend into the cytoplasm and constitute the carboxyl terminal ends of the chains. The α chain is more heavily glycosylated than the β chain. Of the five exons in the α genes, one encodes the signal sequence and two code for the extracellular domains. The transmembrane domain and a portion of the 3′ untranslated segment are encoded by a fourth exon. The remaining part of the 3′ untranslated region is coded for by a fifth exon. Six exons are present in the β genes. They resemble α gene exons 1 through 3. The transmembrane domain and a portion of the cytoplasmic domain are encoded by a fourth exon, the cytoplasmic domain is coded for by the fifth exon, and the sixth exon encodes the 3′ region that is untranslated. B lymphocytes, macrophages, or other accessory cells express MHC class II antigens. Interferon-γ or other agents may induce an aberrant expression of class II antigen

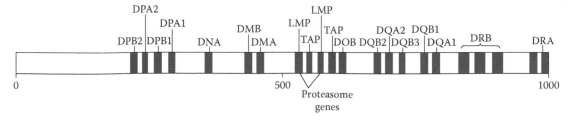

Class II MHC.

C

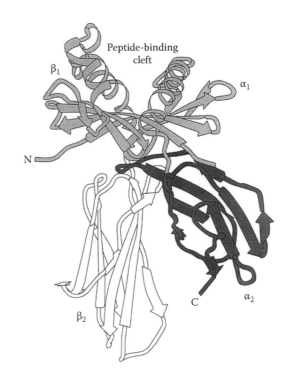

Class II MHC.

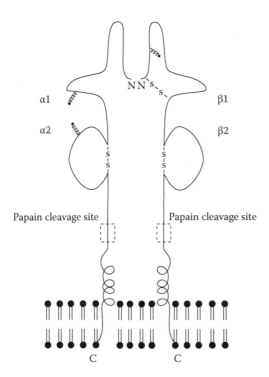

Class II MHC molecules are glycoprotein histocompatibility antigens that play a critical role in immune system cellular interactions. Each class II MHC molecule is comprised of a 32- to 34-kDa α chain and a 29- to 32-kDa β chain, each of which possesses N-like oligosaccharide groups, amino termini that are extracellular, and carboxyl termini that are intracellular. Approximately 70% of both α and β chains are extracellular.

by other types of cells. Antigen-presenting cells (APCs) such as macrophages present antigen at the cell surface to immunoreactive CD4+ helper/inducer T cells in the context of MHC class II antigens. For appropriate presentation, the peptide must bind securely to the MHC class II molecules. Those that do not bind fail to elicit an immune response. Following interaction of the peptide and the CD4+ helper T lymphocyte receptor, the CD4 cell is activated, interleukin-2 (IL2) is released, and the immune response is initiated. In humans, the class II antigens DR, DP, and DQ are encoded by HLA-D-region genes. In mice, class II antigens, designated as Ia antigens, are encoded by I-region genes. The I invariant chain (Ii) represents an essentially nonpolymorphic polypeptide chain associated with MHC class II molecules of humans and mice.

class II region

That part of the major histocompatibility complex (MHC) containing the MHC class II α and β chain genes.

class II transactivator (CIITA)

Refer to MHC class II transactivator.

MHC class II molecular structure.

class II vesicle (CIIV)

A murine B cell membrane-bound organelle that is critical in the major histocompatibility complex (MHC) class II pathway of antigen presentation. It contains all constituents requisite for the formation of peptide antigen and MHC class II molecular complexes, including the enzymes that degrade protein antigens, class II molecules, invariant chain, and HLA-DM.

class III molecules

Substances that include factors B, C2, and C4 that are encoded by genes in the major histocompatibility complex (MHC) region. Although adjacent to class I and class II molecules that are important in histocompatibility, C3 genes are not important in this regard. The 100-kB region is located between HLA-B and HLA-D loci on the short arm of chromosome 6 in humans and between the I and H-2D regions on chromosome 17 in mice. The genes encoding C4 and P-450 21-hydroxylase are closely linked.

class III region

That area of the major histocompatibility complex between the class I and class II regions, called the central MHC. No MHC class I or class II genes are present in this region.

class switching (isotype switching)

A change in the isotype or class of an immunoglobulin synthesized by a B lymphocyte undergoing differentiation.

Immunoglobulin M (IgM) is the main antibody produced first in a primary humoral response to thymus-dependent antigens, with IgG produced later in the response. A secondary antibody response to the same antigen results in the production of only small amounts of IgM but much larger quantities of IgG, IgA, or IgE antibodies. T helper cell lymphokines have a significant role in controlling class switching. Only heavy chain constant regions are involved in switching, with the light chain type and heavy chain variable region remaining the same. The specificity of the antigen-binding region is not altered. Mechanisms of class switching during B cell differentiation include the generation of transcripts processed to separate mRNAs and the rearrangements of immunoglobulin genes that lead to constant region gene segment transposition. Membrane IgM appears first on immature B cells, followed by membrane IgD as cell maturation proceeds. A primary transcript bearing the heavy chain variable region, μ chain constant region, and δ chain constant region may be spliced to form mRNA that codes for each heavy chain. Following stimulation of B cells by antigen and T lymphocytes, class switching is probably attributable to immunoglobulin gene rearrangements. During switching, B cells may temporarily express more than one class of immunoglobulin. Class switching in B cells mediated by interleukin-4 (IL4) is sequential, proceeding from Cμ to Cγ₁ to Cε. IgG₁ expression replaces IgM expression as a consequence of the first switch. IgE expression replaces IgG₁ expression as a result of the second switch. TGF-β and IL5 have been linked to the secretion of IgA.

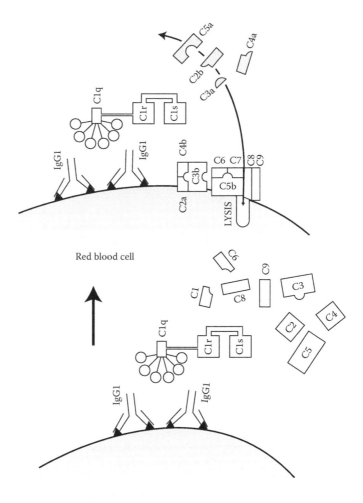

Red blood cell

Classical pathway of complement activation.

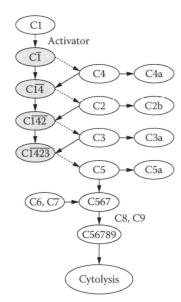

Classical pathway of complement activation.

classical C3 convertase

A surface serine protease comprised of complement components C4b2a, which splits C3 into C3a and C3b. It participates in the classical pathway of complement activation.

classical C5 convertase

Refer to C5 convertase.

classical Hodgkin lymphoma

Classification includes 95% of Hodgkin lymphomas divided into nodular sclerosis, mixed cellularity, lymphocyte-predominant, and lymphocyte-depleted subtypes. Characterized by Reed–Sternberg cells that have a CD30±, CD15⁺, CD20⁻, CD45⁻ immunophenotype.

classical pathway

Refer to classical complement pathway.

classical pathway of complement activation

One of the three complement activation pathways. A mechanism to activate C3 through participation by the serum proteins C1, C4, and C2. Immunoglobulin M (IgM) or a doublet of IgG may bind the C1 subcomponent C1q. Following subsequent activation of C1r and C1s, the two C1s substrates C4 and C2 are cleaved. This yields C4b and C2a fragments that produce C4b2a, known as C3 convertase, and activate opsonization, chemotaxis of leukocytes, increased permeability of vessels, and cell lysis. Activators of the classical pathway include IgM, IgG, staphylococcal protein A, C-reactive protein, and DNA. C1 inhibitor blocks the classical pathway by separating C1r and C1s from C1q. The C4-binding protein also blocks the classical pathway by linking to C4b, separating it from C2a, and permitting factor I to split the C4b heavy chain to yield C4bi, which is unable to unite with C2a, thereby inhibiting the classical pathway.

clathrin

The principal protein enclosing numerous coated vesicles. The molecular structure consists of three 180-kDa heavy chains and three 30- to 35-kDa light chains arranged into typical lattice structures comprised of pentagons or hexagons. These structures encircle the vesicles. Associated with receptor-mediated endocytosis.

Cleveland procedure

A form of peptide map in which protease-digested protein products, with sodium dodecyl sulfate (SDS) present, are subjected to SDS-PAGE. This produces a characteristic peptide fragment pattern that is typical of the protein substrate and enzyme used.

clinical trial

A four-phase process (I through IV) in which a sequence of controlled tests of a drug, vaccine, or treatment of interest is evaluated in human volunteers to establish its safety and efficacy before being recommended for licensing for public use.

CLIP

The processed fragment of invariant chain. In the major histocompatibility complex (MHC) class II transport pathway, the peptide binding groove must be kept free of endogenous peptides. The cell uses one protein, called invariant chain (and its processed fragment CLIP) to block the binding site until needed. HLA-DM facilitates release of CLIP peptides and their exchange for antigenic peptides as they become available. As long as CLIP remains in the binding groove, antigenic peptides cannot bind.

clonal

The exclusive stimulation of only those lymphocyte clones that express receptors for a specific antigen.

clonal anergy

The interaction of immune system cells with an antigen, without a second antigen signal, that is usually needed for a response to an immunogen. This leads to functional inactivation of the immune system cells in contrast to the development of antibody formation or cell-mediated immunity.

clonal balance

In explaining autoimmunity in terms of clonal balance, it is convenient to describe it as an alteration in the helper-to-suppressor ratio with a slight predominance of helper activity. Factors that influence the balance of helper to suppressor cells include aging, steroid hormones, viruses, and chemicals. The genetic constitution of the host and the mechanism of antigen presentation are the two most significant factors that govern clonal balance. Immune response genes associated with major histocompatibility complex (MHC) determine MHC class II antigen expression on cells presenting antigen to helper CD4+ lymphocytes. Thus, the MHC class II genotype may affect susceptibility to autoimmune disease. Other genes may be active as well. Antigen presentation exerts a major influence on the generation of an autoimmune response. Whereas a soluble antigen administered intravenously with an appropriate immunologic adjuvant may induce an autoimmune response leading to immunopathologic injury, the same antigen injected intravenously without the adjuvant may induce no detectable response. Animals rendered tolerant to foreign antigens possess suppressor T lymphocytes associated with the induced unresponsiveness. Thus, self tolerance may be due, in part, to the induction of suppressor T cells. This concept is called clonal balance rather than clonal deletion.

Self antigens are considered to normally induce mostly suppressor rather than helper T cells, leading to a negative suppressor balance in the animal body. Three factors with the potential to suppress immune reactivity against self include nonantigen-specific suppressor T cells, antigen-specific suppressor T cells, and anti-idiotypic antibodies. Suppressor T lymphocytes may leave the thymus slightly before the corresponding helper T cells. Suppressor T cells specific for self antigens are postulated to be continuously stimulated and usually in greater numbers than the corresponding helper T cells.

clonal deletion (negative selection)

The elimination of self-reactive T lymphocytes in the thymus during the development of natural self tolerance. T cells recognize self antigens only in the context of major histocompatibility complex (MHC) molecules. Autoreactive thymocytes are eliminated following contact with self antigens expressed in the thymus before maturation is completed. The majority of CD4+ T lymphocytes in the blood circulation that survive clonal deletion in the thymus fail to respond to any stimulus. This reveals that clonal anergy participates in suppression of autoimmunity. Clonal deletion represents a critical mechanism to rid the body of autoreactive T lymphocytes. This is brought about by minor lymphocyte stimulation (Mls) antigens that interact with the T cell receptor's V β region of the T lymphocyte receptor, thereby mimicking the action of bacterial super antigen. Intrathymic and peripheral tolerance in T lymphocytes can be accounted for by clonal deletion and functional inactivation of T cells reactive against self. In addition to central tolerance that results from clonal deletion of T or B cells, whose antigen receptors identify self antigens with high affinity as a mechanism of negative selection, peripheral tolerance depends on clonal deletion of mature naïve T cells that interact with their homologous self peptide/MHC presented by immature dendritic cells, which leads to the destruction of T cell clones with the potential to induce autoimmunity.

clonal exhaustion

The division of an activated lymphocyte at such a rapid rate in the presence of persistent antigen that its progeny can no longer replicate, *i.e.*, replicative senescence, prior to degeneration of memory cells.

clonal expansion

Antigen-specific lymphocyte proliferation in response to antigenic stimulation that precedes differentiation into effector cells. It is a critical mechanism of adaptive immunity that enables rare antigen-specific cells to proliferate sufficiently to combat the pathogenic microorganisms that provoked the response.

clonal ignorance

Lymphocytes that survive the principal mechanisms of self tolerance and remain functionally competent but are unresponsive to self antigens and do not cause autoimmune reactions.

clonal restriction

An immune response that is limited to the expression of a few lymphoid cell clones.

clonal selection

Antigen-mediated activation and proliferation of members of a clone of B lymphocytes bearing receptors for the antigen or for complexes of major histocompatibility complex (MHC) and peptides derived from the antigen in the case of T lymphocytes. Refer to *clonal selection theory*.

Clonal selection theory.

clonal selection theory

A selective theory of antibody formation proposed by F.M. Burnett, who postulated the presence of numerous antibody-forming cells, each capable of synthesizing its own predetermined antibody. One of the cells, after having been selected by the best-fitting antigen, multiplies and forms a clone of cells that continue to synthesize the same antibody. Considering the existence of many different cells, each capable of synthesizing an antibody of a different specificity, all known facts of antibody formation are easily accounted for. An important element of the clonal selection theory was the hypothesis that many cells with different antibody specificities arise through random somatic mutations during a period of hypermutability early in life. Also early in life, the "forbidden" clones of antibody-forming cells (i.e., the cells that make antibody to the animal's own antigen) are still destroyed after encountering these autoantigens. This process accounts for an animal's tolerance of its own antigens. Antigen would have no effect on most lymphoid cells, but it would selectively stimulate those cells already synthesizing the corresponding antibody at a low rate. The cell surface antibody would serve as receptor for antigen and proliferate into a clone of cells, producing antibody of that specificity. Burnett introduced the forbidden clone concept to explain autoimmunity. Cells capable of forming antibody against a normal self antigen were "forbidden" and eliminated during embryonic life. During fetal development, clones that react with self antigens are destroyed or suppressed. The subsequent activation of suppressed clones reactive with self antigens in later life may induce autoimmune disease. D.W. Talmage proposed a cell selection theory of antibody formation that was the basis for Burnett's clonal selection theory.

clone

A cell or organism that develops from a single progenitor cell and has exactly the same genotype and phenotype of the parent cell. Malignant proliferation of a clone of plasma cells in multiple myeloma represents a type of monoclonal gammopathy. The fusion of an antibody-producing B cell with a mutant myeloma cell *in vitro* by the action of polyethylene glycol to form a hybridoma that is immortal and produces monoclonal antibody is an example of the *in vitro* production of a clone.

cloned DNA

A DNA fragment or gene introduced into a vector and replicated in eukaryotic cells or bacteria.

cloned enzyme donor immunoassay

A homogeneous enzyme immunoassay (EIA) based on the modulation of enzyme activity by bound fragments of β-galactosidase.

cloned T cell line

A lineage of T lymphocytes that grow continuously from a single progenitor cell. Stimulation with antigen from time to time is necessary to maintain their growth. They are used in experimental immunology to investigate T cell function and specificity.

clonotypic

An adjective that defines the features of a specific B cell population's receptors for antigen that are products of a single B lymphocyte clone. Following release from the B cells, these antibodies should be very specific for antigen, have a restricted spectrotype, and possess at least one unique private idiotypic determinant. Clonotypic may also describe the features of a particular clone of T lymphocytes' specific receptor for antigen with respect to idiotypic determinants, specificity for antigen, and receptor similarity from one daughter cell of the clone to another.

Clostridium immunity

Clostridia produce disease by releasing exotoxins. They may produce more than one toxin, and each one is immunologically unique. For example, each of the five types of *Clostridium perfringens* produces a different toxin. Clostridia enter the host by many routes to produce disease. *C. perfringens* gains access through traumatic or surgical wounds to produce gas gangrene and wound infections. The microorganism is aided by a poor blood supply in the area of the wound. Clostridia divide and produce toxins that cause disease. When antibiotics upset the normal bowel flora, *C. difficile* may multiply and induce colitis. The toxins released from this organism act on intestinal epithelial cells and produce diarrhea and chronic inflammation. *C. botulinum* does not grow in the host but forms toxins in contaminated food that when ingested leads to disease.

Most clostridial diseases do not induce protective immunity because the amount of toxin required to produce disease is less than that necessary to induce an immunologic response. Even though systemic immunity does not follow an episode of the disease, tetanus toxoid can induce immunity that may last for 5 years. Tetanus immunoglobulin is also valuable for passive immunization in suspected cases. Antibotulinum toxin antibody is available for laboratory workers. Intravenous administration of γ globulin containing high titers of antibody to *C. difficile* toxin has been useful in the therapy of patients with relapsing *C. difficile* diarrhea.

clotting system

A mixture of cells, their fragments, zymogens, zymogen activation products and naturally occurring inhibitors, adhesive and structural proteins, phospholipids, lipids, cyclic and noncyclic nucleotides, hormones, and inorganic cations, all of which normally maintain blood flow. With disruption of the monocellular layer of endothelial cells lining a vessel wall, the subendothelial layer is exposed, bleeding occurs, and a cascade of events is initiated that leads to clot formation. These homeostatic reactions lead to formation of the primary platelet plug followed by a clot that mainly contains crosslinked fibrin (secondary hemostasis). After the blood vessel is repaired, the clot is dissolved by fibrinolysis. Refer also to coagulation system.

cluster of differentiation (CD)

The designation of antigens on the surfaces of leukocytes by their reactions with clusters of monoclonal antibodies. The antigens are designated as clusters of differentiation (CDs).

clusterin (serum protein SP-40,40)

A complement regulatory protein that inhibits membrane attack complex (MAC) formation by blocking the fluid phase of the MAC. Its substrate is C5b67.

clustering

Monomeric antigens, monovalent lectins, and monovalent antibody to mIg, and other membrane components neither cap on the cell surface nor produce large clusters. Multivalent ligand binding is necessary for clustering and for capping. Clustering, unlike capping, is a passive redistribution process. Spotting or patching does not require a cell to be living or metabolically active. Clustering is affected by the factors that control phenomena occurring in a three-dimensional fluid aqueous phase and also by physicochemical properties of plasma membranes. The outcome of cluster formation is influenced by physiological interactions between the membrane proteins.

CMI

Abbreviation for cell-mediated immunity.

CMK-BRL-1

Chemokine β receptor-like 1 is a member of the G protein-coupled receptor family, the chemokine receptor branch of the rhodopsin family. It is expressed on neutrophils and monocytes but not on eosinophils. It may be found in brain, placenta, lung, liver, and pancreas.

CML

Abbreviation for chronic myelogenous leukemia.

CNS prophylaxis

The intrathecal administration of chemotherapeutic agents or localized CNS and brain irradiation to block tumor cell invasion.

Cμ

An immunoglobulin μ chain constant region. The corresponding exon is designated *Cμ*.

c-*myb*

A protooncogene that codes for the 75- to 89-kDa phosphoprotein designated c-Myb in the nucleus, which immature hematopoietic cells express during differentiation. When casein kinase II phosphorylates Myb at an N terminal site, the union of Myb to DNA and continued activation are blocked. This phosphorylation site is deleted during oncogenic transformation, which permits Myb to combine with DNA.

c-*myb* gene

A gene that encodes formation of a DNA-binding protein that acts during early growth and differentiation stages of normal cells. A c-*myb* gene is expressed mainly in hematopoietic cells, especially bone marrow hematopoietic precursor cells, but it is greatest in the normal murine thymus. The highest c-*myb* expression is in the double-negative thymocyte subpopulation.

c-*myc* gene

Refer to *myc*.

coagglutination

The interaction of immunoglobulin (IgG) antibodies with the surfaces of protein-A-containing *Staphylococcus aureus* microorganisms through their Fc regions, followed by interaction of the Fab regions of these same antibody molecules with surface antigens of bacteria for which they are specific. Thus, when the appropriate reagents are all present, coagglutination will take place in which the Y-shaped antibody molecule will serve as a bridge between staphylococci and the coagglutinated microorganism for which it is specific.

coagulation, invertebrate

A mechanism in higher invertebrates in which lipopolysaccharide combines with a pattern recognition receptor to activate three proteases of a zymogen cascade that leads to crosslinking of coagulogen protein in hemolymph to produce a clot. This halts loss of body fluids and isolates pathogenic microorganisms that may have gained access to the injured site. It may occur after V(D)J recombination and non-homologous end joining repair.

coagulation system

A cascade of interactions among 12 proteins in blood serum that culminates in the generation of fibrin, which prevents bleeding from blood vessels whose integrity has been interrupted.

coated pit

A depression in a cell membrane coated with clathrin. Hormones such as insulin and epidermal growth factor may bind to their receptors in coated pits or migrate toward the pits following binding of the ligand at another site. After the aggregation of complexes of receptor and ligand in the coated pits, they invaginate and bud off as coated vesicles containing the receptor–ligand complexes. These structures, called receptosomes, migrate into cells by endocytosis. Following association with GERL structures, they fuse with lysosomes where receptors and ligands are degraded.

coated vesicle

Vesicles in the cytoplasm usually encircled by a coat of protein-containing clathrin molecules. Coated vesicles originate from coated pits and are important for protein secretion and receptor-mediated endocytosis. Coated vesicles convey receptor–macromolecule complexes from extracellular to intracellular locations. Clathrin-coated vesicles convey proteins from one intracellular organelle to another. Refer also to coated pit.

cobra venom factor (CVF)

A protein in the venom of the Indian cobra, *Naja naja*. It is the equivalent of mammalian C3b and thus can activate the alternative pathway of complement. Mammalian factor I does not inactivate cobra venom, which leads to the production of a stable alternative pathway C3 convertase if CVF is injected intravenously into a mammal. Thus, the injection of cobra venom factor into mammals has been used to destroy complement activity for experimental purposes. A component of cobra venom interacts specifically with the serum complement system, leading to its continuous activation. CVF is a structural and functional analog of complement component C3. It has been employed to decomplement laboratory animals to investigate the biological functions of complement. It has been used in animal experiments involving xenotransplantation to show that complement is a principal contributor to hyperacute rejection of a transplanted organ. It has also been used in antibody conjugates to render monoclonal antibodies cytotoxic.

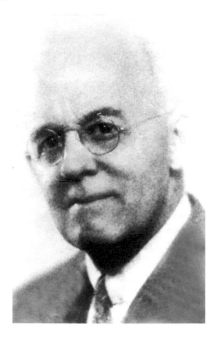

Arthur Fernandez Coca.

Coca, Arthur Fernandez (1875–1959)

American allergist and immunologist. He was a major force in allergy and immunology. He named atopic antibodies and was a pioneer in the isolation of allergens. He and Robert A. Cooke classified allergies in humans.

co-capping

If two molecules are associated in a membrane, capping of one induced by its ligand may lead also to capping of the associated molecule. Antibodies to membrane molecule *x* may induce capping of membrane molecule *y* and *x* if *x* and *y* are associated in the membrane. In this example, the capping of the associated *y* molecule is termed co-capping.

***Coccidioides* immunity**

Immunity against *Coccidioides immitis* depends upon T lymphocytes. IFN-γ plays an important role in protection conferred by the recombinant form of this cytokine in experimental mice. Monocytes have a precise role in limiting infection before a specific immune response develops. Spherules and arthroconidia induce the synthesis of TNFα by human monocytes *in vitro*. TNFα alone or combined with IFN-γ promotes killing of spherules by human monocytes *in vitro*. TNFα and IL6 levels have been shown to be elevated in patients with overwhelming infections by this organism. Antigen overload, specific suppressor T lymphocyte activity from a circulating humoral suppressor substance, may sometimes suppress the T lymphocyte A *Coccidioides*-specific responses in some patients. A positive skin test indicates previous infection. Results usually remain positive for the patient's lifetime. Of all infected individuals, 90% develop antibody responses to *C. immitis*. Mycelial phase antigens are most often used in serodiagnosis. Immunoglobulin M (IgM) forms early but disappears after 6 months, whereas IgG elevated titers may indicate dissemination.

coccidioidin

A *Coccidioides immitis* culture extract used in a skin test for cell-mediated immunity against the microorganism in a manner analogous to the tuberculin skin test.

***coccidiosis* immunity**

Immunity induced by infection is species- and in some instances strain-specific, yet immunization with purified antigens may induce heterologous protection. Immunity is mediated by T cells and is far more significant to resistance than the humoral immune response that is also stimulated. Antibodies act mainly against extracellular parasites to reduce invasion. CD4+ T cells control primary infections, whereas CD8+ lymphocytes are more significant in later stages of infection. There is a vaccine for chickens, but it is expensive.

coding joint

A structure formed when a V gene segment joins imprecisely to a (D)J gene segment in immunoglobulin or T cell receptor genes.

codominant

The expression of both alleles of a pair in a heterozygote. The traits they determine are codominant as in the expression of blood group A and B epitopes in type AB persons.

codominantly expressed

Gene expression when both alleles at one locus are expressed in approximately equal amounts in heterzygotes. The highly polymorphic major histocompatibility complex (MHC) genes, as well as most other genes, manifest this property.

codon

A three-adjacent nucleotide sequence mRNA that acts as a coding unit for a specific amino acid during protein synthesis. The codon controls which amino acid is incorporated into the protein molecule at a certain position in the polypeptide chain. Of 64 codons, 61 encode amino acids, and 3 act as termination codons.

coelomate

An animal possessing a body cavity.

coelomocyte

A circulating or fixed ameboid phagocytic leukocyte that participates in the defense of invertebrate animals that have coeloms by phagocytosis and encapsulation.

Cogan's syndrome

Corneal inflammation (interstitial keratitis) and inflammation of the ear, leading to nausea, vomiting, vertigo, and ringing in the ears. This may be associated with connective tissue disease or may occur following an infection.

cognate antigen

An epitope recognized to be identified by a specific lymphocyte antigen receptor because it was used initially to activate that lymphocyte.

cognate interaction

Processed antigen on a B cell surface interacting with a T cell receptor for antigen resulting in B cell differentiation into an antibody-producing cell.

cognate recognition

Refer to cognate interaction.

Cohn fraction II

γ-Globulin isolated by ethanol fractionation of serum by the method of Cohn.

Cohnheim, Julius (1839–1884)

German experimental pathologist who was the first proponent of inflammation as a vascular phenomenon. (Refer to *Lectures on General Pathology,* 1889.)

coisogenic

Refer to congenic strains.

coisogenic strain

Inbred mouse strain that has an identical genotype except for a difference at one genetic locus. A point mutation in an inbred strain provides the opportunity to develop a coisogenic strain by inbreeding the mouse in which the mutation occurred. The line carrying the mutation is coisogenic with the line not expressing the mutation. Considering the problems associated with developing coisogenic lines, congenic mouse strains were developed as an alternative. Refer to congenic strains.

cold agglutinin

An antibody that agglutinates particulate antigen, such as bacteria or red cells, optimally at temperatures less than 37°C. In clinical medicine, the term usually refers to antibodies against red blood cell antigens as in the cold agglutinin syndrome.

cold agglutinin syndrome

An immune condition in which immunoglobulin M (IgM) autoantibodies agglutinate erythrocytes most effectively at 4°C. Normal individuals may have cold agglutinins in low titer (<1:32). Certain infections such as cytomegalovirus, trypanosomiasis, mycoplasma, malaria, and Epstein–Barr virus, are followed by the development of polyclonal cold agglutinins. These antibodies are of concern only if they are hemolytic. Acquired hemolytic anemia patients with positive direct Coombs' tests should be tested for cold agglutinins. For example, they may have anti-Pr, anti-I, anti-i, anti-Sd^a, or anti-Gd. Aged individuals suffering from monoclonal κ proliferation or simultaneous large cell lymphoma may develop cold agglutinin syndrome. It also occurs in a younger age group in whom anti-I antibodies have been synthesized following an infection with *Mycoplasma pneumoniae* or in whom anti-i antibodies associated with infectious mononucleosis have formed. C3d coats the cells. Agglutination and complement fixation may take place intravascularly in parts of the body exposed to the cold. When the red blood cells with attached complement are warmed to 37°C (normal body temperature), mild hemolysis occurs.

cold antibodies

Antibodies that occur at higher titers at 4°C rather than at 37°C.

cold chain (vaccination)

Continuous refrigeration of a labile vaccine from its preparation and transport to the geographic site where it is to be used.

cold ethanol fractionation

A technique used to fractionate serum proteins by precipitation with cold ethanol. One of the fractions obtained is Cohn fraction II, which contains the immunoglobulins. This method has been largely replaced by more modern and sophisticated techniques.

cold hemagglutinin disease

Refer to cold agglutinin syndrome.

cold hemoglobinuria

Refer to paroxysmal cold hemoglobinuria.

cold hypersensitivity

A localized wheal and flare reaction and bradycardia that follow exposure to low temperatures that induce overstimulation of the autonomic nervous system.

cold-reacting autoantibodies

Cold-reacting autoantibodies represent a special group of both naturally occurring and pathologic antibodies characterized by the unusual property of reacting with the corresponding antigen at low temperature. Those reacting with red blood cells are also called cold agglutinins, although they may also react with other cells. Those with a more restricted range of targets are called cytotoxins.

cold target inhibition

The introduction of unlabeled target cells to inhibit radioisotope release from labeled target cells through the actions of antibody- or cell-mediated immune mechanisms.

cold urticaria

Urticaria that occurs soon after exposure to cold. The lesions are usually confined to the exposed areas. The condition has been observed in patients with underlying conditions that include cryoglobulinemia, cryofibrinogenemia, cold agglutinin disease, and paroxysmal cold hemoglobinuria. Although the mechanism is unknown, cold exposure has been shown to cause the release of histamine and other mediators. Cold sensitivity has been passively transferred in individuals with abnormal proteins. Cryoprecipitates may fix complement and lead to the generation of anaphylatoxin. The condition can be diagnosed by placing ice cubes on the forearm for 4 minutes and observing for the following 10 minutes for the appearance of urticaria when the area is rewarmed. Treatment consists of limiting exposure to cold and the administration of antihistamines such as oral cyproheptadine. Individuals with abnormal protein should have the underlying disease treated.

collagen

A 285-kDa extracellular matrix protein that contains proline hydroxyproline, lysine, hydroxylysine, and glycine 30%. The structure consists of a triple helix of 95-kDa polypeptides forming a tropocollagen molecule that is resistant to proteases. Collagen types other than IV form fibrils with a quarter-stagger overlap between molecules providing a fibrillar structure that resists tension. Several types of collagen have been described, and most of them can be crosslinked through lysine side chains.

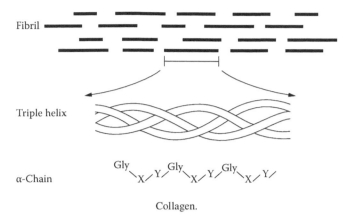

Collagen.

collagen (type I, II, and III) autoantibodies

Autoantibodies found in various autoimmune diseases such as mixed connective tissue disease (MCTD), systemic lupus erythematosus (SLE), progressive systemic sclerosis (PSS), rheumatoid arthritis (RA), and vasculitis. Approximately 85% of SLE patients have antibodies against type I collagen. Type II collagen autoantibodies in rodents and monkeys have led to arthritis. Autoantibodies to types I, II, and III collagen have been identified in adult and juvenile rheumatoid arthritis and relapsing polychondritis. Individuals with hypersensitivity reactions to collagen implants may manifest immunity to native and denatured collagens. Autoantibodies to type II collagen have been associated with RA and relapsing polychondritis patients. Autoimmunity to type II collagen has been hypothesized to have a role in the pathogenesis of RAs. Autoantibodies to type II collagen have also been reported in scleroderma and SLE and possibly in inner ear diseases. Collagen type III antibodies have been found in 44% of SLE patients and 85% of RA patients.

collagen disease and arthritis panel

A cost-effective battery of tests to diagnose rheumatic disease that includes the erythrocyte sedimentation rate and assays for rheumatoid factor (RA test), antinuclear antibody, uric acid levels, and C-reactive protein.

collagen disease/lupus erythematosus diagnostic panel

A battery of serum tests for the diagnosis of collagen vascular disease that yields the most information for the least cost.

collagen-induced arthritis (CIA)

The deliberate injection of DBA/1J mice with type II collagen incorporated into complete Freund's adjuvant to produce arthritis in multiple joints as a consequence of autoimmunity. A murine model of rheumatoid arthritis in humans.

collagen type IV (CIV22)

Anti-collagen type IV is a mouse monoclonal antibody that detects collagen type IV, the major component of the basal lamina. Antibodies to this molecule confirm its presence and reveal the morphological appearance of the structure. Normal tissue stains with this antibody in a fashion consistent with the sites of mesenchymal elements and epithelial basal laminae. Collagen IV can also be useful in the classification of soft tissue tumors; schwannomas, leiomyomas, and their well differentiated malignant counterparts usually immunoreact to this antibody. The vascular nature of neoplasms, hemangiopericytoma, angiosarcoma, and epithelioid hemangioendothelioma can be revealed by this antibody with greater reliability than non-specific stains such as silver reticulum.

collagen type IV autoantibodies

Autoantibodies against collagen type IV that is present in all human basement membranes including those of the kidney, eye, cochlea, lung, placenta, and brain. The triple helical molecules are composed of two α1 chains and one α2 chain in a chicken wire-like network. Four other type IV collagen chains (α3 to α6) form a similar network. Autoantibodies against type IV collagen occur in progressive systemic sclerosis, Raynaud's phenomenon, and scleroderma. Seventy percent of patients with systemic lupus erythematosus (SLE), Raynaud's phenomenon, polyarteritis nodosa, or vasculitides have collagen type IV autoantobodies. Among patients with thromboangiitis obliterans (Burger's disease), 35 to 44% have autoantibodies against types I and IV collagen. Three fourths of patients develop cell-mediated immunity to these two collagens. Autoantibodies to basement membrane and interstitial collagens play a role in the pathogenesis of scleroderma. Autoantibodies to type IV collagen are found also in post-streptococcal glomerulonephritis. Circulating antibodies specific for the NC1 domain of type IV collagen are present in Goodpasture's syndrome and lead to rapidly progressive glomerulonephritis in these subjects. Most Alport syndrome patients lack α3, α4, and α5 chains in their glomerular basement membranes.

collagen vascular diseases

A category of connective tissue diseases in which type III hypersensitivity mechanisms with immune complex of deposition play a major role. These diseases are characterized by inflammation and fibrinoid necrosis in tissues. Patients may manifest involvement of multiple systems, including the vasculature, joints, skin, kidneys, and other tissues. These are classic, systemic autoimmune diseases in most cases. The prototype of this category is systemic lupus erythematosus (SLE). Other disorders included in this category are dermatomyositis, polyarteritis nodosa, progressive systemic sclerosis (scleroderma), rheumatoid arthritis, and mixed connective tissue disease. They are treated with immunosuppressive drugs, especially corticosteroids.

collectin receptor

The receptor of C1q, a subcomponent of the complement component C1.

collectins

A family of structurally related calcium-dependent proteins or sections with collagen-like domains that bind sugars such as mannose-binding protein. Collectins may bind to C1q, thereby activating the complement system, and participate in innate immunity through their actions as microbial recognition receptors. These soluble pattern recognition molecules remove pathogenic microorganisms by opsonization, agglutination, or the lectin pathway of complement activation. Examples include mannose-binding lectin and lung surfactant proteins A and D.

colocalization

Mechanism of differential redistribution of membrane components into patches and caps used to investigate possible interactions between various plasma membrane components or between cell membranes and cytoplasmic structures.

colon antibodies

Immunoglobulin G (IgG) antibodies in the blood sera of 71% of ulcerative colitis patients may be shown by flow cytometry to react with rat colon epithelial cells. Antibodies reactive with a 40-kDa constituent of normal colon extracts have been found

C

in the sera of 79% of ulcerative colitis patients. Antineutrophil cytoplasmic antibodies, distinct from the pANCA of systemic vasculitis and the cANCA of Wegener's granulomatosis, are detectable in 70% of ulcerative colitis patients.

colon autoantibodies

Seventy-one percent of ulcerative colitis (UC) patients have immunoglobulin G (IgG) autoantibodies reactive with rat epithelial cells. A monoclonal antibody against colonic epithelium crossreacted with Barrett epithelium adenocarcinoma and Barrett esophagus epithelium. Other studies revealed shared phenotypic expression of colonic, biliary, and Barrett epithelium. Seventy percent of patients with colitis manifest antibodies reactive with neutrophil cytoplasm distinct from cANCA and pANCA. Of the IgG subclasses of antibodies against colonic antigens, IgG$_4$ and IgG$_1$ have shown the greatest reactivity in separate studies and have differentiated ulcerative colitis patients from Crohn's disease.

colon–ovary tumor antigen (COTA)

A type of mucin demonstrable by immunoperoxidase staining in all colon neoplasms and in some ovarian tumors. COTA occurs infrequently in other neoplasms. Normal tissues express limited quantities of COTA.

colony-forming unit (CFU)

Hematopoietic stem cells and the progeny cells that derive from them. Mature (end-stage) hematopoietic cells in the blood are considered to develop from one CFU. Some progenitor cells are precursors of erythrocytes, others are precursors of polymorphonuclear leukocytes and monocytes, and still others are megakaryocyte and platelet precursors. A gauge of the number of hematopoietic progenitors in a specimen capable of forming a colony comprised of a specific type or types of hematopoietic cells.

colony-forming unit, spleen (CFU-S)

A hematopoietic precursor cell that can produce tiny nodules in the spleens of lethally irradiated mice. These small nodular areas are sites of cellular proliferation. Each arises from a single cell or colony-forming unit. CFU-S cells form colonies of pluripotent stem cells.

colony-stimulating factors (CSFs)

Glycoproteins that govern the formation, differentiation, and function of hematopoietic cells including granulocytes and monomacrophage system cells. CSFs promote the growth, maturation, and differentiation of stem cells to produce progenitor cell colonies. They facilitate the development of functional end-stage cells. They act on cells through specific receptors on target cell surfaces. T cells, fibroblasts, and endothelial cells produce CSFs. Different colony-stimulating factors act on cell line progenitors that include CFU-E (red blood cell precursors), GM-CFC (granulocyte–macrophage colony-forming cells), MEG-CFC (megakaryocyte colony-forming cells), EO-CFC (eosinophil–leukocyte colony-forming cells), T cells, and B cells. CSFs promote the clonal growth of cells and include granulocyte CSF that is synthesized by endothelial cells, macrophages, and fibroblasts. It activates the formation of granulocytes and is synergistic with interleukin-3 (IL3) in the generation of megakaryocytes and granulocytes–macrophages. Endothelial cells, T lymphocytes, and fibroblasts form granulocyte–macrophage CSF, which stimulates granulocyte and macrophage colony formation. It also stimulates megakaryocyte blast cells. Colony-stimulating factor 1 is produced by endothelial cells, macrophages,

The granulocyte colony-stimulating factor (G-CSF) receptor composed of an immunoglobulin domain, a hematopoietin domain, and three fibronectin III domains. The human receptor has two forms: a 25.1 form which has a C kinase phosphorylation site, and a second form in which the transmembrane region has been deleted. The mouse receptor which shares 62.5% homology with the human receptor is similar to the 25.1 form. The human G-CSF receptor has 46.3% sequence homology with the gp130 chain of the IL-6 receptor. The hematopoietin domain contains the binding site for G-CSF, yet proliferative signal transduction requires the membrane-proximal 57 amino acids. Acute phase protein induction mediated by G-CSF involves residues 57 to 96. G-CSF receptors are found on neutrophils, platelets, myeloid leukemia cells, endothelium, and placenta. The human form contains nine potential N-linked glycosylation sites. It is believed that the receptor binds and mediates autophosphorylation of JAK-2 kinase.

and fibroblasts and induces the generation of macrophage colonies. Multi-CSF (IL-3) is produced by T lymphocytes and activates the generation of granulocytes, macrophages, eosinophils, and mast cell colonies. It is synergistic with other factors in activating hematopoietic precursor cells. Renal interstitial cells synthesize erythropoietin, which activates erythroid colony formation.

colostrum

Immunoglobulin-rich first breast milk formed in mammals after parturition. The principal immunoglobulin is IgA with lesser amounts of IgG. It provides passive immune protection of the newborn prior to maturation of its own immune competence.

combination therapy

The use of several antiviral drugs, as in therapy for HIV, in an attempt to circumvent the rapid appearance of mutant

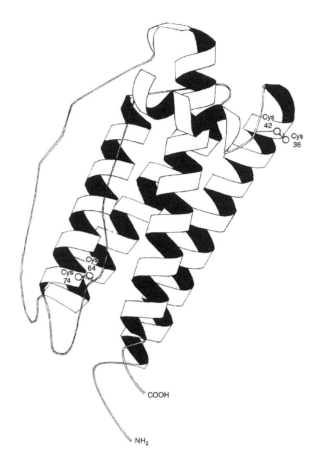

Granulocyte colony-stimulating factor (G-CSF).

viruses that are resistant to one of the drugs in the therapeutic mixture.

combination vaccine

Immunizing preparation that contains immunogens (antigens) from more than one pathogenic microorganism. These vaccines induce protection against more than one disease.

combinatorial diversity

The numerous combinations of variable, diverse, and joining segments that are possible as a consequence of somatic recombination of DNA in the immunoglobulin and TCR loci during B cell or T cell development. It serves as a mechanism for generating large numbers of different antigen receptor genes from a limited number of DNA gene segments.

combinatorial joining

A mechanism for one exon to unite alternatively with several other gene regions, increasing the diversity of products encoded by the gene.

combined immunodeficiency

A genetically determined or primary immunodeficiency that may affect T cell-mediated immunity and B cell (humoral antibody)-mediated immunity. The term is usually reserved for immunodeficiencies that are less profound than severe combined immunodeficiency (SCID). Combined immunodeficiency may occur in both children and adults.

combined prophylactic

Refer to mixed vaccine.

combining site

Refer to antigen-binding site.

commensal mice

Mice that associate closely with humans.

common acute lymphoblastic leukemia antigen (CALLA/CD10) antibody

A useful marker for the characterization of childhood leukemia and B cell lymphomas. This antibody reacts with antigen of lymphoblastic, Burkitt's, and follicular lymphomas and chronic myelocytic leukemias. Also, anti-CD10 detects the antigen of glomerular epithelial cells and the brush border of the proximal tubules; this characteristic may be helpful in interpreting renal ontogenesis in conjunction with other markers. Other nonlymphoid cells that are reactive with anti-CD10 are breast myoepithelial cells, bile canaliculi, neutrophils, and small populations of bone marrow cells, fetal small intestine epithelium, and normal fibroblasts.

common acute lymphocytic leukemia antigen (CALLA)

A 100-kDa surface membrane glycoprotein present on human leukemia cells and, to a lesser degree, on other cells, including granulocytes and kidney cells. It is a zinc metalloproteinase and is classified as CD10/neutral endopeptidase 24.11. Four fifths of non-T cell leukemias express CALLA. Under physiologic conditions, 1% of cells in the bone marrow express CALLA. Its presence is revealed by monoclonal antibodies and flow cytometry using bone marrow or other cells. Bone marrow to be used for autologous transplants may be purged of CALLA-positive lymphocytic leukemia cells by using anti-CALLA monoclonal antibodies and complement. It is a pre-B lymphoblast marker that is the most frequent type of cell in childhood acute lymphocytic leukemia (ALL). The presence of Ia antigen with CALLA portends a favorable prognosis. CALLA may also be positive in Burkitt's lymphomas, B cell lymphomas, and 40% of T cell lymphoblastic lymphomas. All blasts are usually positive, not only for CALLA and the Ia antigen, but also for TdT.

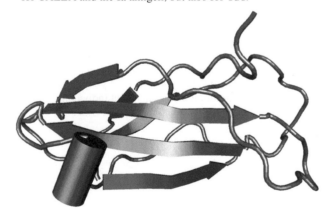

Common γ chain.

common γ chain (γc chain)

An ITAM-containing signal transduction protein that acts as a subunit in IL-2, IL-4, IL-7, IL-9, IL-15, and IL-21 receptors.

common leukocyte antigen (LCA) (CD45)

An antigen shared in common by both T and B lymphocytes and expressed to a lesser degree by histiocytes and plasma cells. By immunoperoxidase staining, it can be demonstrated in sections of paraffin-embedded tissues containing these cell types. Thus, it is a valuable marker to distinguish lymphoreticular neoplasms from carcinomas and sarcomas.

common lymphoid progenitors

Hematopoietic stem cells from which all lymphocytes are derived. Pluripotent hematopoietic stem cells give rise to these progenitors.

C

common mucosal immune system (CMIS)

A network of mucosal defense mechanisms based on the migration of lymphocytes activated in a single mucosal inductive site to multiple effector sites of various mucosal tissues. Refer also to MALT, BALT, GALT, and SALT.

common myeloid progenitor (CMP)

Ancestral descendant of hematopoietic stem cells; precursor of myeloid lineage cells.

common variable antibody deficiency

Refer to common variable immunodeficiency (CVID).

common variable immunodeficiency (CVID)

A relatively common congenital or acquired immunodeficiency that may be familial or sporadic. The familial form may have a variable mode of inheritance. Hypogammaglobulinemia is common to all patients, often with diminished IgA and IgG and occasionally IgM, although all classes of immunoglobulin may be affected. The World Health Organization (WHO) classifies three forms of the disorder: (1) an intrinsic B lymphocyte defect, (2) a disorder of T lymphocyte regulation that includes deficient T helper lymphocytes or activated T suppressor lymphocytes, and (3) autoantibodies against T and B lymphocytes. The majority of patients have intrinsic B cell defects with normal numbers of B cells in the circulation that can identify antigens and proliferate but cannot differentiate into plasma cells. Antibody synthesis is impaired and memory B cells may be undetectable. There may be defects in transmission of T cell help. The ability of B cells to proliferate when stimulated by antigen is evidenced by hyperplasia of B cell regions of lymph nodes, spleen, and other lymphoid tissues, yet differentiation of B cells into plasma cells is blocked. The resulting deficiency of antibody leads to recurrent bacterial infections, as well as intestinal infestation by *Giardia lamblia,* which produces a syndrome that resembles sprue. Noncaseating granulomas occur in many organs. There is an increased incidence of autoimmune diseases such as pernicious anemia, rheumatoid arthritis, and hemolytic anemia. Lymphomas also occur in these immunologically deficient individuals.

competency, immunologic

The capacity of an animal's immune system to generate a response to an immunogen.

competitive binding assay

Serological test in which unknowns are detected and quantified by their ability to inhibit binding of a labeled known ligand to a specific antibody. Also termed competitive inhibition assay.

competitive inhibition assay

A test in which antigens or antibodies are assayed by binding of a known anitbody or antigen to a known amount of labeled antibody or antigen. Known or unknown sources of antibody or antigen are then used as competitive inhibitors. Also termed competitive inhibition assay.

complement (C)

A system of more than 30 soluble and membrane-bound plasma and other body fluid proteins together with many of their cellular receptors and regulatory proteins found in blood and other tissue cells. These proteins play a critical role in aiding phagocytosis of immune complexes that activate the complement system. These molecules and their fragments resulting from the activation process are significant in the regulation of cellular immune responsiveness. Once complement proteins identify and combine with target substance, serine proteases are activated, ultimately leading to the assembly of C3 convertase, a protease on the surface of the target substance. The enzyme cleaves C3, yielding a C3b fragment bound to the target through a covalent linkage. C3b or C3bi fragments bound to phagocytic cell surfaces become ligands for C3 receptors and binding sites for C5. The union of C5b with C6, C7, C8, and C9 generates the membrane attack complex (MAC) that may associate with the lipid bilayer membranes of cells to produce lysis, which is critical in resistance against certain species of bacteria. The complement proteins are significant, nonspecific mediators of humoral immunity. Multiple substances may trigger the complement system. The first of two pathways of complement activation is designated the classical, in which an antigen (e.g., red blood cell) and antibody combine and

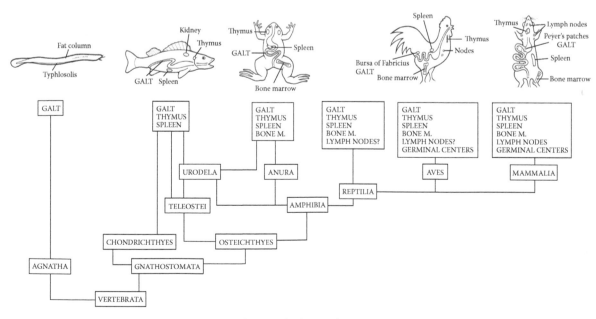

Comparative immunology.

Classical pathway   **Alternative pathway**

Antigen–antibody complex

Recognition unit

C1q

C2   C4

Activation unit — $\overline{C4b, 2a}$ Activation unit

C8

C3a

$\overline{C4a, 2a3b}$ C5

C5a

Activator   Initiation convertase

C3b

Mg^{++} Factor B

C3bB

Properdin (P)   Factor D

$\overline{C3bBb(P)}$ — Activation unit

C3

C3a

$\overline{C3b_2Bb(P)}$

C5b + C6, C7, C8, C9 ⟶ Membrane attack complex formation (lytic unit)

Complement activation.

fix the first subcomponent, designated C1q. This is followed in sequence by C1qrs, 4, 2, 3, 5, 6, 7, 8, and 9 to produce lysis. The alternative pathway does not utilize C1, 4, and 2 components. Bacterial products such as endotoxin and other agents may activate this pathway through C3. Numerous biological activities are associated with complement besides immune lysis, including the formation of anaphylatoxin, chemotaxis, opsonization, phagocytosis, bacteriolysis, hemolysis, and other amplification mechanisms. Complement intermediates can opsonize cells; peptides resulting from complement component cleavage (anaphylatoxins) enhance inflammation and act as chemoattractants. Activation of complement renders immune complexes soluble and facilitates their clearance and promotes antigen presentation, B cell activation, and memory.

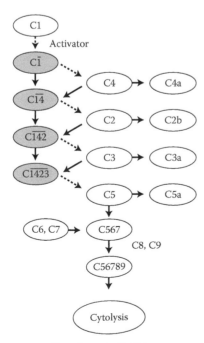

Complement activation.

complement activation

The initiation of a series of reactions involving the complement proteins of plasma that may result in either the death and elimination of a pathogenic microorganism or amplification of the complement cascade effect.

complement components 1-9

Refer to C1-C9.

complement control protein (CCP) modules

Complement activity-regulating proteins that are similar structurally. Refer also to regulators of complement activation (RCA).

complement deficiency conditions

Inherited complement deficiencies are rare. In healthy Japanese blood donors, only 1 in 100,000 persons had no C5, C6, C7, and C8; no C9 was contained in 3 of 1000 individuals. Most individuals with missing complement components do not manifest clinical symptoms. Additional pathways provide complement-dependent functions that are necessary to preserve life. If C3, factor I or any segment of the alternative pathway is missing, the condition may be life threatening with markedly decreased opsonization in phagocytosis. C3 is depleted when factor I is absent. C5, C6, C7, and C8 deficiencies are linked with infections, mainly meningococcal or gonococcal, that usually succumb to the bactericidal action of complement. Deficiencies in classical complement pathway activation are often associated with connective tissue or immune complex diseases. Systemic lupus erythematosus (SLE) may be associated with C1qrs, C2, or C4 deficiencies. Patients with hereditary angioedema (HAE) have a deficiency of C1 inactivator. A number of experimental animals with specific complement deficiencies have been described, such as C6 deficiency in rabbits and C5 deficiency in mice. Acquired complement deficiencies may be caused by either accelerated complement consumption in immune complex diseases with a type III mechanism or by diminished formation of complement proteins as in acute necrosis of the liver.

complement-dependent cytotoxicity test

An assay in which cells bearing surface epitopes are incubated *in vitro* with antibodies of the homologous specificity. After complement is added, cells expressing the antigen

	Classical pathway	Alternative pathway	Lectin pathway
Activated by	binding of antibody molecules (specifically IgM and IgG1, IgG2, IgG3) to a foreign particle	invading micro-organisms	binding of MBP to the mannose groups of carbohydrates on microorganisms
Activation mechanism	antibody-dependent	antibody-independent	antibody-independent
Limb of immunity	Adaptive immune response	Innate immune response	Innate immune response
Components	C1 (C1q, C1r, C1s) to C9	Factors B, D, P, H, I	C1 (C1r, C1s) to C9
Components that initiate enzyme cascade	C1 (q, r, s), C4, C2	C3, B, D	Lectin, MASP1, MASP2, C4, C2
C3 convertase	C4bC2a, C2b	C3bBb	C2b, C4bC2a
C5 convertase	C4bC2aC3b	C3bBbC3b	C4bC2aC3b
Terminal components	C5-C9, MAC (C5b678(9)$_n$)	C5-C9, MAC (C5b678(9)$_n$)	C5-C9, MAC (C5b678(9)$_n$)

B: plasma factor B; D: plasma protease factor D; P: properdin; H: protein H; I: factor I; MBP: mannan-binding protein; MASP: MBP-associated serine protease; MAC: membrane attack complex

Complement activation.

of interest are revealed by the uptake of dye by the fatally injured cells.

complement deviation (Neisser–Wechsberg phenomenon)

Blocking of complement fixation or of complement-induced lysis when excess antibody is present. There is deviation of the complement by the antibody.

complement fixation assay

A serologic test based on the fixation of complement by antigen–antibody complexes. It has been applied to many antigen–antibody systems and was widely used earlier as a serologic test for syphilis.

complement fixation inhibition test

An assay in which a known substance prevents interaction of antibody and antigen, thereby preventing complement uptake and fixation.

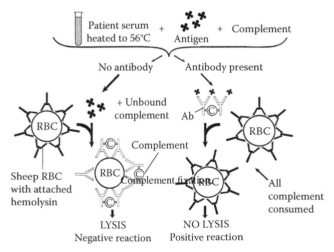

Complement fixation.

complement fixation reaction

The primary union of an antigen with an antibody in the complement fixation reaction takes place almost instantaneously and is invisible. A measured amount of complement

present in the reaction mixture is taken up by complexes of antigen and antibody. The consumption or binding of complement by antigen–antibody complexes serves as the basis for a serologic assay in which antigen is combined with a serum specimen suspected of containing the homologous antibody. Following the addition of a measured amount of complement, which is fixed or consumed only if antibody is present in the serum and has formed a complex with the antigen, sheep red blood cells sensitized (coated) with specific antibody are added to determine whether or not complement has been fixed in the first phase of the reaction. Failure of the sensitized sheep red blood cells to lyse constitutes a positive test, as no complement is available. However, sheep red blood cell lysis indicates that complement was not consumed during the first phase of the reaction, implying that homologous antibody was not present in the serum and complement remains free to lyse the sheep red blood cells sensitized with antibody. Hemolysis constitutes a negative reaction. The sensitivity of the complement fixation test falls between that of agglutination and precipitation. Complement fixation tests may be carried out in microtiter plates, which are designed for the use of relatively small volumes of reagents. The lysis of sheep red blood cells sensitized with rabbit antibody is measured either in a spectrophotometer at 413 nm or by the release of ^{51}Cr from red cells that have been previously labeled with the isotope. Complement fixation can detect either soluble or insoluble antigen. Its ability to detect virus antigens in impure tissue preparations makes the test still useful in diagnosis of virus infections.

complement fixing antibody

An antibody of the immunoglobulin G (IgG) or IgM class that binds complement after reacting with its homologous antigen. It represents complement fixation by the classic pathway. Nonantibody mechanisms and IgA fix complement by the alternative pathway.

complement inhibitor

Protein inhibitor that occurs naturally and blocks the action of complement components; the group includes factor H, factor I, C1 inhibitor, and C4-binding protein (C4BP). Also included among complement inhibitors are heating to 56°C to inactivate C1 and C2; combining with hydrazine and

Three Pathways of Complement System Activation

Parameter	Classical Pathway	Alternative Pathway	Lectin Pathway
Activation	Binding of antibody molecules (specifically IgM and IgG1, IgG2, and IgG3) to foreign particle	Invading microorganisms	Binding of MBP to mannose groups of carbohydrates on microorganisms
Activation mechanism	Antibody-dependent	Antibody-independent	Antibody-independent
Limb of immunity	Adaptive immune response	Innate immune response	Innate immune response
Components	C1 (C1q, C1r, C1s) to C9	Factors B, D, P, H, I	C1 (C1r, C1s) to C9
Components that initiate enzyme cascade	C1 (C1q, C1r, C1s), C2, C4	C3, B, D	Lectin, MASP1, MASP2, C4, C2
C3 convertase	C4b, C2a, C2b	C3bBb	C2b, C4b, C2a
C5 convertase	C4b, C2a, C3b	C3bBb, C3b	C4b, C2a, C3b
Terminal components	C5, C9, MAC (C5b678(9)$_n$)	C5, C9, MAC (C5b678(9)$_n$)	C5, C9, MAC (C5b678(9)$_n$)

B = plasma factor B. D = plasma protease factor D. P = properdin. H = protein H. I = factor I. MBP = mannan-binding protein. MASP = MBP-associated serine protease. MAC: membrane attack complex.

ammonia to block the action of C3 and C4; and the adding of zymosan or cobra venom factor to induce alternate pathway activation of C3, which consumes C3 in the plasma.

complement membrane attack complex

Refer to membrane attack complex.

complement multimer

A doughnut-shaped configuration as a part of the complement reaction sequence.

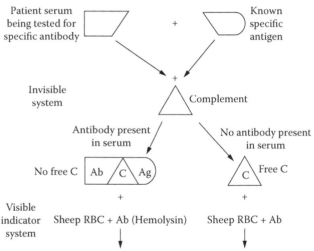

Complement fixation reaction.

complement receptor 1 (CR1)

A membrane glycoprotein found on human erythrocytes, monocytes, polymorphonuclear leukocytes, B cells, a T cell subset, mast cells, and glomerular podocytes. On red cells, CR1 binds C3b or C4b components of immune complexes, facilitating their transport to the mononuclear phagocyte system. It facilitates attachment, endocytosis, and phagocytosis of C3b/C4b-containing complexes to macrophages or neutrophils and may serve as a cofactor for factor-I-mediated C3 cleavage. The identification of CR1 cDNA has made possible the molecular analysis of CR1 biological properties.

complement receptor 2 (CR2)

A receptor for C3 fragments that also serves as a binding site for Epstein–Barr virus (EBV). It is a receptor for C3bi, C3dg, and C3d based on its specificity for their C3d structures. B cells, follicular dendritic cells of lymph nodes, thymocytes, and pharyngeal epithelial cells, but not T cells, express CR2. EBV enters B lymphocytes by way of CR2. The gene encoding CR2 is linked closely with that of CR1. A 140-kDa single polypeptide chain makes up CR2, which has a short consensus repeat (SCR) structure similar to that of CR1. CR2 may be active in B cell activation. Its expression appears restricted to late pre-B cells and to mature B cells. CR2 function is associated with membrane IgM. Analysis of cDNA clones has provided the primary structure of CR2.

complement receptor 3 (CR3)

A principal opsonin receptor expressed by monocytes, macrophages, and neutrophils. It plays an important role in the removal of bacteria and binds fixed C3bi in the presence of divalent cations. It also binds bacterial lipopolysaccharides and β glucans of yeast cell walls. The latter are significant in the ability of granulocytes to identify bacteria and yeast cells. CR3 is an integrin type of adhesion molecule that facilitates the binding of neutrophils to endothelial cells in inflammation. It enables phagocytic cells to attach to bacteria or yeast cells with fixed C3bi, β glucans, or lipopolysaccharides on their surfaces. This facilitates phagocytosis and the respiratory burst. CR3 is comprised of a 165-kDa α glycoprotein chain and a 95-kDa β glycoprotein chain. CR3 appears related to LFA-1 and P-150,95 molecules and shares a β chain with them. All three of these molecules are of critical significance in antigen-independent cellular adhesion, which confines leukocytes to inflammatory areas, among other functions. Deficient surface expression of these molecules occurs in leukocyte adhesion deficiency (LAD), in which patients experience repeated bacterial infections. The primary defect appears associated with the common β chain. Besides C3bi binding, CR3 is of critical significance in IgG- and CR1-facilitated phagocytosis by neutrophils and monocytes. CR3 has a more diverse function than does either CR1 or CR2.

complement receptor 4 (CR4)

Glycoprotein membrane receptor for C3dg on polymorpho-nuclear neutrophils (PMNs), monocytes, and platelets. CR4 facilitates Fc-receptor-mediated phagocytosis and mediates Fc-independent phagocytosis. It consists of a 150-kDa α chain and a 95-kDa β chain. Chromosome 16 is the site of genes that encode the α chain, whereas chromosome 21 is the site of genes that encode the β chain. Tissue macrophages express CR4. It is an integrin with a β chain in common with CR3 and LFA-1.

complement receptor 5 (CR5)

A receptor that binds C3bi, C3dg, and C3d fragments based on its specificity for their C3d component. Reactivity is only in the fluid phase and not when the fragments are fixed. CR5 is the C3dg-dimer receptor. Neutrophils and platelets manifest CR5 activity.

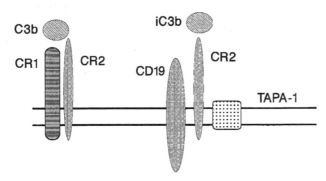

The classical and alternative pathways of the complement system.

complement receptors (CR)

Receptors for products of complement reactions. Proteolytic cleavage of human complement component C3 takes place following activation of the classical or the alternative complement pathway. Following the generation of C3a and C3b, the C3b covalently binds to bacteria, immune complexes, or other targets and then unites with a high affinity receptor termed the C3b/C4b receptor and currently known as CR1. Subsequent proteolytic cleavage of the bound C3b is attributable to factor I and a cofactor. This action yields C3bi, C3dg, and C3c, which interact with specific receptors. CR2 is the C3dg receptor, and CR3 is the C3bi receptor. Proteins on the surfaces of various types of cells identify and unite with complement proteins linked to antigens. Phagocyte surface complement receptors aid the engulfment of complement coated pathogenic microorganisms. CR1, CR2, CR3, CR4 and C1q receptors are examples.

complement receptors, membrane

Receptors expressed on blood cells and tissue macrophages of humans. These include C1q-R (C1q receptor), CR1 (C3b/C4b receptor; CD35), CR2 (C3d/Epstein–Barr virus [EBV] receptor; CD21), CR3 (iC3b receptor; CD11b/CD18), CR4 (C3bi receptor; CD11c/CD18), CR5 (C3dg-dimer receptor), fH-R (factor H receptor), C5a-R (C5a receptor), and C3a/C4a-R (C3a/C4a receptor). Ligands for C receptors generated by either the classic or alternate pathways include fluid phase activation peptides of C3, C4, and C5, designated C3a, C4a, and C5a, which are anaphylatoxins that interact with either C3a/C4a-R or C5a-R and participate in inflammation. Other ligands for C receptors include complement

proteins deposited on immune complexes that are either soluble or particulate. Fixed C4 and C3 fragments (C4b, C3b, C3bi, C3dg, and C3d), C1q, and factor H constitute these ligands. These receptors play a major role in facilitating improved recognition of pathogenic substances. They aid in the elimination of bacteria and soluble immune complexes. Neutrophils, monocytes, and macrophages express C3 receptors on their surfaces. Neutrophils and erythrocytes express immune adherence receptors (CR1) on their surfaces. Four other receptors for CR3 are designated CR2, CR3, CR4, and CR5. Additional receptors for complement components other than C3 and a receptor for C3a are termed C1q-R (C1q receptor), C5a-R (C5a receptor), C3a-R (C3a receptor), and fH-R (factor H receptor).

complement system

A group of more than 30 plasma and cell surface proteins that faciliate the destruction of pathogenic microorganisms by phagocytes or by lysis. Refer to complement.

complementarity

A genetic term that indicates the requirement for more than one gene to express a trait.

complementarity-determining region (CDR)

The hypervariable regions in an immunoglobulin molecule that form the three-dimensional cavity where an epitope binds to the antibody molecule. The heavy and light polypeptide chains each contribute three hypervariable regions to the antigen-binding region of the antibody molecule. Together, they form the site for antigen binding. Likewise, the T cell receptor α and β chains each have three regions with great diversity that are analogous to the CDRs of the immunoglobulin. These hypervariable areas are sites of binding for foreign antigen and self MHC molecular complexes.

complementation

A mechanism whereby a hybrid cell develops the survival capacity of two separate parental cells under different selective circumstances.

complete carcinogen

A cancer-causing agent that can promote all four stages of carcinogenesis.

complete clinical response (hematopoietic neoplasm)

Reduction to nearly zero or ≤ 5% of the number of blasts in a post-treatment patient's blood or bone marrow smear.

complete Freund's adjuvant (CFA)

A suspension of killed and dried mycobacteria suspended in lightweight mineral oil which, when combined with an aqueous phase antigen (such as a water-in-oil emulsion), enhances immunogenicity. CFA facilitates stimulation of both humoral (B cell) and cell-mediated (T cell) limbs of the immune response.

complex allotype

An allotype with multiple amino acid residue positions that are not the same as those of a different allotype at that same locus.

complex release activity

Binding of injected preformed complexes to the endothelial cell membranes immediately after their injection into experimental animals. The amount of such binding decreases with age, favoring deposition of such complexes within tissues.

complotype

A major histocompatibility complex (MHC) class III haplotype. It is a precise arrangement of linked alleles of MHC class III genes that encode C2, factor B, C4A, and C4B MHC

class III molecules in humans. Caucasians have 12 ordinary complotypes that may be in positive linkage disequilibrium.

concanavalin A (con A)

A jack bean (*Canavalia ensiformis*) lectin that induces erythrocyte agglutination and stimulates T lymphocytes to undergo mitosis and proliferate. Con A interacts with carbohydrate residues rich in mannose. Macrophages must be present for T lymphocytes to proliferate in response to con A stimulation. There are four 237-amino acid residue subunits in con A. There is one binding site for saccharide, one for Ca^{2+}, and one for a metallic ion such as Mn^{2+} in each con A subunit. T lymphocytes stimulated by con A release interleukin-2 (IL2). Cytotoxic T lymphocytes stimulated by con A induce lysis of target cells without regard to the antigen specificity of either the effector or target cell. This may be induced by crosslinking of the effector and target cells by con A, which is capable of linking to high-mannose oligosaccharides on target cell surfaces as well as to high-mannose sugars on T cell receptors. Con A binds readily to ordinary cell membrane glycoproteins such as glucopyranosides, fructofuranosides, and mannopyranosides.

concatamer integration

Occurs when the entire genome of vector including the bacterial plasmid is integrated into the host genome.

concomitant immunity

(1) The continued survival of adult worms from a primary infection while the host is demonstrably resistant to reinfection by a secondary challenge of fresh cercariae. (2) In tumor immunology, resistance to a tumor transplanted into a host already bearing that tumor. Immunity to the reinoculated neoplasm does not inhibit growth of the primary tumor. (3) Resistance to reinfection of a host currently infected with that parasite.

concordance rate

A gauge of the incidence of the same disease appearing in two monozygotic or dizygotic twins.

conditional knockout mouse

The rendering of a gene of interest nonfunctional ("knocked out") exclusively at a precise stage of development in a mutant mouse or in a designated cell or tissue following induction by a specific stimulus.

confocal fluorescent microscopy

A technique in which optics are used to form images at very high resolution by having two origins of fluorescent light that join only at one plane of a thicker section.

conformational determinant

An epitope composed of amino acid residues that are not contiguous and represent separated parts of the linear sequence of amino acids brought into proximity to one another by folding of the molecule. A conformational determinant is dependent on three-dimensional structure. Conformational determinants, therefore, are usually associated with native rather than denatured proteins. Antibodies specific for linear determinants and others specific for conformational determinants may give clues as to whether a protein is denatured or native, respectively. Also called discontinuous epitope.

conformational epitope

Discontinuous determinant on a protein antigen formed from several separate regions in the primary sequence of a protein brought together by folding. Antibodies that bind conformational epitopes bind only native folded proteins.

congenic

A mouse line that is identical or almost identical to other inbred stains with the exception of the substitution of an alien allele at a single histocompatibility locus that crosses with a second inbred strain permitting introduction of the foreign allele.

congenic mice

Refer to congenic strains.

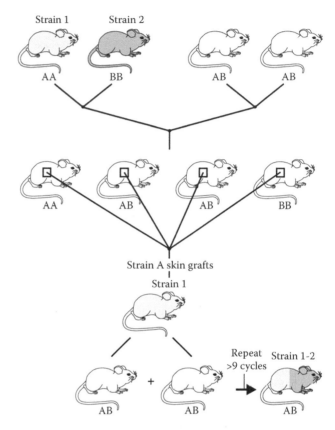

Congenic strains.

congenic strains

Inbred mouse strains that are believed to be genetically identical except for a single genetic locus difference. Congenic strains are produced by crossing a donor strain and a background strain. Repeated backcrossing is made to the background strain, selecting in each generation for heterozygosity at a certain locus. Following 12 to 14 backcrosses, the progeny are inbred through brother–sister matings to yield a homozygous inbred strain. Mutation and genetic linkage may lead to random differences at a few other loci in the congenic strain. Designations for congenic strains consist of the symbol for the background strain followed by a period and then the symbol for the donor strain.

congenic vaccine

An immunogen comprised of polysaccharide bound covalently to proteins. The conjugation of weakly immunogenic, bacterial polysaccharide antigens with protein carrier molecules considerably enhances their immunogenicity. Induces B cell responsiveness against thymus-dependent antigens rather than to thymus-independent antigens. The protein supplies peptide epitopes that activate CD4 T cells to help B cells specific for the

C

polysaccharide. Conjugate vaccines have reduced morbidity and mortality for a number of bacterial diseases in vulnerable populations such as very young or adults with immunodeficiencies. An example of a conjugate vaccine is the *Haemophilus influenzae* 6 polysaccharide polyribosyl-ribitol phosphate vaccine.

congenital agammaglobulinemia

Refer to X-linked agammaglobulinemia.

congenital immunodeficiency

A varied group of unusual disorders with associated auto-immune manifestations, increased incidence of malignancy, allergy, and gastrointestinal abnormalities. These include defects in stem cells, B cells, T cells, phagocytic defects, and complement defects. An example is severe combined immunodeficiency due to various causes. The congenital immunodeficiencies are described under the separate disease categories.

congenital neutropenia

A primary immunodeficiency of innate immunity attributable to mutations in the neutrophil elastase gene complicit in extracellular matrix dissolution. Causes constant neutropenia, i.e., severe congenital neutropenia, or intermittent cyclic neutropenia.

conglutinating complement absorption test

An assay based on the removal of complement from the reaction medium if an antigen–antibody complex develops. This is a test for antibody. As in the complement fixation test, a visible or indicator combination must be added to determine whether any unbound complement is present. This is accomplished by adding sensitized erythrocytes and conglutinin, which is prepared by combining sheep erythrocytes with bovine serum that contains natural antibody against sheep erythrocytes as well as conglutinin. Horse serum may be used as a source of nonhemolytic complement for the reaction. Aggregation of the erythrocytes constitutes a negative test.

conglutination

The strong agglutination of antigen–antibody–complement complexes by conglutinin, a factor present in normal sera of cows and other ruminants. The complexes are similar to EAC1423 and are aggregated by conglutinin in the presence of Ca^{2+}, which is a required cation. Conglutination is a sensitive technique for detecting complement-fixing antibodies.

conglutinin

A bovine serum protein that reacts with fixed C3. It causes the tight aggregation (i.e., conglutination) of red blood cells coated with complement. Conglutinin, which is confined to sera of Bovidae, is not to be confused with immunoconglutinin, which has a similar activity but is produced in other species by immunization with complement-coated substances or may develop spontaneously following activation of complement *in vivo*. Conglutinin reacts with antigen–antibody–complement complexes in a medium containing Ca^{2+}. The N-linked oligosaccharide of the C3bi α chain is its ligand. The phagocytosis of C3bi-containing immune complexes is increased by interaction with conglutinin. Conglutinin contains twelve 33-kDa polypeptide chains that are indistinguishable and are grouped into four subunits. Following a 25-residue amino terminal sequence, there is a 13-kDa sequence that resembles collagen in each chain. The 20-kDa carboxyl-

terminal segments form globular structures that contain disulfide-linked chains.

conglutinin solid-phase assay

A test that quantifies C3bi-containing complexes that may activate complement by either the classical or the alternate pathway.

conjugate

Usually refers to the covalent bonding of a protein carrier with a hapten; may refer to the labeling of a molecule such as an immunoglobulin with fluorescein isothiocyanate, ferritin, or an enzyme used in the enzyme-linked immuno-absorbent assay.

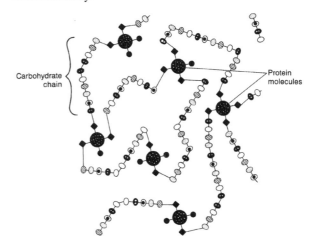

Conjugate vaccine.

conjugated antigen

Refer to conjugate.

connective tissue activating peptide-III (CTAP-III)

A platelet granule peptide derived by proteolytic processing from its CXC chemokine precursor, leukocyte-derived growth factor. It has a powerful effect on fibroblast growth, wound repair, inflammation, and neoplasia. CTAP-III and neutrophil-activating peptide-2 (NAP-2) are heparanases whose growth-promoting activities may be consequences of heparan sulfate solubilization and bound growth factors in extracellular matrix. CTAP-III is a member of the family of molecules known as histamine release factors. In allergic-state, late-phase reactions, CTAP-III may either stimulate or inhibit histamine release based on relative concentration, pattern of release, and responsiveness of basophils and mast cells. The ability of CTAP-III to activate neutrophils is a critical link between platelet activation and neutrophil recruitment in stimulation, which are key features of inflammatory reactions in allergic conditions.

connective tissue disease

One of a group of diseases, formerly known as collagen vascular diseases, that affect blood vessels producing fibrinoid necrosis in connective tissues. The prototype of a systemic connective tissue disease is systemic lupus erythematosus (SLE). Also included in this classification are systemic sclerosis (scleroderma), rheumatoid arthritis, dermatomyositis, polymyositis, Sjögren's syndrome, polyarteritis nodosa, and a number of other disorders believed to have immunological etiologies and pathogenesis. They are often accompanied by the development of autoantibodies such as antinuclear antibodies or antiimmunoglobulin antibodies such as rheumatoid factors.

consensus sequence

The typical nucleic acid or protein sequence where a nucleotide or amino acid residue present at each position is that found most often during comparison of numerous similar sequences in a specific molecular region.

constant domain

The immunoglobulin C_H and C_L regions encoded by the corresponding constant exon. There is only minor variability in the amino acid content of constant domains. A globular compact structure that consists of two antiparallel twisted β sheets. There are differences in the number and the irregularity of the β strands and bilayers in variable (V) and constant (C) subunits of immunoglobulins. C domains have tertiary structures that closely resemble those of the domains comprised of a five-strand β sheet and a four-strand β sheet packed facing one another. However, the C domain does not have a hairpin loop at the edge of one of the sheets. Thus, the C domain has seven or eight β strands rather than the nine that are found in the V domains. Refers also to the constituent domains or constant regions of T cell receptor polypeptides.

constant exon

An exon that encodes the C terminal part of either an immunoglobulin or a T cell receptor protein. The splicing of a C exon at the mRNA level to a rearranged variable (V) exon yields a transcript of a complete immunoglobulin or T cell receptor gene. C exons of the immunoglobulin heavy chain gene locus are comprised of sub-exons.

constant region

That part of an immunoglobulin polypeptide chain that has an invariant amino acid sequence among immunoglobulin chains belonging to the same isotype and allotype. There is a minimum of two and often three or four domains in the constant regions of immunoglobulin heavy polypeptide chains. The hinge region tail end piece (carboxyl terminal region) constitutes part of the constant region in selected classes of immunoglobulin. A few exons encode the constant region of an immunoglobulin heavy chain, and one exon encodes the constant region of an immunoglobulin light chain. The constant region is the location for the majority of isotypic and allotypic determinants. It is associated with a number of antibody functions. T cell receptor α, β, γ, and δ chains have constant regions coded for by three to four exons. Major histocompatibility complex (MHC) class I and II molecules also have segments that are constant regions in that they show little sequence variation from one allele to another. Refers also to the part of a T cell receptor polypeptide chain that does not vary in sequence among different clones and is not involved in antigen binding.

constitutive defense system

See innate or constitutive defense system.

consumption test

An assay in which antigen or antibody disappears from the reaction mixture as a result of its interaction with the homologous antibody or antigen. The result is ascertained by quantifying the amount of unreacted antigen or antibody remaining in the reaction system and comparing it with the quantity of that reagent that was originally present. The antiglobulin consumption test is an example.

contact dermatitis

A type IV, T lymphocyte-mediated hypersensitivity reaction of the delayed type that develops in response to an allergen applied to the skin.

contact hypersensitivity reaction

A type IV delayed-type hypersensitivity reaction in the skin characterized by a delayed-type hypersensitivity (cell-mediated) immune reaction produced by cytotoxic T lymphocytes invading the epidermis. It is often induced by applying a skin-sensitizing simple chemical such as dinitrochlorobenzene (DNCB) that acts as a hapten uniting with proteins in the skin, leading to the delayed-type hypersensitivity response mediated by CD4+ T cells. Although substances such as DNCB alone are not antigenic, they may combine with epidermal proteins that serve as carriers for these simple chemicals acting as haptens. Spongiosis, vesiculation, and pleuritis are present. Poison ivy hypersensitivity is a type of contact hypersensitivity attributable to T cell responses to the chemical antigen pentadecatechol in poison ivy leaves. Langerhans' cells are leukocytes in the epidermis that present antigen to CD4+ T cells. They possess long dendritic processes that course among the epidermal cells, forming a network that is usually encountered by any organism or antigen that penetrates through the stratum corneum barrier. In addition to the cytoplasmic organelles (Birbeck granules), they have membrane antigens that include CD1a major histocompatibility complex (MHC) class II antigens and costimulatory molecules B7-1 and B7-2. They also express adhesion molecules such as E-cadherin, ICAM-1, and LFA-1. The latter two are requisite for their migration to the regional nodes and interaction with T cells.

contact sensitivity (CS) or allergic contact dermatitis

A form of delayed-type hypersensitivity (DTH) reaction limited to the skin and consisting of eczematous changes. It follows sensitization by topical drugs, cosmetics, or other types of contact chemicals. The causative agents, usually simple, low-molecular-weight compounds (mostly aromatic molecules), behave as haptens. The development of sensitization depends on the penetrability of the agent and its ability to form covalent bonds with protein. Part of the sensitizing antigen molecule is thus represented by protein, usually the fibrous protein of the skin. Local skin conditions that alter local proteins, such as inflammation, stasis, and others, facilitate the development of CS, but some chemicals such as penicillin, picric acid, or sulfonamides are unable to conjugate to proteins. It is believed that in this case the degradation products of such chemicals have this property. CS may also be induced by hapten conjugates given by other routes in adjuvants. The actual immunogen in CS remains unidentified. CS may also have a toxic, nonimmunologic component, and frequently both toxic and sensitizing effects can be produced by the same compound. With exposure to industrial compounds, an initial period of increased sensitivity is followed by a gradual decrease in reactivity. This phenomenon is called hardening and may represent a process of spontaneous desensitization. The histologic changes in CS are characteristic. Vascular endothelial cells in skin lesions produce cytokine-regulated surface molecules such as IL-2. IL4 mRNA is strongly expressed in allergic contact dermatitis lesions. IFN-γ mRNA is the predominant cytokine in tuberculin reactions. IL10 mRNA overexpression in atopic dermatitis may facilitate upregulation of humoral responses and downregulation of T_H1 responses. Selected allergic subjects manifest several types of autoantibodies including IgE and β-adrenergic receptor autoantibodies.

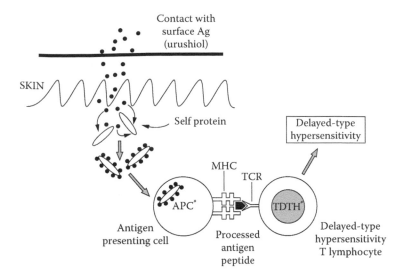

Contact sensitivity to poison ivy plants containing urushiol which induces delayed-type hypersensitivity mediated by CD4+ T cells with skin lesions.

contact system

A system of proteins in the plasma that engage in sequential interactions following contact with surfaces of particles that bear a negative charge, such as glass, or with substances such as lipopolysaccharides, collagen, etc. Bradykinin is produced through their sequential interaction. C1 inhibitor blocks the contact system. Anaphylactic shock, endotoxin shock, and inflammation are processes in which the contact system has a significant role.

continuous epitope

Linear antigenic determinant on proteins. It is contiguous in amino acid sequence and does not require folding of a protein into its native conformation for antibody to bind with it.

contraception, immunological

A method to prevent an undesired pregnancy. Vaccines that induce antibodies and cell-mediated immune responses against either a hormone or gamete antigen significant to reproduction have been developed. Such vaccines control fertility in experimental animals. They have undergone exhaustive safety and toxicological investigations that have shown the safety and reversibility of some of the vaccines and, with the approval of regulatory agencies and ethics commissions, have undergone clinical trials in humans. Six vaccines, three in women and three in men, have completed phase I clinical trials showing their safety and reversibility. One vaccine has successfully completed phase II trials

proving efficacy in females. The trials have determined the titers of antibodies and other immunological features. The fertilized egg makes the hormone hCG. Antibodies that inactivate one or more hormones involved in the production of gametes and sex steroids may be expected to impair fertility. Blocking the action of luteinizing hormone releasing hormone (LHRH) would also inhibit the synthesis of sex steroids. This might prove useful in controlling fertility of domestic animals but would not be acceptable for contraception in humans. Two vaccines against LHRH are in clinical trials for patients with prostate carcinoma. A follicle-stimulating hormone (FSH) vaccine would act at the level of male fertility, as FSH is required for spermatogenesis in primates.

contrasuppression

A part of the immunoregulatory circuit that prevents suppressor effects in a feedback loop. This is a postulated mechanism to counteract the function of suppressor cells in a feedback-type mechanism. Proof of contrasuppressor and suppressor cell circuits awaits confirmation by molecular biologic techniques.

contrasuppressor cell

A T cell that opposes the action of a suppressor T lymphocyte.

control

A specimen of known content used with an unknown specimen during an analysis so the two may be compared.

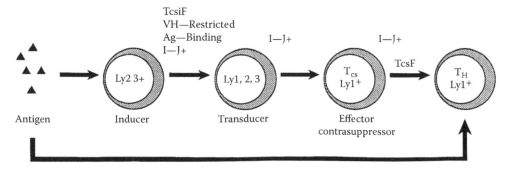

Contrasuppression.

A positive control known to contain the substance under analysis and a negative control known not to contain the substance under analysis are required.

control tolerance

The mechanism that involves the absence or functional inactivation of cells requisite for the initiation of an immune response. These cells are defective or inactivated. Control tolerance affects the afferent limb of the immune response, which is concerned with sensitization and cell proliferation.

convalescent serum

A patient's blood serum sample obtained 2 to 3 weeks following the beginning of a disease. The finding of an antibody titer to a pathogenic microorganism that is higher than the titer of a serum sample taken earlier in the disease is considered to signify infection produced by that particular microorganism. For example, a fourfold or greater elevation in antibody titer would represent presumptive evidence that a particular virus had induced the infection in question.

conventional (holoxenic) animals

Experimental animals exclusive of those raised in a gnotobiotic or germ-free environment.

conventional mouse

A mouse maintained under ordinary living conditions and provided water and food on a regular basis.

convertase

An enzyme that transforms a complement protein into its active form by cleaving it. The generation of C3/C5 convertase is a critical event in complement activation.

Cooke, Robert Anderson (1880–1960)

American immunologist and allergist who was instrumental in the founding of several allergy societies. With Coca, he classified allergies in humans. He also pioneered skin test methods and desensitization techniques.

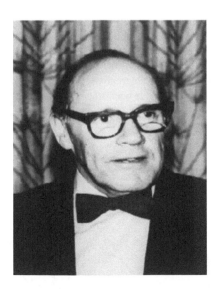

Robin R.A. Coombs.

Coombs, Robin (Robert Royston Amos Coombs, 1921–2006)

British pathologist and immunologist best known for the Coombs' test for detecting immunoglobulin on the surface of a patient's red blood cells. The test was developed in the 1940s to demonstrate autoantibodies on the surfaces of red blood cells that failed to cause agglutination of these

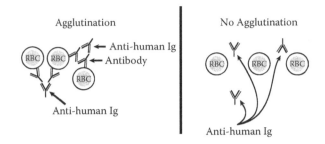

Schematic representation of the mechanism of the Coombs' test.

erythrocytes. It is a test for autoimmune hemolytic anemia. Coombs also contributed much to serology, immunohematology, and immunopathology. (Refer to *The Serology of Conglutination and Its Relation to Disease,* 1961; *Clinical Aspects of Immunology* [with Gell], 1963.)

Coombs' test

An antiglobulin assay that detects immunoglobulin on the surfaces of red blood cells. The test was developed in the 1940s by Robin Coombs to demonstrate autoantibodies on the surfaces of red blood cells that failed to cause agglutination of the cells. In the direct Coombs' test, rabbit antihuman immunoglobulin is added to a suspension of the patient's red cells; if the cells are coated with autoantibody, agglutination results. In the indirect Coombs' test, the patient's serum can be used to coat erythrocytes that are then washed and the anti-immunoglobulin reagent added to produce agglutination if the antibodies in question are present in the serum sample. The Coombs' test has long been a part of an autoimmune disease evaluation of patients. Refer to antiglobulin test.

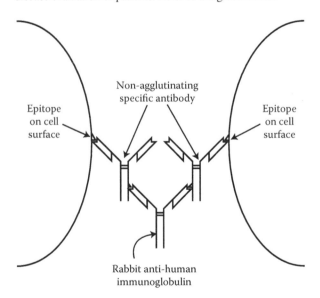

Schematic representation of the mechanisms of antiglobulin used to demonstrate nonagglutinating antibodies on red cell surfaces in autoimmune hemolytic anemia.

Coons, Albert Hewett (1912–1978)

American immunologist and bacteriologist who was an early leader in immunohistochemistry with the development of fluorescent antibodies. Coons, a professor at Harvard, received the Lasker medal in 1959, the Ehrlich prize in 1961, and the Behring prize in 1966.

C

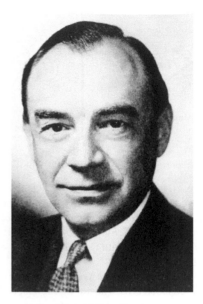

Albert Hewett Coons.

cooperation

Refer to T lymphocyte–B lymphocyte cooperation.

cooperative determinant

Carrier determinant.

cooperativity

The effect observed when two binding sites are linked to their ligand to yield an effect of binding to both that is greater than the sum of each binding site acting independently.

copolymer

A polymer such as a polypeptide comprised of at least two separate chemical specificities such as two different amino acids.

copper and immunity

The copper trace metal is a requisite for a healthy immune system. Copper insufficiency in humans leads to pathologic effects that may include cerebral degeneration in Menkes' syndrome and increased susceptibility to infection among infants who are copper-deficient. In neonatal copper deficiency there is a marked neutropenia associated with infections. Insufficient copper intake among domestic animals leads to diminished bactericidal activity, impairment of neutrophil function, and increased susceptibility to bacterial and fungus infections.

copper deficiency

Trace amounts of copper are requisite for the ontogeny and proper functioning of the immune system. Neonates and malnourished children with copper deficiency may have associated neutropenia and an increased incidence of infection. Antioxidant enzyme levels are diminished in copper deficiency. This may render immunologically competent cells unprotected against elevated oxygen metabolism associated with immune activation.

coprecipitation

The addition of an antibody specific for either the antigen portion or the antibody portion of immune complexes to effect their precipitation. Protein A may be added instead to precipitate soluble immune complexes. The procedure may be employed to quantify low concentrations of radiolabeled antigen that are combined with excess antibody. After soluble complexes have formed, antiimmunoglobulin or protein A is added to induce coprecipitation.

coproantibody

A gastrointestinal tract antibody, commonly of the immunoglobulin A (IgA) class, present in the intestinal lumen or feces.

coral immunity

Syngrafts, i.e., genetically identical grafts, are successful in corals. By contrast, allografts of genetically nonidentical ones are rejected slowly with injury to both donor and recipient. A vestige of adaptive immunity is revealed by limited evidence of immunological memory of a prior rejection episode.

cords of Billroth

Splenic medullary cords.

core (HIV)

Genomic RNA and its associated proteins, the capsid and the matrix.

coreceptor

A cell surface protein that increases the sensitivity of an antigen receptor to antigen by binding to associated ligands and facilitating signaling for activation. CD4 and CD8 are T cell coreceptors that bind nonpolymorphic parts of a major histocompatibility complex (MHC) molecule concurrently with the T cell receptor (TCR) binding to polymorphic residues and the bound peptide. A coreceptor is a structure on the surface of a lymphocyte that binds to a part of an antigen simultaneously with membrane immunoglobulin (Ig) or TCR binding of antigen and transmits signals required for optimal lymphocyte activation. CD4 and CD8 represent T cell coreceptors that bind nonpolymorphic regions of an MHC molecule simultaneously with the binding of the TCR to polymorphic residues and the exhibited peptide. Contact between the pMHC and the T cell receptor is stabilized by the binding, which also seeks protein tyrosine kinases that engage in intracellular signaling. The CD19–CD21–CD81 complex acts as a B cell coreceptor.

corneal response

In an animal that has been previously sensitized to an antigen, the cornea of the eye may become clouded (or develop opacities) after injection of the same antigen into it. Edema and lymphocytic and macrophage infiltration into the area occur. The response has been suggested to represent cell-mediated immunity.

corneal test

Refer to corneal response.

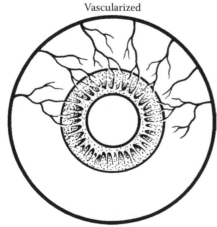

Corneal transplant.

corneal transplantation

A corneal transplantation is different from most other transplants in that the cornea is a "privileged site." Such sites do not have lymphatic drainage. The rejection rate in corneal transplants depends on vascularization; if vascularization occurs, the cornea becomes accessible to the immune system; human leukocyte antigen (HLA) incompatibility increases the risk of rejection if the cornea becomes vascularized. The patient can be treated with topical steroids to cause local immunosuppression. Certain anatomical sites within the animal body provide an immunologically privileged environment that favors the prolonged survival of alien grafts. The potential for development of a blood and lymphatic vascular supply connecting graft and host may be a determining factor in the qualification of an anatomical site as an area that provides an environment favorable to the prolonged survival of a foreign graft. Immunologically privileged sites include: (1) the anterior chamber of the eye, (2) the substantia propria of the cornea, (3) the meninges of the brain, (4) the testes, and (5) the cheek pouch of the Syrian hamster. Foreign grafts implanted in these sites show a diminished ability to induce transplantation immunity in the host. These immunologically privileged sites usually fail to protect alien grafts from the immune rejection mechanism in hosts previously or simultaneously sensitized with donor tissues.

coronavirus immunity

Neutralizing and fusion-inhibiting antibodies are directed mainly against the protein S antigen. Antibodies against HE, N, M, and sM are also significant in neutralization together with complement factors. Among coronavirus antigens, there is high antigenic variability of the S1 subunit of IBV. This subunit induces neutralizing antibodies that bind to discontinuous epitopes. The S2 subunit contains linear epitopes and an amino-dominant region. The S1 subunit of the molecule contains the most immunogenic sites of BCV and MHV. The S2 subunit of MHV also induces neutralizing and fusion-inhibiting antibodies. BCV-specific antibodies against the HE protein participate in neutralization. The M protein of MHV and TGEV stimulate complement-dependent neutralizing antibodies. The TGEV sM protein is involved in neutralization. T lymphocyte responses against SN protein facilitate virus elimination and may confer protection against encephalomyelitis in mice and rats. An immunodominant T cell antigenic site in the N protein of MHV induces neutralizing S protein-specific antibodies.

cortex

The outer or peripheral layer of an organ.

cortical thymic epithelial cells (cTECs)

Refer to thymic epithelial cells.

corticosteroids

Lympholytic steroid hormones, such as cortisone derived from the adrenal cortex, that are potent anti-inflammatory and immunosuppressive agents following their linkage to

Structure of cortisone.

Structure of corticosterone.

Structure of cortisol.

Structure of 6α-methylprednisolone.

Structure of prednisolone.

glucocorticoid receptors and inactivation of transcription factors including NF-KB, AP-1, NF-AT and the STATs. Glucocorticoids such as prednisone or dexamethasone can diminish the size and lymphocyte content of lymph nodes and spleen while sparing proliferating myeloid or erythroid stem cells of the bone marrow. Glucocortoids may interfere with the cell cycle of the activated lymphocyte. They are cytotoxic for selected T lymphocyte subpopulations and able to suppress cell-mediated immunity and antibody synthesis, as well as the formation of prostaglandins and leukotrienes. Corticosteroids may lyse either suppressor or helper T lymphocytes, but plasma cells may be more resistant to their effects. However, precursor lymphoid cells are sensitive to the drugs, which may lead to decreased antibody responsiveness. The repeated administration of prednisone diminishes the concentrations of specific antibodies in the immunoglobulin G (IgG) class whose fractional catabolic rates are increased by prednisone. Corticosteroids interfere with the phagocytosis of antibody-coated cells by

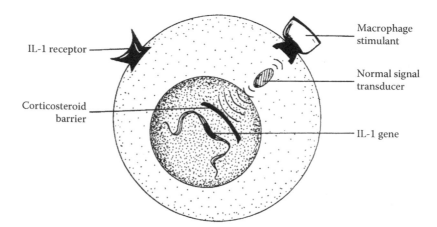

Mechanism of action of corticosteroids.

macrophages. Glucocorticoids have been widely administered for their immunosuppressive properties in autoimmune diseases such as autoimmune hemolytic anemia, systemic lupus erythematosus (SLE), Hashimoto's thyroiditis, idiopathic thrombocytopenic purpura, and inflammatory bowel disease. They are also used in the treatment of various allergic reactions and for bronchial asthma and have been widely used in organ transplantation, especially prior to the introduction of cyclosporine and related drugs. They have been used to manage rejection crises without producing bone marrow toxicity. Long-term usage has adverse effects that include adrenal suppression.

corticotrophin receptor antibodies (CRAs)
Adrenal antibodies that have a role in the pathogenesis of Addison's disease. Corticotrophin receptor antibodies (CRAs) may block adrenocorticotrophic hormone (ACTH) binding to specific receptors on cells of the adrenal cortex. Corticotrophin receptor antibodies of the stimulatory type may be found in Cushing's syndrome attributable to primary pigmented nodular adrenocortical disease.

corticotrophin receptor autoantibodies (CRAs)
Blocking autoantibodies that function by inhibiting adrenocorticotrophic hormone (ACTH) binding to its receptors on adrenal cortical cells. CRAs have high sensitivity specificity and predictive value for idiopathic Addison's disease. Cushing's syndrome due to primary pigmented nodular adrenocortical disease is associated with stimulatory CRAs.

***Corynebacterium diphtheriae* immunity**
Toxins produced by all strains of this organism are identical immunologically; thus antitoxins may neutralize them equally. A single toxoid is used for effective immunization. There is no type-specific immunity. Immunization does not protect against the infection but against the systemic and local effects of the toxin. A high level of immunity is conferred, but it is not complete.

costimulator
An antigen-presenting cell-surface molecule that supplies a stimulus, serving as a second signal, requisite for activation of naïve T lymphocytes, in addition to antigen (the first signal). An example of a costimulator is the B7 molecule on professional antigen-presenting cells that binds to the CD28 molecules on T lymphocytes. Another example is the interaction of CD40 with CD40L on B cells.

costimulatory blockade
Deliberate interruption of costimulatory signal transmission that leads to anergy and antigen-specific T lymphocytes.

costimulatory molecules
Membrane-bound or secreted products of accessory cells that activate signal transduction events in addition to those induced by major histocompatibility complex (MHC)–T cell receptor (TCR) interactions. They are required for full activation of T cells, and it is thought that adjuvants may work by enhancing the expression of costimulator molecules by accessory cells. The interaction of CD28/CTLA-4 with B7 to induce full transcription of IL2 mRNA is an example of a costimulator mechanism.

costimulatory signal
An extra signal requisite to induce proliferation of antigen-primed T lymphocytes. It is generated by the interaction of CD28 on T cells with B7 on antigen-presenting cells or altered self cells. In B cell activation, an analogous second signal is illustrated by the interaction of CD40 on B cells with CD40-L on activated T helper cells.

Coulombic forces
See ionic or Coulombic forces.

counter current electrophoresis
Refer to counter immunoelectrophoresis.

counter electrophoresis
Refer to counter immunoelectrophoresis.

counter immunoelectrophoresis (CIE)
An immunoassay in which antigen and antibody are placed into wells in agar gel, followed by electrophoresis in which the negatively charged antigen migrates toward the antibody, which moves toward the antigen by electroendosmosis. Interaction of antigen and antibody molecules in the gel leads to the formation of a precipitin line. The method has been used to identify serotypes of *Streptococcus pneumoniae*, *Neisseria meningitidis* groups, and *Haemophilus influenzae* type b.

counter migration electrophoresis
Refer to counter immunoelectrophoresis.

coverage (vaccine)
Refer to efficacy.

Cowden syndrome
Increased propensity to develop various neoplasms as a consequence of germline mutations in the tumor suppressor gene PTEN.

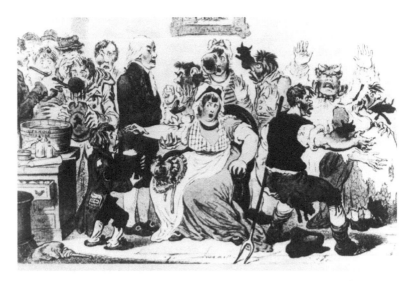

James Gillray's cartoon of the cowpox.

cowpox

A bovine virus disease that induces vesicular lesions on the teats. It is of great historical significance in immunology because Edward Jenner observed that milkmaids who had cowpox lesions on their hands failed to develop smallpox. He used this principle in vaccinating humans with the cowpox preparation to produce harmless vesicular lesions at the site of inoculation (vaccination). This stimulated protective immunity against smallpox (variola) because of shared antigens between the vaccinia virus and the variola virus.

coxsackie

A picornavirus family from Enteroviridiae. Coxsackie A viruses have 23 virotypes and coxsackie B viruses have 6 types. Clinical conditions produced by coxsackie viruses include herpangina, epidemic pleurodynia, aseptic meningitis, summer grippe, and acute nonspecific pericarditis and myocarditis.

CpG nucleotides

Bacterial DNA unmethylated cytidine–guanine sequences that facilitate immune responses acting as an adjuvant. They are believed to enhance DNA vaccine efficacy.

CR, CR1, CR2, CR3, CR4

Abbreviations for complement receptors.

CR1

Refer to complement receptor 1.

CR2

Refer to complement receptor 2.

CR2, type II complement receptor

A coreceptor on B lymphocytes that binds to antigens coated with complement at the same time that membrane immunoglobulin binds an epitope of the antigen.

CR3 deficiency syndrome

Refer to leukocyte adhesion deficiency.

C-reactive protein (CRP)

An acute phase 115-kDA protein. One of the pentraxin proteins in serum. It is comprised of five 206-amino acid

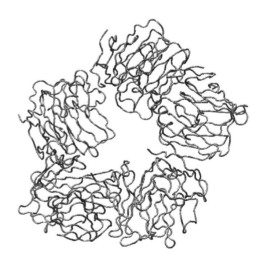

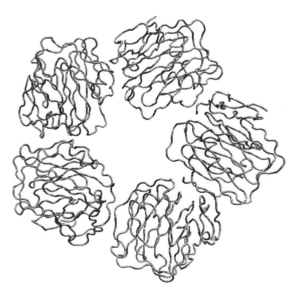

C-reactive protein (CRP).

C

polypeptide subunits that are all the same and arranged in a disk conformation without covalent bonds. Although present in normal individuals in only trace amounts in the plasma, with a median level of <8 μg/mL, inflammation induced by bacterial infection, necrosis of tissue, trauma, or malignant tumors may cause a striking increase in the serum concentration to levels of up to 2000 times the reference range within 48 hours of the inducing condition. CRP is encoded by a gene on chromosome 1. Interleukin-6 (IL6) regulates its production. Only hepatocytes express it. Once the condition that induced its elevation has resolved, the CRP concentration returns to normal within a short time. CRP levels signify the extent of the disease activity. CRP has the greatest sensitivity of any nonspecific test used in screening for organic disease. It is much more reliable than the erythrocyte sedimentation rate (ESR). CRP reacts with phosphoryl choline in the C polysaccharide of *Streptococcus pneumoniae* (pneumococcus) in the presence of Ca^{2+} ions. It binds firmly with platelet-activating factor (PAF). Following CRP binding to its ligands, C-reactive protein may produce effects similar to those of antibodies, such as activation of complement through the classic pathway by binding to C1q, agglutination of particulate ligands, and participation of insoluble ones, as well as neutralization of biological activity.

CREG

Crossreactive group. Public epitope-specific antibodies identify CREGs. *Public* refers to both similar (crossreactive) and identical (public) epitopes shared by more than one human leukocyte antigen (HLA) gene product.

CREST complex

Calcinosis, Raynaud's phenomenon, esophageal dysmotility, sclerodactyly, and telangiectasia associated with mixed connective-tissue disease. The prognosis of CREST is slightly better than that of other connective tissue diseases, but biliary cirrhosis and pulmonary hypertension are complications. CREST patients may develop anticentromere antibodies that may also occur in progressive systemic sclerosis patients, in aged females, or in individuals with HLA-DR1. CREST represents a mild form of systemic sclerosis.

CREST syndrome

A relatively mild clinical form of scleroderma (progressive systemic sclerosis). CREST is an acronym for calcinosis, Raynaud's phenomenon, esophageal dysmotility, sclerodactyly, and telangiectasis. Skin lesions are usually limited to the face and fingers, with only later visceral manifestations. Most (80 to 90%) CREST patients have anticentromere antibodies.

Creutzfeldt–Jakob syndrome

A slow virus infection of brain cells that reveals membrane accumulations.

Crithidia assay

The use of *Crithidia luciliae* hemoflagellates to measure anti-dsDNA antibodies in the sera of systemic lupus erythematosus (SLE) patients by immunofluorescence methods. The kinetoplast of this organism is an altered mitochondrion that is rich in double-stranded DNA.

Crithidia luciliae

A hemoflagellate possessing a large mitochondrion that contains concentrated mitochondrial DNA in a single large network called a kinetoplast. It is used in immunofluorescence assays for the presence of anti-dsDNA antibodies in the blood sera of systemic lupus erythematosus (SLE) patients.

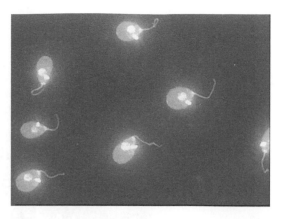

Structural formula for cromolyn

CRM 197

A carrier protein used in vaccines. It is a nontoxic mutant protein related to diphtheria toxin.

Crohn's disease

A condition usually expressed as ileocolitis, but it can affect any segment of the gastrointestinal tract. Crohn's disease is associated with transmural granulomatous inflammation of the bowel wall characterized by lymphocyte, plasma cell, and eosinophil infiltration. Goblet cells and gland architecture are not usually affected. Granuloma formation is classically seen in Crohn's disease, appearing in 70% of patients. The etiology is unknown. *Mycobacterium paratuberculosis* has been found in a few patients with Crohn's disease, although no causal relationship has been established. An immune effector mechanism is believed to be responsible for maintaining chronic disease in these patients. Their serum immunoglobulins and peripheral blood lymphocyte counts are usually normal except for a few diminished T cell counts in selected patients. Helper/suppressor ratios are also normal. Active disease has been associated with reduced suppressor T cell activity, which returns to normal during remission. Patients have complexes in their blood that are relatively small and contain immunoglobulin G (IgG), although no antigen has been identified. The complexes may be merely aggregates of IgG. Complexes in Crohn's disease patients are associated with involvement of the colon and are seen less often in those with the disease confined to the ileum. During active disease, serum concentrations of C3, factor B, C1 inhibitor, and C3b inactivator are elevated but return to normal during remission. Patients with long-standing disease often develop high titers of immunoconglutinins, which are antibodies to activated C3. High-titer antibodies against bacterial antigens such as those of *Escherichia coli* and *Bacteroides* crossreact with colonic goblet cell lipopolysaccharides. Patients' peripheral blood lymphocytes can kill colonic epithelial cells *in vitro*. Colonic mucosa lymphocytes in these patients are also cytotoxic for colonic epithelial cells.

Structural formula for cromolyn.

cromolyn (1,3-*bis*[2-carboxychromon-5-2-hydroxy-propane])

A therapeutic agent that prevents mast cell degranulation. It has proven effective in the therapy of selected allergies, including allergic rhinitis and asthma.

cromolyn sodium

A drug that blocks the release of pharmacological mediators from mast cells and diminishes the symptoms and tissue reactions of type I hypersensitivity (*i.e.,* anaphylaxis) mediated by immunoglobulin E (IgE). Although the mechanism of action of cromolyn sodium remains to be determined, it apparently inhibits the passage of calcium through the cell membrane. It inhibits mast cell degranulation but has no adverse effect on the linkage of IgE to mast cell surfaces or their interactions with antigen. Cromolyn sodium is inhaled as a powder or applied topically to mucous membranes. It is usually used for the treatment of asthma, allergic rhinitis, and allergic conjunctivitis, and it has low cytotoxicity.

cross absorption

The use of crossreacting antigens or crossreacting antibodies to absorb antibodies or antigens, respectively.

cross linking

A process resulting from the joining of multiple identical molecules by the union of multivalent ligands such as antibodies. It may occur with both soluble and cell-surface structures.

cross match testing

An assay used in blood typing and histocompatibility testing to ascertain whether donor and recipient have serum antibodies specific for each other's cells that might hinder successful transfusion of blood products or transplantation of organs or cells. Cross matching reduces the chances of graft rejection by preformed antibodies against donor cell surface antigens, which are usually major histocompatibility complex (MHC) antigens. Donor lymphocytes are mixed with recipient serum, complement is added, and the preparation is observed for cell lysis.

cross matching procedures

The conventional cross matching procedure for organ transplants involves the combination of donor lymphocytes with recipient serum. Three major variables in the standard cross match procedure predominantly affect the reactivity of the cell–serum sensitization: (l) incubation time and temperature, (2) wash steps after sensitization, and (3) the use of additional reagents such as antiglobulin in the test. Variations in these steps can cause wide variations in results. Lymphocytes can be separated into T and B cell categories for cross match procedures conducted at cold (4°C), room (25°C), and warm (37°C) temperatures. These proce-

Cross matching procedure.

dures permit the identification of warm antiT cell antibodies that are almost always associated with graft rejection.

cross presentation

Exogenous peptide antigen presentation on dendritic cell or macrophage MHC class I molecules. There may be fusion of a phagosome containing exogenous antigen with an endoplasmic reticulum-derived vesicle bearing constituents of the endogenous antigen processing apparatus. Peptide regurgitation or peptide interception may also represent a mechanism of cross presentation.

cross priming

Activation or priming of a naïve CD4+ cytotoxic T lymphocyte specific for antigens of a third cell such as a virus-infected cell or tumor cell by a professional antigen-presenting cell (APC). Cross priming takes place when a professional APC ingests an infected cell and the microbial antigens are processed and presented in association with Class I MHC molecules. The professional APC also costimulates the T cells. Also referred to as cross presentation.

crossreacting antibody

An antibody that reacts with epitopes on an antigen molecule different from the one that stimulated its synthesis. The effect is attributable to shared epitopes on the two antigen molecules.

crossreacting antigen

An antigen that interacts with an antibody synthesized following immunogenic challenge with a different antigen. Epitopes shared between these two antigens or epitopes with a similar stereochemical configuration may account for this type of crossreactivity. The presence of the same or a related epitope between bacterial cells, red blood cells, or other types of cells may result in crossreactions of the antigens with an antibody produced against either of them.

crossreaction

The reaction of an antigenic determinant or epitope with an antibody formed against another antigen. The presence of the same epitope on two different antigens and the presence of two similar epitopes on separate antigens may lead to crossreactivity. A laboratory technique used for matching blood for transfusion and organs for transplantation. In blood transfusion, donor erythrocytes are combined with the recipient's serum. Agglutination occurs if antibody in the recipient's serum is specific for donor red cells. This procedure represents the major part of the cross match. In a negative test, the presence of incomplete antibodies may be detected by washing the red blood cells and adding rabbit antihuman globulin. Agglutination signifies the presence of incomplete antibodies. The minor part of the cross match test consists of mixing the recipient's red blood cells with donor serum. This procedure is of less importance than the major cross match because of the limited amount of serum in a unit of blood compared to the red cell volume of the recipient.

crossreactivity

The ability of an antibody or T cell receptor to react with two or more antigens that share an epitope in common.

cross sensitivity

Induction of hypersensitivity to a substance by exposure to another substance containing cross reacting antigens.

cross tolerance

The induction of immunologic tolerance to an antigen by exposure of the host to a separate antigen containing crossreacting epitopes under conditions that favor tolerance induction.

C

crossed immunoelectrophoresis

A gel diffusion method employing two-dimensional immunoelectrophoresis. Protein antigens are separated by gel electrophoresis, followed by the insertion of a segment of the gel into a separate gel into which specific antibodies have been incorporated. The gel is then electrophoresed at right angles to the first electroporesis, forcing the antigen into the gel containing antibody. This results in the formation of precipitin arcs in the shape of a rocket that resemble bands formed in the Laurell rocket technique.

Crotalidae polyvalent immune Fab (ovine) (injection)

Fab fragment of immunoglobulin G (IgG) specific for venom that acts by binding and neutralizing venom toxins, facilitating their redistribution away from target tissues and their elimination from the body.

Crow–Fucase syndrome

Refer to POEMS syndrome.

CRP

Abbreviation for C-reactive protein.

cryofibrinogenemia

Cryofibrinogen in the blood that is either primary or secondary to lymphoproliferative and autoimmune disorders, tumors, and acute or chronic inflammation. Cryofibrinogenemia is often associated with immunoglobulin A (IgA) nephropathy.

cryoglobulin

A serum protein (immunoglobulin) that precipitates or gels when the temperature falls below 37°C. Cryoglobulins undergo reversible precipitation at cold temperatures. Most of them are complexes of immunoglobulin molecules, but nonimmunologic cryoprecipitate proteins such as cryofibrinogen or C-reactive protein–albumin complexes may also occur. When the concentration of cryoglobulins is relatively low, precipitation occurs near 4°C, but if the concentration is greater precipitation occurs at a higher temperature. Cryoglobulins are usually associated with infectious, inflammatory, and neoplastic processes. They are found in different body fluids and also appear in the urine. They are divisible into three groups: Type I cryoglobulins are monoclonal immunoglobulins, usually immunoglobulin M (IgM), associated with malignant B cell neoplasms; type II cryoglobulins consist of mixed cryoglobulins with a monoclonal constituent specific for polyclonal IgG; and type III cryoglobulins are mixed cryoglobulins composed of polyclonal immunoglobulins as immunoglobulin–antiimmunoglobulin complexes. Cryoglobulin is not present in normal serum. Refer to cryoglobulinemia.

cryoglobulinemia

Cryoglobulins in the blood that are usually monoclonal immunoglobulins (IgG or IgM). Polymeric IgG_3 may be associated with cryoglobulinemia, in which the protein precipitates in those parts of the body exposed to cooling. Cryoglobulinemia patients develop embarrassed circulation following precipitation of the protein in peripheral blood vessels. This may lead to ulcers on the skin and to gangrene. More commonly, patients manifest Raynaud's phenomenon following exposure of the hands or other parts of the anatomy to cold. Cryoglobulins may be detected in patients with Waldenström's macroglobulinemia, multiple myeloma, or systemic lupus erythematosus (SLE). Cryoglobulinemias are divisible into three types: type I monoclonal cryoglobulinemia, often associated with a malignant condition (i.e., IgG multiple myeloma, IgM macroglobulinemia, lymphoma or chronic lymphocytic leukemia, and benign monoclonal gammopathy); type II polymonoclonal cryoglobulinemia with mixed immunoglobulin complexes such as IgM–IgG, IgG–IgG, and IgA–IgG that may be linked to connective tissue disease such as rheumatoid arthritis or Sjögren's syndrome or with lymphoreticular disease; and type III mixed polyclonal–polyclonal cryoglobulinemia with IgG and IgM mixtures, rarely including IgA, which is associated with infections, lupus erythematosus, rheumatoid arthritis, Epstein–Barr and cytomegalovirus inclusion virus, Sjögren's syndrome, crescentic and membranoproliferative glomerulonephritis, subacute bacterial infections, biliary cirrhosis, diabetes mellitus, and chronic active hepatitis.

cryopreservation

The technique of freezing tissue or cells or other biological materials so that they remain genetically stable and metabolically inert. Cryopreservation may involve freezing (–80°C) or preservation with dry ice (–79°C) or liquid nitrogen (–196°C).

Cryostat®

A microtome in a refrigerated cabinet used by pathologists to prepare frozen tissue sections for surgical pathologic diagnosis. Immunologists use this method of quick frozen thin sections for immunofluorescence staining by fluorochrome-labeled antibody to identify antigens, antibodies, or immune complexes in tissue sections such as renal biopsies.

cryptantigens

Surface antigens of red cells not normally detectable but demonstrable by microbial enzyme action that leads to the modification of cell surface carbohydrates. Naturally occurring immunoglobulin M (IgM) antibodies in normal serum may agglutinate these exposed antigens.

cryptic epitope

An antigenic determinant concealed from the immune system in health but exposed during inflammation or infection.

***Cryptococcosis neoformans* immunity**

The polysaccharide capsule of *C. neoformans* serves as an antiphagocytic mechanism. It blocks binding sites recognized by phagocytic receptors for β-glucan and mannan that may mediate phagocytosis and secretion of TNFα. The capsule also covers immunoglobulin G (IgG) bound to the cell wall, but it is the site of complement activation in the alternative pathway in which IC3b fragments may facilitate opsonization. Neutrophils, monocytes, and natural killer (NK) cells all show anticryptococcal activity *in vitro*. Nonencapsulated *C. neoformans* generates elevated levels of interleukin-2 (IL2) and interferon-γ (IFN-γ) *in vivo*. The polysaccharide capsule may also induce suppressor T cells that synthesize a factor that inhibits binding of the organism by macrophages. Critical to immunity to this fungus is the recognition of encapsulated *C. neoformans* by antigen-specific mechanisms. A specific immune response is essential to control encapsulated *C. neoformans*. NK and T cells exert their antifungal action against *C. neoformans* independent of oxygen or nitrogen radicals. T cell-mediated immunity is critical for acquired immunity against *C. neoformans*. NK cells have also been shown to play an important role.

Activated T Cell

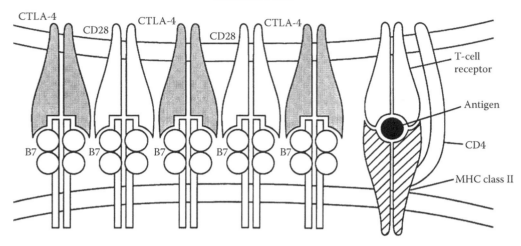

Participation of CTLA-4 molecules during antigen presentation.

cryptodeterminant

Refer to hidden determinant.

Cryptosporidium immunity

Mucosal immunization may prove useful to prevent cryptosporidiosis in AIDS patients. Little is known of the host immune response to *C. parvum*. The infection is increased in severity and duration in immunosuppressed individuals, indicating that a specific mucosal immune response must be induced in the host. Interferon-γ (IFN-γ) limits the infection, whereas CD4⁺ T cells limit the duration of the infection. Thus, both IFN-γ and CD4⁺ T cells are critical to inducing resistance to and resolution of the infection. Interleukin-12 (IL12) activates both natural killer cells and cytotoxic T lymphocytes and induces IFN-γ synthesis. The administration of IL12 prevents *C. parvum* murine infection. This proves that exogenous IL12 therapy can prevent the infection through an IFN-γ-dependent specific immune mechanism and that endogenous IL12 synthesis helps to limit *C. parvum* infection.

crystallographic antibodies

Antibodies against antigenic crystals, such as those found in patients with gout who develop immunoglobulin G (IgG) antibodies against monosodium urate monohydrate (MSUM). These antibodies facilitate crystallization of more MSUM, which can lead to recurrence of gout.

CSIF

Abbreviation for cytokine synthesis inhibitory factor. Refer to interleukin-10.

CSF

Abbreviation for (1) colony-stimulating factor or (2) cerebrospinal fluid.

cSMAC

Central supramolecular activation complex, constituting the center ring of the SMAC. It is composed of activated T cell receptors, pMHC, coreceptors and related kinases, and lipid rafts.

C terminus

The carboxyl terminal end of a polypeptide chain containing a free –COOH group.

CTL

Abbreviation for cytotoxic T lymphocyte.

CTLA-4

Molecule that is homologous to CD28 and expressed on activated T cells. The genes for CD28 and CTLA-4 are closely linked on chromosome 2. The binding of CTLA-4 to its ligand B7 is an important costimulatory mechanism (refer to CD28 and costimulatory molecules). A high affinity receptor for B7 costimulatory molecules on T lymphocytes.

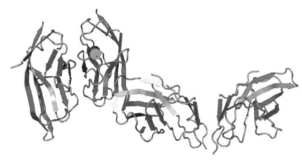

CTLA-4/B7-2 complex.

CTLA-4–Ig

A soluble protein composed of the CD28 homolog CTLA and the constant region of an IgG₁ molecule. It is used experimentally to inhibit the immune response by blocking CD28–B7 interaction.

C-type lectin

The binding of this lectin to carbohydrate ligands is calcium-dependent.

Cu-18

A glycoprotein of breast epithelium. Immunoperoxidase staining identifies this marker in most breast tumors and a few tumors of the ovary and lung. Stomach, pancreas, and colon tumors do not express this antigen.

Cunningham plaque technique

A modification of the hemolytic plaque assay in which an erythrocyte monolayer between a glass slide and cover slip is used without agar for the procedure.

cutaneous anaphylaxis

A local reaction specifically elicited in the skin of an actively or passively sensitized animal. Causes of cutaneous anaphylaxis include an immediate wheal-and-flare response following prick tests with drugs or other substances; insect stings or bites; and contact urticaria in response to food

C

substances such as nuts, fish, or eggs or other substances such as rubber, dander, or other environmental agents. The signs and symptoms of anaphylaxis are associated with the release of chemical mediators, including histamine and other substances, from mast cell or basophil granules following crosslinking of surface immunoglobulin E (IgE) by antigen or nonimmunological degranulation of these cells. The pharmacological mediators act principally on the blood vessels and smooth muscle. The skin may be the site where an anaphylytic reaction is induced or it can be the target of a systemic anaphylactic reaction resulting in itching (pruritus), urticaria, and angiodema.

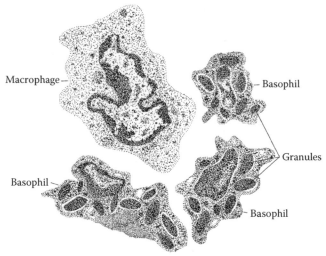

Cutaneous basophil hypersensitivity.

cutaneous basophil hypersensitivity (Jones–Mote hypersensitivity)

A type of delayed (type IV) hypersensitivity in which there is prominent basophil infiltration of the skin immediately beneath the epidermis. It can be induced by the intradermal injection of a soluble antigen such as ovalbumin incorporated into Freund's incomplete adjuvant. Swelling of the skin reaches a maximum within 24 hours. The hypersensitivity reaction is maximal between 7 and 10 days following induction and vanishes when antibody is formed. Histologically, basophils predominate, but lymphocytes and mononuclear cells are also present. Jones–Mote hypersensitivity is greatly influenced by lymphocytes that are sensitive to cyclophosphamide (suppressor lymphocytes).

cutaneous immune system

Adaptive and innate immune system constituents present in the skin that function in concert to detect and respond to environmental antigens. Among the cutaneous immune system constituents are keratinocytes, Langerhans' cells, intraepithelial lymphocytes, dermal lymphocytes, and antigen-presenting cells. Comprises the skin-associated lymphoid tissues (SALT) that can react against invading skin pathogens without obligatory participation by the draining lymph nodes.

cutaneous lymphocyte antigen

HECA-452 epitope expressed on a skin-associated subset of memory T cells that are active in recirculation and homing to skin sites.

cutaneous sensitization

Application of antigen to the skin to induce hypersensitivity.

cutaneous T cell lymphoma

A malignant growth of T lymphocytes that home to the skin, such as mycosis fungoides.

CVID (common variable immunodeficiency)

A relatively common congenital or immune deficiency that may be familial or sporadic. The familial form may have a variable mode of inheritance. Hypogammaglobulinemia is common to all of these patients and usually affects all classes of immunoglobulin, but in some cases only IgG is affected. The World Health Organization (WHO) classifies three forms of the disorder: (1) an intrinsic B lymphocyte defect, (2) a disorder of T lymphocyte regulation that includes deficient T helper lymphocytes or activated T suppressor lymphocytes, and (3) autoantibodies against T and B lymphocytes. Most patients have intrinsic B cell defects with normal numbers of B cells in the circulation that can identify antigens and proliferate but cannot differentiate into plasma cells. The ability of B cells to proliferate when stimulated by antigen is demonstrated by the hyperplasia of B cell regions of lymph nodes, spleen, and other lymphoid tissue; yet, differentiation of B cells into plasma cells is blocked. The deficiency of antibody that results leads to recurrent bacterial infections as well as intestinal infestation by *Giardia lamblia*, which produces a syndrome that resembles sprue. Noncaseating granulomas occur in many organs. The incidence of autoimmune diseases such as pernicious anemia, rheumatoid arthritis, and hemolytic anemia is increased. Lymphomas also occur in these immunologically deficient individuals.

CXC subgroup

A chemokine family in which a disulfide bridge between cysteines is separated by a different amino acid residue (X).

CXCL8

A chemokine formerly called IL-8 and associated with neutrophil extravasation.

CXCR-4

A chemokine receptor, CXCR-4, and its ligand, PBSF/SDF-1, are required for later stages of development of the vascularization of the gastrointestinal tract.

cyanogen bromide

A chemical that specifically breaks methionyl bonds. Approximately one half of the methionine residues in an immunoglobulin G (IgG) molecule (e.g., those in the Fc region) are cleaved by treatment with cyanogen bromide.

cycle-specific drugs

Immunosuppressive and cytotoxic drugs that lead to deaths of mitotic and resting cells.

cyclic adenosine monophosphate (cAMP)

Adenosine 3′,5′-(hydrogen phosphate), a critical regulator within cells. It is produced through the action of adenylate cyclase on adenosine triphosphate and activates protein kinase C. It serves as a "second messenger" when hormones activate cells. Elevated cAMP concentrations in mast cells diminish their response to degranulation signals.

cyclic guanosine monophosphate (cGMP)

Guanosine cyclic 3′,5′-(hydrogen phosphate). A cAMP antagonist produced by the action of guanylatecyclase on guanosine triphosphate. Elevated cGMP concentrations in mast cells accentuate their responses to degranulation signals.

cyclin D1 (polyclonal), rabbit

Anti-cyclin D1 is a rabbit polyclonal antibody that detects cyclin D1, one of the key cell cycle regulators that is a putative proto-oncogene overexpressed in a wide variety of human neoplasms. Cyclins are proteins that govern transitions through distinct phases of the cell cycle by regulating the activity of the cyclin-dependent kinases. In mid to late G1, cyclin D1 shows a maximum expression following growth factor stimulation. It has been successfully employed and is a promising tool for further studies in both cell cycle biology and cancer associated abnormalities. This antibody is useful for separating mantle cell lymphomas (cyclin D1-positive) from SLLs and small cleaved cell lymphomas (cyclin D1-negative).

cyclooxygenase pathway

The method whereby prostaglandins are produced by enzymatic metabolism of arachidonic acid derived from cell membranes, as in type I (anaphylactic) hypersensitivity reactions.

cyclophilins

Cytoplasmic proteins that combine with immunosuppressive therapeutic agents cyclosporin A and tacrolimus. T cell activation is inhibited by the binding of calcineurin by the drug–cyclophilin complex. An 18-kDa protein in the cytoplasm that has peptidyl–prolyl isomerase functions. It has a unique and conserved amino acid sequence that has a broad phylogenetic distribution. It represents a protein kinase with a postulated critical role in cellular activation. It serves as a catalyst in *cis-trans-rotamer* interconversion. It catalyzes phosphorylation of a substrate that then serves as a cytoplasmic messenger associated with gene activation. Genes coding for the synthesis of lymphokines would be activated in helper T lymphocyte responsiveness. Cyclophilin has a high affinity for cyclosporine (CSA), which accounts for the immunosuppressive action of the drug. Inhibition of cyclophilin-mediated activities as a consequence of CSA–cyclophilin interaction may lead to inhibition of the synthesis and release of lymphokines. CSA not only inhibits primary immunization, but it may also halt an ongoing immune response. This has been postulated to occur through inhibition of continued lymphokine release and by suppression of continued effector cell activation and recruitment.

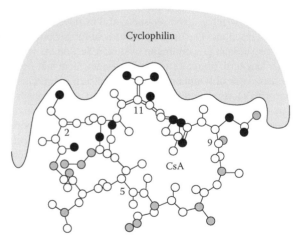

Cyclosporine (CSA) bound to cyclophilin.

cyclophosphamide

(*N,N-bis*-[2-chloroethyl]-tetrahydro-2H-1,3,2-oxazaphosphorine-2-amine-2-oxide), a powerful immunosuppressive drug that is more toxic for B than for T lymphocytes; therefore, it is a more effective suppressor of humoral antibody synthesis than of cell-mediated immune reactions. It is administered orally or intravenously and mediates its

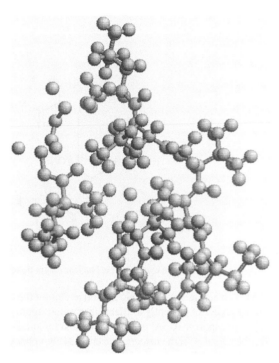

Nuclear magnetic resonance (NMR) structure of cyclosporine A as bound to cyclophilin A.

Structure of cyclosphosphamide.

cytotoxic activity by crosslinking DNA strands. This alkylating action mediates target cell death. It produces dose-related lymphopenia and inhibits lymphocyte proliferation *in vitro*. It destroys proliferating lymphoid cells and may alkylate some resting cells. The greater effect on B than on T cells is apparently related to the lower rate of recovery of B cells. Very large doses of >120mg/kg intravenously over several days may facilitate induction of specific tolerance to a foreign antigen if the drug is administered simultaneously with or immediately following the antigen. Cyclophosphamide is beneficial for the therapy of various autoimmune disorders, including rheumatoid arthritis, systemic lupus erythematosus (SLE)-associated renal disease, Wegener's granulomatosis and other vasculitides, and autoimmune hematologic disorders, including idiopathic thrombocytopenic purpura, pure red cell aplasia, and autoimmune hemolytic anemia. Cyclophosphamide is also used to treat Goodpasture's syndrome and various glomerulonephritides. Its beneficial use as an immunosuppressive agent is tempered by the finding of its significant toxicity, such as its association with hemorrhagic cystitis, suppression of hematopoiesis, gastrointestinal symptoms, etc. It may also increase the chance of opportunistic infections and be associated with an increased incidence of malignancies such as non-Hodgkin lymphoma, bladder carcinoma, and acute myelogenous leukemia.

cyclosporine (cyclosporin A; ciclosporin)

A cyclic endecapeptide of 11 amino acid residues isolated from soil fungi that has revolutionized organ transplantation.

C

Structure of cyclosporine. Nuclear magnetic resonance (NMR) structure of cyclosporine A as bound to cyclophiline A.

Rather than acting as a cytotoxic agent that defines the activity of a number of currently available immmunosuppressive drugs, cyclosporine (CSA) produces an immunomodulatory effect principally on the helper/inducer (CD4) lymphocytes that orchestrate the generation of an immune response. A cyclic polypeptide, CSA blocks T cell help for both humoral and cellular immunity. Functions at an early stage in the antigen-receptor induced differentiation of T cells and inhibits their activation. It binds to cyclophilin, a member of the intracellular class termed immunophilins. Cyclosporine and cyclophilin combine and inhibit cytoplasmic phosphatase, calcineurin, which is requisite for a T cell-specific transcription factor activation. This transcription factor, NF-AT, participates in interleukin (e.g., IL-2) synthesis by activated T cells. *In vitro* studies suggest that cyclosporine inhibits gene transcription of IL-3, IFN-γ, and other products of antigen-stimulated T cells. However, it fails to inhibit the effects of these factors on primed T cells and does not block interaction with antigen. A primary mechanism of action is its ability to suppress interleukin-2 (IL2) synthesis. CSA fails to block activation of antigen-specific suppressor T cells, thereby assisting development of antigen-specific tolerance. Side effects include nephrotoxicity and hepatotoxicity with a possible increase in B cell lymphomas. Some individuals may also develop hypertension. The mechanism of action of CSA appears to include inhibition of the synthesis and release of lymphokines and alteration of expression of major histocompatibility complex (MHC) gene products on the cell surface. CSA inhibits IL2 mRNA formation. This does not affect IL2 receptor expression on the cell surface. Although CSA may diminish the number of low affinity binding sites, it does not appear to alter high affinity binding sites on cell surfaces. CSA inhibits the early increase in cytosolic-free calcium that occurs in beginning activation of normal T lymphocytes. It appears to produce its effect in the cytoplasm rather than on the cell surfaces of lymphocytes. It can reach the cytoplasmic location because of its ability to dissolve in the plasma membrane lipid bilayer. The cytosolic site of action of CSA may involve calmodulin and/or cyclophilin, a protein kinase. Although immunosuppressive action cannot be explained based upon CSA–calmodulin interaction, this association closely parallels the immunosuppressive effect. CSA produces a greater suppressive effect upon class II than

upon class I antigen expression in at least some experiments. While decreasing T helper lymphocytes, the T suppressor cells appear to be spared following CSA therapy. Both sparing and amplification of T lymphocyte suppression have been reported during CSA therapy. CSA is a powerful immunosuppressant that selectively affects CD4+ helper T cells without altering the activity of suppressor T cells, B cells, granulocytes, and macrophages. It alters lymphocyte function, but it does not destroy the cells. Its principal immunosuppressive action is to inhibit IL2 production and secretion. Thus, the suppression of IL2 impairs the development of suppressor and cytotoxic T lymphocytes that are antigen-specific. It has a synergistic immunosuppressive action with corticosteroids. Corticosteroids interfere with IL2 synthesis by inhibiting IL1 release from monocytes and macrophages. Cyclosporine, although water-insoluble, has been successfully employed as a clinical immunosuppressive agent principally in preventing rejection of organ and tissue allotransplants including kidney, heart, lung, pancreas, and bone marrow. It has also been successful in preventing graft-vs.-host reactions. The drug has some nephrotoxic properties that may be kept to a minimum by dose reduction. As with other long-term immunosuppressive agents, there may be increased risk of lymphoma development such as Epstein–Barr (EBV)-associated B cell lymphomas. Cyclosporine is a potent immunosuppressive agent that prolongs survival of allogeneic transplants of skin, kidney, liver, heart, pancreas, bone marrow, small intestine, and lung. The primary effect is on cell-mediated immune responses in allograft rejection, but the compound has some suppressive effect on humoral immunity. It also suppresses delayed type hypersensitivity. The T helper cell is the principal target, although the T suppressor cell may also be suppressed. It inhibits lymphokine production and release, including IL2.

CYNAP antibodies

Cytotoxicity-negative but absorption-positive antibodies that are concerned with human leukocyte antigen (HLA) tissue typing. Most alloantibodies to public epitopes display CYNAP when tested in complement-dependent cytotoxicity assays. Most alloantisera contain public or CREG antibodies, but they act operationally as "private" antibodies because of their CYNAP phenomenon. For this reason, the relative insensitivity of standard CDC, due to CYNAP, has been useful for detecting discrete gene products. Standard CDC is not the recommended procedure for defining HLA molecule-binding specificities. The anti-globulin-augmented CDC (AHG-CDC) more accurately defines the true binding capabilities of alloantisera than do complement-independent assays by overriding the CYNAP phenomenon. CDC is the procedure of choice for HLA antigen detection and HLA antiserum analysis.

CYNAP phenomenon

Refer to CYNAP antibodies.

cytochalasins

Metabolites of various species of fungi that affect microfilaments. They bind to one end of actin filaments and block their polymerization. Thus, they paralyze locomotion, phagocytosis, capping, cytokinesis, etc.

cytochrome *b* deficiency

Refer to chronic granulomatous disease.

cytochrome *c*

Suppression of the anti-apoptotic members or activation of the pro-apoptotic members of the Bcl-2 family leads to altered mitochondrial membrane permeability, resulting in release of cytochrome *c* into the cytosol. In the cytosol or on the surfaces of the mitochondria, cytochrome *c* is bound by the Apaf-1 (apoptotic protease-activating factor) protein that also binds caspase 9 and dATP. Binding of cytochrome *c* triggers activation of caspase 9, which then

accelerates apoptosis by activating other caspases. Release of cytochrome *c* from mitochondria has been established by determining the distribution of cytochrome *c* in subcellular fractions of cells treated or untreated to induce apoptosis. Cytochrome *c* was primarily in the mitochondria-containing fractions obtained from healthy, non-apoptotic cells in the cytosolic non-mitochondria-containing fractions obtained from apoptotic cells. Using mitochondria-enriched fractions from mouse liver, rat liver, or cultured cells demonstrated that release of cytochrome *c* from mitochondria is greatly accelerated by addition of Bax, fragments of Bid, and by cell extracts.

cytokeratin (34βE12), mouse

Anti-cytokeratin (34βE12) mouse monoclonal antibody detects cytokeratin, 34βE12, a high molecular weight cytokeratin that reacts with all squamous and ductal epithelium and stains carcinomas. This antibody recognizes cytokeratins 1,5,10, and 14 found in complex epithelia. Cytokeratin, 34βE12, shows no reactivity with hepatocytes, pancreatic acinar cells, proximal renal tubules or endometrial glands or reactivity with cells derived from simple epithelia. Mesenchymal tumors, lymphomas, melanomas, neural tumors, and neuroendocrine tumors are unreactive with this antibody. Cytokeratin 34βE12 has been shown to be useful in distinguishing prostatic adenocarcinoma from hyperplasia of the prostate.

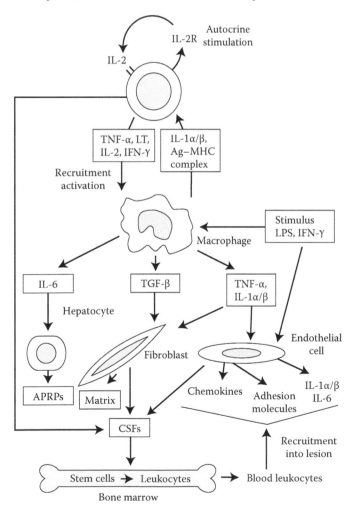

Generation of cytokines (endothelial cells, fibroblasts, T helper lymphocytes, and monocytes/macrophages).

C

cytokeratin 7 (K72), mouse

Anticytokeratin 7 (K72) mouse monoclonal antibody reacts with proteins that are found in most ductal, glandular and transitional epithelium of the urinary tract and bile duct epithelial cells. Cytokeratin 7 distinguishes between lung and breast epithelia that stain positive and colon and prostate epithelial cells that are negative. This antibody also reacts with many benign and malignant epithelial lesions, e.g., adenocarcinomas of the ovary, breast, and lung. Transitional cell carcinomas are positive and prostate cancer is negative. This antibody does not recognize intermediate filament proteins.

cytokine

Leukocytes and other types of cells produce soluble proteins or glycoproteins termed cytokines that serve as chemical communicators between cells. Cytokines are usually secreted, although some may be expressed on cell membranes or maintained in reservoirs in the extracellular matrix. Cytokines include proteins synthesized by cells that affect the actions of other cells. They combine with surface receptors on target cells that are linked to intracellular signal transduction and second messenger pathways. Their effects may be autocrine, acting on cells that produce them, or paracrine, acting on neighboring cells. Cytokines are immune system proteins that are biological response modifiers. They coordinate antibody and T cell immune system interactions and amplify immune reactivity. Cytokines include monokines synthesized by macrophages and lymphokines produced by activated T lymphocytes and natural killer cells. A *monokine* is a cytokine produced by monocytes. It is any one of a group of biologically active factors secreted by monocytes and macrophages that has a regulatory effect on the functions of other cells such as lymphocytes. Monokines include interleukin-1 (IL1), tumor necrosis factor (TNF), α and β interferons (IFNs), and colony-stimulating factors (CSFs). A *lymphokine* is a nonimmunoglobulin polypeptide substance synthesized mainly by T lymphocytes that affects the functions of other cells. It may enhance or suppress an immune response. Lymphokines may facilitate cell proliferation, growth, and differentiation, and they may act on gene transcription to regulate cell function. They exert paracrine or autocrine effects. Many lymphokines have now been described. Well known examples include IL2, IL3, migration inhibitory factor (MIF), and INF-γ. The term *cytokines* includes lymphokines, soluble products produced by lymphocytes, as well as mokines and soluble products produced by monocytes. Lymphokines include IL2 and IL6, INF-γ, granulocyte–macrophage colony-stimulating factor (GM-CSF) and lymphotoxin. MIF, endothelial cells, fibroblasts, and selected other cell types may also synthesize cytokines. Lymphokine research can be traced to the 1960s, when macrophage MIF was described; it is believed to be due to more than one cytokine in lymphocyte supernatants. Lymphotoxin was described in activated lymphocyte culture supernatants in the late 1960s, and lympokines were recognized as cell-free soluble factors formed when sensitized lymphocytes respond to specific antigens. These substances were considered responsible for cell-mediated immune reactions. IL2 was described as T cell growth factor. TNF was the first monocyte-/macrophage-derived cytokine or monokine to be recognized. Other cytokines derived from monocytes include lymphocyte activation factor (LAF), later named interleukin 1 (IL1). It was found to be mitogenic for thymocytes. Immunologists described lymphokines and monokines; virologists described interferons. Interferon is a factor formed by virus-infected cells that are able to induce resistance of cells to infection with homologous or heterologous viruses. Subsequently, IFN-γ, synthesized by T lymphocytes activated by mitogen, was found to be distinct from IFN-α and IFN-β and to be formed by a variety of cell types. CSFs were described as proteins capable of promoting proliferation and differentiation of hematopoietic cells. CSFs promote granulocyte or monocyte colony formation in semisolid media. Proteins that facilitate the growth of nonhematopoietic cells are not usually included with cytokines. Transforming growth factor β (TGF-β) has an important role in inflammation and immunoregulation as well as immunosupressive actions on T cells. Classes of cytokine receptors include the immunoglobin receptor superfamily, the hematopoietic/cytokine receptor superfamily, the nerve growth factor receptor superfamily, the G protein-coupled receptor superfamily and the other family, and the receptor tyrosine or serine kinases plus an unclassified group. Cytokine receptor families are classified according to conserved sequences or folding motifs. Type I receptors share a tryptophan–serine–X–tryptophan–serine (WSXWS) sequence on the proximal extracellular domain. Type I receptors recognize cytokines with a structure of four α-helical strands, including IL2 and G-CSF. Type II receptors are defined by the sequence patterns of type I and type II interferon receptors. Type III serve as receptors for TNF. CD40, nerve growth factor receptor, and Fas protein have sequences homologous to those of type III receptors. A fourth family of receptor has extracellular domains of the immunoglobulin (Ig) superfamily. IL1 receptors as well as some growth factors and colony-stimulating factors have Ig domains. The fifth superfamily of receptors displays a seven-transmembrane α-helical structure. This motif is shared by many of the receptors linked to GTP-binding proteins. A principal feature of cytokines is that their effects are pleiotropic and redundant. Cytokines do not exert a specific effect on one type of target cell. Most of them have a broad spectrum of biological effects on more than one type of tissue and cell. Various cytokines may interact with the same cell type to produce similar effects. Cytokine receptors are grouped into two classes. Class I receptors include those that bind a number of interleukins, including IL2, 3, 4, 6, 7, 9, 11, 12, and 15. Other type I receptors are those for erythropoietin (EPO), growth hormone (GH), granulocyte colony-stimulating factor (G-CSF), granulocyte–macrophage colony-stimulating factor (GM-CSF), leukemia inhibitory factor (LIF), and ciliary neurotrophic factor (CNTF). Class II receptors include those that bind IFN-α/β, IFN-γ, and IL10. Cytokine receptors are usually comprised of multipeptide complexes with a specific ligand-binding subunit and a signal transducer subunit that is class-specific. Receptors for IL3, IL5, and GM-CSF possess a unique a component and a common b signal transducer subunit that account for the redundant effects these molecules have on hematopoietic cells. IL6, CNTF, LIF, oncostatin M (OM), and IL11 belong to a family of receptors that share a gp130 signal tranducer subunit in common, which explains some of the similar functions these molecules have on various tissues. In IL2 signal transduction with respect to T cell growth, IL4, IL7, and IL15 also promote growth of T cells. IL4, IL7, and IL15 use the IL2 receptor γ chain, which accounts for the redundant functions of these cytokines as T cell growth factors. Cytokines have been named on the basis of the cell of origin or of the bioassay used to define them. This system has led to misnomers such as "tumor necrosis factor," which is more appropriately termed an immunomodulator and pro-inflammatory cytokine. The interleukins now number 17, even through IL8 is, in fact, a member of the chemokine cytokine family. The chemokines share a minimum of 25% amino acid homology, are similar in structure, and bind to seven rhodospin superfamily transmembrane spanning receptors. The CC or γ chemokines are encoded by genes on chromosome 17. CXC chemokines attract neutrophils, whereas CC chemokines attract monocytes.

cytokine assays

Tests based on the biological properties, immunological recognition (ELISA or radioimmunoassay), competitive binding to receptor molecule, and inference from transcription of the mRNA. Each method has advantages and disadvantages. Bioassays are quite sensitive and verify biological activity of the cytokine but are not always reproducible or specific. By contrast, immunoassays are reproducible and specific but not nearly as sensitive as bioassays.

cytokine autoantibodies

Autoantibodies that may inhibit cytokine functions and lead to cytokine deficiency. Autoimmune disease may occur, and the action of the cytokine may be inhibited. By contrast, these autoantibodies may serve as cytokine-specific carriers in the circulation. For example, insulin autoantibodies may prolong the release of active insulin to the tissues, leading to hypoglycemia in nondiabetics and a significant decrease in the exogenous insulin requirement in diabetic patients. AIDS patients may develop autoantibodies against IL2, and antibodies against TNFα have been used successfully to treat rheumatoid arthritis. Both normal and inflammatory disease patients may develop autoantibodies against IL1α. Cytokine activity is enhanced even in the presence of cytokine autoantibodies *in vivo* by a mechanism that delays rapid catabolism of cytokines from the circulation. The clinical relevance of cytokine autoantibodies *in vivo* remains to be determined. However, these autoantibodies portend a poor prognosis in any disease. Methods for cytokine autoantibody detection include bioassays, immunometric assays, and blotting techniques.

cytokine inhibitors

Prostaglandins, especially prostaglandin E2 (PGE2), synthesized by monocytes and macrophages, have been suggested to provide feedback inhibition of cytokine synthesis *in vivo*. Cytokine production inhibition is a possible mechanism whereby PGE exerts its anti-inflammatory effect. Treating rats with a monoclonal antibody specific for murine IL6, which mediates the acute phase response, led to increased survival in *Escherichia coli* shock. β-adrenergic agonists increase cAMP levels and THP-1 cells and suppress synthesis of TNFα. A β-adrenergic antagonist can abolish inhibition of TNFα synthesis.

Isoproterenol, a β-adrenergic agonist, inhibits TNFα synthesis. Dexamethasone and cAMP phosphodiesterase (PDE-IV) inhibitors suppress TNFα secretion by lipopolysaccharide (LPS)-activated human monocytes. IL1 receptor antagonist (IL1ra) is the only known natural cytokine antagonist. It inhibits the binding of IL1α and IL1β to their cell surface receptors. Selected antibiotics such as fluoroquinolones, clarithromycin, and tetrandrine inhibit IL1 and TNFα synthesis. Some anti-inflammatory drugs also have cytokine inhibitor capacity.

cytokine receptor classes

Include the immunoglobulin receptor superfamily, the hematopoietic/cytokine receptor superfamily, the nerve growth factor receptor superfamily, the G protein coupled receptor superfamily and the other family, and the receptor tyrosine or serine kinases plus an unclassified group.

cytokine receptor families

A classification system of cytokine receptors according to conserved sequences or folding motifs. Type I receptors share a tryptophan–serine–X–tryptophan–serine (or WSXWS) sequence on the proximal extracellular domains. Type I receptors recognize cytokines with a structure of four α-helical strands, including IL2 and granulocyte colony-stimulating factor (G-CSF). Type II receptors are defined by the sequence patterns of type I and type II interferon receptors. Type III serve as receptors for tumor necrosis factor (TNF) (p55 and p75). CD40, nerve growth factor receptor, and Fas protein have sequences homologous to those of type III receptors. A fourth family of receptors has extracellular domains of the immunoglobulin (Ig) superfamily. IL1 receptors as well as some growth factors and colony-stimulating factors have Ig domains. The fifth family of receptors displays a seven-transmembrane α-helical structure. This motif is shared by many of the receptors linked to GTP-binding proteins.

cytokine receptors

Sites on cell surfaces where cytokines bind, thus leading to new cell activities that include growth, differentiation, and death. Cytokines bind to these high affinity cell surface receptors that share some features in common. They have a high affinity for ligand. Typically a hundred to a few thousand receptors are present per cell. Most cytokine receptors are glycosylated, integral, type I membrane proteins. Functional cytokine receptors are usually complex structures requiring the formation of homologous or heterologous associations between receptor chains. A cytokine receptor group may share chains dubbed "public subunits" and ordinarily engage in signal transduction. Unique chains termed "private subunits" usually determine binding specificity. By contrast, receptors of the chemokine family belong to the serpentine superfamily and span the membrane seven times; they do not appear to form multimeric complexes.

cytokine receptors, soluble

Soluble cytokine receptors include IL1, type I-R, IL1, Type II-R, IL2Rα, IL2Rβ, IL4R, IL5Rα, IL6Rα, gp130 IL6Rβ ciliary neurotrophic factor (CNF)-Rα, and growth hormone R. Most of these function by blocking ligand binding.

cytokine-specific subunit

A multimeric cytokine receptor polypeptide chain that interacts stereospecifically with the target cytokine. It is responsible for the specificity of a receptor for a particular cytokine.

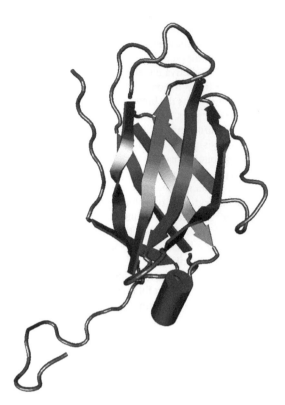

Cytokine/receptor complex.

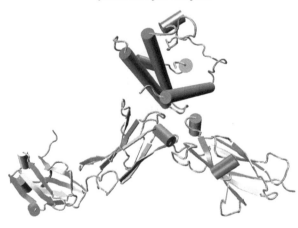

Cytokine/receptor complex.

cytokine synthesis inhibitory factor

Refer to interleukin-10.

cytokine upregulation of HIV coreceptors

HIV-1 virus strains use the chemokine receptors, CCR-5, CXCR-4, or both, to enter cells. Expression of these chemokine receptors may predetermine susceptibility of hematopoietic subsets to HIV-1 infection. Certain cytokines can influence the dynamics of HIV-1 infection by altering chemokine receptor expression levels on hematopoietic cells. During chronic HIV-1 infection, proinflammatory cytokines such as TNF-α and IFN-γ are secreted in excess. IFN-γ increases cell surface expression of CCR-5 by human mononuclear phagocytes and of CXCR-4 by primary hematopoietic cells. In addition, GM-CSF can decrease and IL10 can increase expression of CCR-5. Further research into cytokine-mediated regulation of chemokine receptors may lead to increased understanding of how these receptors affect the pathogenesis of AIDS.

cytolysin

A substance such as perforin that lyses cells.

cytolytic

An adjective describing the property of disrupting a cell.

cytolytic reaction

Cell destruction produced by antibody and complement or perforin released from cytotoxic T lymphocytes.

cytolytic T lymphocytes (CTLs)

Effector T cells that identify and fatally injure target cells exhibiting foreign peptide complexed to MHC class I molecules. Cytotoxic cytokines increased in perforin/granzyme-mediated cytotoxicity represent mechanisms of target cell death.

cytomegalovirus (CMV)

A herpes (DNA) virus group that is distributed worldwide and usually is not a problem, except in individuals who are immunocompromised, such as the recipients of organ or bone marrow transplants and individuals with acquired immune deficiency syndrome (AIDS). Histopathologically, typical inclusion bodies that resemble an owl's eye are found in multiple tissues. CMV is transmitted in the blood. Two classes of antiviral drugs are used to treat human immunodeficiency virus (HIV) infection and AIDS. Nucleotide analogs that inhibit reverse transcriptase activity include azidothymidine (AZT) dideoxyinosine and dideoxycytidine. These analogs may diminish plasma HIV RNA levels for considerable periods but often fail to stop disease progression because of the development of mutated forms of reverse transcriptase that resist these drugs. Viral protease inhibitors are now used to block the processing of precursor proteins into mature viral capsid and core proteins. Currently, a triple-drug therapy consisting of protease inhibitors is used to reduce plasma viral RNA to very low levels in patients treated for more than one year. It remains to be determined whether resistance to this therapy will develop. Disadvantages include their great expense and the complexity of their administration. Antibiotics are used to treat the many infections to which AIDS patients are susceptible. Viral resistance to protease inhibitors may develop after a few days, but resistance to the reverse transcriptase inhibitor zidovudine may only occur after months of administration. Three of four mutations in the viral resistance to zidovudine yet only one mutation can lead to resistance to protease inhibitors.

cytomegalovirus immune globulin intravenous (human, injection)

Indicated for prophylaxis of cytomegalovirus disease associated with transplantation of kidney, lung, liver, pancreas, and heart. Also used to prevent or attenuate primary CMV disease in immunosuppressed recipients of organ and bone marrow transplants.

cytomegalovirus (CMV) immunity

Cytomegalovirus that induces injury only if the host immune response is impaired, which makes it a significant pathogen for fetuses, allograft recipients, and individuals with acquired immune deficiency syndrome (AIDS). Host immune response to CMV is both cell-mediated and humoral. Cytotoxic T lymphocytes are specific for viral structural phosphoproteins. Cell-mediated immunity appears to be the major mechanism that controls CMV replication in murine CMV; however, natural killer (NK) cells are also important. Viral proteins induce a limited humoral

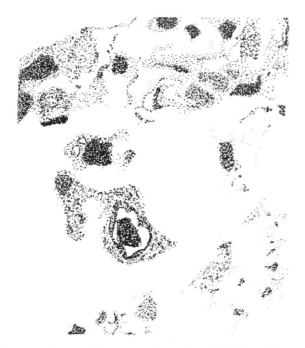

Cytomegalovirus (CMV) nuclear and cytoplasmic inclusions in the lung.

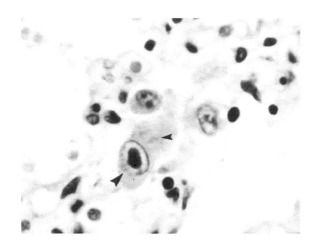

CMV inclusion bodies

▲ Intranuclear

▲ Intracytoplasmic

Cytomegalovirus (CMV).

response to two surface glycoproteins, gB and gH, that are neutralizing domains. Both cell-mediated and humoral immunity are insufficient to block reactivation of latent virus or protect against reinfection from an exogenous source. CMV upregulates adhesion molecules. CMV pneumonitis is immunopathologic. CMV is linked to infection of solid organ grafts and with graft-vs.-host disease after bone marrow transplants. It causes immunosuppression by unknown mechanisms. A live attenuated vaccine strain has no effect on the incidence of CMV infection; a recombinant gB vaccine is in phase I clinical trials.

cytopathic effect (of viruses)

Injurious effects of viruses on host cells produced by various biochemical and molecular mechanisms that are independent of host immunity against the virus. Selected

viruses produce disease even though they have little cytopathic effect because the immune system recognizes and destroys the virus-infected cells.

cytophilic antibody

(1) An antibody that attaches to a cell surface through its Fc region by binding to Fc receptors on the cell surface. For example, immunoglobulin E (IgE) molecules bind to the surfaces of mast cells and basophils in this manner. Murine IgG_1, IgG_{2a}, and IgG_3 bind to mononuclear phagocytic cell surface Fc receptors through their Fc regions. IgG_1 and IgG_3 may also attach through their Fc regions to mononuclear phagocytic cell Fc receptors in humans. Immunoglobulin molecules that bind to macrophage surfaces through their Fc regions represent a type of cytophilic antibody. (2) Described in the 1960s as a globulin fraction of serum adsorbed to certain cells *in vitro* in a manner that allows them to specifically adsorb antigen. Sorkin, in 1963, suggested the possible significance of cytophilic antibody in anaphylaxis and other immunologic and/or hypersensitivity reactions.

cytoplasmic antigens

Immunogenic constituents of cell cytoplasm that induce autoantibody formation in patients with generalized autoimmune diseases who also manifest antinuclear antibodies (ANAs). Thus, anticytoplasmic antibodies are included under the term ANA.

cytosine arabinoside

An antitumor substance that is inactive alone but which, following intracellular conversion to the nucleoside triphosphate, acts as a competitive inhibitor with regard to dCPP of DNA polymerase. It has an immunosuppressive effect on antibody formation in both the primary and secondary immune responses and also depresses the generation of cell-mediated immunity.

cytoskeletal antibodies

Antibodies that are specific for cytoskeletal proteins that include cytokeratins, desmin, actin, titin, vimentin, and tropomyosin. They have been demonstrated in some patients with such diseases as autoimmune diseases, chronic active hepatitis and other liver disease, infection, myasthenia gravis, and Crohn's disease. These antibodies are not helpful in diagnosis.

cytoskeletal autoantibodies

Antibodies specific for cytoskeletal proteins that include microfilaments (actin), microtubules (tubulin), and intermediate filaments (acidic and basic keratins, vimentin, desmin, glial fibrillary acidic protein, peripherin, neurofilaments, α-internexin, nuclear lamins). They are present in low titers in a broad spectrum of diseases, including infection, autoimmune diseases, selected chronic liver diseases, biliary cirrhosis, Crohn's disease, myasthenia gravis, and angioimmunoblastic lymphadenopathy. These antibodies are not useful for diagnosis.

cytoskeleton

A framework of cytoskeletal filaments present in the cell cytoplasm. They maintain the internal arrangement, shape, and motility of the cell. This framework interacts with the membrane of the cell and with organelles in the cytoplasm. Microtubules, microfilaments, and intermediate filaments constitute the varieties of cytoskeletal filaments. Microtubules help to determine cell shape by polymerizing and depolymerizing; they are 24-nm diameter hollow tubes, the walls of which are comprised of protofilaments that contain α and

C

β tubulin dimers. The 7.5-nm diameter microfilaments are actin polymers. In addition to their interactions with myosin filaments in muscle contraction, actin filaments may affect movement or cell shape through polymerization and depolymerization. Microfilaments participate in cytoplasmic streaming, ruffling of membranes, and phagocytosis. They may be responsible for limiting protein mobility in the cell membrane. The proteins of the 10-nm diameter intermediate filaments differ according to the cells in which they occur. Vimentin intermediate filaments occur in macrophages, lymphocytes, and endothelial cells, whereas desmin occurs in muscle and epithelial cells containing keratin.

cytosolic aspartate-specific proteases (CASPases)

Enzymes responsible for the deliberate disassembly of a cell into apoptotic bodies. Caspases are present as inactive proenzymes, most of which are activated by proteolytic cleavage. Caspase-8, caspase-9, and caspase-3 are situated at the pivotal junctions in apoptotic pathways. Caspase-8 initiates disassembly in response to extracellular apoptosis-inducing ligands and is activated in a complex associated with the receptor's cytoplasmic death domains. Caspase-9 activates disassembly in response to agents or insults that trigger release of cytochrome c from the mitochondria and is activated when complexed with dATP, APAF-1, and extramitochondrial cytochrome c. Caspase-3 appears to amplify caspase-8 and caspase-9 signals into a full-fledged commitment to disassembly. Both caspase-8 and caspase-9 can activate caspase-3 by proteolytic cleavage and caspase-3 may then cleave vital cellular proteins or activate additional caspase by proteolytic cleavage. Many other caspases have been described. Caspases are a group of proteases that proteolytically disassemble the cell. Caspases are present in healthy cells as inactive proforms. During apoptosis, most caspases are activated by proteolytic cleavage. Caspase-9, however, may be active without being proteolytically cleaved. Activation is through autoproteolysis or cleavage by other caspases. Cleavage of caspases generates a pro-domain fragment and subunits of approximately 20 and 10 kDa. Active caspases appear to be tetramers consisting of two identical 20 kDa subunits and two identical 10 kDa subunits. Detection of the 20- or 10-kDa subunit by immunoblotting may imply activation of the caspase. Colorimetric and fluorometric assays using fluorogenic peptide substrates can be used to measure caspase activity in apoptotic cells. Caspases cleave substrate proteins at the carboxyl terminus of specific aspartates. Tetrameric peptides with fluorometric or colorimetric groups at the carboxyl terminal have been used to determine the Km values of caspases. Although there is preference for peptides with a certain amino acid (aa) sequence, the aa sequence can have some variance. Caspases also have overlapping preferences for the tetrameric aa sequence (i.e., the same substrates can be cleaved by multiple caspases although one caspase may have a lower Km). Peptides containing groups that form covalent bonds with the cysteine residing at the active site of the caspase are often used to inhibit caspase activities.

cytotoxic

The ability to kill cells.

cytotoxic antibody

Antibody that combines with cell surface epitopes followed by complement fixation, which leads to cell lysis or cell membrane injury without lysis.

cytotoxic CD8 T cells

A T lymphocyte subset that expresses the CD8 coreceptor and recognizes peptide antigen presented in the context of major histocompatibility complex (MHC) class I molecules.

cytotoxic cytokines

Cytokines such as TNF and Ltα that induce fatal injury of cells.

cytotoxic drugs

Agents that kill self-replicating cells such as immunocompetent lymphocytes. Cytotoxic drugs have been used for anticancer therapy as well as for immunosuppression in the treatment of transplant rejection and aberrant immune responses. The four cytotoxic drugs commonly used for immunosuppression include cyclophosphamide, chlorambucil, azathioprine, and methotrexate.

cytotoxic T cells

T lymphocytes that fatally injure other cells. Most are major histocompatibility complex (MHC) class-I-restricted, CD8+ T lymphocytes even though CD4+ T cells may serve as killer cells in some instances. Cytotoxic T cells are significant in host resistance against viruses and other cytosolic pathogens.

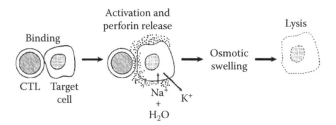

Cytotoxic T lymphocyte (CTL)-mediated target cell lysis.

cytotoxic T lymphocyte (CTL)

A subset of antigen-specific effector T cells that play a principal role in protection and recovery from viral infection, mediate allograft rejection, participate in selected autoimmune diseases, participate in protection and recovery from selected bacterial and parasitic infections, and are active in tumor immunity. They are CD8+, MHC class-I-restricted, nonproliferating, endstage effector cells. However, this classification also includes T cells that envoke one or several mechanisms to produce cytolysis, including perforin/granzyme, FasL/Fas, and tumor necrosis factor α (TNF-α); synthesize various lymphokines by T_H1 and T_H2 lymphocytes; and recognize foreign antigen in the context of MHC either class I or class II molecules.

cytotoxic T lymphocyte precursor (CTLp)

A progenitor that develops into a cytotoxic T lymphocyte after it has reacted with antigen and inducer T cells.

cytotoxicity

The fatal injury of target cells by specific antibody and complement or specifically sensitized cytotoxic T cells, activated macrophages, or natural killer (NK) cells. Dye exclusion tests are used to assay cytotoxicity produced by specific antibody and complement. Measurement of the release of radiolabel or other cellular constituents in the supernatant of the reacting medium is used to determine effector cell-mediated cytotoxicity.

cytotoxicity assays

Techniques to quantify the action of immunological effector cells in inducing cytolysis of target cells. The cell death

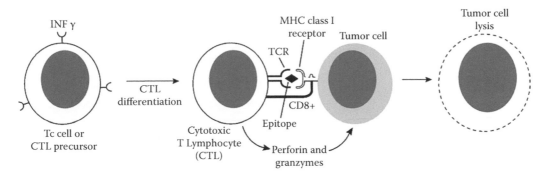

Cytotoxic T lymphocytc (CTL)-mediated tumor lysis.

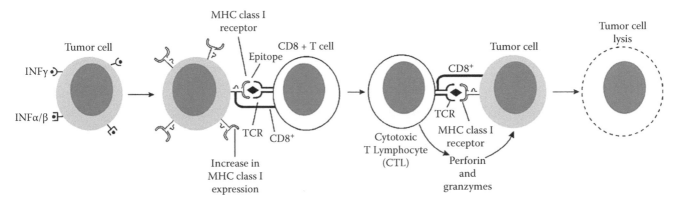

Cytotoxic T lymphocytc (CTL)-mediated killing of tumor cells.

induced can be programmed cell death (apoptosis), in which the nuclear DNA of the dying cell disintegrates and the cell membrane increases in permeability, or the cell death may be the result of necrosis that does not involve active metabolic processes and leads to increased membrane permeability without immediate nuclear disintegration. Cell-mediated cell lysis usually induces apoptosis, whereas antibody and complement usually induce necrosis. Cell death is determined by measurement of increased membrane permeability and by detecting DNA disintegration. The two methods used to determine membrane permeability of cells are dye exclusion, in which Trypan blue is used to stain dead cells but not viable ones, and the chromium release assay, in which target cells are labeled with radioactive ^{51}Cr, which is released from cells that develop increased membrane permeability as a consequence of immune attack. To quantitatively measure either DNA disintegration, ^{125}IUdR or ^{3}H-thymidine can be used to label nuclear DNA.

cytotoxicity tests
(1) Assays for the ability of specific antibody and complement to interrupt the integrity of a cell membrane, which permits a dye to enter and stain the cell. The relative proportion of cells stained, representing dead cells, is the basis for dye exclusion tests. Refer to microlymphocytotoxicity. (2) The ability of specifically sensitized T lymphocytes to kill target cells, the surface epitopes of which are the targets of their receptors. Loss of the structural integrity of the cell membrane is signified by the release of a radioisotope such as ^{51}Cr, which has been taken up by the target cells prior to the test. The amount of isotope released into the supernatant reflects the extent of cellular injury mediated by the effector T lymphocytes.

cytotoxins
Proteins synthesized by cytotoxic T lymphocytes that facilitate target cell destruction. Cytotoxins include perforins and granzymes or fragmentins, and granulysin.

cytotrophic antibodies
Immunoglobulin E (IgE) and IgG antibodies that sensitize cells by binding to Fc receptors on their surface, thereby sensitizing them for anaphylaxis. When the appropriate allergen crosslinks the Fab regions of the molecules, it leads to the degranulation of mast cells and basophils bearing IgE on their surface.

cytotropic anaphylaxis
Form of anaphylaxis caused by antigen binding to reaginic IgE antibodies. The latter are cytotropic; that is, they bind to cells. Cytotropic antibodies (immunoglobulin E [IgE]) bind to specific receptors on the mast cell surface. The receptors are in close proximity to a serine esterase enzyme, causing the release of mast cell granules, and to a natural inhibitor of this enzyme. As long as the surface IgE has not bound antigen, the *status quo* of the cell is maintained. It is believed that binding of the antigen induces a conformational alteration in the IgE, with displacement of the inhibitor from its steric relationship to the enzyme. The inhibition-free enzyme mediates the release. The process requires energy and is Ca^{2+} dependent.

D

d-amino acid polymers

Synthetic peptides (and polypeptides) that are antigenic. They are found very infrequently in living organisms.

D exon

A DNA sequence that encodes a portion of the third hypervariable region of the immunoglobulin heavy chain. It is situated on the 5′ sides of J exons. An intron lies between them. During lymphocyte differentiation, V–D–J sequences that encode the complete variable region of the heavy chain are produced.

D gene

A small segment of immunoglobulin heavy chain and T cell receptor DNA that encodes the third hypervariable regions of most receptors.

D gene region

Diversity region of the genome that encodes heavy chain sequences in the immunoglobulin heavy chain hypervariable region.

D gene segment

The DNA region that codes for the D (or diversity) portion of an immunoglobulin heavy chain or a T lymphocyte receptor β or δ chain. It is the segment that encodes the third hypervariable region situated between the chain regions that the V and J gene segments encode. This part of the heavy chain variable region is frequently significant in determining antibody specificity.

D region

A segment of an immunoglobulin heavy-chain variable region or the β or δ chain of the T lymphocyte receptor coded for by a D gene segment. A few residues constitute the D region in the third hypervariable region in most heavy chains of immunoglobulins. The D (or diversity) region governs antibody specificity and probably T cell receptor specificity, as well.

D3TX mice

More than 95% of female D3TX mice develop autoimmune oophoritis, whereas only 30% of D3TX male mice develop autoimmune orchitis. Following vasectomy, orchitis in D3TX mice increases to over 90%. Because vasectomy is associated with leakage of sperm antigens, the different incidence of orchitis and oophoritis in D3TX mice is believed to indicate a difference in the sequestration between testicular and ovarian antigens.

daclizumab

An immunosuppressive agent that acts as an IL2 receptor antagonist by binding with high affinity to the Tac subunit of the high affinity IL2 receptor complex and blocks IL2 binding. It is highly specific for Tac, which is expressed on activated but not resting lymphocytes. Daclizumab injection inhibits IL2-mediated activation of lymphocytes, which is important in cell-mediated immune responses in allograft rejection. Daclizumab in the circulation impairs the response of the immune system to antigenic challenge.

DAF

Refer to decay-accelerating factor.

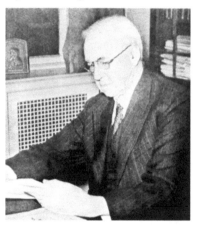

Henry Hallett Dale.

Dale, Henry Hallett (1875–1968)

British investigator who made a wide range of scientific contributions, including work on the chemistry of nerve impulse transmissions, the discovery of histamine, and the development of the Schultz–Dale test for anaphylaxis. He received a Nobel Prize in 1935.

Dalen–Fuchs nodule

A hemispherical granulomatous nodule composed of epithelioid cells and retinal epithelial cells in the choroids

Structure of Heavy Chain Gene From IgM-Producing Cell

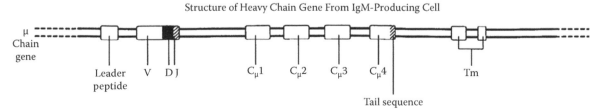

D exon and V segment.

of the eyes in patients with sympathetic ophthalmia and in some other diseases.

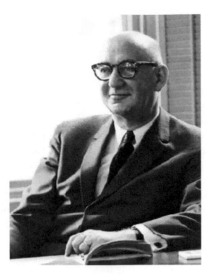

William Dameshek.

Dameshek, William (1900–1969)

Noted Russian-American hematologist who was among the first to understand autoimmune hemolytic anemias. He spent many years as editor-in-chief of *Blood*.

dander antigen

A combination of debris, such as desquamated epithelial cells, microorganisms, hair, and other materials trapped in perspiration and sebum, constantly deleted from the skin. Dander antigens may induce immediate, immunoglobulin E (IgE)-mediated, type I hypersensitivity reactions in atopic individuals.

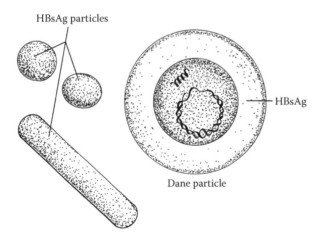

DANE particle.

DANE particle

A 42-nm structure identified by electron microscopy in hepatitis B patients in the acute infective stage. The DANE particle has a 27-nm-diameter icosahedral core that contains DNA polymerase.

danger signals

Molecules from stressed or dying cells or pathogens that unite with pattern recognition molecules of innate response

cells leading to inflammation. Exposure of immature dendritic cells to danger signals leads to their maturation and upregulation of costimulatory molecules, which permits them to activate rather than tolerize T cells. Bacterial CpG DNA, ds and ss viral RNA, inflammatory cytokines and chemokines, internal ROI, products of complement activation, and heat shock proteins are examples of danger signals.

danger theory

Refer to Matzinger danger theory.

Danysz, Jan (1860–1928)

Polish investigator who worked at the Institut Pasteur in Paris. The Danysz neutralization phenomenon was named for him. His wide-ranging interests included viruses that are pathogenic specifically for rodents. He subsequently investigated chemotherapeutic agents.

Danysz phenomenon (Danysz effect)

The addition of toxin to a homologous antitoxin in several fractions with appropriate time intervals between them, resulting in a greater toxicity of the mixture than would occur if the entire sample of toxin was added at once. A greater amount of antitoxin is required for neutralization if the toxin is added in divided doses than if all toxin is added at one time; conversely, less toxin is required to neutralize the given quantity of antitoxin if all toxin is added at one time instead of in divided doses at intervals. This form of reaction has been called the Danysz phenomenon or Danysz effect. Neutralization in the above instances is tested by injection of the toxin–antitoxin mixture into experimental animals. This phenomenon is attributed to the combination of toxin and antitoxin in multiple proportions. The addition of one fraction of toxin to excess antitoxin leads to maximal binding of antitoxin by toxin molecules. When a second fraction of toxin is added, insufficient antitoxin is available to bring about neutralization; therefore, the mixture is toxic due to uncombined excess toxin. Equilibrium is reached after an appropriate time interval. The interaction between toxin and antitoxin is considered to occur in two steps: (1) rapid combination of toxin and antitoxin, and (2) slower aggregation of the molecules.

dapsone

Diaminodiphenyl sulfone, a sulfa drug used in the treatment of leprosy. It has also shown efficacy for prophylaxis of malaria and for therapy of dermatitis herpetiformis.

DARC

Duffy antigen/chemokine receptor. It is a member of the G protein-coupled receptor family, the chemokine receptor branch of the rhodopsin family. It is expressed in erythroid cells in bone marrow. Ligands include the human malarial parasite *Plasmodium vivax*. β chemokine ligands include RANTES; MCP-1 and α chemokine ligands, including IL-8; and MGSA/GRO. DARC is also expressed in endothelial cells lining postcapillary venules and splenic sinusoids in individuals who are Duffy-negative. The receptor is also found in adult spleen, kidney, and brain, and fetal liver and is expressed in K562 and HEL cell lines. Also called erythrocyte chemokine receptor (erythrocyte CKR), RBC chemokine receptor, gpFy, and gpD.

dark zone

That part of a germinal center in secondary lymphoid tissue in which centroblasts undergo rapid division. Site where somatic hypermutation takes place.

DAT

Abbreviation for direct antiglobulin test. Refer to direct Coombs' test.

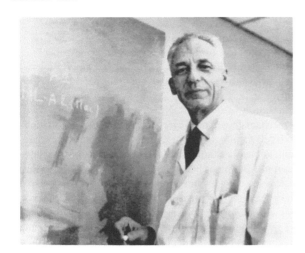

Jean Baptiste Gabriel Dausset.

Dausset, Jean Baptiste Gabriel (1916–)

French physician and investigator. He pioneered research on the human leukocyte antigen (HLA) system and the immunogenetics of histocompatibility. For this work he shared a Nobel prize with Benacerraf and Snell in 1980. (Refer to *Immunohematologie, Biologique et Clinique,* 1956; *HLA and Disease* [with Svejaard], 1977.)

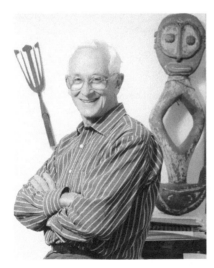

John R. David.

David, John R.

David demonstrated that immune lymphoid cells activated by their corresponding antigens secrete a substance that inhibits macrophage migration, a feature of delayed hypersensitivity. This soluble factor was designated migration inhibitory factor (MIF). David found that MIF had a molecular weight greater than 10,000 Da and was not preformed. Barry R. Bloom and associates proved that lymphocytes synthesized MIF and macrophages were the targets. The description of MIF and its properties was the first demonstration that soluble factors regulate immune responses and play a significant role in intercellular communication.

ddC (dideoxycytidine)

An inhibitor of reverse transcriptase used in AIDS treatment. It resembles ddI.

ddI (2′,3′-dideoxyinosine)

A purine analog that blocks human immunodeficiency virus 1 (HIV-1) *in vivo*. It is transformed into a triphosphorylated substance, ddATP, which blocks HIV reverse transcriptase and suppresses the replication of HIV by inhibiting viral DNA synthesis. Administration of ddI may be followed by an elevation in the CD4+ T helper cells and a significant decrease in p24 antigen, an indicator of HIV activity in the blood. Patients with acquired immune deficiency syndrome (AIDS) tolerate ddI better than they do zidovudine.

DDS syndrome

A hypersensitivity reaction that occurs in 1 in 5000 patients with leprosy who have been treated with dapsone (4,4′-diaminodiphenyl sulfone [DDS]), a drug that prevents folate synthesis by inhibiting the *p*-aminobenzoic acid condensation reaction. Patients develop hemolysis, agranulocytosis, and hypoalbuminemia, as well as exfoliative dermatitis and life-threatening hepatitis.

dead vaccine

Refer to inactivated vaccine.

Dean and Webb titration

Historically important antibody measurement assay. While the quantity of antiserum is held constant, varying dilutions of antigen are added, and the tube contents are mixed. The tube in which flocculation occurs first represents the endpoint. Within the tube, the ratio of antigen to antibody is in optimal proportions.

death by neglect

The mechanism whereby DP thymocytes with T cell receptors that are not functional undergo apoptosis. Also termed death by non-selection.

death by non-selection

Refer to death by neglect.

death domains

Protein molecular structures recognized as participating in protein–protein interactions. The name derives from the original definition related to proteins encoded by genes involved in apoptosis.

death receptor

A molecular configuration of the cell surface which, when engaged, initiates apoptosis. *Fas, TNFR1,* and DR5 are examples.

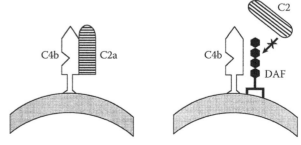

Decay accelerating factor.

decay accelerating factor (DAF)

A cell surface protein that blocks activation of complement on human cells. A 70-kDa membrane glycoprotein of normal human erythrocytes, leukocytes, and platelets that is absent from the red blood cells of paroxysmal nocturnal hemoglobulinuria patients. It facilitates dissociation of classical complement pathway C3 convertase (C4b2a) into C4b and C2a. It also promotes the dissociation of alternative complement pathway C3 convertase (C3bBb) into C3b and Bb. It inhibits C5 convertases (C4b2a3b and C3bBb3b) on the cell surface. DAF reacts with the convertases and destabilizes them by inducing rapid dissociation of a catalytic subunit C2a or Bb. The inhibitory effect of DAF is restricted to C3/C5 convertases bound to host cells; DAF does not inhibit normal complement activation on microbial or immune complex targets. DAF is found on selected mucosal epithelial cells and endothelial cells. It prevents complement cascade amplification on the surfaces of cells to protect them from injury by autologous complement. The physiologic function of DAF may be to protect cells from lysis by serum. DAF competes with C2 for linkage with C4b to block C3 convertase synthesis in the classical pathway. The DAF molecule consists of a single chain bound to the cell membrane by phosphatidylinositol. Paroxysmal nocturnal hemoglobulinuria develops as a consequence of DAF deficiency.

decomplementation

Deliberate inactivation of complement *in vitro* or *in vivo*. To decomplement serum to remove hemolytic action, the specimen may be heated to 56°C for 30 minutes. Other methods for inactivation of complement include the addition of cobra venom factor, zymosan, or other substances that take up complement from the medium in which they are placed. Removal of complement activity in living animals may be accomplished through the injection of cobra venom factor or other substances to use up or inactivate the complement system.

decorating

Term describing the reaction of tissue antigens with monoclonal antibodies, also known as staining in the immunoperoxidase reaction. Thus, a tissue antigen stained with a particular antibody is said to be decorated with that monoclonal antibody. Immunoperoxidase techniques give a reddish-brown color to the reaction product that is read by light microscopic observation.

defective endogenous retroviruses

Partial retroviral genomes that are integrated into host cell DNA and carried as host genes.

defensins

Widely reactive antimicrobial cationic proteins present in polymorphonuclear neutrophilic leukocyte granules. They block cell transport activities and are lethal for Gram-positive and Gram-negative microorganisms. These peptides are rich in cystesine and are found in the skin and in neutrophil granules that function as broad-spectrum antibiotics that kill numerous bacteria and fungi. The inflammatory cytokines, interleukin-1 (IL1) and tumor necrosis factor (TNF), facilitate synthesis of defensins. Defensins (human neutrophil proteins 1–4) are amphipathic, carbohydrate-free, cytotoxic, membrane-active antimicrobial molecules. Three of the defensin peptides (HP-1, HP-2, and HP-3) are nearly identical in sequence. By contrast, the sequences of HP-4, H-5, and HP-6 are very different. HP-1 and HP-2 are chemotactic for monocytes. High concentrations of HP-1 to -4 (25 to 200 μg/mL) manifest antimicrobial and/or viricidal properties *in vitro*. HP-4 has the greatest defensin activity, and HP-3 the least.

deficiency of secondary granules

A rare disorder in which neutrophils are bereft of secondary granules, a condition that has an autosomal-recessive mode of inheritance. Affected individuals show increased incidence of infection by pyogenic microorganisms.

degenerate binding specificity

A form of antigen-binding specificity shown by major histocompatibility complex (MHC) class I and II molecules. Each MHC allotype may bind numerous peptides of different amino acid sequences.

degranulation

A mechanism whereby cytoplasmic granules in cells fuse with cell membranes to discharge the contents from the cells. A classic example is degranulation of mast cells or basophils in immediate (type I) hypersensitivity. In phagocytic cells, cytoplasmic granules combine with phagosomes and release their contents into the phagolysosome formed by their union. The contents of intracytoplasmic granules are released to the outsides of cells, rendering the granules no longer visible microscopically. The discharge may be into a phagosome as well as into the external environment. Degranulation is observed in selected cells that participate in inflammatory and immunological reactions.

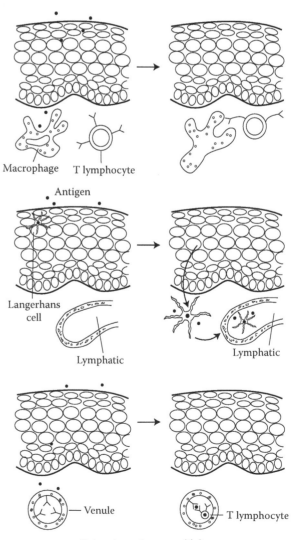

Delayed-type hypersensitivity.

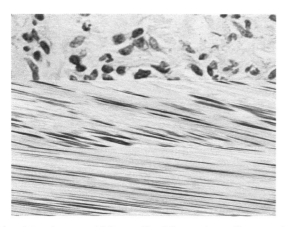

Delayed-type hypersensitivity reaction. Mononuclear cells accumulate around a blood vessel.

delayed-type hypersensitivity (DTH)

Cell-mediated immunity or hypersensitivity mediated by sensitized CD4 T_H1 lymphocytes. There is infiltration by T_H1 cells, macrophages, and basophils, and granuloma formation. Although originally described as a skin reaction that requires 24 to 48 hours to develop following challenge with antigen, current usage emphasizes the mechanism, which is T cell-mediated, as opposed to placing an emphasis on the temporal relationship of antigen injection and host response. The CD4+ T lymphocyte is the principal cell that mediates delayed-type hypersensitivity reactions. To induce a DTH reaction, antigen is injected intradermally in a primed individual. If the reaction is positive, an area of erythema and induration develops 24 to 48 hours following antigen challenge. Edema and infiltration by lymphocytes and macrophages occur at the local site. The CD4+ T lymphocytes identify antigen on Ia-positive macrophages and release lymphokines that entice

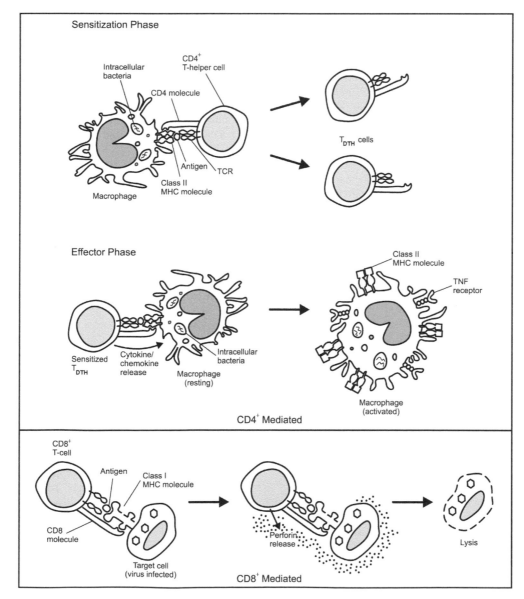

Schematic representation of type IV (cell-mediated) hypersensitivity. The upper frame illustrates tuberculin reactivity in the skin, which is mediated by CD4+ helper/inducer T cells and represents a form of bacterial allergy. The lower frame illustrates the cytotoxic action of CD8+ T cells against a virus-infected target cell that presents antigen via major histocompatibility complex (MHC) class I molecules to its T cell receptor (TCR), resulting in the release of perforin and granzyme molecules leading to target cell lysis.

D

more macrophages to enter the area, where they become activated. Skin tests are used clinically to reveal delayed-type hypersensitivity to infectious disease agents. Skin-test antigens include such substances as tuberculin, histoplasmin, and candidin. Tuberculin or purified protein derivative (PPD), which are extracts of the tubercle bacillus, have long been used to determine whether a patient has had previous contact with the organism from which the test antigen was derived. Delayed-type hypersensitivity reactions are always cell mediated. Thus, they have a mechanism strikingly different from anaphylaxis and the Arthus reaction that occur within minutes to hours following exposure of the host to antigen and are examples of antibody-mediated reactions. DTH is classified as type IV hypersensitivity (Coombs and Gell classification). Delayed-type hypersensitivity may be either permanent, persisting from a month to years after sensitization (as in classic tuberculin-type hypersensitivity), or transient, resembling the permanent type morphologically but disappearing 1 to 2 weeks following induction of sensitization. In the permanent type, the inflammatory reaction remains prominent 72 to 96 hours following intradermal injection of antigen, but the inflammatory reaction disappears 1 to 2 weeks after induction of sensitization in the transient type, in which the inflammatory lesion peaks at 24 hours but disappears by 48 to 72 hours (Jones–Mote hypersensitivity). The activation of T cells in DTH is associated with the secretion of cytokines. Activation of different subsets of T helper (T_H) cells leads to secretion of different types of cytokines. Those associated with a T_H1 CD4+ cellular response profile include interferon γ (IFN-γ), interleukin-2 (IL2), tumor necrosis factor β (TNF-β), TNF-α, granulocyte–macrophage colony-stimulating factor (GM-CSF), and IL3. Cytokines involved in a T_H2 CD4+ cellular response include IL3, IL4, IL5, IL6, IL10, IL13, TNF-α, and GM-CSF. T_H2-type immediate IgE-mediated hypersensitivity immune responses are induced by allergens such as animal dander, dust mites, and pollens, which underlie asthma. Positive tuberculin reactions induce T_H1-type DTH responses associated with T_H1 cytokines. T_H1 immunity may possibly inhibit atopic allergies by repressing T_H2 immune responses.

delayed xenograft rejection

Xenograft failure within days to weeks following transplantation. Attributable to ischemia that is a consequence of graft vascular endothelium hyperactivation caused by binding of anti-galactose-α (1-3) galactose antibodies. Also called acute vascular rejection.

deletional joining

An event during *V(D)J* recombination; both gene segments to be brought into apposition have the same transcriptional orientation.

delivery vehicle

A structure that is both inert and nontoxic and protects vaccine antigens from degradation by nuclease or protease. It may serve also as an adjuvant or increase antigen display. Examples include liposomes, virosomes, ISCOMs, SMAAs, and biodegradables.

delta agent (hepatitis D virus [HDV])

A viral etiologic agent of hepatitis that is a circular, single-stranded incomplete RNA virus without an envelope. It is a 1.7-kilobase virus and consists of a small, highly conserved domain and a larger domain manifesting epitope. HDV is a subviral satellite of the hepatitis B virus (HBV), on which it depends to fit its genome into virions. Thus, the patient

must first be infected with HBV to have HDV. Individuals with the delta agent in their blood are positive for HBsAg, anti-HBC, and often HBe. This agent is frequently present in intravenous drug abusers and may appear in patients with AIDS and in hemophiliacs.

δ chain

The heavy chain of immunoglobulin D (IgD).

denaturation

Changing the secondary and tertiary structures (coiling and folding) of a protein to produce a configuration that is uncoiled or coiled more randomly. Storage causes slow denaturation, but heating or chemical treatment may induce more rapid denaturation of native protein molecules. Denaturation diminishes protein solubility and often abrogates the biologic activity of the molecule. New or previously unexposed epitopes may be revealed as a consequence of denaturation.

dendritic cell immunotherapy

The lack of detectable tumor-specific immune responses in humans led to the use of autologous dendritic cells in active immunotherapy. Dendritic cells are expanded from progenitors *ex vivo*, charged with tumor antigens, and reinfused. Methods are being sought to genetically modify dendritic cells with antigens encoded by viral and nonviral vectors. Dendritic cells might also be used to vaccinate humans at the time a primary tumor is resected. This would permit an immune response to be available to act against metastases not detectable at the time the primary tumor is identified.

dendritic cells

Professional antigen-presenting cells with branched structures that are powerful activators of T cell responses. They are bone marrow-derived and distinct from follicular dendritic cells (DCs) that present antigen to B cells. Immature DCs are capable of antigen uptake and processing but are unable to activate T cells. Mature or activated DCs cells present in secondary lymphoid tissues are able to stimulate T cells. Subsets are derived from both myeloid and lymphoid lineages and comprise conventional and plasmacytoid DCs. Following activation by proinflammatory cytokines, DCs are attracted to draining lymph nodes where they mature and upregulate costimulatory molecule expression. Mature DCs are the only antigen-presenting cells that can activate naïve T cells. Modulated DCs facilitate development of peripheral tolerance. Mononuclear phagocytic cells are found in the skin as Langerhans' cells, in the lymph nodes as interdigitating cells, in the paracortex as veiled cells in the marginal sinuses of afferent lymphatics, and as mononuclear phagocytes in the spleen, where they present antigen to T lymphocytes. Dendritic reticular cells may have nonspecific esterase, Birbeck granules, endogenous peroxidase, possibly CD1, complement receptors CR1 and CR3, and Fc receptors. DCs are sentinels of the immune system. They originate from a bone marrow progenitor, travel through the blood, and are seeded into non-lymphoid tissues. DCs capture and process exogenous antigens for presentation as peptide–major histocompatibility complex (MHC) complexes at cell surfaces and then migrate via the blood and afferent lymph to secondary lymph nodes. In the lymph nodes, they interact with T lymphocytes to facilitate activation of helper and killer T cells. DCs have been named according to their appearance and distribution in the body. During the past decade, DCs have been further characterized by lineage, maturation stage, functional and phenotype characteristics of these stages, and by mechanisms involved in migration and function. DCs are being considered as adjuvants in immunization protocols for antiviral or antitumor immunity. Immature DCs are defined by cell surface markers that represent functional capacity. They express the chemokine receptors CCR-1, CCR-2, CCR-5, CCR-6, (only CD34+ HPC-derived DCs), and CXCR-1, commonly thought to allow DCs to migrate in response to inflammatory chemokines expressed by inflamed tissues. Immature DCs are phagocytic and have high levels of macropinocytosis, allowing them to efficiently process and present antigen on class I molecules. Expression of Fcγ (CD64) and the mannose receptors allows efficient capture of immunoglobulin G (IgG) immune complexes and antigens that expose mannose or fucose residues. The expression of E-cadherin allows DCs to interact with tissue cells and remain in the tissues until activated. Following antigen processing, DCs are remodeled. Fc and mannose receptors are downregulated and the acidic interacellular compartments disappear, resulting in a loss of endocytic activity. During this maturation process, the level of MHC class II molecules and costimulatory molecules are unregulated, and chemokine receptor expression changes. Maturing DCs home to T cell areas of secondary lymph nodes, where they present antigen to naïve T cells. *In vitro* culture of DCs with CD40-L, LPS, and TNF-α generates mature DCs. These cells are very good stimulators of allogeneic T cell proliferation. The DC–T cell interaction is thought to be a two-way interaction. Evidence suggests that T cells interact with DC through CD40 ligation to enhance DC viability and their T cell stimulatory ability. Addition of CD40-L induces DCs to produce interleukin-12 (IL12), which is known to support T_H1 responses. Lipopolysaccharide stimulation generates a weaker *in vitro* immune response than the CD40-L-stimulated DCs.

dendritic epidermal cell

Mouse epidermal cells that are Thy-1 positive and major histocompatibility complex (MHC) class II molecule-negative and possess γδ T cell receptor associated with CD3. This cell is believed to be a variety of bone marrow-derived T lymphocyte separate from Langerhans' cells in the skin.

dendritic epidermal T cells (deTC)

Specialized epidermal γδ T cells present in mice and selected other species but absent from human skin. These cells share a common γδ T cell receptor but their function is unknown.

dengue

An infection produced by the group B flavivirus arbovirus transmitted by the *Stegomyia Aedes aegypti* mosquito. Dengue fever, found in the tropical regions of Africa and America, may either be benign or produce malignant dengue hemorrhagic shock syndrome, in which patients experience severe bone pain (break bone fever). They have myalgia, biphasic fever, headache, lymphadenopathy, and a morbilliform maculopapular rash on the trunk. They also manifest thrombocytopenia and lymphocytopenia.

de novo **pathway of nucleic acid synthesis**

A biosynthetic mechanism whereby new nucleotides are constructed from amino acids. Aminopterin blocks the process.

dense deposit disease

Type II membranoproliferative glomerulonephritis is characterized by the deposition of electron-dense material, often containing C3, in the peripheral capillary basement membrane of the glomerulus. C3 is decreased in the serum

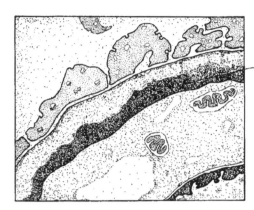

Dense deposits in glomerular capillary basement membrane

Dense deposit disease.

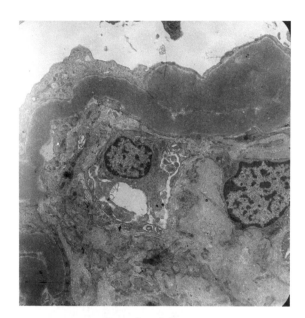

Dense deposit disease.

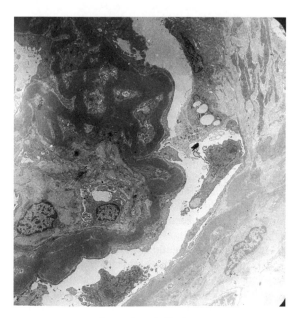

Dense deposit disease.

D

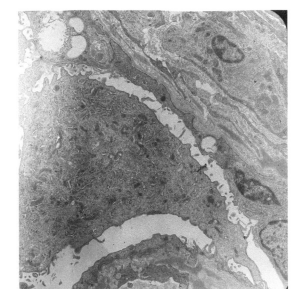

Dense deposit disease.

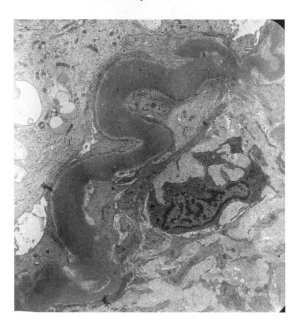

Dense deposit disease.

as a consequence of alternate complement pathway activation. C4 is normal. Sialic acid-rich glomerular basement membrane glycoproteins increase in number. Patients may possess a serum factor, termed nephritic factor, that activates the alternate complement pathway. This factor is an immunoglobulin molecule that reacts with alternate complement pathway-activated components such as the bimolecular C3b and activated factor B complex. Nephritic factor stabilizes alternate pathway C3 convertase.

density gradient centrifugation

The centrifugation of relatively large molecules such as in a solution of DNA with a density gradient substance such as cesium chloride. This method permits the separation of different types of cells as they are centrifuged through a density gradient produced by a substance to

which they are impermeable. A commonly used material is Ficoll–Hypaque. Separation of cells is according to size as they progress through the gradient. When they reach the level where their specific gravity is the same as that of the medium, cell bands of different density are produced. This technique is widely employed to separate hematopoietic cells.

deoxyguanosine

Refer to purine nucleoside phosphorylase (PNP) deficiency.

deoxyribonuclease

An endonuclease that catalyzes DNA hydrolysis.

deoxyribonuclease I

An enzyme that catalyzes DNA hydrolysis to a mono- and oligonucleotide mixture composed of fragments terminating in a 5′-phosphoryl nucleotide.

deoxyribonuclease II

An enzyme that catalyzes DNA hydrolysis to a mono- and oligonucleotide mixture composed of fragments terminating in a 3′-phosphoryl nucleotide.

deoxyribonucleoprotein antibodies

Antibodies reactive with insoluble deoxyribonucleoprotein (DNP) that occur in 60 to 70% of patients with active systemic lupus erythematosus (SLE). Immunoglobulin G (IgG) DNP antibodies, which fix complement, cause the LE cell phenomenon and yield a homogeneous staining pattern.

depot-forming adjuvants

Substances that facilitate an immune response by holding an antigen at the injection site following inoculation. Based on adjuvant-induced granuloma formation that facilitates the slow release of antigen over an extended time and helps attract macrophages and antigen-presenting cells to the site of antigen deposition. To be effective, the adjuvants must be administered with the antigen. Water-in-oil emulsions of the Freund type and aluminum salt (aluminum hydroxide) adjuvants are examples of depot-forming adjuvants. In the past, depot-forming and centrally acting adjuvants were distinguished. However, adjuvant action depends upon far more complicated cellular and molecular mechanisms than the simplistic views of depot formation advanced in the past.

dermatitis herpetiformis (DH)

A skin disease with grouped vesicles and urticaria that is related to celiac disease. Dietary gluten exacerbates the condition and should be avoided to help control it. Most patients (70%) manifest no bowel disease symptoms. Immunoglobulin A (IgA) and C3 granular immune deposits occur along dermal papillae at the dermal–epidermal junction. Groups of papules, plaques, or vesicles appear in a symmetrical distribution on knees, elbows, buttocks, posterior scalp, neck, and superior back region. The disease is chronic unless gluten is deleted from the diet. Neutrophils (PMNs) and fibrin collect at dermal papillae tips, producing microabscesses. Microscopic blisters, which ultimately develop into subepidermal blisters, may develop at the tips of these papillae. These lesions must be distinguished from those of bullous pemphigoid. DH is associated with HLA-B8, HLA-DR3, HLA-B44, and HLA-DR7 haplotypes.

dermatitis venenata

Refer to contact dermatitis.

dermatographism

Wheal-and-flare reaction of the immediate hypersensitivity type induced by scratching the skin. Thus, minor physical trauma induces degranulation of mast cells with the release of the pharmacological mediators of immediate hypersensitivity through physical stimulation. It is an example of an anaphylactoid reaction.

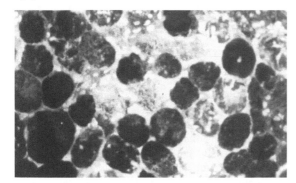

Dermatomyositis.

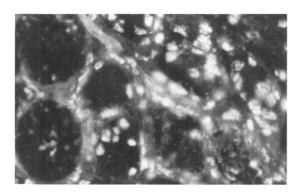

Dermatomyositis.

dermatomyositis

A connective tissue or collagen disease characterized by skin rash and muscle inflammation. It is a type of polymyositis presenting with a purple-tinged skin rash that is prominent on the superior eyelids, extensor joint surfaces, and base of the neck. Weakness, muscle pain, edema, and calcium deposits in the subcutaneous tissue are especially prominent late in the disease. Blood vessels reveal lymphocyte cuffing, and autoantibodies against tRNA synthetases appear in the serum.

dermatopathic lymphadenitis

Benign lymph node hyperplasia that follows skin inflammation or infection.

Dermatophagoides

The house mite genus. Constituents of house mites represent the main allergens in house dust.

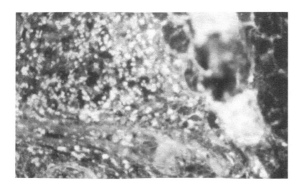

Dermatomyositis. Anti-IgG staining.

Dermatophagoides pteronyssinus

A house dust mite whose antigens may be responsible for house dust allergy in atopic individuals. It is a common cause of asthma.

dermatophytid reaction

Refer to id reaction.

dermis

The skin layer below the epidermis and basement membrane composed of blood vessels, lymphatic vessels, nerve fibers, scattered fibroblasts, macrophages, mast dells, dendritic cells and αβ T cells. The papillary dermis is beneath the basement membrane and the reticular dermis is beneath the papillary dermis. Both papillary and reticular dermis are comprised of collagen and elastin fiber networks in a hyaluronic acid matrix.

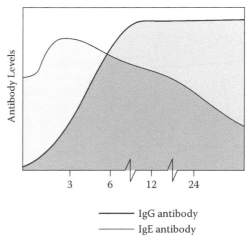

——— IgG antibody
——— IgE antibody

Desensitization.

desensitization

A method of treatment used by allergists to diminish the effects of immunoglobulin E (IgE)-mediated type I hypersensitivity. The mechanism is believed to alter the balance between CD4+ T_h1 and T_h2 cells, thereby switching the antibodies synthesized from IgE to IgG. The allergen to which an individual has been sensitized is repeatedly injected in a form that favors the generation of IgG (blocking) antibodies rather than IgE antibodies that mediate type I hypersensitivity in humans. This method has been used for many years to diminish the symptoms of atopy, such as asthma and allergic rhinitis, and prevent anaphylaxis produced by bee venom. IgG antibodies are believed to prevent antigen interaction with IgE antibodies anchored to mast cell surfaces by intercepting the antigen molecules before they reach the cell-bound IgE. Thus, a type I hypersensitivity reaction of the anaphylactic type is prevented.

desetope

A term that originates from determinant selection. It describes the regions of class II histocompatibility molecules that react with antigen during antigen presentation. Allelic variation permits these contact residues to vary, which is one of the factors in histocompatibility molecule selection of a particular epitope being presented.

designer antibody

A genetically engineered immunoglobulin needed for a specific purpose. The term has been used to refer to chimeric

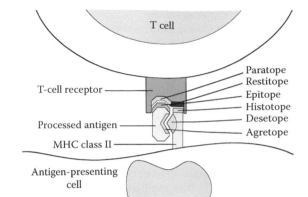

Interaction of major histocompatibility complex (MHC) class II, processed peptide, and T cell receptor molecules during antigen presentation.

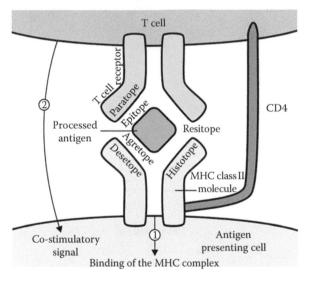

Costimulator for activation of T cells.

from the mouse antibody, while substituting the less immunogenic Fc region of the molecule from a human source. It greatly diminishes the likelihood of an immune response in humans receiving the hybrid immunoglobulin molecules, as most of the mouse immunoglobulin Fc region epitopes have been eliminated through the human Fc substitution.

designer lymphocytes

Lymphocytes into which genes have been introduced to increase the ability of cells to lyse tumor cells. Tumor-infiltrating lymphocytes transfected with these types of genes have been used in experimental adoptive immunotherapy.

desmin

A 55-kDa intermediate filament molecule found in mesenchymal cells that include both smooth and skeletal muscle, endothelial cells of the vessels, and probably myofibroblasts. In surgical pathologic diagnosis, monoclonal antibodies against desmin are useful to identify muscle tumors.

desmin (D33) mouse antibody

An antibody that detects a protein that is expressed by cells of normal smooth, skeletal and cardiac muscle. Light microscopy has suggested that desmin is primarily located at or near the peripheries of Z lines in striated muscle fibrils. In smooth muscle, desmin interconnects cytoplasmic dense bodies with membrane-bound dense plaques. Desmin antibody reacts with leiomyomas, rhabdomyomas, and perivascular cells of glomus tumors of the skin (if they are of myogenic nature). This antibody is basically used to demonstrate the myogenic components of carcinosarcomas and malignant mixed mesodermal tumors.

desmoglein

A protein constituent of desmosomes. A transmembrane glycoprotein that is one of the three components in a complex of epidermal polypeptides formed from the immunoprecipitate of pemphigus foliaceous autoantibodies.

desmosomes

Specialized junctions that connect keratinocytes to one another and guarantee that each keratinocyte layer divides and migrates upward as a unit.

desotope

A term derived from determinant selection. It describes the region of class II histocompatibility molecules that reacts

antibodies produced by linking mouse gene segments that encode the variable region of immunoglobulin with those that encode the constant region of a human immunoglobulin. This technique provides the antigen specificity obtained

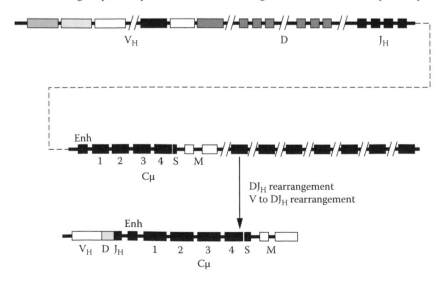

Designer antibody.

D

with the antigen during antigen presentation. Allelic variation permits these contact residues to vary, which is one of the factors in histocompatibility molecule selection of a particular epitope that is being presented.

despecification

A method for reducing the antigenicity of therapeutic antisera prepared in one species and used in another. To render immunoglobulin molecules less immunogenic in a heterologous recipient, they may be treated with pepsin to remove the most immunogenic portion of the molecule (*i.e.,* the Fc fragment) but leave intact the antigen bonding region (*i.e.,* F(ab′)₂ fragments) that retain their antitoxic properties. Had such a treatment been available earlier in the 20th century, serum sickness induced by horse antitoxin administered to human patients as a treatment for diphtheria would have been greatly reduced.

DETC

Dendritic epidermal T cells. Refer to intraepithelial lymphocytes.

determinant groups

Chemical mosaics found on macromolecular antigens that induce an immune response. Also called epitopes.

determinant selection model

Concept that immune response variability to a given antigen among different individuals is attributable to the ability of each person's MHC alleles to successfully bind and present that antigen's determinants.

determinant spreading

An amplification mechanism in inflammatory autoimmune disease in which the initial T lymphocyte response diversifies through induction of T cells against additional autoantigenic determinants. The response to the original epitope is followed by intramolecular spreading, the activation of T lymphocytes for other cryptic or subdominant self determinants of the same antigen during chronic and progressive disease; intermolecular spreading involves epitopes on other unrelated self antigens. A multideterminant protein antigen has dominant, subdominant, and cryptic T cell epitopes. The dominant epitopes are most efficiently processed and presented from native antigen. By contrast, cryptic determinants are inefficiently processed and/or presented. Only by immunization with a peptide that often requires no additional processing can a response to a cryptic determinant be mounted. Subdominant determinants fall between these two types.

deuterostomes

Coelomate-derived animals that developed into the vertebrates.

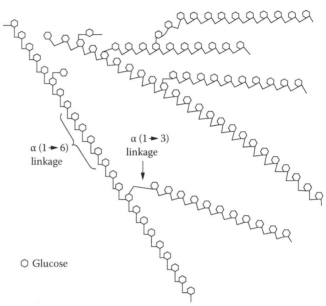

α (1–6) linkages and β (1–3) linkages in dextran molecule.

dextran

Polysaccharides of high molecular weight comprised of d-glucohomopolymers with α glycoside linkages, principally α-1,6 bonds. Dextrans serve as murine B lymphocyte mitogens. Some dextrans may also serve as thymus-independent

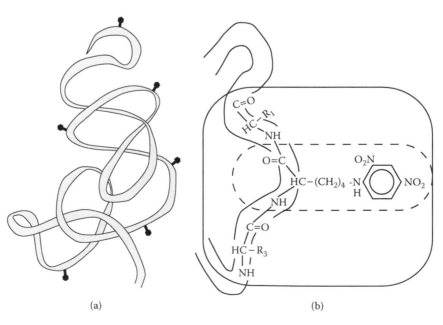

Determinant groups. (a) Conjugated protein with substituents. (b) Broken lines indicate haptenic group. Solid line indicates antigenic determinant.

antigens. Dextrans of relatively low molecular weight have been used as plasma expanders.

dhobi itch

Contact (type IV) hypersensitivity induced by using a laundry-marking ink made from Indian ral tree nuts. It occurs in subjects sensitized by wearing garments marked with such ink. It induces a dermatitis at sites of contact with the ink.

diabetes insipidus

A chronic idiopathic disease due to deficient secretion of vasopressin from the posterior lobe of the pituitary gland. Most cases of diabetes insipidus have a genetic basis or are secondary to recognized conditions that injure or destroy the hypothalamic neurohypophyseal complex, but in some cases an autoimmune response may be the cause. Antibodies have been demonstrated against cells that secrete vasopressin. The biopsy samples from rare cases have been consistent with autoimmune injury as reflected by a lymphocyte–plasma cell infiltrate in the neurohypophysis. Most serological studies for antibodies to vasopressin secreting cells have been reported.

diabetes mellitus

A metabolic disorder caused by the body's failure to synthesize insulin or the inability of its cells to respond to insulin normally. Without insulin, glucose is unable to enter cells and blood sugar levels increase. Characterized by increased thirst and hunger, emaciation, and weakness. Ketoacidosis that develops may lead to a diabetic coma.

diabetes mellitus, insulin-dependent (type 1)

In type I (autoimmune) diabetes mellitus, autoantibodies against islet cells (and insulin) may be identified. Among the three to six genes governing susceptibility to type I diabetes are those encoding the major histocompatibility complex (MHC). Understanding human diabetes has been greatly facilitated by both immunologic and genetic studies in experimental animal models, including nonobese diabetic (NOD) mice and biobreeding (BB) rats. Human type I diabetes mellitus results from autoimmune injury of pancreatic β cells. Specific autoantibodies signal pancreatic β cell destruction. The autoantibodies are against islet cell cytoplasmic, surface antigens, or insulin. Anti-idiotypic

antibodies may also develop against anti-insulin antibodies, possibly leading to antibody blockade of insulin receptors and thereby inducing insulin resistance and β cell exhaustion. Autoantibodies have also been demonstrated against a 64-kDa third islet cell antigen that may represent a primary target of autoimmune reactivity in type I diabetes and has been found in the sera of diabetics before clinical onset of the disease. Human leukocyte antigen (HLA) typing is also useful. DNA sequence analysis has revealed that alleles of HLA-DQ β chain govern diabetes susceptibility and resistance. The amino acid at position 57 has a critical role in disease susceptibility and resistance. Although pancreatic β cells fail to express MHC class II antigens under normal circumstances, they become Ia MHC class II antigen-positive following stimulation by interferon γ (IFN-γ) and tumor necrosis factor (TNF) or lymphotoxin. Pancreatic β cells that are class II-positive may present islet cell autoantigens to T lymphocytes, inaugurating an autoimmune response. Patients at risk for diabetes or prediabetes may benefit from immunosuppressive therapy such as cyclosporine, although most are still treated with insulin. Transplantation of pancreatic islet cells remains a bright possibility in future treatment strategies.

diacylglycerol (DAG)

A substance formed by the action of phospholipase C-γ on inositol phospholipids. DAG serves as an intracellular signaling molecule. It activates cytosolic protein kinase C, which further propagates the signal.

dialysis

The separation of a solution of molecules that differ in molecular weight by employing a semipermeable membrane. Antibody affinity is measured by equilibrium dialysis.

diapedesis

Leukocyte migration from the blood across blood vessel walls into tissue spaces as a consequence of constriction of endothelial cells in the wall. Flattened leukocytes squeeze between the endothelial cells of a post-capillary venule and, through their membranes, into the tissues.

diathelic immunization

Protective immunity induced by injecting antigen into the nipple or teat of a mammary gland.

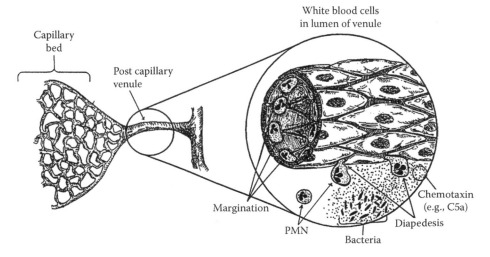

Diapedesis and margination.

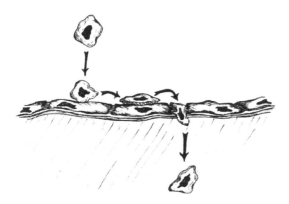

Diapedesis.

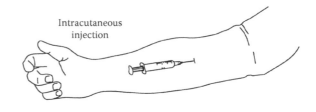

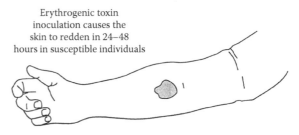

Dick test.

diazo salt

A diazonium salt prepared by diazotization from an arylamine to yield a product with a diazo group. Diazotization has been widely used in the preparation of hapten–carrier conjugates for use in experimental immunology.

diazotization

A method to introduce the diazo group into a molecule. Karl Landsteiner used this technique extensively in coupling low molecular weight chemicals acting as haptens to protein macromolecules serving as carriers. Aromatic amine derivatives can be coupled to side chains of selected amino acid residues to prepare protein–hapten conjugates that stimulate the synthesis of antibodies when used to immunize experimental animals such as rabbits. Some of these antibodies are specific for the hapten, which alone is unable to stimulate an immune response. An aromatic amine reacts with nitrous acid generated through the combination of sodium nitrite with HCL, then the diazonium salt is combined with the protein at a pH that is slightly alkaline. The reaction products include monosubstituted tyrosine and histidine and also lysine residues that are disubstituted.

DIC

Abbreviation for disseminated intravascular coagulation.

Dick test

A skin test to signify susceptibility to scarlet fever in subjects lacking protective antibody against the erythrogenic toxin of *Streptococcus pyogenes*. A minute quantity of diluted erythrogenic toxin is inoculated intradermally. An area of redness (erythema) occurs at the injection site 6 to 12 hours following inoculation of the diluted toxin in individuals who do not have neutralizing antibodies specific for the erythrogenic toxin and are therefore susceptible to scarlet fever. A heat-inactivated preparation of the same diluted toxin is also injected intradermally in the same individual as a control against nonspecific hypersensitivity to other products of the preparation.

differential RNA processing

Derivation of two structural forms of a protein from a single gene at the polyadenylation level. Numerous polyadenylation sites are situated following two or more exons. Primary RNA transcripts of varying lengths, including different exon and intron subsets, will be formed based on the particular site chosen for cleavage and polyadenylation. This process leads to proteins with alternative C terminal amino acid sequences.

differential signaling hypothesis

A proposal that antigens that differ qualitatively may mediate positive and negative selection of thymic T lymphocytes.

differentiation

Process whereby a developing precursor cell or an activated cell achieves functional specialization.

Diazotization.

D

differentiation antigen

Epitope that appears at various stages of development or in separate tissues. This cell surface antigenic determinant is present only on cells of a particular lineage and at a particular developmental stage; it may serve as an immunologic marker. An antigen of protein or carbohydrate composition that is linked only to a particular developmental stage. The inappropriate presence of a differentiation antigen in a tumor cell can render it a tumor-associated antigen.

differentiation factors

Substances that facilitate maturation of cells, such as the ability of interleukin-2 (IL2) to promote the growth of T cells.

diffusion coefficient

Mathematical representation of the diffusion rate of a protein in gel. The diffusion coefficient is useful in determining antigen molecular weight. It is the ratio of diffusion rate to concentration gradient.

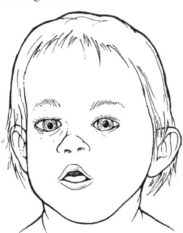

DiGeorge syndrome.

DiGeorge syndrome

A T cell immunodeficiency involving failure of T cell development but normal maturation of stem cells and B lymphocytes. This deficiency is attributable to failure in the development of the thymus, depriving the individual of the mechanism for T lymphocyte development. DiGeorge syndrome is a recessive genetic immunodeficiency characterized by failure of the thymic epithelium to develop. Maldevelopment of the thymus gland is associated with thymic hypoplasia. Anatomical structures derived from the third and fourth pharyngeal pouches during embryogenesis fail to develop, leading to defects in the functions of both the thymus and parathyroid glands. DiGeorge syndrome is believed to be a consequence of intrauterine malfunction. It is not familial. Tetany and hypocalcemia, both characteristics of hypoparathyroidism, are observed in DiGeorge syndrome, in addition to the defects in T cell immunity. Peripheral lymphoid tissues exhibit a deficiency of lymphocytes in thymic-dependent areas. By contrast, the B- or bursa equivalent-dependent areas such as lymphoid follicles show normal numbers of B lymphocytes and plasma cells. Serum immunoglobulin levels are within normal limits, and the immune response is normal following immunization with commonly employed immunogens. A defect in delayed-type hypersensitivity is demonstrated by the failure of affected patients to develop positive skin tests to commonly employed antigens such as candidin or streptokinase and the inability to develop an allograft response. Defective cell-mediated immunity may increase susceptibility to opportunistic infections and render a blood transfusion recipient vulnerable to a graft-vs.-host reaction. There is also minimal or absent *in vitro* responsiveness to T cell antigens or mitogens. The most significant advance has been the identification of microdeletions on human chromosome 22q11 in most DiGeorge syndrome patients. Considerable treatment success has been achieved with fetal thymic transplants and passive administration of thymic humoral factors.

dilution end point

A value expressed as the titer that reflects the lowest amount of an antibody giving a reaction. It is determined by serial dilution of the antibody in serum or other body fluid, while maintaining a constant amount of antigen.

dim

In flow cytometry, indicates the relative fluorescence intensities of cells being analyzed. *Dim* represents the lowest intensity, in contrast to *bright*, which designates the greatest intensity of fluorescence.

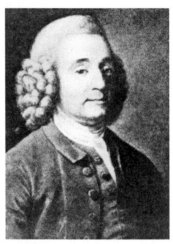

Dr. Dimsdale, a pioneer in smallpox vaccination.

Dimsdale, Dr. Thomas (1712–1800)

Of Hertford, wrote a popular and successful book entitled *The present method of inoculating for the smallpox*. He successfully inoculated Catherine the Great of Russia, her young son, the Grand Duke, and others, which popularized inoculation in Russia.

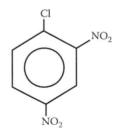

1-chloro-2, 4-dinitrobenzene

Dinitrochlorobenzene.

dinitrochlorobenzene (DNCB)

A substance employed to test capacity to develop a cell-mediated immune reaction. A solution of DNCB is applied to the skin of an individual not previously sensitized against this chemical, where it acts as a hapten, interacting with proteins of the skin. Re-exposure of this same individual to a second application of DNCB 2 weeks after the first challenge results in a T-cell-mediated, delayed-type hypersensitivity (contact dermatitis) reaction. Persons with impaired delayed-type hypersensitivity or cell-mediated immunity may reveal impaired responses. The 2,4-dinitro-1-chlorobenzene interacts with free α amino terminal groups in polypeptide chains and with side chains of lysine, tyrosine, histidine, cysteine, or other amino acid residues.

dinitrofluorobenzene (2,4-dinitro-1-fluorobenzene)(DNFB)

A chemical employed to prepare hapten–carrier conjugates. It inserts the 2,4-dinitrophenyl group into molecules containing free –NH$_2$ groups. When placed on the skin, it leads to contact hypersensitivity.

dinitrophenyl (DNP) group

Designation for 2,4-dinitrophenyl groups that become haptens after they are chemically linked to –NH$_2$ groups of proteins that interact with chlorodinitrobenzene, 2,4-dinitrobenzene sulphonic acid, or dinitrofluorobenzene. These protein carrier–DNP hapten antigens are useful as experimental immunogens. Antibodies specific for the DNP hapten that are generated through immunization with the carrier–hapten complex interact with low molecular weight substances that contain the DNP groups.

diphtheria and tetanus toxoids (adsorbed, injection)

The preparation intended for pediatric use (DT) is indicated for active immunization against diphtheria and tetanus in infants and children from 2 months to 7 years of age, for whom the use of combined vaccine containing pertussis antigen is contraindicated. The vaccine should be administered intramuscularly. The potency of tetanus and diphtheria toxoids has been determined based on immunogenicity studies, with comparison to a serological correlate of protection (0.01 antitoxin units/mL) established by the Panel on Review of Bacterial Vaccines and Toxoids. Results of the study indicated protective levels of antibody were raised in more than 90% of the study population after primary immunization with both components. Booster injections were effective in 100% of individuals with pre-existing antibody responses.

diphtheria and tetanus toxoids and acellular pertussis vaccine (adsorbed [DTaP], injection)

Intended for active immunization against diphtheria, tetanus and pertussis simultaneously in infants and children 6 weeks to 7 years of age (prior to seventh birthday). These preparations combine diphtheria and tetanus toxoids with acellular pertussis bacterial vaccine. The acellular pertussis antigens include pertussis toxin (PT), FHA, and pertactin. Immunization with diphtheria and tetanus toxoid is believed to confer protection lasting 10 years.

Nevertheless, diphtheria toxoid does not prevent carriage of *Corynebacterium diphtheriae* in the pharynx, nose, or skin. Protection against pertussis lasts 4 to 6 years. Serum diphtheria and tetanus antitoxin levels of 0.1 IU/mL and higher are considered protective. Efficacy of the pertussis component does not have a well established correlate of protection.

diphtheria antitoxin

An antibody generated by the hyperimmunization of horses against *Corynebacterium diphtheriae* exotoxin with injections of diphtheria toxoid and diphtheria toxins. When used earlier in the 20th century to treat children with diphtheria, many of the recipients developed serum sickness. It may be employed for passive immunization to treat diphtheria or for short-term protection during epidemics. Presently, pepsin digestion of the serum globulin fraction of the antitoxin yields F(ab′)$_2$ fragments of antibodies that retain their antigen-binding property but lose the highly antigenic Fc region. This process diminishes the development of serum sickness-type reactions and is called despecification.

diphtheria immunization

The repeated administration of diphtheria toxoids as alum-precipitated toxoids (APTs). Toxoid–antitoxin floccules (TAFs) constitute an alternate form for adults who show adverse reactions to adenosine triphosphate (APT). Besides this active immunization procedure, diphtheria antitoxin can also be given for passive immunization in the treatment of diphtheria.

diphtheria toxin

A 62-kDa protein exotoxin synthesized and secreted by *Corynebacterium diphtheriae*. The exotoxin, which is distributed in the blood, induces neuropathy and myocarditis in humans. Tryptic enzymes nick the single-chain diphtheria toxin. Thiols reduce the toxin to produce two fragments. The 40-kDa B fragment gains access to cells through their membranes, permitting the 21-kDa A fragments to enter. Whereas the B fragment is not toxic, the A fragment is toxic and it inactivates elongation factor 2, thereby blocking eukaryocytic protein synthesis. Guinea pigs are especially sensitive to diphtheria toxin, which causes necrosis at injection sites, hemorrhage of the adrenals, and other pathologic consequences. Animal tests developed earlier in the century consisted of intradermal inoculation of *C. diphtheriae* suspensions into the skin of unprotected guinea pigs compared to a control guinea pig that had been pretreated with passive administration of diphtheria antitoxin for protection. In later years, toxin generation was demonstrated *in vitro* by placing filter paper impregnated with antitoxin at right angles to streaks of *C. diphtheriae* microorganisms growing on media in Petri plates. Formalin treatment or storage converts the labile diphtheria toxin into toxoid. A secretory product of *Corynebacterium diphtheriae*, the etiologic agent of diphtheria, produces symptoms of the disease. Immunization requires the use of an inactive form of the toxin (diphtheria toxoid). Refer to diphtheria toxin and diphtheria toxoid.

D

diphtheria toxoid

An immunizing preparation generated by formalin inactivation of *Corynebacterium diphtheriae* exotoxins. This toxoid, used in the active immunization of children against diphtheria, is usually administered as a triple vaccine that includes pertussis microorganisms and tetanus toxoid as a purified toxoid absorbed to hydrated aluminum phosphate (PTAP) or as an alum-precipitated toxoid (APT). Infants immunized with one of these preparations develop active immunity against diphtheria. Toxoid–antitoxin floccules (TAFs) may be administered to adults who demonstrate adverse hypersensitivity reactions to toxoids.

diphtheria vaccine

An immunizing preparation to protect against *Corynebacterium diphtheriae*. Refer to DTaP vaccine.

diploid

A descriptor to indicate dual copies of each autosome and two sex chromosomes in a cell nucleus. The diploid cell has twice the number of chromosomes in a haploid cell.

direct agglutination

The aggregation of particulate antigens such as microorganisms, red cells, or antigen-coated latex particles when they react with specific antibody.

direct allorecognition

The process whereby the T cells of a transplant recipient detect peptide/allo-MHC epitopes on allogeneic graft donor cell surfaces. Refer to allorecognition.

direct amplicon analysis

A technique used in HLA tissue typing for the identification of an unknown HLA allele through discovery of the specific CR primers capable of amplifying a polymorphic region of a gene. Gel electrophoresis and ethidium bromide staining are used to detect the products of amplification.

direct antigen presentation

Cell surface allogeneic major histocompatibility complex (MHC) molecule presentation by graft cells to T lymphocytes of the graft recipient leading to T lymphocyte activation. No processing is required. Direct recognition of foreign MHC molecules is a crossreaction between a normal T cell receptor (TCR) that recognizes self MHC molecules plus foreign antigen and the allogeneic MHC molecule–peptide complex. The powerful T cell response to allografts is due in part to direct presentation.

direct antiglobulin test

An assay in which washed erythrocytes are combined with antiglobulin antibody. If the red cells had been coated with nonagglutinating (incomplete) antibody *in vivo*, agglutination would occur. Examples of this in humans include hemolytic disease of the newborn in which maternal antibodies coat the infant's erythrocytes, and autoimmune hemolytic anemia in which the subject's red cells are coated with autoantibodies. The coating is the basis of the direct Coombs' test.

direct Coombs' test

Refer to direct antiglobulin test.

direct fluorescence antibody method

The use of polyclonal or monoclonal antibodies labeled with a fluorochrome such as fluorescein isothiocyanate that yields an apple-green color by immunofluorescence microscopy, or rhodamine isothiocyanate that produces a reddish-orange color, to identify a specific antigen. This technique

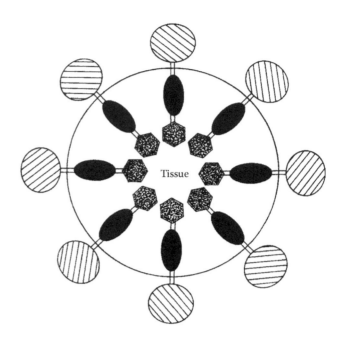

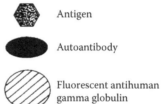

Antigen

Autoantibody

Fluorescent antihuman gamma globulin

Direct fluorescence antibody technique.

is routinely used in immunofluorescence evaluation of renal biopsy specimens and skin biopsy preparations to detect immune complexes comprised of various immunoglobulin classes or complement components.

direct immunofluorescence

The use of fluorochrome-labeled antibody to identify antigens, especially those of tissues and cells. An example is the immunofluorescence evaluation of renal biopsy specimens.

direct pathway of allorecognition

The process whereby a transplant recipient's T cells are stimulated by interactions of their receptors with the transplant donor's dendritic allogeneic HLA molecules.

direct reaction

Skin reaction caused by the intracutaneous injection of viable or nonviable lymphocytes into a host that has been sensitized against donor tissue antigens. This represents a type IV hypersensitivity reaction, which is classified as a delayed-type reaction mediated by T cells. Reactivity is against lymphocyte surface epitopes.

direct staining

A version of the fluorescent antibody staining technique in which a primary antibody has been conjugated with a fluorochrome and applied directly to a tissue sample containing the antigen in question.

direct tag assays

A method in which a tagged antigen or antibody is employed to detect its untagged specific or complementary antibody or antigen.

directional flow

Inhaled microorganisms in dust or droplets greater than 5 μm adhere to the mucosa lining the upper respiratory tract and are swept upward by cilia to the posterior pharynx followed by expectoration or swallowing.

directional selection

A form of natural selection in which older alleles are replaced with newer variants, as in the MHC, leading to change.

discoid lupus erythematosus

A type of lupus erythematosus that involves only the skin, which manifests a characteristic rash. The viscera are not involved. The skin manifests erythematous plaques and telangiectasis with plugging of the follicles. Also called cutaneous lupus erythematosus.

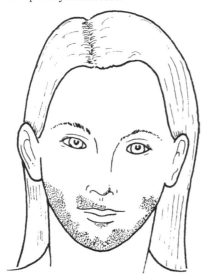

Discoid lupus erythematosus.

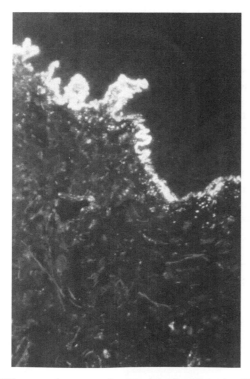

Discoid lupus erythematosus. Immune deposits at dermal–epidermal junction.

discontinuous epitope

Refer to conformational epitope.

disintegrin

Low molecular weight peptide found in several different snake venoms. Disintegrins interrupt integrin function by blocking their interactions with surface receptors. Thus, they function as integrin inhibitory proteins.

disodium cromoglycate

A valuable drug for treating immediate (type I) hypersensitivity reactions, especially allergic asthma. Although commonly used as an inhalant, it may also be administered orally or applied topically to the nose and eyes. Mechanisms of action that have been postulated include mast cell membrane stabilization and bridging of immunoglobulin E (IgE) on mast cell surfaces, thereby blocking bridging by antigen.

disseminated intravascular coagulation (DIC)

A tendency to favor coagulation over fibrinolysis in the blood circulation as a consequence of various factors. In DIC, 30 to 65% of the cases are due to infection. Fast or slow DIC may occur. The fast variety is characterized by acute, fulminant, consumptive coagulopathy with bleeding as a result of Gram-negative substances, massive tissue injury, burns, etc. Deficient or consumed coagulation factors must be replaced in fast DIC. Slow DIC accompanies chronic diseases characterized by thrombosis, microcirculatory ischemia, and end-organ function. Examples include acute promyelocytic leukemia, neoplasia, and vasculitis. The pathogenesis includes endothelial cell damage produced by endotoxins or other agents, activation of platelets, and activation of the intrinsic coagulation pathway. Tissue thromboplastin may be released by trauma or neoplasia, leading to activation of the extrinsic pathway. Patients with DIC have elevated partial thromboplastin time, prothrombin time, fibrinopeptide A, and fibrinogen degradation products along with decreased fibrinogen, factor V, platelets, antithrombin III, factor VIII, and plasminogen. Diffuse cortical necrosis of the kidneys occurs.

dissociation constant

The equilibrium constant for dissociation. This is usually described in enzyme–substrate interactions. If the interaction of enzyme with substrate attains equilibrium prior to catalysis, the Michaelis constant (K_M) represents the dissociation constant. The Michaelis constant is equivalent to the concentration substrate when the reaction velocity is half maximal.

distemper vaccine

An attenuated canine distemper virus vaccine prepared from virus grown in tissue culture or chick embryos.

distribution ratio

The ratio of plasma immunoglobulin to whole-body immunoglobulin.

disulfide bonds

The S–S chemical bonds between amino acids that link polypeptide chains together. Chemical reduction may break these bonds. Disulfide bonds in immunoglobulin molecules are either intrachain or interchain (*i.e.*, linking heavy to light chains and heavy to heavy chains). The different types of bonds in immunoglobulin molecules differ in their ease of chemical reduction.

D

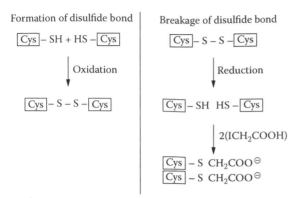

Formation of disulfide bond | Breakage of disulfide bond

Formation of disulfide bonds from the oxidation of two sulfhydryl groups and the breaking of disulfide bonds through reduction, leading to sulfhydryl formation.

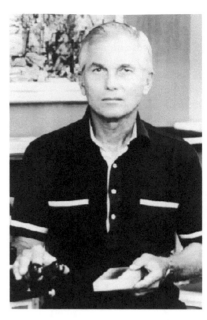

Frank James Dixon.

diversity

The presence of numerous lymphocytes with different antigenic specificities to create a lymphocyte repertoire that is large and varied. Diversity, which is critical to adaptive immune responsiveness, is a consequence of structural variability in antigen-binding sites of lymphocyte receptors for antigen (antibodies and TCRs).

diversity (D) gene segments

Abbreviated coding sequences between the V and constant gene segments in the immunoglobulin heavy chain and T cell receptor β and δ loci together with J segments are recombined somatically with V segments during lymphocyte development. The recombined VDJ DNA encodes the carboxyl terminal ends of the antigen receptor V regions, including the third hypervariable (CDR) regions. D segments used randomly contribute to antigen receptor repertoire diversity.

Dixon, Frank James (1920–2008)

American physician noted for his fundamental contributions to immunopathology, particularly the role of immune complexes in the production of disease. He is also known for his work on antibody formation. Dixon was the founding director of the Research Institute of Scripps Clinic.

DN thymocytes

Double negative thymocytes that fail to express either CD4 or CD8 molecules. Thus, they have a CD4⁻ CD8⁻ surface phenotype. The four DN thymocyte subpopulations are designated DN1 through DN4.

DNA binding motif

A nuclear transcription factor binding site variably present in genomic DNA, such as KB that binds NF-KB and ISRE (interferon-stimulated response element) that binds IRFs.

DNA-dependent RNA polymerase

An enzyme that participates in DNA transcription. With DNA as a template, it catalyzes RNA synthesis from the ribonucleoside-5′-triphosphates.

DNA fingerprinting

A method used to demonstrate short, tandem-repeated highly specific genomic sequences known as mini satellites. The probability that two persons would have the identical DNA fingerprint is only 1 in 30 billion. DNA fingerprinting has greater specificity than restriction fragment length polymorphism (RFLP) analysis. Each individual has a different number of repeats. The insert-free, wild-type M13 bacteriophage identifies the hypervariable mini satellites. The sequence of DNA that identifies the differences is confined to two clusters of 15 base-pair repeats in the protein III gene of the bacteriophage. The specificity of this probe, known as the Jeffries probe, renders it applicable to parentage testing, human genome mapping, and forensic science. RNA may also be split into fragments by an enzymatic digestion followed by electrophoresis. A characteristic pattern for that molecule is produced and aids in identifying it.

DNA laddering

Endonucleases are activated during apoptosis. Activated endonucleases nick genomic DNA at internucleosomal sites to produce DNA fragments. Not all cell types

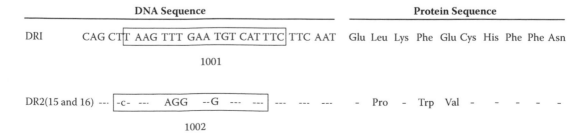

	DNA Sequence	Protein Sequence
DRI	CAG CT|T AAG TTT GAA TGT CAT TTC|TTC AAT	Glu Leu Lys Phe Glu Cys His Phe Phe Asn
	1001	
DR2(15 and 16)	--- |-c- --- AGG --G --- ---| --- --- ---	- Pro - Trp Val - - - - -
	1002	

DNA fingerprinting.

generate uniformly nicked genomic DNA during apoptosis. Following gel electrophoresis, DNA fragments migrate in a pattern resembling a ladder, with individual bands differing by approximately 200 base pairs.

DNA library

A gene library or clone library comprised of multiple nucleotide sequences that are representative of all sections of the DNA in a particular genome. It is a random assemblage of DNA fragments from one organism, linked to vectors and cloned in an appropriate host. This prevents any individual sequence from being systematically excluded. Adjacent clones will overlap, and cloning large fragments helps to ensure that the library will contain all sequences. The DNA to be investigated is reduced to fragments by enzymatic or mechanical treatment, and the fragments are linked to appropriate vectors such as plasmids or viruses. The altered vectors are then introduced into host cells. This is followed by cloning. Transcribed DNA fragments (exons) and nontranscribed DNA fragments (introns or spacers) are part of the gene library. A probe may be used to screen a gene library to locate specific DNA sequences.

DNA ligase

An enzyme that joins DNA strands during repair and replication. It serves as a catalyst in phosphodiester, binding between the 3′-OH and the 5′-PO_4 of the phosphate backbone of DNA.

DNA microarray

A technique in which a different DNA is placed on a small section of a microchip. The microarray is then used to evaluate expression of RNA in normal or neoplastic cells.

DNA nucleotidylexotransferase (terminal deoxynucleotidyl transferase [TdT])

DNA polymerase that randomly catalyzes deoxynucleotide addition to the 3′-OH end of a DNA strand in the absence of a template. It can also be employed to add homopolymer tails. Immature T and B lymphocytes contain TdT. The thymus is rich in TdT, which is also present in the bone marrow. TdT inserts a few nucleotides in T cell receptor and immunoglobulin gene segments at the V–D, D–J, and V–J junctions. This enhances sequence diversity.

DNA polymerase

An enzyme that catalyzes DNA synthesis from deoxyribonucleotide triphosphate by employing a template of either single- or double-stranded DNA. This is known as DNA-dependent (direct) DNA polymerase, in contrast to RNA-dependent (direct) DNA polymerase, which employs an RNA template for DNA synthesis.

DNA polymerase I

DNA-dependent DNA polymerase whose principal function is in DNA repair and synthesis. It catalyzes DNA synthesis in the 5′ to 3′ sense. It also has a proofreading function (3′ → 5′ exonuclease) and a 5′ → 3′ exonuclease.

DNA polymerase II

DNA-dependent DNA polymerase in prokaryotes. It catalyzes DNA synthesis in the 5′ to 3′ sense, has a proofreading function (3′ → 5′ exonuclease), and is thought to play a role in DNA repair.

DNA polymerase III

DNA-dependent DNA polymerase in prokaryotes that catalyzes DNA synthesis in the 5′ to 3′ sense. It is the principal synthetic enzyme in DNA replication. It has a proofreading function (3′ → 5′ exonuclease) and 5′ → 3′ exonuclease activity.

DNA repair

Elimination of DNA mutations to maintain stability of the genome. Facilitated by the NHEJ, homologous recombination, and nucleotide excision pathways.

DNA vaccination

Immunization with plasmid DNA to induce an adaptive immune response against the encoded protein. Bacterial DNA, which is rich in unmethylated CpG dinucleotides, serves as an adjuvant for this kind of vaccination.

DNA vaccine

An immunizing preparation composed of a bacterial plasmid containing a cDNA encoding a protein antigen. The mechanism apparently consists of professional antigen-presenting cells transfected *in vivo* by the plasmid which then express immunogenic peptides that induce specific immune responses. The CpG nucleotides present in the plasmid DNA serve as powerful adjuvants. DNA vaccines may induce strong cytotoxic T lymphocyte responses. This is an immunizing preparation prepared by genetic engineering methods in which the gene that encodes an antigen is inserted into a bacterial plasmid, which is injected into the host. Once inside, the gene employs the nuclear machinery of the host cell to manufacture and express the antigen. In contrast to other vaccines, DNA vaccines may induce cellular as well as humoral immune responses.

DNBS (2,4-dinitrobenzene sulfonate)

A substance employed to generate dinitrophenylated proteins used as experimental antigens. Chemically, DNBS reacts principally with lysine residue-free ε amino groups if an alkaline pH is maintained.

DNCB

Refer to dinitrochlorobenzene.

DNP

Refer to dinitrophenyl group.

DO and DM

Major histocompatibility complex (MHC) class II-like molecules. DO gene expression occurs exclusively in the thymus and on B lymphocytes. DNα and DOβ chains pair to produce the DO molecule. Information related to DM gene products awaits further investigation.

doctrine of original antigenic sin

The immune response against a virus, such as a parental strain, to which an individual was previously exposed may be greater than it is against the immunizing agent, such as type A influenza virus variant. This concept is known as the doctrine of original antigenic sin.

Activity of terminal deoxnucleotidyl transferase (TdT).

D

Doherty, Peter (1940–)

Recipient with Rolf Zinkernagel of the 1996 Nobel Prize for physiology or medicine for their demonstration of major histocompatibility complex (MHC) restriction. In an investigation of how T lymphocytes protect mice against lymphocytic choriomeningitis virus (LCMV) infection, they found that T cells from mice infected by the virus killed only infected target cells expressing a different MHC allele. In the study, murine cytotoxic T cells (CTL) would only lyse virus-infected target cells that were H-2 compatible. This significant finding had broad implications, demonstrating that T cells did not recognize the virus directly but only in conjunction with MHC molecules. Refer also to Zinkernagel, Rolf.

domain

A region of a protein or polypeptide chain that is globular and folded with 40 to 400 amino acid residues. The domain may have a spatially distinct "signature" that permits it to interact specifically with receptors or other proteins. In immunology, domains are the loops in polypeptide chains that are linked by disulfide bonds on constant and variable regions of immunoglobulin molecule light and heavy polypeptide chains or compact T cell receptor (TCR) chain segments composed of amino acids around an S–S bond.

dome

A mucosal lymphoid follicle area comprised of dendritic cells, macrophages, CD4+ T cells, regulatory T cells, and mature B cells that covers a germinal center.

domesticated mouse

A mouse that has adjusted to a captive existence.

dominant negative transgene

A transgene whose product is a protein that is not functional and disrupts the endogenous protein's function or expression.

dominant phenotype

Trait manifested in an individual who is heterozygous at the gene locus of interest.

Donath–Landsteiner antibody

An immunoglobulin specific for P blood group antigens on human erythrocytes. This antibody binds to the patient's red blood cells at cold temperatures and induces hemolysis on warming. It occurs in subjects with paroxysmal cold hemaglobulinemia (PCH). Also called Donath–Landsteiner cold autoantibody.

donor

An individual who offers whole blood, blood products, bone marrow, or an organ to be given to another individual. Individuals who are drug addicts or test positively for certain diseases such as HIV-1 infection or hepatitis B, for example, are not suitable as donors. There are various other reasons for donor rejection not listed here. To be a blood donor, an individual must meet certain criteria, including those pertaining to blood pressure, temperature, hematocrit, pulse, and history. Among the many reasons for donor rejection are low hematocrit, skin lesions, recent surgery, drugs, or positive donor blood tests.

donor cell infusion

The administration of donor bone marrow or hematopoietic stem cells to the recipient of a solid organ transplant to establish chimerism and donor cell acceptance.

dopamine neuron autoantibodies

Autoantibodies against dopamine neurons in the substantia nigra in approximately 78% of cerebrospinal fluid (CSF) from patients with Parkinson's disease and in 3% of normal CSF from subjects with other neurological diseases. Transplantation of adrenal medulla leads to disappearance of the autoantibodies.

dot blot

A rapid hybridization method to partially quantify a specific RNA or DNA fragment found in a specimen without the need for a Northern or Southern blot. After serially diluting DNA, it is "spotted" on a nylon or nitrocellulose membrane and then denatured with NaOH. It is then exposed to a heat-denatured DNA fragment probe believed to be complementary to the nucleic acid fragment to be identified. The probe is labeled with ^{32}P or ^{35}S. When the two strands are complementary, hybridization takes place. This is detected by autoradiography of the radiolabeled probe. Enzymatic, nonradioactive labels may also be employed.

dot DAT

A variation of the Coombs' test known as a dot blot direct antiglobulin test. Immunoglobulin G (IgG) is fixed on a solid-phase support or nitrocellulose membrane. The patient's erythrocytes are incubated on the membrane. This technique eliminates subjective interpretation of results, diminishing the numbers of false positives and false negatives.

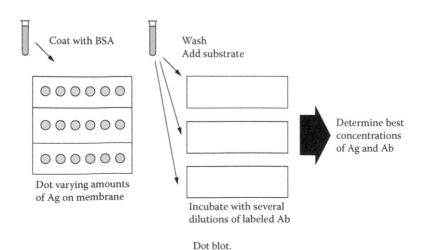

Dot blot.

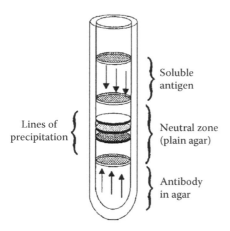

Double diffusion test.

double diffusion test

A test in which soluble antigen and antibody are placed in separate wells of a gel containing electrolyte. The antigen and antibody diffuse toward one another until their molecules meet at the point of equivalence and precipitate, forming a line of precipitation in the gel. In addition to the two-dimensional technique, double immunodiffusion may be accomplished in a tube as a one-dimensional technique. The Oakley–Fulthorpe test is an example of this type of reaction. This technique may be employed to detect whether antigens are similar or different or share epitopes. It may also be used to investigate antigen and antibody purity. Refer also to reaction of identity, reaction of nonidentity, and reaction of partial identity.

double emulsion adjuvant

Water-in-oil-in-water emulsion adjuvant.

double immunodiffusion

A precipitation reaction in gel media in which both antibody and antigen diffuse radially from wells toward each other, thereby forming a concentration gradient. A visible line of precipitation forms as equivalence is reached.

double layer fluorescent antibody technique

An immunofluorescence method to identify antigen in a tissue section or cell preparation on a slide by first covering and incubating it with antibody or serum containing antibody that is not labeled with a fluorochrome. After an appropriate time for interaction, the preparation is washed, and a second application of fluorochrome-labeled antibody such as goat or rabbit antihuman immunoglobulin is applied to the tissue or cell preparation and it is again incubated. This technique has greater sensitivity than does the single layer immunofluorescent method. Examples include applying serum from a patient with Goodpasture's syndrome to a normal kidney section that acts as substrate, incubating and washing, and then covering the preparation with fluorochrome-labeled goat antihuman immunoglobulin G (IgG) to detect antiglomerular basement membrane antibodies in the patient's serum. A similar procedure is used in detecting antibodies against intercellular substance antigens in the serum of patients with pemphigus vulgaris.

double negative (DN) cell

A stage in the development of T lymphocytes in which differentiating α/β T lymphocytes do not possess T cell receptors and do not manifest either the CD4 or the CD8 coreceptor.

double negative thymocyte

Immature T cell that fails to express either CD4 or CD8 molecules. CD4$^-$ CD8$^-$ thymocytes that are few in number and serve as progenitors for all other thymocytes. They represent an intermediate step between pluripotent bone marrow stem cells and immature cells destined to follow T cell development. Significant heterogeneity is present in this cell population. Peripheral extrathymic CD4$^-$ CD8$^-$ T cells have been examined in both skin and spleens of mice, and, like their corresponding cells in the thymus, they express T cell receptor (TCR) $\gamma\delta$ proteins. These double negative cell populations are greatly expanded in certain autoimmune mouse strains such as those expressing the *lpr* or *gld* genes. Available evidence reveals two thymic populations of CD4$^-$ CD8$^-$ cells. Immature double negative bone marrow graft cells have stem cell features. However, double negative cells of greater maturity and without stem cell functions quickly repopulate the thymus. Most double negative thymocytes are in an early stage of development and fail to express antigen receptors.

double positive (DP) cell

A T lymphocyte developmental stage in which differentiating α/β T cells manifest the pre-T cell receptor and both CD4 and CD8 coreceptors.

double positive thymocyte

Cell at an intermediate stage of T lymphocyte development in the thymus that expresses both the CD4 and CD8 coreceptor proteins. These thymocytes also express T cell receptors and are exposed to selection processes that culminate in mature single-positive T lymphocytes that express only CD4 or CD8.

double-stranded DNA antibodies

Antibodies associated with systemic lupus erythematosus (SLE) that may be studied serially using the Farr (ammonium sulfate precipitation) assay to predict activity of the disease and monitor treatment. dsDNA antibody levels are interpreted in conjunction with serum C3 or C4 concentrations. If the dsDNA antibody level doubles or exceeds 30 IU/mL earlier than 10 weeks, an exacerbation of SLE is likely, especially if there is an associated decrease in the serum C4 concentration. This reflects selective stimulation of B cell stimulation known to occur in SLE patients. The Farr assay is more reliable than the enzyme immunoassay method, because the Farr assay measures high avidity antibodies to dsDNA.

double-stranded DNA autoantibodies

Increased concentrations of high affinity, anti-dsDNA (double-stranded DNA) autoantibodies detected by the Farr method to serve as a reliable predictor of systemic lupus erythematosus (SLE). When detected, these antibodies can foretell the development of SLE within a year in approximately two thirds of patients without clinical evidence of SLE. Currently used tests often measure dsDNA autoantibodies of varying affinities that give positive and confusing results in non-SLE patients. Autoantibodies against ssDNA have no clinical significance except as a general screen for autoantibodies. Patients with exacerbations of SLE develop higher concentrations of dsDNA autoantibodies. Doubling of autoantibody levels within 10 weeks, an increase of 30 IU/mL, or an increase of 25% from the lowest value during the preceding 4 months can predict disease exacerbations 90% of the time. In SLE patients with central nervous

D

system involvement, low avidity anti-dsDNA autoantibodies are more common than high avidity anti-dsDNA autoantibodies. Sera from patients suspected of having SLE should be assayed for autoantibodies to dsDNA (Farr technique) and to Sm (enzyme immunoassay with IB confirmation), as either or both of these autoantibodies are essentially diagnostic of SLE.

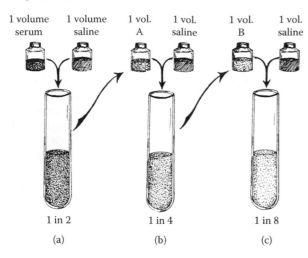

Doubling dilution.

doubling dilution

A technique used in serology to prepare serial dilutions of serum. A fixed quantity (one volume) of physiologic saline is added to each of a row of serological tubes except for the first tube in the row that receives two volumes of serum. One volume of serum from the first tube is added to one volume of saline in the second tube. After thoroughly mixing the contents with the transfer pipette, one volume of the second tube is transferred to the third, and the procedure is repeated down the row. This same volume is then discarded from the final tube after the contents have been thoroughly mixed. Thus, the serum dilution in each tube is double that in the preceding tube. The first tube is undiluted; the second contains a 1:2 dilution; the third, a 1:4; the fourth, a 1:8, etc.

doughnut structure

The assembly and insertion of complement C9 protein monomers into a cell membrane to produce a transmembrane pore that leads to cell destruction through the cytolytic action of the complement cascade.

DP pause

T cell developmental stage during which TCR α genes of the earliest double positive (DP) thymocytes are in the process of TCR α rearrangement on both chromosomes. For 3 to 4 days, a DP cell synthesizes candidate TCR α chains and conducts productivity testing with its existing functional TCRβ chain.

DP thymocytes

Double positive thymocytes that bear both CD4 and CD8 molecules. Thus, their surface phenotype is CD4$^+$ CD8$^+$.

DPT vaccine

A discontinued immunizing preparation that consisted of a combination of diphtheria and tetanus toxoids and killed pertussis microorganisms. It is no longer used in pediatric immunizations because of the superiority of the DTaP vaccine that contains only acellular pertussis microorganisms.

draining lymph node

A lymph node that collects fluid draining through lymphatic channels from an anatomical site of infection before returning to the blood circulation.

Drakeol 6VR™

A purified light mineral oil employed to prepare water-in-oil emulsion adjuvants.

drift

Refer to antigenic drift.

DRiP pathway

Defective ribosomal products pathway. A form of antigen processing whereby misfolded polypeptides are ubiquinated rapidly and digested by standard proteasomes, rendering the resulting DRiP peptides capable of association with MHC class I molecules.

drug allergy

An immunopathologic or hypersensitivity reaction to a drug. Some drugs are notorious for acting as haptens that bind to proteins in the skin or other tissues that act as carriers. This hapten–carrier complex elicits an immune response manifested as either antibodies or T lymphocytes. Any of the four types of hypersensitivity in the Coombs and Gell classification may be mediated by drug allergy. One of the best known allergies is hypersensitivity to penicillin. Antibodies to a drug linked to carrier molecules in the host may occur in autoimmune hemolytic anemia or thrombocytopenia, anaphylaxis, urticaria, and serum sickness. Skin eruptions are frequent manifestations of a T cell-mediated drug allergy.

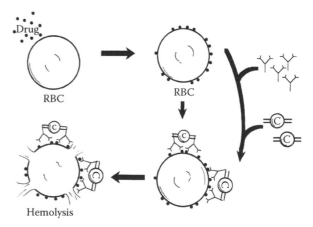

Drug-induced hemolysis.

drug-induced autoimmunity

Some mechanisms in drug-induced autoimmunity are similar to those induced by viruses. Autoantibodies may appear as a result of the helper determinant effect. With some drugs such as hydantoin, the mechanism resembles that of the Epstein–Barr virus (EBV). The generalized lymphoid hyperplasia also involves clones specific for autoantigens. A third form is that seen with α-methyldopa. This drug induces the production of specific antibodies. The drug attaches to cells *in vivo* without changing the surface antigenic makeup. The antibodies, which often have anti-e (Rh series) specificity, combine with the drug on cells, fix complement, and induce a bystander type of complement-mediated lysis. Another form of drug-induced autoimmunity is seen with nitrofurantoin, in which the autoimmunity involves cell-mediated phenomena without evidence of autoantibodies.

drug-induced immune hemolytic anemia

Acquired hemolytic anemia that develops as a consequence of immunological reactions following the administration of certain drugs. Clinically, this anemia resembles autoimmune hemolytic anemia of idiopathic origin. A particular drug may induce hemolysis in one patient, thrombocytopenia in another, neutropenia in yet another, and occasionally combinations of these in a single patient. The drug-induced antibodies that produce these immune cytopenias are cell-specific. Drugs that cause hemolysis by complement-mediated lysis include quinine, quinidine, rifampicin, chlorpropamide, hydrochlorothiazide, nomifensine phenacetin, salicylazosulfapyridine, the sodium salt of *p*-aminosalicylic acid, and stibophen. Drug-dependent immune hemolytic anemia in which the mechanism is extravascular hemolysis may occur with prolonged high dose penicillin therapy or other penicillin derivatives as well as cephalosporins and tetracycline.

drug-induced lupus (DIL)

Drugs that alone can induce a limited form of systemic lupus erythematosus (SLE) include the aromatic amines or hydrazines, the two most common being procainamide and hydralazine. Other drugs that can induce DIL include isoniazid, methyldopa, quinidine, and chlorpromazine. This drug-induced disease remits on discontinuation of the drug. The autoimmune response is very restricted.

DTaP vaccine

Acellular preparation used for protective immunization and composed of diphtheria and tetanus toxoids and acellular pertussis proteins. It is used to induce protective immunity in children against diphtheria, tetanus, and pertussis. Children should receive DTaP vaccine at the ages of 2, 4, 6, and 15 months, with a booster at 4 to 6 years of age. The tetanus and diphtheria toxoids should be repeated at 14 to 16 years of age. The vaccine is contraindicated in individuals who have shown prior allergic reactions to DTaP or in subjects with acute or developing neurologic disease. DTaP vaccine is effective in preventing most cases of the diseases it addresses.

DTH

Delayed-type hypersensitivity. Refer to type IV hypersensitivity.

DTH T cell

CD4⁺ T lymphocyte sensitized against a delayed-type hypersensitivity antigen.

dual tropic HIV

HIV strains capable of infecting macrophages, primary T cells, and cultured immortalized T cell lines.

Duffy blood group

Human erythrocyte epitopes encoded by *Fya* and *Fyb* genes located on chromosome 1. Because these epitopes are receptors for *Plasmodium vivax*, African-Americans who often express the Fy(a-b-) phenotype are not susceptible to the type of malaria induced by this species. A mother immunized through exposure to fetal red cells bearing the Duffy antigens that she does not possess may synthesize antibodies that cross the placenta and induce hemolytic disease of the newborn.

Duncan's syndrome

Marked lymphoproliferation and agammaglobulinemia associated with Epstein–Barr virus infection. The rapidly proliferating B lymphocytes produce neoplasms that may rupture the spleen. This defect in the immune response with susceptibility to infection is inherited as an X-linked recessive disorder. Affected individuals are not able to successfully resist infection by the Epstein–Barr virus.

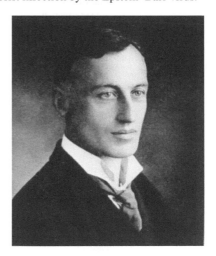

Herbert Durham.

Durham, Herbert (1866–1945)

An English graduate student working in Max von Grüber's laboratory in Vienna in 1896. He studied agglutination of bacteria by the blood and published several papers on the subject.

dust, nuclear (leukocytoclasis)

Extensive basophilic granular material representing karyolytic nuclear debris that accompanies areas of inflammation and necrosis, as in leukocytoclastic vasculitis.

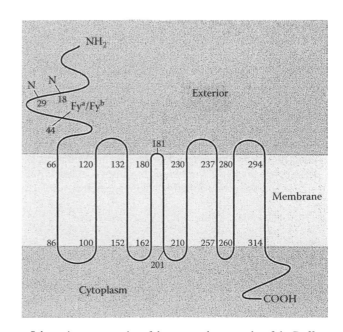

Schematic representation of the proposed topography of the Duffy glycoprotein within the red cell membrane. Numbers represent amino acid residues with the transcription-initiating methionine residue as 1. An extracellular *N*-terminal domain of 65 amino acids containing two *N*-glycosylation sites (N) and the site of the Fya/Fyb polymorphism is follwed by nonmembrane-spanning domains, or alternatively, seven-membrane-spanning domains in common with other chemokine receptors.

Comparison of Combination Diphtheria, Tetanus, and Pertussis Vaccines

Parameter	Diphtheria and Tetanus Toxoids and Whole Cell Pertussis	Diphtheria and Tetanus Toxoids and Acellular Pertussis	Diphtheria and Tetanus Toxoids (Pediatric)	Tetanus and Diphtheria Toxoids (Adult)	Diphtheria and Tetanus Toxoids, Hib Conjugate, and Whole Cell Pertussis
Abbreviation	DTP, DTwP	DTP, DTaP	DT	Td	DTwP-Hib
Manufacturer	Several	Connaught, Lederle	Several	Several	Lederle
Concentration (per 0.5 ml):					
Diphtheria	6.5–12.5 Lfu	6.7–7.5 Lfu	6.6–12.5 Lfu	2 Lfu	6.7 or 12.5 Lfu
Tetanus	5.0–5.5 Lfu	5 Lfu	5.0–7.6 Lfu	2–5 Lfu	5 Lfu
Pertussis	4 u	46.8 µg or 300 HAu	None	None	4 u
Hib	None	None	None	None	None
Packaging	6 or 7.5 ml vial	5.0 or 7.5 ml vial	5 ml vial; 0.5 ml syringe	5 or 30 ml vial; 0.5 ml syringe	5 ml vial
Appropriate age range	2 months to <7 years	18 months to <7 years	2 months to <7 years	7 years to adult	Typically 2 to 15 months
Standard schedule	Five 0.5 ml doses at 2, 4, 6, and 18 months and 4 to 6 years of age	Doses 4 and 5 at 18 months and 4–6 years of age	Three 0.5 ml doses at 2, 4, and 10–16 months of age	Three 0.5 ml doses: the second 4–8 weeks after the first, and the third 6-12 months after the second	Four 0.5 ml doses at 2, 4, 6, and 15 months of age
Routine additional doses	None	None	None	Every 10 years	None
Route	Intramuscular	Intramuscular	Intramuscular	Intramuscular jet	Intramuscular

dye exclusion test

An assay for the viability of cells *in vitro*. Vital dyes such as eosin and Trypan blue are excluded by living cells; however, the loss of cell membrane integrity by dead cells admits the dye that stains the cell. The dye exclusion principle is used in the microlymphocytotoxicity test employed for human leukocyte antigen (HLA) typing in organ transplantation.

dye test

An assay to determine whether an individual has become infected with *Toxoplasma*. Antibody in an infected patient's serum prevents living *Toxoplasma* organisms obtained from infected mouse peritoneum from taking up methylene blue. The organisms do not stain blue if antitoxoplasma antibody is present in the serum.

dysgammaglobulinemia

A pathologic condition associated with selective immunoglobulin deficiency (i.e., depression of one or two classes of serum immunoglobulins and normal or elevated levels of the other immunoglobulin classes). The term also describes antibody-deficient patients whose antibody responses to immunogenic challenge are impaired even though their immunoglobulin levels are normal. Use of the term is discouraged because it is imprecise. Also called dysimmunoglobulinemia.

e allotype

Rabbit immunoglobulin G (IgG) heavy chain or e allotypes are determined by an amino acid substitution at position 309 in C_H2. The e14 allotype heavy chains possess threonine at position 309, whereas e15 allotype heavy chains possess alanine at that location. They are determined by alleles at the *de locus* that encodes rabbit gamma chain constant regions.

E antigen

A hepatitis B virus antigen present in the sera of chronic active hepatitis patients.

E-cadherin

E-cadherin and its associated cytoplasmic proteins α-, β-, and γ-catenin play an important role in epithelial cell–cell adhesion and in the maintenance of tissue architecture. Downregulation or mutation of the E-cadherin/catenin genes can disrupt intercellular adhesion, which may lead to cellular transformation and tumor progression.

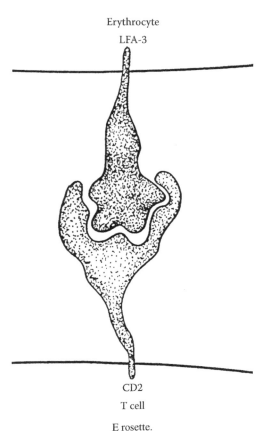

Erythrocyte

LFA-3

CD2

T cell

E rosette.

E rosette

Human T lymphocyte encircled by rings of sheep red blood cells. It was used previously as a method to enumerate T lymphocytes. Refer also to E rosette-forming cell.

E rosette-forming cell

The formation of a complex of sheep red cells encircling a T lymphocyte to form a rosette. This was one of the first methods for enumerating human T cells, as the sheep red cells did not form spontaneous rosettes with human B lymphocytes. This is now known to be due to the presence of the CD2 marker that is a cell adhesion (LFA-2) molecule on T cells. CD2⁺ T cells are now enumerated by the use of monoclonal antibodies and flow cytometry.

E-selectin (endothelial leukocyte adhesion molecule 1 [ELAM-1])

A molecule found on activated endothelial cells that recognizes sialylated Lewis X and related glycans. Its expression is associated with acute cytokine-mediated inflammation. Also called CD62E.

E2A

A transcription factor, critical for B lymphocyte development that is necessary for recombinase-activating gene (RAG) expression and expression of the λ 5 pre-B cell component in B cell development. Also called CD62E.

E5

Murine monoclonal immunoglobulin M (IgM) antibody to endotoxin that has proven safe and capable of diminishing mortality and helping to reverse organ failure in patients with Gram-negative sepsis who are not in shock during therapy. E5 may recognize and combine with lipid A epitope.

E32

A protein formed early in development of B lymphocytes that has a role in immunoglobulin heavy chain transcription.

EA

An erythrocyte (E) coated with a specific antibody (A) that constitutes a technique to measure the activities of Fcγ receptors. Sheep red blood cells with subagglutinating quantities of immunoglobulin G (IgG) antibodies are placed in contact with cells at room temperature. IgG Fc receptor-bearing cells will combine with the EA, resulting in rosette formation.

EAC

Abbreviation for erythrocyte (E), antibody (A), and complement (C), as designated in studies involving the complement cascade. Historically, sheep red blood cells have been combined with antibody specific for them, and lysis is induced only after the addition of complement. This interaction of the three reagents has served as a useful mechanism to study the reaction sequence of the multiple-component complement system, which is often written as EAC1423, etc. EAC may also be employed to reveal the presence of complement receptors 1 through 4. The combination of IgM-coated sheep red blood cells with sublytic quantities of complement to produce EAC provides a mechanism whereby rosettes are formed by cells bearing complement receptors once the EAC is layered onto test cells at room temperature. EAC rosette erythrocytes such as sheep red blood cells, coated or synthesized with antibody and complement, encircle human B lymphocytes to form a rosette. This is based on erythrocyte binding to C3b receptors. This technique has been used in the past to identify B lymphocytes. However, phagocytic cells bearing C3b receptors may also form EAC rosettes. This type of rosette is in contrast to the E rosette that identifies T lymphocytes. B lymphocytes are now enumerated by monoclonal antibodies against the B lymphocyte CD (cluster of differentiation) markers using flow cytometry.

EAE
Acronym for experimental allergic encephalomyelitis.

EAM
Refer to experimental autoimmune myocarditis.

EAMG
Refer to experimental autoimmune myasthenia gravis. The condition can be induced in more than one species of animals by immunizing them with purified AchR from the electric ray (*Torpedo californica*). The autoantigen, nicotinic AchR, is T cell-dependent. The *in vivo* synthesis of anti-AchR antibodies requires helper T cell activity. Antibodies specific for the nicotinic acetylcholine receptors (AchRs) of skeletal muscle react with the postsynaptic membrane at the neuromuscular junction.

early B-cell factor (EBF)
A transcription factor requisite for early B cell development and for RAG expression.

early induced responses
Nonadaptive host responses induced by infectious agents early in infection. The inductive phase of these responses differentiates them from innate immunity, and their failure to involve clonal selection of antigen-specific lymphocytes distinguishes them from adaptive immunity.

early phase reaction
A Type I hypersensitivity elicitation response characterized by the rapid development of clinical symptoms following the release of preformed inflammatory mediators from mast cells undergoing degranulation.

early pro-B cell
Refer to pro-B cell.

early signalosome
The initial TCR signal transduction molecular complex capable of participating in either the immunosome or the telerosome.

EAT
Abbreviation for experimental autoimmune thyroiditis. Includes a murine model for Hashimoto's thyroiditis. There is a strong major histocompatibility complex (MHC) genetic component in susceptibility to Hashimoto's thyroiditis, which has been shown to reside in the IA subregion of the murine MHC (H-2), governing the immune response (Ir) genes to mouse thyroglobulin (MTg). Following induction of EAT with MTg, autoantibodies against MTg appear and mononuclear cells infiltrate the thyroid. Repeated administration of soluble, syngeneic MTg without adjuvant leads to thyroiditis only in the murine haplotype susceptible to EAT. Autoreactive T cells proliferate *in vitro* following stimulation with MTg. The disease can be passively transferred to naïve recipients by adoptive immunization and differentiate into oxytoxic T lymphocytes (T_c) *in vitro*. Thus, lymphoid cells rather than antibodies represent the primary mediator of the disease. *In vitro* proliferation of murine-autoreactive T cells have been found to show a good correlation with susceptibility to EAT and to be dependent on the presence of Thy-1$^+$, Lyt-1$^+$, Ia$^+$, and L3T4$^+$ lymphocytes. Effector T lymphocytes (T_E) in EAT comprise various T cell subsets and Lyt-1 (L3T4) and Lyt-2 phenotypes. T lymphocytes cloned from thyroid infiltrates of patients with Hashimoto's thyroiditis reveal numerous cytotoxic T lymphocytes and clones synthesizing interleukin-2 (IL2) and interferon-γ (IFN-γ). While the T cell subsets participate in pathogenesis of Hashimoto's thyroiditis, autoantibody synthesis appears to aid perpetuation of the disease or result from it.

EAU
Refer to experimental autoimmune uveoretinitis.

EBF (early B cell factor)
A transcription factor requisite for early B cell development and for recombinase-activating gene (RAG) expression.

EBI1
An orphan chemokine receptor expressed on normal lymphoid tissues as well as several B and T lymphocyte cell lines. EBI1 mRNA is detected in Epstein–Barr virus (EBV)-positive B cell lines. The tissue source is EBV-induced cDNA. Also termed BLR2.

EBNA (Epstein–Barr virus nuclear antigen)
Refer to Epstein–Barr nuclear antigen.

ECF-A (eosinophil chemotactic factor of anaphylaxis)
A 500-D acidic polypeptide that attracts eosinophils. Interaction of antigen with immunoglobulin E (IgE) antibody molecules on the surface of mast cells causes ECF-A to be released from the mast cells.

E-cadherin (ECH-6), mouse
Anti-E-cadherin mouse monoclonal antibody detects E-cadherin, an adhesion protein expressed in cells of epithelial lineage. It stains positively in glandular epithelium and in adenocarcinomas of the lung, GI tract, and ovary. It has been useful in distinguishing adenocarcinoma from mesothelioma. It has also been shown to be positive in some thyroid carcinomas.

Echinococcus immunity
The genus *Echinococcus* includes four species of tapeworm parasites, among which is *Echinococcus granulosus*. Its cycle of transmission involves interaction between a definitive host, such as a carnivore, and an intermediate host (herbivore or omnivore). Each host may reveal two morphologically distinct parasite stages. Definitive hosts are infected with the tapeworm stage of *Echinococcus*. Immunological methods have been used to diagnose infection in definitive hosts and to develop a recombinant vaccine that is highly effective in protecting sheep from hydatid infection. Ovine hydatid cyst fluid is rich in antigen. The principal parasite antigens are designated antigen 5 and antigen B. Antibodies against these are useful in immunodiagnosis of hydatid infection in humans; 27- and 94-kDA protein antigens from protoscoleces are recognized by sera of dogs infected with *E. granulosus*; 22-, 30-, and 37-kDA oncosphere antigens are specific for *E. granulosus* and are stage-specific for oncospheres. Little is known regarding cellular responses against *E. granulosus* infection in dogs, but T cells and activated macrophages are believed to play a significant role in cellular immunity against *Echinococcus* in intermediate hosts. With respect to the humoral immune response to infection, dogs form immunoglobulin A (IgA), IgG, and IgM antibodies against *E. granulosus*. IgA antibody against *E. granulosus* is produced in the

intestinal mucosa, but some dogs manifest elevated levels of IgE. IgA, IgE, IgG, and IgM antibodies are synthesized in intermediate hosts infected with this microorganism. Immunodiagnosis can be carried out by ELISA in the definitive host by detecting circulating antibodies specific for the microorganism. Coproantigens of *Echinococcus* may be detected in the feces of infected dogs. The mucosal IgA produced in dogs has little effect on the worms that have the capacity to suppress cytotoxic and effector activity in the region of the scolex. *E. granulosus* is believed to modulate the immune system of the intermediate host through production of cytotoxic substances, immunosuppressive and immunostimulatory cytokines. Concomitant immunity is critical in ensuring the survival of *E. granulosus* in intermediate hosts. This refers to the capacity of established hydatid cysts to avoid the immune system of the intermediate host while inducing an effective immune response against subsequent infection by this microorganism. Concomitant immunity is mediated by antibody and is directed against oncospheres. Killing is induced through an antibody-dependent, complement-mediated lysis of the parasite.

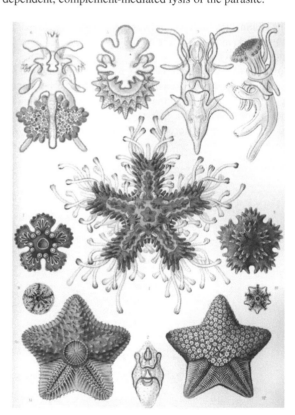

Starfish.

echinoderms

In the starfish, made famous by Metchinkoff's studies of phagocytosis, allograft rejection occurs and is marked by cellular infiltration. There is a significant specific memory response. Cytokine-like molecules similar to interleukin-1 (IL1) and tumor necrosis factor (TNF) have been recognized in echinoderms and other intervertebrates.

ECHO (enteric cytopathogenic human orphan) virus

Comprised of 30 types within the picornavirus family. The virus is cytopathic in cell culture and produces such clinical manifestations in patients as upper respiratory tract infections, diarrhea, exanthema, viremia, and sometimes poliomyelitis and viral meningitis.

eclipsed antigen

An antigen, such as one from a parasite, that so closely resembles host antigens that it fails to stimulate an immune response.

ECRF3

A member of the G protein-coupled receptor family, the chemokine receptor branch of the rhodopsin family, is expressed on T cells. The tissue source is herpesvirus saimiri of the γ-herpesvirus family. *In vitro*, it facilitates calcium efflux. Ligands include MGSA/GRO-α, NAP-2, and IL-8.

ecto-5′-nucleotidase deficiency

A purine metabolism alteration that produces immunodeficiencies of B lymphocytes.

ectopic

The location of expression of a structure or protein away from its normal position in the body or tissue.

eczema

A skin lesion characterized as a weeping eruption consisting of erythema, pruritus with edema, papules, vesicles, pustules, scaling, and possible exudation. It occurs in individuals who are atopic, such as those with atopic dermatitis. Applications to the skin or the ingestion of drugs that may themselves act as haptens may induce this type of hypersensitivity. It may be seen in young children who subsequently develop asthma in later life.

eczema vaccinatum

On occasion, in subjects receiving smallpox vaccination, the virus in the vaccine superinfected areas of skin affected by atopic dermatitis. This led to generalized vaccinia that was severe and frequently fatal. It was also referred to as Kaposi's varicelliform eruption.

eczematoid skin reaction

The appearance of erythematous, vesicular, and pruritic lesions on the skin that resemble eczema but are not due to atopy.

ED$_{50}$

The 50% effective dose. For example, 50% hemolysis can be determined more accurately than can a 100% endpoint.

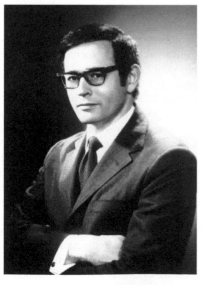

Gerald Maurice Edelman.

E

Edelman, Gerald Maurice (1929–)

American investigator and professor at Rockefeller University who shared a Nobel Prize in 1972 with Porter for their work on antibody structure. Edelman was the first to demonstrate that immunoglobulins are composed of light and heavy polypeptide chains. He also did pioneering work with the Bence–Jones protein, cell adhesion molecules, immunoglobulin amino acid sequences, and neurobiology.

edema

Tissue swelling as a result of fluid extravasation from the intravascular space.

edge artifact

In immunoperoxidase staining of paraffin-embedded tissues, tissue drying may produce nonspecific coloring at the periphery which is an artifact.

edible vaccine

A genetically altered food containing microorganisms or related antigens that may induce active immunity against infection. A plant constituent altered genetically to express an antigen of a pathogen that can be ingested as food.

efalizumab

An immunosuppressive agent used to treat plaque psoriasis. Interacts with CD11a, the α subunit of leukocyte function antigen-1 (LFA-1), which all leukocytes express, and diminishes cell surface expression of CD11a. Inhibits binding of LFA-1 to intercellular adhesion molecule-1 (ICAM-1), inhibiting leukocyte adhesion to other cell types. LFA-1 and ICAM-1 interaction facilitates the initiation and maintenance of multiple processes, including T lymphocyte activation, T lymphocyte adhesion to endothelial cells, and T lymphocyte migration to sites of inflammation, including psoriatic skin.

effector B cell

Refer to effector lymphocyte (effector cell).

effector cells

Lymphocytes capable of eliminating pathogens from the body without further differentiation.

effector function

The nonantigen-binding functions of an antibody molecule that are mediated by the constant regions of heavy chains. These include Fc receptor binding, complement fixation, binding to mast cells, etc. Effector function generally results in removal of antigen from the body, such as in phagocytosis or complement-mediated lysis. The elimination of foreign entities by effector cells through such mechanisms as cytokine secretion, cytotoxicity, and antibody production.

effector lymphocyte

A lymphocyte activated through either specific or non-specific mechanisms to carry out a certain function in the immune response. The differentiated descendants of an activated leukocyte that remove a nonself constituent. Certain effector cells including plasma cells, Th cells, and cytotoxic T lymphocytes require less costimulation than their resting naïve counterparts and express homing and chemokine receptors that are different, thereby permitting excess inflammatory sites. NKT and ILK cells may function as effectors without a need to proliferate. Examples of effector lymphocytes include the natural killer (NK) cell, tumor-infiltrating lymphocyte (TIF), lymphokine-activated killer (LAK) cell, cytotoxic T lymphocyte, helper T lymphocyte, and suppressor T cell. Most commonly, the term

signifies a T lymphocyte capable of mediating cytotoxicity, suppression, or helper function.

effector mechanism

The means whereby post innate and adaptive immune responses destroy and eliminate pathogens from the body.

effector phase

That part of an immune response following recognition and activation phases during which a foreign antigen such as a microbe is inactivated or destroyed.

effector response

An event that follows antigen recognition and binding by antibody, such as complement-mediated lysis.

effector site

An isolated area of the mucosa in which there is differentiation of lymphocytes activated in a mucosal inductive site into effector cells capable of effector functions, such as antibody synthesis.

effector stage (hypersensitivity)

Refer to elicitation.

effector T cell

Refer to effector lymphocyte (effector cell).

efferent lymphatic vessel

The channel through which lymph and lymphocytes exit a lymph node in transit to the blood.

efficacy (vaccine)

Capacity of a vaccine to effectively induce protective immunity against a disease represented by the percentage of vaccinated subjects who develop immunity against the pathogenic microorganism. Frequently evaluated by post-vaccination seroconversion. Referred to also as coverage.

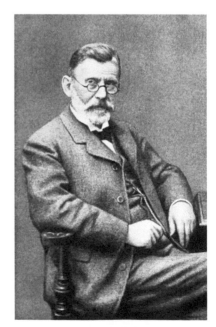

Paul Ehrlich.

Ehrlich, Paul (1854–1915)

Born in Silesia, Germany; graduated from the University of Leipzig as a doctor of medicine. His scientific work included three areas of investigation. He first became interested in stains for tissues and cells and perfected some of the best ones to demonstrate the tubercle bacillus

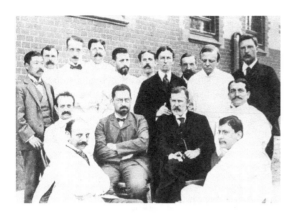

Ehrlich School of Immunology.

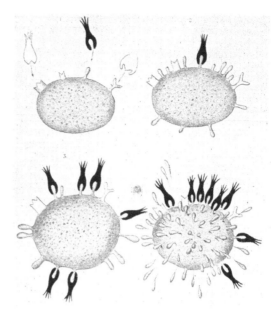

Ehrlich's side chain theory of antibody formation.

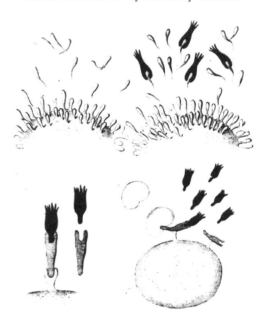

Ehrlich's side chain theory of antibody formation.

and leukocytes in blood. His first immunological studies began in 1890, when he was an assistant at the Institute for Infectious Diseases under Robert Koch. In 1897, Ehrlich published the first practical technique to standardize diphtheria toxin and antitoxin preparations. He proposed the first selective theory of antibody formation, known as the "side-chain" theory, which stimulated much research by his colleagues in attempts to disprove it. He served as director of his own institute in Frankfurt am Main, where he published papers with a number of gifted colleagues, including Dr. Julius Morgenroth on immune hemolysis, and devoted the final phase of his career to the development of chemotherapeutic agents for the treatment of disease. He shared the 1908 Nobel Prize with Metchnikoff for their studies on immunity. Fruits of these labors led to treatments for trypanosomiasis and syphilis (Salvarsan)—the "magic bullet." (Refer to *Collected Studies on Immunity*, 1906; *Collected Papers of Paul Ehrlich*, vol. 3, 1957.)

Ehrlich phenomenon (historical)

The demonstration that the L_0 dose of diphtheria toxin differs from the L_+ dose not by one minimal lethal dose (MLD) as one might anticipate, but by 10 to 100 MLDs, depending on the particular sample. This represents the difference between the dose that causes minimal reactivity and the dose that produces death.

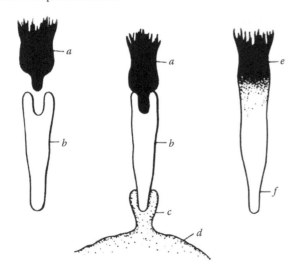

a complement; *b* interbody (immune-body); *c* receptor; *d* part of a cell; *e* toxophore group of the toxin; *f* haptophore group

Ehrlich's diagrams of "toxophore" and "haptophore" groups.

Ehrlich side-chain theory

The first selective theory of antibody synthesis developed by Paul Ehrlich in 1900. Although elaborate in detail, the essential feature of the theory was that cells of the immune system possess the genetic capability to react to all known antigens and that each cell on the surface bears receptors with surface haptophore side chains. On combination with antigen, the side chains are cast off into the circulation, and new receptors replace the old ones. These cast-off receptors represented antibody molecules in the circulation. Although far more complex than this explanation, the importance of the theory was in the amount of research stimulated to try to disprove it. Nevertheless, the theory represented the first effort to account for the importance of genetics in immune responsiveness at a time when Mendel's basic studies had not even yet been "rediscovered" by De Vries.

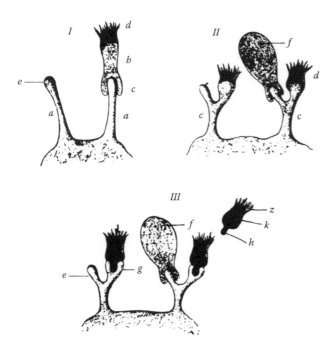

Ehrlich's side chain theory of antibody formation.

EIA

(1) Acronym for exercise-induced anaphylaxis. (2) Acronym for enzyme immunoassay.

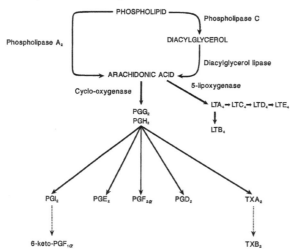

Schematic diagram of eicosanoids.

eicosanoid

An arachidonic acid-derived 20-carbon cyclic fatty acid produced from membrane phospholipids. Eicosanoids and other arachidonic acid metabolites are elevated during shock and following injury and are site specific. They produce various effects including bronchodilation, bronchoconstriction, vasoconstriction, and vasodilation. Eicosanoids include leukotrienes, prostaglandins, thromboxanes, and prostacyclin.

Eisen, Herman Nathaniel (1918–)

American physician whose research contributions range from equilibrium dialysis (with Karush) to the mechanism of contact dermatitis.

ELAM-1 (endothelial leukocyte adhesion molecule 1)

A glycoprotein of the endothelium that facilitates adhesion of neutrophils. Structurally, it has an epidermal growth factor-like domain, a lectin-like domain, amino acid sequence

homology with complement-regulating proteins, and six tandem-repeated motifs. Tumor necrosis factor (TNF), interleukin-1 (IL1), and substance P induce its synthesis. Its immunoregulatory activities include attraction of neutrophils to inflammatory sites and mediating cell adhesion by sialyl–Lewis X, a carbohydrate ligand. It acts as an adhesion molecule or addressin for T lymphocytes that home to the skin.

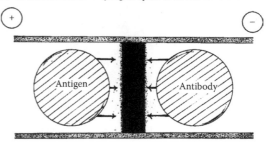

Electroimmunodiffusion.

electroimmunodiffusion

A double-diffusion in-gel method in which antigen and antibody are forced toward one another in an electrical field. Precipitation occurs at the site of their interaction. Refer to Laurell rocket test and rocket immunoelectrophoresis. Also called counter immunoelectrophoresis.

electrophoresis

A method for separating a mixture of proteins based on their different rates of migration in an electrical field. Zone electrophoresis represents a technical improvement in which a stabilizing medium such as cellulose acetate serves as a matrix for buffer and as a structure to which proteins can remain attached following fixation. By this technique, plasma proteins are resolved into five or six major peaks. Zone electrophoresis permits a gross evaluation of the levels of immunoglobulins and other proteins in the serum. In cases of increased levels, electrophoresis indicates whether this involves a general proliferation and hypersecretion by lymphocytes derived from multiple individual cells (polyclonal origin, proteins are heterogeneous) or proliferation and hypersecretion by lymphoid cells derived from a limited number of individual cells (monoclonal origin, proteins are homogeneous).

electrophoretic mobility

The electrophoretic velocity, v, of a charged particle expressed per unit field strength; hence, $u = v/E$, where E is the field strength. The value of u is positive if the particle moves toward the pole of lower potential and negative in the opposite case. The electrophoretic mobility depends only on molecular parameters.

electroporation

A technique to insert molecules into cells through use of brief high-voltage electric pulses. It can be used to insert DNA into animal cells. The electrical discharge produces tiny (nanometers in diameter) pores in the plasma membrane. These pores admit supercoiled or linear DNA.

electrostatic bond

A union attributable to the attraction between charged residues manifesting opposite polarities.

Elek plate

A method to show toxin production by *Corynebacterium diphtheriae* colonies growing on an agar plate. Diphtheria antitoxin impregnated into a strip of filter paper is placed at a right angle

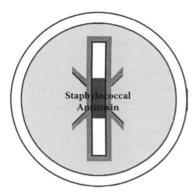

Plasma-agar plate showing
staphylocoagulase effect
inhibited by commercial antitoxin

Elek plate.

to a streak of the microorganisms on the agar plate. Toxin formation by the growing microbes interacts with antitoxin in the filter paper to form a line of precipitation.

elephantiasis

Enlargement of extremities by lymphedema caused by lymphatic obstruction during granulomatous reactivity in filariasis.

elevated IgE, defective chemotaxis, recurrent infection, and eczema

Individuals with the third disorder may manifest several bacterial infections, eczema, abscesses, and pneumonia associated with group A β hemolytic streptococci and *Staphylococcus aureus*. They demonstrate normal functions of both B and T cell limbs of the immune response, although their IgE levels are strikingly elevated, reaching values that are tenfold those of normal individuals. Only chemotactic function is defective, with other parameters of phagocytic cell function within normal limits. No treatment other than antibiotic therapy is available.

elicitation

An overactive, abnormal, secondary response to a sensitizing agent that leads to inflammatory tissue injury. Also referred to as an effector stage. Refer to hypersensitivity and types I through IV hypersensitivities.

ELISA (enzyme-linked immunosorbent assay)

Refer to enzyme-linked immunosorbent assay.

ELISPOT assay

A modification of the enzyme-linked immunosorbent assay (ELISA) that involves the capture of products secreted from cells placed in contact with antigen or antibody fixed to a plastic surface. An enzyme-linked antibody is then used to identify the captured products by cleaving a colorless substrate to yield a colored spot.

eluate

In immunology, a substance such as an antibody obtained by physical or chemical treatment of an antigen–antibody complex. By allowing particulate antigens such as erythrocytes to interact with antibody followed by heating the antibody particle or cell complex to 56°C, the antibody can be dissociated from the particulate antigen and is present in the eluate.

embryonic antigens

Protein or carbohydrate antigens synthesized during embryonic and fetal life that are either absent or formed in only minute quantities in normal adult subjects. Aberrant expression by a tumor cell can render it a tumor-associated antigen. α-Fetoproteins (AFPs) and carcinoembryonic antigens (CEAs) are fetal antigens that may be synthesized once again in large amounts in individuals with certain tumors. Their detection and level during the course of the disease and following surgery to remove a tumor, reducing the substance, may serve as a diagnostic and prognostic indicator of the disease process. Blood group antigens, such as iI, that are reversed in their levels of expression in the fetus and in the adult may show a re-emergence of i antigen in adults with thalassemia and hypoplastic anemia. Cold autoagglutinins specific for i may be found in infectious mononucleosis patients. Common acute lymphoblastic leukemia antigen (CD10) is rarely found on peripheral blood cells of normal subjects, whereas CALLA⁺ cells coexpressing IgM and CD19 molecules may be found in fetal bone marrow and peripheral blood samples. CD10 may be expressed in children with common acute lymphoblastic leukemia.

embryonic stem (ES) cells

Murine embryonic cells that are immortal in culture and retain the capacity to give rise to all cell lineages. They may be altered genetically *in vitro* and introduced into mouse blastocysts to give rise to mutant murine lines. Genes may be deleted in ES cells by homologous recombination to produce mutant ES cells that can give rise to gene knockout mice.

emerging infectious disease

An infection potentially capable of impacting the world population because it is induced by a pathogenic microorganism that has recently emerged or is undergoing alteration.

EMF-1

Embryo fibroblast protein-1 is a chemokine of the α (CXC) family. It has been found in chicken fibroblasts and mononuclear cells, yet no human or murine homolog is known. Cultured chick embryo fibroblasts (CEFs) abundantly express the avian gene 9E3/CEF-4. The EMF-1 gene was isolated from RSV-transformed CEFs identified by differential screening of a cDNA library. EMF-1 is characterized as a chemokine because its sequence resembles that of CTAP-III and PF4. RSV-infected cells represent the tissue source. Fibroblasts in mononuclear cells are the target cells. Expression of EMF-1 together with high collagen levels and its presence in wounded tissues suggest that it has a role in wound response and/or repair. EMF-1 is chemotactic for chicken peripheral blood mononuclear cells.

EMIT

Acronym for enzyme-multiplied immunoassay technique.

emperipolesis

The intrusion or penetration of a lymphocyte into the cytoplasm of another cell followed by passage through the cell. Emperipolesis also describes the movement of one cell within the cytoplasm of another cell.

ENA-78 (epithelial-derived neutrophil attractant-78)

A chemokine of the α family (CXC family). ENA-78 is related to NAP-2, GRO-α, and IL-8. Tissue sources include epithelial cells and platelets. Neutrophils are the target cells. ENA-78 is increased in peripheral blood, synovial fluid, and synovial tissue from rheumatoid arthritis patients. ENA-78 mRNA levels are elevated in acutely rejecting human renal allografts compared with renal allografts that are not being rejected.

ENA antibodies

Antibodies against extractable nuclear antigens. This category includes antibodies to ribonucleoprotein (RNP), presently termed U1 snRNPs (small nuclear ribonucleoproteins) or U1 RNPs, in addition to Sm antibodies that have specificity for Smith antigen. Sm antibodies are associated with systemic lupus erythematosus (SLE), whereas U1 snRNP antibodies in high titer are detected in patients with mixed connective tissue disease. U4/U6 snRNP antibodies are detectable in patients with systemic sclerosis.

ENA autoantibodies

Autoantibodies specific for extractable nuclear antigens. They are small nuclear ribonucleoproteins (snRNPs) and small cellular ribonucleoproteins (scRNPs). U1 snRNP autoantibodies bind to RNP proteins A and C. Sm autoantibodies bind to RNP proteins B'/B, D, and E. scRNP autoantibodies include SS-A/Ro with specificity for 60- and 52-kDa proteins and SS-B/La with specificity for a 48-kDa protein.

encapsulated bacteria

The thick carbohydrate coating or capsule that protects microorganisms such as pneumococci from phagocytosis. Infection-producing encapsulated bacteria cannot be effectively phagocytized and destroyed unless they are first coated with an opsonizing antibody formed in an adaptive immune response and complement.

encapsulation

The reaction of leukocytes to foreign material that cannot be phagocytized because of its large size. Multiple layers of flattened leukocytes form a wall surrounding the foreign body and isolate it within the tissues. This type of reaction occurs in invertebrates including annelids, mollusks, and arthropods. In higher invertebrates, it is mediated by pattern recognition receptors (PRRs), whereby pathogens too large to be phagocytized are encircled by numerous phagocytic cells. Phagocyte reactive oxygen intermediates and lysosomal enzymes then destroy the encapsulated pathogens. In vertebrates, macrophages surround the foreign body, a granuloma is formed, and fibroblasts subsequently appear. A fibrous capsule is formed.

encephalitogenic factors

Myelin basic protein or related molecules found in the brain that can induce experimental allergic encephalomyelitis if administered to experimental animals together with Freund's complete adjuvant. The smallest constituent of myelin that is capable of inducing experimental encephalomyelitis is a nonapeptide (Phe–Leu–Trp–Ala–Glu–Gly–Gln–Lys).

end binders

Selected anticarbohydrate-specific antibodies that bind the ends of oligosaccharide antigens, in contrast to those that bind the sides of these molecules.

end cell

A cell such as a mature plasma cell at the termination point in the maturation pattern of that cell line. End cells do not further divide. They represent the final product of maturation.

end piece (historical)

In the early complement literature, complement activity in the pseudoglobulin fraction of serum was called the end piece, in contrast to the activity in the euglobulin fraction that was called the mid-piece of complement. Current information reveals that what was referred to as the end piece did not contain C1 but did contain all of the C2 and other complement components.

end point

The greatest dilution of an antibody in solution that will still yield an identifiable reaction when combined with antigen. The reciprocal of this dilution represents the titer.

end point immunoassay

A test in which the signal is measured as the antigen–antibody complex reaches equilibrium.

end-stage renal disease (ESRD)

Chronic renal failure. Approximately one third of cases are linked to diabetes mellitus. Kidneys of patients on chronic dialysis ultimately develop ESRD. Proliferation of intravascular smooth muscle induced by ischemia occurs, and there may also be venous thrombosis.

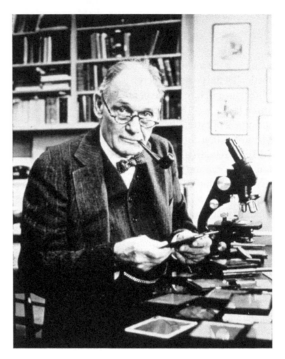

John F. Enders.

Enders, John F. (1897–1985)

An American microbiologist who shared the 1954 Nobel Prize in Medicine with T.H. Weller and F.C. Robbins for discovering that many viruses (specifically poliomyelitis) can be grown in tissue culture and thereby studied and isolated, making possible the production of vaccines.

endocrine

Regulatory molecules such as hormones that reach target cells from the sites of their synthesis through the bloodstream.

endocytic pathway

Membrane-bound vesicles such as endosomes and endolysosomes within cells that harbor hydrolytic enzymes and additional molecules requisite for digestion of internalized substances. Requisite for processing and presentation of exogenous antigen.

endocytic vesicle

Membrane structure derived from the plasma membrane that transports extracellular material into cells.

endocytosis

A mechanism whereby substances are taken into a cell from the extracellular fluid through plasma membrane vesicles. This is accomplished by either pinocytosis or receptor-facilitated endocytosis. In pinocytosis, extracellular fluid is captured within a plasma membrane vesicle. In receptor-facilitated endocytosis, extracellular ligands bind to receptors, and coated pits and coated vesicles facilitate internalization. Clathrin-coated vesicles become uncoated and fuse to form endosomes. Ligand and receptor dissociate within the endosome, and the receptor returns to the cell surface. Endosomes fused with lysosomes form secondary lysosomes where ligand degradation occurs. Low density lipoproteins are handled in this manner.

endogenous

Resulting from conditions within the organism rather than externally caused; derived internally.

endogenous antigen

An epitope that forms in a host cell, such as a protein produced by a virus-infected cell or one infected by an intracellular bacterium.

endogenous antigen processing and presentation

A mechanism whereby cytosolic endogenous antigens are degraded into peptides by proteasomes and bound to MHC Class I molecules in the rough endoplasmic reticulum. This is followed by exhibition of the peptide–MHC Class I complex at the cell surface. This cytosolic antigen processing pathway occurs in nearly all nucleated cell types.

endogenous pyrogen

Cytokine that induces an increase in body temperature, in contrast to an exogenous pyrogen such as an endotoxin from Gram-negative bacteria that elevates body temperature by activating endogenous pyrogen synthesis and release.

endometrial antibodies

Immunoglobulin G (IgG) autoantibodies present in two thirds of women with endometriosis. They react with the epithelial glandular portion but not the stromal component of endometrium. They have been suggested as a possible cause for infertility that occurs in approximately 30 to 40% of women with endometriosis.

endometrial autoantibodies

Immunoglobulin G (IgG) autoantibodies present in 50 to 74% of endometriosis patients. They react with the epithelial (glandular) component and not the stromal component of normal endometrium regardless of menstrual cycle phase. These autoantibodies have been suggested as possible causes of infertility observed in 30 to 40% of endometriosis patients. The sera of endometriotic patients react with both normal and endometriotic tissue. Antibody titer is not correlated with stage of endometriosis or the menstrual cycle phase. Endometriosis patients often manifest lupus anticoagulant (45%), antinuclear antigen reactivity (10 to 25%), and elevated IgG concentrations (95%). They also form antibodies to phospholipids and histones.

endomysial antibodies

Immunoglobulin A (IgA) subclass (IgA EmA) antibodies that are specific for reticulin in smooth muscle endomysium. They are present in essentially all celiac disease (gluten-sensitive enteropathy) patients with villous atrophy and in 60 to 70% of individuals with dermatitis herpetiformis who receive diets with normal gluten content.

endomysial autoantibodies

Immunoglobulin A (IgA) autoantibodies that react with the reticulin constituent of endomysium in primate smooth muscle. These antibodies are present in 70 to 80% of dermatitis herpetiformis (DH) patients on regular

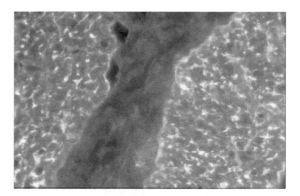

Endomysial autoantibodies.

gluten-containing diets and in all patients with celiac disease (CD), a gluten-sensitive enteropathy with severe villous atrophy. IgA EmA specificity for active gluten-sensitive enteropathy is >98%. IgA EmA is a better predictor for CD than are IgA gliadin autoantibodies (AGA). A positive IgA EmA is confirmatory evidence and indicates the need for intestinal biopsy. IgA AGA and IgA-R1-reticulin autoantibodies (IgA ARA) are present in approximately one quarter of DH patients and in 93 and 44%, respectively, of patients with active CD. The incidence of CD is 10 times greater (with selective IgA deficiency) compared to subjects without selective IgA disease.

endophthalmitis phacoanaphylactica

A condition resulting from the accidental release of lens protein into the blood circulation during cataract removal in humans. This interaction of a normally sequestered antigen (i.e., lens protein) with the host immune system activates an autoimmune response that results in inflammation of the involved eye.

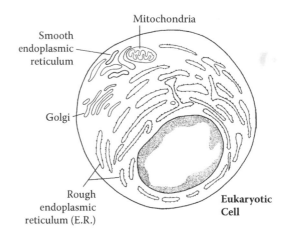

Endoplasmic reticulum.

endoplasmic reticulum

A structure in the cytoplasm comprised of parallel membranes connected to the nuclear membranes. Lipids and selected proteins are synthesized in this organelle. The membrane is continuous and convoluted. Electron microscopy reveals rough endoplasmic reticulum that contains ribosomes on the side exposed to the cytoplasm and smooth endoplasmic reticulum without ribosomes. Fatty acids and phospholipids are synthesized and metabolized in smooth

E

endoplasmic reticulum. Selected membrane and organelle proteins and secreted proteins are synthesized in the rough endoplasmic reticulum. Cells such as plasma cells that produce antibodies or other specialized secretory proteins have abundant rough endoplasmic reticulum in the cytoplasm. Following formation, proteins move from the rough endoplasmic reticulum to the Golgi complex. They may be transported in vesicles that form from the endoplasmic reticulum and fuse with Golgi complex membranes. Once secreted protein reaches the endoplasmic reticulum lumen, it does not have to cross any further barriers prior to exit from the cell.

endoplasmic reticulum autoantibodies

Autoantibodies against trifluoroacetylated (TFA) hepatic proteins in patients who have developed a severe form of halothane-induced hepatitis alluded to be induced by an immune response. The sera of these patients also contain antibodies that recognize various non-TFA-modified proteins that may be present in patients who have been exposed to halothane but do not develop hepatitis. Halothane anesthetic can lead to mild halothane-induced liver damage that is of no clinical significance or can cause the severe form. The clinical significance of antibodies to TNA and non-TFA proteins remains to be determined.

endorphin

An endogenous opioid peptide that links to a cognate receptor; α, β, and γ types exist. The β endorphin is associated with secretion by the pituitary gland and is possibly associated with pain perception.

endosome

A 0.1- to 0.2-μm intracellular vesicle produced by endocytosis. Extracellular proteins are internalized in this structure during antigen processing. The endosome has an acidic pH and contains proteolytic enzymes that degrade proteins into peptides that bind to major histocompatibility complex (MHC) class II molecules. MIICs, a subset of MHC-class-II-rich endosomes, play a critical role in antigen processing and presentation by the class II pathway.

endothelial cell antibodies (ECAs)

Immunoglobulin G (IgG) antibodies present in the sera of systemic lupus erythematosus (SLE) patients that may mediate immunologic injury to blood vessel walls. They may be involved in the pathogenesis of rheumatoid vasculitis. Besides SLE, cytotoxic antibodies reactive with vascular endothelial cells are present in the sera of cardiac allograft recipients undergoing hyperacute rejection despite negative cross matches. ECAs may also be found in patients with hemolytic uremic syndrome, in Kawasaki disease, and in renal allograft recipients who have rejected transplants. Selected patients with Wegener's granulomatosis and with micropolyarteritis may reveal noncytolytic ECAs that are also demonstrable in 44% of dermatomyositis patients, particularly those who also have interstitial lung disease. About 33% of IgA nephropathy patients possess antibodies that show specificity for vascular endothelial cells and for human leukocyte antigen (HLA) class I antigens.

endothelial cell autoantibodies (ECAs)

A heterogeneous family of antibodies that react with various antigens expressed on resting and activated endothelial cells. Some are associated with nephritis in systemic lupus erythematosus (SLE), but ECAs are not

SLE-restricted. Cytotoxic antibodies against vascular endothelial cells have been demonstrated in subjects with hyperacute rejection of cardiac allografts who have had compatible direct lymphocytotoxic crossmatches, in patients who rejected renal allografts, in hemolytic–uremic syndrome, and in Kawasaki disease. ECAs that are not cytolytic have been demonstrated in patients with micropolyarteritis and Wegener's granulomatosis and in approximately 44% of dermatomyositis patients. Serum antibodies that bind to vascular endothelial cells, some with anti-HLA class I specificity, have been demonstrated in about one third of patients with IgA nepropathy. Sera from scleroderma, Wegener's granulomatosis, and microscopic polyarteritis patients mediate antibody-dependent cellular cytoxicity. Cytokine-mediated activation of vascular endothelium is believed to be significant in the pathogenesis of antibody-mediated and cell-mediated entry to blood vessels.

endothelial leukocyte adhesion molecule 1 (ELAM-1)

Facilitates focal adhesion of leukocyte to blood vessel walls. It is induced by endotoxins and cytokines and belongs to the adhesion molecule family. It is considered to play a significant role in the pathogenesis of atherosclerosis and infectious and autoimmune diseases. Neutrophil and monocyte adherence to endothelial cells occurs during inflammation *in vivo*, along with leukocyte margination and migration to areas of inflammation. Endothelial cells activated by interleukin-1 (IL1) and tumor necrosis factor (TNF) synthesize ELAM-1, at least in culture. A 115-kDa chain and a 100-kDa chain comprise the ELAM-1 molecule.

endothelin

A peptide composed of 21 amino acid residues derived from aortic endothelial cells that serves as a powerful vasoconstrictor. A gene on chromosome 6 encodes the molecule. It produces an extended pressor response, stimulates release of aldosterone, inhibits release of renin, and impairs renal excretion. It is elevated in myocardial infarction and cardiogenic shock, major abdominal surgery, pulmonary hypertension, and uremia. It may have a role in the development of congestive heart failure.

endotoxin

A Gram-negative bacterial cell wall lipopolysaccharide (LPS) that is heat stable and causes neutrophils to release pyrogens. It may produce endotoxin or hemorrhagic shock and modify resistance against infection. Endotoxins comprise integral constituents of outer membranes of Gram-negative microorganisms. They are significant virulence factors and induce injury in a number of ways. Toxicity is associated with the lipid A fraction of the molecule composed of a β-1,6-glucosaminyl-glucosamine disaccharide substituted with phosphate groups and fatty acids. LPS has multiple biological properties including the ability to induce fever, lethal action, initiation of both complement and blood coagulation cascades, and mitogenic effects on B lymphocytes. It has the ability to stimulate production of such cytokines as tumor necrosis factor (TNF) and interleukin-1 (IL1) and the ability to clot *Limulus* amebocyte lysate. Cytokines induced by endotoxins cause fever, increased capillary permeability, and possible endotoxic shock. Relatively large amounts of LPS released from Gram-negative bacteria during Gram-negative septicemia may produce endotoxin shock.

endotoxin shock

Circulatory and metabolic collapse following exposure to excessive quantities of cytokines, especially IL1 and TNF, introduced into the blood circulation by macrophages following Gram-negative bacterial infection or their products such as lipopolysaccharide. Falling blood pressure and disseminated intravascular coagulation (DIC) following exposure to relatively large amounts of endotoxin produced during bacterial sepsis with *Escherichia coli*, *Pseudomonas aeruginosa*, or meningococci. DIC leads to the formation of thrombi in small blood vessels and such devastating consequences as bilateral cortical necrosis of the kidneys and blockage of the blood supply to the brain, lungs, and adrenals. When DIC affects the adrenal glands, as in certain meningococcal infections, infarction leads to adrenal insufficiency and death. This is the Waterhouse–Friderichsen syndrome. Referred to also as septic shock.

engraftment

The phase during which transplanted bone marrow manufactures new blood cells.

enhancement

The prolonged survival (or, conversely, the delayed rejection) of tumor or skin allografts in individuals previously immunized or conditioned by passive injection of antibody specific for graft antigens. This is termed immunological enhancement and is believed to be due to a blocking effect by the antibody.

enhanceosome

A multiprotein transactivator complex that unites with an active promoter to initiate or facilitate gene transcription. Refer to SXY-CIITA regulatory system.

enhancer

A segment of DNA containing a group of DNA-binding motifs that can elevate the amount of RNA a cell produces. This DNA sequence activates the beginning of RNA polymerase II transcription from a promoter. Although initially described in the SV40 DNA tumor virus, enhancers have now been demonstrated in the J–C introns of immunoglobulin μ and κ genes. Immunoglobulin enhancers function well in B cells, presumably due to precise regulatory proteins that communicate with the enhancer region.

enhancing antibodies

Blocking antibodies that favor survival of tumor or normal tissue allografts.

enkephalins

A related group of endogenous opioids that are pentamers synthesized in the central nervous system and gastrointestinal tract. They share the initial four amino acids (H–Tyr–Gly–Gly–Phe).

entactin/nidogen

Glomerular basement membrane antigens that may have a possible role in glomerular basement membrane nephritis. Entactin is a 150-kDa glomerular membrane-sulfated glycoprotein that is probably synthesized by endothelial and epithelial cells in the developing kidney. It has a role in cellular adhesion to extracellular material. It is complexed with laminin *in vivo*. Nidogen, also a basement membrane constituent, is a 150-kDa glycoprotein that has binding affinity for laminin. Entactin and nidogen closely resemble one another and may be identical. In one study, serum IgG, IgM, and/or IgA antibodies specific for entactin/nidogen were found in more than 40% of patients with glomerulonephritis.

entactin/nidogen autoantibodies

Autoantibodies against entactin, a 150-kDa sulfated glycoprotein present in the glomerular plasma membrane. Entactin is believed to be synthesized by endothelial and epithelial cells in the developing kidney, but in the mature tissue. It is believed to play a role in cellular adhesion to extracellular material. Laminin and entactin form a complex *in vivo*. Nidogen, another sulfated glycoprotein, was identified in the basement membrane matrix of EHS sarcoma. Nidogen is a 150-kDa glycoprotein and, similar to entactin, reveals an *in vitro* binding affinity for laminin. Subsequent investigations have shown nidogen and entactin to be similar or identical. More than 40% of 206 patients with glomerulonephritis develop immunoglobulin G (IgG), IgM, and/or IgA autoantibodies against entactin/nidogen. Entactin autoantibodies of IgG, IgA, and IgM classes have been found in the sera of system lupus erythematosus (SLE) patients, but IgA entactin autoantibodies are found most frequently in patients with IgA nephropathy.

***Entamoeba histolytica* antibody**

Specific serum antibody that develops in essentially all individuals infected with *E. histolytica*. The antibody responses are composed mainly of immunoglobulin G (IgG) and to a lesser degree IgA. IgM declines quickly, whereas specific IgG remains increased for months or years. Coproantibodies are found in the feces of patients with amebic dysentery, whereas patients with amebic liver abscesses have secretory IgA in their saliva and colostrum. There is little evidence of cellular immunity and granuloma formation in flemebic dysentery ulcers and in amebic liver abscesses. *E. histolytica* trophozoites not only resist normal human leukocytes but in fact kill them. Interferon γ (IFN-γ) induced by antigenic stimulation activates macrophages to kill trophozoites. The organism is potently chemotactic for neutrophils that are killed on contact with the parasite. Lytic enzymes released from dead cells induce tissue injury. IFN-γ- and TNF-α-activated neutrophils are able to kill trophozoites. There have been conflicting reports of the relative complement sensitivity of *E. histolytica*.

enteric neuronal autoantibodies

Immunoglobulin G (IgG) autoantibodies that react strongly with nuclei and weakly with cytoplasm of enteric nuclei of myenteric and submucosal plexuses. They develop in selected patients with the paraneoplastic syndrome marked by intestinal pseudo-obstruction in association with small cell lung carcinoma. These autoantibodies are nonreactive with nuclei of non-neuronal tissue. Myenteric neuronal autoantibodies are specific for enteric neuronal neurofilaments, and they can be detected in scleroderma and visceral neuropathy patients.

enterocytes

Intestinal epithelial cells that actively imbibe nutrients. They bear Toll-like receptors and synthesize cytokines that facilitate intestinal intraepithelial lymphocyte activation.

enterotoxin

A heat-stable bacterial toxin that causes intestinal injury.

envelope

Phospholipid bilayer that encircles a viral core. For example, the HIV-1 viral envelope expresses *gp41 and gp120*.

envelope glycoprotein (Env)

A gene of retroviruses that codes for env envelope glycoprotein (refer to HIV-1 genes). It is present on the plasma membranes of infected cells and on the host-cell-derived membrane coats of viral particles. The NV proteins may be required for viral infectivity. HIV env proteins include gp41 and gp120, which bind to CD4 and chemokine receptors, respectively, on human T lymphocytes and facilitate fusion of viral and T cell membranes.

enzyme immunoassay (EIA)

A technique employed to measure immunochemical reactions based on enzyme catalytic properties. The three widely used techniques include a heterogeneous EIA technique, enzyme-linked immunosorbent assay (ELISA), and two homogeneous techniques: enzyme-multiplied immunoassay technique (EMIT) and cloned enzyme donor immunoassay (CEDIA).

enzyme labeling

A method such as the immunoperoxidase technique that permits detection of antigens or antibodies in tissue sections by chemically conjugating them to an enzyme. By then staining the preparation for the enzyme, antigen or antibody molecules can be located. Refer to immunoperoxidase method.

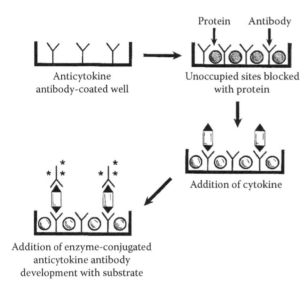

Enzyme-linked immunosorbent assay (ELISA).

enzyme-linked immunosorbent assay (ELISA)

A binder-ligand immunoassay that employs an enzyme linked to either anti-immunoglobulin or antibody specific for antigen and detects either antibody or antigen. This method is based on the sandwich or double-layer technique in which an enzyme rather than a fluorochrome is used as the label. Antibody is attached to the plastic tube, well, or bead surface to which the antigen-containing test sample is added. If antibody is sought in the test sample, the antigen should be attached to the plastic surface. Following antigen–antibody interaction, the enzyme–anti-immunoglobulin conjugate is added. The ELISA test is read by incubating the reactants with an appropriate substrate to yield a colored product that is measured in a spectrophotometer. Alkaline phosphatase and horseradish peroxidase enzymes are often employed. ELISA methods have replaced many radioimmunoassays because of the lower cost and safety, speed, and simplicity to perform.

enzyme-multiplied immunoassay technique (EMIT)

An immunoassay used to monitor therapeutic drugs such as antitumor, antiepileptic, antiasthmatic, and metabolites of cocaine and other agents subject to abuse. It is a one-phase, competitive enzyme-labeled immunoassay.

enzyme replacement therapy

The treatment of a primary immunodeficiency patient, such as one with a genetic deficiency of an enzyme, with a stabilized form of the missing enzyme sufficient to ameliorate disease.

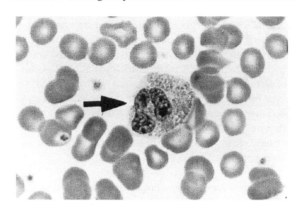

Eosinophil in peripheral blood.

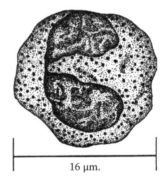

16 μm.

Eosinophil with segmented nucleus.

eosinophil

A polymorphonuclear leukocyte identified in Wright- or Giemsa-stained preparations by staining of secondary granules in the leukocyte cytoplasm as brilliant reddish-orange refractile granules. Cationic peptides are released from these secondary granules when an eosinophil interacts with a target cell and may lead to death of the target. Eosinophils make up 2 to 5% of the total white blood cells in humans. After a brief residence in the circulation, eosinophils migrate into tissues by passing between the lining endothelial cells. They are not believed to return to circulation. The distribution corresponds mainly to areas exposed to the external environment, such as skin, mucosa of the bronchi, and gastrointestinal tract. Eosinophils are elevated during allergic reactions, especially type I immediate hypersensitivity responses, and are also elevated in individuals with parasitic infestations.

eosinophil and neutrophil chemotactic activities

Chemotactic factors for eosinophils and neutrophils (ECA and NCA) are present in bronchoalveolar lavage fluid

(BALF) of selected patients with asthma. ECA induces early atopic dermatitis lesions and is induced by transepidermal permeation of mite allergen. Eosinophils also participate in renal and liver allograft rejection, as reflected by eosinophil cationic protein assays. Eosinophil major basic protein interacts with interleukin-1 (IL1) and transforming growth factor β (TGF-β) to upregulate lung fibroblasts to synthesize IL6 cytokine. When stimulated by C5a, eosinophils produce increased levels of H_2O_2, as assayed by chemiluminescence (CL). Eosinophil activation may also be assayed by flow cytometry. Defective adherence and the migration of neutrophils can be a cause of increased susceptibility to bacterial infection in neonates. The chemotactic cytokine, neutrophil-activating ENA-78 is a proinflammatory polypeptide that shares sequence similarity with IL8 and GRO-α. ENA-78 is a powerful upregulator of MAC-1 cell-surface expression. It is found in cystic fibrosis lung, and its mRNA levels are elevated in human pulmonary inflammation. Flow cytometry and nitroblue tetrazolium reduction can be used to access neutrophil activation.

eosinophil cationic protein (ECP)

An eosinophil, granule, basic, single-chain, zinc-containing protein that manifests cytotoxic, helminthotoxic, ribonuclease, and bactericidal properties. ECP, major basic protein (MBP), eosinophil-derived neurotoxin (EDN), and eosinophil peroxidase (EPO) are the four main eosinophil granule proteins. ECP and MBP induce the release of preformed histamine and synthesis of vasoactive and proinflammatory mediators (PGD_2) from activated human heart mast cells. Acute graft rejection and atopic dermatitis patients manifest provated ECP, whereas systemic sclerosis patients develop increased serum levels of MBP. MBP can act as a cell stimulant and as a toxin. ECP, EPO, EDN, and MBP are versatile in their biological activities that include the capacity to activate other cells including basophils, neutrophils, and platelets. Both enzyme immunoassay (EIA) and flow cytometry have been used to assay intracellular eosinophil proteins in eosinophils from bone marrow and peripheral blood.

eosinophil chemotactic factor

Mast cell granule peptides that induce eosinophil chemotaxis. These include two tetrapeptides: Val–Gly–Ser–Glu and Ala–Gly–Ser–Glu. Histamine also induces eosinophil chemotaxis.

eosinophil differentiation factor (EDF)

A 20-kDa cytokine synthesized by some activated CD4$^+$ T lymphocytes and byb-activated mast cells. Formerly it was called T cell replacing factor or B cell growth factor II. It facilitates B cell growth and differentiation into cells that secrete immunoglobulin A (IgA). It is a costimulator with interleukin-2 (IL2) and IL4 of B cell growth and differentiation. IL5 also stimulates eosinophil growth and differentiation. It activates mature eosinophils to render them capable of killing helminths. Through IL5, T lymphocytes exert regulatory effects on inflammation mediated by eosinophils. Because of its action in promoting eosinophil differentiation, it has been called eosinophil differentiation factor (EDF). IL5 can facilitate B cell differentiation into plaque-forming cells of IgM and IgG classes. In parasitic diseases, IL5 leads to eosinophilia.

eosinophil granule major basic protein (EGMBP)

A polypeptide rich in arginine released from eosinophil granules. It is a powerful toxin for helminths and selected mammalian cells and plays a significant role in late-phase reactions in allergy and asthma and in late-phase skin reactions to allergens such as dust mites. EGMBP is believed to be significant in endomyocardial injury inducted by cardiac localization of eosinophil granule proteins. Interleukin-3 (IL3), granulocyte–macrophage colony-stimulating factor (GM-CSF), and IL5 are eosinophilopoietic cytokines that activate eosinophils and facilitate their survival. These cytokines enhance eosinophil activation in the airways of patients with bronchial asthma which leads to epithelial injury. IFN-α inhibits the release of EGMBP in hypereosinophilic syndrome patients. Immunohistochemistry is used to measure EGMBP from eosinophils infiltrating skin lesions of atopic dermatitis.

eosinophilia

Elevated number of eosinophils in the blood. It occurs in immediate, type I hypersensitivity reactions, including anaphylaxis and atopy, and is observed in patients with parasitic infestations, especially by nematodes.

eosinophilic granuloma

A subtype of a macrophage lineage (histiocytosis X) tumor that contains eosinophils, especially in bone.

eosinophilic myalgia syndrome (EMA)

An intoxication syndrome observed in persons in the United States that appeared to be linked to the consumption of l-tryptophan, proposed by some health advocates as an effective treatment for various disorders such as insomnia, premenstrual syndrome, etc. It was associated with a strain of *Bacillus amyloliquefaciens* employed to produce tryptophan commercially. The inducing agent was apparently an altered amino acid, DTAA (ditryptophan aminal acetaldehyde), a contaminant introduced during manufacture. Clinical manifestations of the syndrome included arthralgia, myopathy, angioedema, alopecia, mobiliform rash, oral ulcers, sclerodermoid lesions, restricted lung disease, fever, lymphadenopathy, and dyspnea, among other features, accompanied by a significant eosinophilia. Interleukin-5 (IL5) was believed to have a role in injury to tissues. Histopathologic examination revealed arteriolitis and sclerosing skin lesions.

eotaxin

A β chemokine family (CC) purified from bronchoalveolar lavage fluid proteins. It has 53% homology with human monocyte chemoattractant protein-1 (MCP-1), 44% with guinea pig MCP-1, 31% with human MIP-1α, and 26% with human RANTES. It is induced locally following transplantation of interleukin-4 (IL4)-secreting tumor cells, suggesting that it may contribute to eosinophil recruitment and antitumor activity of IL4. It has a known human homolog. Eotaxin is expressed by mouse endothelial cells, alveolar macrophages, lung, intestine, stomach, heart, thymus, spleen, liver, testes, and kidney; the target cells are eosinophils. It is constitutively expressed in guinea pig lungs. Its level is increased within 30 minutes after challenge of sensitized guinea pigs with aerosolized antigen in association with eosinophil infiltration. Eotaxin protein can induce accumulation of eosinophils but not neutrophils following intradermal injection. Eotaxin protein administered to guinea pigs in aerosolized form induces eosinophil but not neutrophil accumulation in bronchalveolar fluid. It facilitates chemotaxin eosinophils.

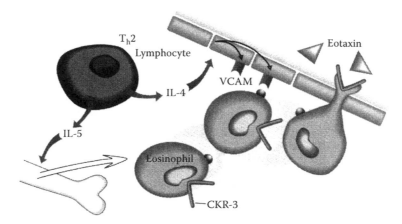

The interaction of cytokines and adhesion molecules in attraction of eosinophils. Recruitment of eosinophils has two separate stages. An increase in circulating eosinophils results from IL5 stimulation of bone marrow growth, differentiation, and release of eosinophils. Attraction of eosinophils to specific tissues presumably involves their adhesion to the endothelium, possible stimulated by IL4-induced expression of VCAM1, followed by chemoattraction by eotaxin and by other nonspecific chemoattractants and activators.

eotaxin-1 and eotaxin-2

CC-chemokines that exert specific action on eosinophils. Referred to as CXCL11 and CXCL24, respectively.

eph receptors and ephrins

The eph receptors constitute the largest known subfamily of receptor tyrosine kinases. The ligands are called ephrins. The ephrin–eph interactions are important in development, especially in cell–cell interactions involved in nervous system patterning (axon guidance) and possibly in cancer.

ephrin/eph

Endothelial cells destined to become arteries express ephrin-B2 while the cognate receptor, eph B4, is expressed on endothelial cells destined to become veins. The ephrin/eph family of cell-surface proteins is important in the cell–cell recognition and signaling of nervous system patterning. Their specific locations on venous versus arterial endothelial cells suggests that the formation of a vascular system may be appreciably more complicated than predicted.

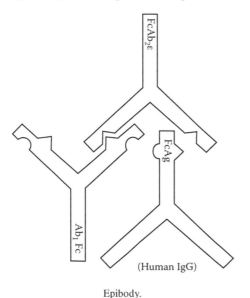

Epibody.

epibody

An anti-idiotypic antibody reactive with an idiotype of a monoclonal, human anti-IgG autoantibody as well as with the human IgG Fc region. These antibodies identify an antigenic determinant associated with the Ser–Ser–Ser sequence. The ability of an epibody to identify an epitope shared by a rheumatoid factor idiotope and an Fcγ epitope demonstrates that this variety of anti-idiotypic antibody may function as a rheumatoid factor.

epidemic

An infectious disease outbreak that affects numerous members of a population.

epidermal growth factor (EGF)

A trisulfated polypeptide consisting of 53 residues. It is a member of the tyrosine kinase family and is related to the *erb* oncogene. EGF has multiple functions, including stimulation of the mitogenic response and facilitation of wound healing, among others. It is present in the saliva of rodents.

epidermal growth factor receptor (EGFR)

A 400-amino-acid protein found in T cell carcinomas, neurons, cornea, fibroblasts, T lymphocytes, liver, vascular endothelium, and placenta. EGFR measurement is used to judge the aggressiveness of such neoplasias as breast cancer.

epidermis

The upper layers of skin that contain principally keratinocytes in addition to skin-associated lymphoid tissue (SALT) constituents but no blood vessels.

epidermolysis bullosa acquisita (EBA)

An uncommon blistering disease characterized by recurrent bullae that heal with scarring. The lesions occur in areas of trauma, especially on the dorsal surfaces of the hands. The split is subepidermal and occurs below the lamina densa of the BMZ. Patients have immunoglobulin G (IgG) autoantibodies that react with various epitopes within the NC1 domain of type VII collagen, the principal constituent of the dermal anchoring fibrils. Dominant epitopes are present in fibronectin-like repeats within the molecule. The disease has an association with HLA-DR2.

epigenetic factors

Factors such as extrachromosomal DNA and environmental stressors that influence the expression of a chromosomally integrated gene.

epithelial cell adhesion molecule (EpCAM)

Considered a pan-carcinoma antigen, EpCAM is highly expressed on a variety of adenocarcinomas of different origins such as breast, ovary, colon, and lung. Its expression in normal tissue is very limited.

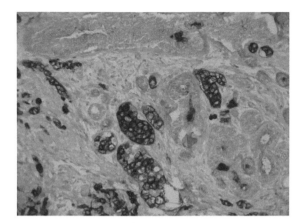

Epithelial membrane antigen—squamous cell carcinoma.

epithelial membrane antigen (EMA)

A marker that identifies, by immunoperoxidase staining, most epithelial cells and tumors derived from them, such as breast carcinomas. However, various nonepithelial neoplasms such as selected lymphomas and sarcomas may also express EMA. Thus, it must be used in conjunction with other markers in tumor identification and/or classification.

epithelial thymic-activating factor (ETAF)

An epithelial cell-culture product capable of facilitating thymocyte growth. The activity is apparently attributable to interleukin-1 (IL1).

epithelioid cell

A particular type of cell characteristic of some types of granulomas such as in tuberculosis, sarcoidosis, leprosy, etc. The cell has poorly defined cellular outlines; cloudy, abundant eosinophilic cytoplasm; and an elongated and pale nucleus. By electron microscopy, the cell shows a few short and slender pseudopodia and well developed cellular organelles. Mitochondria are generally elongated, the Golgi complex is prominent, and lysosomal dense bodies are scattered throughout the cytoplasm. Strands of endoplasmic reticulum, free ribosomes, and fibrils are present in the ground substance. The epithelioid cell derives from the monocyte–macrophage system. Peripheral blood monocytes adhered to cellophane strips and implanted into the subcutaneous tissue of an experimental animal develop into epithelioid cells. Conversion of the macrophage to an epithelioid cell is not preceded by a mitotic division of the macrophage. On the contrary, epithelioid cells are able to divide, resulting in round, small daughter cells that mature in 2 to 4 days, gaining structural and functional characteristics of young macrophages. Material that is taken up by macrophages but cannot be further processed prevents the conversion of epithelioid cells. The lifespan of the epithelioid cell is 1 to 4 weeks.

epitope

An antigenic determinant. It is the simplest form or smallest structural area on a complex antigen molecule that can combine with an antibody or form the major histocompatibility complex (MHC)-binding peptide recognized by T lymphocyte receptors. It must be at least 1 kDa to elicit an antibody response. A smaller molecule such as a hapten may induce an immune response if combined with a carrier protein molecule. Multiple epitopes may be found on large nonpolymeric molecules. Based on x-ray crystallography, epitopes consist of prominently exposed "hill and ridge" regions that manifest surface rigidity. Antigenicity is diminished in more flexible sites. Native and denatured proteins, chemical groups, lipids, carbohydrates, nucleic acids, or other constituents may comprise B cell epitopes. By contrast, T cell epitopes are comprised of a complex of antigenic peptide linked to either MHC class I or class II molecules.

epitope spreading

Increased diversity of the response to autoantigens with time. Immune response against a single epitope induces tissue injury that exposes epitopes previously hidden, thereby activating further lymphocyte clones. Participates in tumor regression, chronic graft rejection and autoimmune responsiveness. Also termed determinant spreading and antigen spreading.

epitype

A family or group of related epitopes.

Epivir®

A synthetic nucleoside analog approved by the U.S. Food and Drug Administration for the treatment of human immunodeficiency virus (HIV). The mechanism of action includes phosphorylation of the drug to its active 5′ triphosphate metabolite that inhibits reverse transcriptase via DNA chain termination after incorporation of the nucleoside analog. Lamivudine is the active component of the drug.

EPO

Refer to erythropoietin.

Epstein–Barr immunodeficiency syndrome

Duncan's X-linked immunodeficiency. This is an X-linked or autosomal-recessive condition associated with congenital cardiovascular and central nervous system defects. Patients may develop fatal infectious mononucleosis. Aplasia of the bone marrow, agammaglobulinemia, and agranulocytosis occur, and the response to mitogens and antigens by B cells is greatly diminished. Natural killer cell activity is decreased, and T cells are abnormal. Patients may develop hepatitis, B cell lymphomas, and immune suppression.

Epstein–Barr nuclear antigen

A molecule that occurs in B cells before virus-directed protein can be found in nuclei of infected cells. Thus, it is the earliest evidence of Epstein–Barr virus infection and can be found in patients with conditions such as infectious mononucleosis and Burkitt's lymphoma.

Epstein–Barr virus (EBV)

A DNA herpes virus linked to aplastic anemia, chronic fatigue syndrome, Burkitt's lymphoma, histiocytic sarcoma, hairy cell leukemia, and immunocompromised patients. EBV may promote the appearance of such lymphoid proliferative disorders as Hodgkin and non-Hodgkin lymphoma, infectious mononucleosis, nasopharyngeal carcinoma, and thymic carcinoma. It readily transforms B lymphocytes and is used in the laboratory for this purpose to develop long-term B lymphocyte cultures. Antibodies produced in patients with EBV infections include those that appear early and are referred to as EA, antibodies against viral capsid antigen (VCA), and antibodies against nuclear antigens (EBNA). EBV selectively infects human B cells by

E

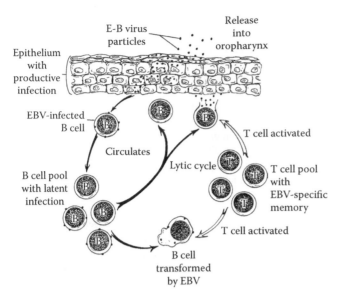

Epstein–Barr virus (EBV)–host interaction.

binding to complement receptor 2 (CR2 or CD21). It causes infectious mononucleosis and establishes a latent infection of B cells that persists for life and is controlled by T cells.

equilibrium constant

A constant that expresses the state of equilibrium reached by molecules in a reversible reaction such as $A + B = AB$. The equilibrium constant may be expressed as a dissociation constant, $K_D = [A][B]/[AB]$ or an association constant, $K_A = [AB]/[A][B]$.

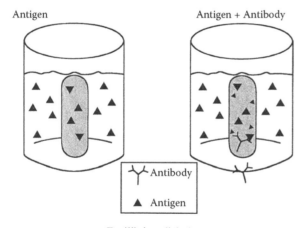

Equilibrium dialysis.

equilibrium dialysis

A method to ascertain the affinity of an antibody for an antigen and its valency. Equilibrium dialysis was developed for the study of primary antibody–hapten interactions. Two cells are separated by a semipermeable membrane, allowing the free passage of hapten molecules but not larger antibody molecules. At time zero (t_0), there is a known concentration of hapten in cell A and antibody in cell B. Hapten from cell A will then diffuse across the membrane into cell B until, at equilibrium, the concentration of free hapten is the same in both cells A and B; that is, the rate of diffusion of hapten from cell A to B is the same as that from cell B to A. Although the concentrations of free hapten are the

same in both cells, the total amount of hapten in cell B is greater because some of the hapten is bound to the antibody molecules. A series of experiments is performed, varying the starting amount of hapten concentration while keeping antibody concentration constant.

equivalence (equivalence point)

In a precipitation reaction *in vitro*, the antigen-to-antibody ratio at which maximal precipitation takes place. The supernatant should not contain free antigen or free antibody, as all of the antigen and antibody molecules react with one another at equivalence.

equivalence zone

Refer to zone of equivalence.

erbA, erbB

Oncogenes expressing tyrosine kinase activity. They are similar in structure to the avian erythroblastosis retrovirus. They code for cell membrane proteins. *erbB* is expressed in breast and salivary gland carcinomas and is a truncated version of epidermal growth factor receptor. Increased copy numbers of the c-*erbB*2 (HER2/neu) gene suggest an unfavorable prognosis for carcinoma of the breast.

ergotype

A T lymphocyte being activated. The injection of antiergotype T cells blocks full-scale activation of T lymphocytes and may prevent development of experimental autoimmune disease in animal models. An example is experimental allergic encephalomyelitis (EAE), in which antiergotype T lymphocytes may prevent full T lymphocyte activation.

erp57

A chaperone molecule that participates in the loading of peptide onto major histocompatibility complex (MHC) class I molecules in the endoplasmic reticulum.

erythema

Redness of the skin caused by dilatation of blood vessels lying near the surface.

erythema marginatum

Immune-complex-induced vasculitis in the subcutaneous tissues associated with rheumatic fever.

erythema multiforme

Skin lesions resulting from subcutaneous vasculitis produced by immune complexes. They are frequently linked to drug reactions. A lesion is identified by a red center encircled by an area of pale edema that is encircled by a red or erythematous ring. This gives it a target appearance. Erythema multiforme usually signifies a drug allergy or may be linked to systemic infection. Lymphocytes and macrophages infiltrate the lesions. When involvement and sloughing of the mucous membranes are present, the lesions are considered quite severe and even life threatening. This form is called the Stevens–Johnson syndrome.

erythema nodosum

Slightly elevated erythematous nodules that develop on the shins and sometimes the forearm and head and are very painful. They represent subcutaneous vasculitis involving small arteries. The phenomenon is associated with infection and is produced by antigen–antibody complexes. Erythema nodosum may be an indicator of inflammatory bowel disease, histoplasmosis, tuberculosis, sarcoidosis, or leprosy. It can follow the use of certain drugs. Although claimed in the past to be due to antigen–antibody deposits in the walls of small venules, the immunologic mechanism may involve type IV (delayed-type) hypersensitivity in the small venules.

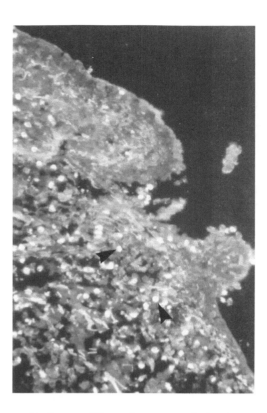

Erythema multiforme. Immunocytes in dermis.

Neutrophils, macrophages, and lymphocytes infiltrate the subcutaneous fat.

erythroblastosis fetalis

A human fetal disease induced by immunoglobulin G (IgG) antibodies passed across the placenta from mother to fetus that are specific for fetal red blood cells, leading to their destruction. Although not often a serious problem until the third pregnancy, the escape of fetal red blood cells into the maternal circulation, especially at the time of parturition, produces a booster response in the mother of the IgG antibody that produces an even more severe reaction in the second and third fetus. The basis for this reaction is an isoantigen such as RhD antigen not present in the mother but present in the fetal red cells and inherited from the father. Clinical consequences of this maternal–fetal blood group incompatibility include anemia, jaundice, kernicterus, hydrops fetalis, and even stillbirth. Preventive therapy now includes administration of anti-D antiserum (RhIG) within 72 hours following parturition. This antibody combines with the fetal red cells dumped into the mother's circulation at parturition and dampens production of a booster response. This is an antibody-mediated type II hypersensitivity reaction. May also be called Rh disease.

erythrocyte

Red blood cell.

erythrocyte agglutination test

Refer to hemagglutination test.

erythrocyte autoantibodies

Autoantibodies against erythrocytes. They are of significance in the autoimmune form of hemolytic anemia and are usually classified into cold and warm varieties by the thermal range of their activity.

erythroid progenitor

An immature cell that leads to the production of erythrocytes and megakaryocytes, but no other blood cell types.

erythropoiesis

The formation of erythrocytes or red blood cells.

erythropoietin

A 46-kDa glycoprotein produced by the kidney, more specifically by cells adjacent to the proximal renal tubules, based on the presence of oxygen-sensitive substances such as heme in the kidneys. It stimulates red blood cell production by combining with erythroid precursor receptors to promote mature red cell development. Erythropoietin formation is increased by hypoxia. It is useful in the treatment of various types of anemia.

***Escherichia coli* immunity**

Immunoglobulin M (IgM) and IgG antibodies are formed against O, H, and K antigens of *E. coli* of the diarrhea-producing strains in infants. Secretory IgA specific for *E. coli* diminishes the adherence of diarrhea-producing *E. coli* in the intestines of infants. Secretory IgA in breast milk also offers significant protection of infants through passive immunity. Secretory IgA may be specific for LT enterotoxins and for colonization factor antigens.

essential mixed cryoglobulinemia

A condition that is identified by purpura (skin hemorrhages), joint pains, impaired circulation in the extremities on exposure to cold (Raynaud's phenomenon), and glomerulonephritis. Renal failure may result. Polyclonal immunoglobulin G (IgG), IgM, and complement are detectable as granular deposits in the glomerular basement membranes. The cryoprecipitates containing IgG and IgM may also contain hepatitis B antigen, as this condition is frequently a sequela of hepatitis B.

estradiol

In diagnostic immunology, a marker identifiable in breast carcinoma tissue by monoclonal antibody and the immunoperoxidase technique that correlates, to a limited degree, with estrogen receptor activity in cytosols from the same preparation.

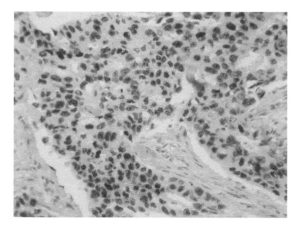

Estrogen receptor—carcinoma of the breast.

estrogen/progesterone receptor protein

Monoclonal antibodies against estrogen receptor protein and progesterone receptor protein permit identification of tumor cells by their preferential immunoperoxidase staining for these markers, whereas stromal cells remain unstained. This method is claimed by some to be superior to cytosol assays in evaluating the clinical response to hormones.

etanercept (injection)

Binds specifically to TNF, inhibiting its interaction with cell surface TNF receptors. TNF is a naturally occurring cytokine involved in inflammatory and immune responses, and plays a significant role in the inflammatory processes of rheumatoid arthritis, juvenile rheumatoid arthritis, and ankylosing spondylitis along with the resulting joint pathology. A dimeric fusion protein comprised of human IgG_1 constant regions (CH_2, CH_3, and hinge, but not CH_1) fused with the TNF receptor. A soluble form of the p75 TNF receptor that can anchor to two TNF molecules. It blocks the binding of both TNF α and TNF β to cell surface TNF receptors, rendering TNF biologically inactive and inhibiting TNF-α-mediated inflammation. Etanercept can also modulate biological responses induced or regulated by TNF including adhesion molecule expression and serum levels of cytokines. It is used for adult rheumatoid arthritis, polyarticular-course juvenile RA, and psoriatic arthritis.

euglobulin

A type of globulin that is insoluble in water but dissolves in salt solutions. In the past, it was used to designate the part of serum protein that could be precipitated by 33% saturated ammonium sulfate at 4°C or by 14.2% sodium sulfate at room temperature. Euglobulin is precipitated from the serum proteins at low ionic strength.

eukaryote

A cell or organism with a real nucleus containing chromosomes encircled by a nuclear membrane.

evasion strategies

Methods imposed by a pathogen to circumvent or compromise a host's immune response.

everolimus

A proliferation-signal inhibitor that is useful in diminishing rejection in cardiac allotransplantation.

EVI antibodies

Found in Chagas' disease, autoantibodies to endocardium, vascular structures, and interstitial of striated muscles. The target is laminin but the relevance is in doubt, because other diseases produce antilaminin antibodies that do not produce the unique pathology seen in Chagas' disease.

exchange transfusion

Replacement of the entire blood volume of a patient with donor blood. This is done to remove toxic substances such as those formed in kernicterus in infants with erythroblastosis fetalis or to remove anti-Rh antibodies causing hemolytic disease of a newborn.

excitation filter

A filter in a fluorescent microscope that permits only light of a specific excitation wavelength (e.g., ultraviolet) to pass through.

exercise and immunity

Exercise leads to altered distribution and function of immunocompetent cells. This is related in part to changes in hormone release, blood flow distribution, and other factors that affect immune system function. Vigorous exercise leads to immediate leukocytosis. Exercise-induced immunosuppression or immunoenhancement may affect disease risk. Absolute numbers of $CD3^+$, $CD8^+$, and $CD16^+/C56$ (natural killer, NK) cells increase after exercise, and B lymphocytes also rise with acute exercise, but these increases

return to pre-exercise levels within a few hours following cessation of exercise. The $CD4^+/CD8^+$ lymphocyte helper/suppressor ratio diminishes soon after exercise, attributable to increased CD8 counts. Acute exercise is followed by increase in the concentration and *in vitro* cytolytic activity of $CD16^+/CD56^+$ cells, but exhaustive exercise leads to a decrease in the cytolytic activity of NK cells. Exercise also leads to cytokine release, such as the elevation of interleukin-6 (IL6) but not IL1. After exercise, TNF-γ and granulocyte–macrophage colony-stimulating factor (GM-CSF) are essentially undetectable. IL2 levels also decrease following exercise. Increased urinary concentrations of IFN-γ, TNF-α, and IL6 have been demonstrated following long distance running. Exercise has little functional impact on immune effector cells. The response of lymphocytes to T cell mitogens such as phytohemagglutinin (PHA) and concanavalin A (con A) is diminished immediately after exercise but returns to normal within 24 hours. The proliferative response to B cell mitogens such as lipopolysaccharide (LPS) and mixed T and B cell mitogens such as PWM increases following exercise. Antibody synthesis is not much affected by limited exercise. Immunoglobulin G (IgG), IgM, and IgA levels, as well as the ability to synthesize antibody to tetanus toxoid antigen, are not compromised by exercise. Exercise prior to exposure to infection diminishes morbidity or mortality, yet exercise during an infection produces the reverse effect. Prolonged intense exercise is followed by some immunosuppression. The immune parameters altered by physical exercise are related to the neuroendocrine changes such as those that occur in response to physical or psychological stress.

exercise-induced asthma

An attack of asthma brought on by exercise.

exoantigen

Released antigen.

exocytosis

The release of intracellular vesicle contents to the exterior of a cell. The vesicles make their way to the plasma membrane, with which they fuse to permit the contents to be released to the external environment. Examples include immunoglobulin released from plasma cells and mast cell degranulation, which releases histamine and other pharmacological mediators of anaphylaxis to the exterior of the cell. Cytokines may also be released from cells of this process.

exogenous

Externally caused rather than resulting from conditions within the organism; derived externally.

exogenous antigen

An epitope that occurs outside the host's body, such as a bacterial toxin.

exogenous antigen processing and presentation

Epitopes that originate outside the animal body are taken up by antigen-presenting cells, degraded via the endocytic pathway and bound to MHC class II molecules in an endolysosomal vesicle. This is followed by exhibition of the peptide-MHC class II complex at the cell surface. This pathway is confined almost exclusively to antigen-presenting cells.

exon

That segment of a strand of DNA responsible for coding. This continuous DNA sequence in a gene encodes the amino acid sequence of the gene product. Exons are buttressed on both ends by introns, which are noncoding regions of DNA. The coding sequence is transcribed in mature mRNA and subsequently translated into proteins. Exons produce folding regions, functional regions, domains, and subdomains. Introns, which are junk DNA, are spliced out. They constitute the turns or edges of secondary structures.

exotoxins

An extracellular product of pathogenic microorganisms. Exotoxins are 3- to 500-kDa polypeptides produced by such microorganisms as *Corynebacterium diphtheria,* *Clostridium tetani,* and *C. botulinum. Vibrio cholerae* produces exotoxins that elevate cyclic adenosine monophosphate (cAMP) levels in intestinal mucosa cells and increase the flow of water and ions into the intestinal lumen, producing diarrhea. Exotoxins are polypeptides released from bacterial cells and are diffusible, thermolabile, and able to be converted to toxoids that are immunogenic but not toxic. Bacterial exotoxins are either cytolytic, acting on cell membranes, or bipartite (A–B toxins), linking to a cell surface through the B segment of the toxin and releasing the A segment only after the molecule reaches the cytoplasm, where it produces injury. Some may serve as superantigens.

experimental allergic encephalomyelitis

An autoimmune disease induced by immunization of experimental animals with preparations of brain or spinal cord incorporated into Freund's complete adjuvant. After 10 to 12 days, perivascular accumulations of lymphocytes and mononuclear phagocytes surround the vasculature of the brain and spinal cord white matter. Demyelination may also be present, worsening as the disease becomes chronic. The animals often develop paralysis. The disease can be passively transferred from a sick animal to a healthy one of the same strain with T lymphocytes, but not with antibodies. The mechanism involves T cell receptor interaction with an 18-kDa myelin basic protein molecule, which is an organ-specific antigen of nervous system tissue. The CD4+ T lymphocyte represents the phenotype that is reactive with myelin basic protein. The immune reaction induces myelinolysis, wasting, and paralysis. Peptides derived from myelin basic protein (MBP) may be used to induce experimental allergic encephalomyelitis in animals. This experimental autoimmune disease is an animal model for multiple sclerosis and postvaccination encephalitis in humans.

experimental allergic neuritis

An experimental disease induced by injecting rats with peripheral nerve incorporated into Freund's complete adjuvant. P2 antigen is involved. Lymphocytes and macrophages infiltrate the sciatic nerve, and paralysis may develop.

experimental allergic orchitis

An experimental autoimmune disease induced by injecting experimental animals with isogeneic or allogeneic testicular tissue incorporated into Freund's complete adjuvant.

experimental allergic thyroiditis

An autoimmune disease produced by injecting experimental animals with thyroid tissue or extract or thyroglobulin incorporated into Freund's complete adjuvant. It represents an animal model of Hashimoto's thyroiditis in humans, with mixed extensive lymphocytic infiltrate. Another animal model is the spontaneous occurrence of this disease in the obese strain of chickens as well as in Buffalo rats.

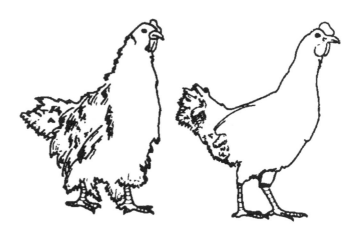

Experimental allergic thyroiditis (EAT).

experimental autoimmune encephalymyelitis

Autoimmune demyelinating central nervous system disease in animal models induced by immunizing rats with myelin basic protein from the myelin sheath of nerves, incorporated into Freund's adjuvant. CD4+ T lymphocytes with specificity for myelin sheath proteins secrete cytokines that mediate the disease.

experimental autoimmune myasthenia gravis (EAMG)

Myasthenia gravis (MG) is an autoantibody-mediated autoimmune disease. Experimental forms of MG were made possible through the ready availability of AChR from electric fish. Monoclonal antibodies were developed, followed by molecular cloning techniques that permitted definition of the AChR structure. EAMG can be induced in more than one species of animals by immunizing them with purified AChR from the electric ray (*Torpedo californica*). The autoantigen, nicotinic AChR, is T cell-dependent. The *in vivo* synthesis of anti-AChR antibodies requires helper T cell activity. Antibodies specific for the nicotinic AChR of skeletal muscle react with the postsynaptic membrane at the neuromuscular junction.

experimental autoimmune myocarditis (EAM)

Murine model of human autoimmune myocarditis. Infection of A/J and BALB/c mice with coxsackie Bc virus or immunization of susceptible mice with cardiac myosin may lead to development of EAM.

experimental autoimmune neuritis (EAN)

A condition induced in mammalian species by immunization with peripheral nervous system (PNS) myelin, purified PNS myelin proteins, or synthetic peptides of PNS antigens, myelin basic protein, the PO glycoprotein, and the P2 protein. EAN develops 10 to 14 days after immunization with ascending paraparesis and paralysis. CD4+ T cells and macrophages infiltrate PNS tissue. Macrophages cause demyelination. Autoantibodies to myelin may also play a role in EAN pathogenesis.

experimental autoimmune oophoritis

Ovarian autoimmune disease induced by immunization with synthetic peptides of mouse CP3, a glycoprotein with sperm receptor activity located in the zona pellucida of developing and mature oocytes. A single subcutaneous injection of ZP3 peptide incorporated into Freund's complete adjuvant can induce the disease in (C57B1/6 × A/J)S₁ hybrid mice. It is marked by ovarian inflammation that may be followed by ovarian follicle loss and ovarian atrophy.

E

The infiltrating lymphocytes are comprised mainly of CD4⁺ T lymphocytes. There are also many macrophages, and immunoglobulin G (IgG) is found in the zona pellucida.

experimental autoimmune sialoadenitis (EAS)

An animal model used to investigate the pathogenesis of salivary gland injury in Sjögren's syndrome. It may be induced in LEW rats by immunization with allogeneic or syngeneic submandibular gland tissue in complete Freund's adjuvant and *Bordetella pertussis*. Autoantibodies are produced against antigens of salivary ducts as well as mononuclear cell infiltration of salivary tissues, comprised of CD4⁺, CD8⁺, and B lymphocytes. Injury of glands is acute, yet tissue damage resolves spontaneously 4 to 5 weeks after immunization. CD4⁺ T lymphocytes play a critical role in EAS induction.

experimental autoimmune thyroiditis (EAT)

A murine model for Hashimoto's thyroiditis. Susceptibility to Hashimoto's thyroiditis has a strong major histocompatibility complex (MHC) genetic component, which has been shown to reside in the *IA* subregion of the murine MHC (H-2), governing the immune response (*Ir*) genes to mouse thyroglobulin (MTg). Induced by immunizing CBA/J mouse substrains with Freund's complete adjuvant with whole thyroglobulin protein or its peptides. Following induction of EAT with MTg, autoantibodies against MTg appear, and mononuclear cells infiltrate the thyroid. Repeated administration of soluble, syngeneic MTg without adjuvant leads to thyroiditis only in the murine haplotype susceptible to EAT. Autoreactive T cells proliferate *in vitro* following stimulation with MTg, passively transfer the disease to naïve recipients by adoptive immunization and differentiate into cytotoxic T lymphocytes (T$_c$) *in vitro*. Thus, lymphoid cells rather than antibodies represent the primary mediators of the disease. *In vitro* proliferation of murine-autoreactive T cells was found to show a good correlation with susceptibility to EAT and was dependent on the presence of Thy-1⁺, Lyt-1⁺, Ia⁺, and L3T4⁺ lymphocytes. Effector T lymphocytes (T$_E$) in EAT comprise various T cell subsets and Lyt-1 (L3T4) and Lyt-2 phenotypes. T lymphocytes cloned from thyroid infiltrates of patients with Hashimoto's thyroiditis reveal numerous cytotoxic T lymphocytes and clones synthesizing IL-2 and IFN-γ. While the T cell subsets participate in the pathogenesis of Hashimoto's thyroiditis, autoantibody synthesis appears to aid perpetuation of the disease or result from it.

experimental autoimmune uveitis (EAU)

A disease of the neural retina and related tissues induced by immunization with purified retinal antigens. It is a model for various human ocular inflammatory diseases, possibly autoimmune, that are accompanied by immunologic responses to ocular antigens. The most frequently used are retinal soluble antigen (S-Ag), the interphotoreceptor retinoid-binding protein (IRBP), and rhodopsin. Immunization with these antigens incorporated into complete Freund's adjuvant leads to injury of the photoreceptor cell layer of the retina. Histopathologically, inflammatory cells infiltrate the retina, and the photoreceptors are injured. Also called experimental autoimmune uveoretinitis.

experimental tolerance

Antigen-specific suppression of an immune response induced by the inoculation of a mature animal with a nonimmunogenic form of the antigen through the usual manner of immunization or an immunogenic form of the antigen through a nonimmunogenic route of administration.

extended haplotype

Linked alleles in positive linkage disequilibrium situated between and including HLA-DR and HLA-B of the major histocompatibility complex (MHC) of humans. Examples of extended haplotypes include the association of B8/DR3/SCO1/GLO2 with membranoproliferative glomerulonephritis and of A25/B18/DR2 with complement C2 deficiency. Extended haplotypes may be consequences of crossover suppression through environmental influences together with selected HLA types, leading to autoimmune conditions. The B27 relationship to *Klebsiella* is an example. Polymerase chain reaction (PCR) amplification and direct sequencing help identify a large number of allelic differences and specific associations of extended haplotypes with disease. Extended haplotypes are more informative than single polymorphisms. Some diseases associated with extended haplotypes include Graves' disease, pemphigus vulgaris, type I (juvenile onset) psoriasis, insulin-dependent diabetes mellitus, celiac disease, and autoimmune hepatitis.

extracellular antigen

Refer to exogenous antigen.

extracellular pathogen

A pathogenic microorganism that reproduces in the interstitial fluid, blood or lumens of the respiratory, urogenital, and gastrointestinal tracts rather than entering host cells.

extramedullary plasmacytoma

A plasma cell dyscrasia in which the malignant plasma cells have moved beyond the bone marrow and entered other tissues.

extramedullary tissues

Tissues and organs other than lymphoid tissues or bone marrow.

extranodal lymphoma

A lymphoma of diffuse lymphoid tissue, such as gut-associated lymphoid tissue.

extrathymic T cell development

Development and maturation of T lymphocytes in tissues external to the thymus gland.

extravasation

The movement of fluid and cells from the circulating blood into the surrounding tissues without interrupting the integrity of vessel walls, as in inflammation. The process consists of margination and diapedesis.

extrinsic allergic alveolitis

Inflammation in the lung produced by immune reactivity, mainly of the granulomatous type, to inhaled antigens such as dust, bacteria, molds, grains, and other substances. Also called farmer's lung.

extrinsic apoptotic pathway

Refer to apoptosis.

extrinsic asthma

An asthma caused by antigen-antibody reactions. It has two mutually non-exclusive forms: (1) atopic, involving immunoglobulin E (IgE) antibodies, and (2) nonatopic, involving either antibodies other than IgE or immune complexes. The atopic form usually begins in childhood and is preceded by other atopic manifestations such as paroxysmal rhinitis, seasonal hay fever, or infantile eczema. A familial history is usually obtainable. Other environmental agents may sometimes be recognized in the nonatopic form. Patients with extrinsic asthma respond favorably to bronchodilators.

exudate
Fluid containing cells and cellular debris that have escaped from blood vessels and have been deposited in tissues or on tissue surfaces as a consequence of inflammation. In contrast to a transudate, an exudate is characterized by a high content of proteins, cells, or solid material derived from cells.

exudation
The passage of blood cells and fluid containing serum proteins from the blood into the tissues during inflammation.

E

F

F-actin

Actin molecules in a dual-stranded helical polymer. Together with the tropomyosin–tropinin regulatory complex, F-actin constitutes the thin filaments of skeletal muscle.

f allotype

A rabbit immunoglobulin A (IgA) subclass α heavy-chain allotype. Allelic genes at the *f* locus encode five *f* allotypes designated f69 through f73. More than one allotypic determinant is associated with each allotype.

f-Met peptides

Bacterial tripeptides such as formyl–Met–Leu–Phe that are chemotactic for inflammatory cells, inducing leukocyte migration.

F protein

A 42-kDa protein in the cytoplasm of murine hepatocytes. It occurs in F.1 and F.2 allelic forms in separate inbred murine strains.

F_1 hybrid

The first generation of offspring after a mating between genetically different parents, such as from two different inbred strains.

F_1 hybrid disease

A graft-vs.-host reaction that takes place after the F_1 hybrid is injected with immunologically competent lymphoid cells from a parent. Whereas the hybrid is immunologically tolerant to the histocompatibility antigens of the parent, the injected T lymphocytes from the parent react against antigens of the other parent that are expressed in tissues of the F_1 hybrid, producing the graft-vs.-host-like reactivity. The severity of the reaction depends on the histocompatibility differences between the two parents of the F_1 hybrid.

F_1 hybrid resistance

A condition that results when two inbred mouse strains are crossed and a bone marrow graft from either of the parents is rejected by the F_1 offspring. Attributable to variation in NK inhibitory receptor expression by F1 natural (NK) cells.

F_2 generation

The second generation of offspring produced following a specific mating.

Fab fragment

Fragment, antigen-binding. A product of papain digestion of an immunoglobulin G (IgG) molecule. It is comprised of one light chain and the segment of heavy chain on the N terminal side of the central disulfide bond. The light and heavy chain segments are linked by interchain disulfide bonds. Its weight is 47 kDa and its sedimentation coefficient is 3.5 S. The Fab fragment has a single antigen-binding site. Each IgG molecule has two Fab regions.

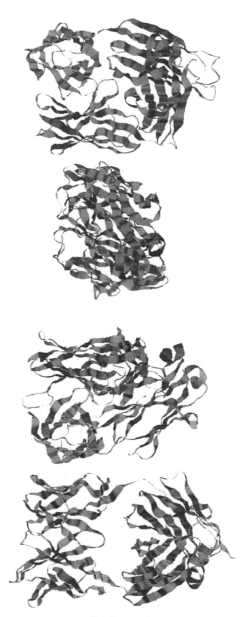

Fab fragment.

Fab′ fragment

A product of reduction of an F(ab′)$_2$ fragment that results from pepsin digestion of immunoglobulin G (IgG). It is comprised of one light chain linked by disulfide bonds to the N terminal segment of the heavy chain. The Fab′ fragment has a single antigen-binding site. Each F(ab′)$_2$ fragment has two Fab′ fragments.

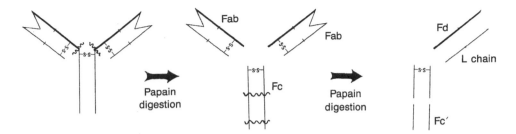

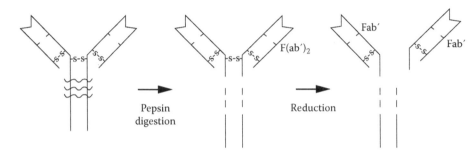

The Fab fragment is composed of one light chain and the variable and C_H1 regions of a heavy chain. They are united by disulfide bonds and have a single binding site for antigen. The heavy chain part of a Fab fragment is referred to as Fd. Further digestion with papain yields an Fc′.

Pepsin digestion of an IgG molecule leading to formation of $F(ab')_2$ intermediate fragments with reduction to the formation of Fab′ fragments.

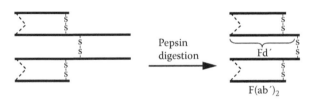

$F(ab')_2$ fragment containing 2 Fd′ heavy chain portions.

F(ab′)₂ fragment

A product of pepsin digestion of an immunoglobulin G (IgG) molecule. This 95-kDa immunoglobulin fragment has a valence or antigen-binding capacity of two that renders it capable of inducing agglutination or precipitation with homologous antigen. However, the functions associated with the Fc region of the intact IgG molecule, such as complement fixation and attachment to Fc receptors on cell surfaces, are missing. Pepsin digestion occurs on the carboxyl terminal side of the central disulfide bond at the hinge region of the molecule which leaves the central disulfide bond intact. The C_H2 domain is converted to minute peptides, yet the C_H3 domain is left whole, and the two C_H3 domains comprise the pFc′ fragment.

Fab″ fragment

Refer to F(ab′)₂ fragment.

Fabc fragment

A 5-S intermediate fragment produced by partial digestion of immunoglobulin G (IgG) by papain in which only one Fab fragment is cleaved from the parent molecule in the hinge region. This leaves the Fabc fragment, which is composed of a Fab region bound covalently to an Fc region and is functionally univalent.

Facb fragment

Abbreviation for fragment antigen and complement binding. The action of plasmin on immunoglobulin G (IgG) molecules denatured by acid cleaves C_H3 domains from both heavy chain constituents of the Fc region. This yields a bivalent fragment functionally capable of precipitation and agglutination with an Fc remnant still capable of fixing complement.

FACS®

Refer to fluorescence-activated cell sorter.

factor B

An alternative complement pathway component. It is a 739-amino-acid residue, single-polypeptide chain that combines with C3b and is cleaved by factor D to produce alternative pathway C3 convertase. Cleavage by factor D is at an arginine–lysine bond at position 234 to 235 to yield an amino terminal fragment Ba. The carboxyl-terminal fragment termed Bb remains attached to C3b. C3bBb is C3 convertase, and C3bBb3b is C5 convertase of the alternative complement pathway. The Bb fragment is the enzyme's active site. Factor B has three short homologous, 60-amino acid residue repeats and four attachment sites for N-linked oligosaccharides. Alleles for human factor B include *BfS* and *BfF*. The factor B gene is located in the major histocompatibility complex (MHC) situated on the short arm of chromosome 6 in humans and on chromosome 17 in mice. Also called C3 proactivator.

factor D

An alternative complement activation pathway serine esterase. It splits factor B to produce Ba and Bb fragments. It is also called C3 activator convertase.

factor D deficiency

An extremely rare genetic deficiency of factor D which has an X-linked or autosomal-recessive pattern of inheritance. The sera of affected patients contain only 1% of the physiologic amounts of factor D, which renders them susceptible to repeated infection by *Neisseria* microorganisms. The sera of heterozygotes contain half the physiologic levels of factor D, but they have no clinical symptoms related to this deficiency.

factor H

A regulator of complement in the blood under physiologic conditions. Factor H is a glycoprotein in serum that unites

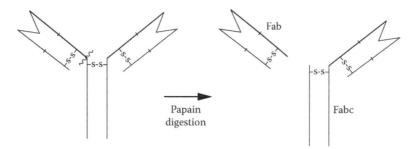

Generation of Fabc fragment by papain digestion of IgG in which one Fab region is cleaved, leaving an Fabc fragment consisting of the Fc region and one Fab region of the molecule bearing a single antigen-binding site.

with C3b and facilitates dissociation of alternative complement pathway C3 convertase, designated C3bBb, into C3b and Bb. Factor I splits C3b if factor H is present. In humans, factor H is a 1231-amino-acid residue, single polypeptide chain. It is comprised of 20 short homologous repeats composed of about 60 residues present in proteins that interact with C3 or C4. Factor H is an inhibitor of the alternative complement pathway. Previously called β-1H globulin.

factor H deficiency
Extremely rare genetic deficiency of factor H that has an autosomal-recessive mode of inheritance. Only 1% of the physiologic level of factor H is present in the sera of affected individuals, which renders them susceptible to recurrent infections by pyogenic microorganisms. People who are heterozygotes have 50% of normal levels of factor H in their sera and show no clinical effects.

factor H receptor (fH-R)
A receptor that initial studies have shown to be comprised of a 170-kD protein expressed by Raji cells and tonsil B cells. Neutrophils, B lymphocytes, and monocytes express fH-R activity.

factor I
A serine protease that splits the α chain of C3b to produce C3bi and the α chain of C4b to yield C4bi. Factor I splits a 17-amino-acid residue peptide termed C3f, if factor H or complement receptor 1 are present, from the C3b α chain to yield C3bi. Factor I splits the C3bi, if complement receptor I or factor H are present, to yield C3c and C3dg. Factor I splits the C4b α chain, if C4-binding protein is present, to yield C4bi. C4c and C4d are produced by a second splitting of the α chain of C4bi. Factor I is a heterodimeric molecule. It is also called C3b/C4b inactivator.

factor I deficiency
Very uncommon genetic deficiency of C3b inactivator that has an autosomal-recessive pattern of inheritance. Less than 1% of the physiologic level of factor I is present in the sera of affected subjects, which renders them susceptible to repeated infections by pyogenic microorganisms. These individuals also reveal deficiencies of factor B and C3 in their serum, as these components are normally split *in vivo* by alternative pathway C3 convertase (C3bBb), which factors I and H inhibit under physiologic conditions. These patients may develop urticaria because of the formation of C3a, which induces the release of histamine.

factor P (properdin)
A key participant in the alternative pathway of complement activation. It is a globulin, but not an immunoglobulin, that combines with C3b and stabilizes alternative pathway C3 convertase (C3bB) to produce C3bBbP. Factor P is a 3- or 4-polypeptide chain structure.

factor VIII
A coagulation protein produced by endothelial cells, which makes it a useful marker for vascular tumors. It is demonstrable by immunoperoxidase staining. Megakaryocytes and platelets also stain for factor VIII.

facultative phagocytes
Cells such as fibroblasts that may show phagocytic properties under special circumstances.

FAE
Refer to follicle-associated epithelium.

Faenia rectivirgula
The most frequently encountered inhalant in farmer's lung disease, the most common type of hypersensitivity pneumonitis in the United States. This agent or its

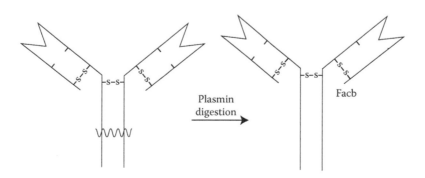

Generation of Facb fragment through plasmin digestion of an IgG molecule.

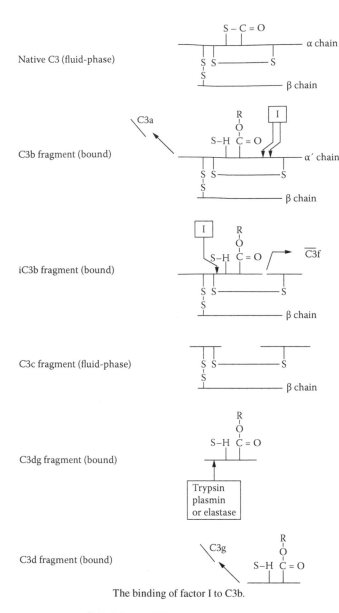

Native C3 (fluid-phase)

C3b fragment (bound)

iC3b fragment (bound)

C3c fragment (fluid-phase)

C3dg fragment (bound)

C3d fragment (bound)

The binding of factor I to C3b.

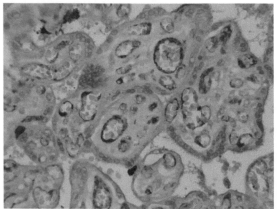

Factor VIII—placenta

antigens induce interleukin-1 (IL1) synthesis by alveolar machrophages and facilitate increased secretion of tumor necrosis factor-α (TNF-α) from alveolar macrophages and monocytes, revealing cytokine participation in the

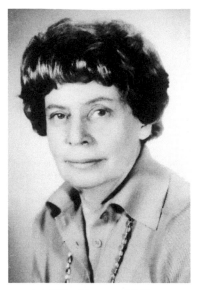

Astrid Elsa Fagraeus–Wallbom.

pathogenesis of hypersensitivity pneumonitis. Precipitin antibodies are formed in a number of the subjects.

Fagraeus–Wallbom, Astrid Elsa (1913–)

Swedish investigator noted for her doctoral thesis that provided the first clear evidence that immunoglobulins are made in plasma cells. (Refer to *Antibody Production in Relation to the Development of Plasma Cells*, 1948.)

familial Mediterranean fever (FMF)

An autoinflammatory primary immunodeficiency attributable to inherited mutations of marenostrin, an inflammatory regulator.

FANA

An abbreviation for fluorescent antinuclear antibody.

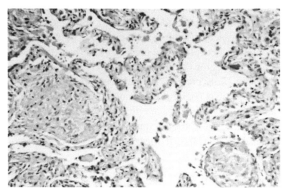

Farmer's lung.

farmer's lung

A pulmonary disease of farm workers who are exposed repeatedly to organic dust and fungi such as the *Aspergillus* species. It occurs as an extrinsic allergic alveolitis or hypersensitivity pneumonitis in nonatopic subjects. It is mediated by IgG_1. Antibodies specific for moldy hay, in which a number of fungi grow readily, are manifest in 90% of individuals. These include *Microspora vulgaris* and *Micropolyspora faeni*. The pathogenesis is believed to involve a type III hypersensitivity mechanism with the deposition of immune complexes in the lung. IgG antibodies interact with large particles of inhaled allergen

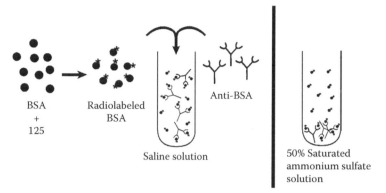

Farr technique.

in the alveolar wall of the lung. This leads to inflammation that impairs gas exchange by the lungs. Patients become breathless within hours after inhaling the dust and may develop interstitial pneumonitis with cellular infiltration of the alveolar walls where monocytes and lymphocytes are prominent. This may lead to pulmonary fibrosis following chronic inflammation, peribronchiolar granulomatous reaction, and foreign-body-type giant cell reactions. Corticosteroids are used for treatment. Interaction of the immunoglobulin G (IgG) antibodies with the inhaled allergen in the alveoli wall of the lung leads to inflammation and compromised gas exchange.

Farr technique

An assay to measure primary binding of antibody with antigen as opposed to secondary manifestations of antibody–antigen interactions such as precipitation, agglutination, etc. It is a quantitation of an antiserum's antigen-binding properties and is appropriate for antibodies of all immunoglobulin classes and subclasses. The technique is limited to the assay of antibody against antigens soluble in 40% saturated ammonium sulfate solution, in which antibodies precipitate. Following interaction of antibody with radiolabeled antigen, precipitation in ammonium sulfate separates the bound antigen from the free antigen. The quantity of radiolabeled antigen that has reacted with antibody can be measured in the precipitate. The antibody dilution that precipitates part of the ligand reflects the antigen-binding ability.

Fas

Fas (AP0-1/CD95) is a member of the tumor necrosis factor (TNF) receptor superfamily. Fas ligand (FasL) is a member of the TNF family of type 2 membrane proteins. Soluble FasL can be produced by proteolysis of membrane-associated Fas. Ligation of Fas by FasL or anti-Fas antibody can induce apoptotic cell death in cells expressing Fas. Fas is a member of the TNF receptor family that is expressed on selected cells, including T cells, and renders them susceptible to apoptotic death mediated by cells expressing Fas ligand, a member of the TNF family of proteins on the cell surface.

Fas ligand

Binding to Fas initiates the death pathway of apotosis in Fas-bearing cells. Fas-mediated killing of T lymphocytes is critical for the maintenance of self tolerance. Fas gene mutations can lead to systemic autoimmune disease. Fas ligand (FasL) is a member of the tumor necrosis factor

(TNF) family of proteins expressed on the cell surfaces of activated T lymphocytes. Binding of FasL to Fas initiates the signaling pathway that leads to apoptotic cell death of the cell expressing Fas. FasL gene mutations may lead to systemic autoimmune disease in mice.

Fas pathway

An apoptotic pathway leading to death of Fas-expressing cells, which is induced by ligation of the death receptor Fas by FasL. FADD, caspase-8 and the caspase-3 cascade mediate signal transduction of this pathway.

fascin (55k-2), mouse

Fascin is a very sensitive marker for Reed–Sternberg cells and variants in nodular sclerosis, mixed cellularity and lymphocyte depletion Hodgkin disease. It is uniformly negative in lymphoid cells, plasma cells, and myeloid cells. Fascin is positive in dendritic cells. This marker may be helpful in distinguishing between Hodgkin disease and non-Hodgkin lymphoma in difficult cases. Also, the lack of expression of fascin in the neoplastic follicles in follicular lymphoma can be helpful in distinguishing these lymphomas from reactive follicular hyperplasia in which the number of follicular dendritic cells is normal or increased.

Fasciola immunity

An inflammatory response in the liver is associated with primary infection of a host with the liver fluke Fasciola hepatica. The cellular infiltrate includes neutrophils, eosinophils, lymphocytes, and macrophages. A significant eosinophilia occurs in the peritoneal cavity and the blood. There is no cellular response encircling the juvenile flukes. Numerous macrophages and fibroblasts occur in injured areas in the chronic phase of a primary infection. This is followed by liver fibrosis, which is accompanied by numerous CD8+ and αβ-TCR+ T cells. Numerous lymphocytes and eosinophils infiltrate larger bile ducts, and in cattle a granulomatous reaction is followed by bile duct calcification. Resistance to reinfection follows primary infection of cattle, rats, and possibly humans, but fails to occur in sheep and mice. The failure of sheep to develop resistance against reinfection may be associated with cellular immune deficiencies. Products released from F. hepatica may adversely affect the host immune response, such as cathepsin proteases, which flukes secrete and which may cleave immunoglobulins, thereby inhibiting attachment to host effector cells. Other immunosuppressive molecules may be toxic to host cells.

F

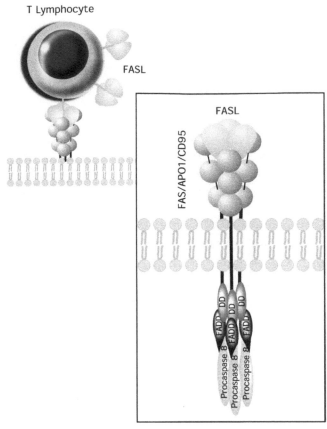

Fas Is a member of the tumor necrosis factor (TNF) receptor superfamily and contains a cytoplasmic death domain (DD) required for Induction of apoptosis. *Fas* ligand (*FasL*)-Induced receptor trimerization aggregates the DD of *Fas* and recruites the adaptor protein FADD and procaspase 8. Following activation of caspase 8, the DD-Induced complex can trigger subsequent events of apoptosis.

FasL/Fas cytotoxicity

A cytotoxic sequence that commences with crosslinking of target cell *Fas* by *FasL* on the effector cell. This does not require macromolecular synthesis or extracellular calcium. *FasL* crosslinks *Fas* triggering signals that lead to a target cell apoptotic response. *Fas* crosslinking leads to activation of intracellular caspases.

FasL/Fas toxicity

Cytotoxic sequence that commences with crosslinking of target cell *Fas* by *FasL* on the effector cell. This does not require macromolecular synthesis or extracellular calcium. *FasL* crosslinks *Fas* triggering signals that lead to a target

cell apoptotic response. Fas crosslinking leads to activation of intracellular caspases.

fatty acids and immunity

Dietary lipids exert significant effects on antigen-specific and -nonspecific immunity. These effects are related to total and fat-derived energy intake, synthesis of multiple eicosanoids, and alterations in cell membrane content. Eicosanoids are biologic mediators with multiple effects on immune cells. Their oversynthesis contributes to the development of chronic and acute inflammatory, autoimmune, atherosclerotic, and neoplastic diseases. Feeding a fish oil (n3 PUFA) diet leads to recovery of splenic T cell blastogenesis, diminished secretion of PGE_2 by splenic cells, and diminished splenic suppressor activity. PUFA–immune system interactions are guided by the rate at which they are converted to eicosanoids. Dietary n3 PUFAs diminish autoimmune, inflammatory, and atherosclerotic disease severity by diminishing the synthesis of n6 PUFA-derived eicosanoids and cytokines. The increased eicosanoids found in shock and trauma can induce immunosuppression in humans. Supplementation of the diet with n3 PUFA may protect from immunosuppression following trauma. Dietary fish oil supplements also improve joint tenderness in rheumatoid arthritis patients. Dietary supplements of n3 PUFAs such as linoleic acid or fish oil significantly inhibit the mixed lymphocyte reaction, which reflects graft survival. Linoleic acid is the only fatty acid needed to facilitate proliferation maturation of immunoglobulin-secreting cells. n3 PUFAs may suppress B cell function by displacing linoleic acid and arachidonic acid. Cell membrane lipids play a critical role in both primary and secondary immune responses against an immunogenic challenge or to an infection.

Fb fragment

Immunoglobulin G (IgG) fragment that is the product of subtilisin digestion. It is composed of the C_H1 and C_L (constant) domains of the Fab fragment.

FcαR

The two FcαR molecules are designated FcαR (CD89) and FcαRb. FcαR represents the high affinity receptor for IgA and is comprised of an α chain that binds IgA and FcRγ chain dimer. It is expressed in five splice variants found on eosinophils, monocytes, and alveolar macrophages. Neutrophils employ the FcαR molecule in ADCC. FcαRb possesses sequences that aid secretion but do not possess the transmembrane and cytoplasmic domains found in FcαR.

Fc fragment (fragment crystallizable)

A product of papain digestion of an immunoglobulin G (IgG) molecule. Also called Fc region or Fc piece. It is

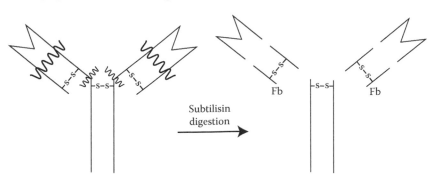

Formation of Fb fragments by digestion of IgG molecules with subtilisin.

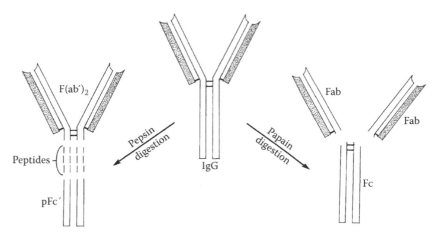

Fc fragment.

comprised of two C terminal heavy chain segments
(C_H2, C_H3) and a portion of the hinge region linked by the
central disulfide bond and noncovalent forces. This 50-kDa
fragment is unable to bind antigen, but it has multiple
other biological functions, including complement fixation,
interaction with Fc receptors on cell surfaces, and placental transmission of IgG. One Fc fragment is produced by
papain digestion of each IgG molecule. The Fc region of an
intact IgG molecule mediates effector functions by binding
to cell surface receptors or C1q complement protein.

FcμR
IgM Fc receptors have been described but remain to be
well characterized.

Fc piece
Refer to Fc fragment.

Fc receptor
A structure on the surfaces of some lymphocytes, macrophages, or mast cells that specifically binds the Fc region
of immunoglobulin, often when the Fc is aggregated.
Effector cells express isoforms FcαcR, FcγR, or FcεR and
activate signaling that mediates receptor-mediated endocytosis, phagocytosis, and ADCC in addition to neutrophil
and mast cell degranulation with the release of inflammatory mediators and cytokines. Numerous FcRs belong to the
immunoglobulin (Ig) superfamily and contain ITAMs. The
Fc receptors for immunoglobulin G (IgG) are designated
FcγR. Those for IgE are designated FcεR. IgM and IgD
Fc receptors have yet to be defined. Neutrophils, eosinophils, mononuclear phagocytes, B lymphocytes, selected T
lymphocytes, and accessory cells bear Fc receptors for IgG
on their surfaces. When the Fc region of immunoglobulin
binds to the cation permease Fc receptor, there is an influx
of Na^+ or K^+ that activates phagocytosis, H_2O_2 formation,
and cell movement by macrophages.

Fc receptors on human T cells
Fc receptors (FcRs) are carried on 95% of human peripheral
blood T lymphocytes. On about 75% of the cells, the FcRs
are specific for immunoglobulin M (IgM); the remaining
20% are specific for IgG. The FcR-bearing T cells are also
designated T_M and T_G or Tμ and Tγ. The T_M cells act as
helpers in B cell function. They are required for the B cell
responses to pokeweed mitogen (PWM). In cultures of B
cells with PWM, the T_M cells also proliferate, supporting
the views on their helper effects. Binding of IgM to FcR of

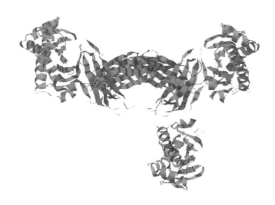

Fc (IgG) receptor (neonatal).

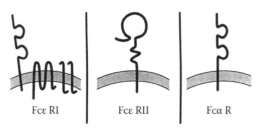

Fcα and Fcε receptors.

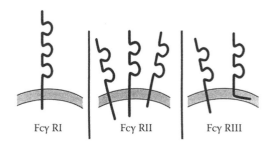

Fcγ receptors.

T_M cells is not a prerequisite for helper activity. In contrast
to the T_M cells, the T_G cells effectively suppress B cell differentiation. They act on the T_M cells, and their suppressive

F

effect requires prior binding of their Fc–IgG receptors by IgG immune complexes. T_M and T_G cells differ in a number of ways. Circulating T_G cells may be present in increased numbers, often accompanied by a reduction in the circulating number of T_M cells. Increased numbers of T_G cells are seen in cord blood and in some patients with hypogammaglobulinemia, sex-linked agammaglobulinemia, IgA deficiency, Hodgkin disease, and thymoma, to mention only a few.

Fc region
Refer to Fc fragment.

Fc′ fragment
A product of papain digestion of immunoglobulin G (IgG). It is comprised of two noncovalently bonded C_H3 domains that lack the terminal 13 amino acids. This 24-kDa dimer consists of the region between the heavy-chain amino acid residues 14 through 105 from the carboxyl terminal end. Normal human urine contains minute quantities of Fc′ fragment.

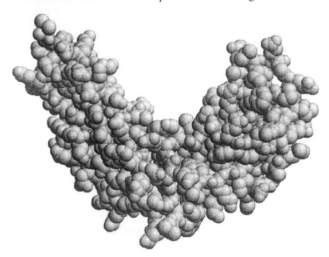

FcεRI.

Fcε receptor (FcεR)
Mast cell and leukocyte high affinity receptor for the Fc region of immunoglobulin E (IgE). When immune complexes bind to Fcε receptors, cells may respond by releasing the mediators of immediate hypersensitivity such as histamine and serotonin. Modulation of antibody synthesis may also occur. The two varieties of Fcε receptors are designated FcεRI and FcεRII (CD23). FcεRI represents a high affinity receptor found on mast cells and basophils, anchors monomeric IgE to the cell surface, and possesses 1α, 1β, and 2γ chains. FcεRII represents a low affinity receptor found on mononuclear phagocytes, B lymphocytes, eosinophils, and platelets. Subjects with increased IgE in the serum have elevated numbers of FcεRII on their cells. FcεRII is a 321-amino-acid, single polypeptide chain that is homologous with asialoglycoprotein receptor. FcεRI and FcεRII are the two subtypes. Blood basophils and tissue mast cells are the principal sites of FcεRI, which is the high affinity receptor. Allergic individuals also express it on Langerhans' cells, eosinophils, and monocytes. Its tetrameric molecular structure is composed of α and β polypeptides and a dimer of the FcRγ chain and αβ(γ)2 molecule that contains ITAM. There is also an ITAM in the cytoplasmic domain of the β chain. FcεRI binds to monomeric IgE. The interaction of multivalent antigen with multiple IgE molecules on the mast cells surface leads to aggregation of the FcεRI configurations

causing degranulation of mast cells, releasing vasoactive amines that produce local inflammation and allergy symptoms. FcεRII (CD23) is comprised of one transmembrane chain and demonstrates less affinity for IgE than does FcεRI. Its lectin-binding domain facilitates its interaction with selected carbohydrates on cells. FcεRII is found on monocytes, eosinophils, B and T cells, but not mast cells or basophils. The FcεRIIA isoform is found mainly on B cells, although its function is unknown. It is believed to bind to the B cell co-receptor molecule CD19. The FcεRIIB molecule is found on monocytes and eosinophils, which enables them to fatally injure target cells coated with IgE through an ADCC mechanism. This isoform induces NO and IL-10 synthesis by monocytes and macrophages.

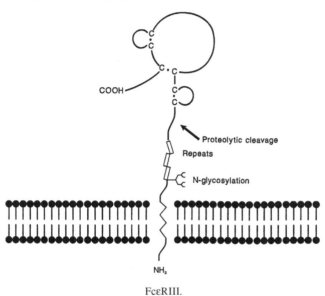

FcεRIII.

Fcε receptor (FcεRI)
A mast cell, basophil and activated eosinophil surface receptor that combines with free IgE with high affinity. Specific antigen interaction with the cell-bound IgE molecules leading to crosslinkage results in cell activation and degranulation.

Fcγ receptor (FcγR)
Receptor for the Fc region of IgG. B and T lymphocytes, natural killer cells, polymorphonuclear leukocytes, mononuclear phagocytes, and platelets contain FcγR. When these receptors bind immune complexes, the cells may produce leukotrienes and prostaglandins, modulate antibody synthesis, increase consumption of oxygen, activate oxygen metabolites, and become phagocytic. The three types of Fcγ receptors include FcγRI, FcγRII (CD32), and Fc RIII (CD16). FcγRI represents a high affinity receptor found on mononuclear phagocytes; in humans, it binds IgG_1 and IgG_3. FcγRII and FcγRIII represent low affinity IgG receptors. Neutrophils, monocytes, eosinophils, platelets, and B lymphocytes express FcγRII on their membranes. Neutrophils, natural killer cells, eosinophils, macrophages, and selected T lymphocytes express FcγRIII on their membranes in humans and bind IgG_1 and IgG_3. Patients with paroxysmal nocturnal hemoglobulinuria have deficient FcγRIII on their neutrophil membranes.

Fcγ receptors
Cell surface structures that are specific for IgG antibody Fc regions. These receptors are different for subclasses of IgG.

Fcγ R

The three principal R types of FcRγ include Fcγ RI, Fcγ RII, and Fcγ RIII that differ in their ITAMs/ITIMs content, which determines their role in effector cell activation and in their IgG affinity. Fcγ R I (CD64), the high affinity IgG receptor, is expressed exclusively on activated granulocytes and is upregulated by inflammatory cytokines. Fcγ R I is comprised of an α chain that binds IgG and and FcRγ homodimer that contains ITAMs. Fcγ R I unites with the C terminal region of a single H chain comprising the Fc region of an IgG molecule. It has the greatest affinity for IgG1 or IgG3 antibodies. Thus, these IgG, subtypes are excellent opsonins. Fcγ R I interacts with IgG, leading to inflammatory cytokine secretion and macrophage and monocyte induced target cell lysis through an ADCC mechanism. It also results in the generation of superoxide by neutrophils. Fcγ RII (CD32) has broader expression but lower affinity for noncomplexed IgG molecules than does Fcγ RI. Fcγ RII reacts only with aggregated IgG that is bound to a multivalent antigen. It is comprised of a single transmembrane chain. Phagocytes, as well as megakaryocytes and platelets, express Fcγ RIIA, which contains ITAM. IgG union with Fcγ RIIA leads to a respiratory burst in neutrophils and causes platelets to secrete inflammatory molecules. Fcγ RIIB contains ITIM rather than an ITAM sequence. It is expressed by lymphoid and myeloid cells. It is believed that this receptor in B cells may signal the cell to decrease antibody synthesis when a critical level of antibody has become bound to surface Fcγ R IIB molecules. Macrophages, monocytes, neutrophils, megakaryocytes and platelets express Fcγ RIIC receptors, which possess an ITAM and show only low binding affinity for IgG. The Fcγ RIII receptor (CD16) manifests low IgG affinity. The Fcγ RIIIA isoform is comprised of an IgG binding α chain and an ITAM-containing FcRγ chain dimer. Phagocytes and NK cells are the principal sites of Fcγ RIIIA expression. This isoform may be found also on B cells, mast cells, Langerhans' cells, and γδ T cells. The only FcR found on NK cells is Fcγ RIIIA, which has a classic FcR transmembrane region that facilitates NK cell induced ADCC and degranulation of mast cells. Neutrophils alone express the Fcγ RIIIB isoform, which is comprised of a single-chain protein without transmembrane chains or ITAMs. Phosphatidyl inositol residues fix Fcγ RIIIB in the membrane. Neutrophils employ Fcγ R III receptors to convey a requirement for vigorous phagocytosis.

Fcγ RI

Represents a high affinity receptor found on mononuclear phagocytes. In humans it binds IgG1 and IgG3.

Fcγ RII

A membrane protein designated as CD32 that serves as a receptor for the Fc regions of immunoglobulin G (IgG) molecules.

Fcγ RIII

Fcγ RII and Fcγ RIII represent low affinity IgG receptors. In humans, neutrophils, monocytes, eosinophils, platelets, and B lymphocytes express Fcγ RII on their membranes. Neutrophils, natural killer cells, eosinophils, macrophages, and selected T lymphocytes express Fcγ RIII on their membranes and bind IgG1 and IgG3. Paroxysmal nocturnal hemoglobulinuria patients have deficient Fcγ RIII on their neutrophil membranes.

FcRn (neonatal)

Fc receptors expressed by neonatal intestinal cells that bind IgG in breast milk. They facilitate its passage into the neonatal intestinal lumen and also aid IgG transport in the adult intestine and placenta. Also called Brambell receptor.

FDCs

Refer to follicular dendritic cells.

Fd fragment

The heavy chain portion of a Fab fragment produced by papain digestion of an immunoglobulin G (IgG) molecule. It is on the N terminal side of the papain digestion site.

Fd piece

Refer to Fd fragment.

Fd' fragment

The heavy chain portion of an Fab' fragment produced by reduction of the F(ab')$_2$ fragment that results from pepsin digestion of IgG. It is comprised of V_H1, C_H1, and the heavy chain hinge region. Fd contains 235 amino acid residues.

Fd' piece

Refer to Fd' fragment.

FDNB (1-fluoro-2-4-dinitrobenzene)

Refer to dinitrofluorobenzene (DNFB).

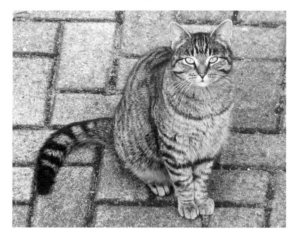

Feline immunity.

feline immunity

Although peripheral lymphoid tissues and thymus glands of cats are comparable to those of other mammals, they possess a population of pulmonary intravascular macrophages that may cause the animals to manifest increased susceptibility to septic shock mediated by macrophage-derived tumor necrosis factor. Forty to 45% of feline peripheral blood lymphocytes are B cells, and 32 to 41% are T cells; 20% of feline peripheral blood cells are null cells considered to be natural killer (NK) cells. Both T helper and T suppressor activities have been described. Feline interleukin-1 (IL1) and IL2 as well as IL6 have been identified, although the physical and chemical properties of the latter are different from those of the human and mouse interleukins. Interferons α, β, and γ have been characterized and resemble those of other species. Although all immunoglobulin isotypes of other species are recognized in cats, neither IgE nor IgD has been formally identified. Cats also have secretory IgA with a J-chain that resembles equivalent molecules of other species. Although cats do not respond to tuberculin, they develop good delayed hypersensitivity responses (viral antigens) in the skin to dinitrochlorobenzene and to BCG vaccine, but the delayed-type response is less intense than in other species. The granulomatous reaction to tuberculosis is essentially the same as in other mammals. The major histocompatibility complex (MHC) is designated FLA and is not polymorphic. The FLA system contains 10 to 20 class I gene loci, only two of which are expressed. They manifest five class II gene loci, only three of which are expressed. The lack of MHC polymorphism renders bone marrow transplantation very successful in this species. Cats possess all major complement components at levels equivalent to those in other mammals. The principal target organ for anaphylaxis in the cat is the lung, where serotonin released from mast cells is the principal mediator. Flea bite dermatitis is the most frequent allergic skin disease of cats. Feline blood group antigens are designated A and B. In the United States, 99% of cats belong to group A and 1% to group B. Spontaneous autoimmune diseases in cats include hemolytic anemia, hyperthryoidism, thrombocytopenic purpura, pemphigus vulgaris, pemphigus foliaceous, myasthenia gravis, systemic lupus erythematosus, and arthritis. Cats only rarely have immunodeficiencies. Chediak–Higashi syndrome is the most common congenital defect in immune function. The leukocytes manifest large lysosomal granules, but susceptibility to infection is not increased. Colostral immunoglobulins are not passively transferred in cats. Secondary immunodeficiencies are attributable usually to feline leukemia virus (FeLV) infection, which often induces severe immunodeficiency in infected animals. Feline immunodeficiency virus (FIV) is a lentivirus that infects both domestic and wild cats. It leads to depletion of CD4⁺ T lymphocytes and resembles human AIDS. The virus receptor is mediated through fCD9 rather than fCD4. There is polyclonal stimulation of B cells and of fCD8⁺ T cells. The disease terminates in an AIDS-like condition. Cats also develop plasmacytomas, although they are not common.

Felton phenomenon

Specific immunologic unresponsiveness or paralysis induced by the inoculation of relatively large quantities of pneumococcal polysaccharide into mice.

Felty's syndrome

A type of rheumatoid arthritis in which patients develop profound leukopenia and splenomegaly.

feral mouse

A mouse that returns to the wild from its former commensal existence.

Fernandez reaction

An early (24- to 48-hour) tuberculin-like delayed-type hypersensitivity reaction to lepromin observed in tuberculoid leprosy; a skin test for leprosy.

ferritin

An iron-containing protein that is electron dense and serves as a source of stored iron until it is needed for the synthesis of hemoglobulin. It is an excellent antigen and is found in abundant quantities in horse spleen. Ferritin's electron-dense quality makes it useful for labeling antibodies or for identifying and localizing antigens in electron microscopic preparations.

ferritin labeling

The conjugation of ferritin to antibody molecules to render them visible in histologic or cytologic specimens observed by electron microscopy. Antibodies may be labeled with

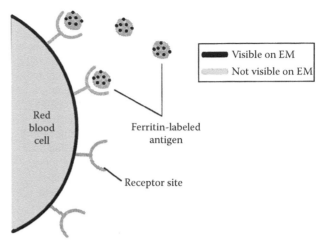

Ferritin labeling.

ferritin by use of a crosslinking reagent such as toluene-2,4-diisocyanate. The ferritin-labeled antibody may be reacted directly with the specimen, or ferritin-labeled antiimmunoglobulin may be used to react with unlabeled specific antibody attached to the target tissue antigen.

fertilizin

A glycoprotein present as a jelly-like substance surrounding sea urchin eggs. It behaves as an antigen-like substance from the standpoint of valence. Sperm, which contain proteinaceous antifertilizin, agglutinate into clumps when combined with soluble fertilizin, which is dissolved from eggs by acidified seawater.

fetal antigen

A fetal or oncofetal antigen expressed as a normal constituent of embryos and not in adult tissues. It is re-expressed in neoplasms of adult tissues, apparently as a result of derepression of the gene responsible for its formation.

fetal–maternal tolerance

Among mammals, a mother's tolerance for her fetus that expresses allogeneic paternal MHC molecules. A fetus implanted into the uterus represents a tissue graft that avoids rejection. Its survival is facilitated by immune privilege and other factors.

fetal thymic organ culture (FTC)

The culture *in vitro* of thymic tissue excised from a fetal mouse. The thymus in culture retains the capacity to facilitate T lymphocyte development.

fetus allograft

Success of the haplo-nonidentical fetus as an allograft was suggested in the 1950s by Medawar, Brent, and Billingham to rely on four possibilities: (1) the conceptus might not be immunogenic, (2) pregnancy might alter the immune response, (3) the uterus might be an immunologically privileged site, and (4) the placenta might represent an effective immunological barrier between mother and fetus. Further studies have shown that transplantation privilege afforded the fetal–placental unit in pregnancy depends on intrauterine mechanisms. The pregnant uterus has been shown not to be an immunologically privileged site. Pregnancies usually are successful in maternal hosts with high levels of pre-existing alloimmunity. The temporary status has focused on specialized features of fetal trophoblastic cells that facilitate transplantation protection. Fetal trophoblast protects itself from maternal cytotoxic attack by failing to express on placental villous cytotrophoblasts and syncytiotrophoblasts any classical polymorphic histocompatibility complex (MHC) class I or II antigens. Constitutive human leukocyte antigen (HLA) expression is also not induced by known upregulators such as interferon-γ. Thus, classical MHC antigens are not expressed throughout gestation. Extravillous cytotrophoblast cells selectively express HLA-G, a nonclassical MHC class I antigen that has limited genetic polymorphism. HLA-G may protect the cytotrophoblast population from MHC-nonrestricted natural killer (NK) cell attack. The trophoblast also protects itself from maternal cytotoxicity during gestation by expressing a high level of complement regulatory proteins on its surface such as membrane cofactor protein (MCP; CD46), decay-accelerating factor (DAF; CD55), and membrane attack complex inhibitory factor (CD59). The maternal immune system recognizes pregnancy (i.e., the fetal trophoblast) in a manner that results in cellular, antibody, and cytokine responses that protect the fetal allograft. CD56-positive large granular lymphocytes may be regulated by hormones in the endometrium that control their function. They have been suggested to be a form of NK cell in arrested maturation, possibly due to persistent expression of HLA-G on target invasive cytotrophoblast. Contemporary studies have addressed cytokine interactions at the fetal–maternal tissue interface in pregnancy. HLA-G or other fetal trophoblast antigens have been postulated to possibly stimulate maternal lymphocytes in endometrial tissue to synthesize cytokines and growth factors that act in a paracrine manner beneficial to trophoblast growth and differentiation. This has been called the immunotrophism hypothesis. Other cytokines released into decidual tissue include colony-stimulating factors (CSFs), tumor necrosis factor α (TNF-α), IL6, and transforming growth factor β (TGF-β). Fetal syncytiotrophoblast has numerous growth factor receptors. Thus, an extensive cytokine network is present within the uteroplacental tissue that offers both immunosuppressive and growth-promoting signals. In humans, IgG is selectively transported across the placenta into the fetal circulation following combination with transporting Fcγ receptors on the placenta. This transfer takes place during the 20th to the 22nd week of gestation. Maternal HLA-specific alloantibody that is specific for the fetal HLA type is bound by nontrophoblastic cells expressing fetal HLA antigens, including macrophages, fibroblasts, and endothelium within the villous mesenchyme of placental tissue, thereby preventing these antibodies from reaching the fetal circulation. Maternal antibodies against any other antigen of the fetus will likewise be bound within the placental tissues to a cell expressing that antigen. The placenta acts as a sponge to absorb potentially harmful antibodies. Exceptions to placental trapping of deleterious maternal IgG antibodies include maternal IgG antibodies against RhD antigen and certain maternal organ-specific autoantibodies.

Feulgen reaction

A standard method that detects DNA in tissues.

fever

An increase in the body temperature above normal. Attributable to cytokines released during infection.

fibrillarin antibodies

Antibodies against fibrillarin found in about 8% of patients with diffuse and limited scleroderma. Fibrillarin is a 34-kDa protein constituent of U3 ribonucleoprotein (U3-RNP).

Mercuric chloride induces autoantibodies against U3 small nuclear ribonucleoprotein in susceptible mice.

fibrillarin autoantibodies

Antibodies discovered in 4 to 9% of patients with scleroderma. Fibrillarin is the main 34-kDa component of U3 ribonucleoprotein (U3-RNP). Fifty-six percent of black patients with diffuse cutaneous scleroderma compared with only 14% of black patients with limited cutaneous scleroderma and white patients with diffuse and limited cutaneous scleroderma (5% and 4%, respectively) had antifibrillarin autoantibodies in their sera. Mercuric chloride can induce fibrillarin antibodies in mouse strains that recognize the same epitopes as fibrillarin antibodies found in scleroderma patients and are mainly of the immunoglobulin G (IgG) class. The demonstration that selected human leukocyte antigen (HLA) haplotypes occur at a greater frequency in patients with fibrillarin antibodies suggests a genetic predisposition to develop these autoantibodies. Indirect immunofluorescence and immunoblotting are the methods of choice for antifibrillarin antibody detection.

fibrin

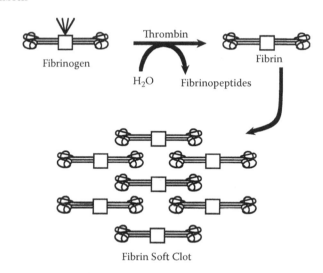

Fibrin.

Protein responsible for the coagulation of blood. It is formed through the degradation of fibrinogen into fibrin monomers. Polymerization of the nascent fibrin molecules (comprising the α, β, and γ chains) occurs by end-to-end as well as lateral interactions. The fibrin polymer is envisaged as having two chains of the triad structure lying side by side in a staggered fashion in such a way that two terminal nodules are associated with the central nodule of a third molecule. The chains may also be twisted around each other. The fibrin polymer thus formed is stabilized under the action of a fibrin-stabilizing factor, another component of the coagulation system. Fibrinogen may also be degraded by plasmin. In this process, a number of intermediates, designated as fragments X, Y, D, and E, are formed. These fragments interfere with polymerization of fibrin by binding to nascent intact fibrin molecules, thus causing a defective and unstable polymerization. Fibrin is also cleaved by plasmin into similar but shorter fragments, collectively designated fibrin degradation products. Of course, any excess of such fragments will impair the normal coagulation process,

F

an event with serious clinical significance. Abzymes, such as thromboplastin activator linked to an antibody specific for antigens in fibrin that are not present in fibrinogen, are used clinically to lyse fibrin clots obstructing coronary arteries in myocardial infarction patients.

fibrinogen

Fibrinogen is one of the largest plasma proteins, with a molecular weight of 330 to 340 kDa, and is composed of more than 3000 amino acid residues. The concentration in the plasma ranges between 200 and 500 mg/l00 mL. The molecule contains 3% carbohydrate, about 28 to 29 disulfide linkages, and one free sulfhydryl group. Fibrinogen exists as a dimer and can be split into two identical sets composed of three different polypeptide chains. Fibrinogen is susceptible to enzymatic cleavage by a variety of enzymes. The three polypeptide chains of fibrinogen are designated Aα, Bβ, and γ. By electron microscopy, the dried fibrinogen molecule shows a linear arrangement of three nodules 50 to 70 Å in diameter connected by a strand about 15 Å thick.

fibrinoid necrosis

Tissue death in which there is a smudgy eosinophilic deposit that resembles fibrin microscopically and camouflages cellular detail. It is induced by proteases released from neutrophils that digest the tissue and cause fibrin deposition. Fibrinoid necrosis is seen in tissues in a number of connective tissue diseases with immune mechanisms. An example is systemic lupus erythematosus (SLE). Fibrinoid necrosis is classically seen in the walls of small vessels in immune complex vasculitis such as occurs in the Arthus reaction.

fibrinopeptides

Peptides released by the conversion of fibrinogen into fibrin. Thrombin splits fragments from the N terminal regions of Aα and Bβ chains of fibrinogen. The split fragments are called fibrinopeptide A and B, respectively, and are released in the fluid phase. They may be further degraded and apparently have vasoactive functions. The release rate of fibrinopeptide A exceeds that of fibrinopeptide B, and this differential release may play a role in the propensity of nascent fibrin to polymerize.

fibronectin

An adhesion-promoting dimeric glycoprotein found abundantly in connective tissues and basement membranes. The tetrapeptide, Arg–Gly–Asp–Ser, facilitates cell adhesion to fibrin, Clq, collagens, heparin, and type I-, II-, III-, V-, and VI-sulfated proteoglycans. Fibronectin is also present in plasma and on normal cell surfaces. Approximately 20 separate fibronectin chains are known. They are produced from the fibronectin gene by alternative splicing of the RNA transcript. Fibronectin is comprised of two 250-kDa subunits joined near their carboxyl terminal ends by disulfide bonds. The amino acid residues in the subunits vary in number from 2145 to 2445. Fibronectin is important in contact inhibition, cell movement in embryos, cell-substrate adhesion, inflammation, and wound healing. It may also serve as an opsonin.

fibrosis

The formation of fibrous tissue, as in repair or replacement of parenchymatous elements. A process that leads to the development of a type of scar tissue at a site of chronic inflammation.

FICA (fluoroimmunocytoadherence)

The use of column chromatography to capture antigen-binding cells.

ficin

A substance employed to delete sialic acid from cell surfaces, which is especially useful in blood grouping to decrease the ζ potential and facilitate otherwise poorly agglutinating antibodies. Erythrocytes treated with ficin reveal enhanced expression of Kidd, Ii, Rh, and Lewis antigens. The treatment destroys MNSs, Lutheran, Duffy, Chido, Rodgers, and Tn, among other antigens.

Ficoll™

A 400-kDa water-soluble polymer composed of sucrose and epichlorohydrin. It is employed in the manufacture of Ficoll–Hypaque, a density gradient substance used to separate and purify mononuclear cells by centrifugation following removal of the buffy coat.

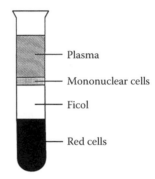

Schematic representation of Ficoll-Hypaque technique of cell separation.

Ficoll–Hypaque

A density gradient medium used to separate and purify mononuclear cells by centrifugation.

FIGE

Field inversion gel electrophoresis. Refer to pulsed-field gradient gel electrophoresis.

filarial immunity

Increased levels of parasite-specific antibodies are synthesized following filarial infection. Subjects with asymptomatic microfilaremic infections develop high titers of filarial-specific immunoglobulin G$_4$ (IgG$_4$) antibodies, yet patients with chronic lymphatic obstruction develop mainly IgG$_1$, IgG$_2$, and IgG$_3$. Most infected subjects develop antifilarial IgE antibodies. IgE and IgG4 antibodies are usually directed against the same epitopes and are regulated by interleukin-4 (IL4) and IL13. Little or no proliferative response to parasite antigens occurs in lymphocytes from asymptomatic microfilaremia individuals. This lack of T cell reactivity is parasite antigen-specific, as responsiveness to nonparasite antigens and mitogens is unaffected. Asymptomatic microfilaremic subjects are unable to produce interferon (IFN) or IFN-γ but retain the ability to synthesize IL4 and IL5. Subjects with chronic lymphatic pathology synthesize IFN-γ, IL4, and IL5 following exposure to the parasite antigen. IL10 modulates the synthesis of IFN-γ in microfilaremia. Prenatal exposure to microfilarial stage antigens can lead to long-term anergy to filarial antigens once naturally infected. Protective immunity can be induced by attenuated larvae or by repeated infections. Individuals who develop resistance to new infection while maintaining adult parasites acquire concomitant immunity. The few individuals who remain free of infection in spite of long-term residence in high endemic areas are said to have putative immunity.

F

filariasis

Infection by filaria such as *Wuchereria bancrofti*.

filovirus immunity

No effective immune responses are associated with fatal filovirus infections that cause fulminating hemorrhagic fever with severe shock syndrome and high mortality in humans and nonhuman primates. Antibodies that develop in monkeys against Ebola–Reston virus are nonprotective. No significant role for neutralizing antibodies has been found for viral clearance. Extensive alterations of the parafollicular regions in the spleen and lymph nodes lead to destruction of antigen-presenting dendritic cells, pointing to disruption of cell-mediated immunity during filoviral hemorrhagic fever. Besides these cytolytic effects, the high carbohydrate content of these viruses may suppress immune reactivity. A nonstructural glycoprotein (GP) secreted from cells infected with the Ebola virus may interfere with an immune response against the virus. A fragment of spike GP released by infected cells may have a similar action. Filovirus GP possesses a sequence motif homologous to an immunosuppressive domain of retroviral glycoproteins. Filoviruses are now known to induce immunosuppression in the infected host which contributes to the rapid course and severity of the infection. Even though little neutralizing antibody can be detected in human convalescent sera, it is believed that passive immunization with antibodies against Ebola virus afford some benefit in treatment. No vaccines for humans are presently available.

fimbria

Hair-like filaments. They are adhesins that facilitate attachment to host cells.

fimbrial antigens

Epitopes of hair-like structures termed fimbriae or pili on Gram-negative bacteria.

final serum dilution

A serological term to designate the titration end point. It is the precise dilution of serum reached following combination with all components needed for the reaction (i.e., the addition of antigen and complement to the diluted serum).

fingerprinting, DNA

A method to demonstrate short, tandem-repeated, highly specific genomic sequences known as minisatellites. The probability that two persons would have the identical DNA fingerprint is only 1 in 30 billion. DNA fingerprinting has greater specificity than restriction fragment length polymorphism (RFLP) analysis. Each individual has a different number of repeats. The insert-free, wild-type M13 bacteriophage identifies the hypervariable minisatellites. The sequence of DNA that identifies the differences is confined to two clusters of 15-base-pair repeats in the protein III gene of the bacteriophage. The specificity of this probe, known as the Jeffries probe, renders it applicable to human genome mapping, parentage testing, and forensic science. RNA may also be split into fragments by enzymatic digestion followed by electrophoresis. A characteristic pattern for that molecule is produced and aids in identifying it.

Finn, Ronald

Dr. Ronald Finn, analyzing Kleihauer's slides, realized that if the blood of a new mother that contained many dark fetal cells could be treated so that no fetal cells appeared, she

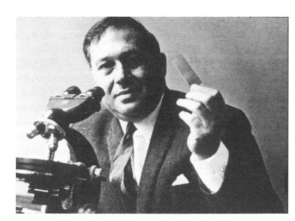

Ronald Finn.

would be spared Rh sensitization and her next baby would not be ill.

first-set rejection

Acute form of allograft rejection in a nonsensitized recipient. It is usually completed in 12 to 14 days. It is mediated by type IV (delayed-type) hypersensitivity to graft antigens.

first-use syndrome

An anaphylactoid reaction that may occur in some hemodialysis patients during initial use of a dialyzer. It may be produced by dialyzer material or by residual ethylene oxide used for sterilization.

FISH (fluorescence *in situ* hybridization)

A method to determine ploidy by examining interphase (nondividing) nuclei in cytogenetic and cytologic samples.

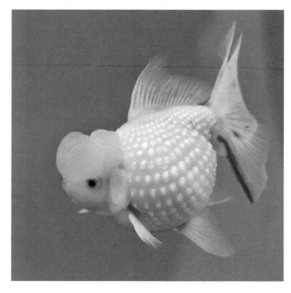

Fish immunity.

fish immunity

Primary and secondary lymphoid tissues of fish are found in the thymus, kidney, and spleen. Immune cells are also found in the skin and mucous membranes. The gills play an important role in antigen uptake, because they contain lymphoid and antibody-secreting cells. Fish have no lymph nodes or gut-associated lymphoid tissues. The thymus is found in the gill chamber as a paired organ. The fish thymus resembles the mammalian thymus in structure and function and contains lymphocytes and some epithelial-type cells and macrophages. It represents the primary lymphoid organ. Fish thymocytes resemble T lineage cells in mammals. The anterior tip of the kidney consists largely of lymphoreticular and hematopoietic tissues. It is the principal antibody-synthesizing tissue. The fish spleen is comprised mostly of red pulp sinuses; the white pulp is poorly differentiated. The fish kidney and spleen have melanomacrophage centers. These may be analogs of germinal centers in mammals. Fish have T- and B-like lymphocytes. The B-like population possesses surface immunoglobulin similar to mammalian B lymphocytes. Although the fish T-like lymphocyte antigen receptor has not yet been characterized, it is postulated to be homologous to the mammalian T cell receptor. Monocytes and macrophages as well as granulocytes that participate in inflammatory responses have been identified in fish. Mast cells have not been demonstrated, but a granulocytic cell with eosinophilic granules that otherwise resembles a mast cell has been described along with natural cytotoxic cells. Fish demonstrate both humoral and cell-mediated immunity, which is temperature-dependent. Some species respond very slowly immunologically after antigenic challenge at 4°C yet exhibit a maximal response at 12°C. The optimal temperature varies from one species to another. An IgM-like antibody is the only immunoglobulin class present. It is a tetrameric molecule, and in some species it is monomeric. Secretory IgM has also been described. Two types of light chains comparable to κ and λ light chains of vertebrates and heavy chains of different molecular masses have been described. The kinetics of the antibody response in fish resembles that in higher vertebrates. Fish also demonstrate cell-mediated immunity that includes production of lymphokines, yet no fish cytokine has yet been characterized. Fish have shown evidence for interferon γ, IL1, IL2, colony-stimulating factor, transforming growth factor β, and tumor necrosis factor. Immunological memory involving both humoral and cell-mediated responses has been described. Memory antibody responses in fish are usually lower than in mammals, and memory is temperature-dependent. Immunological tolerance has also been shown in some species. Vaccines are available to protect fish against the main bacterial and viral diseases. Three methods of fish vaccination include injection, immersion, and oral. Injection vaccinations stimulate protective immunity. Immersion vaccination involves placing the fish in water containing formalin-killed broth culture vaccines and immunizing them through immersion for 1 minute in the vaccine, which enters through the gills. Vaccine absorption through the hind intestine leads to protective immunity in certain species.

FITC (fluorescein isothiocyanate)

A widely used fluorochrome for labeling antibody molecules. It may also be used to label other proteins. Fluorescein-labeled antibodies are popular because they appear apple-green under ultraviolet irradiation, permitting easy detection of antigens of interest in tissues and cells. FITC fluoresces at 490 and 520 nm. FITC-labeled antibodies are useful for the demonstration of immune deposits in both skin and kidney biopsies.

fixed drug eruption

A hypersensitivity reaction to a drug that appears at the same local site on the body surface regardless of the route by which the drug is administered. The lesion is a clearly

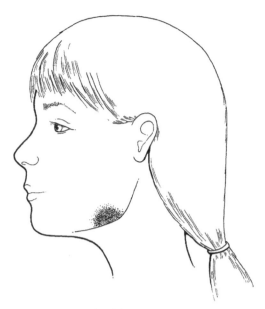

Fixed drug eruption.

circumscribed plaque that is reddish-brown or purple and edematous. It may be covered by a bulla. Common sites of occurrence include the extremities, hands, and glans penis. Drugs that may induce this reaction include sulfonamides, barbiturates, quinine, and tetracycline, among other substances. There is hydropic degeneration of the basal layer.

FK506

Refer to tacrolimus.

FKBP (FK-binding protein)

An immunophilin protein that binds FK506. A rotamase enzyme with an amino acid sequence that closely resembles that of protein kinase C. It serves as a receptor for both FK506 and rapamycin. Cyclophilins that bind tacrolimus (FK506) are FK-binding proteins. Refer also to cyclophilins.

Structure of FK506.

flagellar antigen

Epitopes of flagella in an organelle that renders some bacteria motile. Also called H antigens.

flagellin

A protein that is a principal constituent of bacterial flagella. It consists of 25- to 60-kDa monomers that are arranged into helical chains that wind around a central hollow core.

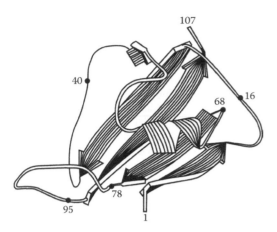

Ribbon model of FKBP.

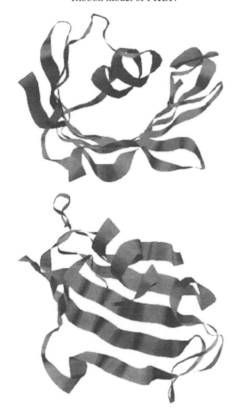

Atomic structure of FKBP–rapamycin, an immunophilin–immunosuppressant complex.

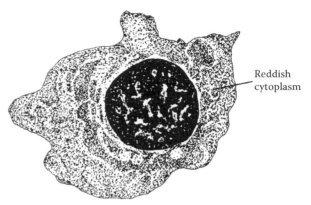

Flame cell.

Polymeric flagellin is an excellent thymus-independent antigen. Mutations may occur in the central part of a flagellin monomer, which has a variable sequence.

flame cells

Plasma cells whose cytoplasm stains intensely eosinophilic and contains glycoprotein globules. Flame cells occur in immunoglobulin A (IgA) myelomas especially, but also in Waldenström's macroglobulinemia and in the leptomeninges of patients with African trypanosomiasis near neutrophil aggregates.

flavivirus immunity

Yellow fever, dengue, Japanese encephalitis, and tick-borne encephalitis are the most important of the flavivirus group. The E protein plays a critical role in infection and immunity, as it possesses cellular receptor-binding determinants, membrane fusion activity, and epitopes for neutralizing antibodies. Macrophages clear the viremia, yet antiviral function may be affected by their state of activation and levels of virus-specific antibodies. West Nile virus infection is associated with impaired natural killer (NK) cell function that may be related to major histocompatibility complex (MHC) class I antigen expression on virus-infected cells and may represent an immune escape mechanism. Virus-specific antibodies provide protection against flavivirus disease. Anti-E protein antibodies are protective in various species and are believed to play a major role in immunity and natural infections. Previous infections are thought to ameliorate or protect from subsequent infections with heterologous viruses by inducing the formation of group-specific antibodies. Flavivirus NS1 protein stimulates protective antibodies. Antibody-dependent cellular cytotoxicity (ADCC) occurs in dengue fever. Cellular immunity is believed to be required for control of infection, as T cells adoptively transferred into unimmunized mice can protect them against lethal encephalitis. Antibody-enhanced infection of mononuclear phagocytes occurs in dengue fever. Primary dengue infection sensitizes serotype cross-reactive memory T lymphocytes for activation during the secondary infection, leading to inflammatory cytokine release that facilitates the development of capillary leak syndrome. CD4 and CD8 cytotoxic lysis of virus-infected cells has been observed in dengue fever. Dengue antigen stimulates CD4+ T cells to synthesize interferon γ. Memory responses are primed for major activation during secondary infections. The YF17D strain of yellow fever virus was the first live-attenuated vaccine for this virus family. It has proven safe and highly effective for inducing long-lasting immunity. Other members of this virus group are also candidates for vaccine development. Tick-borne encephalitis virus vaccine is a formalin-inactivated preparation that is highly effective in producing few side effects. Vaccination against Japanese encephalitis has included both inactivated and live attenuated viruses.

FLIP/FLAM

FLIP/FLAM is highly homologous to caspase-8. It does not, however, contain the active site required for proteolytic activity. FLIP appears to compete with caspase-8 binding to the cytosolic receptor complex, thereby preventing the activation of the caspase cascade in response to members of the tumor necrosis factor (TNF) family of ligands. The exact *in vivo* influence of the inhibitor of apoptosis (IAP) family of protein on apoptosis is not clear.

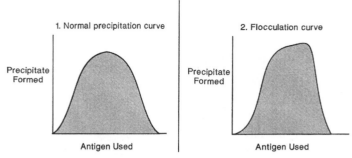

Flocculation.

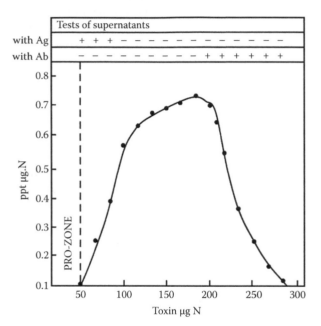

Flocculation curve of Pappenheimer and Robinson.

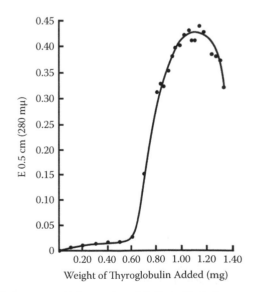

Flocculation curve with human thyroglobulin and homologous antibody.

flocculation

A variant of the precipitin reaction in which soluble antigens interact with antibody to produce precipitation over a relatively narrow range of antigen-to-antibody ratios; also used in the past to refer to flocculation aggregation of such lipids as cardiolipin and others in serological tests for syphilis, but these reactions are more correctly referred to as agglutination rather than flocculation. Flocculation differs from the classic precipitin reaction in that insoluble aggregates are not formed until a greater amount of antigen is added than would be required in a typical precipitin reaction. If the antibody (or total protein) precipitated is plotted against antigen added, the plot does not extrapolate to the origin. In flocculation reactions, excess antibody and excess antigen inhibit precipitation. Thus, precipitation occurs only over a narrow range of antibody-to-antigen ratios. Soluble antigen–antibody complexes are formed in both antigen and antibody excess. Horse antisera commonly give flocculation reactions (for example, antisera to diphtheria toxin and certain streptococcal toxins). The peculiar aspects of the flocculation reaction must be attributed to the reacting antibodies as opposed to the antigen, which gives a typical precipitin reaction with rabbit antisera. For many years, this reaction was known as the toxin–antitoxin type of curve because it was observed with horse antibodies against diphtheria and tetanus toxins. In recent years, it has been observed with sera from some patients with Hashimoto's thyroiditis. These patients develop autoantibodies against human thyroglobulin. This antithyroglobulin antibody may give a classic precipitin curve, but some individuals develop flocculation types of antibody responses against the antigen.

flow cytometry

An analytical technique to phenotype cell populations. It requires a special apparatus, termed a flow cytometer, that can detect fluorescence on individual cells in suspension and thereby ascertain the number of cells that express the molecule binding a fluorescent probe. Cell suspensions are incubated with fluorescent-labeled monoclonal antibodies or other probes, and the quantity of probe bound by each cell in the population is assayed by passing the cells one at a time through a spectrofluorometer with a laser-generated incident beam. Sample cells flow single file past a narrowly focused excitation light beam that is used to probe the cell properties of interest. As the cells pass the focused excitation light beam, each cell scatters light and may emit fluorescent light, depending on whether or not it is labeled with a fluorochrome or is autofluorescent. Scattered light is measured in both the forward and perpendicular directions relative to the incident beam. The fluorescent emissions of the cell are measured in the perpendicular directions by a photosensitive detector. Measurements of light scatter and fluorescent emission intensities are used to characterize each cell as it is processed. Flow cytometry is a fast, accurate way to measure multiple characteristics of a single cell simultaneously. These objective measurements are made one cell at a time, at routine rates of 500 to 4000 particles per second in a moving fluid stream. A flow cytometer measures relative size (FSC), relative granularity or internal complexity (SSC), and relative fluorescence. Three-color flow cytometry is used to analyze blood cells by size, cytoplasmic granularity, and surface markers labeled with different fluorochromes. Flow cytometry serves as the basis

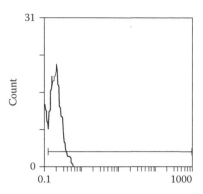

Negative flow crossmatch.

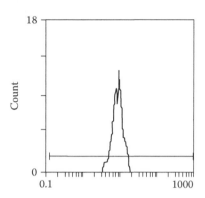

Positive flow crossmatch.

for numerous very different, highly specialized assays. It is a multifactorial analysis technique and provides the capability for performing many of these assays simultaneously.

Flt3 ligand

A hematopoietic growth factor significant in NK cell development. It is related to the macrophage colony-stimulating factor, which binds to a receptor termed fms. Thus Flt3 is a receptor termed fms-like tyrosine kinase 3, and Flt3-L is its ligand. Flt3-L is synthesized by bone marrow stromal cells.

fludarabine

A nucleoside precursor that becomes a purine analogue known as F-ara-A following injection into a human or other animal. F-ara-A enters and accumulates in cells in a phosphorylated form (F-ara-Appl), which inhibits cell proliferation mainly by blocking ribonucleotide reductase and DNA polymerase. Its incorporation into DNA inhibits DNA ligase, while incorporation into RNA blocks transcription. An anticancer drug used to treat low-grade leukemias and lymphomas, it has been used in transplantation to facilitate graft acceptance when used in combination with low doses of other immunosuppressive drugs. Toxicity is relatively low.

fluid mosaic model

A fluid lipid molecular bilayer in the plasma membrane and organelle membranes of cells. This structure permits membrane proteins and glycoproteins to float. The lipid molecules are situated in a manner that arranges the polar heads toward the outer surfaces and their hydrophobic side chains project into the interior. There can be lateral movement of molecules in the bilayer plain or they may rotate on their long axes. This is the Singer–Nicholson fluid mosaic. The bilayer consists of glycolipids and phospholipids. Amphipathic lipids and globular proteins are spaced throughout the membrane. The fluid consistency permits movement of the receptors, proteins, and glycoprotein laterally.

FluMist®

Contains live attenuated influenza viruses that reproduce in the nasopharynx of the recipient and are present in respiratory secretions.

fluorescein

A yellow dye that stains with brilliant apple-green fluorescence when excited. Its isothiocyanate derivative is widely employed to label proteins such as immunoglobulins that are useful in diagnostic medicine as well as in basic science research.

fluorescein isothiocyanate (FITC)

A widely used fluorochrome for labeling antibody molecules. It may also be used to label other proteins. Fluorescein-labeled antibodies are popular because they

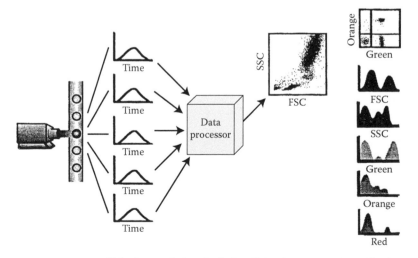

Flow cytometry is a fast, accurate way to measure multiple characteristics of a single cell simultaneously. These objective measurements are made one cell at a time at routine rates of 500 to 4000 particles per second in a moving fluid stream. A flow cytometer measures relative size (FSC), relative granularity or internal complexity (SSC), and relative fluorescence. Three-color flow cytometry is used to analyze blood cells by size, cytoplasmic granularity, and surface markers labeled with different fluorochromes.

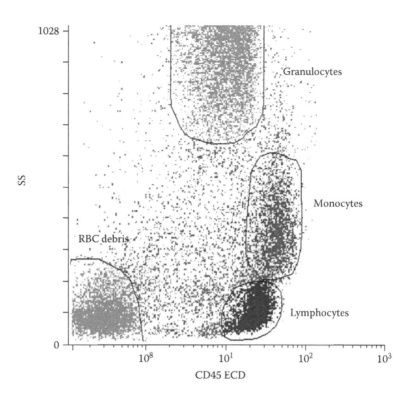

Flow cytometric analysis of normal peripheral blood.

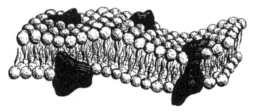

Fluid mosaic model.

Structure of fluorescein.

Structure of fluorescein isothiocyanate (FITC).

appear apple-green under ultraviolet irradiation, permitting easy detection of antigens of interest in tissues and cells. FITC fluoresces at 490 and 520 nm. FITC-labeled antibodies are useful for the demonstration of immune deposits in both skin and kidney biopsies.

fluorescein-labeled antibody

An antibody tagged with a fluorescein derivative such as fluorescein isothiocyanate. These antibodies are useful for localizing antigens in tissues and cells by their brilliant apple-green fluorescence under ultraviolet light.

fluorescence

Emission of light of one wavelength by a substance irradiated with light of a different wavelength.

fluorescence-activated cell sorter (FACS)

An instrument designed to measure the size, granularity, and fluorescence of cells attributable to bound fluorescent antibodies as individual cells flow in a stream

past photodetectors. Single-cell analysis by this method is termed flow cytometry, and the device that makes the measurements and/or sorts cells is termed a flow cytometer or cell sorter. The flow cytometry fluorescence detectors are connected to computer-controlled electromagnetic deflector plates programmed to deposit a cell with a particular fluorescent signal due to bound fluorochrome-tagged antibody of a particular wavelength (color) and intensity to a specific collection tube.

fluorescence enhancement

Increased fluorescence of certain substances after their combination with antibody. This is attributable to changing the substance from an aqueous milieu to the hydrophobic surroundings of the antibody combining site.

fluorescence microscopy

A special microscope that uses ultraviolet light to illuminate a tissue or cell stained with a fluorochrome-labeled substance such as an antibody against an antigen of interest in the tissue. When returning from an excited state to a ground state, the tissue emits fluorescent light that permits the observer to localize an antigen of interest in the tissue or cell.

fluorescence quenching

A method to ascertain association constants of antibody molecules interacting with ligands. It results from excitation

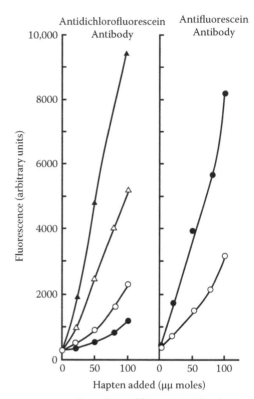

Quenching of fluorescein (○) and
dichlorofluorescein (●) fluorescence by homologous
and cross-reacting rabbit antibody.
Dichloro-fluorescein (▲) and fluorescein fluorescence (△) in
buffer alone are shown in the left-hand figure.

Titration curves using fluorescence quenching.

energy transfer by which certain electronically excited residues in protein molecules such as tryptophan and tyrosine
transfer energy to a second molecule bound to the protein.
Maximum emission is a wavelength of approximately 345
nm. The attachment of the acceptor molecule need not be
covalent. This transfer of energy occurs when the absor-
bance spectrum of the acceptor molecule overlaps that of
the emission spectrum of the donor and takes place via
resonance interaction. The two molecules need not contact
directly for energy transfer. If the acceptor molecule is
nonfluorescent, diminution of energy occurs through non-
radiation processes. Conversely, if the acceptor molecule
is fluorescent, the transfer of radiation to it results in its
own fluorescence (sensitized fluorescence). Fluorescence
quenching techniques can provide very sensitive quantitative data on antibody–hapten interactions.

fluorescence treponemal antibody test
Refer to FTA–ABS test.

Rhodamine B isothiocyanate is a reddish-orange fluorochrome used to label
immunoglobulins or other proteins for use in immunofluorescence studies.

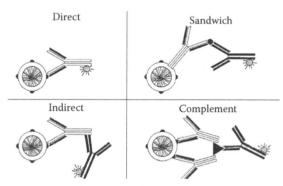

Rhodamine disulfonic acid is a red fluorochrome used in
immunofluorescence.

Lissamine rhodamine (RB200) is a fluorochrome that produces
orange fluorescence. Interaction with phosphorus pentachloride
yields a reactive sulfonyl chloride that is useful for labeling protein
molecules to be used in immunofluorescence staining.

Fluorescent antibody technique.

fluorescent antibody
An antibody molecule to which a fluorochrome such as
fluorescein isothiocyanate has been conjugated.

fluorescent antibody technique
An immunofluorescence method in which antibody labeled
with a fluorochrome such as fluorescein isothiocyanate (FITC)
is used to identify antigen in tissues or cells when examined by
ultraviolet light used in fluorescence microscopy. In addition
to the direct technique, antigens in tissue sections treated with
unlabeled antibody can be counterstained with fluorescein-
labeled antiimmunoglobulin to localize antigen in tissues by the
indirect immunofluorescence method.

fluorescence *in situ* hybridization (FISH)
A technique in which whole cells or a chromosomal spread
on a microscope slide are exposed to a fluorescently labeled
DNA probe. Subsequent microscopic examination of the
whole chromosome or a specific part may reveal tumori-
genic chromosomal translocations that are clearly visible
by this technique. Multiple probes tagged with separate
fluorochromes may be used simultaneously.

fluorescent protein tracing
Fluorescent dyes are used in place of nonfluorescent dyes
because they are detectable in much lower concentrations.

F

Radioactive labeling is usually employed if the substance to be detected is present in minute amounts. Fluorescent labeling, however, provides simplicity of technique and precise microscopic observation of fluorescence. Fluorescent microscopic preparations require several hours and permit localization at the cellular level, whereas autoradiograms require a longer period and are localized at the tissue level. Either fluorescein (apple-green fluorescence) or rhodamine (reddish-orange fluorescence) compounds may be used for tracing.

fluorochrome

A label such as fluorescein isothiocyanate or rhodamine isothiocyanate used to label antibody molecules or other substances. A fluorochrome emits visible light of a defined wavelength upon irradiation with light of a shorter wavelength such as ultraviolet light.

fluorodinitrobenzene

Refer to dinitrofluorobenzene (DNFB).

fluorography

A method used to identify radiolabeled proteins following their separation by gel electrophoresis. A fluor such as diphenyl oxazole is incorporated into the gel, where it emits photons on exposure to a radioisotope. After drying, the gel is placed on x-ray film in the dark.

FLU/v

A newly developed vaccine against influenza that focuses on parts of the virus that do not mutate from year to year. Murine studies show that 57% of mice given the new vaccine survived lethal doses of the flu compared with no mice that received a controlled flu vaccine. This new vaccine purportedly protects permanently against all strains of influenza including bird flu. Current vaccines only protect against specific strains for a limited time. Investigators attempt to predict which version will be prominent in the forthcoming flu season. Because of the propensity for the influenza virus to mutate, the vaccine for a particular year may not be as effective as hoped, and new vaccines must be developed each flu season. FLU/v can be produced faster and more easily than traditional vaccines.

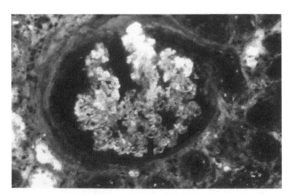

Fluorescence of focal segmental glomerulosclerosis.

fog fever

An episode of acute respiratory distress in cows approximately 7 days after their removal to a pasture where hay has been recently cut. They may die within 1 day, developing pulmonary edema with extensive emphysema. This disease may present as an atopic allergy in sensitized animals exposed to grass proteins, pollen, and fungal spores. A nonimmunologic intoxication has also been suggested as a cause. Cattle may also suffer a reaction that resembles farmer's lung in humans if they have been fed hay containing *Micropolyspora faeni* spores. Precipitating antibodies are present in their sera.

follicle

Circular or oval areas of lymphocytes in lymphoid tissues rich in B cells. They are present in the cortices of lymph nodes and in the splenic white pulp. Primary follicles contain small and medium-sized B lymphocytes. They are demonstrable in lymph nodes prior to antigenic stimulation. Once a lymph node is stimulated by antigen, secondary follicles develop. They contain large B lymphocytes in the germinal centers, where tingible body macrophages (those phagocytizing nuclear particles) and follicular dendritic cells are present.

follicle-associated epithelium (FAE)

Epithelium overlying single or aggregated lymphoid follicles that facilitate transcytosis via the presence of M cells.

follicular B cells

Lymphoid follicle mature B cells in secondary lymphoid tissue that are activated by Td antigens and generate memory B cells as well as short- and long-lived plasma cells.

follicular center cell lymphoma

A mature B cell malignancy.

follicular center cells

B lymphocytes in germinal centers (secondary follicles).

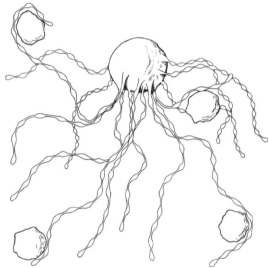

Schematic representation of follicular dendritic cell.

follicular dendritic cell

Cells manifesting narrow cytoplasmic processes that interdigitate between densely populated areas of B lymphocytes in lymph node follicles and in spleen. Antigen–antibody complexes adhere to the surfaces of follicular dendritic cells and are not generally endocytosed but are associated with the formation of germinal centers. These cells are bereft of class II histocompatibility molecules, although Fc receptors, complement receptor 1, and complement receptor 2 molecules are demonstrable on their surfaces. They display antigens on their surfaces for B cell recognition and participate in the activation and selection of B cells expressing high-affinity membrane immunoglobulin during affinity maturation.

follicular hyperplasia

Lymph node enlargement associated with an increase in follicle size and number. Germinal centers are usually present in the follicles. Follicular hyperplasia is often a postinfection reactive process in lymph nodes.

follicular lymphoma

The most common form of non-Hodgkin lymphoma in the United States, comprising approximately 45% of adult lymphomas. The neoplastic cells closely resemble normal germinal center B cells. They resemble normal follicular center B cells, expressing CD19, CD20, CD10, and monotypic surface immunoglobulin. CD5 is not expressed, which differentiates follicular lymphoma from B cell chronic lymphocytic leukemia (CLL), small lymphocytic lymphoma (SLL), and mantle cell lymphoma. Follicular lymphoma cells express BCL2 protein, in contrast to normal follicular center B cells that are BCL2-negative. A 14;18 translocation is characteristic of follicular lymphoma, in which juxtaposition of the IgH locus on chromosome 14 and the BCL2 locus on chromosome 18 occurs.

food allergy

Type I (anaphylactic) or type III (antigen–antibody complex) hypersensitivity mechanism responses to allergens or antigens in ingested foods may lead to intestinal distress, producing nausea, vomiting, and diarrhea, along with edema of the buccal mucosa, generalized urticaria, or eczema. Food categories associated with allergies in some individuals include eggs, fish, nuts, peanuts, soy, and wheat. Atopic sensitization to cow's milk is the most common food allergy; casein is the major allergenic and antigenic protein in cow's milk. Both skin tests and RAST tests using the appropriate allergen or antigen may identify individuals with a particular food allergy.

food and drug additive reactions

Urticaria and angioneurotic edema are the main symptoms.

footprinting

A method to ascertain the DNA segment (or segments) that binds to a protein. Radiolabeled double-stranded DNA is combined with the binding protein to yield a complex that is exposed to an endonuclease that cuts the molecules once and at random. The digested DNA is electrophoresed in polyacrylamide gel together with a control DNA sample (treated similarly, but without added protein) to permit separation of fragments differing in length by one nucleotide. Autoradiography of the material reveals a series of bands representing the DNA fragments. In the area of protein binding, the DNA is spared from digestion, and no corresponding bands appear compared to the control. The protected area's specific location can be ascertained by running a DNA sequencing gel in parallel.

footprints

Macrophages filled with *Mycobacterium leprae* without caseation necrosis. A similar situation may be observed in anergic Hodgkin disease patients and in AIDS patients infected with *M. avium-intercellulare.*

forbidden clone theory

According to this hypothesis, self-reactive lymphocyte clones are eliminated in the thymus during embryonic life, but subsequent mutation may permit the reappearance of self-reactive clones of lymphocytes that induce autoimmunity.

foreign gene

See transgenic mice.

formol toxoids

A toxoid generated by the treatment of an exotoxin such as diphtheria toxin with formalin. Although first used nearly a century ago, it was subsequently modified to contain an adjuvant such as an aluminum compound to boost immune responsiveness to the toxoid. It was later replaced with the so-called triple vaccine for diphtheria, pertussis, and tetanus.

formyl–methionyl–leucyl–phenylalanine (F–Met–Leu–Phe)

A synthetic peptide that is a powerful chemotactic attractant for leukocytes, facilitating their migration. It may also induce neutrophil degranulation. It resembles chemotactic factors released from bacteria. Following interaction with neutrophils, leukocyte migration is enhanced, and complement receptor 3 molecules are increased in cell membranes.

Forssman antibody

An antibody specific for the Forssman (heterogenetic) antigen. Human serum may contain Forssman antibody as a natural antibody.

Forssman antigen

A heterophil or heterogenetic glycolipid antigen that stimulates the synthesis of anti-sheep hemolysin in rabbits. Its broad phylogenetic distribution spans both animal and plant kingdoms. The antigen is present in guinea pig and horse organs, but not in their red blood cells. In sheep, it is found exclusively in erythrocytes. Forssman antigen occurs in both red blood cells and organs in chickens. It is also present in goats, ostriches, mice, dogs, cats, spinach, and *Bacillus anthracis* and on the gastrointestinal mucosa of a limited number of people. It is absent in rabbits, rats, cows, pigs, cuckoos, beans, and *Salmonella typhi*. Forssman substance is ceramide tetrasaccharide. The Forssman antigen contains *N*-acylsphingo-sine (ceramide), galactose, and *N*-acetylgalactosamine. As originally defined, it is present in guinea pig kidney and is heat-stable and alcohol-soluble. Forssman antigen-containing tissue is effective in absorbing the homologous antibody from serum. Antibodies to the Forssman antigen occur in the sera of patients recovering from infectious mononucleosis.

Forssman, Magnus John Karl August (1868–1947)

Swedish professor for whom the heterophile antigen was named, following his discovery and work with that protein.

forward-angle light scatter (FALS)

In flow cytometry, particle size is measured by the amount of scattered light (0.5 to 2 degrees) detected as the focused laser beam encounters the cell and continues as scattered light to the forward-angle light scatter detector.

forward genetics approach

Mutating a gene in an experimental animal to prove that gene's role in a particular disease and determining whether the mutation produces the disease of interest.

Foscarnet.

foscarnet

An investigational drug used to combat cytomegalovirus-induced pneumonia, hepatitis, colitis, and retinitis in AIDS patients rendered nonresponsive to gancyclovir, which is frequently used to treat cytomegalovirus infection.

Foxp3

A member of the forkhead/winged helix family of transcriptional regulators that act as master regulators in regulatory T cell development and function. Human FOXP3 genes contain eleven coding exons. The FOXP3 gene maps to chromosome Xp11.23. In IPEX, the X-linked syndrome of immunodysregulation, polyendocrinopathy, and enteropathy, the FOXP3 gene is mutated. The mutations occur in the forkhead domain of FOXP3, suggesting that the mutations may disrupt critical DNA interactions. A Foxp3 mutation, consisting of a frameshift mutation that results in protein lacking the forkhead domain, leads to "scurfy" in mice. This is an X-linked recessive mouse mutant that is lethal in hemizygous males 16 to 25 days after birth. These mice have over-proliferation of CD4+ T lymphocytes, extensive multiorgan infiltration, and increases in multiple cytokines. This phenotype resembles the lack of expression of CTLA-4, TGF-beta, human disease IPEX, or deletion of the Foxp3 gene in mice. The pathology in scurfy mice is apparently a consequence of the inability to regulate properly CD4+ T cell function. Mice over-expressing the Foxp3 gene have diminished numbers of T cells that reveal poor proliferative and cytolytic responses and only weak IL2 production even though thymic development is normal. Histologically, the peripheral lymphoid organs, especially lymph nodes, lack cells.

F:P ratio

Fluorescence-to-protein ratio that expresses the ratio of fluorochrome to protein in an antibody preparation labeled with the fluorochrome.

FPR

N-formyl peptide receptor (FPR) is a member of the G protein-coupled receptor family, the chemokine receptor branch of the rhodopsin family. Tissue sources include HL-60 cells differentiated with Bt2 cAMP. Undifferentiated HL-60 cells transfected with FPR bound FMLP with two affinities. COS7 cells transfected with FPR bound FMLPK-Pep12 with low and high affinity. The receptor is expressed in neutrophils. Dibutyryl cAMP includes FPR transcription in HL-60 cells.

Fracastoro, Girolamo (1478–1553)

A physician who was born in Verona and educated at Padua. His interests ranged from poetry to geography. He proposed the theory of acquired immunity and was a leader in the early theories of contagion. (Refer to *Syphilis sive Morbus Gallicus*, 1530; *De Sympathia et Antipathia Rerum*, 1546; *De Contagione*, 1546.)

fractional catabolic rate

The total plasma immunoglobulin percentage catabolized daily. Predicted from the half-life of plasma or from the excretion rate of catabolized immunoglobulin products in urine.

fragmentins

Serine esterases present in cytotoxic T cell and natural killer cell cytoplasmic granules. The introduction of fragmentins into the cytosol of a cell causes apoptosis as the DNA in the nucleus is fragmented into 200-base-pair multimers. Also called granzymes.

framework regions (FRs)

Relatively invariant regions within variable domains of immunoglobulins and T cell receptors that constitute a

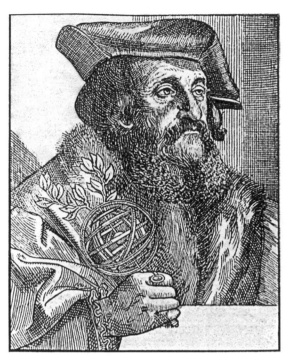

Girolamo Fracastoro.

protein scaffold for hypervariable regions interacting with antigen. Amino acid sequences in variable regions of heavy or light immunoglobulin chains other than the hypervariable sequences. There is much less variability in the framework region than in the hypervariable region. Two β-pleated sheets opposing one another comprise the structural features of the framework regions of an antibody domain. Polypeptide chain loops join the β-pleated sheet strands. The framework regions contribute to the secondary and tertiary structures of the variable region domain, although they are less significant than the hypervariable regions for the antigen-binding site. The framework region forms the folding part of the immunoglobulin molecule. Light chain FRs are found at amino acid residues 1 to 28, 38 to 50, 56 to 89, and 97 to 107. Heavy chain FRs are present at amino acid residues 1 to 31, 35 to 49, 66 to 101, and 110 to 117.

Francisella immunity

The causative agent of tularemia, *Francisella tularensis*, may induce two forms of the disease: ulceroglandular tularemia, borne by vectors or induced by contact with infected animals, and respiratory tularemia, caused by inhalation of contaminated dust. A powerful antibody response occurs during infection with this microorganism and is detectable by agglutination, ELISA, or other techniques. The antibodies appear at the end of the second or during the third week of infection. They persist for several years following recovery. Immunoglobulin M (IgM) antibodies do not appear before IgG antibodies and may even be present for years following recovery. Cell-mediated immunity in tularemia is demonstrated by a delayed-type hypersensitivity test or by *in vitro* activation of T cells. Cell-mediated immunity against *F. tularensis* is requisite for host protection. The microorganism's capsule protects it against lysis by complement and affords resistance to intracellular killing by polymorphonuclear leukocytes. Attenuated strains of the microorganism, termed *F. tularensis* LVS, are easily killed by polymorpho-nuclear leukocytes and are susceptible to hydrochloric acid and hydrogen peroxide produced as a result of the oxidative burst. No significant toxins are produced by *F. tularensis.* T-cell-mediated immunity can prevent fulminating disease. Infection or vaccination with live attenuated bacteria can induce host protection against tularemia.

freemartin

The female of dizygotic cattle twins; the other twin is a male. Their placentas are fused *in utero,* causing them to be exposed to each other's cells *in utero* prior to the development of immunologic maturity. This renders the animals immunologically tolerant of each other's cells and prevents a twin from rejecting grafts from the other twin. The female has reproductive abnormalities and is sterile.

Frei test

A tuberculin type of delayed hypersensitivity skin test employed to reveal delayed-type hypersensitivity in lymphogranuloma venereum patients. Following intradermal injection of lymphogranuloma venereum virus, an erythematous and indurated papule develops after 4 days.

Freund, Jules (1890–1960)

Hungarian physician who later worked in the United States. He made many contributions to immunology, including his work on antibody formation, studies on allergic encephalomyelitis, and the development of Freund's adjuvant. He received the Lasker Award in 1959.

Freund's adjuvant

A water-in-oil emulsion that facilitates or enhances an immune response to antigen incorporated into the adjuvant. There are two forms. Complete Freund's adjuvant (CFA) consists of lightweight mineral oil that contains killed, dried mycobacteria. With the aid of an emulsifying agent such as Arlacel A, antigen in an aqueous phase is incorporated into the oil phase containing mycobacteria. This emulsion is then used as the immunogen. Incomplete Freund's adjuvant (IFA) differs from the complete form only in that it does not contain mycobacteria. In both cases, the augmenting effect depends on and parallels the magnitude of the local inflammatory lesion, essentially a non-necrotic monocytic reaction with fibrous encapsulation. Whereas the complete form facilitates stimulation of both T and B limbs of the immune response, the incomplete variety enhances antibody formation but does not stimulate cell-mediated immunity except for transient Jones–Mote reactivity. The adjuvant principle in mycobacteria is the cell wall wax D fraction. CFA does not potentiate the immune response to the so-called thymus-independent antigens such as pneumococcal polysaccharide or polyvinylpyrrolidone. CFA may be combined with normal tissues and injected into animals of the type supplying the tissue to induce autoimmune diseases such as thyroiditis, allergic encephalomyelitis, or adjuvant arthritis.

Freund's adjuvant, complete

Refer to Freund's adjuvant.

Freund's adjuvant, incomplete

Refer to Freund's adjuvant.

front typing

In blood typing for transfusion, antibodies of known specificity are used to identify erythrocyte ABO antigens. Differences between front and back typing may be attributable to acquired group B or B subtypes, diminished

Front Typing		Back Typing			Interpretation
Reaction of Cells Tested with		Reaction of Serum Tested Against			
Anti-A	Anti-B	A Cells	B Cells	O Cells	ABO Group
O	O	+	+	O	O
+	O	O	+	O	A
O	+	+	O	O	B
+	+	O	O	O	AB

+ = agglutination
O = no agglutination

ABO blood grouping by front and back typing.

immunoglobulins, anti-B and anti-A₁ antibody polyagglutination, rouleau formation, cold agglutinins, Wharton's jelly, or two separate cell populations.

frustrated phagocytosis

The inability of a phagocyte to engulf a target particle because of its large size or fixation in a tissue, which leads to the external release of lysosomal contents, resulting in localized tissue injury.

FTA–ABS (fluorescence treponema antibody absorption)

A serological test for syphilis that is very sensitive (i.e., approaching 100%) in the diagnosis of secondary, tertiary, congenital, and neurosyphilis.

FTA–ABS test

An assay for specific antibodies to *Treponema pallidum* in the sera of patients suspected of having syphilis. Before combining serum with killed *T. pallidum* microorganisms fixed on a slide, the serum is first absorbed with an extract of Reiter's treponemes to remove group-specific antibodies. After washing, the specimen is covered with fluorescein-labeled antihuman globulin, followed by examination by fluorescence microscopy with ultraviolet light. Demonstration of positive fluorescence of the target microorganisms reveals specific antibody present in the serum. The greater specificity and sensitivity of this test make it preferable to the previously used FTA-200 assay.

FTY720

An investigational immunosuppressive drug, which is a synthetic analogue of the fungal toxin known as myriocin and synthesized by *Isaria sinclairii*, which inhibits the serine palmitoyltransferase enzyme needed for the *de novo* production of sphingolipids and sphingosine. This drug has no effect on innate immune system cells, making it more desirable than other immunosuppressive drugs that might facilitate opportunistic infections.

Fudenberg, Hugh (1928–)

Prolific author and editor of immunology research articles and books. Research interests have included immunoglobulins, cell-mediated immunity, suppressor T cells, and neuroimmunology, among others.

full chimerism

The state in which all of an individual's hematopoietic cells are of donor origin. This results when a bone marrow or hematopoietic stem cell transplant is performed following myeloablative conditioning to eliminate all the recipient's hematopoietic cells.

functional affinity

Association constant for a bivalent or multivalent antibody's interaction with a bivalent or multivalent ligand. The

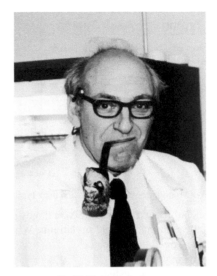

Dr. H. Hugh Fudenberg.

multivalent reactivity may enhance the affinity of multiple antigen–antibody reactions. Avidity has a similar connotation, but it is a less precise term.

functional antigen

Refer to protective antigen.

functional immunity

Refer to protective immunity.

fungal immunity

Nonspecific immune mechanisms of a host that form a first line of defense against fungal infections include the mechanical barriers provided by the skin and mucous membranes, competition by normal bacterial flora for nutrients, and the respiratory tract's mucociliary clearance mechanism. Fungi are not lysed by the terminal components of the complement system and specific antibody, but complement components serving as opsonins facilitate phagocytosis of fungi by phagocytic cells. Fungi are powerful activators of the alternative complement system. Neutrophils are very significant in protection against various mycoses, including disseminated candidiasis and invasive aspergillosis.

Monocytes and resident macrophages vary in their ability to kill fungi. Few specific antifungal activities of activated human macrophages have been demonstrated. Bronchoalveolar macrophages play an important role in the immune response to inhaled fungi. Natural killer (NK) cells inhibit the growth of *C. neoformans* and *P. brasiliensis in vitro*. NK cells have also been shown to clear cryptococcus from mice. Specific antibodies are of little use in host defense against most mycoses, but specific cell-mediated immunity is paramount for a protective immune response to *C. neoformans* disease and dimorphic fungi. It is also important for protection against dermatophyte infections. Cell-mediated immunity plays an important role in protection against mucocutaneous candidiasis. AIDS patients have a high incidence of fungal infections. Cytokines formed in a specific cell-mediated immune response facilitate the antifungal action of NK cells, nonspecific T lymphocytes, and neutrophils. Cytokines such as tumor necrosis factor (TNF), granulocyte–macrophage colony-stimulating factor (GM-CSF), and interleukin-12 (IL12) released during a cell-mediated immune response may activate effector cells to kill fungi. Immunosuppressive cytokines such as IL10 and transforming growth factor β (TGF-β) are also formed in response to fungal infection. Severe fungal infections usually occur in profoundly immunosuppressed patients who have diminished responses to immunization. Defects in host immunity associated with fungal infections are being identified in order that cytokines such as interferon-γ (IFN-γ) may be administered to chronic granulomatous disease patients and GM-CSF may be administered to neutropenic patients. Monoclonal antibodies against capsular glucuronoxylomannan have been given to patients with cryptococcosis.

fungi

Single-celled and multicellular eukaryotic microorganisms such as yeast and molds. They readily invade and colonize a host with compromised immunity, producing a variety of diseases. Immunity to fungi involves both cell-mediated and humoral immune responses.

1. Chimeric antibody — Rodent variable

Human constant

2. Reshaped humanized antibody with specificity of original rodent antibody.

Rodent hypervariable

Human framework

Human constant

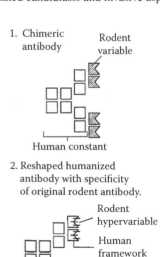

3. Antibody-toxin/enzyme chimeric molecule

F(ab′)₂

Fc replaced by enzyme or toxin

4.

Single domain antibody

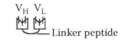

5. Single-chain Fv molecule created by linked V domains from an L and an H chain

V_H V_L

Linker peptide

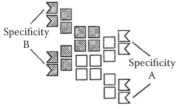

6. Bi-specific antibody created by protein engineering

Heavy chain

Specificity A

Specificity B

Light chain

7. Bi-specific antibodies created by protein engineering

Specificity B

Specificity A

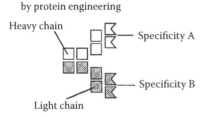

Genetically engineered antibodies.

fusin

A receptor present on CD4$^+$ T lymphocytes and selected other human cells that is linked to a G protein and is believed to be requisite for human immunodeficiency virus (HIV) fusion with target cells.

Fusobacterium immunity

F. nucleatum adheres to lymphocytes through lectin-like ligands to facilitate other activity or exert an immunosuppressive effect on them. The latter enhances the pathogenicity of the microorganism. Patients with periodontal disease, peritonsillar cellulitis and abscesses, infectious mononucleosis, and acute streptococcal, nonstreptococcal, and recurrent tonsilitis manifest increased levels of antibodies against protein antigens of *F. nucleatum*. Antibodies against these outer membrane proteins may point to a pathogenic role for this microorganism in these infections. Delayed-type hypersensitivity to *F. necrophorum* has been induced in mice, and leukotoxin-specific antibodies have been found in cattle. Natural infection or vaccination with a toxoid does not always protect against reinfection. This microorganism is believed to be a weak immunogenic pathogen.

Fv fragment

An antibody fragment consisting of the N terminal variable segments of both heavy (V$_H$) and light (V$_L$) chain domains that are joined by noncovalent forces. The fragment has one antigen-binding site.

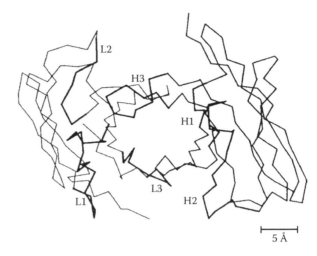

Fv region.

Fv region

The N terminal variable segments of both the heavy and light chains in each Fab region of an immunoglobulin molecule with a four-chain unit structure.

fyn

Refer to lck, fyn, ZAP (phosphotyrosine kinases in T cells).

G

G protein

Proteins that bind guanosine triphosphate (GTP) and convert it to guanosine diphosphate (GDP) during cell signal transduction. These heterotrimeric proteins are active when GTP occupies the guanine binding site and inactive when it anchors GDP. The two types of G proteins include the trimeric (α, β, γ) receptor-associated G protein and the small G proteins, including Ras and Raf, which function downstream of numerous transmembrane signaling events. Trimeric GTP-binding proteins are associated with parts of numerous cell surface receptors in the cytoplasm, including chemokine receptors.

G protein-coupled receptor family

Receptors for lipid inflammatory mediators, hormones, and chemokines that employ associated trimeric G proteins for intracellular signaling.

GAD-65

A major autoantigen in insulin-dependent diabetes mellitus. It is expressed primarily in human β cells.

gag

The retroviral HIV-1 gene that encodes the heterogeneous p24 protein of the virus core.

GALT

Abbreviation for gut-associated lymphoid tissues. Refer also to MALT.

γ globulin

Obsolete designation for immunoglobulin. γ Globulins are serum proteins that show the lowest mobility toward the anode during electrophoresis when the pH is neutral. The γ globulin fraction contains immunoglobulins. It is the most cationic of the serum globulins.

γ globulin fraction

The electrophoretic fraction of serum in which most of the immunoglobulin classes are found.

γ heavy chain disease

γ Heavy chain disease, also called Franklin's disease, is a very rare syndrome in which the myeloma cells synthesize γ heavy chains only. Clinically, this disease affects mostly older individuals; onset is gradual or sudden. The patients may be weak, have fever and malaise, and demonstrate lymphadenopathy over time. Swelling of the uvula and edema of the palate may be consequences of lymphoid tissue involvement of the nasopharynx and Waldeyer's ring. Lymph nodes affected may include those of the axilla, mediastinum, tracheobronchial tree, and abdomen. Fever and enlargement of the spleen and liver may follow infection. The disease may last from several months to 5 years and usually leads to death, although remission has been described in occasional patients. The blood serum contains proteins with electrophoretic peaks that correspond in mobility to the homogeneous (Bence–Jones negative) proteins present in the urine. An elevated sedimentation rate, mild anemia, thrombocytopenia, leukopenia, and

sometimes eosinophilia occur. Abnormal plasma cells and lymphocytes may appear in the blood and occasionally be manifested as plasma cell leukemia. To confirm the diagnosis of γ heavy chain disease, one must demonstrate a spike with the electrophoretic mobility of a fast γ or β globulin reactive with antiserum against γ heavy chains, but not with κ or λ light chains. Numerous deletions in γ chains vary in location but often include most of the variable region and the total C_H1 segment, with continuation of the normal sequence where the hinge region begins. Whereas patients with Franklin's disease demonstrate heavy γ chains in both serum and urine, the other immunoglobulin levels are diminished. Light chain synthesis totally fails in all individuals. Thus, γ heavy chain disease may mimic lymphomas of one type or another (as well as multiple myeloma, toxoplasmosis, and histoplasmosis) and may be associated occasionally with tuberculosis, rheumatoid arthritis, and various other conditions.

γ interferon

Refer to interferon γ.

γ macroglobulin

Obsolete term for immunoglobulin M (IgM).

$\gamma\delta$ T cell receptor (TCR)

A heterodimer comprised of TCRγ and δ chains together with the CD3 complex. Antigens include *MICA/MICB*, Hsps, T10/22 proteins, altered phospholipids, lipoproteins, phosphorylated oligonucleotides, pyrophosphate-like epitopes, alkylamines, peptides, pathogens, or whole proteins. Selected $\gamma\delta$ TCRs can recognize *CD1c*. Double-negative CD4$^-$ CD8$^-$ T cells may express CD3-associated $\gamma\delta$ TCRs. $\gamma\delta$ TCRs may be capable of reacting with polymorphic ligand(s). The initial receptor to be expressed during thymic ontogeny is the $\gamma\delta$ TCR. Cells lacking $\gamma\delta$ TCR expression may subsequently rearrange α and β chains, resulting in $\alpha\beta$ TCR expression. Thus, a single cell never normally expresses both receptors. Cells expressing the $\alpha\beta$ TCR mediate helper T cell and cytotoxic T cell functions. Whereas $\gamma\delta$ TCRs are expressed on double negative cells only, $\alpha\beta$ TCRs may be present on CD4$^+$ or CD8$^+$. The $\gamma\delta$ TCR apparently can function in the absence of major histocompatibility complex (MHC) molecules, in contrast to the association of CD4$^+$ with MHC class II or CD8$^+$ with MHC class I recognition by cells expressing $\alpha\beta$ TCRs. $\gamma\delta$-TCR-expressing cells may protect against microorganisms entering through the epithelium in the skin, lung, intestines, etc. $\gamma\delta$-TCR-bearing cells constitute a majority of T cells during thymic ontogeny and in mouse epidermis. Whether the epidermis and/or epithelium of the skin can function as sites for T cell education and maturation is unknown. $\gamma\delta$ TCR represents an evolutionary precursor of the $\alpha\beta$ TCR, as reflected by the relatively low percentages of cells expressing $\gamma\delta$ TCRs in adults and the fact that cells expressing the $\alpha\beta$ TCRs carry out the principal immunologic functions.

G

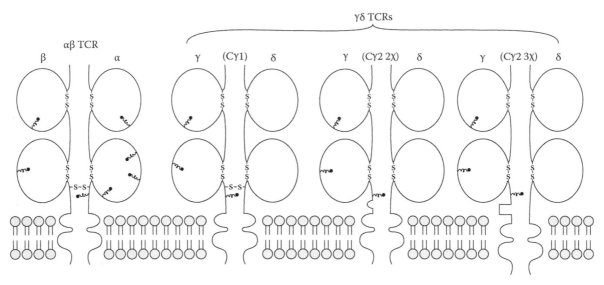

T cell receptor (TCR) showing αβ and γδ receptors.

The diversity of the γδ TCRs and lymphokine synthesis by cells expressing the γδ TCRs attest to the significance of the cells in the immune system. Little is known concerning the types of antigen recognized by γδ TCRs. They fail to recognize peptide complexes bound to polymorphic MHC molecules.

γδ T cells

Early T lymphocytes that express γ and δ chains comprising the T cell receptor of the cell surface. They comprise only 5% of the normal circulating T cells in healthy adults. γδ T cells home to the lamina propria of the gut. Their function is not fully understood. γδ T lymphocytes recognize antigens or pathogens in their natural and unprocessed states. They respond more rapidly than do αβ T cells to antigen and proliferate less than the latter. γδ T cells require negligible or no conventional costimulation. They have been called sentinels of innate immunity and represent a link to the adaptive immune system.

γM globulin

Obsolete term for IgM.

gammopathy

An abnormal increase in immunoglobulin synthesis. Gammopathies that are monoclonal usually signify malignancy such as multiple myeloma, Waldenström's disease, heavy chain disease, or chronic lymphocytic leukemia. Benign gammopathies occur in amyloidosis and monoclonal gammopathy of undetermined etiology. Inflammatory disorders are often accompanied by benign polyclonal gammopathies. These include rheumatoid arthritis, lupus erythematosus, tuberculosis, cirrhosis, and angioimmunoblastic lymphadenopathy.

gancyclovir (9-[2-hydroxy-1(hydroxymethyl) ethoxymethyl] guanine)

An antiviral drug used for the therapy of immunocompromised patients infected with cytomegalic inclusion virus. Five days of gancyclovir therapy has proven effective for clearing cytomegalovirus (CMV) from the blood, urine, and respiratory secretions. It has been used successfully to treat CMV retinitis, gastroenteritis, and hepatitis. Drug resistance may develop. The drug may induce neutropenia

and thrombocytopenia as side effects. It has not proven very effective in AIDS or bone marrow transplant patients.

ganglioside autoantibodies

Autoantibodies to the monosialogangliosides GM_1, GM_2, and GM_3 are present in Guillain–Barré syndrome (GBS), multiple sclerosis (MS), rheumatic disorders with neurologic involvement, motor neuron diseases (MNDs), and various neoplasms. These autoantibodies crossreact with one or more polysialogangliosides, including GD_{1a}, GD_{1b}, GD_2, GD_3, GT_{1a}, GT_{1b}, and GQ_{1b}. Cross or polyreactivity patterns lend some clinical specificity to the antiganglioside response in GBS, Miller–Fisher syndrome (MFS), MNDs, and other neurological diseases that include schizophrenia, AIDS dementia complex, and neuropsychiatric–systemic lupus erythematosus (SLE).

Gardasil®

A human papillomavirus (HPV) vaccine comprised of four strains of HPV, a virus transmitted through the skin via sexual contact. Protects against two strains of HPV that cause approximately 70% of cervical cancer cases. It also protects against two additional strains that are responsible for approximately 90% of genital wart cases. It is considered safe and effective for 9- to 26-year old females. Clinical trials proved Gardasil 100% effective against HPV strains 16 and 18, the etiologic agents for 70% of cervical cancer cases. It was 99% effective against HPV strains 6 and 11 that induce 90% of genital wart cases. The CDC indicates that more than 20 million people have HPV infections. Eighty percent of females are infected by the time they reach 50 years of age and 50% of sexually active individuals have HPV. Refer to human papillomavirus recombinant vaccine.

gas gangrene antitoxin

Antibodies found in antisera against exotoxins produced by *Clostridium perfringens*, *C. septicum*, and *C. oedematiens*, bacteria that may cause gas gangrene. In the past, this antiserum was used with antibiotics and surgical intervention in the treatment of wounds with potential for gas gangrene.

gastric cell cAMP-stimulating autoantibodies

These autoantibodies have been detected in young males with long-standing duodenal ulcer disease, a family history of this condition, and poor responsiveness to H2-receptor antagonists; however, other investigators have failed to confirm these results.

gastrin-producing cell antibodies (GPCAs)

Antibodies present in 8 to 16% of antral (type B) chronic atrophic gastritis patients. GPCAs may lead to diminished gastrin secretion and fewer gastrin-producing cells in antral gastritis. There are no parietal cell antibodies present, and GPCAs are not linked to pernicious anemia. GPCAs in type B gastritis are different from gastric fundus parietal cell antibodies that have been linked to fundal mucosal atrophy in type A gastritis.

gastrin-producing cell autoantibodies (GPCAs)

Autoantibodies found in 8 to 16% of patients with antral (type B) chronic atrophic gastritis, which primarily affects the antral mucosa. Parietal cell autoantibodies (PCA) are not present, and the autoantibodies are not associated with pernicious anemia or polyendocrinopathy. The GPCAs are believed to be responsible for the diminished gastrin secretion and fewer gastrin-producing cells in antral gastritis. PCAs are found only in patients with normal antral mucosa. By contrast, GPCAs are present only in patients with normal antral mucosa or mild antral gastritis but not in individuals with moderate or severe antral gastritis. *Helicobacter pylori* has a world-established association with antral (type B) gastritis and peptic ulcer disease, but antibodies against *H. pylori* are not helpful for monitoring the disease.

gastrin receptor antibodies

These antibodies are claimed to be present in 30% of pernicious anemia patients by some investigators, but this finding has not been confirmed. Gastric receptor antibodies may inhibit gastrin binding and have been demonstrated to bind gastric parietal cells.

***GATA-2* gene**

A gene that encodes a transcription factor required for the development of lymphoid, erythroid, and myeloid hematopoietic cell lineages.

gatekeeper effect

Contraction of endothelium mediated by immunoglobulin E (IgE), permitting components of the blood to gain access to the extravascular space as a consequence of increased vascular permeability.

gay bowel syndrome

A constellation of gastrointestinal symptoms in homosexual males related to both infectious and noninfectious etiologies before the acquired immune deficiency syndrome (AIDS) epidemic. Clinical features include alterations in bowel habits, condyloma acuminata, bloating, flatulence, diarrhea, nausea, vomiting, adenomatous polyps, fistulas, fissures, hemorrhoids, and perirectal abscesses, among many other features. Associated sexually transmitted infections include syphilis, herpes simplex, gonorrhea, and *Chlamydia trachomatis*. Numerous other microbial species identified include human papilloma virus, *Campylobacter* organisms, hepatitis A and B, cytomegalovirus, and parasites such as *Entamoeba histolytica*. Treatment varies with the etiology of gay bowel syndrome manifestations.

GCDFP-15 (23A3)

Gross cystic disease fluid protein-15 is a 15,000-Da glycoprotein localized in the apocrine metaplastic epithelium lining breast cysts and in apocrine glands in the axilla, vulva, eyelid and ear canal. Approximately 70% of breast carcinomas stain positive with antibody to GCDFP-15. Colorectal carcinomas and mesotheliomas do not stain with this antibody. Lung adenocarcinoma rarely stains with this antibody.

GCP-2 (granulocyte chemotactic protein-2)

Granulocyte chemotactic protein-2 is a chemokine of the α (CXC) family. Osteosarcoma cells can produce both human GCP-2 and interleukin-8 (IL8). The bovine homolog of human CP-2 has been demonstrated in kidney tumor cells. Human and bovine GCP-2 are chemotactic for human granulocytes and activate postreceptor mechanisms that cause the release of gelatinase B, which portends a possible role in inflammation and tumor cell invasion. Tissue sources include osteosarcoma cells and kidney neoplastic cells. Granulocytes are the target cells.

G-CSF

Granulocyte colony-stimulating factor. A biological response modifier that facilitates formation of granulocytes in the bone marrow. It was first licensed by the U.S. Food and Drug Administration in 1991 and may be useful to reactivate granulocyte production in the marrow of irradiated or chemotherapy-treated patients. The genes for G-CSF are found on chromosome 17. Endothelial cells, macrophages, and fibroblasts produce G-CSF, which functions synergistically with IL3 in stimulating bone marrow cells. G-CSF induces differentiation and clonal extinction in certain myeloid leukemia cell lines. It promotes almost exclusively the development of neutrophils from normal hematopoietic progenitor cells.

GEF

Refer to guanine-nucleotide exchange factor.

gel

A semisolid substance prepared from seaweed agar that was widely used in bacteriology and is now used in immunology for diffusion of antigen and antibody in Ouchterlony-type techniques, electrophoresis, immunoelectrophoresis, and related methods.

gel diffusion

A method to evaluate antibodies and antigens based upon their diffusion in gels toward one another and their reaction at the point of contact in the gel.

gel filtration chromatography

This method permits the separation of molecules on the basis of size. Porous beads are allowed to swell in buffer, water, or other solutions and are packed into a column. The molecular pores of the beads permit the entry of some molecules and exclude others on the basis of size. Molecules larger than the pores pass through the column and emerge with the void volume. Because the solute molecules within the beads maintain a concentration equilibrium with solutes in the liquid phase outside the beads, molecular species of a given weight, shape, and degree of hydration move as a band. Gel chromatography using spherical agarose gel particles is useful in the exclusion of immunoglobulin M (IgM), which is present in the first peak. Of course, other molecules of similar size, such as macroglobulins, are also present in this peak. IgG is present in the second peak, but the fractions of the leading side are contaminated by IgA and IgD.

gemtuzumab

A humanized IgG4 monoclonal antibody that contains a κ light chain specific for CD33, a sialoadhesion protein

G

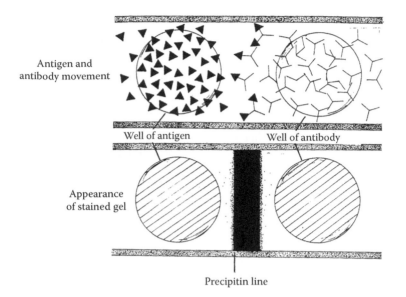

Antigen and
antibody movement

Well of antigen   Well of antibody

Appearance
of stained gel

Precipitin line

Gel diffusion.

present on leukemic blast cells in most acute myelogenous
leukemia patients. Toxicities include myelosuppression,
including neutropenia, hepatotoxicity, and hypersensitivity
reactions.

gene amplification
One of more duplications of a gene or its chromosomal
region to yield many copies of that gene in the genome.

gene bank
DNA library.

gene cloning
The use of recombinant DNA technology to replicate genes
or their fragments.

gene conversion
Recombination of two homologous genes in which a local
segment of one gene is replaced by a homologous segment
of a second gene. In avian species and lagomorphs, gene
conversion facilitates immunoglobulin receptor diversity
principally through homologous, inactive V gene segments
exchanging short sequences with an active, rearranged
variable-region gene.

gene conversion hypothesis
Method by which alternative sequences can be introduced
into major histocompatibility complex (MHC) genes
without reciprocal crossover events. This mechanism may
account for the incredible polymorphism of alleles. The
alternative sequences may include those found in the class
I-like genes and pseudogenes present on chromosome 6.
Hypothetically, gene conversion was an evolutionary event
as well as an ongoing one, giving rise to new mutations,
therefore new alleles, within a population.

gene diversity
Determination of the extent of an immune response to a
particular antigen or immunogen by mixing and matching of exons from variable, joining, diversity, and constant
region gene segments. S. Tonegawa received a Nobel Prize
for revealing the mechanism of the generation of diversity
in antibody formation.

gene escape mutant
A pathogenic microorganism that avoids host immune
response or drug therapy by causing a mutation in a gene

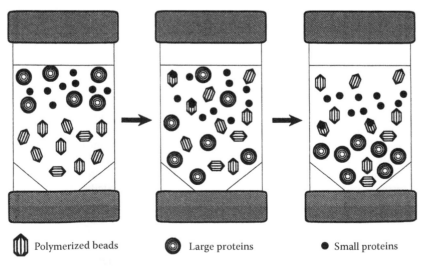

⬜ Polymerized beads   ◉ Large proteins   ● Small proteins

Gel filtration chromatography.

encoding a protein that is responsible for either antigenicity or drug susceptibility, respectively.

gene family

Genes that encode proteins with similar structures and frequently with similar functions.

gene gun

An apparatus that forces tiny plasmid-coated gold particles into the cytoplasm of living cells, which synthesize the antigen encoded by the plasmid. Used for experimental vaccination.

gene knockout

Gene disruption by homologous recombination. It may refer to a cell or animal in which the function of a specific gene is purposely eliminated by replacing the normal gene with an inactive mutant gene.

gene mapping

Gene localization or gene order. Gene localization can be in relationship to other genes or to a chromosomal band. The term may also refer to the ordering of gene segments.

gene rearrangement

Genetic shuffling that results in elimination of introns and the joining of exons to produce mRNA. Gene rearrangement within a lymphocyte signifies its dedication to the formation of a single cell type via immunoglobulin synthesis by B lymphocytes or production of a β chain receptor by T lymphocytes. Neoplastic transformation of lymphocytes may be followed by the expansion of a single clone of cells detectable by Southern blotting.

gene segments

Multiple short DNA sequences in immunoglobulin and T cell receptor genes that can undergo rearrangements in many combinations to yield a vast diversity of immunoglobin or T cell receptor polypeptide chains. A gene segment is a short, germline sequence of DNA derived from the variable (V) diversity (D) or joining (J) families. It combines randomly by way of V(D)J recombination with one or two other gene segments to form a V exon in either Ig or TCR loci. Gene segments do not possess RNA splice donor and acceptor sites.

gene therapy

The introduction of a normal functional gene into cells of the bone marrow to correct a genetic defect. Also termed somatic

gene therapy because it does not affect germline genes. A mechanism to achieve a therapeutic effect by transferring new genetic information into affected cells or tissues or into accessory cells. Adenosine deaminase deficiency has been successfully treated by this method. The technique also applies to patients with neoplasms or degenerative syndrome.

generalized anaphylaxis

The signs and symptoms of anaphylactic shock manifest within seconds to minutes following the administration of an antigen or allergen that interacts with specific immunoglobulin E (IgE) antibodies bound to mast cell or basophil surfaces, causing the release of pharmacologically active mediators that include vasoactive amines from their granules. Symptoms may vary from transient respiratory difficulties (due to contraction of the smooth muscle and terminal bronchioles) to even death.

generalized vaccinia

A condition observed in some children vaccinated against smallpox with vaccinia virus. Numerous vaccinia skin lesions occurred in children who had primary immunodeficiencies in antibody synthesis. Although usually self-limited, children who also had atopic dermatitis in addition to the generalized vaccinia often died.

generative lymphoid organ

An organ in which lymphocytes arise from immature precursor cells. The principal generative lymphoid organ for T cells is the thymus, and for B cells it is bone marrow.

genetic code

The codons (nucleotide triplets) correlating with amino acid residues in protein synthesis. The nucleotide linear sequence in mRNA is translated into the amino acid residue sequence.

genetic immunization

The inoculation of plasmid DNA encoding a protein into muscle for the purpose of inducing an adaptive immune response. For reasons yet to be explained, the plasmid DNA is expressed and induces T cell responses and antibody formation to the protein that the DNA encoded.

genetic knockout

A technique to introduce precise genetic lesions into the mouse genome to cause gene disruption and generate an animal model with a specific genetic defect. Specific defects

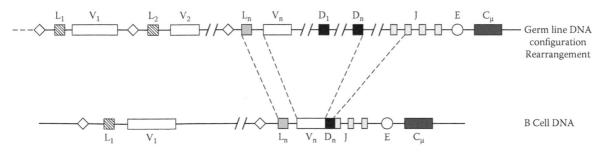

= Promoter
L = Leader sequence
V = Variable region
D = Diversity regions
J = Junction regions
C = Constant region coding block
E = Enhancer sequence

Immunoglobulin gene rearrangement.

G

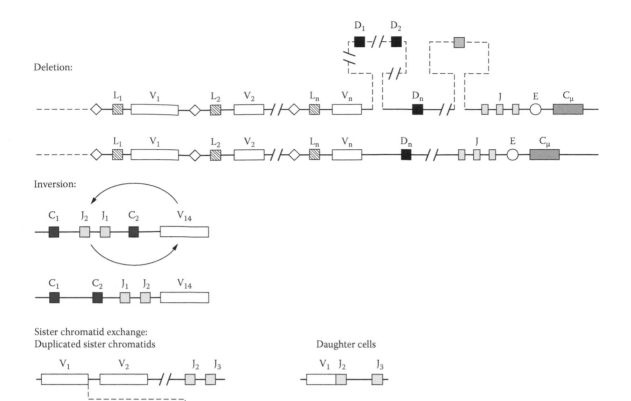

Immunoglobulin gene rearrangement.

may be introduced into any murine gene by permitting investigation of this alteration *in vivo*. Technological advances that made this possible include using homologous recombination to introduce defined changes into the murine genome and the reintroduction of genetically altered embryonic stem cells into the murine germline to produce mutant mouse strains.

genetic polymorphism
Variation in a population attributable to the existence of two or more alleles of a gene.

genetic switch hypothesis
A concept that predicts a switch in the gene governing heavy chain synthesis by plasma cells during immune response ontogeny.

genome
All genetic information contained in a cell or in a gamete; the total genetic material found in the haploid set of chromosomes.

genomic DNA
DNA found in the chromosomes. Refer to DNA.

genomics
Study of an organism's complete genome.

genotype
The genetic makeup of an organism. It constitutes the combined genetic constituents inherited from both parents and refers to the alleles present at one or more specific loci. When referring to microinjected transgenes, mice can be

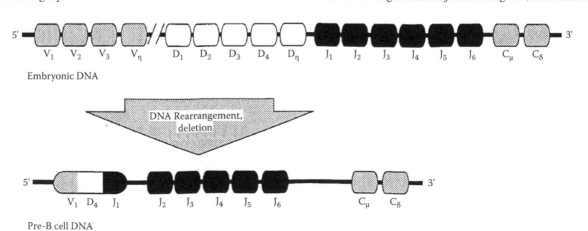

Gene rearrangement.

homozygous (transgene present on only one chromosome in a pair) or wild type (transgene not present on either chromosome in a pair). When referring to knockout mice, the correct term is *homozygous* (and sometimes they are called null mice).

germ-free animal

An animal such as a laboratory mouse raised under sterile conditions so that it is free from exposure to microorganisms and is not exposed to larger organisms. Germ-free animals have decreased serum immunoglobulin and lymphoid tissues that are not fully developed. Their diets may also be controlled to avoid exposure to food antigens. Most difficult is the ability to maintain a virus-free environment for these animals.

germline

Unaltered genetic material that is transmitted from one generation to the next through gametes. An individual's germline genes are those present in the zygote from which it arose. The term refers to non-rearranged genes rather than those rearranged for the production of immunoglobulin or T cell receptor (TCR) molecules.

germ theory of disease

The concept that pathogenic microorganisms including bacteria, fungi, parasites, and viruses visible only with the aid of a microscope or electron microscope cause specific diseases.

germline configuration

The arrangement of immunoglobulin and T cell receptor genes in the DNA of germ cells and in almost all somatic cells in which somatic recombination has not taken place.

germline diversity

The inheritance of multiple gene segments that encode V domains of antigen receptors. This form of diversity is distinguished from that generated during gene rearrangement or following receptor gene expression that is generated somatically.

germline diversity of antigen receptors

The inheritance of multiple gene segments that encode V domains. This is in contrast to the diversity arising from gene rearrangement or following receptor gene expression, which is somatically generated.

germline organization

The inherited arrangement of variable, diversity, joining, and constant region gene segments of antigen receptor loci in nonlymphoid cells or in immature lymphocytes. The germline organization in developing T or B lymphocytes is modified by somatic recombination to form functional immunoglobulin or T cell receptor genes.

germline theory

A concept to explain antibody diversity by postulating that each antibody is encoded in a separate germline gene.

germinal center

Germinal (or follicular) centers in lymph node and lymphoid aggregates within primary follicles of lymphoid tissues following antigenic stimulation. A germinal center is a site of intense B cell proliferation, selection, maturation, and death in secondary lymphoid tissue. Germinal centers develop around follicular dendritic cell networks when activated B cells migrate into lymphoid follicles. The mixed cell population in the germinal center is comprised of B lymphoblasts (cleaved and transformed lymphocytes), follicular dendritic cells, and numerous tingible body-containing macrophages. Germinal centers seen in various pathologic states include "burned out" germinal centers

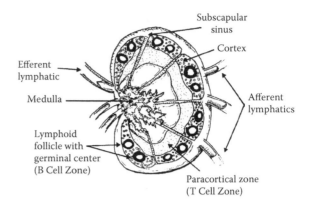

Germinal center.

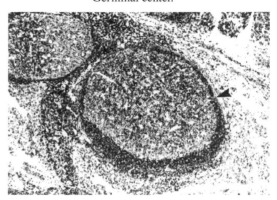

Germinal center.

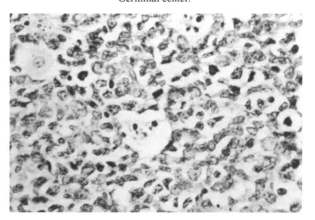

Tingible body macrophages in germinal center.

composed of accumulations of pale histiocytes and scattered immunoblasts; "progressively transformed" center that shows "starry sky" patterns containing epithelioid histiocytes, dendritic reticulum cells, increased T lymphocytes, and mantle zone lymphocytes; and "regressively transformed" germinal centers that are relatively small, have few lymphocytes, and reveal an onion-skin layering of dendritic reticulum cells, vascular endothelial cells, and fibroblasts. Germinal centers are sites of isotype switching, somatic hypermutation and affinity maturation.

germinal follicle

Refer to germinal center.

Gershon, Richard K. (1932–1983)

One of the first to demonstrate the suppressor role of the T cell. The suppressor T cell was described as a subpopulation of lymphocytes that diminish or suppress antibody

G

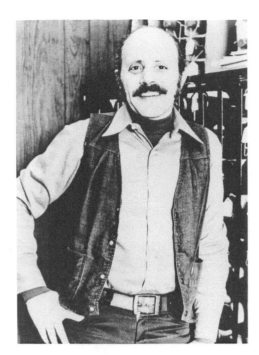

Richard K. Gershon.

formation by B cells or downregulate the ability of
T lymphocytes to mount a cellular immune response. The
inability to confirm the presence of receptor molecules on
their surfaces has cast a cloud over the suppressor cell, but
functional suppressor cell effects are indisputable.

Ghon complex

The combination of a pleural surface-healed granuloma
or scar on the middle lobe of the lung, together with hilar
lymph node granulomas. The Ghon complex signifies
healed primary tuberculosis.

giant cell arteritis

Inflammation of the temporal artery in middle-aged
subjects; it may become systemic arteritis in 10 to 15%
of affected subjects. Blindness may occur eventually in
some of them. Nodular swelling of the entire artery wall
is present. Neutrophils, mononuclear cells, and eosinophils may infiltrate the wall with production of giant cell
granulomas.

glatiramer acetate (injection)

An immunosuppressive agent, whose mechanism of action
in multiple sclerosis (MS) patients is not fully understood. It
is believed to act by modifying immune processes responsible for the pathogenesis of MS. This belief is based on
studies of experimental allergic encephalomyelitis (EAE),
frequently used as an experimental animal model of MS.
Studies suggest that the agent induces glatiramer acetate-
specific suppressor T cells and activates them in the periphery. Its ability to also alter naturally occurring immune
responses remains undetermined.

***gld* gene**

Murine mutant gene on chromosome 1. When homozygous,
the *gld* gene produces progressive lymphadenopathy and
lupus-like immunopathology.

gld mouse

A natural mouse mutant expressing the FasL mutation
develops an autoimmune disease that resembles human SLE
and ALPS.

Gleevec

Imatinib mesylate, a drug that inhibits the activity of
selected kinases that include the chimeric Bcr-Abl kinase in
chronic myelogenous leukemia.

gliadin autoantibodies

Autoantibodies used to screen persons at risk for developing celiac disease (CD) and other gluten-sensitive
enteropathies including dermatitis herpetiformis (DH) and
to monitor patient adherence to a gluten-free diet (GFD).
Gliadins constitute a type of protein present in the glutens
of wheat and rye grains. In genetically susceptible subjects, α-gliadins activate CD, a gastrointestinal disorder
in which jejunal mucosa is flattened. Immunoglobulin G
(IgG) antigliadin antibodies (AGAs) are more sensitive
(~100%) than IgA AGA (~50%), and IgA AGAs are more
specific (~95%) than IgG AGAs (~60%). Both isotypes of
the autoantibodies increase significantly during a challenge
with gluten. Perhaps even months prior to clinical relapse,
CD is 10 times more frequent in subjects with selective IgA
deficiency. Enzyme immunoassay (EIA) is the method of
choice to detect AGAs in CD.

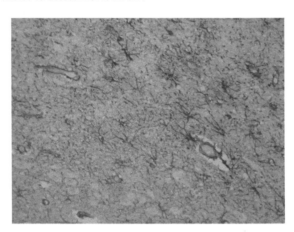

Glial fibrillary acidic protein—brain.

glial fibrillary acidic protein (GFAP)

An intermediate filament protein constituent of astrocytes
that is also abundant in glial cell tumors. The immunoperoxidase technique employing monoclonal antibodies against
the GFAP is used in surgical pathologic diagnosis to identify tumors based on their histogenetic origin.

Glick, Bruce

Demonstrated the role of the bursa of Fabricius in the production of antibodies and the division of labor in lymphocyte populations.

globulin

Serum proteins composed of α, β, and γ globulins and
classified on the basis of their electrophoretic mobility. All
three globulin fractions demonstrate less anodic mobility than albumin. α Globulins have the greatest negative
charge, whereas γ globulins have the least. Originally,
globulins were characterized based on their insolubility
in water (i.e., euglobulins) or sparing solubility in water

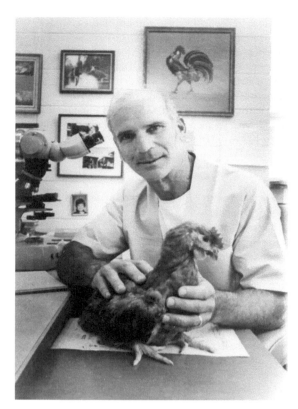

Bruce Glick.

(pseudoglobulins). Globulins are precipitated in half-saturated ammonium sulfate solution.

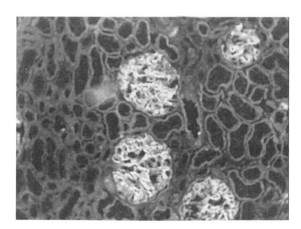

Glomerular basement membrane (GBM) autoantibodies.

glomerular basement membrane (GBM) autoantibodies

Autoantibodies against the noncollagenous portion (NC1) of the α3 chain of type IV collagen present in both GBM and alveolar basement membranes are revealed by enzyme immunoassay (EIA) in Goodpasture's syndrome. NC1 antibodies comprise 1% of the total immunoglobulin M (IgM) in patients with this syndrome, and 90% of these autoantibodies are specific for the α3 (IV) chain. Antibodies to the other α (IV) chains occur in 80% of the patients. Both CXC and CC chemokines are associated with glomerular polymorphonuclear neutrophil and monocyte/macrophage infiltration in glomerulonephritis induced by GBM antibody.

Sixty percent of human anti-GBM nephritis patients reveal antibody deposits along tubule basement membranes and manifest tubulointerstitial injury. Ten to 35% of patients with Goodpasture's syndrome develop pANCA with myeloperoxidase antibody activity. ANCA and GBM antibodies may appear together in the sera of patients with rapidly progressive glomerulonephritis (RPGN) associated with GBM disease and systemic vasculitis.

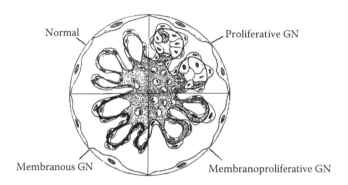

Types of glomerulonephritis.

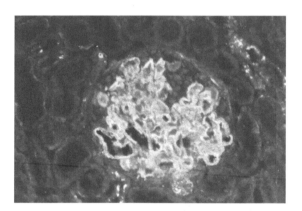

Glomerulonephritis (GN).

glomerulonephritis (GN)

A group of diseases characterized by glomerular injury. Immune mechanisms are responsible for most cases of primary glomerulonephritis and many of the secondary glomerulonephritis group. More than 70% of glomerulonephritis patients have glomerular deposits of immunoglobulins, frequently with complement components. Antibody-associated injury may result from the deposition of soluble circulating antigen–antibody complexes in the glomerulus or by antibodies reacting in the glomerulus with antigens intrinsic to the glomerulus or with molecules planted within the glomerulus. Cytotoxic antibodies may also cause glomerular injury. Goodpasture's syndrome is an example of a disease in which antibodies react directly with the glomerular basement membrane, interrupting its integrity and permitting red blood cells to pass into the urine. Antigen–antibody complexes such as those produced in systemic lupus erythematosus (SLE) may be deposited in the walls of the peripheral capillary loops, especially in subendothelial locations, leading to various manifestations of glomerulonephritis, depending on the stage of the disease. In membranoproliferative glomerulonephritis type I, IgG and C3 are found deposited in the glomerulus, whereas in dense deposit disease (membranoproliferative glomerulonephritis type II), C3 alone is demonstrable in the dense deposits within capillary walls. The types of primary glomerulonephritis include acute diffuse proliferative GN, rapidly progressive (crescentic) GN, membranous GN, lipoid nephrosis, focal segmental glomerulosclerosis, membranoproliferative GN, IgA nephropathy, and chronic GN. Secondary diseases affecting the glomeruli include SLE, diabetes mellitus, amyloidosis, Goodpasture's syndrome, polyarteritis nodosa, Wegener's granulomatosis, Henoch–Schönlein purpura, and bacterial endocarditis.

glucocorticoids (GCs)

Glucocorticoids are powerful immunosuppressive and antiinflammatory drugs that have lympholytic properties. They reduce circulating lymphocytes and monocytes, in addition to suppressing interleukin-1 (IL1) and IL2 production. Glucocorticoid administration diminishes the size and lymphoid content of the lymph nodes and spleen. Glucocorticoids are cytotoxic to selected T cell subsets, but their immunologic effects are probably attributable to their capacity to modify cellular functions rather than to direct cytotoxicity. Cellular immunity is affected more than is humoral immunity. Continuous administration increases the fractional catabolic rate of IgG, the principal class of antibody immunoglobulin. Glucocorticoid therapy usually abrogates DTH T cell-mediated contact hypersensitivity. However, chronic use produces adverse effects, including increased susceptibility to infection, bone fractures, diabetes, and cataracts. GCs act by binding to cytoplasmic GC receptor that regulates transcription of cytokine genes associated with inflammation. GCs regulate expression of the cytokines TNF-α, granulocyte–macrophage colony-stimulating factor (GC-CSF), IL1, IL2, IL3, IL4, IL5, IL6, and IL8. IL1, IL6, and TNF-α induce GC release in a prostaglandin–corticotropin-releasing, hormone-dependent manner from the hypothalamic–pituitary–adrenal axis. GCs are powerful inhibitors of nitric oxide synthase induction and induce the expression of the 37-kDa immunomodulator, lipocortin-1, in PMNLs and macrophages. Lipocortin is a powerful inhibitor of phospholipase A$_2$, which releases arachidonic acid for proinflammatory eicosanoid synthesis. GCs downregulate expression of the eosinophil chemokine RANTES. Endogenous GCs (corticosterone) inhibit neutrophil chemotaxis in inflammatory cholestasis. GCs also induce a prolonged increase in plasma cortisol.

glucose-6-phosphate dehydrogenase deficiency

Occasionally, individuals of both sexes have been shown to have no glucose-6-phosphate dehydrogenase in their leukocytes. This could be associated with deficient NADPH with diminished hexose monophosphate shunt activity and reduced formation of hydrogen peroxide in leukocytes, which are unable to kill microorganisms intracellularly, as described in chronic granulomatous disease (CGD). Clinical aspects resemble those in CGD, except that glucose-6-phosphate dehydrogenase deficiency occurs later and affects both sexes, in addition to being associated with hemolytic anemia. Although the nitroblue tetrazolium (NBT) test is within normal limits, glucose-6-phosphate dehydrogenase activity is deficient, the killing curve is altered, formation of H$_2$O$_2$ is abnormal, and oxygen consumption is inadequate. No effective treatment is available.

glutamic acid decarboxylase autoantibodies (GADs)

Autoantibodies associated with a rare neurological disorder known as stiff man syndrome (SMS) and with insulin-dependent diabetes mellitus (IDDM). Autoantibodies in the sera of SMS patients react with denatured GADs on immunoblots. By contrast, antibodies in IDDM patients react only with native (nondenatured) GADs by immunoprecipitation. In SMS, the frequency of GAD autoantibodies ranges from 60 to 100%; in IDDM, the frequency ranges from 25 to 79%. GAD autoantibodies are almost always present with islet cell antibodies (ICA) and may represent a constituent of ICA.

gluten-sensitive enteropathy (celiac sprue, nontropical sprue)

A disease that results from defective gastrointestinal absorption due to hypersensitivity to cereal grain storage proteins, including gluten or its product gliadin, present in wheat, barley, and oats. Diarrhea, weight loss, and steatorrhea occur. It is characterized by villous atrophy and malabsorption in the small intestine. It occurs mostly in Caucasians and occasionally in African-Americans, but not in Asians, and is associated with HLA-DR3 and DR7. The disease may be limited to the intestines or associated with dermatitis herpetiformis, a vesicular skin eruption. Antigliadin antibodies which are immunoglobulin A (IgA) are formed, and lymphocytes and plasma cells appear in the lamina propria in association with villous atrophy. Diagnosis is made by showing villous atrophy in a small intestinal biopsy. Administering a gluten-free diet leads to resolution of the disease.

GlyCAM-1

A vascular addressin molecule resembling mucin that is present on high endothelial venules in lymphoid tissues. L-selectin molecules on lymphocytes in the peripheral blood bind GlyCAM-1 molecules, causing the lymphocytes to exit the blood circulation and enter the lymphoid tissues.

glycocalyx

A thick layer of mucin-like molecules in the apical membranes of the brush borders of intestinal epithelial cells. It possesses hydrolytic enzymes and has a negative charge that repels pathogenic microorganisms.

glycosyl phosphatidylinositol (GPI)-linked membrane antigens

A class of cell surface antigens attached to membranes by glycosyl phosphatidylinositol. Monoclonal antibody studies indicate that in both human and murine subjects GTI-linked antigens are capable of stimulating T cells and sometimes B cells. Structurally, they are diverse. See also Ly-5 and Qa-2.

Gm allotype

A genetic variant determinant of the human immunoglobulin G (IgG) heavy chain. Allelic genes that encode the γ1, γ2, and γ3 heavy chain constant regions encode the Gm allotypes. They were recognized by the ability of sera from rheumatoid arthritis patients containing anti-IgG rheumatoid factor to react with them. Gm allotypic determinants are associated with specific amino acid substitution in different γ chain constant regions in humans. IgG subclasses are associated with certain Gm determinants. For example, IgG$_1$ is associated with G$_1$m(1) and G$_1$m(4), and IgG$_3$ is associated with G$_3$m(5). Although the majority of Gm allotypes are restricted to the IgG-γ chain Fc region,

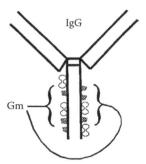

Locations of Gm marker specificities on the Fc region of an IgG molecule.

a substitution at position 214 of C_H1 of arginine yields the $G_1m(4)$ allotype, and a substitution at this same site of lysine yields $G_1m(17)$. For Gm expression, the light chain part of the molecule must be intact.

GM₁ autoantibodies

A principal sialic acid-containing glycolipid enriched in peripheral and central nervous system myelin (i.e., Schwann cells and oligodendrocytes). It participates in the recognition of cells, compaction of myelin, signal transduction, and chemokine binding. Autoantibodies are specific for the terminal sialic acid and/or the galactosyl (β1–3) N-acetylgalactosamine epitope of GM₁. GM₁ antibodies are present in amyotrophic lateral sclerosis (ALS), Guillain–Barré syndrome (GBS), and other motor neuron diseases (MNDs) including chronic inflammatory demyelinating polyradiculoneuropathy (CIDP) and multifocal motor neuropathy (MMN). Sensorimotor neuropathies with plasma cell dyscrasia (monoclonal gammopathy) are associated with IgM GM₁ paraproteins at frequencies of 50 to 60%. Acute peripheral neuropathy patients may demonstrate IgG GM₁ antibodies, especially following infection with *Campylobacter jejuni*. There may be molecular mimicry between gangliosides and bacterial lipopolysaccharides (LPSs). Enzyme immunoassay (EIA) detection of GM₁ antibody reveals 50% sensitivity and 80% specificity for motor neuron diseases. These antibodies may also be associated with systemic infections and autoimmune diseases with neurologic involvement.

GM-CSF

Abbreviation for granulocyte–macrophage colony-stimulating factor. A growth factor for hematopoietic cells that is synthesized by lymphocytes, monocytes, fibroblasts, and endothelial cells. It has been prepared in recombinant form to stimulate production of leukocytes in patients with AIDS and to initiate hematopoiesis following chemotherapy of bone marrow recipients. Patients with anemia and malignant neoplasms may also derive benefit from GM-CSF administration. It is a cytokine that induces the proliferation, differentiation, and functional activation of hematopoietic cells and has an established role in clinical medicine. GM-CSF is produced by T lymphocytes, macrophages, fibroblasts, and endothelial cells that have been stimulated by antigen, lectin, interleukin-1 (IL-1), lipopolysaccharide, tumor necrosis factor α, and phorbol ester. Human and mouse GM-CSFs contain 124 and 127 amino acids, respectively. The mature protein is preceded by a 17-amino-acid leader sequence. GM-CSF has been shown by x-ray crystallography to combine a two-stranded anti-parallel β sheet with an open bundle of four α helices. A single copy of 2.5 kb contains four exons and three introns. In the mouse, it has been mapped to chromosome 11, and in the human to the long arm of chromosome 5. It induces proliferation and differentiation for granulocyte, monocyte, and eosinophil progenitors and enhances the function of mature effector cells. It enhances the function of granulocytes and macrophages in immune responses. Its biological effects are mediated through binding to specific cell surface receptors of low or high affinity on hematopoietic cells. *In vivo*, GM-CSF is a potent stimulator of hematopoiesis. Its administration is usually well tolerated but may be associated with bone pain and influenza-like symptoms including fever, flushing, malaise, myalgia, arthralgia, anorexia, and headache that usually resolve with continued administration. Higher doses of GM-CSF may lead to capillary leak syndrome. GM-CSF has been used to support chemotherapy and to manage cytopenias associated with HIV infection. Low doses can elevate neutrophil counts. It has been used as a supportive agent to manage secondary infections following chemotherapy for AIDS-related non-Hodgkin lymphoma. GM-CSF has been used following autologous bone marrow transplantation to reduce neutropenia, the occurrence of serious infection, and the use of antibiotics. It has also been used to mobilize peripheral blood progenitor cells for collection by apheresis and subsequent transplantation.

Gm marker

Refer to Gm allotype.

gnotobiotic

An animal or environment in which all the microorganisms are known. A germ-free animal or an animal contaminated with one microorganism may be considered gnotobiotic. In addition to animal models, the so-called "bubble boy" who suffered severe combined immunodeficiency (SCID) survived for 8 years in a plastic bubble that enclosed his gnotobiotic, germ-free environment.

goblet cells

Cells of the intestinal epithelium that produce mucus, which facilitates mucosal immunity.

gold compounds

Gold suppresses or prevents, but does not cure, arthritis and synovitis. It is taken up by macrophages, leading to inhibition of phagocytosis and possibly lysosomal enzyme activity. It diminishes concentrations of rheumatoid factor and immunoglobulins. Its exact mode of action in RA is unknown. It may diminish synovial inflammation and retard cartilage and bone destruction. Its therapeutic effects occur slowly.

gold therapy

A treatment for arthritis that inhibits oxidative degradation of membrane proteins and lipids and counteracts singlet oxygen produced as free radicals. It is administered in such forms as aurothioglucose and gold sodium thiomalate. Gold may induce such gastrointestinal symptoms as nausea and vomiting, diarrhea, and abdominal pain and such renal symptoms as nephrotic syndrome and proteinuria, as well as skin rashes, hepatitis, or blood dyscrasias. Renal biopsy may reveal IgG and C3 in a "moth-eaten" pattern in the glomerular basement membrane, as well as "feathery crystals" in the renal tubules.

G

Golgi apparatus

A stack of vesicles enclosed by membranes found within a cell that serves as a site of glycosylation and packaging of secreted proteins. It is part of the GERL complex.

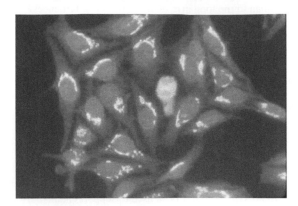

Golgi autoantibodies.

Golgi autoantibodies

Autoantibodies against Golgi apparatus cisternal and vesicular membranes are very rare. Golgi apparatus is a target of heterogenous autoantibodies with specificity for certain autoantigens that include golgin 95, golgin 160, golgin 97, golgin 180, macrogolgin, and GCp372. Immunofluorescence using Hep-2 cells is the technique employed to detect the Golgi autoantibodies, but no diagnostic significance has yet been correlated with disease activity.

Golgi complex

Tubular cytoplasmic structures that participate in protein secretion. The complex consists of flattened membranous sacs (cisternae) arranged on top of each other. These are also associated with spherical vesicles. Proteins arriving from the rough endoplasmic reticulum are processed in the Golgi complex and sent elsewhere in cells. Proteins handled in this manner include those that are secreted constitutively such as immunoglobulins, those of the membrane, those stored in secretory granules to be released on command, and lysosomal enzymes.

gonococcal complement fixation test

A complement fixation test that uses as antigen an extract of *Neisseria gonorrhoea*. It is of little value in diagnosing early cases of gonorrhea that appear before the generation of an antibody response but may be used to identify late manifestations in untreated individuals.

Good, Robert Alan (1922–2003)

American immunologist and pediatrician who made major contributions to studies of the ontogeny and phylogeny of the immune response. Much of his work focused on the role of the thymus and the bursa of Fabricius in immunity. (Refer to *The Thymus in Immunobiology,* 1964; *Phylogeny of Immunity,* 1966.)

Goodpasture, Ernest W. (1886–1960)

Professor and chair of pathology at Vanderbilt University Medical School, for whom Goodpasture's syndrome is named. He was a pioneer in virology and had a distinguished career in basic medical research and as an administrator. He also served as dean of the Vanderbilt Medical School.

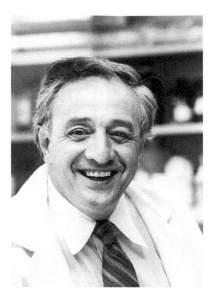

Robert Alan Good.

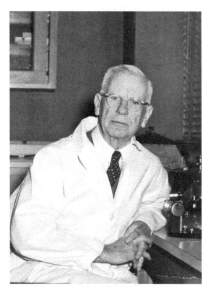

Ernest W. Goodpasture.

Goodpasture's antigen

An antigen found in the noncollagenous part of type IV collagen. It is present in human glomerular and alveolar basement membranes, making them targets for injury-inducing, anti-GBM (glomerular basement membrane) antibodies in the sera of patients with Goodpasture's syndrome. Interestingly, individuals with Alport's (hereditary) nephritis do *not* have the Goodpasture antigen in their basement membranes. Thus, renal transplants stimulate anti-GBM antibodies in such patients.

Goodpasture's syndrome

An autoimmune disease mediated by Type II hypersensitivity in which autoantibodies target collagen epitopes present in kidney and lung basement membranes. It is a disease with pulmonary hemorrhage (coughing up blood) and glomerulonephritis (blood in the urine) induced by antiglomerular basement membrane autoantibodies that also interact with alveolar basement membrane antigens. A linear

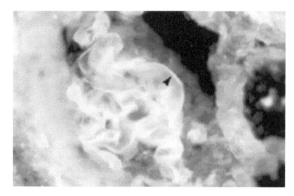

Goodpasture's syndrome. Stained with anti-glomerular basement membrane (anti-GBM) antibody.

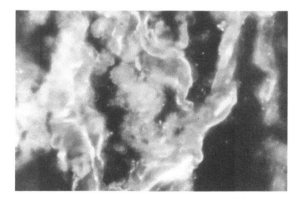

Goodpasture's syndrome. Stained with anti-glomerular basement membrane (anti-GBM) antibody.

Goodpasture's syndrome. Stained with anti-lung alveolar basement membrane antibody.

pattern of immunofluorescent staining confirms interaction of the immunoglobulin G (IgG) antibodies with basement membrane antigens in the kidney and lung, leading to membrane injury with pulmonary hemorrhage and acute (rapidly progressive or crescentic) proliferative glomerulonephritis. Pulmonary hemorrhage may precede hematuria. In addition to linear IgG, membranes may reveal linear staining for C3.

GOR autoantibodies

GOR autoantibodies are detected in approximately 80% of patients with HCV-RNA-positive chronic hepatitis C infection, in fewer than 10% of chronic HBV or alcohol misuse cases, and in approximately 2% of normal subjects. These autoantibodies recognize an epitope of the sequence GRRGQKAKSNPNRPL, which is common to a presumed core gene product of HCV and a host nuclear component. GOR autoantibodies are detected also in most HCV-antibody-positive patients with LKM-1-autoantibody-positive autoimmune hepatitis type 2b.

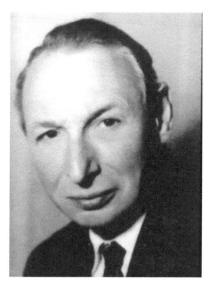

Peter Alfred Gorer.

Gorer, Peter Alfred (1907–1961)

British pathologist. With Snell, he discovered the H-2 murine histocompatibility complex. Most of his work was in transplantation genetics. He identified antigen II and described its association with tumor rejection. (Refer to *The Gorer Symposium*, 1985.)

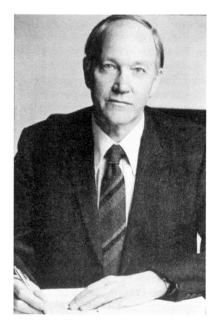

James Gowans.

Gowans, James (1924–)

British physician and investigator whose principal contribution to immunology was the demonstration that lymphocytes recirculate via the thoracic duct, which radically changed the understanding of the role lymphocytes play in immune reactions. He also investigated lymphocyte function. He served as director of the MRC Cellular Immunobiology Unit, Oxford, 1963.

gp41

A human immunodeficiency virus (HIV) glycoprotein that anchors gp120 in the HIV envelope.

gp120

A surface 120-kDa glycoprotein of human immunodeficiency virus type 1 (HIV-1) that combines with the CD4 receptor on T lymphocytes and macrophages. The principal envelope protein of HIV, which binds to host cell receptors and expresses immunodominant epitopes. Synthetic soluble CD4 molecules have been used to block gp120 antigens and spare CD4+ lymphocytes from becoming infected. The *env* gene, which mutates frequently, encodes gp120, thereby interfering with host efforts to manufacture effective or protective antibodies.

gp160 vaccine

A vaccine that contains a cloned segment of the envelope protein of HIV-1. It activates both humoral and cellular immunity against HIV products during early infection with HIV-1 and diminishes the rate at which CD4+ T lymphocytes are lost.

GPLA

The guinea pig major histocompatibility complex (MHC). Two loci encode MHC class I molecules: *GPLA-B* and *GPLA-S*. The *GPLA-Ia* locus encodes MHC class II molecules. Complement protein factors B, C2, and C4 are encoded by other loci. The genes are *BF* (factor B), C2, C4, *Ia*, *B*, and *S*.

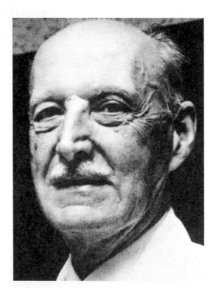

Pierre Grabar.

Grabar, Pierre (1898–1986)

French-educated immunologist born in Kiev who served as chef de service at the Institut Pasteur and as director of the National Center for Scientific Research, Paris. Best known for his work with Williams in the development of immunoelectrophoresis. He studied antigen–antibody interactions and developed the "carrier" theory of antibody function. He was instrumental in reviving European immunology in the era after World War II.

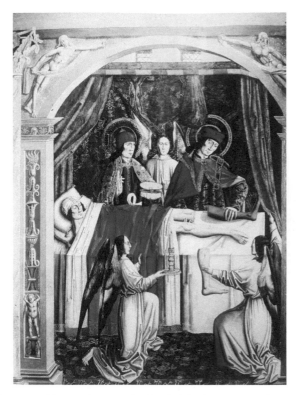

St. Cosmas and St. Damian transplanting the leg of a Moor onto the stump of a young man who lost his leg.

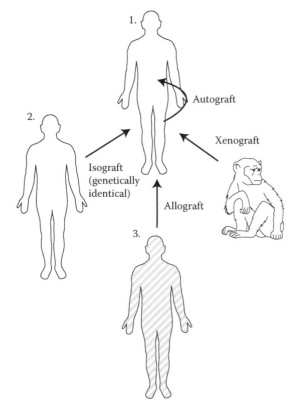

Types of grafts.

graft

The transplantation of a tissue or organ from one site to another within the same individual or between individuals of the same or a different species.

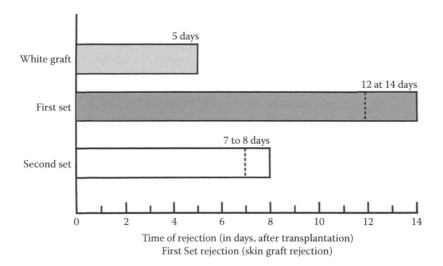

First Set rejection (skin graft rejection)

Types of skin graft rejection.

graft arteriosclerosis

Intimal smooth muscle cell proliferation that occludes graft arteries. It may occur 6 to 12 months following transplantation and leads to chronic rejection of vascularized organ grafts. It is probably attributable to a chronic immune response to alloantigens of the vessel wall. It is also termed accelerated arteriosclerosis.

graft facilitation

Prolonged graft survival attributable to conditioning of the recipient with IgG antibody, which is believed to act as a blocking factor. It also decreases cell-mediated immunity. This phenomenon is related to immunologic enhancement of tumors by antibody and has been referred to as immunological facilitation (*facilitation immunologique*).

graft rejection

The immunologic destruction of transplanted tissues or organs between two members or strains of a species differing at the major histocompatibility complex (MHC) for that species (i.e., HLA in humans and H-2 in mice). The rejection is based upon both cell-mediated and antibody-mediated immunity against cells of the graft by the histoincompatible recipient. First-set rejection usually occurs within 2 weeks after transplantation. The placement of a second graft with the same antigenic specificity as the first in the same host leads to rejection within 1 week and is termed second-set rejection. This demonstrates the presence of immunological memory learned from the first experience with the histocompatibility antigens of the graft. When the donor and recipient differ only at minor histocompatibility loci, rejection of the transplanted tissue may be delayed, depending upon the relative strength of the minor loci in which they differ. Grafts placed in a hyperimmune individual, such as those with preformed antibodies, may undergo hyperacute or accelerated rejection. Hyperacute rejection of a kidney allograft by preformed antibodies in the recipient is characterized by formation of fibrin plugs in the vasculature as a consequence of the antibodies reacting against endothelial cells lining vessels, complement fixation, polymorphonuclear neutrophil attraction, and denuding of the vessel wall, followed by platelet accumulation and fibrin

plugging. As the blood supply to the organ is interrupted, the tissue undergoes infarction and must be removed.

graft-vs.-host disease (GVHD)

Disease produced by the reaction of immunocompetent T lymphocytes of the donor graft that are histoincompatible with the tissues of the recipient into which they have been transplanted. Attributable to MHC or MiHA mismatching. For the disease to occur, the recipient must be immunologically immature, immunosuppressed by irradiation or drug therapy, or tolerant to the administered cells. The grafted cells must be immunocompetent. Patients develop skin rash, fever, diarrhea, weight loss, hepatosplenomegaly, and aplasia of the bone marrow. The donor lymphocytes infiltrate the skin, gastrointestinal tract, and liver. The disease may be either acute or chronic. Murine GVHD is called runt disease, secondary disease, or wasting disease. Both allo- and autoimmunity associated with GVHD may follow bone marrow or hematopoietic stem cell transplantation. Of patients receiving HLA-identical bone marrow transplants, 20 to 50% still manifest GVHD, with associated weight loss, skin rash, fever, diarrhea, liver disease, and immunodeficiency. GVHD may be either acute, which is an alloimmune disease, or chronic, which consists of both allo- and autoimmune components. The conditions requisite for the GVH reaction include genetic differences between immunocompetent cells in the marrow graft and host tissues, immunoincompetence of the host, and alloimmune differences that promote proliferation of donor cells that react with host tissues. In addition to allogenic marrow and hematopoietic stem cell grafts, the transfusion of nonirradiated blood products to an immunosuppressed patient or intrauterine transfusion from mother to fetus may lead to GVHD. GVHD is most common in bone marrow and hematopoietic stem cell transplantation but rare in solid organ transplants.

graft-vs.-host reaction (GVHR)

The reaction of a graft containing immunocompetent T cells against alloantigens of the genetically dissimilar tissues of an immunosuppressed recipient. Criteria requisite for a GVHR include: (1) histoincompatibility between the

G

donor and recipient, (2) passively transferred immunologically reactive cells, and (3) a recipient host who has been either naturally immunosuppressed because of immaturity or genetic defect or deliberately immunosuppressed by irradiation or drugs. The immunocompetent grafted cells are especially reactive against rapidly dividing cells. Target organs include the skin, gastrointestinal tract (including the gastric mucosa), liver, and lymphoid tissues. Patients often develop skin rashes and hepatosplenomegaly and may have aplasia of the bone marrow. GVHR usually develops within 7 to 30 days following the transplant or infusion of the lymphocytes. Prevention of the GVHR is an important procedural step in several forms of transplantation and may be accomplished by irradiating the transplant. The clinical course of GVHR may take a hyperacute, acute, or chronic form, as seen in graft rejection.

graft-vs.-leukemia (GVL)

Bone marrow or stem cell transplantation as therapy for leukemia. Partial genetic incompatibility between donor and recipient is believed to facilitate elimination of residual leukemia cells by NK cells and T lymphocytes from the allogeneic transplant. This is a very desirable consequence of MiHA and MHC mismatches between recipient and donor. Also termed graft-vs.-tumor effect.

Gram-negative bacteria

Microorganisms with thin cell walls that contain peptidoglycan and lipopolysaccharide (LPS) that stain red in the Gram staining technique.

Gram-positive bacteria

Microorganisms with thick cell walls that contain peptidoglycan and lipotechoic and techoic acids that stain purple in the Gram staining technique.

granular cells

Hemocytes that express PRR in higher invertebrates that facilitate wound healing and coagulation to entrap pathogenic microorganisms. They also synthesize bactericidal proteins and opsonins that aid encapsulation by phagocytic cells. Also termed hemostatic cells.

granule exocytosis pathway

A mechanism used by armed cytotoxic T lymphocytes (CTLs) to kill target cells. Following conjugate formation and T cell receptor activation, the CTL repositions its Golgi apparatus, permitting its preformed cytotoxic granules to fuse with the CTL membrane. The granule contents, comprised of perforin and granzymes, are exocytosed in the direction of the target cell membrane, which leads to target cell apoptosis.

granulocyte antibodies

Immunoglobulin G (IgG) and/or IgM antibodies present in approximately 33% of adult patients with idiopathic neutropenia. They are also implicated in the pathogenesis of drug-induced neutropenia, febrile transfusion reactions, isoimmune neonatal neutropenia, Evans syndrome, primary autoimmune neutropenia of early childhood, systemic lupus erythematosus, Graves' disease, the neutropenia of Felty syndrome and selected other autoimmune diseases.

granulocyte autoantibodies

Autoantibodies against granulocytes that serve as the principal cause of autoimmune neutropenia (AIN). Autoantibodies to the neutrophil-specific antigens of the NA system are associated with this condition. Fifty percent of patients with systemic lupus erythematosus (SLE) have

granulocyte autoantibodies, which are also found in febrile, non-hemolytic transfusion reactions, transfusion-associated acute lung injury, and alloimmune neonatal neutropenia (ANN). Granulocyte autoantibodies on the neutrophil surface can be detected by immunofluorescence (GIFT), enzyme immunoassay (EIA), radioimmunoassay (RIA), or flow cytometry (FC) or indirectly by detection of autoantibody effects. Granulocyte autoantibodies are mainly of the IgG isotype. Flow cytometry is preferred for assay of these autoantibodies.

granulocyte chemotactic protein-2 (GCP-2)

A chemokine of the α family (CXC family). Osteosarcoma cells can produce both human GCP-2 and interleukin-8 (IL8). The bovine homolog of human CP-2 has been demonstrated in kidney tumor cells. Human and bovine GCP-2 are chemotactic for human granulocytes and activate post-receptor mechanisms that cause the release of gelatinase B, which portends a possible role in inflammation and tumor cell invasion. Tissue sources include osteosarcoma cells and kidney neoplastic cells. Granulocytes are the target cells.

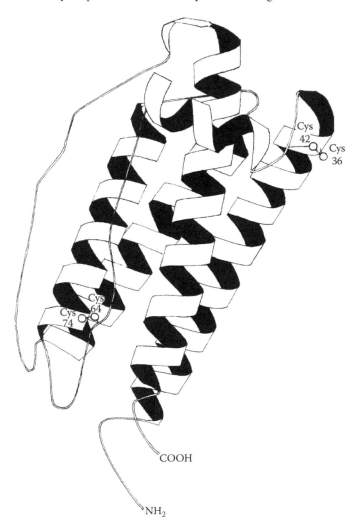

Granulocyte colony-stimulating factor (g-CSF).

granulocyte colony-stimulating factor (g-CSF)

A cytokine synthesized by activated T lymphocytes, macrophages, and endothelial cells at infection sites that causes bone marrow to increase the production and mobilization of polymorphonuclear neutrophils to replace those spent by inflammatory processes.

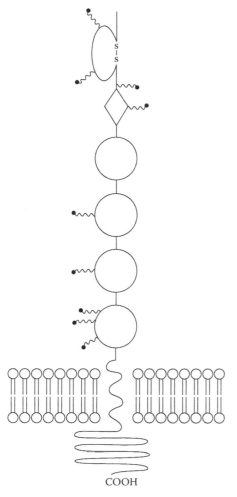

The G-CSF receptor composed of an immunoglobulin domain, a hematopoietin domain, and three fibronectin III domains. The two forms of the human receptor are the 25.1 form that has a C kinase phosphorylation site and a second form in which the transmembrane region has been deleted. The mouse receptor that shares 62.5% homology with the human receptor is similar to the 25.1 form. The human G-CSF receptor has 46.3% sequence homology with IL5 receptor's gp130 chain. The hematopoietin domain contains the binding site for G-CSF, yet proliferative signal transduction requires the membrane proximal 57 amino acids. Acute phase protein induction mediated by G-CSF involves residues 57 to 96. G-CSF receptors are found on neutrophils, platelets, myeloid leukemia cells, endothelium, and placenta. The human form contains nine potential N-linked glycosylation sites. It is believed that the receptor binds and mediates autophosphorylation of JAK-2 kinase.

granulocyte–macrophage colony-stimulating factor (GM-CSF)

A cytokine that participates in the growth and differentiation of myeloid and monocytic lineage cells including dendritic cells, monocytes, macrophages, and granulocyte lineage cells.

granulocyte–monocyte colony-stimulating factor

A cytokine synthesized by activated T lymphocytes, macrophages, stromal fibroblasts, and endothelial cells that leads to increased production of neutrophils and monocytes in the bone marrow. GM-CSF also activates macrophages

and facilitates the differentiation of Langerhans' cells into mature dendritic cells.

granulocytes

Leukocytes of the myeloid series with irregularly shaped, multilobed nuclei with large intracellular granules that contain hydrolytic enzymes capable of destroying micro-organisms. The term refers to the three types of polymorphonuclear leukocytes that differ mainly in the staining properties of their cytoplasmic granules. The three types are classified as neutrophils, eosinophils, and basophils. They are all mature myeloid-series cells and have different functions. Granulocytes constitute 58 to 71% of the leukocytes in the blood circulation. Refer to the individual cells for details.

granulocyte-specific antinuclear antibodies

Autoantibodies that react with the nuclei of neutrophils to produce a homogeneous staining pattern by immunofluorescence. They do not react with Hep-2 cells or liver substrates. These antibodies are claimed to be present in patients with active rheumatoid arthritis with vasculitis and/or neutropenia and in 17% of juvenile rheumatoid arthritis patients. Granulocyte-specific antinuclear antibodies may be correlated with erosive joint disease.

granulocyte-specific antinuclear autoantibodies (GS-ANAs)

Specific antinuclear autoantibodies that react with neutrophil nuclei or cytoplasm in a homogeneous pattern but not with other substrates used for ANA detection. The exact histone target antigens of GS-ANAs remain to be determined. GS-ANAs are found in the sera of patients with active rheumatoid arthritis (RA) and with vasculitis and/or neutropenia in frequencies approaching 75%, and in 90% of Felty's syndrome. They are found in only 41% of effectively managed RA patients and in 17% of juvenile rheumatoid arthritis. GS-ANAs correlate well with erosive joint disease. They can be demonstrated in five immunoglobulin isotypes with mostly immunoglobulin G (IgG) and IgM in RA and Felty's syndrome. Indirect immunofluorescence is the preferred method of detection.

granulocytopenia

An abnormally low number of blood granulocytes.

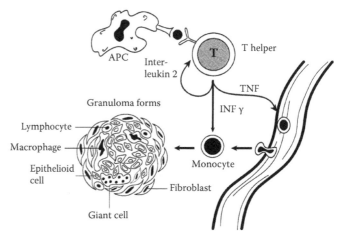

Granuloma.

granuloma

A tissue reaction characterized by altered macrophages (epithelioid cells), lymphocytes, and fibroblasts caused by

G

hyperactivated macrophages that fuse together to isolate a persistent pathogenic microorganism or nondegradable foreign body. It also contains CD4+ and CD8+ T lymphocytes. Its production is dependent on TNF synthesized by activated T_H1 effector lymphocytes. The cells form microscopic masses of mononuclear cells. Giant cells form from some of these fused cells. Granulomas may be of the foreign body type, such as those surrounding silica or carbon particles, or of the immune type, which encircle particulate antigens derived from microorganisms. Activated macrophages trap antigen, which may cause T cells to release lymphokines, causing more macrophages to accumulate. This process isolates the microorganism. Granulomas appear in cases of tuberculosis and develop under the influence of helper T cells that react against *Mycobacterium tuberculosis.* Some macrophages and epithelioid cells fuse to form multinucleated giant cells in immune granulomas. Neutrophils and eosinophils may also be present occasionally. Necrosis may develop. It is a delayed-type hypersensitivity reaction that persists as a consequence of the continuous presence of foreign body or infection.

granulomatous hepatitis
Granulomatous inflammation of the liver.

granulopoietin
A 45-kDa glycoprotein produced by monocytes that governs granulocyte formation in the bone marrow. Also called colony-stimulating factor.

granulysin
A cytotoxic T cell granule protein capable of perturbing a membrane, as when perforin leads to pore formation in a target cell membrane.

granzymes
Serine esterases released from large granular lymphocyte (LGL) and cytotoxic T lymphocyte (CTL) granules that contribute to fatal injuries of target cells subjected to the cytotoxic action of perforin. Antigranzyme antibodies inhibit target cell lysis. Serine esterase enzymes are present in the granules of cytotoxic T lymphocytes and natural killer (NK) cells. Also called fragmentins.

Graves' disease (hyperthyroidism)
Thyroid gland hyperplasia with increased thyroid hormone (thyroxine) secretion that produces signs and symptoms of hyperthyroidism. Patients may develop immunoglobulin G (IgG) autoantibodies against thyroid-stimulating hormone (TSH) receptors. This autoantibody is termed long-acting thyroid stimulator (LATS). When the LATS IgG antibody binds to the TSH receptor, it has a stimulatory effect on thyroid-promoting hyperactivity. This IgG autoantibody can cross the placenta and produce transient hyperthyroidism in a newborn infant. The disease has a female predominance.

gravity and immunity
Space flight has been associated with the development of neutrophilia, slight T cell lymphopenia, and diminished blastogenic responsiveness of T cells in post-flight blood samples. Eosinophilia has been noted. Lymphopenia has been marked by decreased numbers of T cells and natural killer (NK) cells. Changes have also been observed in post-flight concentrations of immunoglobulins, complement components, lysozyme, interferon, and α_2-macroglobulin. There is a modest depression in cell-mediated immunity after both short and long space flights. Human NK cells diminish and reveal decreased cytotoxic activity after both

long and short flights. Delayed-type dermal hypersensitivity (DTH) reactions decrease or even disappear during prolonged residence in space. Immunoglobulin A (IgA) and IgM have risen, but IgG has remained constant during long space flights. No defects in humoral immunity have been noted. Interleukin-2 (IL2) and interferon synthesis by lymphocytes has decreased significantly in both human and rodents after long flights.

gross cystic disease fluid protein 15 (GCDFP-15) antigen
A 15-kDa glycoprotein that is demonstrable with immunoperoxidase staining and expressed by primary and metastatic breast carcinomas with apocrine features and extramammary Paget's disease. Normal apocrine sweat glands, eccrine glands (variable), minor salivary glands, bronchial glands, metaplastic breast epithelium, benign sweat gland tumors of skin, and submandibular serous cells express GCDFP-15 antigen.

group agglutination
In the serologic classification of microorganisms, the identification of group-specific antigens rather than species-specific antigens by the antibody used for serotyping.

growth factors
Messenger molecules synthesized by leukocytes and nonleukocytes, inducibly or constitutively, rather than by glands. They may induce or sustain proliferation of multiple cell types. Cytokines that facilitate the growth and proliferation of cells. Examples include platelet-derived growth factor, erythropoietin, interleukin-2 (T cell growth factor), and many others.

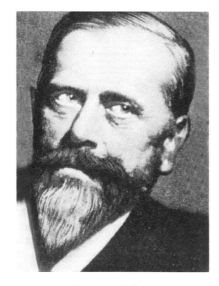

Max von Grüber.

Grüber, Max von (1853–1927)
Professor of hygiene at Vienna and Munich, who studied bacterial agglutination by the blood in collaboration with Herbert Durham, a graduate student from England.

guanine–nucleotide exchange factors (GEFs)
Proteins that can disengage bound guanosine diphosphate (GDP) from small G proteins. This permits guanosine triphosphate (GTP) to bind and activate the G protein.

Guillain–Barré syndrome
An autoimmune disease due to interaction of autoantibody with peripheral nerve antigens. It is a type of idiopathic

polyneuritis in which autoimmunity to peripheral nerve myelin leads to diminished electrical impulse transmission, resulting in muscle weakness and paralysis. It is often self-limiting and is associated with recovery from infection by selected pathogens. It is characterized by chronic demyelination of peripheral nerves.

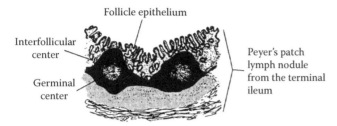

GALT (gut-associated lymphoid tissue).

gut-associated lymphoid tissue (GALT)

Lymphoid tissue situated in the gastrointestinal mucosa and submucosa. It constitutes the gastrointestinal immune system. GALT is present in the appendix, tonsils, and Peyer's patches subjacent to the mucosa. GALT represents the counterpart of bronchial-associated lymphoid tissue (BALT) and consists of radially arranged and closely packed lymphoid follicles that impinge upon the intestinal epithelium, forming dome-like structures. In GALT, specialized epithelial cells overlie the lymphoid follicles, forming a membrane between the lymphoid cells and the lumen. These cells are called M cells and are believed to be gatekeepers for molecules passing across. Other GALT components include IgA-synthesizing B cells and intraepithelial lymphocytes such as CD8+ T cells, as well as the lymphocytes in the lamina propria that include CD4+ T lymphocytes, B lymphocytes that synthesize IgA, and null cells. Refer also to MALT.

GVH

Refer to graft-vs.-host reaction (GVHR) and graft-vs.-host disease (GVHD).

GVH disease

Refer to graft-vs-host disease.

H

H-2 complex

Murine major histocompatibility complex. Comprised of K, P, A, E, S, D, Q, T, and M loci that contain multiple genes. Refer to H-2 histocompatibility system.

H-2 histocompatibility system

The major histocompatibility complex of the mouse. H-2 genes are located on chromosome 17. They encode somatic cell surface antigens and the host immune response (*Ir* genes). Each of these has a length of 600 base pairs. The H-2 complex has four regions, designated K, I, S, and D. K region genes encode class I histocompatibility molecules designated K. I region genes encode class II histocompatibility molecules designated I-A and I-E. S region genes encode class III molecules designated C2, C4, factor B, and cytochrome P-450 (21-hydroxylase). D region genes encode class I histocompatibility molecules designated D and L. Antigens that represent the H-2 type of a particular inbred strain of mice are encoded by H-2 alleles. Thus, differences in the antigenic structures of inbred mice of differing H-2 alleles are critical in the acceptance or rejection of tissue grafts exchanged. K, D, and L subregions of H-2 correspond to A, B, and C subregions of human leukocyte antigen (HLA). The I-A and I-E regions are equivalent to the human HLA-D region.

H-2 locus

The mouse major histocompatibility region on chromosome 17.

H-2 restriction

Major histocompatibility complex (MHC) restriction involving the murine H-2 MHC.

H-2D

A murine H-2 major histocompatibility complex (MHC) locus whose products are class I antigens. The *H2D* gene has multiple alleles.

H-2I region

A murine H-2 major histocompatibility complex (MHC) region where the genes encoding class II molecules are found.

H-2K

A murine H-2 major histocompatibility complex (MHC) locus. Genes at this locus, which has multiple alleles, encode MHC class I antigens.

H-2L

Murine class I histocompatibility antigen found on spleen cells that serves as a target epitope in graft rejection.

H65-RTA

An immunosuppressant used clinically in the treatment of acute graft-vs.-host disease and rheumatoid arthritis. H65-RTA is an immunoconjugate consisting of anti-CD5 monoclonal antibody coupled to a cytotoxic enzyme. It leads to inhibition of protein synthesis, cell depletion, and lymphocyte activation.

H7

A pharmacological agent used to study T cell activation. Its target is protein kinase C.

H antigens

(1) Epitopes on flagellae of enteric bacteria that are motile and Gram-negative. The H designation is from the German *Hauch*, which means breath, and refers to the production of films on agar plates that resemble breathing on glass. In the Kaufmann–White classification scheme for *Salmonella*, H antigens serve as the basis for the division of microorganisms into phase I and phase II, depending on the flagellins they contain. A single cell synthesizes only one type of flagellin. Phase variation may result in a switch to production of the other type which is genetically controlled. (2) An ABO blood group system antigen also called H substance. (3) Histocompatibility antigen.

H chain (heavy chain)

A principal constituent of immunoglobulin molecules. Each immunoglobulin is comprised of at least one 4-polypeptide chain monomer that consists of two heavy and two light polypeptide chains. The two heavy chains are identical in

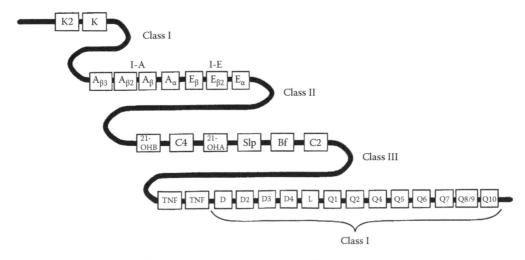

H-2 histocompatibility system is the major histocompatibility complex (MHC) in the mouse.

any one molecule, as are the two light chains. Refer also to heavy chain.

H chain disease

A variant of multiple myeloma in which immunoglobulin free heavy chains are demonstrable in serum. This condition, characterized by free H chains in the serum but not free light chains, is called heavy chain disease.

H substance

A basic carbohydrate of the human ABO blood group system structure. Most people express this ABO-related antigen. The body fluids of secretor individuals contain soluble H substance.

H_1, H_2 blocking agents

Refer to antihistamine.

H1 receptors

Histamine receptors on vascular smooth muscle cells through which histamine mediates vasodilation.

H2 receptors

Histamine receptors on different types of tissue cells through which histamine mediates bronchial constriction in asthma, gastrointestinal constriction in diarrhea, and endothelial constriction resulting in edema.

HA-1A

Human monoclonal immunoglobulin M (IgM) antibody specific for the lipid A domain of endotoxin. It can prevent deaths of laboratory animals that have Gram-negative bacteremia and endotoxemia. In clinical trials, HA-1A has proven safe and effective for the treatment of patients with sepsis and Gram-negative bacteremia, whether or not they are in shock, but not in those with focal Gram-negative infections.

HAART

A regimen comprised of at least two different types of antiretroviral drugs as a cocktail to treat HIV-infected patients. Refer to highly active antiretroviral therapy.

haemolin

A protein that occurs in soluble form in hemolymph and as a membrane-bound protein on phagocytic hemocyte surfaces. Soluble haemolin serves as an opsonin on whole pathogens or lipopolysaccharide (LPS) and facilitates phagocytosis.

Haemophilus b conjugate vaccine (injection)

Induces protective antibody to _Haemophilus_ b polysaccharide. A preexisting titer of antibody to HbPs of 0.15 mcg/mL correlates with protection. Data from a Finnish field trial in children 18 to 71 months of age suggests that a titer of >1 µg/mL 3 weeks after vaccination is linked to long-term protection. Linkage of _Haemophilus_ b saccharides to a protein such as CRM[197] converts the saccharide (HbO) to a T-dependent (HbOC) antigen and leads to enhanced antibody response to the saccharide in infants that primes for an anamnestic response and is mainly IgG. The response to _ActHIB_ is a classic T-dependent immune response. IgG is the main isotype of anticapsular PRP antibody induced by _ActHIB_. A prominent booster response has been shown in children 12 months of age or older who previously received two or three doses. Bactericidal activity against _H. influenzae_ type b is present in serum after immunization and correlates statistically with the anti-PRP antibody response induced by _ActHIB_. Antibody to _H. influenzae_ capsular polysaccharide (anti-PRP) titers of >1 µg/mL after vaccination with unconjugated PRP vaccine correlated with long-term protection against invasive _H. influenzae_ type b disease in children older than 24 months of age. _ActHIB_ induced anti-PRP levels

greater than or equal to 1 µg/mL in 90% of infants after the primary series and in 98% of infants after a booster dose.

Haemophilus immunity

Serum bactericidal activity to _Haemophilus influenzae_ serotype b (Hib) is associated with protection from infection. This effect is mediated by antibody to the capsule. Antibody to the PRP polysaccharide capsule protects against invasive infection. Two-year-olds have only low titers of anticapsular antibodies and are susceptible to reinfection and episodes of Hib meningitis. NTHI strains of the organism demonstrate antigenic heterogeneity of surface antigens among strains. Infection does not induce protective immunity from infection by NTHI strains following otitis media attributable to an NTHI strain. Serum bactericidal antibody associated with protection develops. The immune response is strain-specific, rendering the child susceptible to infection with other strains of NTHI. The immune response is strain-specific with reactivity directed to the immunodominant surface epitopes on the P2 OMP. _H. influenzae_ LOS is a principal toxin against which humoral immune responses are directed. The mucosal immune response to NTHI remains to be defined. Conjugate vaccines developed to prevent invasive infections by Hib have been very successful in preventing the infectious disease. High titers of serum IgG specific for Hib capsular polysaccharide are associated with increased bactericidal and protective activity. Linking the PRP capsular polysaccharide to protein carriers has yielded a conjugate vaccine that is effective in protecting infants against invasive Hib infections.

Haemophilus influenzae type b vaccine (HB)

An immunizing preparation that contains purified polysaccharide antigen from _H. influenzae_ microorganisms and a carrier protein. It diminishes the risks of epiglottitis, meningitis, and other diseases induced by _H. influenzae_ during childhood.

Hageman factor (HF)

A zymogen in plasma that is activated by contact with a surface or by the kallikrein system at the beginning of the intrinsic pathway of blood coagulation. This is an 80-kDa plasma glycoprotein which, following activation, is split into α and β chains. When activated, it is a serine protease that transforms prekallikrein into kallikrein. HF is coagulation factor XII.

hairpin loop

The looped structure of hairpin DNA.

hairy cell leukemia

A B lymphocyte leukemia in which the B cells have characteristic cytoplasmic filopodia.

half-life ($T_{1/2}$)

The time required for a substance to be diminished to one half of its earlier level by degradation or decay; by catabolism, as in biological half-life; or by elimination. In immunology, $T_{1/2}$ refers to the time in which an immunoglobulin remains in the blood circulation. For IgG, the half-life is 20 to 25 days; for IgA, 6 days; for IgM, 5 days; for IgD, 2 to 8 days; and for IgE, 1 to 5 days.

halogenation

Halogen binding to the cell wall of a microorganism with resulting injury to the microbe.

halothane antigens

Antigenic determinants that result from the action of halothane on rabbit and rat liver cell components. Also referred to as TFA antigens.

HALV (human AIDS–lymphotrophic virus)

A designation proposed to replace Montagnier's LAV and Gallo's HTLV-III designations for the AIDS virus; the HIV designation for human immunodeficiency virus was subsequently chosen instead.

HAM

HTLV-1-associated myelopathy.

HAM-1 and HAM-2

Histocompatibility antigen modifier. Two murine genes that determine formation of permeases that are antigen transporters (oligopeptides) from the cytoplasm to a membrane-bound compartment where antigen complexes with major histocompatibility complex (MHC) class I and class II molecules. In humans, the equivalents of HAM-1 and -2 are referred to as ATP-binding cassette transporters.

HAM test

Refer to paroxysmal nocturnal hemoglobulinuria (PNH).

HAMA

Human anti-mouse antibody. A group of murine monoclonal antibodies administered to selected cancer patients in research treatment protocols stimulates synthesis of anti-mouse antibodies in the recipients. The murine monoclonal antibodies are specific for human tumor cell epitopes. The anti-mouse response affects the continued administration of the monoclonal antibody preparation. The hypersensitivity induced can be expressed as anaphylaxis, subacute allergic reaction, delayed-type hypersensitivity, rash, urticaria, flu-like symptoms, gastrointestinal disorders, dyspnea, hypotension, and renal failure.

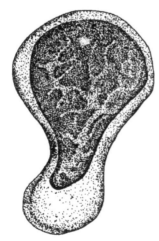

Hand-mirror cell.

hand-mirror cell

A lymphocyte in which the nucleus represents the mirror and the cytoplasm has extended into a uropod that resembles the handle of a mirror. Cells with this morphology may be found in both benign and neoplastic hematopoietic conditions. They may represent immature T lymphocytes, large granular lymphocytes such as natural killer cells, or atypical lymphocytes such as those seen in infectious mononucleosis. However, hand-mirror cells are most frequently found in acute lymphocytic leukemia of FAB L1 or L2 subtypes. They may also be seen in cases of multiple myeloma, lymphosarcoma, Hodgkin disease, acute myelogenous leukemia of the FAB M5a subtype, and acute and chronic lymphocytic leukemia. Hand-mirror cells in lymphocytic leukemia may be associated with defective immune function.

Hand–Schuller–Christian disease

A macrophage lineage neoplasm (histiocytosis X) that mainly affects bone.

HANE (hereditary angioneurotic edema)

A condition induced by C1q esterase inhibitor (C1q-INH) deficiency in which immune complexes induce uptake of activated C1, C4, and C2. This may be activated by trauma, cold, vibration, or other physical stimuli, histamine release, or menstruation. HANE induces nonpitting swelling that is neither pruritic nor urticarial and reaches a peak within 12 to 18 hours. It occurs on the face, extremities, toes, fingers, elbows, knees, gastrointestinal mucosa, and oral pharynx. It can produce edema of the epiglottis, which is fatal in approximately one third of the cases. Patients may have nausea and abdominal pain with vomiting. Four types have been described, two of which are congenital. In type I, which accounts for 85% of cases, C1q-INH is diminished to 30% of normal. In the type II variant, the product of the gene is present but does not function properly; type II may be acquired or autoimmune. The acquired type is associated with certain lymphoproliferative disorders such as Waldenström's macroglobulinemia, IgA myeloma, chronic lymphocytic leukemia, and other types of B cell proliferation. The autoimmune type is linked to IgG_1 autoantibodies. C1s activation is unregulated.

Hanganitziu–Deicher antigen

An altered ganglioside present in certain human neoplasms (CD3, GM_1, and terminal 4NAcNeu).

haploid

A single copy of each autosome and one sex chromosome constitutes one set of unpaired chromosomes in a nucleus. The term may also refer to a cell containing this number of chromosomes.

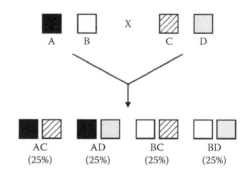

Each set of alleles is referred to as a haplotype.

haploidentical transplant

The sharing of one HLA haplotype between donor and recipient who differ in the second HLA haplotype.

haplotype

Phenotypic characteristic encoded by closely linked genes on one chromosome inherited from one parent. Each individual inherits two haplotypes, one from each parent. The term frequently describes several major histocompatibility complex (MHC) alleles on a single chromosome. Selected haplotypes are in strong linkage disequilibrium between alleles of different loci. According to Mendelian genetics, 25% of siblings share both haplotypes.

hapten

A relatively small molecule that alone is unable to elicit an immune response when injected into an animal but is capable of reacting *in vitro* with an antibody specific for it.

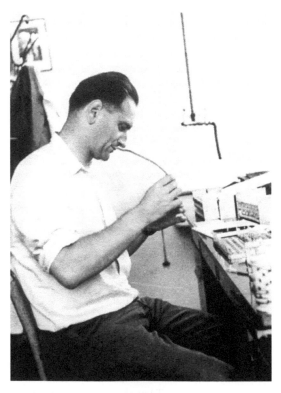

Hapten- carrier conjugate.

Only when complexed to a carrier molecule prior to administration can a hapten induce an immune response. Haptens usually bear only one epitope. The conjugation of a hapten to a carrier macromolecule can enable it to enduce a hapten-specific B and T cell response. Pneumococcal polysaccharide is an example of a larger molecule that may act as a hapten in rabbits but as a complete antigen in humans.

hapten–carrier conjugate

The combination of a small molecule covalently linked to a large immunogenic carrier molecule.

hapten conjugate response

The response to hapten conjugates requires two populations of lymphocytes: T and B cells. The cells producing the antibodies are derived from B cells. T cells act as helpers in this process. B cell preparations, depleted of T cells, cannot respond to hapten conjugates. The T cells are responsive to the carrier portion of the conjugate, although in some cases they also recognize the hapten. The influence of the carrier on the ensuing response is called carrier effect. The experimental design for demonstrating the carrier effect involves adoptive transfer of hapten-sensitive B cells and of T cells primed with one or another carrier. The primed cells are those that have already had an opportunity to encounter the antigen.

hapten inhibition test

An assay for serological characterization or elucidation of the molecular structure of an epitope by blocking the antigen-binding site of an antibody specific for the epitope with a defined hapten.

hapten X

Refer to CD15.

HAR

Refer to hyperacute graft rejection.

harderian gland

A tear-secreting gland in the orbit of the eye in mammals and birds. Immunoglobulin G (IgG), IgM, and secretory IgA may originate from this location in birds.

Milan Hasek.

Hasek, Milan (1925–1985)

Czechoslovakian scientist whose contributions to immunology include investigations of immunologic tolerance and the development of chick embryo parabiosis. Hasek also made fundamental contributions to transplantation biology.

Hashimoto's disease (Hashimoto's thyroiditis)

Autoimmune thyroiditis that usually occurs in women past the age of 40. Thyroid gland inflammation is characterized

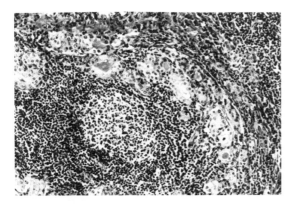

Hashimoto's thyroiditis.

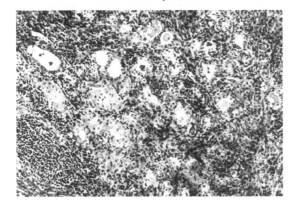

Hashimoto's thyroiditis.

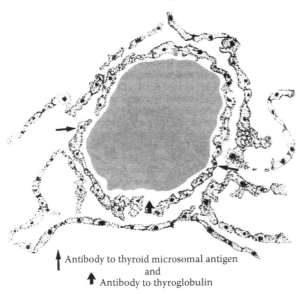

↑ Antibody to thyroid microsomal antigen
and
↑ Antibody to thyroglobulin

Hashimoto's thyroiditis.

by lymphocyte, plasma cell, and macrophage infiltration and often formation of lymphoid germinal centers. The thyroid becomes firm and enlarged. There is lymphocytic infiltration and oxyphilic alteration of the thyroid follicular epithelium. Thyroid follicles exhibit permanent germinal centers, and the thyroid epithelium is atrophied. Autoantibodies against thyroid peroxidase (microsomal antibodies), thyroglobulin, and colloid are demonstrable. The antibodies against thyroid-specific antigens recruit natural killer (NK) cells to the thyroid, leading to tissue injury and inflammation. Destruction of thyroid follicular cells by a cell-mediated

response leads to insufficient synthesis of thyroxine, producing hypothyroidism. Even though the thyroid gland increases in size, the acinar epithelium is continually destroyed. Thus, the principal pathogenesis is by autoimmune mechanisms. The disease leads to a decrease in thyroid function. This is considered to be an organ-specific autoimmune disease. Hormonal replacement therapy is used for treatment. Also called chronic autoimmune thyroiditis.

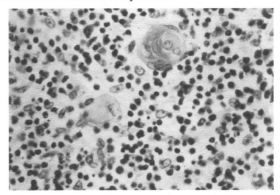

Hassall's corpuscles.

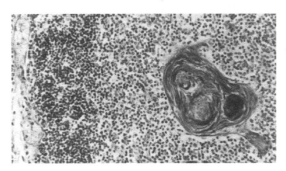

Normal thymus. This child's thymus shows the dense cortex composed predominantly of lymphocytes and the less dense medulla with fewer lymphocytes. Note the Hassall's corpuscle.

Hassall's corpuscles

Epithelial cell whorls in the medulla of the thymus. They are thought to produce thymic hormones. Whereas the center may exhibit degeneration, cells at the periphery may reveal endocrine secretion granules.

HAT medium

A growth medium used in tissue culture of animal cells that contains hypoxanthine, aminopterin, and thymidine and is used to selectively isolate hybrid cells. Aminopterin, a folic acid antagonist, blocks nucleic acid *de novo* synthesis but does not have this effect for synthesis by the salvage pathway mechanism. Hypoxanthine and thymidine are substances from which nucleic acid can be synthesized by the second mechanism. The enzymes hypoxanthine-guanine phosphoribosyl transferase (HGPRT) and thymidine kinase are requisite for the salvage pathway. Thus, HAT medium cannot sustain cells lacking these enzymes, as nucleic acid synthesis is totally inhibited. However, hybrid cells produced from each of the two cell lines whose enzyme defects are different can survive and grow in HAT medium. This makes it a useful selective medium for hybrid cells. It is widely employed in hybridoma production, as it permits myeloma cell–lymphocyte hybrids to survive. Nonfused myeloma cells die for lack of HGPRT, and unfused lymphocytes die because of their very limited proliferative capacity. The hybrid cell that survives in HAT medium receives the missing enzymes from the lymphocyte and proliferative capacity from the myeloma cell.

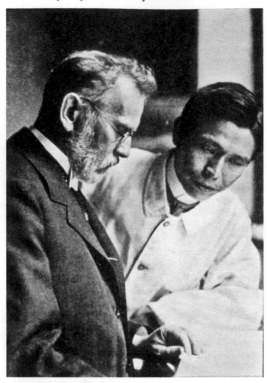

Sachahiro Hata (right) with P. Ehrlich (left).

HAT selection

Refer to HAT medium.

Hata, Sachahiro

Co-discoverer, with his mentor, Paul Ehrlich, of the first specific treatment for syphilis. They developed the arsenical compound numbered 606 and named salvarsan.

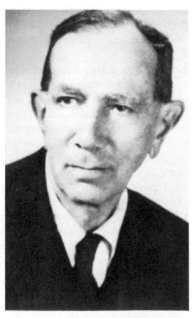

Felix Haurowitz.

Haurowitz, Felix (1896–1988)

A noted protein chemist from Prague who later moved to the United States. He investigated the chemistry of hemoglobins. In 1930 (with Breinl) he advanced the instruction theory of antibody formation. (Refer to *Chemistry and Biology of Proteins,* 1950; *Immunochemistry and Biosynthesis of Antibodies,* 1968.)

Hausen, Harald zur

Nobel Laureate in Physiology or Medicine (2008). German investigator who discovered that some types of human papilloma virus (HPV) cause cervical cancer.

HAV

Acronym for hepatitis A virus.

hay fever

Allergic rhinitis, recurrent asthma, rhinitis, and conjunctivitis in atopic individuals who inhale allergenic (antigenic) materials such as pollens, animal dander, house dust, etc. These substances do not induce allergic reactions in nonatopic (normal) individuals. Hay fever is a type I immediate hypersensitivity reaction mediated by homocytotrophic IgE antibodies specific for the allergen for which the individual is hypersensitive. Hay fever is worse during seasons when airborne environmental allergens are most concentrated.

HBcAg

Hepatitis B core antigen. This 27-nm core can be detected in hepatocyte nuclei.

HBeAg

Hepatitis B nucleocapsid constituent of relatively low molecular weight that signifies an infectious state when it appears in serum.

HBIG (hepatitis B immunoglobulin)

A preparation of donor-pool-derived antibodies against hepatitis B virus (HBV). It is heat treated and shown not to contain human immunodeficiency virus (HIV). HBIG is given at the time when individuals are exposed to HBV and 1 month thereafter. Low-titer (1:128) and high-titer (1:100,000) preparations are available.

HBLV (human B lymphotropic virus)

Herpesvirus 6.

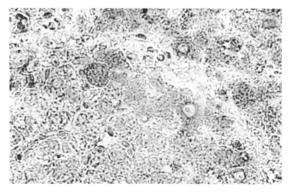

HBs antigen in liver cells.

HBsAg

Hepatitis B virus envelope or surface antigen.

HBV

Acronym for hepatitis B virus.

HBx

A regulatory gene of hepatitis B that codes for the production of an HBx protein that is a transcriptional transactivator of viral genes. It modifies expression of the host gene.

In transgenic mouse-induced hepatomas, it may promote development of hepatocellular carcinoma.

HCC-1

A β chemokine (CC family) isolated from the hemofiltrates of chronic renal failure patients. HCC-1 has 46% sequence identity with MIP-1α and MIP-1β, and 29 to 37% with the remaining human β chemokines. In contrast to other β chemokines, HCC-1 is expressed constitutively in normal spleen, liver, skeletal and heart muscle, gut, and bone marrow. It reaches significant concentrations (1 to 80 nM) in plasma. It is expressed by monocytes and hematopoietic progenitor cells.

hCG (human choriogonadotrophic hormone)

A glycoprotein comprised of lactose and hexosamine that is synthesized by syncytiotrophoblast, fetal kidney, and liver-selected tumors. It may be measured by radioimmunoassay or enzyme-linked immunosorbent assay (ELISA). It is elevated in patients with various types of tumors, such as carcinoma of the liver, stomach, breast, pancreas, lungs, kidneys, and renal cortex, and conditions such as lymphoma, leukemia, melanoma, and seminoma.

HCT

Abbreviation for hematopoietic cell transplant.

HD$_{50}$

An uncommon designation for CH$_{50}$, the hemolytic complement activity of a serum sample.

HDN

Hemolytic disease of the newborn.

heaf test

A type of tuberculin test in which an automatic multiple puncture device with six needles is used to administer the test material by intradermal inoculation. The multiple needles advance 2 to 3 mm into the skin. Also called Tine test.

heart–lung transplantation

A procedure that has proven effective for the treatment of primary respiratory disease with dysfunction of gas exchange and alveolar mechanics, together with a secondary elevation in pulmonary vascular resistance, and in primary high-resistance circulatory disorder associated with pulmonary vascular disease.

heat-aggregated protein antigen

Partial denaturation of a protein antigen by mild heating. This diminishes the protein's solubility, but causes it to express new epitopes. An example is the greater reactivity of rheumatoid factor (e.g., IgM anti-IgG autoantibody) with heat-aggregated γ globulin than with unheated γ globulin.

heat inactivation

Loss of biological activity through heating. Heating a serum sample at 56°C in a water bath for 30 minutes destroys complement activity through inactivation of C1, C2, and factor B. By diminishing the heat to 52°C for 30 minutes, only factor B is destroyed, whereas C1 and C2 remain intact. This inactivates the alternative complement pathway but not the classical pathway. Immunoglobulin G (IgG), IgM, and IgA are resistant to incubation in a 56°C water bath for 30 minutes, whereas IgE antibodies are destroyed by this temperature.

heat-labile antibody

An antigen-specific immunoglobulin that loses its ability to interact with antigen following exposure to heating at 56°C for 30 minutes.

heat shock protein antibodies

Antibodies of the immunoglobulin M (IgM), IgG, and IgA classes specific for a 73-kDa chaperonin that belongs to the hsp70 family present in the sera of approximately 40% of systemic lupus erythematosus (SLE) patients and in 10 to 20% of individuals with rheumatoid arthritis. Antibodies specific for the 65-kDa heat shock protein derived from mycobacteria show specificity for rheumatoid synovium. RA synovial fluid T cells specific for a 65-kDa mycobacterial heat shock protein have been reported to be inversely proportional to the disease duration.

heat shock proteins (HSPs)

A restricted number of highly conserved cellular proteins that increase during metabolic stress such as exposure to heat, inflammation, or tumor transformation. Inside cells, HSPs escort peptides from the proteasome to TAP in the course of endogenous antigen processing. Stressed cells may release HSPs as "danger signals" linking Toll-like receptors. They may facilitate exogenous antigen processing and cross presentation. Heat shock proteins affect assembly into protein complexes, proper protein folding, protein uptake into cellular organelles, and protein sorting. The main group of HSPs are 70-kDa proteins. Heat shock (stress) proteins are expressed by many pathogens and are classified into four families based on molecular size: HSP90, HSP70, HSP60, and small HSP (<40 kDa). Mycobacterial HSP65 antibodies are found in rheumatoid arthritis, atherosclerosis, multiple sclerosis, Alzheimer's disease, and Parkinson's disease. Enzyme immunoassay (EIA) is the method of choice for their detection but there is no known clinical significance for HSP antibodies.

heavy chain (H chain)

An immunoglobulin polypeptide chain that designates the class of immunoglobulin. The five immunoglobulin classes are based upon the heavy chains they possess and are IgM, IgG, IgA, IgD, and IgE. Each four-chain immunoglobulin molecule or four-chain monomeric unit of IgM contains two heavy chains and two light chains fastened together by disulfide bonds. The variable region of the heavy chain, designated V$_H$, is located at the amino terminus. Adjacent to this is the first constant region, designated C$_H$1 through C$_H$3 or C$_H$4 domains, based on immunoglobulin class. Heavy chain antigenic determinants determine not only the immunoglobulin class but also the subclass.

heavy chain class

Immunoglobulin heavy polypeptide chain primary (antigenic) structure present in all members of a species that is different from the other heavy chain classes. Primary structural features governing immunoglobulin heavy chain class are located in the constant region. Lowercase Greek letters such as μ, γ, α, δ, and ε designate the heavy chain class.

heavy chain class (isotype) switching

The mechanism whereby a B cell changes the class (or isotype) of antibodies it synthesizes from immunoglobulin M (IgM) to IgG, IgE, or IgA, without altering the antigen-binding specificity of the antibody. Helper T lymphocyte cytokines and CD40 ligand regulate heavy chain class switching, which involves B cell VDJ segment recombination with downstream heavy chain gene segments.

heavy chain diseases

Monoclonal gammopathies or paraproteinemias associated with lymphoproliferative disease and characterized by excess synthesis of Fc fragments of immunoglobulins that appear in the serum and/or urine. The most common is the α heavy chain disease (Seligmann's disease)

in which patients produce excess incomplete α chains of
IgA$_1$ molecules. It mainly affects Sephardic Jews, Arabs,
and other Mediterranean residents, as well as subjects in
South America and Asia. It may appear in childhood or
adolescence as a lymphoproliferative disorder associated
with the respiratory tract or gastrointestinal tract. Patients
may manifest malabsorption, diarrhea, steatorrhea, hepatic
dysfunction, weight loss, lymphadenopathy, hypocalcemia,
and extensive mononuclear infiltration. α Heavy chain
disease may either spontaneously remit or respond favorably to treatment with antibiotics; it may require chemotherapy in some cases. δ Heavy chain disease has been
reported in an elderly male demonstrating abnormal plasma
cell infiltration of the bone marrow along with osteolytic
lesions. γ Heavy chain disease (Franklin's disease) occurs
in older men, and may induce death rapidly (within weeks)
or last for years. Death usually takes place within 1 year
because of infection. Patients develop lymphoproliferation
with fever, anemia, fatigue, angioimmunoblastic lymphadenopathy, hepatosplenomegaly, eosinophilic infiltrates,
leukopenia, lymphoma, autoimmune disease, or tuberculosis. Serum IgG$_1$ is elevated. γ Heavy chain disease has been
treated with cyclophosphamide, vincristine, and prednisone.
μ Heavy chain disease is a rare condition affecting middle-
aged to older individuals. Some patients may ultimately
develop chronic lymphocytic leukemia. μ Heavy chain disease is characterized by lymphadenopathy, hepatosplenomegaly, infiltration of the bone marrow by vacuolated plasma
cells, and frequently elevated synthesis of κ light chain.

heavy chain subclass

Within an immunoglobulin heavy chain class, differences
in primary structure associated with the constant region
that can further distinguish these heavy chains of the same
class are designated as subclasses. These differences are
based on primary or antigenic structure. The heavy chain
subclasses are designated γ$_1$, γ$_2$, γ$_3$, etc.

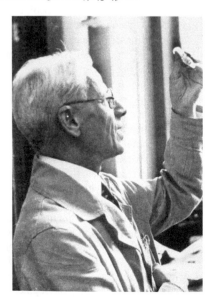

Michael Heidelberger.

Heidelberger, Michael (1888–1991)

An American considered the father of immunochemistry.
He began his career as an organic chemist. His contributions to immunology include the perfection of quantitative

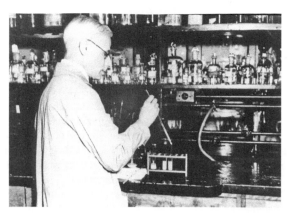

Michael Heidelberger, who purified the first component of complement
and showed that complement was real, had weight, and contained protein.

immunochemical methods and the immunochemical char-
acterization of pneumococcal polysaccharides. His contri-
butions to immunologic research are legion. He received the
Lasker Award, the National Medal of Science, the Behring
Award, the Pasteur Medal, and the French Legion of Honor.
(Refer to *Lectures on Immunochemistry,* 1956.)

Helicobacter pylori immunity

Both circulating and local humoral antibody responses follow *H. pylori* colonization of the gastric mucosa. During the
prolonged mucosal infection, IgG$_1$ and IgG$_4$ and often IgG$_2$
antibodies are detectable but IgG$_3$ and IgM antibodies only
rarely. IgA antibodies are usually also present. The initial
IgM response is followed later by IgA with conversion to
IgG 22 to 33 days after infection. IgA antibodies are found
at the local mucosal level and are secreted into the gastric
juice. IgG produced locally is rapidly inactivated when it
reaches the gastric juice. A systemic IgG response is present
throughout the infection and diminishes, only prolonging
successful therapy. If the infection reappears, the IgG antibody titer rises. The specificity of circulating host antibody
against *H. pylori* varies greatly. This is attributable in part to
variations in host response and to a lesser degree to antigenic
diversity of the microorganisms such as variation in the Vac
A and Cag A proteins. Most infected subjects synthesize
antibodies against numerous antigens, including the urease
subunits, the flagellins, and the 54-kDa HSP60 homolog.
Antibodies usually develop to Vac A and Cag A polypeptides if they are present in the infecting strain. Although of
variable complexity, the antigens all include urease. Plasma
cells, lymphocytes, and monocytes infiltrate the superficial
layers of the lamina propria in *H. pylori*-associated gastritis.
Half of the mature B cells and infiltrate are B cells producing mostly IgA but also IgG and IgM. These cells produce
antibodies specific for *H. pylori* and are mostly of the CD8$^+$
subset, although CD4$^+$ T cells are also increased, as well
as γδ T cells. Gastric epithelial cells aberrantly express
HLA-DR during *H. pylori* infection, which is also associated
with elevated synthesis of IL1, IL6, and TNF-α in the gastric
mucosa. *H. pylori* induces IL1, IL6, and TNF-α in the gastric
mucosa. It also induces IL8 expression in gastric epithelium
which induces neutrophil chemotaxis; 92% of non-Hodgkin
lymphoma cases affecting the stomach are associated with
H. pylori infection. The bacteria may engage in immune
avoidance by continually losing highly antigenic materials
such as urease and flagella sheaths from the bacterial surface,

thereby diminishing the effectiveness of bound antibodies. The immune response may also be downregulated during infection as antigen-specific responsiveness of local and circulating T cells is diminished. The complexity of the disease makes development of effective vaccines difficult. An oral subunit vaccine used with a mucosal adjuvant has protected animal models. Thus immunotherapy may be a future option for prevention.

helminth

A parasitic worm. Infections by helminths induce a T_H2-regulated immune response associated with inflammatory infiltrates rich in eosinophils and IgE synthesis.

helper CD4+ T cells

CD4+ T lymphocytes that facilitate antibody formation by B cells following antigenic challenge. T_H2 T cells that synthesize cytokines IL-4 and IL-5 represent the most efficient helper T cells in contrast to other helper CD4+ T cells.

helper/suppressor ratio

The ratio of CD4+ helper/inducer T lymphocytes to CD8+ suppressor/cytotoxic T lymphocytes. This value normally ranges between 1.5 and 2.0; however, in certain virus infections (notably AIDS), the ratio becomes inverted as a consequence of greatly diminished CD4+ lymphocytes and either stationary or elevated levels of CD8+ lymphocytes. Inversion of the ratio continues as the clinical situation deteriorates. Eventually, the CD4+ cells may completely disappear in an AIDS patient. Other conditions in which the helper/suppressor (CD4/CD8) ratio is decreased include other viral infections such as herpes, cytomegalovirus, Epstein–Barr virus, and measles, graft-vs.-host disease, lupus erythematosus with renal involvement, severe burns, exercise, myelodysplasia, acute lymphocytic leukemia in remission, severe sunburn, exercise, and loss of sleep. Elevated ratios may occur in such conditions as atopic dermatitis, Sezary syndrome, psoriasis, rheumatoid arthritis, primary biliary cirrhosis, lupus erythematosus without renal involvement, chronic autoimmune hepatitis, and type I insulin-dependent diabetes mellitus.

helper T cells

CD4+ helper/inducer T lymphocytes that represent a subset of T cells critical to induction of an immune response to a foreign antigen. Antigen is presented by an antigen-presenting cell, such as a macrophage, in the context of self major histocompatibility complex (MHC) class II antigen and interleukin-1 (IL1). Once activated, the CD4+ T cells express IL2 receptors and produce IL2 molecules that can act in an autocrine fashion by combining with the IL2 receptors and mediating the CD4+ cells to proliferate. Differentiated CD4+ lymphocytes synthesize and secrete lymphokines that affect the functions of other cells of the immune system such as CD8+ cells, B cells, and natural killer (NK) cells. B cells differentiate into plasma cells that synthesize antibody. Activated macrophages participate in delayed-type hypersensitivity (type IV) reactions. Cytotoxic T cells also develop. Murine monoclonal antibodies are used to enumerate CD4+ T lymphocytes by flow cytometry.

hemadsorption inhibition test

A red blood cell suspension is added to a tissue culture infected with a hemagglutinating virus. Viral hemagglutinin, expressed at the tissue culture cell surfaces, facilitates the hemadsorption of erythrocyte aggregates to the tissue culture surfaces. Antiviral antibody added to the culture

prevents this hemadsorption, which serves as the basis for testing for antiviral antibody.

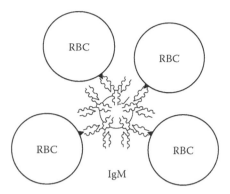

Hemagglutination.

hemagglutination

The aggregation of red blood cells by antibodies, viruses, lectin, or other substances.

hemagglutination inhibition reaction

A serological test based upon inhibiting the aggregation of erythrocytes bearing antigen. It may be employed for diagnosis of such viral infections as rubella, variola–vaccinia, rubeola, herpes zoster, herpes simplex types I and II, cytomegalovirus, and Epstein–Barr virus. It is also used in the diagnosis of adenovirus, influenza, coronavirus, parainfluenza, mumps, and such viral diseases as St. Louis, Eastern, Venezuelan, and Western equine encephalitides. It has also been used in diagnosing various bacterial and parasitic diseases.

hemagglutination inhibition test

An assay for antibody or antigen based on the ability to interfere with red blood cell aggregation. Certain viruses are able to agglutinate red blood cells. In the presence of antiviral antibody, the ability to agglutinate erythrocytes is inhibited, thus serving as a basis to assay the antibody.

hemagglutination test

An assay based upon the aggregation of red blood cells into clusters either through the action of antibody specific for their surface epitopes or through the action of a virus that possesses a hemagglutinin as part of its structure and does not involve antibody.

hemagglutinin

A red blood cell agglutinating substance. Antibodies, lectins, and some viral glycoproteins may induce erythrocyte agglutination. In immunology, hemagglutinin usually refers to an antibody that causes red blood cell aggregation in physiological salt solution either at 37°C (warm hemagglutinins) or at 4°C (cold hemagglutinins).

hematocytes

Cells resembling leukocytes that appear in invertebrate hemolymph.

hematogones

Early precursor B cells that express cell surface antigens such HLA-DR, CD10, CD19, and CD20. Morphologically they appear as small compact lymphocytes.

hematopoiesis

The development of the cellular elements of the blood including erythrocytes, leukocytes, and platelets from pluripotent stem cells in the bone marrow and fetal liver. Various cytokine growth factors are synthesized by bone marrow. Stromal cells, T cells, and other types of cells regulate hematopoiesis.

hematopoietic cells

Erythrocytes and leukocytes.

hematopoietic cell transplant (HCT)

The inoculation of hematopoietic stem cells from the peripheral blood, induced from the bone marrow, or occasionally from umbilical cord blood of a histocompatible donor into a recipient with an injured immune system.

hematopoietic chimerism

A successful bone marrow transplant leads to a state of hematological and/or immunological chimerism in which donor-type blood cells coexist permanently with host-type tissues, without manifesting alloreactivity to each other. Usually incomplete or mixed hematopoietic chimerism is generated after bone marrow transplantation in which both host-type and donor-type blood cells can be detected in the recipient. Not only is immune reactivity against donor type cells an obstacle to bone marrow engraftment, but the problem of graft-vs.-host disease (GVHD) mediated by donor T cells reactive against host antigens is also present. Refer to chimera.

hematopoietic-inducing microenvironment (HIM)

An anatomical location in which the cells and cellular factors requisite for the generation of hematopoietic cells may be found.

hematopoietic lineage

A series of cells that develop from hematopoietic stem cells and yield mature blood elements.

hematopoietic stem cell (HSC)

An undifferentiated bone marrow cell that serves as a precursor for multiple cell lineages. A common pluripotent hematopoietic precursor capable of self-renewal or commitment to differentiation into the common myeloid precursor that is the parent cell of a myeloid lineage (myelopoiesis) or a common lymphoid progenitor that leads to cells of the lymphoid lineage (lymphopoiesis). These cells are also demonstrable in the yolk sac and later in the liver in the fetus.

hematopoietic stem cell transplantation

Used to reconstitute hematopoietic cell lineages and treat neoplastic diseases. Twenty-five percent of allogenic marrow transplants in 1995 were performed using hematopoietic stem cells (HSCs) obtained from unrelated donors. Because only 30% of patients requiring allogenic marrow transplants had siblings that were human leukocyte antigen (HLA)-genotypically identical, it became necessary to identify related or unrelated potential marrow donors. It was found that complete HLA compatibility between donor and recipient is not absolutely necessary to reconstitute patients immunologically. Transplantation of unrelated marrow is accompanied by an increased incidence of graft-vs.-host disease (GVHD). Removal of mature T lymphocytes from marrow grafts decreases the severity of GVHD but often increases the incidence of graft failure and disease relapse. HLA-phenotypically identical marrow transplants among relatives are often successful. HSC transplantation provides a method to reconstitute hematopoietic cell lineages with normal cells capable of continuous self renewal. The principal complications of HSC transplantation are GVHD, graft rejection, graft failure, prolonged immunodeficiency, toxicity from radio-chemotherapy given pre-and post-

transplantation, and GVHD prophylaxis. Methotrexate and cyclosporin A are given to help prevent acute GVHD. Chronic GVHD may also become a serious complication that involves the skin, gut, and liver, and an associated sicca syndrome. Allogeneic HSC transplantation often involves older individuals and unrelated donors. Thus, blood stem cell transplantation represents an effective method for the treatment of patients with hematologic and nonhematologic malignancies and various types of immunodeficiencies. The *in vitro* expansion of a small number of CD34+ cells stimulated by various combinations of cytokines appears to produce hematopoietic reconstitution when reinfused after a high-dose therapy. Recombinant human hematopoietic growth factors (HGFs; cytokines) may be given to counteract chemotherapy-treatment-related myelotoxicity. HGF increases the number of circulating progenitor and stem cells which is important for the support of high-dose therapy in autologous and allogeneic HSC transplantation. Both the bone marrow and umbilical cord blood serve as sources for hematopoietic stem cells.

hematopoietic system

Those tissues and cells that generate peripheral blood cells.

hematopoietic tumor

The malignant transformation of immune system cells.

hematopoietins

Factors that facilitate the growth and development of blood cells.

hematoxylin bodies

Nuclear aggregates of irregular shape found in areas of fibrinoid change or fibrinoid necrosis in systemic lupus erythematosus patients. These homogeneous-staining nuclear masses contain nuclear protein and DNA, as well as anti-DNA. They are probably formed from injured cell nuclei that interacted with antinuclear antibodies *in vivo*. Hematoxylin staining imparts a bluish-purple color to hematoxylin bodies. They may be viewed in the kidneys, lymph nodes, spleen, lungs, atrial endocardium, synovium, and serous membranes. Hematoxylin bodies of the tissue correspond to LE cells of the peripheral blood.

hematuria

Macroscopic or microscopic blood in the urine from any cause, whether glomerular basement membrane injury or renal stones, for example.

hemocyanin

A blood pigment that transports oxygen in invertebrates. In immunology, hemocyanin of the keyhole limpet has been widely used as an experimental antigen.

hemocytoblast

A bone marrow stem cell.

hemolymph

Invertebrate circulatory system liquid that conveys nutritious molecules and waste products throughout the body of the organism.

hemolysin

A complement-fixing antibody that lyses erythrocytes in the presence of complement and acts with complement to produce an interruption in the membrane integrity of red blood cells, causing disruption. Historically, the term refers to rabbit anti-sheep erythrocyte antibody used in the visible part of a complement fixation test. Microbial products such as streptolysin O may disrupt (lyse) red blood cells in agar medium.

hemolysis

Interruption of the cellular integrity of red blood cells that may be immune- or nonimmune-mediated. Clinically, immune hemolysis may be IgM-mediated when immunoglobulins combine with red blood cell surfaces for which they are specific, such as the ABO blood groups, and activate complement to produce lysis. This results in the release of free hemoglobin in the intravascular space with serious consequences. By contrast, hemolysis mediated by IgG in the extravascular space may be less severe. Indirect bilirubin is elevated, as the liver may not be able to conjugate the bilirubin in case of massive hemolysis. Lactate dehydrogenase is elevated, and hemoglobin appears in the blood and urine. Urobilinogen is elevated in both urine and feces. Hemolysis may be also attributable to the action of enzymes or other chemicals on cell membranes. It can also be induced by such mechanisms as placing the red cells in a hypotonic solution.

hemolytic anemia

A disease characterized by diminished circulating erythrocytes as a consequence of their destruction based either on an intrinsic abnormality, as in sickle cell anemia and thalassemia, or as a consequence of membrane-specific antibody and complement (Type II hypersensitivity). Certain infections such as malaria are also associated with hemolytic anemia. Free hemoglobin in serum may lead to renal problems.

hemolytic anemia of the newborn

Refer to hemolytic disease of the newborn.

hemolytic disease of the newborn (HDN)

A fetus with RhD⁺ red blood cells can stimulate an RhD⁻ mother to produce anti-RhD immunoglobulin G (IgG) antibodies that cross the placenta and destroy the fetal red blood cells when a sufficient titer is obtained. This is usually not until the third pregnancy with an Rh⁺ fetus. At parturition, the RhD⁺ red blood cells enter the maternal circulation and subsequent pregnancies provide a booster to this response. With the third pregnancy, a sufficient quantity of high-titer antibody crosses the placenta to produce considerable lysis of fetal red blood cells. This may lead to erythroblastosis fetalis (hemolytic disease of the newborn). Seventy percent of HDN cases are due to RhD incompatibility of the mother and fetus. Exchange transfusions may be required for treatment. Two other antibodies against erythrocytes that may likewise be a cause for transfusion exchange include anti-Fyᵃ and Kell. As bilirubin levels rise, the immature blood–brain barrier permits bilirubin to penetrate and deposit on the basal ganglia. Anti-D antibody passively injected into the mother following parturition unites with the RhD⁺ red cells, leading to their elimination by the mononuclear phagocyte system. Also termed *erythroblastosis fetalis*.

hemolytic plaque assay

A technique to identify and enumerate cells synthesizing antibodies. Typically, spleen cells from a mouse immunized against sheep red blood cells are combined with melted agar or agarose in which sheep erythrocytes are suspended. After gentle mixing, the suspension is distributed into Petri plates, where it gels. This is followed by incubation at 37°C, after which complement is added to the dish from a pipette. Thus, the sheep erythrocytes (SRBCs) surrounding cells secreting immunoglobulin M (IgM) antibody against SRBCs are lysed by the added complement, producing a clear zone of hemolysis resembling the effect produced by β hemolytic streptococci on blood agar. IgG antibody against sheep erythrocytes can be identified by adding anti-IgG antibody to aid lysis by complement. Whereas modifications of this method have been used to identify cells producing antibodies against a variety of antigens or haptens conjugated to the sheep red cells, it can also be used to ascertain the immunoglobulin class secreted. Refer to figure for Jerne plaque assay.

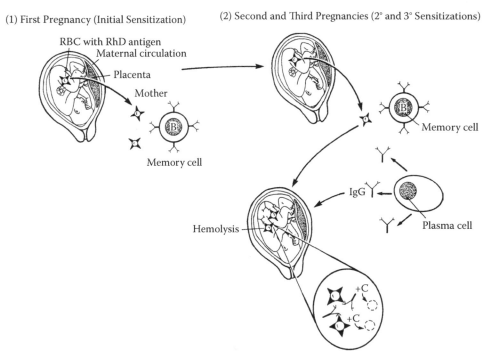

(1) First Pregnancy (Initial Sensitization)

(2) Second and Third Pregnancies (2° and 3° Sensitizations)

RBC with RhD antigen
Maternal circulation
Placenta
Mother
Memory cell
Memory cell
Hemolysis
IgG
Plasma cell
+C
+C

Representation of the mechanism of hemolytic disease of the newborn.

H

hemolytic system

The visible phase of a complement fixation test in which sheep red blood cells (SRBCs) combine with their homologous antibody and are added to a system in which antigen is mixed with patient serum, presumed to contain specific antibody, followed by complement. If antibody is present in the patient's serum and combines with the antigen, the added complement is fixed and is no longer available to react with antibody-coated sheep red cells, which are added as the second phase or visible reaction. Lysis indicates the presence of free complement from the first phase of the reaction, indicating that antibody against the antigen in question is not present in the patient's serum. By contrast, no hemolysis indicates the presence of the antibody. The hemolytic system may also be used to describe a reaction in which erythrocytes are combined with their homologous antibody. The addition of all nine components of complement together with calcium and magnesium ions followed by incubation at 37°C results in immune lysis (hemolysis).

hemophagocytic syndrome (HPS)

A primary immunodeficiency attributable mainly to a granule exocytosis pathway defect of cytotoxic T lymphocytes. Also referred to as hemophagocytic lymphohistiocytosis.

hemophilia

An inherited coagulation defect attributable to blood clotting factor VIII, factor IX, or factor XI deficiency. Hemophilia A patients are successfully maintained by the administration of exogenous factor VIII, which is now safe. Before mid-1985, factor products transmitted several cases of AIDS when factor VIII was accidentally extracted from the blood of HIV-positive subjects. Hemophilia B patients are treated with factor IX. Hemophilia A and B are X-linked; hemophilia C is autosomal.

Hemophilus influenzae vaccine

Refer to Hib.

hemopoietic resistance (HR)

Transplantation of allogeneic, parental, or xenogeneic bone marrow or leukemia cells into animals exposed to total body irradiation often results in the destruction of the transplanted cells. The mechanism causing the failure of the transplant appears similar for all three types of cells. This phenomenon, designated hemopoietic resistance (HR), has a genetic basis and mechanism different from conventional transplantation reactions against solid tumor allografts. It does not require prior sensitization and apparently involves the cooperation of natural killer (NK) cells and macrophages, both resistant to irradiation. The NK cells have the characteristics of null cells; macrophages play an accessory cell role. The cooperative activity seems to represent *in vivo* surveillance against leukemogenesis.

hemostatic plug

The immediate response to a vessel wall injury is the adhesion of platelets to the injury site and the growth by further aggregation of platelets of a mass that tends to obstruct (often incompletely) the lumen of the damaged vessel. This platelet mass is called a hemostatic plug. The exposed basement membranes at the sites of injury are the substrate for platelet adhesion, but deeper tissue components may have a similar effect. Far from being static, the hemostatic plug has a continuous tendency to break up with new masses re-formed immediately at the original site.

Henoch–Schoenlein purpura

A systemic form of small vessel vasculitis that is characterized by arthralgias, nonthrombocytopenic purpuric skin lesions, abdominal pain with bleeding, and renal disease. Immunologically, immune complexes containing IgA activate the alternate pathway of complement. Patients may present with upper respiratory infections preceding onset of the disease. Certain drugs, food, and immunizations have also been suspected as etiologic agents. The disease usually occurs in children 4 to 7 years of age, although it can occur in adults. Histopathologically, diffuse leukocytoclastic vasculitis involves small vessels. The submucosa and subserosa of the bowel may be sites of hemorrhage. There may be focal or diffuse glomerulonephritis in the kidneys. Children may manifest lesions associated with the skin, gastrointestinal tract, or joints, whereas in adults the disease is usually associated with skin findings. The skin lesions begin as a pruritic urticarial lesion that develops into a pink maculopapular spot, which matures into a raised and darkened lesion. The maculopapular lesion may ultimately resolve in 2 weeks without leaving a scar. Patients may also have arthralgias associated with the large joints of the lower extremities. Skin biopsy reveals the vasculitis, and immunofluorescence examination shows immunoglobulin A (IgA) deposits in vessel walls, in accord with a diagnosis of Henoch–Schoenlein purpura.

HEP

Acronym for high egg passage, which signifies multiple passages of rabies virus through eggs to achieve attenuation for preparation of a vaccine appropriate for use in immunizing cattle.

heparan sulfate

A glycosaminoglycan that resembles heparin and is comprised of the same disaccharide repeating unit; it is a smaller molecule and less sulfated than heparin. An extracellular substance, heparin sulfate is present in the lungs and arterial walls and on numerous cell surfaces.

heparin

A glycosaminoglycan comprised of two types of disaccharide repeating units. One is composed of d-glucosamine and d-glucuronic acid, and the other is composed of d-glucosamine and l-iduronic acid. Heparin is extensively sulfated and is an anticoagulant. It unites with an antithrombin III, which can unite with and block numerous coagulation factors. It is produced by mast cells and endothelial cells. It is found in the lungs, liver, skin, and gastrointestinal mucosa. Based on its anticoagulant properties, heparin is useful for treatment of thrombosis and phlebitis.

hepatitis A

A picornavirus, also called enterovirus 72. It is spread from person to person via the fecal–oral route or by consumption of contaminated water or food.

hepatitis A (inactivated, injection)

For active immunization of individuals 12 months of age and older against disease caused by hepatitis A virus (HAV). Primary immunization should be administered at least 2 weeks before expected exposure to HAV. Primary immunization of children and adolescents (12 months to 18 years) consists of a single dose of 720 enzyme-linked immunosorbent assay (ELISA) units in 7.5 mL and a booster dose (720 units in 0.5 mL) should be administered 6 to 12 months later. For adults, primary immunization consists of a single dose of 1440 ELISA units in 1 mL and a booster dose (1440 units in 1 mL) should be administered 6 to 12 months later.

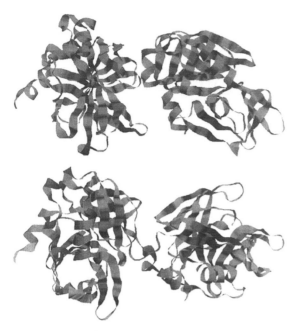

Hepatitis A virus 3C proteinase.

hepatitis A, inactivated and hepatitis B, recombinant vaccine (injection)

For active immunization of individuals 18 years of age or older against disease caused by hepatitis A virus (HAV) and infection by all known subtypes of hepatitis B virus (HBV). Vaccination may not protect 100% of recipients. Hepatitis D (delta virus) fails to occur in the absence of HVB infection. Thus, this vaccine also protects against hepatitis D.

hepatitis A virus immunity

Protective immunity is conferred by circulating antibodies that can be passively transferred. Recovery from hepatitis A virus infection is associated with lifelong protective immunity against reinfection. Pooled human immunoglobulin (HNIG) has been used since World War II to prevent hepatitis A virus infection and is 90% effective if administered prior to exposure. Three inactivated cell-culture-derived hepatitis A virus vaccines have been developed to induce circulating antibodies to antigens present on the virus surface. These vaccines are safe, very immunogenic, and protect against infection.

hepatitis B

A DNA virus that is relatively small and has four open reading frames. The S gene codes for hepatitis B surface antigen (HBsAg). The P gene codes for a DNA polymerase. An X gene and a core gene code for hepatitis B core antigen (HBcAG), and the precore area codes for HBeAg.

hepatitis B immune globulin (human, injection)

Indicated for post-exposure hepatitis B prophylaxis such as acute exposure to blood containing HBsAg, perinatal exposure of infants born to HBsAg-positive mothers, sexual exposure to an HBsAg-positive individual, or household exposure to persons with acute HBV infection.

hepatitis B surface antigen (HBsAg) antibody

A murine monoclonal antibody specific for the HBsAg phenotype.

hepatitis B vaccine

The human-plasma-derived hepatitis B vaccine (Heptavax-B) developed in the 1980s was unpopular because of the fear of AIDS related to any injectable

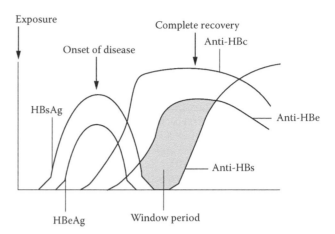

Hepatitis B virus and its antigens.

product derived from human plasma. The vaccine was replaced by a recombinant DNA vaccine (Recombivax™) prepared in yeast (*Saccharomyces cervesiae*). It is very effective in inducing protective antibodies in most recipients. Nonresponders are often successfully immunized by intracutaneous vaccination.

hepatitis B vaccine (recombinant, injection)

For immunization against infection caused by all known subtypes of hepatitis B virus, one of several that produce systemic infection with major pathology in the liver. These include hepatitis A virus, hepatitis D virus, and hepatitis C and E viruses (previously referred to as non-A, non-B hepatitis viruses). Hepatocellular carcinoma is a serious complication of hepatitis B virus infection. Reliable studies have linked chronic hepatitis B infection with hepatocellular carcinoma. Eighty percent of primary liver neoplasms are induced by hepatitis B virus infection. The CDC has recognized hepatitis B vaccine as the first anticancer vaccine because it can prevent primary liver cancer.

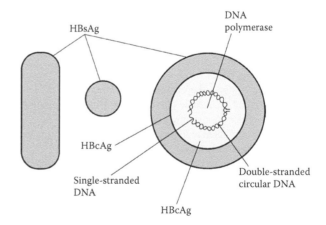

Hepatitis B virus and its antigens.

hepatitis B virus immunity

Hepatitis B virus (HBV) infection leads to chronic liver disease and hepatocellular carcinoma (HCC). The virus is not believed to cause direct cytopathic injury of liver cells. Liver injury is likely due to host immune response. During acute hepatitis B infection, immunoglobulin M (IgM) anti-

HBc, a thymus-independent response, appears in the early phases of the infection together with hepatitis B surface antigen (HBsAg) and HBeAg. Anti-pre-S1 also appears early in the infection, together with a potent major histocompatibility complex (MHC) class-I-restricted cytolytic T lymphocyte (CTL) response specific for numerous epitopes of the structural and nonstructural proteins of the virus. CTLs are critical for viral clearance as are cytokines, interferon (IFN-γ), and tumor necrosis factor (TNF-α). In the early phase of acute hepatitis B, nucleocapsid antigens, hepatitis B core antigen (HBcAg), and HBeAG induce a powerful MHC class-II-restricted T helper cell proliferative response. The MHC class II locus DRB1*-1302 is associated with recovery. The CD4 response has a significant role in recovery. When the virus is eliminated from the liver, HBeAg is lost from the serum and anti-HBe is detected. A short time thereafter, HBsAg is lost and anti-HBs antibodies appear. The immune response fails to eliminate HBV in selected patients who become chronically infected. HBsAg isolated from infected serum or created by recombinant DNA technology represents a successful immunogen in inducing protective immunity against HBV infection.

hepatitis B virus protein X

Refer to HBx.

hepatitis C virus immunity

Hepatitis C virus (HCV)-infected subjects develop specific antibodies whose clinical and biological significance remains to be determined. They are not protective. Most anti-HCV positive sera are also RT–PCR (reverse transcription–polymerase chain reaction)-positive. Antibodies to the envelope glycoproteins may have neutralizing activity. The cellular immune response against recombinant viral antigens has been investigated in proliferation and cytotoxicity assays. Chronic progressive liver disease may be linked to T_H2 cytokine profiles from liver-derived T cells. HCV-specific cytotoxic CD8$^+$ T cells have been found in HCV-infected patients. HCV escapes surveillance by the immune system by altering its antigenic determinants. Problems for vaccine development include diversity of HCV genotypes and subtypes in the hypervariability of HCV species within the host.

hepatitis D virus

Refer to δ agent.

hepatitis E virus (HEV)

Enteric non-A, non-B hepatitis. A single-stranded RNA virus that has an oral–fecal route of transmission and can introduce epidemics under poor sanitary conditions where drinking water is contaminated and the population is poorly nourished.

hepatitis E virus immunity

Immunity against hepatitis E virus (HEV), a self-limiting disease that resembles hepatitis A, consists of an immunoglobulin M (IgM) antibody response against HEV in the acute phase of the disease. Once a peak titer is reached, it declines to undetectable levels 5 months after the immune response begins. IgG titers reach their height during the early convalescent phase and decline during the following months. Half of post-infection patients reveal undetectable levels of HEV-specific IgG although some still reveal IgG antibodies 2 to 14 years following infection. HEV-specific IgG antibodies prevent reinfection and clinical hepatitis E in young adults.

hepatitis (immunopathology panel)

Assays that are very useful for establishing the clinical and immune status of a patient believed to have hepatitis. The

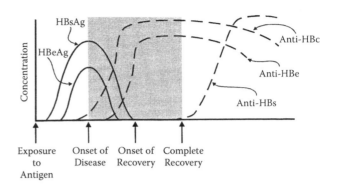

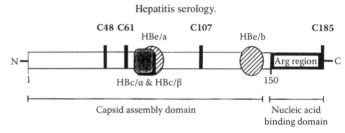

Hepatitis serology.

HBV core polypeptide. The 185-residue p21.5 polypeptide (genotype A) is shown with the amino terminus (N) at the left and the carboxyl terminus (C) at the right. The open region depicts the hydrophobic assembly domain (a.a.s 1–149; open); the Arg-rich nucleic acid binding region is also known as the protamine domain (a.a.s 150–185; shaded). Hatched ovals indicate the approximate locations of the HBe/a and HBe/b antigenic determinants. The shaded rectangle portrays the capsid-specific HBc/α and HBc/β epitopes that supposedly overlap HBe/a. Also indicated are the four Cys residues 48, 61, 107, and 185 (vertical bars).

	150	160	170	180
w.t.	TTVV RRRDRGR sPRRRTP sPRRRRSQ sPRRRRSQ SRESQC			
	I	II	III	IV
Δ172	TTVV RRRDRGR sPRRRTP sPRRRRSQ S			
Δ162	TTVV RRRDRGR sPRRRT			
Δ157	TTVV RRRDRGR Sqc			
Δ149	TTVV			
Δ149R4	TTVV RRRR			

The protamine region of p21.5 contains four Arg-rich repeats that mediate interactions between the core protein and nucleic acid. Shown are the C terminal amino acid sequences (residues 150–185) of wild-type (w.t.) p21.5 (top) and a series of truncated core proteins with defined endpoints.

panel for acute hepatitis may include hepatitis B surface antigen (HBsAg), antibody to hepatitis B core antigen (anti-HBc), anti-hepatitis B surface antigen (anti-ABs), anti-hepatitis A (IgM), anti-HBe, and anti-hepatitis C. The panel for chronic hepatitis (carrier) includes all but the anti-hepatitis A test.

hepatitis, non-A, non-B (C) (NANBH)

The principal cause of hepatitis that is transfusion-related. Risk factors include intravenous drug abuse (42%), unknown risk factors (40%), sexual contact (6%), blood transfusion (6%), household contact (3%), and health professional occupations (2%). In the United States, 150,000 cases per year are reported. Of those, 30 to 50% become chronic carriers and 20% develop cirrhosis. Parenteral NANBH is usually hepatitis C, and enteric NANBH is usually hepatitis E.

hepatitis serology

Hepatitis B antigens and antibodies against them. Core antigen is designated HBc. The HBc particle is comprised of double-stranded DNA and DNA polymerase. It has an association with HBe antigens. Core antigen signifies persistence of replicating hepatitis B virus. Anti-HBc antibody is a serologic indicator of hepatitis B. It is an immunoglobulin M (IgM) antibody that increases early and is still detectable 20 years post-infection. The IgM anti-HBc antibody assay is the best for acute hepatitis B. The HBe antigen (HBeAG) follows the same pattern as HBsAg antigen. When found, it signifies a carrier state. Anti-HBe increases as HBe decreases. Anti-HBe appears in patients who are recovering and may last for years after the hepatitis is resolved. The first antigen detectable following hepatitis B infection is surface antigen (HBsAg). It is detectable a few weeks before clinical disease and is highest with the first appearance of symptoms. It disappears 6 months from infection. Antibody to HBs increases as the HBsAg levels diminish. Anti-HBs is often detectable for the lifetime of the individual.

hepatitis vaccines

The vaccine used to actively immunize subjects against hepatitis B virus contains purified hepatitis B surface antigen. Current practice uses an immunogen prepared by recombinant DNA technology (Recombivax). The antigen preparation is administered in three sequential intramuscular injections to individuals such as physicians, nurses, and other medical personnel who are at risk. Temporary protection against hepatitis A is induced by the passive administration of pooled normal human serum immunoglobulin, which protects against hepatitis A virus for a brief time. Antibody for passive protection against hepatitis must be derived from the blood sera of specifically immune individuals.

hepatocyte-stimulating factor

A substance indistinguishable from interleukin-6 (IL6), classified as a monokine, that stimulates hepatocytes to produce acute phase reactants.

hepatosplenomegaly

Liver and spleen enlargement attributable to an expanded lymphocyte population.

herbimycin A

An inhibitor of T cell activation. Its target is the Sre family of protein tyrosine kinases.

Herceptin®

Refer to trastuzumab.

herd immunity

Nonspecific factors along with specific immunity may have a significant role in resistance of a group (herd) of humans or other animals against an infectious disease agent. Elimination of reservoirs of the disease agent may be as important as specific immunity in diminishing disease incidence among individuals. Herd immunity also means that an epidemic will not follow infection of a single member of the herd or group if other members are immune to that particular infectious agent. The successful vaccination of most members of a population against a selected pathogen may protect nonimmune individuals in the group, whose vulnerability is diminished because the pathogen cannot become established in the vaccinated population.

hereditary angioedema (HAE)

A disorder in which recurrent attacks of edema persisting for 48 to 72 hours occur in the skin and gastrointestinal and respiratory tracts. It is nonpitting and life-threatening if laryngeal edema becomes severe enough to obstruct the airway. Swelling of the epiglottis may lead to suffocation. Edema in the jejunum may be associated with abdominal cramps and bilious vomiting. Edema of the colon may lead to watery diarrhea. No redness or itching is associated with edema of the skin. Tissue trauma of no apparent initiating cause may induce an attack. HAE is due to decreased or absent C1 inhibitor (C1 INH). It is inherited in an autosomal-dominant fashion. Heterozygotes for the defect develop the disorder. Greatly diminished C1 INH levels (5 to 30% of normal) are found in affected individuals. Activation of C1 leads to increased cleavage of C4 and C2, decreasing their serum levels during an attack. C1 INH is also a kinin system inactivator. The C1 INH deficiency in HAE permits a kinin-like peptide produced from C2b to increase vascular permeability, leading to the manifestations of HAE. Some have proposed that bradykinin may represent the vasopermeability factor. Hereditary angioedema has been treated with ε aminocaproic acid and transexamic acid, but they do not elevate C1 INH or C4 levels. Anabolic steroids such as danazol and stanozolol, which activate C1 INH synthesis in affected individuals, represent the treatment of choice.

hereditary angioneurotic edema (HANE)

Refer to hereditary angioedema.

hereditary ataxia telangiectasia

Refer to ataxic telangiectasia.

hereditary complement deficiencies

Associated with defects in activation of the classical pathway that lead to increased susceptibility to pyogenic infections. A deficiency of C3 produces a defect in activation of both the classical and alternative pathways that leads to an increased frequency of pyogenic infections that may prove fatal. Other characteristics are defective opsonization and phagocytosis. Defects of alternate pathway factors D and P lead to impaired activation of the alternative pathway with increased susceptibility to pyogenic infections. Deficiencies of C5 through C9 are associated with defective membrane attack complex (MAC) formation and lysis of cells, including bacteria. This produces increased susceptibility to disseminated *Neisseria* infection.

herpes gestationis (HG)

A very pruritic blistering condition of the skin characterized by vesicles and bullae that develop in rare cases of pregnancy. HG is rare in black subjects and is associated with HLA-DR3 and DR4. By light microscopy, a subepidermal bulla with eosinophils may be identified in a few cases. Edema of the papillary dermis, lymphohistiocytic infiltrate with eosinophils in perivascular regions, spongiosis, liquefactive degeneration, and possible necrosis in the epidermis are present. The eruption occurs usually in the second or third trimester of pregnancy and appears as hive-like plaques, blisters, or vesicles. Immunofluorescence reveals C3 at the dermal–epidermal junction in nearly all cases, and IgG in 25% of biopsies. Circulating IgG antibody binds to the herpes gestationis antigen, a 180-kDa epidermal protein in the skin basement membrane.

herpes gestationis (HG) antibodies

Antibodies present in 89% of HG sera that are incomplete Freund's adjuvant (IFA)-positive and in sera of 47% of patients with bullous pemphigoid. These antibodies are not

H

found in physiologic pregnancy. Direct immunofluorescence may be used to demonstrate immunoglobulin G (IgG) antibodies against the basement membrane zone in 30 to 50% of HG cases. By contrast, C3 is demonstrable at the skin basement membrane zones in almost 100% of cases. Use of the sensitive immunoblotting method permits identification of antibodies against the hemidesmosome constituents of the basement membrane zones in the skin of 90% of HG subjects.

herpes gestationis (HG) autoantibodies

Autoantibodies from patients with herpes gestationis (HG) and bullous pemphigoid (BP) react with epidermal hemidesmosome 230- and 180-kDa proteins, respectively, helping to anchor basal keratinocytes to the lamina densa of the basement membrane. Although not present in normal pregnancy, HG autoantibodies are found in 71 to 89% of positive HG sera and in 47 to 53% of BP sera. Immunoglobulin G (IgG) autoantibodies to the basement membrane zone (BMZ) are revealed by direct immunofluorescence in 30 to 50% of cases, whereas C3 is detected at the BMZ of perilesional skin in approximately 100% of HG. With immunoblotting, serum antibodies to heterogeneous hemidesmosomal components of the BMZ can be detected in about 90% of HG patients. The MCW-1 antigenic site that comprises a part of the noncollagenous domain is believed to be involved in subepidermal blister formation. Patients with HG and their relatives face increased risk for development of other autoimmune conditions such as Graves' disease.

herpes simplex virus 1 and 2 (HSV-1 and HSV-2) polyclonal antibody

An antibody used to identify specific and qualitative localization of herpes simplex virus (HSV) types 1 and 2 in formalin-fixed, paraffin-embedded or frozen tissue sections.

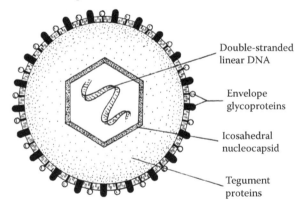

Double-stranded linear DNA

Envelope glycoproteins

Icosahedral nucleocapsid

Tegument proteins

Herpesvirus.

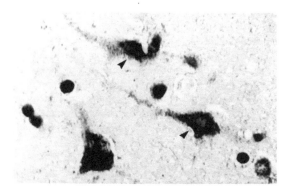

Herpes simplex in the brain.

HSV-1 is most often acquired during early childhood by non-venereal means and causes gingivostomatitis (fever blisters). HSV-2 is usually acquired by venereal contact but can also be acquired by a neonate from an infected mother's genital tract at the time of delivery. HSV-2 causes herpes genitalis.

herpes simplex virus immunity

The two related subtypes of herpes simplex virus (HSV) are designated HSV-1 and HSV-2. The viruses are named human herpesviruses 1 and 2, respectively. The immune response to HSV has been investigated mainly in mouse, rabbit, and guinea pig models. Genetic resistance of a host animal is a result of several mechanisms, such as the effective killing actions of macrophages and natural killer (NK) cells and interferon synthesis. NK cells and interferon activity can restrict an infection but cannot clear the virus, which depends on the host-specific immune response. Both antibody and T cell immunity are induced. Antibodies interact with the virus, infected-cell glycoproteins, capsid proteins, and selected infected-cell polypeptides. In mice, passively transferred antibodies against HSV can protect from lethal doses of the virus. Antibody alone is insufficient to clear virus from the nervous system or the periphery; it may retard virus spread through the nervous system. Antibody activities of HSV-specific antibody *in vitro* include virus neutralization, complement-mediated cytotoxicity, and antibody-dependent cell-mediated cytotoxicity (ADCC). Reactivation and recurrence or reinfection with HSV in humans often occurs in the presence of high titers of neutralizing antibodies, which reveals that the antibody has failed to protect. T cells are vital in HSV infections. The cytotoxic T lymphocyte response to HSV is mediated by CD8+ T lymphocytes in both humans and mice. CD4+ major histocompatibility complex (MHC) class-II-restricted lymphocytes are involved in the delayed-type hypersensitivity response to HSV; CTL activity and T cells help in antibody production. CD4+ T cells are critical for clearance of the virus. The T_H1 subset is protective. HSV survives for many years in the host through establishment of a latent infection without discernible protein expression. The efficacy of avirulent or inactivated virus and subunit vaccines has not been definitely established in human trials. Animal trials have revealed that protection can be induced with glycoprotein D using recombinant *Salmonella* introduced orally.

herpesvirus

A DNA virus family that contains a central icosahedral core of double-stranded DNA and a trilaminar lipoprotein envelope that is 100 nm in diameter and has a nucleus 30 to 43 nm in diameter. Herpesviruses may persist for years in a dormant state. Six types have been described. HSV-1 (herpes simplex virus 1) can account for oral lesions such as fever blisters. HHV-2 (human herpesvirus 2) produces lesions below the waistline and is sexually transmitted. It may produce venereal disease of the vagina and vulva, as well as herpetic ulcers of the penis. HHV-3 (herpes varicella zoster) occurs clinically as an acute form known as chickenpox or as a chronic form termed shingles. HHV-4 (Epstein–Barr virus), HHV-5 (cytomegalovirus), and HHV-6 (human B cell lymphotrophic virus) are the other types.

herpesvirus-6 immunity

Humoral immune responses during primary infection include an immunoglobulin M (IgM) response. Secondary infection is associated with an increase in IgG titer as well as a recrudescence of IgM reactivity. The humoral immune response is strongly cross reactive among HHV-6 variants. The T cell response to infection remains to be elucidated.

herpesvirus-8 immunity

Antibodies specific for a latent HHV-8 antigen and to a recombinant structural antigen present in patients with Kaposi's sarcoma or those at risk for developing this disease. Strong evidence links HHV-8 and the pathogenesis of Kaposi's sarcoma. Antibodies to HHV-8 antigens occur more often in HIV-uninfected homosexual men than in the general population including blood donors. Antibodies to undefined structural HHV-8 antigens are present in one quarter of all blood donors in North America; yet, antibodies to the recombinant capsid-related and latent HHV-8 proteins are present in 0 to 2% of blood donors in North America and Northern Europe.

herpes zoster

A viral infection that occurs in a band-like pattern according to distribution in the skin-involved nerves. It is usually a reactivation of the virus that causes chickenpox.

Herxheimer reaction

A serum sickness (type III) form of hypersensitivity that occurs following the treatment of selected chronic infectious diseases with an effective drug. When the microorganisms are destroyed in large numbers in the blood circulation, a significant amount of antigen is released from the disrupted microbes that tend to react with preformed antibodies in the circulation. This type of reaction has been described after the use of effective drugs to treat syphilis, trypanosomiasis, and brucellosis.

heteroantibody

An autoantibody with the ability to cross react with an antigen of a different species.

heteroantigen

An antigen that induces an immune response in a species other than the one from which it was derived.

heteroclitic antibody

An antibody with greater affinity for a heterologous epitope than for the homologous one that stimulated its synthesis.

heterocliticity

The preferential binding by an antibody to an epitope other than the one that generated synthesis of the antibody.

heteroconjugate

Hybrids of two different antibody molecules.

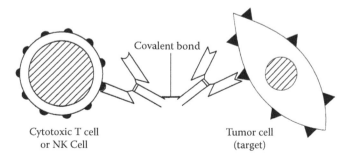

Covalent bond

Cytotoxic T cell
or NK Cell

Tumor cell
(target)

Heteroconjugate antibodies.

heteroconjugate antibodies

Antibodies against a tumor antigen coupled covalently to an antibody specific for a natural killer (NK) cell or cytotoxic T lymphocyte surface antigen. These antibodies facilitate binding of cytotoxic effector cells to tumor target cells. Antibodies against effector cell surface markers may also

be coupled covalently with hormones that bind to receptors on tumor cells. Hybrids of two different antibody molecules.

heterocytotropic antibody

An antibody that has a greater affinity when fixed to mast cells of a species other than the one in which the antibody is produced. Frequently assayed by skin-fixing ability, as revealed through the passive cutaneous anaphylaxis test. Interaction with the antigen for which these "fixed" antibodies are specific may lead to local heterocytotrophic anaphylaxis.

heterodimer

A molecule comprised of two components that are different but closely joined structures, such as a protein comprised of two separate chains. Examples include the T cell receptor comprised of either α and β chains or γ and δ chains and class I along with class II histocompatibility molecules.

heterogeneic

Refer to xenogeneic.

heterogeneous nuclear ribonuleoprotein (9RA-33) autoantibodies

Heterogeneous nuclear ribonucleoprotein (hnRNP) autoantibodies are associated mainly with rheumatoid arthritis (RA), systemic lupus erythematosus (SLE), and mixed connective tissue disease (MCTD) and less often with other connective tissue diseases. The role of these autoantibodies in the pathogenesis of the diseases cited is unknown. RA-33 autoantibodies have been correlated with severe erosive arthritis in lupus patients. They appear early in the course of the disease, thus rendering them valuable in the diagnosis of early RA, especially rheumatoid factor (RF-negative RA). Both enzyme immunoassay (EIA) and immunoblotting techniques have been used to detect these antibodies.

heterogenetic antibody

Refer to heterophile antibody.

heterogenetic antigen

Refer to heterophile antigen.

heterograft

Refer to xenograft.

heterokaryon

The formation of a hybrid cell by fusion of two or more separate cells that are not genetically identical, leading to a cell with two nuclei and a single cytoplasm. Cell fusion may be accomplished through the use of polyethylene glycol or ultraviolet light-inactivated Sendai virus.

heterologous

In transplantation biology, refers to an organ or tissue transplant from one species to a recipient belonging to another species (i.e., a xenogeneic graft). It also refers to a material from a foreign source.

heterologous antigen

A cross reacting antigen.

heterologous vaccine

A vaccine that induces protective immunity against pathogenic microorganisms that it does not contain. The microorganisms present in the heterologous vaccine possess antigens that cross react with those of the pathogenic agent absent from the vaccine. Measles vaccine can stimulate protection against canine distemper. Vaccinia virus was used in the past to induce immunity against smallpox because the agents of vaccinia and variola share antigens in common.

heterophile antibody

An antibody found in an animal of one species that can react with erythrocytes of a different and phylogenetically

H

unrelated species. The antibody is often an immunoglobulin M (IgM) agglutinin. Heterophile antibodies are detected in infectious mononucleosis patients who demonstrate antibodies reactive with sheep erythrocytes. To differentiate this condition from serum sickness, which also is associated with high titers of heterophile antibodies, the serum sample is absorbed with beef erythrocytes that contain Forssman antigen. This treatment removes the heterophile antibody reactivity from the sera of infectious mononucleosis patients.

heterophile antigen

An antigen (epitope) present in divergent animal species, plants, and bacteria that manifests broad cross reactivity with antibodies of the heterophile group. Heterophile antigens induce the formation of heterophile antibodies when introduced into a species in which they are absent. Heterophile antigens are often carbohydrates.

heterospecific

Showing specificity for a species other than the one from which the substance in question was derived.

heterotopic

The placement of an organ or tissue graft in an anatomic site other than the one where it is normally located.

heterotopic graft

A tissue or organ transplanted to an anatomic site other than the one where it is usually found under natural conditions—for example, the anastomosis of the renal vasculature at an anatomical site that would situate the kidney in a place other than the renal fossa, where it is customarily found.

heterotypic vaccine

Refer to heterologous vaccine.

heterozygosity

The presence of different alleles at one or more loci on homologous chromosomes.

heterozygous

Descriptor for individuals possessing two different alleles of a particular gene.

HEV

Refer to high endothelial venules.

Hewson, William (1739–1774)

British physician credited as the "father of hematology."

Heymann antigen

A 330-kDa glycoprotein (GP330) present on visceral epithelial cell basal surfaces in coated pits and on tubular brush borders. It participates in production of experimental nephritis in rats. See also Heymann glomerulonephritis.

Heymann glomerulonephritis

An experimental model of membranous glomerulonephritis induced by immunizing rats with proximal tubule brush border preparations containing subepithelial antigen or Heymann factor, a 330-kDa protein incorporated in Freund's adjuvant. The rats produce antibodies against brush border antigens and membranous glomerulonephritis is induced. Autoantibodies combine with shed epithelial cell antigen. The union of antibody with Heymann antigen, distributed in an interrupted manner along visceral epithelial cell surfaces, leads to subepithelial electron-dense, granular deposits. Immunoglobulins and complement are deposited in a granular rather than linear pattern along the glomerular basement membrane, as revealed by immunofluorescence. The glomerulonephritis results from interaction

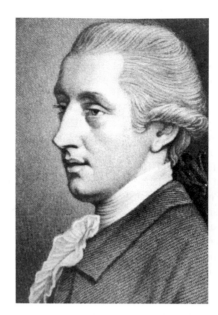

William Hewson.

of anti-brush border antibody with the 330-kDa glycoprotein, which is fixed but discontinuously distributed on the bases of visceral epithelial cells and is cross reactive with brush border antigens. Heymann nephritis closely resembles human membranous glomerulonephritis.

Heymann's nephritis

Refer to Heymann glomerulonephritis.

HGG

Abbreviation for human γ globulin.

HGP-30

An experimental vaccine for AIDS that employs a synthetic HIV core protein, p17.

HHV

Human herpesvirus.

Hib (*Hemophilus influenzae* type b)

A microorganism that induces infection, mostly in infants below 5 years of age. Approximately 1,000 deaths among 20,000 annual cases are recorded. A polysaccharide vaccine (Hib Vac) was of only marginal efficacy and poorly immunogenic. By contrast, anti-Hib vaccine that contains capsular polysaccharide of Hib bound covalently to a carrier protein such as polyribosylribitol–diphtheria toxoid (PRP-D) induces a very high level of protection, for example, 94% in one cohort of Finnish infants. PRP–tetanus toxoid has induced 75% protection, and PRP–diphtheria toxoid vaccine is claimed to be 88% effective.

hidden determinant

An epitope on a cell or molecule that is unavailable for interaction with either lymphocyte receptors or the antigen-binding region of antibody molecules because of stereochemical factors. These hidden or cryptic determinants neither react with lymphocyte or antibody receptors nor induce an immune response unless an alteration in the steric configuration of the molecule causes the epitope to be exposed.

HIG

Acronym for human immune globulin.

high-dose tolerance

Specific immunologic unresponsiveness induced by the repeated administration of large doses of antigen (tolerogen) if the substance is a protein or a massive single dose if the

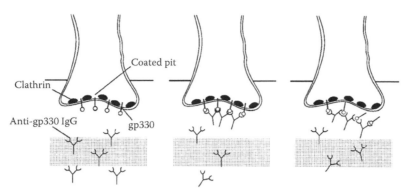

Heymann's glomerulonephritis.

substance is a polysaccharide to immunocompetent adult animals. Although no precise inducing dose of antigen can be defined, usually in high-dose tolerance the antigen level exceeds 10^4 mol antigen per kilogram of body weight. Also called high-zone tolerance.

high endothelial postcapillary venules

Lymphoid organ vessels that are especially designed for circulating lymphocytes to gain access into the parenchyma of an organ. They contain cuboidal endothelium that permits lymphocytes to pass between the cells into the tissues. Lymphocyte recirculation from the blood to the lymph occurs through these vessel walls.

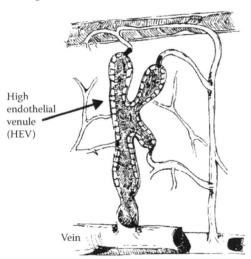

High endothelial venules (HEVs).

high endothelial venules (HEVs)

Postcapillary venules of lymph node paracortical areas. They also occur in Peyer's patches that are components of gut-associated lymphoid tissue (GALT). Their specialized columnar cells bear receptors for antigen-primed lymphocytes. They signal lymphocytes to leave the peripheral blood circulation. These cuboidal cells express adhesion molecules that promote adherence and transendothelial passage of naïve lymphocytes. A homing receptor for circulating lymphocytes is found in lymph nodes.

high responder

A mouse, guinea pig, or other inbred strain that mounts pronounced immune responses to selected antigens in comparison to the responses of other strains including so-called low responder strains. Immune response (IR) genes encode this capability.

high titer, low avidity antibodies (HTLAs)

Antibodies that induce erythrocyte agglutination at high dilutions in the Coombs' antiglobulin test. These antibodies cause only weak agglutination and are almost never linked to hemolysis of clinical importance. Examples of HTLA antibodies are anti-Bg^a, -Cs, -Ch, -Kna, -JMH, -Rg, and -Yk, among others.

high-zone tolerance

Antigen-induced specific immunosuppression with relatively large doses of protein antigens (tolerogens). B cell tolerance usually requires high antigen doses. High-zone tolerance is relatively short lived. Called also high-dose tolerance. Refer to high-dose tolerance.

higher vertebrates

Animals with backbones, including the agnatha (jawless fish such as lampreys); Chondrichthyes (cartilaginous jawed fish such as skates, sharks and rays); Osteichthyes (bony jawed fish including lobe-finned, ray-finned, and advanced bony fishes such as salmon); amphibians (frogs, toads, and salamanders); reptiles (crocodiles and snakes); birds; and mammals that include such divergent species as mice and humans.

highly active antiretroviral therapy (HAART)

The combined use of reverse transcriptase inhibitors and a viral protease inhibitor for HIV infection. This therapy can diminish virus titers to undetectable levels for more than a year and slow the progression of HIV disease. The combination slows the development of drug-resistant mutant viruses that arise when a lone drug is used.

highly polymorphic

Units of inheritance (i.e., genes) possessing numerous alleles for which most subjects in a population are heterozygous.

hinge region

An area of an immunoglobulin heavy chain situated between the first constant domain and the second constant domain (C_H1 and C_H2) in an immunoglobulin (Ig) polypeptide chain. The high content of proline residues in this region provides considerable flexibility to this area, which enables the Fab region of an immunoglobulin molecule to combine with cell surface epitopes it might not otherwise reach. Fab regions of an Ig molecule can rotate on the hinge region. The angle between the two Fab regions of an IgG molecule may extend up to 180°. In addition to the proline residues, one or several half cysteines may be associated with the interchain disulfide bonds. Enzyme action by papain or pepsin occurs near the hinge region. Whereas γ, α, and δ chains contain hinge regions, μ and ε chains do not. The 5′ part of the C_H2 exon encodes the human and

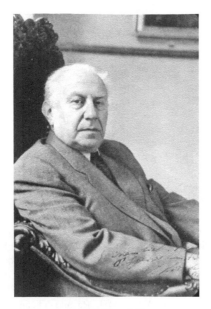

Ludwik Hirszfeld.

mouse α chain hinge region. Four exons encode the γ-3 chains of humans, and two exons encode human δ chains.

Hirszfeld, Ludwik (1884–1954)
Hirszfeld and Emil von Dungern studied the genetics of blood groups.

histaminase
A common tissue enzyme, termed diamine oxidase, that transforms histamine into imidazoleacetic acid, an inactive substance.

histamine
A biologically active amine (i.e., δ-aminoethylimidazole) with a molecular weight of 111 kDa that induces contraction of the smooth muscles of human bronchioles and small blood vessels, increased capillary permeability, and increased secretion by the mucous glands of the nose and bronchial tree. It is a principal pharmacological mediator of immediate (type I) hypersensitivity (anaphylaxis) in humans and guinea pigs. Although found in many tissues, it is especially concentrated in mast cells of the tissues and basophils of the blood. It is stored in their cytoplasmic granules and is released following cross linking of immunoglobulin E (IgE) antibodies by a specific antigen on their surfaces. It is produced by the decarboxylation of histidine through the action of histidine decarboxylase. When histamine combines with H_1 receptors, smooth muscle contraction and increased vascular permeability may result. Combination with H_2 receptors induces gastric secretion and blocks mediator release from mast cells and basophils. It may interfere with suppressor T cell function. Histamine attracts eosinophils that produce histaminase, which degrades histamine.

histamine release assay
In 4 to 13% of allergic patients, the immunoglobulin E (IgE)-mediated release of histamine from basophils depends on cytokines. These anti-IgE-non-releasers respond to f–Met–Leu–Pro (FMLP), which bypasses the IgE receptor pathway. Histamine release assays are valuable when skin testing and RAST function suboptimally, especially in patients with urticaria and atopic dermatitis in whom only a weak correlation between IgE and disease is apparent. Histamine release assays may be informative in patients with urticaria, asthma, and atopic dermatitis.

histamine release factors (HRFs)
Protein cytokines that cause release of histamine from basophils and mast cells. The 12-kDa HRF is similar to connective-tissue-activating peptide III (CTAP-III) and its degradation product, neutrophil-activating peptide 2 (NAP-2). The sera of patients with chronic idiopathic urticaria (CIU) contain a histamine-releasing factor in the IgG fraction of serum that correlates with disease activity.

The synthesis of histamine, a principal mediator of immediate (Type I) hypersensitivity reactions.

histamine-releasing factor

A lymphokine produced from antigen-stimulated lymphocytes that induces the release of histamine from basophils.

histiocyte

A tissue macrophage that is fixed in the tissues such as connective tissues. Histiocytes are frequently found around blood vessels and are actively phagocytic. They may be derived from monocytes in the circulating blood.

histiocytic lymphoma

A misnomer for large cell lymphomas, principally B cell tumors. The term *histiocytic lymphoma* more accurately describes a lymphoma of macrophage lineage.

histiocytosis X

A descriptor for neoplasms of macrophage lineage. Included in this category are Letterer–Siwe disease, Hand–Schüller–Christian disease, and eosinophilic granuloma of bone.

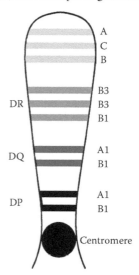

Human chromosome 6.

histocompatibility

Tissue compatibility, as in the transplantation of tissues or organs from one member to another of the same species (allograft) or from one species to another (xenograft). The genes that encode antigens that should match if a tissue or organ graft is to survive in a recipient are located in the major histocompatibility complex (MHC) region on the short arm of chromosome 6 in humans and on chromosome 17 in mice. MHC class I and class II antigens are important in tissue transplantation. The greater the match between donor and recipient, the more likely a transplant is to survive. For example, a six-antigen match implies sharing of two HLA-A antigens, two HLA-B antigens, and two HLA-DR antigens between donor and recipient. Even though antigenically dissimilar grafts may survive when a powerful immunosuppressive drug such as cyclosporine is used, the longevity of the graft is still improved by having as many antigens match as possible.

histocompatibility antigen

One of a group of genetically encoded antigens present on tissue cells that provoke a rejection response if the tissue containing them is transplanted to a genetically dissimilar recipient. These antigens are detected by typing lymphocytes on which they are expressed. They are encoded in humans by genes at the human leukocyte antigen (HLA) locus on the short arm of chromosome 6. In mice, they are encoded by genes at the H-2 locus on chromosome 17.

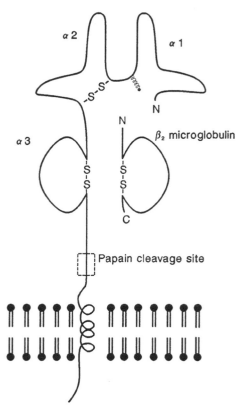

Hand-mirror cell.

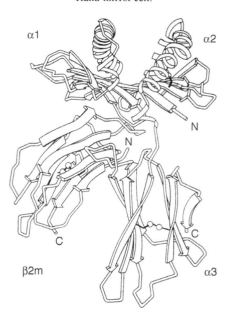

Schematic representation of the three-dimensional structure of the external domains of a human class I HLA molecule based on x-ray crystallographic analysis. The β strands are depicted as thick arrows and the α helices as spiral ribbons. Disulfide bonds are shown as two interconnected spheres. The α_1 and α_2 domains interact to form the peptide-binding cleft. Note the immunoglobulin-fold structure of the α_3 and α_2 microglobulin.

histocompatibility locus

The specific site on a chromosome where the histocompatibility genes that encode histocompatibility antigens are located. There are major histocompatibility loci such as human leukocyte antigen (HLA) in humans and H-2 in

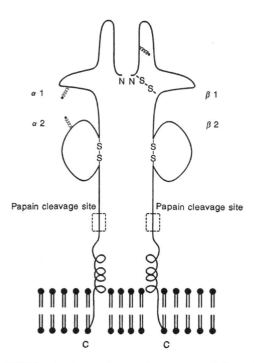

Class II MHC molecules are glycoprotein histocompatibility antigens that play a critical role in immune system cellular interactions. Each class II MHC molecule is comprised of a 32- to 34-kDa α chain and a 29- to 32-kDa β chain, each of which possesses N-linked oligosaccharide groups, amino termini that are extracellular, and carboxyl termini that are intracellular. Approximately 70% of both α and β chains are extracellular.

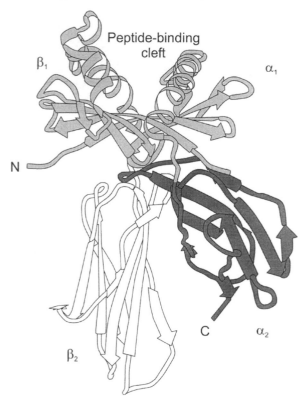

MHC class II molecular structure.

mice, across which incompatible grafts are rejected within 1 to 2 weeks, and several minor histocompatibility loci with more subtle antigenic differences, across which only slow, low-level graft rejection reactions occur.

histocompatibility testing

Determination of the major histocompatibility complex (MHC) class I and class II tissue types of both donor and recipient prior to organ or tissue transplantation. In humans, HLA-A, HLA-B, and HLA-DR types are determined, followed by cross matching donor lymphocytes with recipient serum prior to transplantation. A mixed lymphocyte culture (MLC) is necessary for bone marrow transplantation, in conjunction with molecular DNA typing. The MLC may also be requested in living related organ transplants. As in renal allotransplantation, serum samples of organ recipients are tested for percent reactive antibodies, which reveals whether they have been presensitized against HLA antigens of organs for which they may be the recipients.

histone antibodies

Antibodies of the immunoglobulin G (IgG) class against H2A–H2B histones detectable in essentially all procainamide-induced lupus patients manifesting symptoms. They are also present in approximately one fifth of systemic lupus erythematosus (SLE) patients and in procainamide-treated persons who do not manifest symptoms. Antibodies against H2A, H2B, and H2A–H2B complex react well with histone fragments resistant to trypsin. By contrast, antibodies in the sera of SLE patients manifest reactivity for intact histones but not with their fragments. In lupus induced by hydralazine, antihistone antibodies react mainly with H3 and H4 and their fragments that are resistant to trypsin.

histone autoantibodies ((non-H2A–H2B)–DNA)

H1–H4 autoantibodies of the immunoglobulin M (IgM) isotype are broadly reactive and frequently found in patients with systemic lupus erythematosus (SLE) and in normal persons taking various medications. Patients with localized scleroderma (40 to 60%) and those with generalized morphea (80%) demonstrate autoantibodies against histones H1, H2A, and H2B. Systemic sclerosis patients (29%) and diffuse cutaneous systemic sclerosis patients (44%) reveal histone H1 autoantibodies associated with the severity of pulmonary fibrosis in systemic sclerosis. Autoantibodies against histone (H2A–H2B)–DNA complexes are seen more frequently in scleroderma-related disorders than in SLE. Elevated IgA antibodies against all H1, H2A, H2B, H3, and H4 are detectable in IgA nephropathy, primary glomerulonephritis, membranous glomerulonephritis, and idiopathic nephrotic syndrome. The serum histone autoantibody titer is also positively correlated with the extent of dementia in Alzheimer's disease.

histone (H2A–H2B)–DNA complex autoantibodies

Immunoglobulin G (IgG) autoantibodies against histones develop in drug-induced lupus (DIL) in the absence of other autoantibodies. They show high reactivity with histone H2A–H2B dimers, when induced by procainamide. The autoantibodies diminish when the drug is discontinued. IgM autoantibodies against histone H1–H4 are found frequently in systemic lupus erythematosus (SLE) and in persons receiving a variety of medications. Autoantibodies against histone (H2A–H2B)–DNA complexes are generated in DIL attributable to procainamide, quinidine, acebutolol, penicillamine, and isoniazid but not methyldopa. H2A and H2B histone linear epitopes are identified by separate histone autoantibody populations associated with SLE, DIL, juvenile rheumatoid arthritis, and scleroderma.

Histoplasma immunity

Cell-mediated immunity is the main host defense against infection with *Histoplasma capsulatum*. The specific cell-

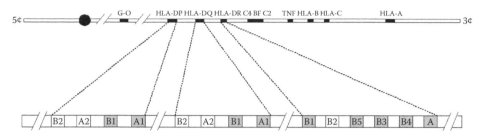

Short arm of human chromosome 6.

mediated response in humans occurs in lymphoid organs and other tissues 7 to 18 days following exposure to conidia. This leads to initiation of the healing of lesions and organs with the formation of granulomas having central necrosis. Lymph nodes that drain sites of infection are large and encapsulate and may calcify. Delayed-type hypersensitivity responses to histoplasmin are detectable a month after infection. Macrophages and neutrophils may harbor *H. capsulatum.* Yeasts and conidia that are not coated with opsonins bind to epitopes of the lymphocyte-function-associated antigen 1 (CD11a/CD18), complement receptor type III (CD11b/CD18), and the P-150–195 complex (CD11c/CD18) of adhesion-promoting receptors on human macrophages. Yeast binding requires divalent cations. Human macrophages form hydrogen peroxide. *Histoplasma* yeasts fail to induce a respiratory burst when phagocytosed. Antigen-specific CD4+ T lymphocytes mediate both protective immunity and delayed-type hypersensitivity. Cytokines that influence the outcome of infection in naïve animals include interleukin 12 (IL12) and tumor necrosis factor α (TNF-α). IL3, granulocyte–macrophage colony-stimulating factor (GM-CSF), and macrophage CSF activate human macrophages to block yeast cell growth. There is no licensed vaccine for *H. capsulatum,* but its heat shock protein system may be a promising candidate for a future vaccine.

histoplasmin

An extract from cultures of *Histoplasma capsulatum* that is injected intradermally, in the same manner as the tuberculin test, to evaluate whether an individual has cell-mediated immunity against this microorganism.

histoplasmin test

A skin test analogous to the tuberculin skin test, which determines whether an individual manifests delayed-type hypersensitivity (cell-mediated) immunity to *Histoplasma capsulatum,*

the causative agent of histoplasmosis in humans. A positive skin test implies a current or earlier infection with *H. capsulatum.*

histotope

That portion of a major histocompatibility complex (MHC) class II molecule that reacts with a T lymphocyte receptor.

Hitchens, A. Parker

First chairman of the American Association of Immunologists Council, father of the association's constitution and bylaws and the force behind development of an association journal.

HIV

Abbreviation for human immunodeficiency virus.

HIV-1 genes

The *gag* gene encodes the structural core proteins p17, p24, p15, and p55 precursor. The *pol* gene encodes a protease that cleaves *gag* precursors. It also encodes reverse transcriptase, which produces proviral DNA from RNA, and an integrase necessary for proviral insertion. The *env* gene encodes gp160 precursor, gp120, and gp41 in mature proteins; gp120 binds CD4 molecules; and gp41 is needed for fusion of the virus with the cell; the function of *vpr* is unknown; *vif* encodes a 23-kDa product that is necessary for infection of cells by free virus and is not needed for infection from cell to cell; *tat* encodes a p14 product that binds to viral long terminal repeat (LTR) sequence and activates viral gene transcription; *rev* encodes a 20-kDa protein product required for post-transcriptional expression of *gag* and *env* genes; *nef* encodes a 27-kDa protein that inhibits human immunodeficiency virus (HIV) transcription and slows viral replication; and *vpu* encodes a 16-kDa protein product that may be required for assembly and packaging of new virus particles.

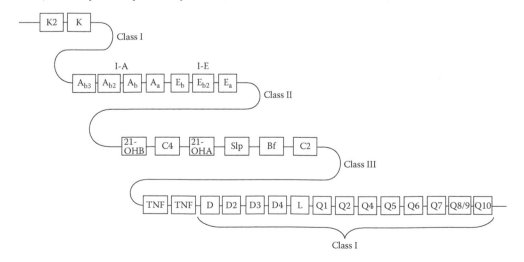

H-2 complex on chromosome 17 of a mouse.

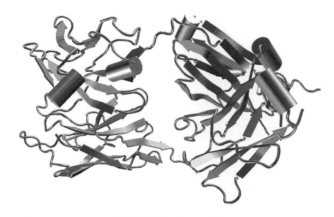

Anti HIV-1 protease Fab.

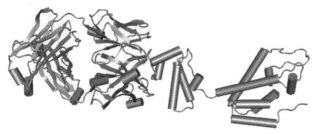

HIV-1 capsid protein (P24).

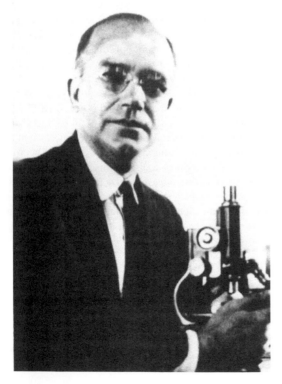

A. Parker Hitchens.

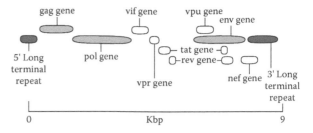

Human immunodeficiency virus 1 (HIV-1) genes..

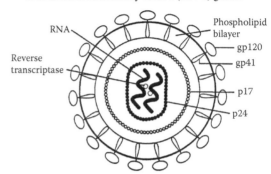

HIV-1 virus structure.

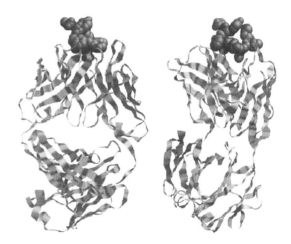

IgG/gp120 complex.

HIV-1 virus structure

Human immunodeficiency virus 1 (HIV-1) is composed of two identical RNA strands that constitute the viral genome. These are associated with reverse transcriptase and p17 and p24, which are core polypeptides. These components are all enclosed in a phospholipid membrane envelope derived from the host cell. Proteins gp120 and gp41 encoded by the virus are anchored to the envelope.

HIV-2

Human immunodeficiency virus 2 (HIV-2) was previously named HTLV-IV, LAV-2, and SIV/AGM. This virus was first discovered in individuals from western Africa who showed aberrant reactions to HIV-1 and simian immunodeficiency virus (SIV). It shows greater sequence homology (70%) with SIV/membrane attack complex (MAC) than with HIV-1 (40% sequence homology). It has only 50% conservation for *gag* and *pol*; the remaining HIV genes are even less conserved. It has p24, gp36, and gp140 structural antigens. Its clinical course resembles that of AIDS produced by HIV-1, but it is confined principally to western Africa and is transmitted principally through heterosexual promiscuity.

HIV-2V

Human immunodeficiency virus 2 (HIV-2) that possesses *X-ORF* and *VPX*, both of which are unique to it.

HIV coreceptors

Human immunodeficiency virus 1 (HIV-1) virus strains use the chemokine receptors CCR-5 or CXCR-4 or both to enter cells. Expression of these receptors may predetermine susceptibility of hematopoietic subsets to HIV-1 infection.

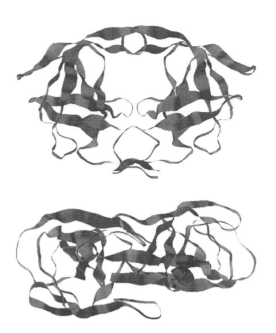

Nuclear magnetic resonance (NMR) image of human immunologic deficiency virus 1 (HIV-1) protease.

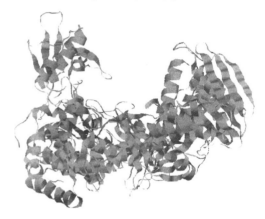

Human immunodeficiency virus 1 (HIV-1) reverse transcriptase.

Certain cytokines can influence the dynamics of HIV-1 infection by altering chemokine receptor expression levels on hematopoietic cells. During chronic HIV-1 infection, proinflammatory cytokines such as tumor necrosis factor α (TNF-α) and interferon γ (IFN-γ) are secreted in excess. IFN-γ increases cell surface expression of CCR-5 by human mononuclear phagocytes and of CXCR-4 by primary hematopoietic cells. In addition, GN-CSF can decrease and interleukin-10 (IL10) can increase expression of CCR-5. Further research into cytokine-mediated regulation of chemokine receptors may lead to increased understanding of how these receptors affect the pathogenesis of AIDS.

HIV infection

Recognition of infection by the human immunodeficiency virus (HIV) is through seroconversion. Following conversion to positive reactivity in an antibody screening test, a western blot analysis is performed to confirm the result of positive testing for HIV. HIV mainly affects the immune system and the brain. It affects the CD4+ lymphocytes that are necessary to initiate an immune response by interaction with antigen-presenting cells, and thus deprives other cells of the immune system from receiving a supply of interleukin-2 (IL2) through CD4+ lymphocyte stimulation, leading to a progressive decline

in immune system function. HIV transmission is by sexual contact, through blood products, or occurs horizontally from mother to young. Although first observed in male homosexuals, it later became a major problem of intravenous drug abusers and ultimately has become more serious in the heterosexual population, affecting increasing numbers of women and men. Clinically, individuals may develop acute HIV mononucleosis that usually occurs 2 to 6 weeks following infection, although it may occur later. The main symptoms include headache, fever, malaise, sore throat, and rash. Patients may develop pharyngitis; generalized lymphadenopathy; a macular or urticarial rash on the face, trunk, and limbs; and hepatosplenomegaly. The severity of the symptoms may vary. Acute HIV infection may also induce neurologic diseases including meningitis, encephalitis, and other manifestations. Some individuals may not develop symptoms or illness for years. Others develop AIDS-related complex (ARC), which represents progressive immune dysfunction. Symptoms include fever, night sweats, weight loss, chronic diarrhea, generalized lymphadenopathy, herpes zoster, and oral lesions. Individuals with ARC may progress to AIDS or death may occur in the ARC stage. ARC patients do not revert to an asymptomatic condition. Other individuals may develop persistent generalized lymphadenopathy (PGL) characterized by enlarged lymph nodes in the neck, axilla, and groin. The Centers for Disease Control (CDC) set up criteria for the diagnosis of AIDS that include the individuals who develop certain opportunistic infections and neoplasms, HIV-related encephalopathy, and HIV-induced wasting syndrome. The most frequent opportunistic infections in AIDS patients include *Pneumocystis carinii,* which produces pneumonia, and *Mycobacterium avium-intracellulare,* among other microorganisms. The most frequent tumor found in AIDS patients is Kaposi's sarcoma. At present, AIDS is 100% fatal.

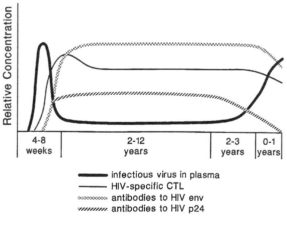

HIV serology..

hives

A wheal-and-flare reaction of the anaphylactic type produced in the skin as a consequence of histamine produced by activated mast cells. The reaction is accompanied by edema, erythema, and pruritus. *Hives* is a synonym for urticaria.

HL

Abbreviation for Hodgkin lymphoma.

HLA

Acronym for human leukocyte antigen. The HLA histocompatibility system in humans represents a complex of major histocompatibility complex (MHC) class I molecules

H

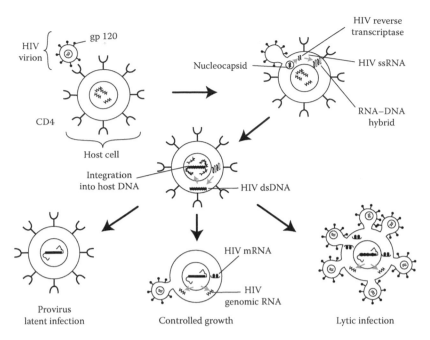

Human immunodeficiency virus (HIV) infection.

distributed on essentially all nucleated cells of the body and MHC class II molecules that are distributed on B lymphocytes, macrophages, and a few other cell types. These are encoded by genes at the MHC. The HLA locus in humans is found on the short arm of chromosome 6. This has now been well defined. In addition to encoding surface isoantigens, genes at the HLA locus also encode immune response (IR) genes. The class I region consists of HLA-A, HLA-B, and HLA-C loci, and the class II region consists of the D region, which is subdivided into HLA-DP, HLA-DQ, and HLA-DR subregions. Class II molecules play an important role in the induction of an immune response, as antigen-presenting cells must complex an antigen with class II molecules to present it in the presence of interleukin-1 (IL1) to CD4+ T lymphocytes. Class I molecules are important in the presentation of intracellular antigen to CD8+ T lymphocytes and for effector

functions of target cells. Class III molecules encoded by genes located between those that encode class I and class II molecules include C2, BF, C4a, and C4b. Class I and class II molecules play an important role in organ and tissue transplantation. The microlymphocytotoxicity assay is used for HLA-A, -B, -C, -DR, and -DQ typing. The primed lymphocyte test is used for DP typing. Uppercase letters designate individual HLA loci, such as HLA-B. Alleles are designated by numbers, such as in HLA-B*0701.

HLA-A

A class I histocompatibility antigen in humans. It is expressed on nucleated cells of the body. Tissue typing to identify an individual's HLA-A antigens employs lymphocytes.

HLA-A, HLA-B, and HLA-C

The highly polymorphic human major histocompatibility complex (MHC) class I genes.

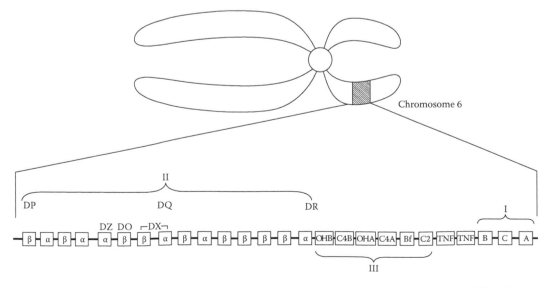

HLA is an abbreviation for human leukocyte antigen. The HLA locus in humans is found on the short arm of chromosome 6. The class I region consists of HLA-A, HLA-B, and HLA-C loci, and the class II region consists of the D region which is subdivided into HLA-DP, HLA-DQ, and HLA-DR subregions.

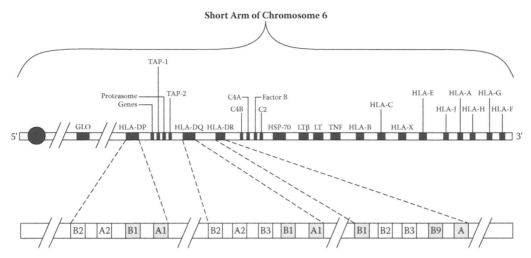

MHC genes encode the major histocompatibility antigens that are expressed on cell membranes. MHC genes in the mouse are located at the H-2 locus on chromosome 17, whereas the MHC genes in man are located at the HLA locus on the short arm of chromosome 6.

HLA allelic variation

Genomic analysis has identified specific individual allelic variants to explain HLA associations with rheumatoid arthritis, type I diabetes mellitus, multiple sclerosis, and celiac disease. A minimum of six α and eight β genes are arranged in distinct clusters, termed HLA-DR, -DQ, and -DP, within the HLA class II genes. DO and DN class II genes are related, but map outside DR, DQ, and DP regions. The two types of dimers along the HLA cell surface HLA-DR class II molecules consist of either DRα polypeptide associated with DRβ$_1$ polypeptide or DR with DRβ$_2$ polypeptide. Structural variation in class II gene products is linked to functional features of immune recognition, leading to individual variations in histocompatibility, immune recognition, and susceptibility to disease. The two types of structural variations are (1) among DP, DQ, and DR products in primary amino acid sequence by as much as 35% and (2) individual variations attributable to different allelic forms of class II genes. The class II polypeptide chain possesses domains that are specific structural subunits containing variable sequences that distinguish among class II α genes or class II β genes. These allelic variation sites have been suggested to form epitopes that represent individual structural differences in immune recognition.

HLA-B

A class I histocompatibility antigen in humans that is expressed on nucleated cells. Tissue typing to define HLA-B antigens employs lymphocytes.

HLA-B27-related arthropathies

Joint diseases that occur with increased frequency in individuals who are HLA-B27 antigen-positive. Juvenile rheumatoid arthritis, ankylosing spondylitis, Reiter's syndrome, *Salmonella*-related arthritis, psoriatic arthritis, and *Yersinia* arthritis belong to this group.

HLA-C

A class I histocompatibility antigen in humans that is expressed on nucleated cells. Lymphocytes are employed for tissue typing to determine HLA-C antigens. HLA-C antigens play little or no role in graft rejection.

HLA class I

Refer to MHC genes and class I MHC molecules.

HLA class I molecules

The term used to describe MHC class I molecules in humans.

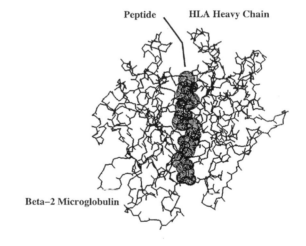

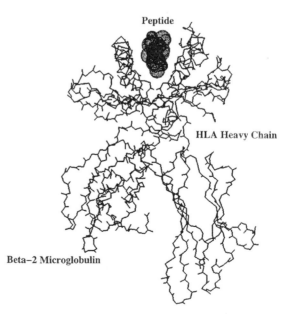

A schematic backbone structure of human class I histocompatibility antigen (HLA-A 0201) complexed with a decameric peptide from hepatitis B nucleocapsid protein (residues 18–27). Determined by x-ray crystallography..

H

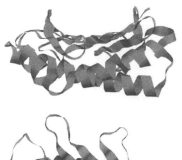

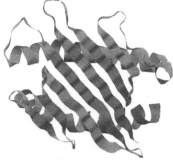

Human class I histocompatibility antigen (HLA-A 0201) complexed with a decameric peptide from calreticulin HLA-A 0201. Human recombinant extracellular fragment expressed in *Escherichia coli*; peptide synthesis based on sequence of human calreticulin.

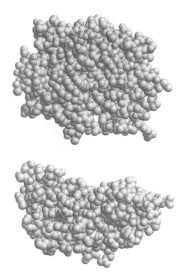

Class I histocompatibility antigen HLA-B*2705 complexed with nonapeptide arg–arg–ile–thr–leu–lys (theoretical model).

HLA class II
Refer to MHC genes and class II MHC molecules.

HLA class II molecules
The term used to describe MHC class II molecules in humans.

HLA class III
Refer to MHC genes and class III MHC molecules.

HLA-D region
The human major histocompatibility complex (MHC) class II region comprised of three subregions designated DR, DQ, and DP. Multiple genetic loci are present in each of these. Each of the DN (previously DZ) and DO subregions is comprised of one genetic locus. Each HLA class II molecule is composed of one α chain and one β chain that constitute a heterodimer. Genes within each subregion encode the α and β chains of a particular class II molecule. Class II genes that encode α chains are designated A, and class II genes that encode β

chains are designated B. A number is used following A or B if a particular subregion contains two or more A or B genes.

HLA disease association
Certain human leukocyte antigen (HLA) alleles occur in higher frequencies in individuals with particular diseases than in the general population. This type of data permits estimation of the relative risk of developing a disease with every known HLA allele. For example, a strong association exists between ankylosing spondylitis, an autoimmune disorder involving the vertebral joints, and the major histocompatibility complex (MHC) class I allele HLA-B27. A strong association exists between products of the polymorphic class II alleles HLA-DR and -DQ and certain autoimmune diseases, because MHC class II molecules are of great importance in the selection and activation of CD4[+] T lymphocytes that regulate the immune responses against protein antigens. For example, 95% of Caucasians with insulin-dependent (type I) diabetes mellitus have HLA-DR3 or HLA-DR4 or both. A strong association of HLA-DR4 with rheumatoid arthritis also exists. Numerous other examples are the targets of current investigations, especially in extended studies employing DNA probes. Calculation of the relative risk (RR) and absolute risk (AR) can be found elsewhere in this dictionary.

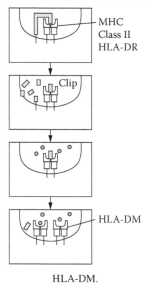

HLA-DM.

HLA-DM
Invariant MHC class II molecule that facilitates the loading of antigenic peptides onto major histocompatibility complex (MHC) class II molecules in humans. As a result of proteolysis of the invariant chain, a small fragment called the class-II-associated invariant chain peptide (CLIP) remains bound to the MHC class II molecule. CLIP is replaced by antigenic peptides; however, this does not occur in the absence of HLA-DM. The HLA-DM molecule present in endosomal compartments plays some part in removal of CLIP and in the loading of antigenic peptides. Although HLA-DM is structurally similar to MHC class II molecules, it is not polymorphic.

HLA-DO
A negative modulator of HLA-DM-mediated MHC class II peptide loading. By stably associating with HLA-DM, the catalytic action of HLA-DM on class II peptide loading is inhibited. Therefore, HLA-DO affects the peptide

TABLE 8.1
Characteristics of HLA Molecules

Name	Previous Equivalents	Molecular Characteristics
HLA-A	–	Class I α-chain
HLA-B	–	Class I α-chain
HLA-C	–	Class I α-chain
HLA-E	E, 6.2	Associated with class I 6.2-kB Hind III fragment
HLA-F	F, 5.4	Associated with class I 5.4-kB Hind III fragment
HLA-G	G, 6.0	Associated with class 6.0 Hind III fragment
HLA-H	H, AR, 12.4	Class I pseudogene associated with 5.4-kB Hind III fragment
HLA-J	cda 12	Class I pseudogene associated with 5.9-kB Hind III fragment
HLA-K	HLA-70	Class I pseudogene associated with 7.0-kB Hind III fragment
HLA-L	HLA-92	Class I pseudogene associated with 9.2-kB Hind III fragment
HLA-DRA	DRα	DR α chain
HLA-DRB1, DR3, DR4, DR5, etc.	DRβI, DR1B	DR β1 chain determining specificities
DR1, DR2 HLA-DRB2	DRβII	Pseudogene with DR β-like sequences
HLA-DRB3 Dw26	DRβIII, DR3B	DR β3 chain determining DR52 and Dw24, Dw25 specificities
HLA-DRB4	DRβIV, DR4B	DR β4 chain determining DR53 specificities
HLA-DRB5	DRβIII	DR β5 chain determining DR51 specificities
HLA-DRB6	DRBX, DRBσ	DRB pseudogene found on DR1, DR2, and DR10 haplotypes
HLA-DRB7	DRBψ1	DRB pseudogene found on DR4, DR7 and DR9 haplotypes
HLA-DRB8	DRBψ2	DRB pseudogene found on DR4, DR7 and DR9 haplotypes
HLA-DRB9	M4.2 β exon	DRB pseudogene, isolated fragment
HLA-DQA1	DQα1, DQ1A	DQ α chain as expressed
HLA-DQB1	DQβ1, DQ1B	DQ β chain as expressed
HLA-DQA2	DXα, DQ2A	DQ α-chain-related sequence, not known to be expressed
HLA-DQB2	DXβ, DQ2B	DQ β-chain-related sequence, not known to be expressed
HLA-DQB3	DVβ, DQB3	DQ β-chain-related sequence, not known to be expressed
HLA-DOB	DOβ	DO β chain
HLA-DMA	RING6	DM α chain
HLA-DMB	RING7	DM β chain
HLA-DNA	DZα, DOα	DN α chain
HLA-DPA1	DPα1, DP1A	DP α chain as expressed
HLA-DPB1	DPβ2, DP2B	DP β chain as expressed
HLA-DPA2	DPα2, DP2A	DP α-chain-related pseudogene
HLA-DPB2	DPβ2, DP2B	DP β-chain-related pseudogene
TAP-1	RING4, Y3, PSF1	ABC (ATP binding cassette) transporter
TAP-2	RING11, Y1, PSF2	ABC (ATP binding cassette) transporter
LMP2	RING12	Proteasome-related sequence
LMP7	RING10	Proteasome-related sequence

repertoire presented to the immune system by MHC class II molecules.

HLA-DP subregion

The site of two sets of genes designated HLA-DPA1 and HLA-DPB1 and the pseudogenes HLA-DPA2 and HLA-DPB2. DP α and DP β chains, encoded by the corresponding genes DPA1 and DPB1, unite to produce the DP αβ molecule. DP antigen or type is determined principally by the very polymorphic DP β chain, in contrast to the much less polymorphic DP α chain. DP molecules carry DPw1–DPw6 antigens.

HLA-DQ subregion

Two sets of genes, designated DQA1 and DQB1 and DQA2 and DQB2, are found in this region. DQA2 and DRB2 are pseudogenes. DQ α and DQ β chains, encoded by DQA1 and DQB1 genes, unite to produce the DQ αβ molecule. Although both DQ α and DQ β chains are polymorphic, the DQ β chain is the principal factor in determining the DQ antigen or type. DQ αβ molecules carry DQw1–DQw9 specificities.

HLA-DR antigenic specificities

Epitopes on DR gene products. Selected specificities have been mapped to defined loci. HLA serologic typing requires the identification of a prescribed antigenic determinant on a particular HLA molecular product. One typing specificity may be present on many different molecules. Different alleles at the same locus may encode these various HLA

H

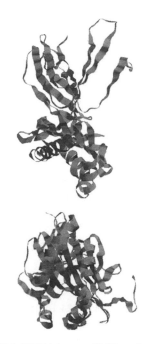

HLA-DR1 histocompatibility antigen.

molecules. Monoclonal antibodies are now used to recognize certain antigenic determinants shared by various molecules bearing the same HLA typing specificity. Monoclonal antibodies have been employed to recognize specific class II alleles with disease associations.

HLA-DR subregion

The site of one HLA-DRA gene. Although the DRB gene number varies with DR type, the usual number is three DRB genes, termed DRB1, DRB2, and DRB3 (or DRB4). The DRB2 pseudogene is not expressed. The DR α chain encoded by the DRA gene can unite with products of DRB1 and DRB3 (or DRB4) genes that are the DR β-1 and DR β-3 (or DR β-4) chains. This yields two separate DR molecules, DR αβ-1 and DR αβ-3 (or DR αβ-4). The DRβ chain determines the DR antigen (DR type), as it is very polymorphic, whereas the DRα chain is not. DR αβ-1 molecules carry DR specificities DR1–DRw18. Yet, DR αβ-3 molecules carry the DRw52, and the DR αβ-4 molecules carry the DRw53 specificity.

HLA-E

Human leukocyte antigen (HLA) class I nonclassical molecule. Relatively invariant human MHC class I molecules that serve as ligands for NK cell receptors.

HLA-F

Human leukocyte antigen (HLA) class I nonclassical molecule. Believed to be a peptide-binding molecule that may reach the cell surface where it would be capable of interacting with LIR1 (ILT2) and LIR2 (ILT4) receptors, thereby altering the activation thresholds of immune effector cells. A predominantly empty, intracellular, TAP-associated MHC class Ib protein with a restricted expression pattern.

HLA-G

HLA-G either is nonpolymorphic or has very limited polymorphism. It is a nonclassical (class Ib) major histocompatibility complex (MHC) molecule expressed in immune-privileged tissues. It is a class I HLA antigen with extensive variability in the α-2 domain. It is found on trophoblasts (i.e., placenta cells and trophoblastic neoplasms). HLA-G is expressed only on cells such as placental

extravillous cytotrophoblasts, and choriocarcinoma that fail to express HLA-A, -B, and -C antigens. HLA-G expression is most pronounced during the first trimester of pregnancy. Fetal trophoblasts do not express the class Ia MHC molecule's HLA-A and HLA-B, allowing the fetus to escape the maternal T cell response. Evidence suggests that HLA-G protects the fetus from attack by natural killer (NK) cells, macrophages, and monocytes by interacting with the inhibitory receptors on leukocyte immunoglobulin-like receptor 1 (LIR-1 or ILT-2), leukocyte immunoglobulin-like receptor 2 (LIR02 or ILT-4), and killer immunoglobulin-like receptor 2DL4 (KIR2DLA). Trophoblast cells expressing HLA-G at the maternal–fetal junction may protect the semiallogeneic fetus from "rejection." Prominent HLA-G expression suggests maternal immune tolerance. HLA-G exerts tolerogenic functions involved in transplant acceptance as well as in tumoral and viral immune escape.

HLA-H

A pseudogene found in the major histocompatibility complex (MHC) class I region that is structurally similar to HLA-A but is nonfunctional due to the absence of a cysteine residue at position 164 in its protein product and the deletion of the codon 227 nucleotide.

HLA complex

Alternate name for human major histocompatibility complex (MHC).

HLA locus

The major histocompatibility locus in humans.

HLA nonclassical class I genes

Genes located within the major histocompatibility complex (MHC) class I region that encode products that can associate with β_2 microglobulin; however, their function and tissue distribution are different from those of HLA-A, -B, and -C molecules. Examples include HLA-E, -F, and -G. Only HLA-G is expressed on cell surfaces. Whether these HLA molecules are involved in peptide binding and presentation like classical class I molecules remains uncertain.

HLA oligotyping

A recently developed method using oligonucleotide probes to supplement other histocompatibility testing techniques. Whereas serological and cellular methods identify phenotypic characteristics of human leukocyte antigen (HLA) proteins, oligotyping defines the genotype of the DNA that encodes HLA protein structure and specificity. Thus, oligotyping can identify a DNA type even when a failure of expression of HLA genes renders serological techniques ineffective.

HLA tissue typing

The identification of major histocompatibility complex (MHC) class I and class II antigens on lymphocytes by serological and cellular techniques. The principal serological assay is microlymphocytotoxicity using a microtiter plate containing predispensed antibodies against human leukocyte antigen (HLA) specificities to which lymphocytes of unknown specificity plus rabbit complement and vital dye are added. Following incubation, the wells are scored according to the relative proportion of cells killed. This method is employed for organ transplants such as renal allotransplants. For bone marrow transplants, mixed lymphocyte reaction procedures are performed to determine the relative degree of histocompatibility or histoincompatibility between donor and recipient. Serological tests have been largely replaced by DNA typing procedures employing

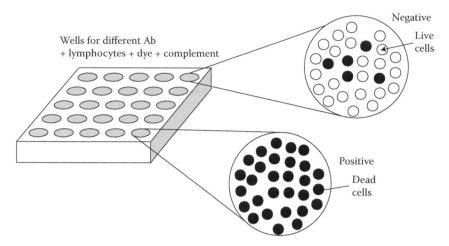

Wells for different Ab
+ lymphocytes + dye + complement

Negative
Live cells

Positive
Dead cells

HLA tissue typing.

polymerase chain reaction (PCR) methodology and DNA or oligonucleotide probes, especially for MHC class II typing. Class I typing involves reactions between lymphocytes to be typed with HLA antisera of known specificity in the presence of complement. Cell lysis is detected by phase or fluorescence microscopy. This is important in parentage testing, disease association, transfusion practices, and transplantation. HLA-A, -B, -C antigens should be defined by at least one of the following: (1) at least two different sera if both are monospecific, (2) one monospecific and two multispecific antisera, (3) at least three multispecific antisera if all multispecific types are used. Class II typing detects HLA-DR antigens using purified B cell preparations. It is based on antibody-specific, complement-dependent disruption of the membranes of lymphocytes. Cell death is demonstrated by the penetration of dye into the membrane. Class II typing is more difficult than type II methods and complement toxicity. At least three antisera must be used if all are monospecific, and at least five antisera must be used for multispecific sera.

HLA type
Both HLA class I and HLA class II allotypes expressed by an individual.

HLA supertype
Human MHC alleles with overlapping peptide-binding repertoires. The three HLA class I supertypes described include A2, A3, and B7.

Hm-1
Designation for the Syrian hamster major histocompatibility complex (MHC). MHC class II genes have been recognized.

Hodgkin disease
A type of lymphoma that involves the lymph nodes and spleen, causing a replacement of the lymph node architecture with binucleated giant cells known as Reed–Sternberg cells, reticular cells, neutrophils, eosinophils, and lymphocytes. Both lymphadenopathy and splenomegaly are present. Patients manifest deficiencies of cell-mediated immunity that cause tuberculin type skin tests to be negative. By contrast, their B cell functions are not altered. They may exhibit increases in suppressor cell activity and their susceptibility to opportunistic infections is increased. Antigen-presenting cells resembling dendritic cells apparently represent the transformed cell type. Hodgkin lymphoma, characterized by a predominance of lymphocytes, has a much better prognosis

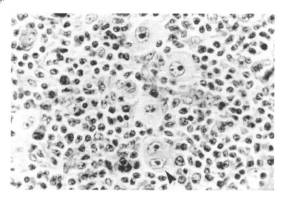

Hodgkin lymphoma; Hodgkin cell and Reed Sternberg cell.

than does the nodular sclerosis variety of the disease in which the predominant cell type is nonlymphoid. Associated with transformed germinal center B cells.

Hof
German word for courtyard that refers to the perinuclear clear zone adjacent to the nuclei of plasma cells. Lymphoblasts and Reed–Sternberg cells may also exhibit *hof zones*.

"hole in the repertoire" model
A concept that proposes that an animal failing to respond to a given antigen is bereft of the requisite T cell specificity attributable to tolerance mechanisms. The relevant foreign peptide/self MHC combination is considered to closely resemble a self peptide/self MHC combination in the subject, leading to deletion of any T cell clones that would respond to the antigen as autoreactive during negative selection in the thymus or tolerization in the periphery. Thus, a "hole" exists in the individual's T cell repertoire compared with the T cell repertoire of a responder.

holoxenic
An animal raised under ordinary conditions as opposed to an axenic or gnotobiotic animal.

homeostasis
In immunology, the maintenance of a constant and physiologic number of lymphocytes with a diverse repertoire even in the presence of new lymphocytes and exponential expansion of individual clones that follows immunogenic stimulation.

homing
The differential migration of lymphocytes or other leukocytes to specific tissues or organs.

H

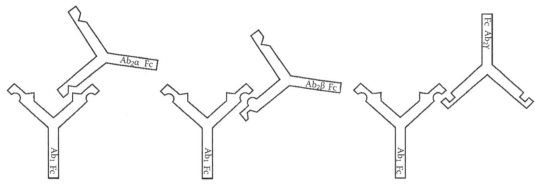

Homobody.

homing cell adhesion molecule (H-CAM)

Also known as CD44, gp$^{90\,hermes}$, GP85/Pgp-1, and ECMRIII. H-CAM is a lymphocyte transmembrane glycoprotein with a molecular weight of 85 to 95 kDa expressed in macrophages, granulocytes, fibroclasts, endothelial cells, and epithelial cells. H-CAM has been found to bind to extracellular matrix molecules such as collagen and hyaluronic acid. It is also an important signal transduction protein during lymphocyte adhesion, as it has been demonstrated that phosphorylation by kinase C and acylation by acyl-transferases enhance the interactions of H-CAM with cytoskeletal proteins.

homing receptors

Molecules on cell surfaces that direct traffic of the cells to precise locations in other tissues or organs. For example, lymphocytes bear surface receptors that facilitate their attachment to high endothelial cells of postcapillary venules in lymph nodes. Adhesion molecules present on lymphocyte surfaces enable lymphocytes to recirculate and home to specific tissues. Homing receptors bind to ligands termed addressins found on endothelial cells in affected vessels. L-selectin on naïve lymphocytes binds to GlyCAM-1 molecules on high endothelial venules.

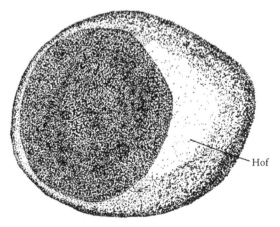

Homobody.

homobody

An idiotypic determinant of an antibody molecule with a three-dimensional structure that resembles antigen. Also called internal image of antigen. For example, anti-idiotypic antibodies of this type of insulin receptor may partially mimic the action of insulin.

homocytotrophic antibody

An antibody that attaches better to animal cells of the same species in which it is produced than to animal cells of a different species. The term usually refers to an antibody that becomes fixed to mast cells of an animal of the same species, resulting in anaphylaxis with the release of pharmacological mediators of immediate hypersensitivity. These include histamines and other vasoactive amines when the mast cells degranulate.

homodimer

A protein composed of dual peptide chains that are identical.

homogenicity

The composition from like parts, elements, or characteristics.

homograft

Allograft (i.e., an organ or tissue graft) from a donor to a recipient of the same species.

homograft reaction

An immune reaction generated by a homograft (allograft) recipient against the graft alloantigens. Also called an allograft reaction.

homograft rejection

Allograft rejection. An immune response induced by histocompatibility antigens in the donor graft that are not present in the recipient. This is principally a cell-mediated type of immune response.

homokaryon

A cell that is multinucleate as a consequence of the fusion of two or more genetically identical cells.

homologous

Arising from the same source, for example, an organ allotransplant from one member to a recipient member of the same species (e.g., renal allotransplantation in humans).

homologous antigen

An antigen (immunogen) that stimulates the synthesis of an antibody and reacts specifically with it.

homologous chromosomes

A pair of chromosomes containing the same linear gene sequences, each derived from one parent.

homologous disease

Refer to allogeneic disease and graft-vs.-host disease (GVHD).

homologous recombination

The exchange of DNA fragments between two DNA molecules or chromatids of paired chromosomes (during crossing over) at the site of identical nucleotide sequences. Employed to introduce a mutated version of a gene into mass embryonic stem cells to produce a knockout mouse or a mouse manifesting a knock-in transgene.

homologous recombination pathway

A DNA repair pathway that employs homologous DNA to repair major gaps in double-stranded DNA in an "error-free" manner. Associated with the BLM gene (refer to Bloom syndrome).

homologous restriction factor (HRF)

An erythrocyte surface protein that prevents cell lysis by homologous complement on its surface. It bears a structural resemblance to C8 and C9.

homologous vaccine

Autogenous vaccine.

homology region

A 105- to 115-amino-acid residue sequence of heavy or light chains of immunoglobulins that have primary structures resembling other corresponding sequences of the same size. A homology region has a globular shape and an intrachain disulfide bond. The exons that encode homology regions are separated by introns. Light polypeptide chain homology regions are termed V_L and C_L. Heavy chain homology regions are designated V_H, C_H1, C_H2, and C_H3.

homology unit

A structural feature of an immunoglobulin domain.

homopolymer

A molecule comprised of repeating units of only one amino acid.

homotransplantation

Homograft (i.e., allograft) transplantation.

homozygote

An organism whose genotype is characterized by two identical alleles of a gene.

homozygous

Containing two copies of the same allele.

homozygous typing cell (HTC) technique

An assay that employs a stimulator cell that is homozygous at the HLA-D locus. The HTC incorporates only a minute amount of tritiated thymidine when combined with a homozygous cell in the MLR. This implies that the HTC shares HLA-D determinants with the other cell type. By contrast, when an HTC is combined with a nonhomozygous cell, much larger amounts of tritiated thymidine are incorporated. Many variations between these two extremes are noted in actual practice. HTCs are frequently obtained from the progeny of marriages between cousins.

homozygous typing cells (HTCs)

Cells obtained from a subject who is homozygous at the HLA-D locus. HTCs facilitate MLR typing of the human D locus.

Hood, Leroy

Pioneer in immunogenetics and molecular biology. His work with Tonegawa proved that three separate DNA segments must be combined to complete the heavy chain variable region sequence of immunoglobulin. They found yet another diversity (D) group of DNA segments in addition to the V and J segments. Hood went on to demonstrate mutations in these gene segments. The elegant body of scientific evidence elucidated finally solved one of immunology's most mystifying conundrums.

hook effect

An artifact that may be seen in the immunoradiometric assay (IRMA) when a hormone assayed is present in very high concentration. The excess amount cannot be measured by the detector system because it will have reached its

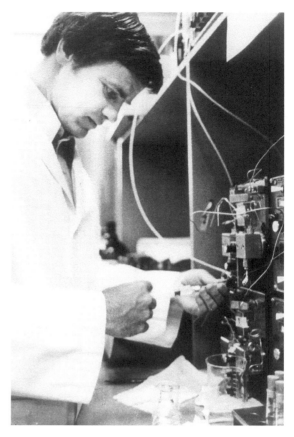

Leroy Hood.

theoretical limit. The diminished counts with the labeled antibody at the elevated hormone concentration yield spuriously low results. Thus, IRMA is not an appropriate method for assaying hormones present in relatively high concentrations, such as gastrin, prolactin, or hCG. The hook effect requires measurement of two separate concentrations to establish linearity.

hookworm immunity

Hookworms in humans induce various antibody responses that may be assayed by ELISA or the radioimmunoassay technique. There is a prominent immune response to excretory–secretory (ES) products and surface antigens, as well as a sharp rise in specific immunoglobulin isotypes during infection. Marked elevation of total serum immunoglobulin E (IgE) occurs in human hookworm disease; the remaining additional immunoglobulin in the circulation is not specific for parasite antigens. Serum IgA may be diminished during hookworm disease, because hookworm proteases are able to digest host IgA. The greater the burden of worms, the more intense the antibody response to adult antigens. Subjects who have fewer worms develop higher titers of antilarval antibodies that increase the resistance to larval challenge. Hookworms induce T_H2-type responses together with specific IgE antibodies against ES products and eosinophilia. Evidence is lacking to support the concept that T_H2-dependent immunity plays a major role in host-protective immunity against hookworms. Little is known concerning cellular responses to hookworms. Eosinophilia is a common finding in hookworm infection. Production of superoxide is increased, and chemotaxis of eosinophils from infected donors is enhanced; yet, the eosinophilia has

H

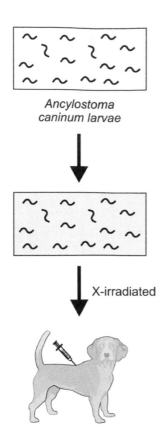

Ancylostoma caninum larvae

↓

X-irradiated

↓

Hookworm vaccine.

not been linked to host-protective immunity to hookworms. No vaccines are available for immunization against hookworm disease in humans.

hookworm vaccine

A live vaccine to protect dogs against the hookworm, *Ancylostoma caninum.* The vaccine is comprised of x-irradiated larvae to halt their development to adult forms.

hormone immunoassays

Multiple hormones, such as thyroid-stimulating hormone, human growth hormone, insulin, glucagon, and many others, may be measured by an immunoassay using radioactively labeled reagents or through enzyme color reactions using the ELISA technique. Labeled and unlabeled hormones, are allowed to compete for binding sites with antihormone antibody. This step is followed by the separation of bound from unbound hormones by one of several techniques.

hormones

Messenger chemical molecules synthesized in the body by an organ, cells of an organ, or diffusely located cells, which have a precise regulatory action on the functions of certain organs or organs on cell types. Substances secreted by various endocrine glands and transported in the blood stream to target organs on which their effects are produced. Also applied to various substances not produced by special glands but having a similar action.

horror autotoxicus (historical)

A term coined by Paul Ehrlich (*circa* 1900) to account for an individual's failure to produce autoantibodies against his own self constituents even though they are excellent antigens or immunogens in other species. This lack of immune reactivity against self was believed to protect against autoimmune disease. It was also postulated to be a fear of poisoning or destroying one's self. Abrogation of horror autotoxicus leads to autoimmune disease. Horror autotoxicus was later (1959) referred to as self tolerance by F.M. Burnett.

horse serum sensitivity

An allergic or hypersensitive reaction in a human or other animal receiving antitoxin or antithymocyte globulin generated by immunization of horses whose immune serum is used for therapeutic purposes. Classic serum sickness is an example of this type of hypersensitivity that first appeared in children receiving diphtheria antitoxin early in the 20th century.

host-vs.-graft disease (HVGD)

The humoral and cell-mediated immune response of a recipient host to donor graft antigens.

hot antigen suicide

The labeling of an antigen with a powerful radioisotope such as ^{131}I proves lethal upon contact with antigen-binding cells that have receptors specific for it. This leads to a failure to synthesize antibodies specific for that antigen, provided the antigen-binding and antibody-synthesizing cells are one and the same. Hot antigen suicide supports the clonal selection theory of antibody formation.

hot spot

A hypervariable region in DNA that encodes the variable region of the heavy (V_H) and light (V_L) polypeptide chains of an immunoglobulin (Ig) molecule. Also designated complementarity-determining regions (CDRs), they are the areas for specific antigen binding. They also determine the idiotype of an immunoglobulin molecule. The remaining background support structures of the heavy and light polypeptide chains are termed framework regions (FRs). The κ and λ light chain hot spots are situated near amino acid residues 30, 50, and 95. Also called hypervariable regions.

house dust allergy

Type I immediate hypersensitivity reaction in atopic individuals exposed to house dust in which the principal allergen is *Dermatophagoides pteronyssinus,* the house dust mite. The condition is expressed as a respiratory allergy with the atopic subject manifesting either asthma or allergic rhinitis.

HPV

Human papilloma virus. A human virus that has the potential to be oncogenic and occurs most frequently in individuals with multiple sexual partners. HPV has 46 genotypes. The virus can be demonstrated by *in situ* hybridization in proliferations of epithelial cells that are benign, such as condyloma accuminatum, or malignant, such as squamous cell carcinoma of the uterine cervix. Whereas HPV types 6 and 11 are not usually premalignant, HPV types 16, 18, 31, 33, and 35 are linked to cervical intraeptithelial neoplasia (CIN), cervical dysplasia, and anogenital cancer. HPV is predicted to induce derepression as a neoplastic mechanism. HPV encodes E6, a viral protein that combines with the tumor suppressor protein p53.

HR

Abbreviation for hypersensitive response.

HSA

Abbreviation for human serum albumin, an antigen commonly used in experimental immunology.

HSC

Abbreviation for hematopoietic stem cell.

HSC mobilization

The inoculation of a donor with G-CSF or GM-CSF to induce hematopoietic stem cell proliferation in the bone marrow. These cells subsequently spill over from the stimulated bone marrow into the peripheral blood from which they can be harvested for use in hematopoietic stem cell transplantation by leukapheresis.

HSV

Herpes simplex virus.

HTLA (human T lymphocyte antigen)

An obsolete term for human T lymphocyte antigen; it has been replaced by a cluster of differentiation (CD) designations.

HTLA antibody

High titer, low avidity antibody.

HTLV (human T lymphocyte virus)

Human T cell leukemia virus. A retrovirus that infects human CD4+ T lymphocytes and produces adult T cell leukemia.

HTLV-IV

A human retrovirus isolated from western Africa that is related to HIV-1 and HIV-2 but appears to be nonpathogenic.

human chorionic gonadotropin (hCG)

A hormone synthesized by placental syncytiotrophoblasts that serves as a marker demonstrable by immunoperoxidase staining in trophoblastic neoplasms (e.g., choriocarcinomas). Germ cell and nontrophoblastic neoplasms, such as various carcinomas, may express hCG.

human diploid cell rabies vaccine (HDCV)

An inactivated virus vaccine prepared from fixed rabies virus grown in human diploid cell tissue culture.

human immune globulin (HIG)

A pooled globulin preparation from the plasma of donors who are negative for human immunodeficiency virus (HIV). It is used in the treatment of primary immunodeficiencies such as severe combined immunodeficiency (SCID), Burton's disease, and combined variable immunodeficiency and in cases of idiopathic thrombocytopenic purpura. The method of production is extraction by cold ethanol fractionation at acid pH. Viruses are inactivated, allowing the safe administration of HIG to patients without risk of HIV, HAV, HBV, or non-A, non-B hepatitis.

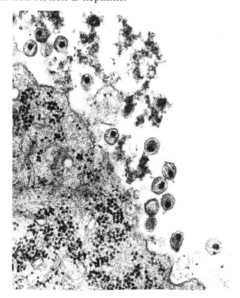

Electron micrograph of human immunodeficiency virus (HIV). (Courtesy of Dr. Tom Folks, Centers for Disease Control, Atlanta, GA.)

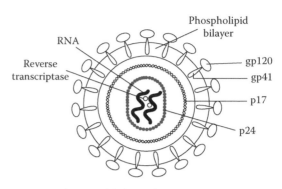

Human immunodeficiency virus (HIV-1) structure.

human immunodeficiency virus (HIV)

A retrovirus that induces acquired immune deficiency syndrome (AIDS) and associated disorders. It was previously designated HTLV-III, LAV, and ARV. It infects CD4+ T lymphocytes, mononuclear phagocytes carrying CD4 molecules on their surfaces, follicular dendritic cells, and Langerhans' cells. HIV produces profound immunodeficiency affecting both humoral and cell-mediated immunity. CD4+ helper/inducer T lymphocytes progressively decrease until they are finally depleted in many patients. Polyclonal activation of B lymphocytes with elevated synthesis of immunoglobulins may be present. The immune response to the virus is not protective and does not improve the patient's condition. The virus is composed of an envelope glycoprotein (gp160), which is its principal antigen. It has a gp120 external segment and a gp41 transmembrane segment. CD4 molecules on CD4+ lymphocytes and macrophages serve as receptors for gp120 of HIV. It has an inner core that contains RNA and is encircled by a lipid envelope. It contains structural genes designated *env*, *gag*, and *pol* that encode the envelope protein, core protein, and reverse transcriptase, respectively. HIV also possesses at least six additional genes (e.g., *tat*) that regulate virus replication. HIV can increase production of viral protein several thousandfold. The *rev* gene encodes proteins that block transcription of regulatory genes; *vif (sor)* is the virus infectivity gene whose product increases viral infectivity and may promote cell-to-cell transmission; *nef* is a negative regulatory factor that encodes a product that blocks replication of the virus; and *vpr* (viral protein R) and *vpu* (viral protein U) genes have also been described. No successful vaccine has yet been developed, although several types are under investigation.

human leukocyte antigen (HLA)

The major histocompatibility complex (MHC) in humans that contains the genes that encode the polymorphic MHC class I and class II molecules as well as other important genes.

human leukocyte antigen (HLA) complex

The major histocompatibility complex (MHC) of humans.

human milk-fat globulin (HMFG)

Human milk glycoprotein on secretory breast cell surfaces. Many breast and ovarian carcinomas are positive for HMFG.

human papillomavirus recombinant vaccine (quadrivalent, injection)

Females 9 to 26 years of age should be vaccinated to prevent disease caused by human papillomavirus (HPV) types 6, 11, 16 and 18. Diseases caused by these virus types include cervical cancer, genital warts (condyloma acuminata), and precancerous or dysplastic lesions including

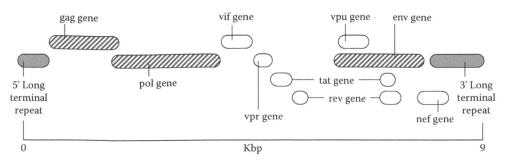

Human immunodeficiency virus (HIV-1) genes.

cervical adenocarcinoma *in situ* (AIS), cervical intraepithelial neoplasia (CIN), vulvar intraepithelial neoplasia (VIN), vaginal intraepithelial neoplasia (VAIN), and CIN grade 1. Quadrivalent HPV (types 6, 11, 16 and 18) recombinant vaccine should be given intramuscularly as three separate 0.5 mL doses according to the following schedule: first dose at the elected date; second dose 2 months after first dose; third dose 6 months after first. Refer also to Gardasil®.

human SCID (hu-SCID) mouse

Because SCID (severe combined immunodeficiency) mice have no functioning immune systems, xenogeneic transplantation can be accomplished with little or no graft rejection. This has led to the establishment of a chimeric construct in which a functional human immune system can be established within an SCID mouse (hu-SCID). This model permits the evaluation of many important aspects of human immune-mediated pathology. Other applications of the hu-SCID model include the study of human infectious diseases and the validation of novel immune-targeted therapies. Currently, immune-mediated human diseases are being re-created in hu-SCID mice.

human T lymphocyte

A human T lymphocyte encircled by rings of sheep red blood cells (SRBCs) is referred to as an E rosette and was used as a method to enumerate T lymphocytes.

humanization

The genetic engineering of murine hypervariable loop specificity into human antibodies. The DNA encoding hypervariable loops of murine monoclonal antibodies or V regions selected in phage display libraries is inserted into the framework regions of human immunoglobulin genes. This technique permits the synthesis of antibodies of a particular specificity without inducing an immune response in the human subject treated with them.

humanize

To substitute, through genetic engineering, the CDR loops in a human antibody molecule with the corresponding murine antibody CDR sequences of a given specificity.

humanized antibody

An engineered antibody produced through recombinant DNA technology. A humanized antibody contains the antigen-binding specificity of an antibody developed in a mouse, whereas the remainder of the molecule is of human origin. To accomplish this, hypervariable genes that encode the antigen-binding regions of a mouse antibody are transferred to the normal human gene that encodes an immunoglobulin molecule that is mostly human but expresses the antigen-binding specificity of the mouse antibody in the variable region of the molecule. This greatly diminishes any immune response to the antibody molecule as a foreign protein by the human host, while retaining the desired functional capacity of reacting with the specific antigen.

humoral

The antibody limb of the immune response, in contrast to the cell-mediated limb, together with the action of complement. Thus, immunity based on antibodies or antibodies and complement is produced and referred to as humoral immunity. Humoral immunity of the antibody type represents the products of the B cell system.

humoral antibody

Antibody found in the blood plasma, lymph, and other body fluids. Humoral antibody, together with complement, mediates humoral immunity, which is based upon soluble effector molecules.

humoral immune response

Host defense mediated by antibody molecules found in the plasma, lymph, and tissue fluids. This type of immunity protects against extracellular bacteria in foreign micromolecules. Humoral immunity may be transferred passively with antibodies or serum containing antibodies.

humoral immunity

Immunity attributable to specific immunoglobulin antibody and present in the plasma, lymph, other body fluids, and tissues. The antibody may also adhere to cells in the form of cytophilic antibodies. Antibody- or immunoglobulin-mediated immunity acts in conjunction with complement proteins to produce beneficial (protective) or pathogenic (hypersensitivity-tissue injuring) reactions. Antibodies that are the messengers of humoral immunity are derived from B cells. For purposes of discussion, humoral immunity is separated from so-called cellular or T-cell-mediated immunity; however, the two cannot be clearly distinguished because antibodies and T cells often participate in immune reactions together. However, the classification of humoral separate from cellular immunity is useful in understanding and explaining biological mechanisms.

hump

Immune deposits containing IgG and C3, as well as the alternate complement pathway components, properdin, and factor B, that occur in post-infectious glomerulonephritis on the subepithelial sides of peripheral capillary basement membranes. They resolve within 4 to 8 weeks of the infection in most individuals. They may also occur in selected other nonstreptococcal post-infectious glomerulonephritides.

Hunter, John (1728–1793)

British surgeon, the "father of experimental surgery," was intrigued by the possibility of transplantation and was

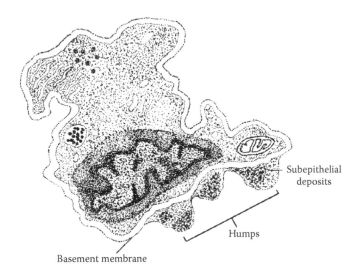

Hump.

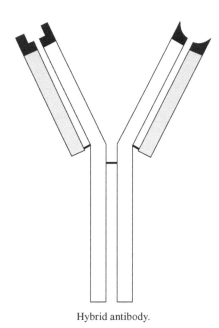

Hybrid antibody.

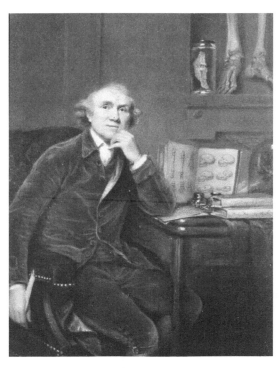

John Hunter.

successful in replacing a premolar tooth some hours after it had been knocked out. He believed he was successful in transplanting a human tooth into the comb of a cock, a specimen still on view at the Hunterian Museum.

HUT 78

The original designation for a cell line derived from a patient with mycosis fungoides (now termed H-9) that was susceptible to infection with HIV-1 virus; it greatly aided HIV-1 culture *in vitro*.

HV regions

Refer to hypervariable regions.

H-Y

A male-specific transplantation antigen. Females of some but not all inbred mouse strains can reject skin grafts from males of the same syngeneic strain. By contrast, male-to-male, female-to-female, and female-to-male grafts succeed. This finding

indicates the presence of a minor histocompatibility antigen gene on the Y chromosome that is H-Y. It is a weak transplantation antigen compared to the major mouse histocompatibility complex (MHC) designated H-2. Several H-Y epitopes have been identified in mice and one in humans. H-Y peptide epitopes are derived from several linked genes.

hybrid antibody

An immunoglobulin molecule that may be prepared artificially but may never occur in nature. Each of two antigen-binding sites is of a different specificity. If immunoglobulin G (IgG) whole molecules or F(ab')$_2$ fragments prepared from them are subjected to mild reduction, the central disulfide bond is converted to sulfhydryl groups. A preparation of half molecules or F(ab') fragments is produced. If either of these is reoxidized, hybrid molecules will constitute some of the products. These can be purified by passing over immunoadsorbents containing bound antigen of the appropriate specificity. Hybrid antibodies are monovalent and do not induce precipitation. They may be used in labeling cell surface antigens in which one antigen-binding site of the molecule is specific for cell surface epitopes and the other combines with a marker that renders the reaction product visible.

hybrid cell

A cell produced when two cells fuse and their nuclei fuse to form a heterokaryon. Although hybrid cell lines can be established from clones of hybrid cells, they lack stability and delete chromosomes, but they are nevertheless useful for gene mapping. Hybrid cell lines can be isolated by using HAT (hypoxanthine, aminopterin, and thymidine) as a selective medium.

hybrid hapten

A hydrophobic type of hapten that lies within the folds of a protein carrier away from the aqueous solvent, creating a new spatial structure.

hybrid resistance

The resistance of members of an F$_1$ generation of animals to growth of a transplantable neoplasm from either one of the parent strains.

H

hybridoma

A hybrid cell produced by the fusion of an antibody-secreting cell isolated from the spleen of an animal immunized against that particular antigen with a mutant myeloma cell of the same species that no longer secretes its own protein product. Polyethylene glycol is used to effect cell fusion. Antibody-synthesizing cells provide the ability to produce a specific monoclonal antibody. The mutant myeloma cell line confers immortality upon the hybridoma. If the nucleotide synthesis pathway is inhibited, the myeloma cells become dependent on hypoxanthine guanine phosphoribosyl transferase (HGRPT) and the salvage pathway. The antibody-synthesizing cells provide the HGPRT, and the mutant myeloma cell enables endless reproduction. Once isolated through use of a selective medium such as HAT (hypoxanthine, aminopterin, and thymidine), hybridoma cell lines can be maintained for relatively long periods. Hybridomas produce specific monoclonal antibodies that may be collected in great quantities for use in diagnosis and selected types of therapy.

hybridoma, T cell

The immortalization of normal T lymphocytes by fusion with continuously replicating tumor cells. Fusion randomly immortalizes T lymphocytes regardless of their antigen specificity and genetic restrictions to form a T cell hybridoma. This represents one of two methods to isolate and propagate T cell lines in clones of defined specificity. The other technique is to span clones of normal immune T lymphocytes stimulated with appropriate antigens and antigen-presenting cells. The hybridoma technique holds the advantage over T cell cloning in the relative ease of securing relatively large numbers of T cells of interest and their biologically active products. Lymphokines and other regulatory molecules together with their nRNA and DNA represent T cell hybridoma products. This technology has also facilitated evaluation of T cell receptors and their antigen recognition mechanisms. The adoptive (passive) transfer of autoantigen-specific T cell hybridomas in mice can induce autoimmune diseases.

Hydrogen bonding shown in dotted lines.

hydrogen bonds

Formed between hydrogen atoms covalently linked to an electronegative atom and a second electronegative atom containing an unshared pair of electrons. The hydrogen atom becomes electron-deficient through polarization of its electron cloud toward the electronegative atom covalently bonded to it, allowing for an electrostatic attraction to a relatively negative second electronegative atom. The contribution of hydrogen bonding to the stability of the complex is minor compared to the other forces involved and decreases with the sixth power of the distance between interaction groups.

hydrophilic

A water-soluble substance. A cell membrane or protein that contains hydrophilic groups on its surface that attract water molecules.

hydrophobic

A substance that is insoluble in water. Protein or membrane hydrophobic groups are situated inside these structures away from water.

hydrophobic bond

A bond generated in an aqueous medium when polar water molecules thrust hydrophobic, nonpolar chemical groups together in an effort to generate the minimum nonpolar surface area possible, thereby maximizing the entropy of the water molecules.

hydrops fetalis

A hydropic condition that occurs in newborns who may appear puffy and plethoric; it may be induced by immune or nonimmune mechanisms. In the immune type, the mother synthesizes immunoglobulin G (IgG) antibodies specific for antigens of the offspring, such as anti-RhD erythrocyte antigen. These IgG antibodies pass across the placenta into the fetal circulation, causing hemolysis. Nonimmune hydrops results from various etiologies not discussed here.

hydroxychloroquine

Hydroxychloroquine, also known as 2-[(4-[7-chloro-4-quinolyl]amino)ethyl-amino]ethanol sulfate, is an antimalarial agent that has immunosuppressive properties. It is believed to suppress intracellular antigen processing and loading of peptides onto MHC class II molecules through elevation of the pH of lysosomal and endosomal compartments. Thus, T cell activation is decreased. It has been used in the treatment of selected autoimmune disorders such as rheumatoid arthritis and systemic lupus erythematosus and in the prevention of graft-vs.-host disease.

hydroxychloroquine sulfate (oral)

An antirheumatic agent used in the treatment of lupus erythematosus and rheumatoid arthritis in patients who have not responded satisfactorily to standard treatments. It is also used to treat malaria.

17-hydroxycorticosteroids (17-OHCSs)

Adrenal steroid hormones synthesized by the action of 17-hydroxylase, including cortisone, cortisol, 11-deoxycortisol, and tetrahydro derivatives of 17-hydroxylase. 17-OHCS presence in the urine indicates the functional status of adrenal glands and catabolic rates. 17-OHCSs are elevated in Cushing's disease, obesity, pregnancy, and pancreatitis but decreased in hypopituitarism and Addison's disease.

hygiene hypothesis

The concept that extreme measures to prevent exposure of infants to disease-producing microorganisms results in failure of the immature immune system to become activated. This is claimed to lead to Th2 responses that may predispose a subject to hypersensitivity and/or autoimmunity. Thus, increased hygienic conditions, vaccination, and antibiotic therapy are claimed to prevent children's immune systems from becoming accustomed to interacting with infectious disease agents in the environment.

hyperactivated macrophage

Refer to macrophage.

hyperacute graft rejection (HAR)

Accelerated allograft rejection attributable to preformed antibodies in the circulation of the recipient that are

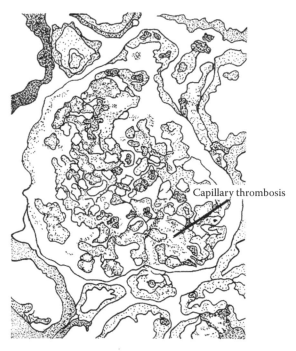

Hyperacute rejection of renal allograft.

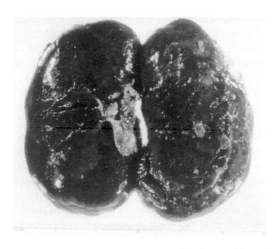

Hyperacute rejection of renal allotransplant showing swelling and purplish discoloration. This is a bivalved transplanted kidney. The allograft was removed within a few hours following transplantation.

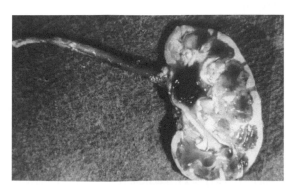

A bivalved transplanted kidney showing hyperacute rejection. There is extensive pale cortical necrosis. This kidney was removed 5 days after transplantation.

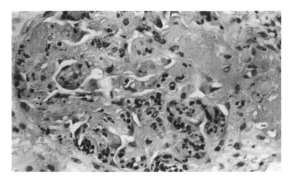

Microscopic view of hyperacute rejection showing a necrotic glomerulus infiltrated with numerous polymorphonuclear leukocytes. H&E stained section 25×.

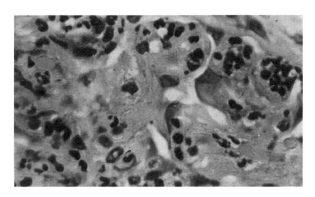

High-power view of hyperacute rejection showing necrotic glomerulus. There are large numbers of polymorphonuclear leukocytes present. Extensive endothelial cell destruction is apparent. H&E stained section 50×.

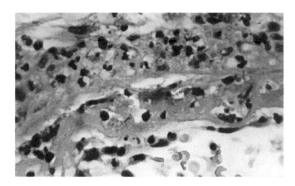

Microscopic view of hyperacute rejection showing necrosis of the wall of a small arteriole.

specific for antigens of the donor. Produced by complement activation induced by preformed antibodies that recognize allogeneic epitopes on the graft vasculature. These antibodies react with antigens which may be HLA class I antigens or ABO blood group antigens of endothelial cells lining capillaries of the donor organ. The reaction sets in motion a process that culminates in fibrin plugging of the donor organ vessels, resulting in ischemia and loss of function and necessitating removal of the transplanted organ. A type II hypersensitivity mechanism.

hyperacute xenograft rejection

An antigraft immune response mediated by human natural antibodies that crossreact with porcine xenograft endothelial cells expressing glycolipid and glycoprotein galactose-α (1-3) galactose.

hypereosinophilia

Markedly elevated numbers of eosinophils in the peripheral blood.

hypergammaglobulinemia

Elevated serum γ globulin (immunoglobulin) levels. A polyclonal increase in immunoglobulins in the serum occurs in any condition involving continuous stimulation of the immune system, such as chronic infection, autoimmune disease, systemic lupus erythematosus (SLE), etc. Hypergammaglobulinemia may also result from a monoclonal increase in immunoglobulin production, as in multiple myeloma, Waldenström's macroglobulinemia, and other conditions associated with the formation of monoclonal immunoglobulins. Repeated immunization may also induce hypergammaglobulinemia.

hypergammaglobulinemic purpura

Purpura hyperglobulinemia.

hyper-IgD with periodic fever syndrome

An autoinflammatory primary immunodeficiency associated with increased serum IgD. Attributable to mutations in mevalonate kinase, an enzyme that participates in cholesterol biosynthesis.

hyper-IgE syndrome

A primary immunodeficiency of unknown etiology and associated with remarkably elevated circulating levels of IgE.

hyper-IgM syndrome (HIGM)

Related primary immunodeficiencies associated with normal to markedly elevated levels of circulating IgM but very diminished or absent levels of the remaining immunoglobulin isotypes. Monoclonal antibodies against CD40 surface protein of B cells induce isotype switching in the presence of appropriate costimulatory cytokines. CD40L is a surface molecule transiently expressed on activated T cells mostly of the CD4+ subpopulation. Mutations of CD40L account for the X-linked form of the disease.

hyperimmune

A descriptor for an animal with a high level of immunity that is induced by repeated immunization of the animal to generate large amounts of functionally effective antibodies, in comparison to animals subjected to routine immunization protocols, perhaps with fewer boosters.

hyperimmunization

Successive administration of an immunogen to an animal to induce the synthesis of antibody in relatively large amounts. This procedure is followed in the preparation of therapeutic antisera by repeatedly immunizing animals to render them hyperimmune.

hyperimmunized individual

A person who has formed alloantibodies against an antigen to which he or she was previously exposed, such as a prior allograft, blood transfusion, or pregnancy. May sometimes be attributable to natural antibodies specific for antigenic determinants of pathogens that cross react with allogeneic donor antigens of a graft.

hyperimmunoglobulin E syndrome (HIE)

A condition characterized by markedly elevated immunoglobulin E (IgE) levels (above 5000 IU/mL). The patients have early eczema and repeated abscesses of the skin, sinuses, lungs, eyes, and ears. *Staphylococcus aureus, Candida albicans, Haemophilus influenzae, Streptococcus*

pneumoniae, and group A hemolytic streptococci are among the more common infectious agents. The principal infection produced by *S. aureus* and *C. albicans* is a "cold abscess" of the skin. The failure of IgE to fix complement and therefore cause inflammation at the infection site is characteristic. IgG antibodies against IgE form complexes that bind to mononuclear phagocytes, resulting in monokine release that induces calcium resorption from bone. As calcium is lost from the bone, osteoporosis results, leading to bone fractures. Patients with HIE have diminished antibody responses to vaccines and to major histocompatibility antigens. They may be anergic, and *in vitro* challenge of their lymphocytes with mitogens or antigens leads to diminished responsiveness. The CD8+ T lymphocyte population in the peripheral blood also decreases. The disease becomes manifest in young infants, shows no predilection for males versus females, and is not hereditary. Also called Job's syndrome.

hyperimmunoglobulin M syndrome

An immunodeficiency disorder in which the serum immunoglobulin M (IgM) level is normal or elevated. By contrast, the serum IgG and IgA levels are strikingly diminished or absent. Patients have repeated infections and may develop neoplasms in childhood. This syndrome may be transmitted in an X-linked or autosomal-dominant fashion. It may also be related to congenital rubella. The condition is produced by failure of T lymphocytes to signal IgM-synthesizing B cells to switch to IgG- and IgA-producing cells. In this X-linked disease in boys who are unable to synthesize immunoglobulin isotypes other than IgM, the gene encoding the CD40 ligand is defective. The T$_H$ cells fail to express CD40L. These patients do not develop germinal centers or displaced somatic hypermutation. They do not form memory B cells and are subject to pyogenic bacterial and protozoal infections.

hyperplasia

An increase in the cell number that leads to an increase in organ size. It is often linked to a physiological reaction to a stimulus and is reversible.

hypersensitive response (HR)

An antipathogen response in plants produced by *avr-R* system activation that leads to alterations in Ca+ flux, MAPK activation, and NO and ROI formation. There is rapid necrosis of plant cells in contact with the pathogen. This process prevents spread of the pathogen and releases hydrolytic enzymes that facilitate injury to the pathogen's structural integrity.

hypersensitivity

Increased reactivity or increased sensitivity by an animal body to an antigen to which it has been previously exposed. The term is often used as a synonym for allergy, which describes a state of altered reactivity to an antigen. Hypersensitivity has been divided into categories based upon whether it can be passively transferred by antibodies or by specifically immune lymphoid cells. The most widely adopted current classification is that of Coombs and Gell, which designates immunoglobulin-mediated hypersensitivity reactions as types I, II, and III and lymphoid-cell-mediated (delayed-type) hypersensitivity/cell-mediated immunity as a type IV reaction. *Hypersensitivity* generally represents the "dark side," signifying the undesirable aspects of an immune reaction, whereas *immunity* implies a desirable effect.

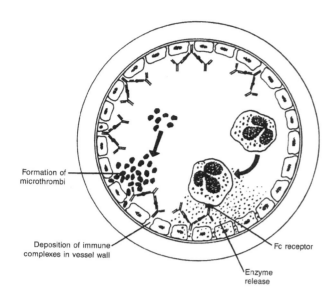

Schematic representation of the formation and deposition of immune complexes in vessel walls in type III hypersensitivity.

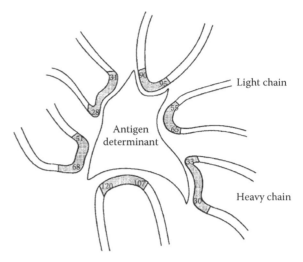

The structure of the six hypervariable regions of an antibody.

hypersensitivity angiitis
Small vessel inflammation most frequently induced by drugs.

hypersensitivity diseases
Disorders medicated at least in part by immune mechanisms such as autoimmune diseases in which autoantibodies react with basement membranes such as the kidney, lung, and skin or in which autoantibodies react against cell constituents such as DNA as in systemic lupus erythematosus (SLE). Any of the four mechanisms of hypersensitivity reaction may participate in the production of a hypersensitivity disease.

hypersensitivity pneumonitis
Lung inflammation induced by antibodies specific for substances that have been inhaled. Within hours of inhaling the causative agent, dyspnea, chills, fever, and coughing occur. Histopathology of the lung reveals inflammation of alveoli in the interstitium with obliterating bronchiolitis. Immunofluorescence examination reveals deposits of C3. Hyperactivity of the lungs to airborne immunogens or allergens may ultimately lead to interstitial lung disease. An example is farmer's lung, which is characterized by malaise, coughing, fever, tightness in the chest, and myalgias. Of the numerous syndromes and associated antigens that may induce hypersensitivity pneumonitis, humidifier lung (thermophilic actinomycetes), bagassosis (*Thermoactinomyces vulgaris*), and bird fancier's lung (bird droppings) are well known. Types of hypersensitivity pneumonitis caused by *Penicillium* species include cheese worker's disease, humidifier lung, woodman's disease, and cork worker's disease.

hypersensitivity reaction
Refer to hypersensitivity.

hypersensitivity vasculitis
An allergic response to drugs, microbial antigens, or antigens from other sources, leading to an inflammatory reaction involving small arterioles, venules, and capillaries.

hyperthyroidism
A metabolic disorder attributable to thyroid hyperplasia with an elevation in thyroid hormone secretion. Also called Graves' disease.

hypervariable regions
A minimum of four sites of great variability that are present throughout the heavy and light chain V regions. They govern the antigen-binding sites of antibody molecules. The grouping of these hypervariable residues into areas governs both conformation and specificity of the antigen-binding sites upon folding of the protein molecules. Hypervariable residues are also responsible for variations in idiotypes between immunoglobulins produced by separate cell clones. Those parts of the variable region that are not hypervariable are called framework regions (FRs). Hypervariable regions are also called complementarity-determining regions (CDRs; refer to hot spot). The term also refers to portions of T cell receptors (TCRs) that constitute antigen-binding sites. Each antibody heavy chain and light chain and each TCR α chain and β chain possesses three hypervariable loops, also called CDRs. Most of the variability between different antibodies or TCRs is present within these loops.

hypocomplementemia
Diminished complement in the blood. It can arise from a number of diseases in which immune complexes fix complement *in vivo,* leading to decreases in complement proteins. Examples include active cases of systemic lupus erythematosus (SLE), proliferative glomerulonephritis, and serum sickness. Protein-deficient patients may also have diminished plasma complement protein levels.

hypocomplementemic glomerulonephritis
Decreased complement in the blood during the course of chronic progressive glomerulonephritis, in which C3 is deposited in the glomerular basement membrane of the kidney.

hypocomplementemic vasculitis urticarial syndrome
A type of systemic inflammation with leukocytoclastic vasculitis. Diminished serum complement levels and urticaria are present.

hypogammaglobulinemia
Deficient levels of IgG, IgM, and IgA serum immunoglobulins that may be attributable to decreased synthesis or increased loss. Hypogammaglobulinemia can be physiologic in neonates. It may be a manifestation of congenital or acquired antibody deficiency syndromes. Several types are described and include Bruton's

disease, a congenital type, and an acquired type such as in chronic lymphocytic leukemia. Human γ globulin is used for treatment.

hypogammaglobulinemia of infancy

A temporary delay in immunoglobulin synthesis during the first 12 or even 24 months of life. This delay leads only to a transient physiologic immunodeficiency following catabolism of maternal immunoglobulins passed to the infant.

hyposensitization

A technique to decrease responsiveness to antigens acting as allergens in individuals with immediate (type I) hypersensitivity to them. Because the reaction is mediated by immunoglobulin E (IgE) antibodies specific for the allergen becoming fixed to the surface of the patient's mast cells, the aim of this mode of therapy is to stimulate the production of IgG-blocking antibodies that will combine with the allergen before it reaches the mast cell-bound IgE antibodies. This is accomplished by graded administration of an altered form of the allergen that favors the production of IgG rather than IgE antibodies. In addition to intercepting allergen prior to its interaction with IgE, the IgG antibodies may also inhibit further production of IgE. The subcutaneous inoculation of progressively increasing quantities of purified allergen on a regular basis for 3 to 5 years leads to the synthesis of allergen-specific IgG4, which fails to trigger mast cell degranulation instead of the production of allergen-specific IgE.

hypothalamic–pituitary–adrenal (HPA) axis

The neural system pathway that is responsible for the "fight or flight" acute stress response. Activation of the HPA by extreme stress leads to excessive glucocorticoid synthesis, suppressed inflammatory responses, and increased susceptibility to infections.

hypothyroid

Markedly diminished synthesis of thyroid hormone by the thyroid gland.

H-Y antigen

An epitope detected by cell-mediated and humoral immune responses of homogametic persons against heterogametic subjects of the same species, which are otherwise genetically identical. Such responses have been shown in mammals, birds, and amphibians.

H-Y system

Genes on the Y chromosome encode H-Y antigens that are "self" when expressed in males amd "non-self" when expressed in females who are otherwise genetically identical.

I-309

A chemokine of the β (CC) family. It is secreted by activated T lymphocytes and is a chemoattractant for monocytes. Its primary structure reveals two characteristics not present in other β chemokines: two extra cysteine residues in a single *N*-linked glycosylation site located in the middle of the β strand that constitutes the proposed dimer interface. Tissue sources include T lymphocytes, human mast cells, HMC-1, and murine mast cell lines. Target cells include monocytes, macrophages, neutrophils, basophils, and microglial cells.

I invariant (Ii)

Refer to invariant chain.

I-K

Abbreviation for immunoconglutinin.

I region

In the mouse, the DNA segment of the major histocompatibility complex (MHC) where the gene that encodes MHC class II molecules is located. The 250-kb I region consists of I-A and I-E subregions. The genes designated pseudo Aβ3, Aβ2, Aβ1, and Aβ are located in the 175-kb I-A subregion. The genes designated Eβ2 and Eα are located in the 75-kb I-E subregion. Eβ1 is located where the I-A and I-E subregions join. The S region contains the Eβ3 gene.

Ia antigen (immune-associated antigen)

Product of major histocompatibility complex (MHC) class I region genes that encodes murine cellular antigens. In humans, the equivalent antigens are designated HLA-DR and are encoded by MHC class II genes. B lymphocytes, monocytes, and activated T lymphocytes express Ia antigens.

iatrogenic

A disease or injury resulting from therapy by a medical practitioner.

IBD

Abbreviation for inflammatory bowel disease.

ibuprofen

Its chemical name is (+)-2-(*p*-isobutylphenyl)propionic acid. An antiinflammatory drug used in the therapy of patients with rheumatoid arthritis, ankylosing spondylitis, and juvenile rheumatoid arthritis.

iC3B (inactivated C3b)

Also designated C3bi.

iC3b-Neo

Complement component C3 expresses a neoepitope not present on native C3 or C3 degradation products following activation or cleavage by C3 convertases of the classical or alternative pathways. Increased iC3b concentrations have been found in septic shock, transplant rejection, and in some patients with systemic lupus erythematosus (SLE). Localized elevations have been found in atherosclerotic lesions, suggesting a role for complement in atherosclerosis. The clinical significance of iC3b determination has not yet been determined.

iC4b

Synonym for C4bi.

ICA512 (IA-2)

A protein tyrosine phosphatase-like molecule that belongs to a group of transmembrane molecules. It was discovered by screening islet expression libraries with human insulin-dependent diabetes mellitus sera. IA-2 and phogrin are the two homologs. The IA-2 antigen is expressed in islets and in the brain.

ICAM-1 (intercellular adhesion molecule 1)

A γ interferon-induced protein necessary for the migration of polymorphonuclear neutrophils into areas of inflammation.

ICAM-2

Refer to intercellular adhesion molecule 2.

ICAM-3

Refer to intercellular adhesion molecule 3.

iccosomes (immune-complex-coated antibodies)

Small membrane fragments coated with immune complexes that fragment off follicular dendritic cell processes in lymphoid follicles early in a secondary or subsequent antibody response. Iccosomes budding from follicular dendritic cells can unite with B cell receptors through the presence of

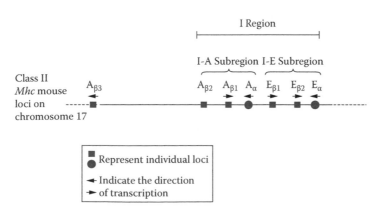

In the mouse, the I region is the DNA segment of the major histocompatibility complex, where the genes that encode MHC class II molecules are located.

specific antigen. The antigen from iccosomes taken up by B cells can be presented on MHC class II molecules to a T helper cell.

ICOS

A CD28-related protein that develops on activated T lymphocytes and is able to enhance T cell responses. Licos, the ligand to which it binds, is distinct from B7 molecules.

IDDM

Abbreviation for insulin-dependent diabetes mellitus.

identity, reaction of

Refer to reaction of identity.

identity testing

See paternity testing.

idiopathic thrombocytopenic purpura

An autoimmune disease in which antiplatelet autoantibodies destroy platelets. Splenic macrophages remove circulating platelets coated with immunoglobulin G (IgG) autoantibodies at an accelerated rate. Thrombocytopenia occurs even though the bone marrow increases platelet production, which can lead to purpura and bleeding. The platelet count may fall below 20,000 to 30,000/μL. Antiplatelet antibodies are detectable in the serum and on platelets. Platelet survival is decreased. Splenectomy is recommended in adults. Corticosteroids facilitate a temporary elevation in the platelet count. This disease is characterized by decreased blood platelets, hemorrhage, and extensive thromboic lesions.

idiosyncrasy

A quantitatively abnormal response usually not corresponding to the pharmacological action of a drug. The response does not have an immunological mechanism.

idiotope

An epitope or antigenic determinant in the hypervariable region of the N terminus of an immunoglobulin molecule, T cell receptor molecule, or on the V region of an antibody molecule. This type of antigenic determinant is present on immunoglobulin molecules synthesized by one clone or a few clones of antibody-producing cells. It can activate the synthesis of antibodies following administration to a member of the same species.

idiotype (Id)

A segment of an immunoglobulin or antibody molecule that determines its specificity for antigen and is based upon the multiple combinations of variable (V), diversity (D), and joining (J) exons. The Id is located in the Fab region, and its expression usually requires participation of the variable regions of both heavy and light chains, namely the Fv fragments that contain antigen-combining sites. The antigen-binding specificity of the combining site may imply that all antibodies produced by an animal in response to a given immunogen have the same Id. This is not true, however, as the antibody response is heterogeneous. A major Id usually represents 20 to 70% of the specific antibody response; the remainder carries different Ids that may crossreact with the major Id. Crossreacting idiotypy represents the extent of heterogeneity among the antibodies of a given specificity. The unique antigenic determinants that govern the Id of an immunoglobulin molecule occur on the products of either a single or several clones of cells synthesizing immunoglobulins. This unique idiotypic determinant is sometimes called a private Id that appears in all V regions

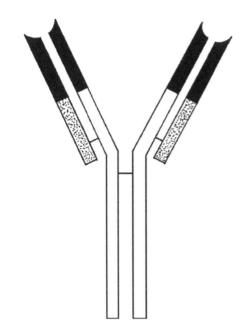

The idiotype (in black) is determined by the variable regions of heavy and light chains of an immunoglobulin molecule.

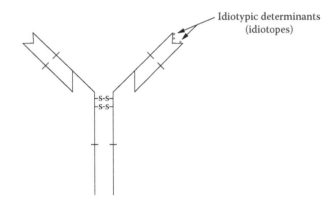

Idiotypic determinants (idiotypes).

of immunoglobulin molecules whose amino acid sequences are the same. Shared Ids are known as public idiotype determinants. They may appear in a relatively large number of immunoglobulin molecules produced by inbred strains of mice or other genetically identical animals in response to a specific antigen. The localization of Ids in the antigen-binding site of the V region of the molecule is illustrated by the ability of haptens to block or inhibit the interaction of anti-idiotypic antibodies with their homologous antigenic markers or determinants in the antigen-binding regions of antibody molecules.

idiotype network

The interaction of idiotypes and anti-idiotypes that leads to the regulation of antibody synthesis or of lymphoid cells bearing receptors that express these idiotypic specificities. Responses of one or a few lymphocyte clones to antigen leads to idiotype expansion and anti-idiotype responses that downregulate the antigen-specific response.

idiotype network theory

Refer to network theory.

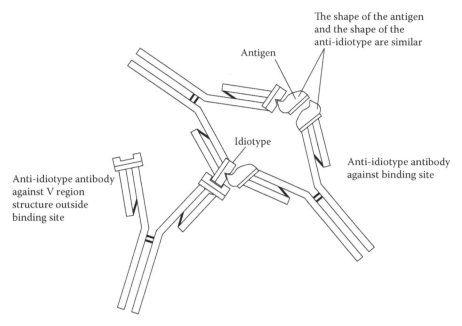

Idiotype network.

Antigen

The shape of the antigen
and the shape of the
anti-idiotype are similar

Idiotype

Anti-idiotype antibody
against V region
structure outside
binding site

Anti-idiotype antibody
against binding site

idiotype suppression

The inhibition of idiotype antibody production by suppressor T lymphocytes activated by antiidiotype antibodies.

idiotype vaccine

Antibody preparation that mimics antigens at the molecular level. These vaccines induce immunity specific for the antigens they mimic. They are not infectious to recipients, are physiologic, and can be used in place of many antigens, e.g., the idiotype vaccine related to *Plasmodium falciparum* circumsporozote (CS) protein.

idiotypic determinant

Refer to epitope.

idiotypic specificity

Characteristic folding of the antigen-binding site, thereby exposing various groups that, by their arrangement, confer antigenic properties to the immunoglobulin V region. Antibodies against a specific antigen usually carry both a few predominant idiotypes and other similar, but not identical, crossreacting idiotypes. The proportion between the two indicates the degree of heterogeneity of the antibody response in a given individual.

id reaction

Dermatophytid reaction. A sudden rash linked to, but anatomically separated from, an inflammatory reaction of the skin in a sensitized individual with the same types of lesions elsewhere. The hands and arms are usual sites of id reactions that are expressed as sterile papulovesicular pustules. They may be linked with dermatophytosis such as tinea capitis or tinea pedis. They may also be associated with stasis dermatitis, contact dermatitis, and eczema.

IE

Acronym for immunoelectrophoresis.

IEF

Acronym for isoelectric focusing.

IEP

Acronym for immunoelectrophoresis.

i-exons

Leader-like sequences present in the C_H region of the IgH locus, where transcription of germline C_H transcripts requisite for switch recombination begins.

IFE

Acronym for immunofixation electrophoresis.

IFN

Acronym for interferon.

IFN-α

Abbreviation for interferon-α.

IFN-β

Abbreviation for interferon-β.

IFN-γ

Abbreviation for interferon-γ.

Igα/Igβ complex

A B cell receptor complex accessory heterodimer needed to transduce intracellular signaling activated by mIg interaction with antigen. Igα and Igβ cytoplasmic tails contain ITAMs.

Ig domain

Refer to immunoglobulin domain.

IGF-II

Insulin-like growth factor-II (IGF-II). A fetal growth factor expressed at high levels in many tissues during fetal and early postnatal development but only in the central nervous system thereafter.

Ig

Abbreviation for immunoglobulin.

Igα and Igβ

Proteins on the B cell surface that are noncovalently associated with cell surface immunoglobulin M (IgM) and IgD. They link the B cell antigen receptor complex to intracellular tyrosine kinases. Anti-Ig binding leads to their phosphorylation. Igα and Igβ are requisite for expression of IgM and IgD on B cell surfaces. Disulfide bonds link Igα and Igβ pairs that are associated noncovalently with the membrane Ig cytoplasmic tail to form the B cell receptor complex (BRC). The Igα and Igβ cytoplasmic domains bear immunoreceptor tyrosine-based activation motifs (ITAMs) that participate in early signaling when antigens activate B cells.

Igα/Igβ (CD79a/CD79b)

The Igα/Igβ heterodimer interacts with immunoglobulin heavy chains for signal transduction. In the pro-B cell stage, rearrangement of the immunoglobulin heavy chain gene leads to expression of surface membrane immunoglobulin (mIgμ). mIgμ associates with Igα/Igβ and surrogate light chain in pre-B cells or ordinary light chains in B cells to form the precursor B cell receptor and B cell receptor, respectively. Igα and Igβ are expressed before immunoglobulin heavy chain gene rearrangement. They are products of mb-1 and B29 genes, respectively. Allelic exclusion is mediated through signal transduction via Igα and Igβ and depends on intact tyrosine residues.

IgA

Refer to immunoglobulin A.

IgA deficiency

Refer to immunoglobulin A deficiency.

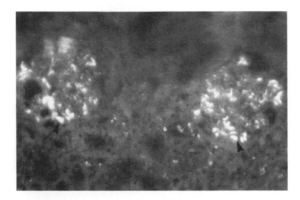

IgA nephropathy. Granular immune deposits in mesangial areas.

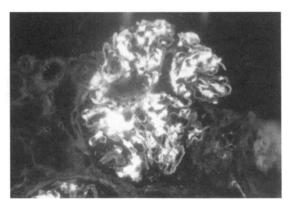

IgA nephropathy (Berger's disease). Granular immune deposits containing IgG, IgA, and C3 in mesangial areas.

IgA nephropathy (Berger's disease)

A type of glomerulonephritis in which prominent IgA-containing immune deposits are present in mesangial areas. Patients usually present with gross or microscopic hematuria and often mild proteinuria. Mesangial widening or proliferation may be observed by light microscopy; however, immunofluorescence microscopy demonstrating IgA and C3 fixed by the alternative pathway is requisite for diagnosis.

Electron microscopy confirms the presence of electron-dense deposits in mesangial areas. Half of the cases progress to chronic renal failure over a 20-year course.

IgA paraproteinemia

Myeloma in which the paraimmunoglobulin belonging to the IgA class occurs in only about one fifth of affected patients. IgA myeloma patients are reputed to have lower survival rates than those patients affected with IgG myeloma, but this claim awaits confirmation. IgA myeloma may be associated with myeloma cell infiltration of the liver leading to jaundice and altered liver function tests. It is frequently associated with hyperviscosity syndrome, which may be related to the ability of IgA molecules to polymerize and form complexes with such substances as haptoglobin, α-1 antitrypsin, β lipoprotein, antihemophilic factor, and albumin.

IgD

Refer to immunoglobulin D.

IgE

Refer to immunoglobulin E.

IgG

Refer to immunoglobulin G.

IgG index

The ratio of IgG and albumin synthesis in the brain and in peripheral tissues. It is increased in multiple central nervous system infections, inflammatory disorders, and neoplasms.

IgG-induced autoimmune hemolysis

Two fifths of cases of this hemolysis are secondary to other diseases such as neoplasia including chronic lymphocytic leukemia and ovarian tumors. This hemolysis may also be secondary to connective tissue diseases such as lupus erythematosus, rheumatoid arthritis, and progressive systemic sclerosis. Patients experience hemolysis leading to anemia with fatigue, dizziness, palpitations, exertion dyspnea, mild jaundice, and splenomegaly. They manifest positive Coombs' antiglobulin tests. Their erythrocytes appear as spherocytes and schistocytes, and evidence of erythrophagocytosis is present. Erythroid hyperplasia of the bone marrow and lymphoproliferative disease may be present. Glucocorticoids and blood transfusions are used for treatment. Approximately 66% improve after splenectomy but often relapse. Three quarters of these individuals survive for a decade.

IgG myeloma subclasses

The most frequent myeloma paraimmunoglobulin is IgG-κ, which belongs to the IgG_1 subclass most commonly and to the IgG_4 subclass only rarely. IgG_3 paraimmunoglobulins are associated with increased serum viscosity, which leads to aggregates that are related to concentration and may be associated with serum cryoglobulin. In IgG paraimmunoglobulin myeloma, the serum concentration of IgG may reach 2000 mg/dL. Concomitantly there is a reduction in other immunoglobulins. Because the IgG myeloma paraimmunoglobulin belongs to one heavy-chain subtype, the Gm allotypes are restricted in a manner similar to the restriction of light chains to either the κ or λ type.

IgG subclass deficiency

Decreased or absent IgG_2, IgG_3, or IgG_4 subclasses. Total serum IgG is unaffected because it is 65 to 70% IgG_1. Deletion of constant heavy chain genes or defects in isotype switching may lead to IgG subclass deficiency. IgG_1 and IgG_3 subclasses mature faster than IgG_2 or IgG_4. Patients have recurrent respiratory infections and recurring pyogenic sinopulmonary infections with *Hemophilus influenzae*, *Staphylococcus aureus*, and *Streptococcus pneumoniae*. Some patients manifest features of autoimmune disease, such as systemic lupus erythematosus (SLE). IgG$_2$–IgG$_4$ deficiency is often associated with recurrent infections or autoimmune disease. IgG$_2$ deficiency is reflected as recurrent sinopulmonary infections and nonresponsiveness to polysaccharide antigens such as those of *Pneumococcus*. A few individuals have IgG$_3$ deficiency and develop recurrent infections. In IgG$_4$-deficient patients, recurrent respiratory infections and autoimmune manifestations also occur. The diagnosis is established by the demonstration of significantly lower levels of at least one IgG subclass in the patient compared with IgG subclass levels in normal age-matched controls. γ Globulin is the treatment choice. Very infrequently, C gene segment deletions may lead to IgG subclass deficiency.

IgM
Refer to immunoglobulin M.

IgM, 7S
Monomeric IgM.

IgM deficiency syndrome
An infrequent condition characterized by diminished activation of complement and decreased B lymphocyte membrane 5-ecto nucleotidase. Patients manifest heightened susceptibility to pulmonary infections, septicemia, and tumors.

IgM index
Reflects total IgM formation in the blood–brain barrier. The index is elevated in infectious meningoencephalomyelitis and may also be increased in central nervous system lupus erythematosus (SLE) and multiple sclerosis (MS).

IgM paraproteinemia
Occasional cases of IgM myeloma occur and are characterized by infiltration of the bone marrow by plasmacytes, numerous osteolytic lesions, and occasionally bleeding diathesis. IgM myeloma is distinct from true Waldenström's macroglobulinemia but is rare compared with the IgG and IgA types. Myelomas associated with the minor classes of immunoglobulin IgD and IgE occur with even less frequency than do the IgM myelomas.

IgR
A second class of immunoglobulin protein in *Raja kenojei*.

IgT
An obsolete term for the T lymphocyte antigen receptor that was incorrectly considered an immunoglobulin of a special class. IgT should not be confused with IgG.

IgW
An immunoglobulin isotype of sharks.

IgX
An immunoglobulin isotype of *Xenopus*.

IgY
An immunoglobulin isotype of *Xenopus*.

Ii
Refer to invariant chain.

Ii antigens
Two nonallelic carbohydrate antigens (epitopes) on the surface membranes of human erythrocytes. They may also occur on some nonhematopoietic cells. The i epitope is found on fetal erythrocytes and red cell blood precursors. The I antigen is formed when aliphatic galactose-*N*-acetyl-glucosamine is converted to a complex branched structure. I represents the mature form and i the immature form. Mature erythrocytes express I. Antibodies against i antigen are hemolytic in cases of infectious mononucleosis.

iIELs
Abbreviation for intestinal intraepithelial lymphocytes.

I-J
An area of the murine I region predicted to encode for a suppressor cell antigen. Recombinant mouse strains were used to show that the I-J gene locus maps to a region between the I-A and I-E loci of the H-2 complex. Monoclonal antibodies against I-J react with antigen-specific suppressor T cells that secrete suppressive factors. The anti-I-J specific antibodies react with an epitope among the suppressor cell factors. I-J determinant is associated with a 13-kDa protein known as the glycosylation-inhibiting factor that has suppressive activity.

Ikaros
A transcription factor requisite for all lineages of lymphoid cells to develop.

IL
Abbreviation for interleukin.

IL1
Abbreviation for interleukin-1.

IL1 Ra
Abbreviation for IL1 receptor antagonist.

IL1 receptor antagonist (IL1ra)
Refer to interleukin-1 receptor antagonist (IL1ra).

IL2
Abbreviation for interleukin-2.

IL2/LAK cells
Interleukin-2 lymphokine-activated killer (LAK) cells. Natural killer (NK) cells that express only the p70 and not the p55 receptor for IL2, are incubated with IL2, converting them into an activated form referred to as LAK cells. The IL2/LAK combination has been used to treat cancer patients through adoptive immunotherapy, which has been successful in inducing transient regression of tumors in selected cases of melanoma, colorectal carcinoma, non-Hodgkin lymphoma, and renal cell carcinoma, as well as regression of metastases in the livers and lungs of some patients. Transient defective chemotaxis of neutrophils may be present and patients often develop capillary leak syndrome, producing pulmonary edema. Patients may also develop congestive heart failure.

IL2 receptor (CD25)
Refer to interleukin-2 receptor (IL2R).

IL3
Abbreviation for interleukin-3.

IL4
Abbreviation for interleukin-4.

Ii Antigens

Phenotype	Antigen Expression	
	I	i
I adult	Strong	Very weak
I cord	Weak	Strong
i adult	Very weak	Strong

IL5

Abbreviation for interleukin-5.

IL6

Abbreviation for interleukin-6.

IL7

Abbreviation for interleukin-7.

IL7Rd

cDNA that encodes the receptor for IL7, known as IL7Rα, has been cloned from both humans and mice.

IL8

Abbreviation for interleukin-8.

IL8RA

Abbreviation for interleukin-8 receptor, type A.

IL8RB

Abbreviation for interleukin-8 receptor, type B.

IL9

Abbreviation for interleukin-9.

IL10

Abbreviation for interleukin-10.

IL11

Abbreviation for interleukin-11.

IL12

Abbreviation for interleukin-12.

IL13

Abbreviation for interleukin-13.

IL14

Abbreviation for interleukin-14.

IL15

Abbreviation for interleukin-15.

IL16

Abbreviation for interleukin-16.

IL17

Abbreviation for interleukin-17.

IL18

Abbreviation for interleukin-18.

IL19

Abbreviation for interleukin-19.

IL20

Abbreviation for interleukin-20.

IL21

Abbreviation for interleukin-21.

IL22

Abbreviation for interleukin-22.

IL23

Abbreviation for interleukin-23.

IL24

Abbreviation for interleukin-24.

IL25

Abbreviation for interleukin-25.

IL26

Abbreviation for interleukin-26.

IL27

Abbreviation for interleukin-27.

IL28

Abbreviation for interleukin-28.

IL29

Abbreviation for interleukin-29.

IL30

Abbreviation for interleukin-30.

IL31

Abbreviation for interleukin-31.

IL32

Abbreviation for interleukin-32.

IL33

Abbreviation for interleukin-33.

IL34

Abbreviation for interleukin-34.

imbritumomab tiuxetan

An anti-CD20 murine monoclonal antibody labeled with isotopic yttrium (^{90}Y) or indium (^{111}In). Isotopic radiation provides the antitumor activity. It is used in the treatment of patients with relapsed or refractory low-grade, follicular, or B cell non-Hodgkin lymphoma.

ImD$_{50}$

The antigen (or vaccine) dose capable of successfully immunizing 50% of a particular animal test population.

IMiDs

Immunomodulatory derivatives of thalidomide designed to be even more effective than thalidomide in regulating cytokines and affecting T cell proliferation.

immature B cells

B lymphocytes in which heavy and light chain variable-region gene rearrangement has occurred with expression of surface IgM, but not surface IgD.

immature B lymphocyte

A B cell that has rearranged a heavy and light chain variable-region gene and expresses surface IgM, but not surface IgD. It arises from bone marrow precursors that fail to proliferate or differentiate following exposure to antigen. By contrast, it undergoes apoptosis and is functionally unresponsive. This mechanism plays a role in the negative selection of B cells specific for self antigens in the bone marrow.

immature dendritic cells

Cells that exit the various body tissues in which they are present only in response to an inflammatory mediator or an infection. They take up antigen but fail to express costimulatory molecules and are unable to act as professional antigen-presenting cells to naïve T cells.

immediate hypersensitivity

Antibody-mediated hypersensitivity. In humans, this homocytotrophic antibody is IgE and in certain other species IgG$_1$. The IgE antibodies are attached to mast cells through their Fc receptors. Once the Fab regions of the mast cell-bound IgE molecules interact with specific antigen, vasoactive amines are released from the cytoplasmic granules as described under type I hypersensitivity reactions. The term *immediate* is used to indicate that this type of reaction occurs within seconds to minutes following contact of a cell-fixed IgE antibody with antigen. Skin tests and RAST are useful for detecting immediate hypersensitivity in humans, and passive cutaneous anaphylaxis reveals immediate hypersensitivity in selected other species. Examples of immediate hypersensitivity in humans include the classic anaphylactic reaction to penicillin administration, hay fever, and environmental allergens such as tree and grass pollens, bee stings, etc.

immediate reaction

The onset of hypersensitivity within seconds to minutes following exposure to antigen. It is attributable to preformed antibodies in the blood circulation, such as IgE antibodies in humans, which mediate anaphylaxis. Refer also to immediate hypersensitivity reactions.

immediate spin cross match

A test for incompatibility between donor erythrocytes and recipient serum. This assay reveals ABO incompatibility in most cases but is unable to identify immunoglobulin G (IgG) alloantibodies against erythrocyte antigens.

immobilization test

A method for the identification of antibodies specific for motile microorganisms by determining the ability of antibody to inhibit motility. This may be attributable to adhesion or agglutination of the microorganisms' flagella or cell wall injury when complement is present.

immune

Having natural or acquired resistance to a disease. A subclinical infection with a causative agent or deliberate immunization with antigenic substances prepared from it may render a host immune. Because of immunological memory, the immune state is heightened upon second exposure to an immunogen. A subject may become immune as a consequence of having experienced and recovered from an infectious disease.

immune adherence

Attachment of antigen–antibody complexes or of antibody-coated bacteria or other particles carrying C3b or C4b to complement receptor 1 (CR1)-expressing cells. Erythrocytes of primates, B cells, T cells, phagocytic cells, and glomerular epithelial cells all express CR1. It is absent on the erythrocytes of other mammals but is found on their thrombocytes. Immune adherence facilitates the elimination of antigen–antibody complexes from the blood circulation, especially through their attachment to red blood cells and platelets followed by uptake by phagocytic cells through CR 3.

immune adherence receptor

Synonym for complement receptor 1.

immune antibody

An antibody induced by transfusion or other immunogenic challenge in contrast to a natural antibody such as an isohemagglutinin against ABO blood group substances found in humans.

immune cell cryopreservation

The use of glycerol and dimethylsufoxide (DMSO) to cryopreserve bone marrow for transplantation first involves freezing at a constant rate of 1°C min^{-1} to –79°C, followed by storage for a 6-month period. Dye exclusion is used to test cells for viability after thawing. Lymphocytes have been cryopreserved for *in vitro* studies using 15% DMSO and stored in liquid nitrogen (–196°C) for 3 months followed by an assay for viability.

immune cell motility

Migration of immune cells is a principal host defense mechanism for the recruitment of leukocytes to inflammatory sites in the development of cell-mediated immunity. The induction of migratory responses follows the interaction of signal molecules with plasma membrane receptors, initiating cytoskeletal reorganization and changes in cell shape. Motile responses may be random, chemokinetic, chemotactic, or haptotactic. Random migration of unstimulated motility and chemokinetic migration (i.e., stimulated random movement of cells without a stimulus gradient) are motile responses that are not consistently directional. By contrast, directional responses include those that are chemotactic and haptotactic. They take place when cells are subjected to a signal gradient, and the cells migrate toward an increasing concentration of the stimulus. The various motile responses may participate in the mobilization of immune cells to sites of inflammation.

immune clearance

Refer to immune elimination.

immune complex coated bodies

Refer to iccosomes.

immune complex disease (ICD)

As described for the type III hypersensitivity reaction, the fates of antigen–antibody complexes depend in part on their size. The larger insoluble immune complexes are removed by the mononuclear phagocyte system. The smaller complexes become lodged in the microvasculature such as the renal glomeruli. They may activate the complement system and attract polymorphonuclear neutrophils, initiating an inflammatory reaction. The antigen of an immune complex may be from microorganisms such as streptococci leading to subepithelial deposits in renal glomeruli in post-streptococcal glomerulonephritism, or they may be endogenous, such as DNA or nuclear antigens in systemic lupus erythematosus (SLE). Diphtheria antitoxin prepared in horses induced serum sickness when the foreign horse serum proteins stimulated antibodies in human recipients. Immune complex disease is characterized clinically by fever, joint pain, lymphadenopathy, eosinophilia, hypocomplementemia, proteinuria, purpura, and urticaria, among other features. Laboratory techniques to detect immune complexes include the solid-phase Clq assay, the Clq-binding assay, the Raji cell technique, and the staphylococcal protein assay, among other methods. Most autoimmune diseases have type III (antigen–antibody complex)-mediated mechanisms. Connective tissue diseases such as SLE, polyarteritis nodosa, progressive systemic sclerosis, dermatomyositis, rheumatoid arthritis, and others fall within this category. Viral infections such as hepatitis B, cytomegalovirus, infectious mononucleosis, dengue, and neoplasias such as carcinomas and melanomas, may be associated with immune complex formation. Refer to type III hypersensitivity reaction.

immune complex glomerulonephritis

Inflammation induced by antigen–antibody complexes deposited in the renal glomeruli leading to impairment of renal function.

immune complex pneumonitis

A type III, immune complex, Arthus-type reaction in the pulmonary alveoli.

immune complex reaction

Type III hypersensitivity in which antigen–antibody complexes fix complement and induce inflammation in tissues such as capillary walls.

immune complexes

The product of interaction between antigen and antigen-specific antibody (refer also to antigen–antibody complex); a macromolecular complex of antibody molecules that are bivalent and antigen molecules that are multivalent and may also contain complement components. Because antigens and antibodies can combine in multiple proportions, the complexes range from large (more easily removed by the mononuclear phagocyte system) to small soluble complexes that deposit in small blood vessel walls, leading to inflammation and tissue injury. Refer also to type III hypersensitivity.

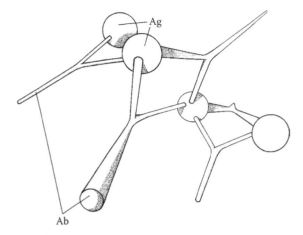

Immune complex disease.

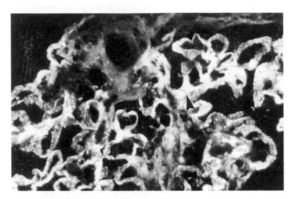

Immune complexes in renal glomerulus.

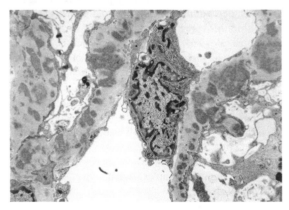

Immune complex disease (ICD). Electron dense deposits.

immune costimulatory molecules

B7-1 and B7-2 and the CD28 and CTLA-4 receptors constitute one of the dominant costimulatory pathways that regulate T and B cell responses. Although both CTLA-4 and CD28 can bind to the same ligands, CTLA-4 binds to B7-1 and B7-2 with a 20- to 100-fold higher affinity than CD28 and is involved in the downregulation of the immune response. B7-1 is expressed on activated B cells, activated T cells, and macrophages. B7-2 is constitutively expressed on interdigitating dendritic cells, Langerhans' cells, peripheral blood dendritic cells, memory B cells, and germinal center B cells. Both human and mouse B7-1 and B7-2 can bind to either human or mouse CD28 and CTLA-4, suggesting that conserved amino acids form the B7-1/ B7-2/CD28/CTLA-4 critical binding sites.

immune cytolysis

Complement-induced destruction or lysis of antibody-coated target cells such as tumor cells. Immune cytolysis of red blood cells is referred to as immune hemolysis. Immune cytolysis also involves the destruction of target cells by cytotoxic T lymphocytes or natural killer (NK) cells (including K cells) through the release of perforins.

immune deviation

Antigen-mediated suppression of the immune response may selectively affect delayed-type hypersensitivity (DTH), leaving certain types of immunoglobulin responses relatively intact and unaltered. This selective suppression of certain phases of the immune response to an antigen without alteration of others is termed immune deviation. It may involve conversion of a T cell response involving T_H1 cytokines that induce cell-mediated immunity to a T_H2 cytokine response that induces synthesis of selected antibody isotypes. Split tolerance or immune deviation offers an experimental model for dissection of the immune response into its component parts. It is necessary to use an antigen capable of inducing formation of humoral antibody and development of delayed-type hypersensitivity to induce immune deviation. Because it is essential that both humoral and cellular phases of the immune response be directed to the same antigenic determinant group, defined antigens are required. Immune deviation selectively suppresses delayed-type hypersensitivity and IgG_2 antibody production. By contrast, immunologic tolerance affects both IgG_1 and IgG_2 antibody production and delayed-type hypersensitivity. For example, prior administration of certain protein antigens to guinea pigs may lead to antibody production. However, the subsequent injection of antigen incorporated into Freund's complete adjuvant leads to deviation from the expected heightened, delayed-type hypersensitivity and formation of IgG_2 antibodies to result in little of either, i.e., negligible delayed-type hypersensitivity and suppression of IgG_2 formation. Recent advances in understanding of cytokines and T cell subsets have rekindled interest in immune deviation with the delineation of the T_H1 and T_H2 subsets of CD4+ effector T lymphocytes, and a cellular framework for immune deviation is available. Powerful cell-mediated (DTH) responses occur when T_H1 cells secreting interleukin-2 (IL2) and interferon γ (IFN-γ) are preferentially activated under the influence of macrophage-derived IL12. By contrast, synthesis of most antibody classes is favored by stimulation of IL4-secreting T_H2 cells. Cross-inhibition of T_H2 cells by IFN-γ and T_H1 cells by IL4 and IL10 reinforces deviation down one rather than the other T cell pathway.

immune elimination

Accelerated removal of an antigen from the blood circulation following its interaction with specific antibody and elimination of antigen–antibody complexes through the mononuclear phagocyte system. A few days following antigen administration, antibodies appear in the circulation and eliminate the antigen at a much more rapid rate than the rate in nonimmune individuals. Splenic and liver macrophages express Fc receptors that bind antigen–antibody complexes and also complement receptors, which bind those immune

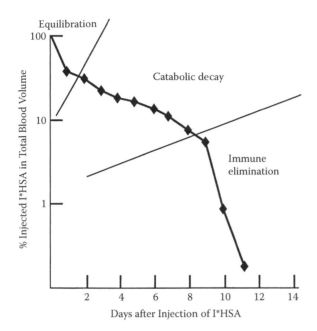

Immune elimination.

complexes that have already fixed complement. This is followed by removal of immune complexes through the phagocytic actions of mononuclear phagocytes. Immune elimination also describes an assay to evaluate the antibody response by monitoring the rate at which a radiolabeled antigen is eliminated in an animal with specific (homologous) antibodies in the circulation.

immune exclusion

Prevention of antigen entry into the body by the products of a specific immune response, such as the blocking of access by an antigen to the body by mucosal surfaces when secretory IgA specific for the antigen is present.

immune globulin, human (intravenous, IVEEGAM EN)

Indicated for replacement therapy in individuals with primary immunodeficiency syndromes including congenital agammaglobulinemia, common variable immunodeficiency, X-linked agammaglobulinemia (with or without hyper IgM) and Wiskott–Aldrich syndrome. Patients with severe combined immunodeficiency have an impairment of antibody synthesis and T cell defects. Thus, they may benefit from replacement therapy with immune globulin even though the therapy does not correct their basic cellular defects. Immune globulin IV (human) is very effective in providing high levels of circulating antibodies within a short time when intramuscular injections are contraindicated. It has also been used for Kawasaki syndrome and has other unlabeled uses including post-transfusion purpura, Guillain-Barré syndrome, and chronic inflammatory demyelinating polyneuropathy. It is also useful in treatment of selected autoimmune diseases such as rhesus hemolytic disease, factor VIII deficiencies, bullous pemphigoid, rheumatoid arthritis, Sjögren's syndrome, type I diabetes mellitus, IgG4 subclass deficiencies, intractable epilepsy (possibly caused by IgG2 subclass deficiency), cystic fibrosis, trauma, thermal injury (e.g., severe burns), cytomegalovirus infection, neuromuscular disorders, prophylaxis of infections associated with bone marrow transplantation, and GI protection (i.e., oral administration).

immune hemolysis

The lysis of erythrocytes through the action of specific antibody and complement.

immune inflammation

Reaction to injury mediated by an adaptive immune response to antigen. Neutrophils and macrophages responding to T cell cytokines may comprise the inflammatory cellular infiltrate.

immune interferon

Synonym for interferon-γ.

immune modulation

Refer to immunomodulation.

immune modulator

An agent that alters the level of an immune response.

immune network hypothesis of Jerne

The antigen-binding sites (paratopes) of antibody molecules are encoded by variable region genes and have idiotopes as phenotypic markers. Each paratope recognizes idiotopes on a different antibody molecule. Interaction of idiotypes with anti-idiotypes is physiologic idiotypy and is shared among immunoglobulin (Ig) classes. This comprises antibodies produced in response to the same antigen. The idiotypic network consists of the interaction of idiotypes involving free molecules as well as B and T lymphocyte receptors. Idiotypes are considered central in immunoregulation involving autoantigens.

immune–neuroendocrine axis

A bidirectional regulatory circuit exists between the immune and neuroendocrine systems that affect each other. Receptors for neurally active polypeptides, neurotransmitters, and hormones are present on immune system cells, whereas receptors reactive with products of the immune system may be identified on nervous system cells. Neuroendocrine hormones have variable immunoregulatory effects mediated through specific receptors. Neurotransmitter influence on cell function is determined in part by the receptor-linked signal amplification associated with second messenger systems. Neuroimmunoregulation is mediated either through a neural pathway involving pituitary peptides and adrenal steroid hormones or through a second pathway consisting of direct innervation of immune system tissues. The thymus, spleen, bone marrow, and perhaps other lymphoid organs contain afferent and efferent nerve fibers. Adrenocorticotrophic hormone (ACTH), endorphins, enkephalins, and adrenal cortical steroids derived from the pituitary represent one direction for modulating the immune response. For example, prolactin (PRL) regulates lymphocyte function. Stimulated lymphocytes or nonstimulated macrophages may produce neuroendocrine hormone-related peptides, ACTH, and endorphins. The participation of these substances in a stress response represents the opposite direction of regulation. Thymic hormones may also induce an endocrine response. Neuroendocrine hormones may exert a positive or negative regulatory effect on macrophages that play a key role in both inflammation and immune responsiveness. Leukocyte mediators are known to alter both central nervous system and immune system functions. Interleukin-1 (IL1) acts on the hypothalamus to produce fever and participates in antigen-induced activation. IL1 is synthesized by macrophages and plays a major role in inflammation and immune responsiveness. Substance P (SP) has been postulated to have an effect in hypersensitivity

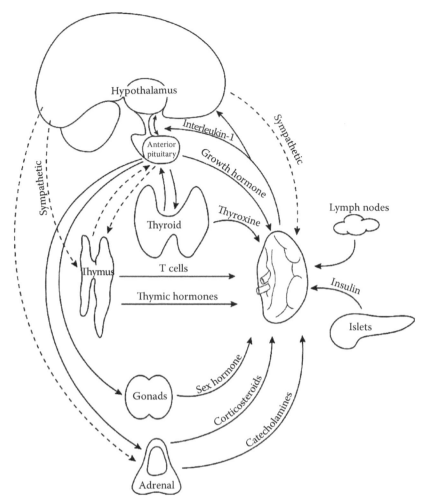

Immune–neuroendocrine axis.

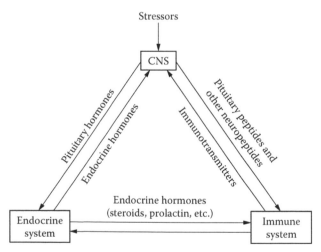

Interactions of endocrine, central nervous, and immune systems.

diseases including arthritis and asthma. The nervous system may release SP into joints in arthritis and into the respiratory tract in asthma, perpetuating inflammation. SP has also been found to participate in immune system functions such as the induction of monocyte chemotaxis in *in vitro* experiments. Through their effect on mast cells, enkephalins influence hypersensitivity reactions. Enkephalins have been shown to diminish antibody formation against cellular and soluble immunogens and to diminish passive cutaneous anaphylaxis. Mast cells, which can be stimulated by either immunologic or nonimmunologic mechanisms, may be significant in immune regulation of neural function.

immune neutropenia

Neutrophil degradation by antibodies (leukoagglutinins) that are specific for neutrophil epitopes. Penicillin, other drugs and blood transfusions may induce immune neutropenia. The condition may be associated with such autoimmune disorders as systemic lupus erythematosus (SLE) and may occur in neonates through passage of leukoagglutinins from mother to young.

immune paralysis

Refer to immunologic paralysis.

immune privilege

Refer to immunologically privileged sites.

immune response

Reaction to challenge by an immunogen. The response is expressed as antibody production and/or cell-mediated immunity or immunologic tolerance. Immune response may follow stimulation by a wide variety of agents such as pathogenic microorganisms, tissue transplants, or other antigenic substances deliberately introduced for a number of purposes. Infectious agents may also induce inflammatory reactions characterized by the production of chemical mediators at the site of injury. In addition to the adaptive immune response described above, animals have innate or natural immunity present from birth and designed to protect the host from injury or infection without previous contact with the infectious agent or antigen. It includes such protective factors as the skin, mucous membranes, lysozyme in tears, stomach acid, and other factors. Phagocytes, natural killer cells, and complement represent key participants in natural innate immunity. The immune response consists of a recognition stage in which the inducing agent is identified as nonself or dangerous to self and an effector stage aimed at elimination of the immunogen.

immune response (Ir) genes

Genes that regulate immune responsiveness to synthetic polypeptide and protein antigens as demonstrated in guinea pigs and mice. This property is transmitted as an autosomal-dominant trait that maps to the major histocompatibility complex (MHC) region. Ir genes control helper T lymphocyte activation required for the generation of antibodies against protein antigens. T lymphocytes with specific receptors for antigen fail to recognize free or soluble antigens, but they do recognize protein antigens noncovalently linked to products of MHC genes termed MHC class I and class II molecules. The failure of certain animal strains to respond may be due to ineffective antigen presentation in which processed antigen fails to bind properly to MHC class II molecules or to an ineffective interaction between the T cell receptor and the MHC class II–antigen complex.

immune serum

An antiserum containing antibodies specific for a particular antigen or immunogen. Such antibodies may confer protective immunity.

immune serum globulin

Injectable immunoglobulin that consists mainly of IgG extracted by cold ethanol fractionation from pooled plasma from up to 1000 human donors. It is administered as a sterile $16.5 \pm 1.5\%$ solution to patients with immunodeficiencies and as a preventive against certain viral infections including measles and hepatitis A.

immune stimulatory complexes

Refer to ISCOMs.

immune suppression

Decreased immune responsiveness as a consequence of therapeutic intervention with drugs or irradiation or arising from a disease process that adversely affects the immune response, such as acquired immune deficiency syndrome (AIDS).

immune surveillance

The policing function of immune system cells to identify and destroy clones of transformed cells prior to their development into neoplasms and to destroy tumors after they develop. Indirect evidence for this concept has included observations that the incidence of neoplasia increases with age-associated decrease in immune competence, the development of tumors in T cell-deficient subjects, and increased incidence of tumor development in deliberately immunosuppressed individuals, such as those receiving organ allotransplants.

immune system

The molecules, cells, tissues, and organs associated with adaptive immunity, such as the host defense mechanisms, mainly against infectious agents.

Microorganism	Cell Type
Extracellular bacteria	Polymorphonuclear neutrophils (PMNs)
Parasites	Eosinophils
Intracellular microorganisms (i.e., mycobacteria or fungi)	Macrophages
Viruses	Lymphocytes, NK cells

Nonspecific cellular defense.

immune system anatomy

The lymphocyte is the cell responsible for immune response specificity. The human mature lymphoid system is comprised of 2×10^{12} lymphocytes and various accessory cells that include epithelial cells, monocytes/macrophages, and other antigen-presenting cells. Accessory cells are requisite for both maturation and effector functions of lymphocytes. The thymus is the site of maturation of T cells, and the bone marrow is the maturation site of B cells. These two tissues comprise the primary lymphoid organs. The secondary lymphoid organs consist of the cervical lymph nodes, ancillary lymph nodes, spleen, mesenteric lymph nodes, and inguinal lymph nodes. Mature lymphocytes migrate from the central lymphoid organs by way of the blood vessels to the secondary or peripheral tissues and organs, where they respond to antigen. Peripheral lymphoid tissues comprise the spleen and lymph nodes and mucosa-associated lymphoid tissue (MALT) associated with the respiratory, genitourinary, and gastrointestinal tracts making up 50% of the lymphoid cells of the body. MALT consists of the adenoids, tonsils, and mucosa-associated lymphoid cells of the respiratory, genitourinary, and gastrointestinal tracts, and Peyer's patches in the gut.

immune tolerance

Refer to immunologic tolerance.

immunity

Acquired or innate resistance or protection from a pathogenic microorganism or its products or from the effects of toxic substances such as snake or insect venom.

immunity deficiency syndrome

Synonym for immunodeficiency.

immunity in prokaryotes

Numerous antimicrobial agents synthesized and released extracellularly by bacteria exert specific effects on bacteria. They include (1) enzymatically synthesized antibiotics, (2) post-translationally modified peptide antibiotics, (3) protein antibiotics such as bacteriocins, protein exotoxins, and bacteriolytic enzymes, and (4) intemperate or temperate bacterial viruses. Once these agents are inside bacterial cells they must remain unchanged to exert their actions. Bacteriocins released by bacteria may inhibit the growth of other sensitive closely related bacteria. The strain producing the bacteriocin is usually able to resist its effect through specific immunity peptides or proteins.

immunity to extracellular bacteria

Neutrophil (PMN), monocyte, and tissue macrophage phagocytosis leads to rapid microbial action against ingested microbes from the extracellular environment. The capacity of a microorganism to resist phagocytosis and digestion in phagocytic cells is a principal feature of its virulence.

Vaccine	Birth	2 months	4 months	6 months	12 months	15 months	18 months	4–6 years	11–12 years	14–16 years
Hepatitis B	HB-1	HB-2		HB-3						
Diphtheria, Tetanus, Pertussis		DTP	DTP	DTP	DTP or DTaP at ≥ 15 months			DTP or DTaP	Td	
H. influenzae type b		Hib	Hib	Hib	Hib					
Measles, mumps, and rubella		OPV	OPV	OPV				OPV		
Measles, mumps, and rubella					MMR				MMR or MMR	

Childhood immunization schedule recommended by U.S. Public Health Service, January 1996.

Complement activation represents a significant mechanism for ridding the body of invading microorganisms.

immunization

The deliberate administration of an antigen or immunogen to induce active immunity that is often protective, as in the case of immunization against antigenic products of infectious disease agents.

immunize

To deliberately administer an antigen or immunogen for the purpose of inducing active immunity that is often protective, as in the case of immunization against antigenic products of infectious disease agents. As a consequence of contact between the antigen or immunogen and immunologically competent cells of the host, specific antibodies and specifically reactive immune lymphoid cells are induced to confer a state of immunity.

immunizing dose (ImD$_{50}$)

In vaccine standardization, the ImD$_{50}$ is that amount of immunogen requisite to immunize 50% of the test animal population, as determined by appropriate immunoassay.

immunoablation

The deliberate destruction of immune competence to condition a patient for organ transplantation or treat refractory autoimmune diseases.

immunoabsorbent

A gel or other inert substance employed to absorb antibodies from a solution or purify them.

immunoabsorption

The use of a solid phase system to which antibody or antigen is bound for the removal of complementary antigen or antibody from a mixture by adherence to the insoluble support to which the antigen or antibody is bound.

immunoadsorbents

Specific antibodies that are chemically bound to solid supports. When a mixture containing antigen is poured over the solid support, antigen is bound noncovalently to the immunoadsorbent, from which it may be isolated after treating the sorbent–ligand complex with a denaturing agent.

immunoassay

A test that measures antigen or antibody. When choosing an immunoassay technique, one should keep in mind the differing levels of sensitivity of various methods. Whereas immunoelectrophoresis is relatively insensitive, requiring 5,000 to 10,000 ng/mL for detection, the enzyme-linked immunoabsorbent assay (ELISA), radioimmunoassay (RIA), and immunofluorescence may detect less than 0.001 ng/mL. Between these two extremes are agglutination, which detects 1,000 to 10,000 ng/mL, and complement fixation, which detects 5 ng/mL.

immunoaugmentive therapy (IAT)

An approach to tumor therapy practiced by selected individuals in Mexico, Germany, and the Bahamas that is not based on scientific fact and is of unproven efficacy or safety. Concoctions of tumor cell lysate and blood serum from tumor-bearing patients and from normal individuals are injected into cancer patients, ostensibly to provide tumor antibody, "blocking" and "deblocking" proteins. The method is not based on a scientifically approved protocol and is of very doubtful value. Treatment preparations are often contaminated with microorganisms.

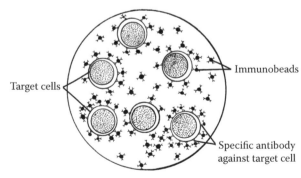

Immunobeads.

immunobeads

Minute plastic spheres with a coating of antigen (or antibody) that may be aggregated or agglutinated in the presence of the homologous antibody. Immunobeads are used also for the isolation of specific cell subpopulations such as the separation of B cells from T cells that is useful in major histocompatibility complex (MHC) class II typing for tissue transplantation.

immunobiology

A branch of biological science concerned with the molecular and cellular bases of self–nonself recognition, immune responsiveness including host defense against infection, and immunologic tolerance.

immunoblast

Lymphoblast.

immunoblastic lymphadenopathy

Refer to angioimmunoblastic lymphadenopathy (AILA).

immunoblastic sarcoma

A lymphoma comprised of immunoblast-like cells that are divided into B and T cell immunoblastic sarcomas. Both are malignant lymphomas. B cell immunoblastic sarcoma is characterized by large immunoblastic plasmacytoid cells and Reed–Sternberg cells. This is the most frequent lymphoma in individuals with natural immunodeficiency or suppression of the immune system or who manifest immunoproliferative disorders such as angioimmunoblastic lymphadenopathy or autoimmune diseases such as Hashimoto's thyroiditis, α chain disease, etc. The disease has a poor prognosis. T cell immunoblastic sarcoma is less frequent than the B cell variety. The tumor cells are large and have a clear cytoplasm containing round to oval nuclei with fine chromatin. One to three nucleoli are present amid lobulation and nuclear folding. Other cells present include plasma cells and histiocytes. Patients with mycosis fungoides who develop polyclonal gammopathy and general lymphadenopathy may develop a T cell immunoblastic sarcoma.

immunoblot (western blot)

The interaction between labeled antibodies and proteins separated by gel electrophoresis and absorbed or blotted on nitrocellulose paper. Refer to western blot.

immunoblotting

A method to identify antigens via polyacrylamide gel electrophoresis (PAGE) of a protein mixture containing the antigen. PAGE separates the components according to their electrophoretic mobility. After transfer to a nitrocellulose filter by electroblotting, antibodies labeled with enzyme or radioisotope and specific for the antigen in question are incubated with the cellulose membrane. After washing to remove excess antibody that does not bind, substrate can be added if an enzyme was used, or autoradiography can be used if a radioisotope was used to determine where the labeled antibodies were bound to homologous antigen. Also called western blotting.

immunochemistry

The branch of immunology concerned with the properties of antigens, antibodies, complement, T cell receptors, major histocompatibility complex (MHC) molecules, and all the molecules and receptors that participate in immune interactions *in vivo* and *in vitro*. Immunochemistry aims to identify active sites in immune responses and define the forces that govern antigen–antibody interaction. It is also concerned with the design of new molecules such as catalytic antibodies and other biological catalysts. Also called molecular immunology.

immunocompetent

A mature functional lymphocyte that can recognize a specific antigen and mediate an immune response. The term also may refer to the immune status of a human or other animal to indicate the ability to respond immunologically to an immunogenic challenge.

immunoconglutination

Aggregation of C3bi- or C4bi-coated erythrocytes or bacteria by antibodies to C3bi or C4bi, produced by immunizing animals with erythrocytes or bacteria that have interacted with antibody and complement. The antibody is termed immunoconglutinin; it resembles conglutinin in its activity but should not be confused with it. Autoantibodies specific for C3bi or C4bi may develop as a result of an infection and produce immunoconglutination.

immunoconglutinin

An autoantibody, usually of the immunoglobulin M (IgM) class, that is specific for neoantigens in C3bi or C4bi. It may be stimulated during acute and chronic infections caused by bacteria, viruses, or parasites and in chronic inflammatory disorders. The level is also increased in many autoimmune diseases and after immunization with various immunogens. C3 nephritic factor is an example of an immunoconglutinin. Also called *immune conglutinin,* it should not be confused with conglutinin. Refer also to immunoconglutination.

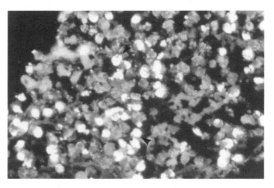

Immunocytes in reticular dermis.

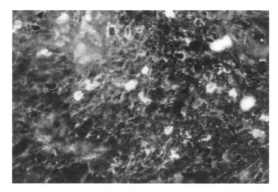

Immunocytes in dermis.

immunoconjugate

A chimeric protein product of the linkage of a whole monoclonal antibody or one of its structural derivatives to another molecule either chemically or at the DNA level. Refer to immunocytokine, immunoradioisotope, and immunotoxin.

immunocyte

Literally "immune cell." A term sometimes used by pathologists to describe plasma cells in stained tissue sections (e.g., in the papillary or reticular dermis in erythema multiforme).

immunocytoadherence

A method to detect cells with surface immunoglobulin, either synthesized or attached through Fc receptors. Red blood cells coated with the homologous antigen are mixed with the immunoglobulin-bearing cells and result in rosette formation. A laboratory assay is employed to identify antibody-bearing cells by the formation of rosettes comprised of red blood cells and antibody-bearing cells.

immunocytochemistry

The visual recognition of target molecules and tissues and cells by a specific reaction of antibody with antigen through the use of antibodies labeled with indicator molecules. By tagging an antibody with a fluorochrome, color-producing enzyme, or metallic particle, the target molecules can be identified.

immunocytokine (ICK)

An immunoconjugate in which a monoclonal antibody or one of its derivatives is bound to a cytokine. Designed to deliver antitumor cytokines to a tumor site during cancer treatment.

immunodeficiency

A failure in humoral antibody or cell-mediated limbs of the immune response. If attributable to intrinsic defects in T and/or B lymphocytes, the condition is termed a primary immunodeficiency. If the defect results from loss of antibody and/or lymphocytes, the condition is a secondary immunodeficiency. The term may refer also to defective leukocyte–bactericidal immunity as in chronic granulomatous disease, or may be associated with deficiencies of the complement system.

immunodeficiency, acquired

A decrease in the immune response to immunogenic (antigenic) challenge as a consequence of numerous diseases or conditions that include acquired immune deficiency syndrome (AIDS), chemotherapy, immunosuppressive drugs such as corticosteroids, psychological depression, burns, nonsteroidal antiinflammatory drugs, radiation, Alzheimer's disease, celiac disease, sarcoidosis, lymphoproliferative disease, Waldenström's macroglobulinemia, multiple myeloma, aplastic anemia, sickle cell disease, malnutrition, aging, neoplasia, diabetes mellitus, and numerous other conditions.

immunodeficiency animal models

Common murine models of immunodeficiency include the mouse strains designated SCID, Motheaten, Viable Motheaten, Nude, Lipopolysaccharide, X-Linked Immunodeficiency, Complement Deficient, Beige, Dominant Spotting, Steel, and Wasted. These models are critical for revealing how genetic abnormalities affect immune competence.

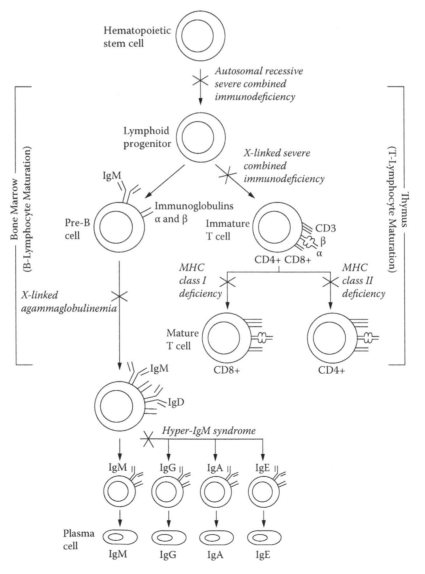

Congenital immunodeficiencies.

immunodeficiency associated with hereditary defective response to Epstein–Barr virus

An immunodeficiency that develops in previously healthy subjects with normal immune systems who develop primary Epstein–Barr virus infections. They develop elevated numbers of natural killer cells in the presence of a lymphopenia. The condition is serious, and its acute stage may lead to B cell lymphoma, failure of the bone marrow, or agammaglobulinemia. The disease may be fatal. The condition was first considered to have an X-linked recessive mode of inheritance recurring only in males, but it has now been found in occasional females. The term Duncan's syndrome is often used to describe the X-linked variety of this condition.

immunodeficiency, congenital

A varied group of unusual disorders with associated autoimmune manifestations, increased incidence of malignancy, allergy, and gastrointestinal abnormalities. These include defects in stem cells, B cells, T cells, phagocytic defects, and complement defects. An example is severe combined immunodeficiency (SCID) due to various causes. The congenital immunodeficiencies are described under the separate disease categories.

immunodeficiency disorders

Conditions characterized by decreased immune function. They may be grouped into four principal categories based on recommendations from a committee of the World Health Organization: antibody (B cell) deficiency, cellular (T cell) deficiency, combined T cell and B cell deficiencies, and phagocyte dysfunction. The deficiency may be congenital or acquired. It can be secondary to an embryologic abnormality or an enzymatic defect or may be attributable to an unknown cause. Types of infections produced and the physical findings are characteristic of the type of disease. Screening tests identify a number of these conditions, whereas others have unknown etiologies. Antimicrobial agents for the treatment of recurrent infections, immunotherapy, bone marrow transplantation, enzyme replacement, and gene therapy are all modes of treatment.

immunodeficiency from hypercatabolism of immunoglobulin

Serum levels of immunoglobulins fluctuate according to their rates of synthesis and catabolism. Although many immunological deficiencies result from defective synthesis of immunoglobulins and lymphocytes, immunoglobulin levels in serum can decline as a consequence of increased catabolism or loss into the gastrointestinal tract or other areas. Defective catabolism may affect one to several immunoglobulin classes. For example, in myotonic dystrophy, only IgG is hypercatabolized. In contrast to the normal levels of IgM, IgA, IgD, IgE, and albumin in the serum, the IgG concentration is markedly diminished. Synthesis of IgG in these individuals is normal, but the half-lives of IgG molecules are reduced as a consequence of increased catabolism. Patients with ataxia telangiectasia and those with selective IgA deficiency have antibodies directed against IgA that remove this class of immunoglobulin. Patients with the rare condition known as familial hypercatabolic hypoproteinemia demonstrate reduced IgG and albumin levels in the serum and slightly lower IgM levels, but the IgA and IgE concentrations are either normal or barely increased. Although synthesis of IgG and albumin in such patients is within normal limits, the catabolism of these two proteins is greatly accelerated.

immunodeficiency from severe loss of immunoglobulins and lymphocytes

The gastrointestinal and urinary tracts are two sources of serious protein loss in disease processes. The loss of integrity of the renal glomerular basement membrane or renal tubular disease or both may result in loss of immunoglobulin molecules into the urine. Because the small IgG molecules pass through in many situations, leaving larger IgA molecules in the intravascular space, all immunoglobulins are not lost from the serum at the same rate. More than 90 diseases that affect the gastrointestinal tract have been associated with protein-losing gastroenteropathy. This may be secondary to inflammatory or allergic disorders or disease processes involving the lymphatics. In intestinal lymphangiectasia associated with lymphatic blockage, lymphocytes and proteins are lost. Lymphatics in the small intestine are dilated. Intestinal lymphangiectasia patients show defects in both humoral and cellular immune mechanisms. The major immunoglobulins are diminished to less than half of normal. IgG is affected more than IgA and IgM; they are more affected than IgE.

immunodeficiency with B cell neoplasms

B cell leukemias can be classified as pre-B cell, B cell, or plasma cell neoplasms. They include Burkitt's lymphoma, Hodgkin disease, and chronic lymphocytic leukemia (CLL). Neoplasms of plasma cells are associated with multiple myeloma and Waldenström's macroglobulinemia. Many of these conditions are associated with hypogammaglobulinemia and a diminished capacity to form antibodies in response to the administration of an immunogen. In CLL, more than 95% of individuals have malignant leukemic cells that are identifiable as B lymphocytes expressing surface immunoglobulin. These patients frequently develop infections and have autoimmune manifestations such as autoimmune hemolytic anemia. CLL patients may have secondary immunodeficiencies that affect both B and T limbs of the immune response. Diminished immunoglobulin levels are due primarily to diminished synthesis.

immunodeficiency with partial albinism

A type of combined immunodeficiency characterized by decreased cell-mediated immunity and deficient natural killer cells. Patients develop cerebral atrophy and aggregation of pigment in melanocytes. This disease, which leads to death, has an autosomal-recessive mode of inheritance.

immunodeficiency with T cell neoplasms

Almost one third of patients with acute lymphocytic leukemia (ALL), individuals with Sézary syndrome, and a very few patients with chronic lymphocytic leukemia (CLL) develop a malignant type of proliferation of lymphoid cells. Sézary cells are poor mediators of T cell cytotoxicity, but they can produce migration inhibitory factor (MIF)-like lymphokines. Sézary cells produce neither immunoglobulin nor suppressor substances, but they exert a helper effect for immunoglobulin synthesis by B cells. In mycosis fungoides, skin lesions contain T lymphocytes; an increase in the number of null cells in the blood occurs with a simultaneous decrease in the numbers of B and T cells. T cell immunity is decreased, but IgA and IgE may be elevated. Whereas ALL patients show major defects in cell-mediated or humoral (antibody) immunity, a few manifest profound reductions in their serum immunoglobulin concentrations. This has been suggested to be due to malignant expansion of their T suppressor lymphocytes.

immunodeficiency with thrombocytopenia

Synonym for Wiskott–Aldrich syndrome.

immunodeficiency with thrombocytopenia and eczema (Wiskott–Aldrich syndrome)

An X-linked recessive disease characterized by thrombocytopenia, eczema, and susceptibility to recurrent infections, sometimes leading to early death. The lifespan of young boys is diminished as a consequence of extensive infection, hemorrhage, and sometimes malignant disease of the lymphoreticular system. Infectious agents affecting these individuals include the Gram-negative and Gram-positive bacteria, fungi, and viruses. The thymus is normal morphologically, but there is a variable decline in cellular immunity that is thymus-dependent. The lymph node architecture may be altered as paracortical areas become depleted of cells with progression of the disease. IgM levels in serum are low, but IgA and IgG may be increased. Isohemagglutinins are usually undetectable in the serum. Patients may respond normally to protein antigens, but show defective responsiveness to polysaccharide antigens. There is decreased immune responsiveness to lipopolysaccharides from enteric bacteria and B blood group substances.

immunodeficiency with thymoma

An abnormality in B cell development with a striking decrease in B cell numbers and immunoglobulins in selected patients with thymoma. Their cell-mediated immunity progressively decreases as the disease continues. Most patients develop chronic sinopulmonary infections. Approximately 20% develop thrombocytopenia, and about 25% have splenomegaly. Immunoglobulin class alterations are variable. Skin test reactivity and responsiveness to skin allografts are decreased. Patients have few or no lymphocytes expressing surface immunoglobulin. The disease is due to a stem cell defect. The preferred treatment is γ globulin administration.

immunodiagnosis

The use of antibody assays, immunocytochemistry, identification of lymphocyte markers, and other techniques to diagnose infectious diseases and malignant neoplasms.

immunodiffusion

A method in which antigen and antibody are placed in wells at different sites in agar gel and are permitted to diffuse toward each other. The formation of precipitin lines at their points of contact in the agar gel signifies a positive reaction, showing that the antibody is specific for the antigen in question. Multiple variations of this technique have been described.

immunodominance

The immune response-generating capacity of the part of an epitope on an antigen molecule that serves as an immunodominant area providing the principal binding energy for reaction with a paratope on an antibody molecule or with a T cell receptor for antigen. The hapten portion of a hapten–carrier complex is often the immunodominant part of the molecule. Immunodominance refers to the region of an antigenic determinant that is the principal binding site for antibody.

immunodominant epitope

The antigenic determinant on an antigen molecule that binds or fits best with the antibody or T cell receptor specific for it.

immunodominant site

Refer to immunodominant epitope.

Immunodrug Platform™

A virus bacteria chimera developed by Marten Bachmann of Cytos Biotechnology in 2006. A segment from mycobacterial DNA long known to induce a strong immune response is incorporated into virus-like particles. Packaging the DNA inside the virus-like particles protects it from degradation and delivers it to dendritic cells that influence T cell responses. This preparation induces an antiallergenic response whether or not it is combined with an offending allergin prior to injection.

immunodysregulation, polyendocrinopathy, enteropathy X-linked (IPEX) syndrome

An autoimmune disease that is X-linked and associated with inflammation of numerous tissues and the synthesis of autoantibodies specific for antigens of the pancreatic islets, thyroid and adrenal glands, smooth muscle, intestine, and kidney. It is attributable to a mutation of the FOXP3 transcription factor requisite for IL2 expression and the generation and function of T regulatory cells.

immunoelectroadsorption

A quantitative assay for antibody using a metal-treated glass slide to adsorb antigen followed by antibody from serum. Adsorption is facilitated by an electric current. Measurement of the antibody layer's thickness reflects the serum concentration.

immunoelectron microscopy

Traditionally, the use of antibodies labeled with ferritin to study the ultrastructures of subcellular organelles and, more recently, the use of immunogold labeling and related procedures for the identification and localization of antigens by electron microscopy.

immunoelectroosmophoresis

Refer to counter immunoelectrophoresis.

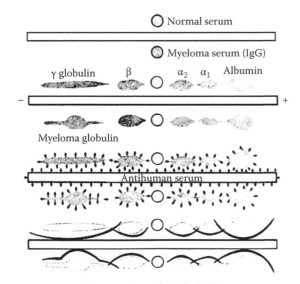

Immunoelectrophoresis (IEP).

immunoelectrophoresis (IEP or IE)

A method to identify antigens on the basis of their electrophoretic mobility, diffusion in gel, and formation of precipitation arcs with specific antibody. Electrophoresis in gel is combined with diffusion of a specific antibody in a gel medium containing electrolyte to identify separated antigenic substances. This allows determination of the presence or absence of immunoglobulin molecules of various classes in a serum sample. One percent agar containing electrolyte is layered onto microscope slides and allowed to gel, and patterns of appropriate troughs and wells are cut in the solidified medium. Antigen to be identified is placed in the circular wells cut into the agar medium. This is followed by electrophoresis that permits separation of the antigenic components according to their electrophoretic mobility. Antiserum is placed in a long trough in the center of the slide. After antibody has diffused through the agar toward each separated antigen, precipitin arcs form where the antigen and antibody interact. Abnormal amounts of immunoglobulins result in changes in the shape and position of precipitin arcs when compared with the arcs formed by antibody against normal human serum components. With monoclonal gammopathies, the arcs become broad, bulged, and displaced. The absence of immunoglobulin classes such as those found in certain immunodeficiencies can also be detected with IEP.

immunoenhancement

Increasing or contributing to the level of immune response by various specific and nonspecific means such as immunization.

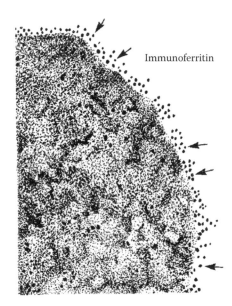

Immunoferritin method. A ferritin-conjugated anti-A globulin treated group A red cell. The binding of ferritin particles to the surface of the erythrocyte denotes the site of the antigen.

immunoferritin method

A technique to aid detection by electron microscopy of sites where antibody interacts with antigen of cells and tissues. Immunoglobulin may be conjugated with ferritin, an electron-dense marker, without altering its immunological reactivity. These ferritin-labeled antibodies localize molecules of antigen in subcellular areas. Electron-dense ferritin permits visualization of antibody binding to homologous antigen in cells and tissues by electron microscopy. In addition to ferritin, horseradish-peroxidase-labeled antibodies may also be adapted for use in immunoelectron microscopy.

immunoferritin technique

A method that involves the labeling of antibody molecules with an electron-dense material (e.g., ferritin), rendering

their site of attachment to cell or tissue antigen visible when observed by electron microscopy. In addition to this direct method, the use of ferritin-labeled antiimmunoglobulin can detect unlabeled antibody bound to tissue antigen by indirect "sandwich" immunoferritin methodology.

immunofixation

A method to identify antigen in a protein mixture that has been electrophoresed in agarose gel. Antibodies are applied to the gel, which is then rinsed to remove excess reactants, and the preparation is stained to reveal precipitates of antigen and antibody.

immunofixation electrophoresis (IFE)

The application of specific antibodies to a gel in which the antigen has been electrophoresed. Precipitation occurs at the location where antibodies interact with the electrophoresed homologous antigen. The method is used to identify specific antigenic components that might otherwise be camouflaged because of close similarity of molecules not otherwise discernible by conventional immunoelectrophoresis.

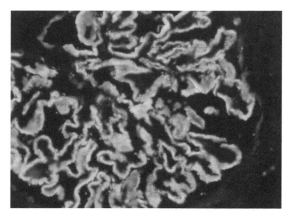

Fluorescence antibody method showing immune deposits in glomerulonephritis.

immunofluorescence

A method for the detection of antigen or antibody in cells or tissue sections through the use of fluorescent labels (fluorochromes) by fluorescent light microscopic examination. The most commonly used fluorochromes are fluorescein isothiocyanate, which imparts an apple-green fluorescence, and rhodamine B isothiocyanate, which imparts a reddish-orange tint. This method, developed by Albert Coons in the 1940s, has a wide application in diagnostic medicine and research. In addition to antigens and antibodies, complements and other immune mediators may also be detected by this method. It is based on the principle that, following adsorption of light by molecules, cells or tissues dispose of their increased energy by various means, such as emission of light of longer wavelength. Fluorescence is the process whereby emission is of relatively short duration (10^{-6} to 10^{-9} seconds) for return of the excited molecules to the ground state. The active groups in protein that allow them to attach fluorochromes include free amino and carboxyl groups at the ends of each polypeptide chain, many free amino groups and lysine side chains, many free carboxyl groups in asparatic and glutamic acid residues, the guanidino group of arginine, the phenolic group of tyrosine, and the amino groups of histidine and tryptophan. Labeling antibody molecules with fluorochromes does not alter their antigen-binding specificity. Several immunofluorescence techniques are available. In the direct test, smears of the substance to be examined are fixed with heat or methanol and followed by flooding with a fluorochrome–antibody conjugate. This is followed by incubating in a moist chamber for 30 to 60 minutes at 37°C, after which the smear is washed first in buffered saline for 5 to 10 minutes and then in tap water for another 5 to 10 minutes. The washing procedures remove uncombined conjugated globulin. After adding a small drop of buffered glycerol and a cover slip, the smear may be examined with a fluorescence light microscope. In the indirect test, which is more sensitive, a smear or tissue section is first flooded with unlabeled antibody specific for the antigen sought. After washing, fluorescein-labeled antiimmuno-globulin of the species of the primary antibody is layered over the section. After appropriate incubation and washing, the section is cover slipped and examined as in the direct method. Variations such as complement staining are also available. The indirect method is more sensitive and considerably less expensive; one fluorochrome-labeled antiimmu-noglobulin may be used with multiple primary antibodies specific for a battery of antigens. The technique is widely used to diagnose and classify renal diseases and bullous skin diseases and study cells and tissues in connective tissue disorders such as systemic lupus erythematosus (SLE).

immunofluorescent "staining" of C4d

In peritubular capillaries of renal allograft biopsies, immu-nofluorescent "staining" of C4d reveals a humoral component of allograft rejection.

immunogen

A substance that can induce a humoral antibody and/or cell-mediated immune response rather than immunological tolerance. *Immunogen* and *antigen* are sometimes used interchangeably, but the term signifies the ability to stimulate an immune response and react with its products (e.g., antibodies). By contrast, some use *antigen* to describe a substance that reacts with antibody. The principal immunogens are proteins and polysaccharides, whereas lipids may serve as haptens.

immunogenetics

The branch of immunology concerned with genetic analysis of molecules with specific relevance for the immune system. The term previously referred to the use of antibodies specific for genetically polymorphic molecules used to analyze genetic traits including blood group antigens and major histocompatibility complex (MHC) proteins.

immunogenic

The capacity to induce humoral antibody and/or cell-mediated immune responsiveness, but not immunological tolerance. Immunogenicity depends on characteristics of the immunogen and on the injected animal's genetic capacity to respond to the immunogen. To be immunogenic, a substance must be foreign to the recipient. Significant molecular size and complexity of the immunogen along with host factors such as previous exposure to the immunogen and immuno-competence are all critical factors in immunogenicity.

immunogenic carbohydrates

Carbohydrates are important in various immunological processes that include opsinization and phagocytosis of micro-organisms, and cell activation and differentiation. They exert their effects through interaction with carbohydrate-binding proteins or lectins that have a widespread distribution in mammalian tissues including the immune system. Immunogenic carbohydrates are usually large polymers of glucose (glucans and lentinans), mannose (mannans), xylose, (hemicelluloses), fructose (levans), or mixtures of these sugars. Complex carbohydrates may stimulate the immune system by activating macrophages with fungal glycans or stimulating T cells with lentinan. Acemannin activates microphages and T cells, thereby influencing both cellular and humoral immunity. Glucans stimulate immunity against bacterial diseases by activating macrophages and stimulating their lysosomal and phagocytic activities. Complex carbohydrates may activate the immune systems of patients or experimental animals with neoplastic diseases. Some mannans and glucans are powerful anticancer agents. Lentinin, derived from edible mushrooms, exerts antineoplastic effects against several allogeneic and syngeneic tumors without mediating cytotoxicity of the tumor cells. Mannans derived from yeast also produce significant antitumor effects, as do levans that activate macrophages and B and T cells as well. Pectin is a galactose-containing carbohydrate concentrated in citrus that causes an antitumor effect.

immunogenicity

The ability of an antigen serving as an immunogen to induce an immune response in a particular species of recipient. Immunogenicity depends on a number of physical and chemical characteristics of the immunogen (antigen) and on the genetic capacity of the host.

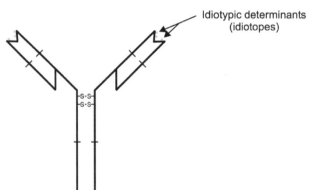

Schematic representation of idiotypes present on an immuno-globulin molecule.

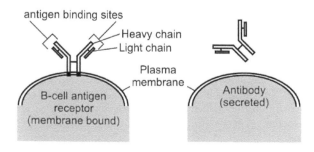

Schematic representation of an antigen receptor on the plasma membrane of a B cell.

immunoglobulin

A mature B cell product synthesized in response to stimulation by an antigen. Antibody molecules are immuno-globulins of defined specificity produced by plasma cells.

The immunoglobulin molecule consists of heavy (H) and light (L) chains fastened together by disulfide bonds. The molecules are subdivided into classes and subclasses based on the antigenic specificities of the heavy chains. Heavy chains are designated by lower case Greek letters (μ, γ, α, δ, and ε), and the immunoglobulins are designated IgM, IgG, IgA, IgD, and IgE, respectively. The three major classes are IgG, IgM, and IgA, and the two minor classes are IgD and IgE that together comprise less than 1% of the total immunoglobulins. The two types of light chains (κ and λ) are present in all five immunoglobulin classes, although only one type is present in an individual molecule. IgG, IgD, and IgE have two H and two L polypeptide chains, whereas IgM and IgA consist of multimers of this basic chain structure. Disulfide bridges and noncovalent forces stabilize immunoglobulin structures. The basic monomeric unit is Y-shaped, with a hinge region rich in proline and susceptible to cleavage by proteolytic enzymes. Both H and L chains have constant regions at their carboxyl termini and variable regions at their amino termini. The two heavy chains are alike, as are the two light chains, in all immunoglobulin molecules. Approximately 60% of human immunoglobulin molecules have κ light chains, and 40% have λ light chains. The five immunoglobulin classes are termed isotypes based on the heavy chain specificity of each immunoglobulin class. Two IgA and IgG classes are further subdivided into subclasses based on H chain differences. The four IgG subclasses are designated as IgG_1 through IgG_4, and the two IgA subclasses are designated IgA_1 and IgA_2. Digestion of IgG molecules with papain yields two Fab and one Fc fragments. Each Fab fragment has one antigen-binding site. By contrast, the Fc fragment has no antigen-binding site but is responsible for fixation of complement and attachment of the molecule to a cell surface. Pepsin cleaves the molecule toward the carboxyl terminal end of the central disulfide bond, yielding an $F(ab')_2$ fragment and a pFc' fragment. $F(ab')_2$ fragments have two antigen-binding sites. L chains have a single variable and constant domain, whereas H chains possess one variable and three to four constant domains. Secretory IgA is found in body secretions such as saliva, milk, and intestinal and bronchial secretions. IgD and IgM are present as membrane-bound immunoglobulins on B cells, where they interact with antigen to activate B cells. IgE is associated with anaphylaxis, and IgG, which is the only immunoglobulin capable of crossing the placenta, is the major human immunoglobulin.

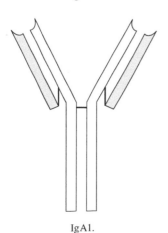

IgA1.

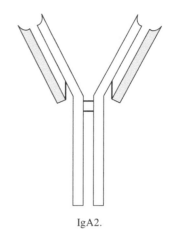

IgA2.

Secretory IgA that consists of two IgA monomers, a J chain, and a secretory piece that is believed to protect the molecule from enzymatic digestion in the gut.

immunoglobulin A (IgA)

Immunoglobulin A (IgA) comprises 5 to 15% of the serum immunoglobulins and has a half-life of 6 days. It has a molecular weight of 160 kDa and a basic four-chain monomeric structure; however, it can occur as a monomer, dimer, trimer, or multimer. It contains α heavy chains and κ or λ light chains. The two subclasses of IgA are designated IgA_1 and IgA_2. In addition to monomeric serum IgA, a dimeric secretory or exocrine variety appears in body secretions and provides local immunity. For example, the Sabin oral polio vaccine stimulates secretory IgA antibodies in the gut that provide effective immunity against poliomyelitis. IgA-deficient individuals have an increased incidence of respiratory infections associated with a lack of secretory IgA in the respiratory system. Secretory or exocrine IgA appears in colostrum, intestinal, and respiratory secretions; saliva; tears; and other secretions.

immunoglobulin A deficiency

The most frequent human immunodeficiency that affects 1 in 600 persons in the United States. Even though the B cells of these individuals have IgA on their surfaces, they do not differentiate into plasma cells that secrete IgA. IgA levels are decreased from a normal value of 76 to 390 mg/dL to a value below 5 mg/dL. Almost half develop anti-IgA antibodies that are subclass-specific. IgA-deficient individuals with heightened susceptibility to infection by pyogenic microorganisms also are deficient in IgG_2 and often IgG_4. The administration of a blood transfusion to IgA-deficient patients possessing anti-IgA antibodies can lead to anaphylactic shock due to IgE antibodies specific for IgA or to a fatal hemolytic transfusion reaction. Patients may also

Ig	IgG	IgM	IgA	IgD	IgE
Serum concentration (mg/dl)	800–1700	50–190	140–420	0.3–0.4	<0.001
Total Ig (%)	85	5–10	5–15	< 1	< 1
Complement fixation	+	++++	–	–	–
Principal biological effect	Resistance-opsonin; secondary response	Resistance-precipitin; primary response	Resistance prevents movement across mucous membranes	?	Anaphylaxis
Principal site of action	Serum	Serum	Secretions	?; receptor for B cells	Mast cells
Molecular weight (kDa)	154	900	160 (+dimer)	185	190
Serum half-life (days)	23	5	6	2–3	2–3
Antibacterial lysis	+	+++	+	?	?
Antiviral lysis	+	+	+++	?	?
H-chain class	γ	μ	α	δ	ε
Subclass	γ1 γ2 γ3 γ4		α1 α2		

Human immunoglobulins and their properties.

have intestinal lymphangiectasia, arthritis, gluten-sensitive enteropathy, allergies, and myotonic dystrophy. They may also develop low molecular weight IgM antibodies against food substances such as milk. Other clinical features may include sinopulmonary infections, cirrhosis, and autoimmune disease. IgA deficiency is detectable in approximately three fourths of ataxia telangiectasia patients. Intravenous immune globulin with only minute quantities of IgA may be beneficial to these patients.

immunoglobulin α chain

A 58-kDa, 470-amino-acid residue heavy polypeptide chain that confers class specificity on immunoglobulin A molecules. The chain is divisible into three constant domains, designated C_H1, C_H2, and C_H3, and one variable domain, designated V_H. A hinge region is situated between C_H1 and C_H2 domains. An additional segment of 18 amino acid residues at the penultimate position of the chain contains a cysteine residue where the J chain can be linked through a disulfide bond. The IgA subclass is divisible into IgA_1 and IgA_2 subclasses, reflecting two separate α chain isotypes. The α-2 chain has two allotypes designated A2m(1) and A2m(2) and does not have disulfide bonds linking H to L chains. Subclass-specific residues are found in a number of positions in C_H1, the hinge region, and C_H2, where α-1 and α-2 chains differ but α-2 chains are the same. Differences in the two α chains are found in two C_H1 and five C_H3 positions. Thus, humans have three varieties of α heavy chains.

immunoglobulin class

The subdivision of immunoglobulin molecules based on antigenic and structural differences in the Fc regions of their heavy polypeptide chains. Immunoglobulin molecules belonging to a particular class have at least one constant region isotypic determinant in common. The different classes such as IgG, IgM, and IgA designate separate isotypes. Because the light chains of immunoglobulin molecules are one of two types, the heavy chains determine immunoglobulin class. There is about 30% amino acid sequence homology among the five immunoglobulin heavy chain constant regions in humans. Heavy chains (or isotypes) also differ in carbohydrate content. Immunization of a nonhuman species

with human immunoglobulin provides antisera that may be used for class or isotype determination. IgG is divided into four subclasses, and IgA is divided into two subclasses.

immunoglobulin class switching

Refer to isotype switching, switch, switch cells, switch region, and switch site.

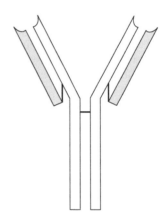

Immunoglobulin D (IgD) structure showing a four-chain monomeric unit that consists of two δ heavy chains and either two kappa (κ) or two lambda (λ) light chains.

immunoglobulin D (IgD)

Immunoglobulin D (IgD), which has a molecular weight of 185 kDa, comprises less than 1% of serum immunoglobulins. It has the basic four-chain monomeric structure with two δ heavy chains (molecular weight 63,000 Da each) and either two κ or two λ light chains (molecular weight 22,000 Da each). The half-life of IgD is only 2 to 3 days, and its role in immunity remains elusive. Surface membrane IgD serves with IgM as an antigen receptor on mature naïve B cell membranes.

immunoglobulin deficiency with elevated IgM

Antibody deficiency characterized by heightened susceptibility to infection by pyogenic microorganisms. Whereas IgM and IgD levels are elevated in the serum, the IgA and IgG concentrations are greatly diminished or not detectable. Patients often manifest IgM autoantibodies against neutrophils and platelets. The only immunoglobulins secreted

Variable heavy (V_H) and light (V_L) chain regions on an antibody.

by B cells in this X-linked recessive immunodeficiency syndrome are IgM and IgD.

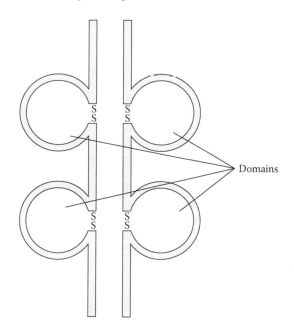

Domain structures of light and heavy polypeptide chains, the subunits of immunoglobulin molecules.

immunoglobulin δ chain

A 64-kDa, 500-amino acid residue, heavy polypeptide chain consisting of one variable region designated V_H and a three-domain (designated C_H1, C_H2, and C_H3) constant region. Human δ chains also have a 58-amino acid residue hinge region. Two exons encode the hinge region. IgD is very susceptible to the action of proteolytic enzymes at its hinge region. Two separate exons encode the membrane

component of the δ chain. A distinct exon encodes the carboxyl terminal portion of the human δ chain that is secreted. The human δ chain contains three N-linked oligosaccharides. Two δ chains and two light chains, either κ or λ, fastened together by disulfide bonds constitute an IgD molecule.

immunoglobulin domain

An immunoglobulin heavy or light polypeptide chain structural unit composed of approximately 110 amino acid residues. Immunoglobulin functions may be linked to certain domains. There is much primary and three-dimensional structural homology among immunoglobulin domains. A particular exon may encode an immunoglobulin domain. In addition to immunoglobulins, these three-dimensional globular structural motifs may also be identified in T cell receptors and major histocompatibility complex (MHC) molecules. The amino acid residues are folded into a sandwich-like structure consisting of two β-pleated sheets, each layer of which is comprised of three to five strands of anti-parallel polypeptide chains fastened together by a disulfide bond. Immunoglobulin domains may be designated as V-like or C-like based on their homology to immunoglobulin V or C domains.

immunoglobulin E (IgE)

IgE constitutes less than 1% of the total immunoglobulins and has a half-life of approximately 2.5 days. This antibody has a four-chain unit structure with two ε heavy chains (molecular weight 75,000 Da each) and either two κ or two λ light chains per molecule (total molecular weight 190 kDa). IgE does not precipitate with antigen *in vitro* and is heat labile. IgE is responsible for anaphylactic hypersensitivity in humans. It is elevated and plays a beneficial role in parasitic infections.

immunoglobulin ε chain

A 72-kDa, 550-amino acid residue, heavy polypeptide chain comprised of one variable region designated V_H and a

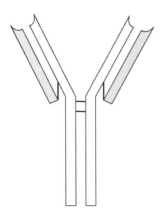

Immunoglobulin E (IgE) molecule.

four-domain (designated C_H1, C_H2, C_H3, and C_H4) constant region. This heavy chain does not possess a hinge region. In humans, the ε heavy chain has 428-amino-acid residues in the constant region. The ε chains have no carboxyl terminal portions. Two ε heavy polypeptide chains, together with two κ or two λ light chains fastened together by disulfide bonds, comprise an IgE molecule.

immunoglobulin evolution

Like mammalian immunoglobulins, dogfish and shark immunoglobulins contain two light and two heavy polypeptide chains that express charge diversity. Shark immunoglobulin most closely resembles mammalian IgM. All vertebrates synthesize antibodies that have classic immunoglobulin structures. They consist of two kinds of polypeptide chains that are linked covalently by disulfide bonds and are polydisperse in charge. Immunoglobulins of all classes of vertebrates derived from the primitive jawed fish (placoderms) are now known, such as those from elasmobranches that include sharks and rays; teleost fish that include goldfish; amphibians that include bullfrogs and *Xenopus*; reptiles; and birds. All of these synthesize antibodies comparable to the IgM isotypes of mammals. The IgM molecules of bony fish teleosts occur as tetramers rather than pentamers. Lungfish, amphibians, reptiles, and birds develop other classes of immunoglobulins characterized by distinct heavy chains that resemble γ chains. Distinct immunoglobulin monomers of amphibians, reptiles, and birds have larger heavy chains than the mammalian γ chain and may represent gene duplications. These non-IgM immunoglobulins are designated IgY (amphibians, reptiles, chickens). Other distinct immunoglobulin classes are present in amphibians (IgX), lungfish (IgN), reptiles (IgN), and birds (IgN). Light chains are designated as κ or λ, and their relative frequencies vary from one species to another. Sharks possess a second major immunoglobulin class termed IgW or IgNARC (new antigen receptor from cartilaginous fish). It has a heavy chain that possesses one variable and six constant domains and may be the primitive immunoglobulin in evolution. IgW variable domains are similar to those of heavy chains but differ in that they vary in sequence consistent with diversity through recognized many antigens. Two genes are requisite early in T and B cell development for recombination of variable, diversity, and joining segments of immunoglobulin light and heavy chains and T cell

receptor chains to take place. The most primitive living vertebrates, the cyclostomes (hagfish and lampreys) synthesize antibodies equivalent to those of higher vertebrates in their possession of heavy and light polypeptide chains, disulfide covalent bonding, and charge dispersity.

immunoglobulin fold

An immunoglobulin domain's three-dimensional configuration. An immunoglobulin fold has a sandwich-like structure comprised of two β-pleated sheets that are nearly parallel. One sheet has four antiparallel chain segments, and the other has three. Approximately 50% of the amino acid residues of the domain are in the β-pleated sheets. The other 50% are situated in polypeptide chain loops and terminal segments. The turns are sites of invariant glycine residues. Hydrophobic amino acid side chains are situated between the sheets.

immunoglobulin fragment

A term reserved for products that result from the action of proteolytic enzymes on immunoglobulin molecules. Intrachain disulfide bonds can be severed by reduction in the presence of denaturing agents such as urea, guanidine, or detergents. Peptide bonds in intact domains are not easily split by proteolytic enzymes. Light chains can be cleaved at the V–C junction, giving rise to large segments that correspond to the V_L and C_L domains. Similar cleavage of the heavy chain is more difficult to achieve. Papain cleaves H chains at the N terminus of the H–H disulfide bonds, giving two individual portions of the terminus of the molecule, called Fab, and the fragment of the C terminus region, Fc, which is crystallizable. In contrast, pepsin cleaves H chains at the C terminus of the H–H disulfide bonds; thus, the two Fab fragments will remain joined and are called $F(ab')_2$. Pepsin degrades the C_H2 domains but splits the C_H3 domains, which remain noncovalently bonded in dimeric form and are called pFc′. Further digestion of the pFc′ with papain results in smaller dimeric fragments called Fc′. Plasmin has been found to cleave the immunoglobulin molecule between C_H2 and C_H3, giving rise to a fragment designated Facb. The heavy chain portion of the Fab, designated Fd, and the heavy chain portion of the Fab′ fragment, designated Fd′, result from the breakdown of an $F(ab')_2$ fragment produced by pepsin digestion of the IgG molecule. The Fv fragment consists of the variable domain of heavy and light chains on an immunoglobulin molecule where antigen binding occurs.

immunoglobulin function

Links an antigen to its elimination mechanism (effector system). Antibodies induce complement activation and cellular elimination mechanisms that include phagocytosis and antibody-dependent, cell-mediated cytotoxicity (ADCC). This type of activation usually requires antibody molecules clustered together on a cell surface rather than as free unliganded antibody. Antibodies can combine with virus particles to render them noninfectious *in vitro* through neutralization. IgG catabolism is regulated by IgG concentration. All immunoglobulin classes can be expressed on B cell surfaces, where they act as antigen receptors, although this is mainly a function of IgM and IgD. Surface immunoglobulin has an extra C terminal sequence compared to secreted immunoglobulin containing linker, transmembrane, and cytoplasmic segments.

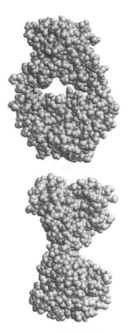

IgG1 Fab fragment.

immunoglobulin G (IgG)

Immunoglobulin G (IgG) comprises approximately 85% of the immunoglobulins in adults. It has a molecular weight of 154 kDa based on two light chains of 22,000 Da each and two heavy chains of 55,000 Da each. It has the longest half-life (23 days) of the five immunoglobulin classes, crosses the placenta, and is the principal antibody in the anamnestic or booster response. IgG shows high avidity or binding capacity for antigen, fixes complement, stimulates chemotaxis, and acts as an opsonin to facilitate phagocytosis.

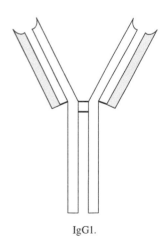

IgG1.

immunoglobulin γ chain

A 51-kDa, 450-amino acid residue heavy polypeptide chain comprised of one variable V_H domain and a constant region with three domains designated C_H1, C_H2, and C_H3. The hinge region is situated between C_H1 and C_H2. The four subclasses of IgG in humans have four corresponding γ chain isotypes, designated γ-1, γ-2, γ-3, and γ-4. IgG_1, IgG_2, IgG_3, and IgG_4 have differences in their hinge regions and differ in the number and position of disulfide bonds that

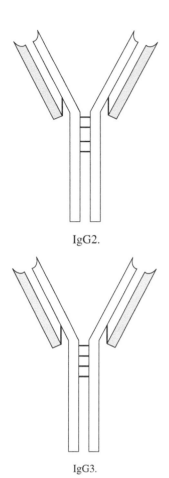

IgG2.

IgG3.

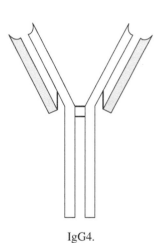

IgG4.

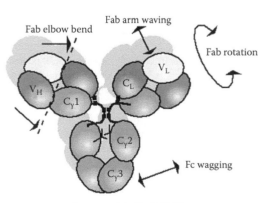

Immunoglobulin G (IgG).

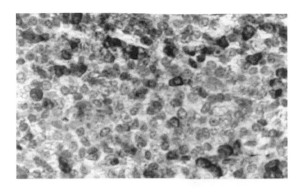

Photomicrograph of immunoglobulin G-producing cells (immuno peroxidase staining).

link the two γ chains in each IgG molecule. There is only a 5% difference in amino acid sequence among human γ chain isotypes, exclusive of the hinge region. Cysteine residues, which make it possible for inter-heavy (γ) chain disulfide bonds to form, are found in the hinge area. IgG_1 and IgG_4 have two inter-heavy chain disulfide bonds, IgG_2 has four, and IgG_3 has 11. Proteolytic enzymes such as papain and pepsin cleave an IgG molecule in the hinge region to produce Fab and $F(ab')_2$ and Fc fragments. Four murine isotypes have also been described. Two exons encode the carboxyl terminal region of the membrane γ chain. Two γ chains, together with two κ or λ light chains, fastened together by disulfide bonds, comprise an IgG molecule.

immunoglobulin gene superfamily

Refer to immunoglobulin superfamily.

immunoglobulin genes

Genes that encode heavy and light polypeptide chains of antibody molecules are found on different chromosomes (i.e., chromosome 14 for heavy chain, chromosome 2 for κ light chain, and chromosome 22 for λ light chain). The DNA of the majority of cells does not contain one gene that encodes a complete immunoglobulin heavy or light polypeptide chain. Separate gene segments that are widely distributed in somatic cells and germ cells come together to form these genes. In B cells, gene rearrangement leads to the creation of an antibody gene that codes for a specific protein. Somatic gene rearrangement also occurs with the genes that encode T cell antigen receptors. Gene rearrangement of this type permits the great versatility of the immune system in recognizing a vast array of epitopes. Three forms of gene segments join to form an immunoglobulin light chain gene. The three types include light chain variable region (*VL*), joining (*JL*), and constant region (*CL*) gene segments. *VH*, *JH*, and *CH* as well as *D* (diversity) gene segments assemble to encode the heavy chain. Heavy and light chain genes have a closely similar organizational structure. There are 100 to 300 *V*κ genes, 5 *J*κ genes, and a single *C*κ gene on the κ locus of chromosome 2. There are 100 *VH* genes, 30 *D* genes, 6 *JH* genes, and 11 *CH* genes on the heavy chain locus of chromosome 14. Several *V*λ, six *J*λ, and six *C*λ genes are present on the λ locus of chromosome 22 in humans. *VH* and *VL* genes are classified as *V* gene families, depending on the sequence homology of their nucleotides or amino acids.

immunoglobulin heavy chain

A 51- to 71-kDa polypeptide chain present in immunoglobulin molecules that serves as the basis for dividing immunoglobulins into classes. The heavy chain is comprised of three to four constant domains, depending upon class, and one variable domain. In addition, a hinge region is present in some chains. There is approximately 30% homology, with respect to amino acid sequence, among the five classes of immunoglobulin heavy chain in humans. The heavy chain of IgM is μ; of IgG, γ; of IgA, α; of IgD, δ; and of IgE, ε. Heavy chain constant regions are responsible for such effector functions as complement activation and phagocyte engagement.

immunoglobulin heavy-chain-binding protein (BiP)

A 77-kDa protein that combines with selected membrane and secretory proteins. It is believed to facilitate their passage through the endoplasmic reticulum.

immunoglobulin κ chain

A 23-kDa, 214-amino acid residue polypeptide chain composed of a single variable region and a single constant region. It is one of the two types of light polypeptide chain present in all five immunoglobulin classes. Approximately 60% of light immunoglobulin chains in humans are κ with wide variations of their percentages in other species. Whereas κ chains are virtually absent in immunoglobulins of dogs, they comprise the vast majority of murine immunoglobulin light chains. κ light-chain allotypes in humans are termed Km1, Km1,2, and Km3.

immunoglobulin λ chain

A 23-kDa, 214-amino acid residue polypeptide chain with a single variable region and a single constant region. λ chains represent one of two light polypeptide chains comprising all five classes of immunoglobulin molecules. Approximately 40% of immunoglobulin light chains in humans are λ. Wide variations in percentages are observed in other species. For example, the great majority of immunoglobulin light chains in horses and dogs are λ, whereas they constitute only 5% of murine light chains. Constant region differences exist among λ light chains of mice and humans, and the molecules are divided into four isotypes in humans. A different *C* gene segment encodes the separate constant regions defining each λ light chain isotype. The human λ light chain isotypes are designated Kern–Oz+, Kern+Oz–, and Mcg.

immunoglobulin light chain

A 23-kDa, 214-amino acid polypeptide chain comprised of a single constant region and a single variable region; the chain is present in all five classes of immunoglobulin molecules. The two types of light chains are designated κ and λ. They are found in association with heavy polypeptide chains and in immunoglobulin molecules and are fastened to these structures through disulfide bonds. Approximately 60% of antibodies in humans contain κ light chains and 40% contain λ light chains.

immunoglobulin-like domain

A 100-amino-acid residue structure found in selected β-sheet-rich proteins with intrachain disulfide bonds. It is found in immunoglobulins, interleukin-1 and interleukin-6, T cell receptors, and platelet-derived growth factors. Structural regions of proteins that are similar to the immunoglobulin domain, but are present in various other proteins.

immunoglobulin M (IgM)

Immunoglobulin M (IgM) comprises 5 to 10% of the total immunoglobulins in adults and has a half-life of 5 days. It

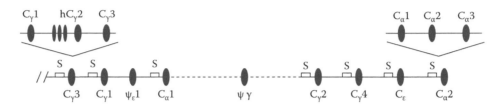

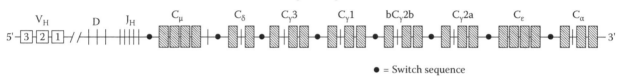

Immunoglobulin genes.

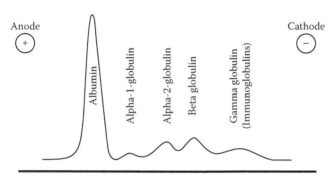

● = Switch sequence

Mouse immunoglobulin gene.

Electrophoresis of serum protein showing the gammaglobulin region that contains the immunoglobulins.

is a pentameric molecule with five four-chain monomers joined by disulfide bonds and a J chain, with a total molecular weight of 900 kDa. Theoretically, this immunoglobulin has ten antigen-binding sites. IgM is the most efficient immunoglobulin in fixing complement. A single IgM pentamer can activate the classic pathway. Monomeric IgM is found with IgD on B lymphocyte cell surfaces, where it serves as a receptor for antigen. It is the first immnoglobulin expressed on the B cell surface and the first antibody secreted in an immune response. Because IgM is relatively large, it is confined to intravascular locations. IgM is particularly important for immunity against polysaccharide antigens on the exterior of pathogenic microorganisms. It

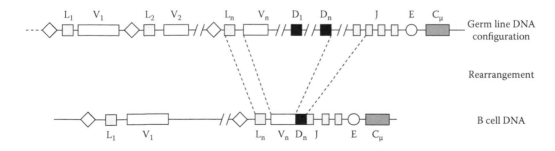

◇ = Promoter
L = Leader sequence
V = Variable regions
D = Diversity regions
J = Junction regions
C = Constant region coding block
E = Enhancer sequence

Immunoglobulin gene rearrangement.

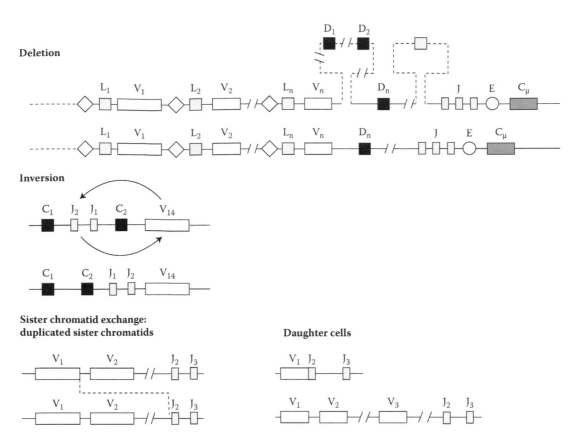

Deletion

Inversion

Sister chromatid exchange:
duplicated sister chromatids   **Daughter cells**

Immunoglobulin gene rearrangement (see previous figure for key).

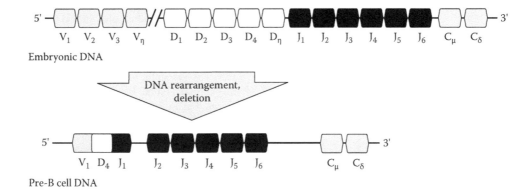

Embryonic DNA

DNA rearrangement, deletion

Pre-B cell DNA

Immunoglobulin gene rearrangement (see previous figure for key).

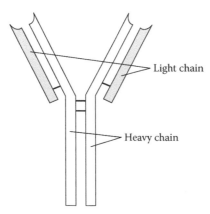

Immunoglobulin heavy chains that are fastened to each other or to light poly-peptide changes by disulfide bonds.

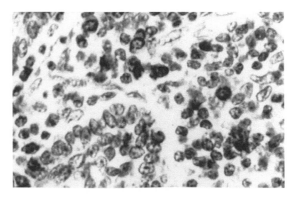

Photomicrograph of immunoglobulin κ light chain "staining" by immunoperoxidase.

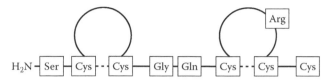

Kappa light chain showing domain structure.

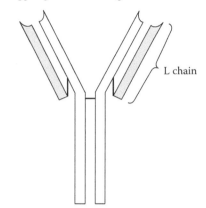

Immunoglobulin light chain.

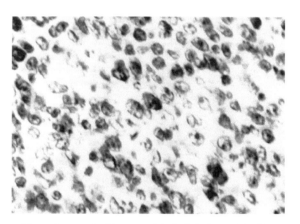

Photomicrograph of immunoglobulin λ light "staining" by immunoperoxidase.

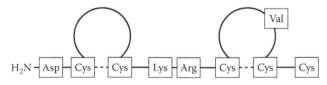

Lambda light chain showing domain structure.

also promotes phagocytosis and bacteriolysis through its complement activation activity.

immunoglobulin monomer

The basic unit of immunoglobulin, comprised of two heavy chains and two light chains.

immunoglobulin μ chain

A 72-kDa, 570-amino acid heavy polypeptide chain composed of one variable region designated V_H and a constant region with four domains designated C_H1, C_H2, C_H3, and C_H4. The μ chain does not have a hinge region. A "tail piece" is located at the carboxyl terminal end of the chain. It is composed of 18 amino acid residues. A cysteine residue at the penultimate position of a carboxyl terminal region of the μ chain forms a disulfide bond that joins to the J chain.

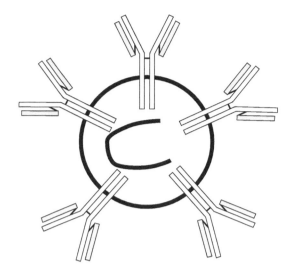

Pentameric immunoglobulin M (IgM) consisting of five 7S monomers composed of two heavy and two light polypeptide chains each and one J chain per molecule.

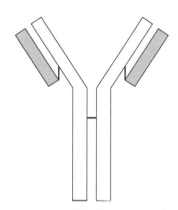

Monomeric immunoglobulin M (IgM) that contains two heavy chain and two κ or two λ light chains.

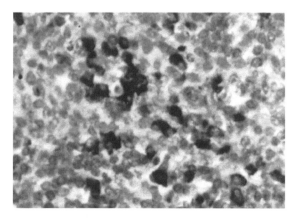

Photomicrograph of IgM-producing cells (immunoperoxidase staining).

The μ chain of humans has five *N*-linked oligosaccharides. Secreted IgM ($μ_s$) and membrane IgM ($μ_m$) and μ chain differ only in the final 20 amino acid residues at the carboxyl terminal end. The membrane form of IgM has 41 different residues substituted for the final 20 residues in the secreted form. A 26-residue region of this carboxyl terminal section

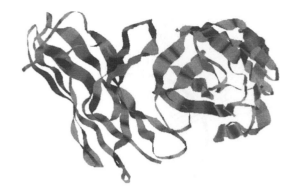

IgM Fv fragment.

Ig	IgG	IgM	IgA	IgE	IgD
H-chain class	γ	μ	α	ε	δ
Subclass	γ₁ γ₂ γ₃ γ₄		α₁ α₂		

Heavy chain designations of immunoglobulins that determine class and their subdivisons that determine subclass.

in the membrane form of IgM apparently represents the hydrophobic transmembrane part of the chain.

immunoglobulin staining

Demonstrable by immunoperoxidase staining of plasma cell and B lymphocyte cytoplasm in frozen or paraffin-embedded sections. B-5 fixative is preferable to formalin for

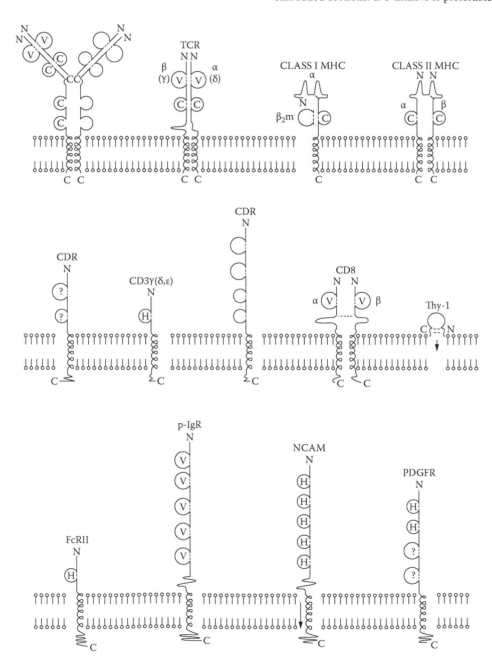

Immunoglobulin superfamily.

demonstration of intracellular IgG or light chains in paraffin sections. Monoclonal cytoplasmic staining for either κ or λ light chains aids the diagnosis of B cell lymphomas.

immunoglobulin structure

Refer to immunoglobulin.

immunoglobulin subclass

The subdivision of immunoglobulin classes according to structural and antigenic differences in the constant regions of their heavy polypeptide chains. All molecules in a subclass must express the isotypic antigenic determinants unique to that class, but they also express other epitopes that render that subclass different from others. Immunoglobulin G (IgG) has four subclasses designated IgG_1, IgG_2, IgG_3, and IgG_4. Whereas there is only 30% identity among the five immunoglobulin classes, the similarity among IgG subclasses is three times that. The IgA class is divisible into two subclasses, but the remaining three immunoglobulin classes have not been further subdivided into subclasses. The structural differences in subclasses are exemplified by the variations and number of inter-heavy chain disulfide bonds that the four IgG subclasses possess. The function of immunoglobulin molecules differs from one subclass to another, as exemplified by the inability of IgG_4 to fix complement.

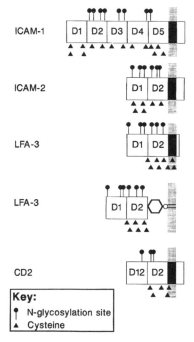

Immunoglobulin superfamily adhesion receptors.

immunoglobulin superfamily

Several molecules that participate in the immune response and show similarities in structure, causing them to be named the immunoglobulin supergene family. Included are CD2, CD3, CD4, CD7, CD8, CD28, T cell receptor (TCR), major histocompatibility complex (MHC) class I and class II molecules, leukocyte function-associated antigen 3 (LFA-3), the IgG receptor, and a dozen other proteins. These molecules share in common an immunoglobulin-like domain with a length of approximately 100 amino acid residues and a central disulfide bond that anchors and stabilizes antiparallel β strands into a folded structure resembling immunoglobulin. Immunoglobulin

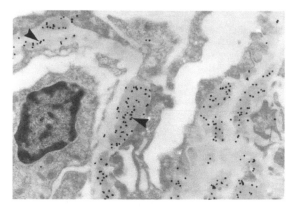

Immunogold labeling.

superfamily members may share homology with constant or variable immunoglobulin domain regions. Various molecules of the cell surface with polypeptide chains whose folded structures are involved in cell-to-cell interactions belong in this category. Single-gene and multigene members are included. Protein molecules sharing 15% amino acid homology with immunoglobulin proteins and possessing one or more immunoglobulin domains belong to this large molecular family.

immunogold labeling

A technique to identify antigens in tissue preparations by electron microscopy. Incubating sections with primary antibody is followed by treatment with colloidal gold-labeled anti-IgG antibody. Electron-dense particles are localized at sites of antigen–antibody interactions.

immunogold silver staining (IGSS)

An immunohistochemical technique to detect antigens in tissues and cells by light microscopy. IGSS offers higher labeling intensity than most other methods when examined in a bright field or in conjunction with polarized light. The technique successfully stains tissue sections from paraffin wax, resin, or cryostat preparations. It is also effective for cell suspensions or smears, cytospin preparations, cell cultures, or tissue sections. Both l- and 5-nm gold conjugates are used for light microscopy. The l-nm particles are advantageous in studies of cell penetration. In immunogold silver staining, primary antibody is incubated with tissues or cells to localize antigens that are identified with gold-labeled secondary antibodies and silver enhanced.

immunohematology

The study of blood group antigens and antibodies and their interactions in health and disease. Both the cellular elements and the serum constituents of the blood have distinct profiles of antigens. There are multiple systems of blood cell groups, all of which may stimulate antibodies and interact with them. These may be associated with erythrocytes, leukocytes, or platelets.

immunohistochemistry

A method to detect antigens in tissues that employs an enzyme-linked antibody specific for antigen. The enzyme degrades a colorless substrate to a colored insoluble substance that precipitates where the antibody and, therefore, the antigen are located. Identification of the site of the colored precipitate and the antigen in the tissue section is accomplished by light microscopy. Diagnostic pathology services routinely offer approximately 100 antigens

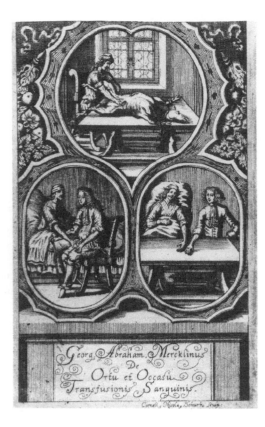

Engraved title page from G.A. Mercklin's *Tractatio Med. Curiosa de Ortu et Sanguinis* (1679). This is one of the best early depictions of blood transfusion. (Courtesy of the Cruse Collection, Middleton Library, University of Wisconsin, Madison.)

identified by immunoperoxidase technology that are used in diagnosis.

immunoincompetence

Inability to produce a physiologic immune response. For example, patients with acquired immune deficiency syndrome (AIDS) become immunoincompetent as a consequence of destruction of their helper/inducer (CD4+) T lymphocyte population. Infants born without thymus glands and experimental animals thymectomized at birth are immunologically incompetent. Children born with severe combined immunodeficiency (SCID) due to one or several causes are unable to mount appropriate immune responses. Immunoincompetence may involve either the B cell limb as in Bruton's hypogammaglobulinemia or the T cell limb as in patients with DiGeorge's syndrome.

immunoinformatics

A subset of bioinformatics focusing on the field of immunology. Immunoinformatics applications are of increasing significance to immunological research. The major findings of structural, functional, and regulatory aspects of molecular immunology, coupled with rapid accumulation of immunological data, have been complemented by the development of more sophisticated computational solutions for immunological research. Immunology is a combinatorial science. The immune system is intertwined with all other body systems. Bioinformatics applications are well developed for some immunological areas, including databases, genomic applications, study of T cell epitopes, modeling immune systems and, to a lesser degree, the analysis of allergenicity of proteins. Also called computational immunology; includes theoretical immunology.

immunoinhibitory genes

Selected human leukocyte antigen (HLA) genes that appear to protect against immunological diseases. Their mechanisms of action are in dispute.

immunoisolation

The enclosure of allogeneic tissues, such as pancreatic islet cell allografts, within a membrane that is semipermeable but does not induce an immune response. Substances of relatively low molecular weight can reach the graft through the membrane, while it remains protected from immunologic rejection by the host.

immunologic (or immunological)

Aspects of a subject that fall under the purview of the scientific discipline of immunology.

immunologic adjuvant

A substance that enhances an immune response, either humoral or cellular, or both, to an immunogen (antigen).

immunologic barrier

An anatomical site that diminishes or protects against immune response. Term refers principally to immunologically privileged sites where grafts of tissue may survive for prolonged periods without undergoing immunologic rejection, based mainly on the lack of adequate lymphatic drainage in these areas. Examples include prolonged survival of foreign grafts in the brain.

immunologic colitis

An ulcerative condition that may involve the entire colon but does not significantly affect the small intestine. Neutrophil, plasma cell eosinophil infiltration of the colonic mucosa occurs, followed by ulceration of the surface epithelium, loss of goblet cells, and formation of crypt abscess. The etiology is unknown. An immune effector mechanism is believed to maintain chronic disease in these patients whose serum immunoglobulins and peripheral blood lymphocyte counts usually are normal. Complexes present in the blood are relatively small and contain immunoglobulin G (IgG), although no antigen has been identified. The complexes may be merely aggregates of IgG. Patients have diarrhea with blood and mucus in stools. The signs and symptoms are intermittent, and the severity of colon lesions varies. The lymphocytes are cytotoxic for colon epithelial cells. Antibodies against *Escherichia coli* may cross react with colonic in these patients; however, whether such antibodies play a role in etiology and pathogenesis remains to be proven.

immunologic competence

The capability to mount an immune response.

immunologic enhancement (tumor enhancement)

The prolonged survival, and conversely the delayed rejection, of a tumor allograft in a host as a consequence of contact with a specific antibody. Antitumor antibodies may produce paradoxical effects. Instead of eradicating a neoplasm, they may facilitate its survival and progressive growth in the host. Both peripheral and central mechanisms have been postulated. Coating of tumor cells with antibody was presumed in the past to interfere with the ability of specifically reactive lymphocytes to destroy them, but a central effect in suppressing cell-mediated immunity, perhaps through suppressor T lymphocytes, is also possible. Enhancing antibodies are blocking antibodies that favor survival of tumor or normal tissue allografts.

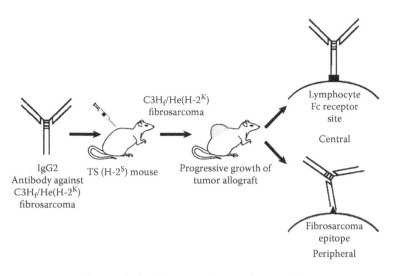

Immunologic enhancement (tumor enhancement).

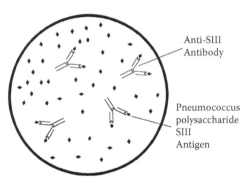

Schematic view of antigen excess

Immunologic (or immune) paralysis.

immunologic facilitation (facilitation immunologique)

Slightly prolonged survival of certain normal tissue allografts (e.g., skin) in mice conditioned with isoantiserum specific for the graft.

immunologic paralysis

Immunologic unresponsiveness induced by the injection of large doses of pneumococcal polysaccharide into mice, where it is metabolized slowly. Any antibody that is formed is consumed and is not detectable. The pneumococcal polysaccharide antigen remains in the tissue of recipients for months, during which time they produce no immune response to the antigen. Immunologic paralysis is much easier to induce with polysaccharide than with protein antigens. It is highly specific for the antigen used for its induction. Felton's first observation of immunologic paralysis preceded the demonstration of acquired immunologic tolerance by Medawar et al.

immunologic tolerance

An active but carefully regulated response of lymphocytes to self antigens. Autoantibodies are formed against a variety of self antigens. Maintenance of self tolerance is a quantitative process. When comparing the ease with which T and B cell tolerance may be induced, it was found that T cell tolerance is induced more rapidly and lasts longer than B cell tolerance. For example, T cell tolerance may be induced in a single day, whereas B cells may require 10 days for induction. In addition, 100 times more tolerogen may be required for B cell tolerance than for T cell tolerance. The duration of tolerance is much greater in T cells (e.g., 150 days) compared to that in B cells, which is only 50 to 60 days. T suppressor cells are also very important in maintaining natural tolerance to self antigens; for example, they may suppress T helper cell activity. Maintenance of tolerance is considered to require the continued presence of specific antigens. Low antigen doses may be effective in inducing tolerance in immature B cells, leading to clonal abortion, but T cell tolerance does not depend upon the level of maturation. Another mechanism of B cell tolerance is cloning exhaustion, in which the immunogen activates all of the B lymphocytes specific for it, leading to maturation of cells and transient antibody synthesis, thereby exhausting and diluting the B cell response. Another mechanism of B cell tolerance is antibody-forming cell blockade. Antibody-expressing B cells are coated with excess antigen, rendering them unresponsive to the antigen.

immunological contraception

A method to prevent an undesired pregnancy. Vaccines that induce antibodies and cell-mediated immune responses against either a hormone or gamete antigen significant to reproduction have been developed. Such vaccines control fertility in experimental animals. They have undergone exhaustive safety and toxicological investigations which have shown the safety and reversibility of some of the vaccines and with approval of regulatory agencies and ethics commissions, have undergone clinical trials in humans. Six vaccines, three in women and three in men, have completed phase I clinical trials showing their safety and reversibility. One vaccine has successfully completed phase II trials, proving efficacy in females. The trials determined the titers of antibodies and other immunological features. A fertilized egg makes the hormone hCG. Antibodies that inactivate one or more hormones involved in the production of gametes and sex steroids may be expected to impair fertility. Blocking the action of LHRH would also inhibit the synthesis of sex steroids. This may prove useful in controlling fertility of domestic animals but would not be acceptable for contraception in humans. Two vaccines against LHRH are in clinical trials in prostate carcinoma patients. An FSH vaccine would act at the level of male fertility since FSH is required for spermatogenesis in primates.

immunological deficiency state

Immunodeficiency.

immunological escape

A mechanism of escape in which tumors that are immunogenic continue to grow in immunocompetent syngeneic hosts in the presence of a modest *in vivo* antitumor immune response. Escape mechanisms may facilitate evasion of a fatal tumoricidal response and render tumors incapable of inducing such a response. Failure of tumor antigen presentation by major histocompatibility complex (MHC) class I molecules, lack of costimulation, and downregulation of tumor-destructive immune responses by tumor antigens, immune complexes, and molecules such as TGF-β and P15E are all believed to contribute to the inefficiency of tumor immunity.

immunological ignorance

A type of tolerance to self in which a target antigen and lymphocytes capable of reacting with it are both present simultaneously in an individual without an autoimmune reaction occurring. Peripheral tolerance to self constituents present in such small quantities that immature dendritic cells rather take them up and present them to cognate T cells. The abrogation of immunologic ignorance may lead to autoimmune disease.

immunological inertia

Specific immunosuppression related to paternal histocompatibility antigens during pregnancy, such as suppression of maternal immune reactivity against fetal histocompatibility antigens.

immunological infertility

Infertility in 12 to 25% of cases in which couples experience infertility even though they manifest no significant abnormalities upon physical examination. These cases of unexplained infertility may be caused by autoimmune responses to organ-specific antigens of the reproductive tract of both males and females and isoimmune reactions of females against semen components. Immune responses may cause or contribute to infertility in approximately 10% of these couples.

immunological memory

The effectiveness of protective immunity against an infectious agent depends on the ability of the immune system to retain a memory of the original infective agent in order to provide an enhanced immune response on re-exposure to the same agent. This mechanism usually prevents overt infection and a fatal outcome; however, not all consequences of immune memory are beneficial. A second infection with the dengue virus may be more severe than the first. Another detrimental effect of immunity is sensitization to an allergen that leads to a hypersensitivity reaction. During a primary immune response to an infectious agent, each antigen-specific lymphocyte clone activated produces numerous memory lymphocytes of identical specificity and greater affinity. A second attack by the same pathogen leads to a secondary immune response when memory lymphocytes are activated, which leads to more rapid and efficient elimination of the invading pathogen. Immunologic memory is specific for a particular antigen and is long lasting. Immunological memory is governed by many factors, with both B and T cells contributing to it. Immunological memory depends upon interactions between memory T cells and memory B cells.

immunological reaction

In vivo or *in vitro* responses of lymphoid cells to an antigen they have not previously encountered or for which they are already primed or sensitized. An immunological reaction may consist of antibody formation, cell-mediated immunity, or immunological tolerance. The humoral antibody and cell-mediated immune reactions may mediate either protective immunity or hypersensitivity, depending on various conditions.

immunological rejection

The destruction of an allograft or even a xenograft in a recipient host whose immune system has been activated to respond to the foreign tissue antigens.

immunological suicide

The use of an antigen deliberately labeled with high-dose radioisotope to kill a subpopulation of lymphocytes with receptors specific for that antigen following antigen binding.

immunological synapse

The nanometer-scale gap between a T cell and an antigen-presenting cell, which is the site of interaction between a T cell antigen receptor and major histocompatibility complex (MHC) molecule–peptide complex that initiates the adaptive immune response. Refer to SMAC (supramolecular activation complex).

immunological unresponsiveness

Failure to form antibodies or develop a lymphoid cell-mediated response following exposure to immunogen (antigen). Immunosuppression that is specific for only one antigen, with no interference with the responses to all other antigens, is termed immunological tolerance. By contrast, the administration of powerful immunosuppressive agents such as azathioprine, cyclosporine, or total body irradiation causes generalized immunological unresponsiveness to essentially all immunogens to which the host is exposed.

immunologically activated cell

An immunologically competent cell following its interaction with antigen. This response may be expressed as lymphocyte transformation, immunological memory, cell-mediated immunity, immunologic tolerance, or antibody synthesis.

immunologically competent cell

A lymphocyte, such as a B cell or T cell, that can recognize and respond to a specific antigen.

immunologically privileged sites

Certain anatomical sites within the animal body provide an immunologically privileged environment that favors the prolonged survival of alien grafts. The potential for development of a blood and lymphatic vascular supply connecting graft and host may be a determining factor in the qualification of an anatomical site as an area that provides an environment favorable to the prolonged survival of a foreign graft. Immunologically privileged areas include (1) the anterior chamber of the eye, (2) the substantia propria of the cornea, (3) the meninges of the brain, (4) the testis, and (5) the cheek pouch of the Syrian hamster. Foreign grafts implanted in these sites show a diminished ability to induce transplantation immunity in the host. Immunologically privileged sites usually fail to protect alien grafts from the immune rejection mechanism in hosts previously or simultaneously sensitized with donor tissues. The capacity of cells expressing Fas ligand to cause deletion of activated lymphocytes provides a possible explanation for the phenomenon of immune privilege. Animals with a deficiency in either Fas ligand or the Fas receptor fail to manifest significant immune privilege. Both epithelial cells of the eye and

Sertoli cells of the testes express Fas ligand. Immune privilege is a consequence not only of the lack of an inflammatory response but also the immune consequences of the accumulation of apoptotic immune cells within a tissue. Immune cell apoptosis may be a signal to terminate inflammation. Apoptotic cell accumulation during an immune response may activate the development of cells that function to downregulate or suppress further immune activation. Thus, immunosuppression by physical barriers, hormone secretion, low numbers of dendritic cells, immune deviation, immunosuppressive cytokines, or Fas killing may facilitate the induction of immunological privilege.

immunologist

A person who makes a special study of immunology.

immunology

The branch of biomedical science concerned with the responses of organisms to immunogenic (antigenic) challenges, the recognition of self from nonself, and all the biological (*in vivo*), serological (*in vitro*), physical, and chemical aspects of immune phenomena.

immunolymphoscintigraphy

A method to determine the presence of tumor metastasis in lymph nodes. Antibody fragments or monoclonal antibodies against specific tumor antigens are radiolabeled and then detected by scintigraphy.

immunomagnetic technique

The use of magnetic microspheres to sort, isolate, or identify cells with specific antigenic determinants.

immunomodulation

Therapeutic alteration of the immune system by the administration of biological response modifiers such as lymphokines or antibodies against cell surface markers bound to a toxin such as ricin.

immunomodulator

An agent that alters the level of an immune response.

immunopathic damage

Collateral injury to host tissues induced by cytokines and effector cells released in the course of an immune response.

immunonephelometry

A test that measures light scattered at a 90° angle to a laser or light source as it is passes through a suspension of minute complexes of antigen and antibody. Measurement is made at 340 to 360 nm using a spectrophotometer.

immunoosmoelectropheresis

Refer to counter immunoelectrophoresis.

immunoparasitology

Immunologic aspects of the interactions between animal parasites and their hosts.

immunopathic

Injury to cells, tissues, or organs induced by either humoral (antibodies) or cellular products of an immune response.

immunopathology

The study of disease processes that have immunological etiology or pathogenesis involving either humoral antibody (from B cells) and complement or T-cell-mediated or cytokine mechanisms. Immunologic injury of tissues and cells may be mediated by any of the four types of hypersensitivity (described separately).

immunoperoxidase method

Nakene and Pierce in 1966 first proposed that enzymes be used in the place of fluorochromes as labels for antibodies.

Horseradish peroxidase (HRP) is the enzyme label most widely employed. The immunoperoxidase technique permits the demonstration of antigens in various types of cells and fixed tissues. This method has certain advantages: (1) conventional light microscopy is used, (2) stained preparations may be kept permanently, (3) the method may be adapted for use with electron microscopy of tissues, and (4) counterstains may be employed. The disadvantages include: (1) the demonstration of relatively minute, positively staining areas is limited by the resolution of the light microscope, (2) endogenous peroxidase may not have been completely eliminated from the tissue under investigation, and (3) diffusion of products results from enzyme reactions away from the area where antigen is localized. The peroxidase–antiperoxidase (PAP) technique employs unlabeled antibodies and a PAP reagent. It has proven highly successful for demonstrating antigens in paraffin-embedded tissues as an aid in surgical pathologic diagnosis. Tissue sections preserved in paraffin are first treated with xylene; after deparaffinization they are exposed to a hydrogen peroxide solution that destroys the endogenous peroxidase activity in tissue. The sections are next incubated with normal swine serum, which suppresses nonspecific binding of immunoglobulin molecules to tissues containing collagen. Thereafter, the primary rabbit antibody against the antigen to be identified is reacted with the tissue section. Unbound primary antibody is removed by rinsing the sections that are then covered with swine antibody against rabbit immunoglobulin. This so-called linking antibody will combine with any primary rabbit antibody in the tissue. It is added in excess, which causes one of its antigen-binding sites to remain free. After washing, the PAP reagent is placed on the section, and the antibody portion of this complex, which is raised in rabbits, will be bound to the free antigen-binding site of the linking antibody on the sections. The unbound PAP complex is then washed away by rinsing. To read the sections microscopically, it is necessary to add a substrate of hydrogen peroxide and aminoethylcarbazole (AEC), which permits the formation of a visible product that may be detected with a light microscope. The AEC is oxidized to produce a reddish-brown pigment that is not water soluble. Peroxidase catalyzes the reaction. Because peroxidase occurs only at sites where the PAP is bound via linking antibody and primary antibody to antigen molecules, the antigen is identified by the reddish-brown pigment. The tissue sections can then be counterstained with hematoxylin or other suitable dye, covered with mounting medium and cover slips, and read by conventional light microscopy. The PAP technique has been replaced, in part, by the avidin–biotin complex (ABC) technique.

immunophenotyping

The use of monoclonal antibodies and flow cytometry to reveal cell surface or cytoplasmic antigens that yield information that may reflect clonality and cell lineage classification. This type of data is valuable clinically in aiding the diagnosis of leukemias and lymphomas through the use of a battery of B cell, T cell, and myeloid markers. However, immunophenotyping results must be used only in conjunction with morphologic criteria when reaching a diagnosis of leukemia or lymphoma.

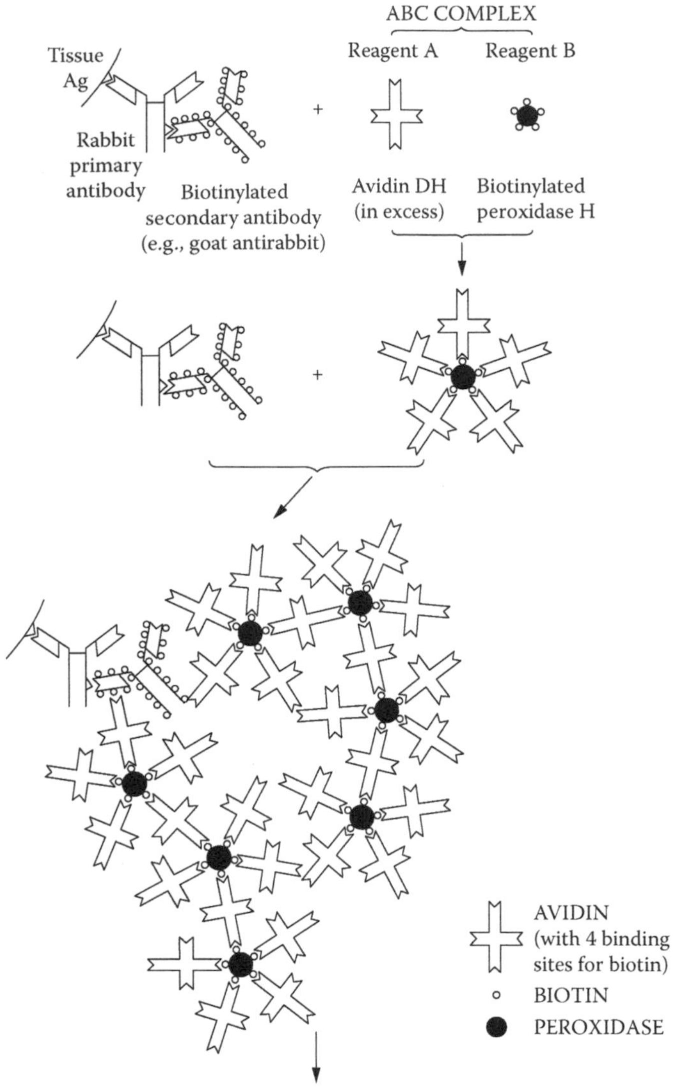

Immunoperoxidase method. Development in chromogenic hydrogen donor and hydrogen peroxide. (The reaction product is seen as a reddish brown or brown granular deposit depending upon the chromogenic hydrogen donor used.)

immunophilins (*Tacrolimus* and *Rapamycin sirolimus*)

High-affinity receptor proteins with peptidyl-prolyl *cis–trans* isomerase activity that combine with such immunosuppressants as cyclosporin A, FK506, and rapamycin. They prevent the activity of rotamase by blocking conversion between *cis* and *trans* rotamers of the peptide and protein substrate peptidyl–prolylamide bond. Immunophilins are important in transducing signals from the cell surface to the nucleus. Immunosuppressants have been postulated to prevent signal transduction mediated by T lymphocyte receptors which blocks nuclear factor activation in activated T lymphocytes. Cyclophilin- and FK506-binding proteins represent immunophilins. Drug–immunophilin complexes are implicated in the mechanism of action of the immunosuppressant drugs, cyclosporin, FK506, and rapamycin.

immunophysiology

The physiologic basis of immunologic processes.

immunopotency

The capability of a part of an antigen molecule to function as an epitope and induce the synthesis of specific antibodies.

immunopotentiation

Facilitation of the immune response usually with the aid of adjuvants such as muramyl dipeptide, Freund's adjuvant, synthetic polynucleotides, or other agents. Biological response modifiers, cloned cytokines, and purified immunoglobulins have been used as immunopotentiating agents.

immunoprecipitation

A method to recover or isolate an antigen molecule from solution by uniting it with an antibody and rendering the antigen–antibody complex insoluble through interaction with an anti-antibody or through coupling the first antibody to an insoluble support such as a particle or bead. A common technique used for identifying protein–protein interactions. IP is usually performed using a primary antibody together with a second antibody resin or protein A or G resin. After IP, a western blot is used to detect any possible proteins associated with the target protein. Used to isolate or detect antigens present in complex mixtures of proteins in solution.

immunoproliferative small intestinal disease (IPSID)

Mediterranean lymphoma α heavy chain disease. A varied group of disorders in which there is monoclonal synthesis of immunoglobulin heavy chain (often α). Light chains are not produced. The variable region and often the C_H1 constant region may be missing. Whereas the monoclonal protein usually elevated is the α chain, some cases may manifest γ or μ chain elevations. Patients experience weight loss, pain in the abdomen, diarrhea, and malabsorption. Expansion of the mesenteric lymphoid tissue and the proximal small intestine occurs, accompanied by clubbing of the fingers. Tetracyclines are the recommended treatments.

immunoprophylaxis

Disease prevention through the use of vaccines to induce active immunization or antisera to induce passive immunization.

immunoproteasome

Refer to proteasome.

immunoprotein

An immunologically active protein, such as one that serves as a target for immunological probes or therapy.

immunoradioisotope

An immunoconjugate used in radioimmunotherapy in which a monoclonal antibody or monoclonal antibody derivative is bound to a radioisotope capable of destroying a tumor cell on contact.

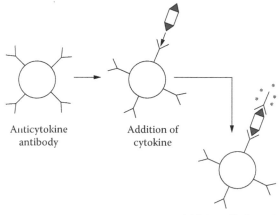

Anticytokine antibody   Addition of cytokine

Addition of iodinated monoclonal antibody

Immunoradiometric assay (IRMA).

immunoradiometric assay (IRMA)

A quantitative method to assay certain plasma proteins based on a "sandwich" technique using radiolabeled antibody rather than radiolabeled hormone competing with hormone from a patient in the radioimmunoassay (RIA).

immunoradiometry

A radioimmunoassay method in which the antibody rather than the antigen is radiolabeled.

immunoreactant

Any substance, including immunoglobulins, complement components, and antigens involved in immune reactions.

immunoreaction

The reaction of antibody with antigen.

immunoreceptor tyrosine-based activation motif (ITAM)

Amino acid sequences in the intracellular portions of signal-transducing cell surface molecules that are sites of tyrosine phosphorylation and association with tyrosine kinases and phophotyrosine-binding proteins that participate in signal transduction. Examples include Igα, Igβ, CD3

chains, and several Ig Fc receptors. Following receptor–ligand binding and phosphorylation, docking sites are formed for other molecules that participate in maintaining cell-activating, signal transduction mechanisms.

immunoreceptor tyrosine-based inhibition motif (ITIM)

Motifs with effects that oppose those of immunoreceptor tyrosine-based activation motifs (ITAMs). These amino acids in the cytoplasmic tails of transmembrane molecules bind phosphate groups added by tyrosine kinases. This six-amino acid (isoleucine–X–tyrosine–X–X–leucine) motif is present in the cytoplasmic tails of immune system inhibitory receptors that include FcγRIIB on B lymphocytes and the killer inhibitory receptors (KIR) on natural killer (NK) cells. Following receptor–ligand binding and phosporylation on the tyrosine residue, a docking site is formed for protein tyrosine phosphatases that inhibit other signal transduction pathways, thereby negatively regulating cell activation.

immunoregulation

Control of the immune response, usually by its own products such as the idiotypic network of antibody regulation described by Niels Jerne, feedback inhibition of antibody formation by antibody molecules, T cell receptor interaction with antibodies specific for them, and the effects of immunosuppressive and immunoenhancing cytokines on the immune response in addition to other mechanisms. Refers to control of both humoral and cellular limbs of the immune response by mechanisms such as antibody feedback inhibition, the immunoglobulin idiotype–anti-idiotype network, helper and suppressor T cells, and cytokines. Results of these immunoregulatory interactions may lead to either suppression or potentiation of one or the other limb of the immune response.

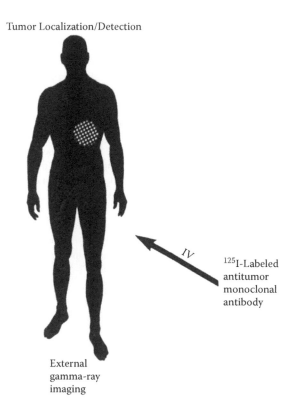

Tumor Localization/Detection

IV

^{125}I-Labeled antitumor monoclonal antibody

External gamma-ray imaging

Immunoscintigraphy.

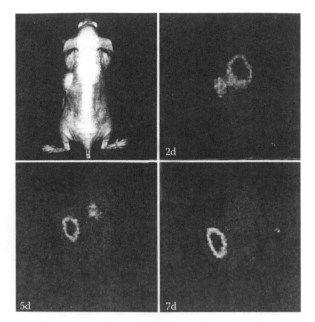

Immunoscintigraphy (nude mouse) with a ^{131}I-labeled monoclonal antibody. The mouse shown bears a human colon carcinoma in its left flank. The scintigrams were recorded 2, 5, and 7 days after injection. While the second picture shows mainly the blood pool and little of the tumor, the tumor is the major imaged spot in the body after 5 days; after 7 days, only the tumor is recognizable.

immunoscintigraphy

The formation of two-dimensional images of the distribution of radioactivity in tissues following the administration of antibodies labeled with a radionuclide that are specific for tissue antigens. A scintillation camera is used to record the images.

immunoselection

The selective survival of cells due to their diminished surface antigenicity, which permits these cells to escape the injurious effects of antibodies or immune lymphoid cells.

immunosenescence

The age-associated decrease of the immune system and host defenses. Cell-mediated immunity declines in the elderly, who develop secondary decreases in humoral immunity. Elderly persons may have defective host defenses that place them at a greater risk for developing infectious diseases and may manifest increased risks of morbidity and mortality from infectious diseases.

immunosome

The complete membrane complex of antigen-stimulated T cell receptor, CD3 chains, costimulatory and adhesion molecules, coreceptors, and other signaling molecules linked with the lipid rafts of activated T cells.

immunosuppression

Decreased or abolished immune responsiveness. Can be mediated by immunosuppressive cytokines, immunosuppressive drugs, anti-cytokine antibodies or antibodies against lymphocytes. (1) The deliberate administration of drugs, such as cyclosporine, azathioprine, corticosteroids, FK506, or rapamycin, or the administration of specific antibody, or the use of irradiation to depress immune reactivity in recipients of organ or bone marrow allotransplants. (2) Profound depression of immune responses in patients

with certain diseases such as acquired immune deficiency syndrome (AIDS), in which the helper/inducer (CD4+) T lymphocytes are destroyed by the human immunodeficiency virus 1 (HIV-1). In addition to these examples of nonspecific immunosuppression, antigen-induced specific immunosuppression is associated with immunologic tolerance.

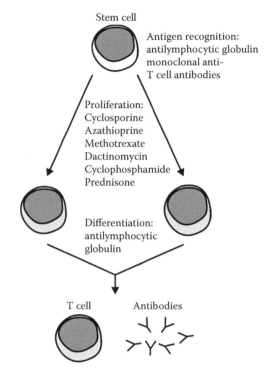

Immunosuppressive drugs: a summary.

immunosuppressive agent

A drug such as cyclosporine, FK506, rapamycin, azathioprine, or corticosteroids; an antibody such as antilymphocyte serum; or irradiation that produces mild to profound depression of a host's ability to respond to an immunogen (antigen), as in the conditioning of an organ allotransplant recipient. Substances that inhibit adaptive immune responses may be used also to treat autoimmune diseases.

immunosuppressive cytokines

Cellular chemical mediators such as IL10 and TGFβ that diminish immune system cell activation by hindering intracellular signaling pathways.

immunosuppressive drugs

Therapeutic substances that diminish immune responses by inhibiting lymphocyte homing receptors. Costimulation, proliferation, activation-induced cell death (AICD), or leukocyte function or trafficking. May also decrease cytokine or chemokine expression or antigen uptake by dendritic cells. Inhibit adaptive immune responses.

immunosurveillance

The monitoring function by cells of the immune system in recognizing, reacting against, and fatally injuring aberrant cells (e.g., neoplastic cells) that arise by somatic mutation and express new antigens (neoantigens). Immunosurveillance is believed to be mediated by the cellular limb of the immune response. Indirect evidence in support of the concept includes (1) increased incidence of tumors in aged individuals who have decreased immune competence, (2) increased tumor incidence in children with T cell immunodeficiencies, and (3) the development of neoplasms (lymphomas) in a significant number of organ and bone marrow transplant recipients who have been deliberately immunosuppressed.

immunotactoid glomerulopathy

A renal malady characterized by glomerular deposits of fibrillar material comprised of 10- to 48.9-nm microfibrils or microtubules as viewed by electron microscopy. These deposits are not birefringent when stained with Congo red and examined by polarizing light microscopy; this differentiates them from amyloid. Usually, no extraglomerular fibrillar deposits are present, differentiating the condition from amyloid or light chain deposition. It is not associated with concomitant systemic disease such as cryoglobulinemia or systemic lupus erythematosus. The condition typically affects middle-aged males who may manifest hypertension, nephritic range proteinuria, and microscopic hematuria.

immunotherapy

A treatment mechanism in which therapy is aimed at targets of the immune system that include antigen-presenting cells, activated T cells, macrophages, and B cells. The term also refers to the therapeutic use of immunological reagents such as antibodies, T cells, or their modifications. Both types have been applied to animal models of autoimmune diseases, and attempts are in progress to apply immunotherapy to human autoimmune diseases. A principal goal of immunotherapy is to selectively diminish the unwanted immune response but retain protective immune mechanisms. Selective immunosuppression involves the induction of immunologic tolerance, which is antigen-induced specific immunosuppression. Oral tolerance also shows promise. Trials are being conducted with peptide-induced tolerance, peptide–MHC complexes, and TCR peptides. Bystander suppression, nonspecific immune suppression, and antibody-dependent immunotherapy are other treatment modalities.

immunotoxicology

The study of adverse effects on the immune system that result directly or indirectly from occupational, environmental, or therapeutic exposure to chemicals (including drugs), biologic materials, and in some cases physiologic factors, referred to as agents.

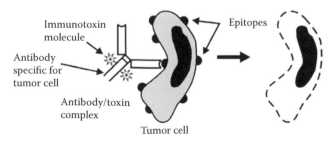

Immunotoxin.

immunotoxin

The linkage of a monoclonal antibody or monoclonal antibody derivative specific for target cell antigens with a cytotoxic substance such as the ricin toxin to yield an immunotoxin. Upon parenteral injection, its antibody portion directs the immunotoxin to the target and its toxic portion destroys target cells on contact. Among its uses is the purging

of T cells from hematopoietic cell preparations used for bone marrow transplantation. An immunotoxin is produced by the union of a monoclonal antibody or one of its fractions with a toxic molecule such as a radioisotope, bacterial or plant toxin, or chemotherapeutic agent. The antibody portion is intended to direct the molecule to antigens on a target cell, such as those of a malignant tumor. The purpose of the toxic portion of the molecule is to destroy the target cell. Contemporary methods of recombinant DNA technology have permitted the preparation of specific hybrid molecules for use in immunotoxin therapy. Immunotoxins may have difficulty reaching the intended target tumor, may be quickly metabolized, and may stimulate the development of antiimmunotoxin antibodies. Crosslinking proteins may likewise be unstable. Immunotoxins have potential for antitumor therapy and as immunosuppressive agents.

immunotoxin-induced apoptosis

Immunotoxins are cytotoxic agents usually assembled as recombinant fusion proteins composed of a targeting domain and a toxin. The targeting domain controls the specificity of action and is usually derived from an antibody Fv fragment, a growth factor, or a soluble receptor. The protein toxins are obtained from bacteria e.g., *Pseudomonas* endotoxin (PE) or diphtheria toxin (DT), or from plants, e.g., ricin. Immunotoxins have been studied as treatments for cancer, graft-vs.-host disease, autoimmine diseases, and AIDS. The PE and DT act via the ADP ribosylation of elongation factor 2, thereby inactivating it. This results in the arrest of protein synthesis and subsequent cell death. These toxins can also induce apoptosis, although the mechanism is unknown. Two common features of apoptotic cell death are the activation of a group of cysteine proteases called caspases and the caspase-catalyzed cleavage of so-called "death substrates" such as the nuclear repair enzyme poly (ADP-ribose) polymerase (PARP).

immunotyping

Refer to immunophenotyping.

inaccessible antigens

Refer to hidden determinant (epitope).

inactivated poliovirus vaccine

An immunizing preparation prepared from three types of inactivated polioviruses. Also called Salk vaccine.

inactivated vaccine

An immunizing preparation that contains microorganisms such as bacteria or viruses that were killed to stop their replication while preserving their protection-inducing antigens. Formaldehyde, phenol, and β-propiolactone have been used to inactivate viruses. Formaldehyde, acetone, phenol, and heating have been used to kill bacteria for use in vaccines.

inactivated virus vaccine

Refer to killed virus vaccine.

inactivation

A term used mostly by immunologists to signify loss of complement activity in a serum sample treated with hydrazine or heated to 56°C for 30 minutes. Inactivation also applies to chemical or heat treatment of pathogenic microorganisms in a manner that preserves their antigenicity for use in inactivated vaccines.

inbred mouse strain

Refer to inbred strain.

inbred strain

Laboratory animals developed by sequential brother–sister matings. After 20 generations, the animals (e.g., mice) are said to be inbred. They are homozygous at approximately 98% of genetic loci. This homogeneity at the histocompatibility loci permits successful grafting without rejection among members of the inbred strain. Recessive deleterious genes may become homozygous during inbreeding, leading them to manifest their negative effects with respect to such factors as growth rate, susceptibility to disease, or fertility, thus limiting the number of possible inbred generations. An additional problem is the development of sublines of an inbred strain caused by mutations and evolutionary factors.

inbreeding

The mating of animals of a species that are genetically more similar to one another than to members of that same species selected by chance or at random in the population. Deliberate inbreeding of experimental animals is carried out to induce genetic uniformity or homozygosity. Raising inbred strains of mice for laboratory investigation involves brother–sister matings for 20 or more generations; thereafter, the progeny are said to be inbred.

incompatibility

Dissimilarity between the antigens of a donor and recipient as in tissue allotransplantation or blood transfusions. The transplantation of a histoincompatible organ or the transfusion of incompatible blood into a recipient may induce an immune response against the antigens not shared by the recipient and produce injurious consequences.

incomplete antibody

A nonagglutinating antibody that must have a linking agent such as anti-IgG to reveal its presence in an agglutination reaction. Refer to Coombs' test.

incomplete Freund's adjuvant (IFA)

A lightweight mineral oil (without mycobacteria) that when combined with an aqueous phase antigen such as a water-in-oil emulsion enhances the humoral or antibody (B cell) limb of the immune response. It does not facilitate T-cell-mediated immune responsiveness.

incubation time

Interlude between an initial infection and disease onset.

index of variability

Refer to Wu–Kabat plot.

indinavir sulfate

Inhibitor of human immunodeficiency virus (HIV) protease.

indirect agglutination (passive agglutination)

The aggregation or agglutination of a specific antibody with carrier particles such as latex or tanned red blood cells to which antigens have been adsorbed or with *bis*-diazotized red blood cells to which antigens have been linked chemically. Refer to passive agglutination.

indirect allorecognition

Refer to indirect antigen presentation.

indirect antigen presentation

In organ or tissue transplantation, the mechanism whereby donor allogeneic major histocompatibility complex (MHC) molecules present microbial proteins. The recipient's professional antigen-presenting cells process the allogeneic MHC proteins. The resulting allogeneic MHC peptides are presented, in association with recipient (self) MHC molecules to host T lymphocytes. By contrast, recipient T cells recognize unprocessed allogeneic MHC molecules on the surfaces of the graft cells in direct antigen presentation.

indirect antiglobulin test

A method to detect incomplete (nonagglutinating) antibody in human serum. Following incubation of red blood cells or other cells possessing the antigen for which the incomplete antibodies of interest are specific, rabbit anti-human globulin is added to the antibody-coated cells that have first been washed. If agglutination results, incomplete agglutinating antibody is present in the serum with which the antigen-bearing red cells have been incubated.

indirect complement fixation test

A complement fixation assay for antibodies that are unable to fix guinea pig complement. It involves the addition of a rabbit antibody of established guinea pig complement-fixing capacity to an antigen–(avian)–antibody–guinea pig complement complex. This is followed by the addition of a visible hemolytic system. Cell lysis indicates the initial presence of avian antibody.

indirect Coombs' test

Refer to indirect antiglobulin test.

indirect fluorescence antibody technique

A method to identify antibody or antigen using a fluorochrome-labeled antibody that combines with an intermediate antibody or antigen rather than directly with the antibody or antigen sought. The indirect test has a greater sensitivity than the direct fluorescence antibody technique. It is often referred to as the sandwich or double-layer method.

indirect hemagglutination test

Refer to passive agglutination test.

indirect immunofluorescence

The interaction of unlabeled antibody with cells or tissues expressing antigen for which the antibody is specific, followed by treatment of this antigen–antibody complex with fluorochrome-labeled antiimmunoglobulin that interacts with the first antibody, forming a so-called sandwich.

indirect staining

An immunofluorescence staining technique in which the primary antibody is unlabeled with fluorochrome, yet its

Indinavir sulfate.

interaction with antigen is detected by the use of a fluoro-chrome-labeled antibody specific for the primary antibody.

indirect tag assays

A two-step method in which the union of antigen with antibody is monitored by tagging a third constituent that unites with the unlabeled antigen–antibody pair. This third component is usually a secondary antibody, protein A or G, or the biotin–avidin system.

indirect template theory (historical)

A variation of the template hypothesis postulating that instructions for antibody synthesis were copied from the antigen configuration into the DNA encoding the specific antibody. This was later shown to be untenable and is of historical interest only.

indolent

A tumor in which the transformed cells undergo relatively slow growth and progression of the neoplasm is gradual.

indomethacin

Indomethacin (1-[4-chlorobenzylyl]-5-methoxy-2-methyl-1H-indole-3-acetic acid) is a drug that blocks synthesis of prostaglandin. It is used for therapy of rheumatoid arthritis and ankylosing spondylitis and may counter the effects of suppressor macrophages.

induced fit

The theory that an antigen may affect conformation of the antigen-binding site of an antibody molecule or T cell receptor to render a better fit with antigen. The same concept applies to peptide binding in MHC class I and II protein grooves.

inducer

A substance that promotes cellular differentiation, such as a colony-stimulating factor.

inducer determinant

Hapten determinant.

inducer T lymphocyte

A cell required for the initiation of an immune response. The inducer T lymphocyte recognizes antigens in the context of major histocompatibility complex (MHC) class II molecules. It stimulates helper, cytotoxic, and suppressor T lymphocytes, whereas helper T cells activate B cells. The human leukocyte common antigen variant, termed 2H4, occurs on the inducer T cell surface, and 4B4 surface molecules are present on CD4$^+$ helper T cells. CD4$^+$ T lymphocytes must be positive for either 4B4 or for 2H4.

inducible nitric oxide synthase (iNOS)

A mechanism of macrophages or various other cells to activate NO synthesis in response to numerous stimuli. This mechanism represents a principal mechanism of host resistance against murine intracellular infection and may occur in humans as well. Enzyme generated principally in phagocytes by products of microbes or proinflammatory cytokines. Transforms arginine to citrulline and nitric oxide, which is toxic to pathogens that have been endocytosed.

inductive phase

The time between antigen administration and detection of immune reactivity.

inductive site

Small patches of mucous membrane that overlie organized lymphoid follicles and contain M cells. A localized mucosal area where antigen induces a primary adaptive immune response.

inert particle agglutination tests

Assays that employ particles of latex, bentonite, or other inert materials to adsorb soluble antigen on their surfaces to test for the presence of specific antibody in the passive agglutination test. The particles coated with adsorbed antigen agglutinate if antibody is present. An example is the rheumatoid arthritis (RA) test in which pooled human immunoglobulin G (IgG) is adsorbed to latex particles that agglutinate if combined with a serum sample containing rheumatoid factor (i.e., anti-IgG autoantibody).

infantile agammaglobulinemia

Synonym for X-linked agammaglobulinemia.

infantile sex-linked hypogammaglobulinemia

Antibody deficiency syndrome that is sex linked and occurs in males following the disappearance of passively transferred antibodies from the mother following birth. Serum immunoglobulin concentrations are relatively low, and antibody synthesis is defective, giving rise to recurring bacterial infections. Cell-mediated immunity remains intact.

infection

A consequence of the adherence and penetration by a pathogen into a host body through successful avoidance of innate host defense mechanisms, allowing the infectious agent to reproduce.

infection allergy

T cell-mediated, delayed-type hypersensitivity associated with infection by selected microorganisms such as *Mycobacterium tuberculosis,* representing type IV hypersensitivity to antigenic products of microorganisms inducing a particular infection. This hypersensitivity also develops in brucellosis, lymphogranuloma venereum, mumps, and vaccinia. Also called infection hypersensitivity.

infection or bacterial allergy

A hypersensitivity, especially of the delayed T cell type, that develops in subjects infected with certain microorganisms such as *Mycobacterium tuberculosis* and certain pathogenic fungi.

infection hypersensitivity

Tuberculin-type sensitivity that is more evident in some infections than others. It develops with great facility in tuberculosis, brucellosis, lymphogranuloma venereum, mumps, and vaccinia. The sensitizing component of the antigen molecule is usually protein, although polysaccharides may induce delayed reactivity in cases of systemic fungal infections such as those caused by *Blastomyces, Histoplasma,* and *Coccidioides.*

infectious bursal agent

A virus infection of cells in the bursa of Fabricius in young chicks, leading to destruction of the bursa and most of the antibody-producing capability of the animal.

infectious mononucleosis

A disease of teenagers and young adults characterized by sore throat, fever, and enlarged lymph nodes. Atypical large lymphocytes with increased cytoplasm, which is also vacuolated, are found in the peripheral blood and have been shown by immunophenotyping to be T cells that are apparently responding to Epstein–Barr virus (EBV)-infected B lymphocytes. Lymphocytosis, neutropenia, and thrombocytopenia are also present. Patients also develop heterophile antibodies that agglutinate horse, ox, and sheep red blood cells as revealed by the Paul–Bunnell test. Infectious mononucleosis is the most common condition caused by

EBV. Splenomegaly and chemical hepatitis may also be present.

infectious mononucleosis syndromes

Conditions induced by viruses that produce an acute and striking peripheral blood monocytosis and lead to symptoms resembling those of infectious mononucleosis induced by Epstein–Barr virus. Examples include herpes virus, cytomegalovirus, HIV-1, HHV-6, and *Toxoplasma gondii* infections.

infectious tolerance

A state in which induced peripheral tolerance to a given antigen is transmitted from an anergic T cell population to a population of normal T cells that are rendered tolerant to the same antigen. This phenomenon may be mediated by regulatory T cells. Infectious tolerance was described in the 1970s. Animals rendered tolerant to foreign antigens were found to possess suppressor T lymphocytes associated with the induced unresponsiveness. Thus, self tolerance was postulated to be based on the induction of suppressor T cells. Noel Rose referred to this concept as clonal balance rather than clonal deletion. Self antigens are considered to normally induce mostly suppressor rather than helper T cells, leading to a negative suppressor balance in the animal body. Three factors with the potential to suppress immune reactivity against self include nonantigen-specific suppressor T cells, antigen-specific suppressor T cells, and anti-idiotypic antibodies. Rose suggested that suppressor T lymphocytes leave the thymus slightly before the corresponding helper T cells. Suppressor T cells specific for self antigens are postulated to be continuously stimulated and usually in greater numbers than the corresponding helper T cells.

infertility, immunological

Infertility in 12 to 25% of cases in which infertile couples are unable to conceive even though they manifest no significant abnormalities upon physical examination. These cases of unexplained infertility may be caused by autoimmune responses to organ-specific antigens of the reproductive tracts of both males and females and isoimmune reactions of females against semen components. Immune responses may cause or contribute to infertility in approximately 10% of these couples.

inflammation

A defense reaction of living tissue to injury. Plays an integral role in both innate and adaptive immunity. Inflammatory cells phagocytize antigen, generate chemical signals that facilitate wound healing, and secrete cytokines and chemokines that attract and regulate lymphocytes. The literal meaning of the word is burning, and it originates from the cardinal symptoms of *rubor, calor, tumor,* and *dolor,* the Latin terms equivalent to redness, heat, swelling, and pain, respectively. Inflammation is beneficial for the host and essential for survival of the species, although in some cases the response is exaggerated and may be itself injurious. Inflammation is the result of multiple interactions that have as a first objective localization of the process and removal of the irritant. This is followed by a period of repair. Inflammation is not necessarily of an immunologic nature, although immunologic reactions are among the immediate causes inducing inflammation and the immunologic status of the host determines the intensity of the inflammatory response. Inflammation tends to be less intense in infants, whose immune systems are not fully mature. The causes of inflammation are numerous and include living microorganisms such as pathogenic bacteria and animal parasites that act mainly by the chemical poisons they produce and less by mechanical irritation; viruses that become offenders after they multiply in the host and cause cell damage; and fungi that grow at the surface of the skin but produce little or no inflammation in the dermis. Other causes of inflammation include physical agents such as trauma, thermal and radiant energy, and chemical agents that represent a large group of exogenous or endogenous causes including immunologic offenders. Mediators of inflammation include kinins, acute phase proteins, leukotrienes, prostaglandins, and vasoactive amines including histamine. Refer to inflammatory response.

inflammatory bowel disease (IBD)

A general term that applies to ulcerative colitis, Crohn's disease, and idiopathic inflammatory bowel disease that resembles the other two. There is a hereditary predisposition to IBD. Intestinal epithelial cells express HLA-DR (MHC class II) antigens in Crohn's disease, ulcerative colitis, and infectious colitis patients that may render the antigens capable of becoming autoantigen-presenting cells. Inflammatory bowel disease patients may become sensitized to cow's milk antigens, developing IgG and IgM antibodies against this protein. Leukotrienes have been shown to be of greater significance than prostaglandins in mediating inflammation in ulcerative colitis. Mucocutaneous conditions such as oral ulcers, epidermolysis bullosa acquisita, erythema nodosa, etc., and eye diseases such as uveitis and iridocyclitis may be associated with IBD. Some IBD patients may also have cirrhosis, chronic active hepatitis, or joint involvement such as ankylosing spondylitis. IBD patients may have abdominal pain, fever, and diarrhea. Granulomas may develop in the gut wall, and lymphocytes that stain for IgA in the cytoplasm are often abundant. Autoantibodies reactive with fetal colon antigens may be present. IBD develops in gene knockout mice lacking interleukin-2 (IL2), IL10, or the TCR-α chain. Inflammation is mediated in part through the action of cytokines that include IL1α, IL1β, IL6, or tumor necrosis factor α (TNF-α). IL1α and IL1β induce fever, stimulate acute phase protein synthesis, and activate the immune system. TNF-α and IL6 enhance cellular catabolism, induce acute phase proteins, and stimulate pyrogenic activity. TNF-α can induce IL1 and IL6. TNF-α and IL2 stimulate prostaglandin I_2 (PGIL$_2$), prostaglandin E (PGE$_2$), and platelet-activating factor (PAF) secretion.

inflammatory CD4 T cell

Armed effector T$_H$1 cell that synthesizes interferon γ (IFN-γ) and tumor necrosis factor (TNF) cytokines when it recognizes antigen. Its principal function is to activate macrophages. Selected T$_H$1 cells may also mediate cytotoxicity.

inflammatory cells

Cells of the blood and tissues that participate in acute and chronic inflammatory reactions. They include polymorphonuclear neutrophils, eosinophils, and macrophages.

inflammatory macrophage

A macrophage in a peritoneal exudate induced by thioglycolate broth or mineral oil injection into the peritoneal cavity of an experimental animal.

inflammatory mediator

A substance that participates in an inflammatory reaction.

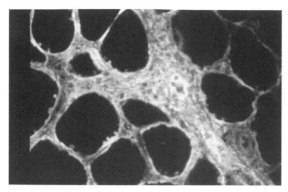

Inflammatory myopathy. Both regenerating and atrophic fibers are present with fibrosis.

inflammatory myopathy

Occurs after necrosis and phagocytosis of muscle fibers with inflammatory cells.

inflammatory response

Acute inflammation represents an early defense mechanism to contain an infection and prevent its spread from the initial focus. When microbes multiply in host tissues, two principal defense mechanisms mounted against them are antibodies and leukocytes. The three major events in acute inflammation are (1) dilation of capillaries to increase blood flow; (2) changes in the microvasculature structure, leading to escape of plasma proteins and leukocytes from the circulation; and (3) leukocyte emigration from the capillaries and accumulation at the site of injury. Widening of interendothelial cell junctions of venules or injury of endothelial cells facilitates the escape of plasma proteins from the vessels. Neutrophils attached to the endothelium through adhesion molecules escape the microvasculature and are attracted to sites of injury by chemotactic agents. This is followed by phagocytosis of microorganisms that may lead to their intracellular destruction. Activated leukocytes may produce toxic metabolites and proteases that injure endothelium and tissues when they are released. Activation of the third complement component (C3) is also a critical step in inflammation. Multiple chemical mediators of inflammation derived from either plasma or cells have been described. Mediators and plasma proteins such as complement are present as precursors that require activation to become biologically active. Mediators derived from cells are present as precursors in intracellular granules such as histamine and mast cells. Following activation, these substances are secreted. Other mediators such as prostaglandins may be synthesized following stimulation. These mediators are quickly activated by enzymes or other substances such as antioxidants. A chemical mediator may also cause a target cell to release a secondary mediator with a similar or opposing action. Besides histamine, other preformed chemical mediators in cells include serotonin and lysosomal enzymes. Those that are newly synthesized include prostaglandins, leukotrienes, platelet-activating factors, cytokines, and nitric oxide. Chemical mediators in plasma include complement fragments C3a and C5a and the C5b–9 sequence. Three plasma-derived factors—kinins, complement, and clotting factors—are involved in inflammation. Bradykinin is produced by activation of the kinin system. It induces arteriolar dilation and increased venule permeability through contraction of endothelial cells and extravascular smooth muscle. Activation of bradykinin precursors involves activated factor XII (Hageman factor) generated by its contact with injured tissues. During clotting, fibrinopeptides produced during the conversion of fibrinogen to fibrin increase vascular permeability and are chemotactic for leukocytes. The fibrinolytic system participates in inflammation through the kinin system. Products produced during arachidonic acid metabolism also affect inflammation. These include prostaglandins and leukotrienes that can mediate essentially every aspect of acute inflammation.

infliximab

A human–mouse chimeric IgG$_1$ monoclonal antibody comprised of human constant (Fc) regions and murine variable regions. Neutralizes biological activity of TNF-α by binding with high affinity to the soluble and and transmembrane forms of TNF-α and blocks binding of TNF-α with its receptors. It fails to neutralize TNF-β. TNF-α induces proinflammatory cytokines, such as IL1 and IL6; enhancement of leukocyte migration by increasing endothelial layer permeability; and expression of adhesion molecules by endothelial cells and leukocytes. It is associated with activation of neutrophil and eosinophil functional activity and induction of acute phase reactants. Infliximab prevents disease in transgenic mice that develop polyarthritis as a consequence of constitutive expression of human TNF-α, and leads to healing of eroded joints when administered after the disease has begun. It is used in the treatment of Crohn's disease, ulcerative colitis, rheumatoid arthritis, ankylosing spondylitis, and psoriatic arthritis.

influenza hemagglutinin

An influenza-virus-coated glycoprotein that binds selected carbohydrates on human cells, the initial event in viral infection. Antigenic shift results from changes in the hemagglutinin.

influenza viruses

Infectious agents that induce an acute, febrile respiratory illness often associated with myalgia and headache. The classification of influenza A viruses into subtypes is based on their hemagglutinin (H) and neuraminidase (N) antigens. Three hemagglutinin (H1, H2, and H3) and two neuraminidase (N1 and N2) subtypes are the principal influenza A virus antigenic subtypes that produce disease in humans. Due to antigenic change (antigenic drift), infection or vaccination by one strain provides little or no protection against subsequent infection by a distantly related strain of the same subtype. Influenza B viruses undergo less frequent antigenic variation.

influenza virus immunity

Influenza A viruses undergo changes in their surface hemagglutinin (HA) and neuraminidase (NA) glycoproteins leading to repeated epidemics and pandemics. Mucosal immunoglobulin A (IgA) and serum IgG antibodies are specific for the HA molecule, neutralize virus infectivity, and mainly confer resistance to reinfection. This is the reason for vaccination against epidemic strains with killed virus. The antibody response to HA is subtype-specific, but antigenic drift facilitates escape of infectious virus from antibody-mediated destruction. Five protective antigenic sites are present on the globular head of the HA molecule. Antibodies against neuraminidase fail to prevent infection but diminish spread of the virus. Enzyme-active centers on each of the four subunits of

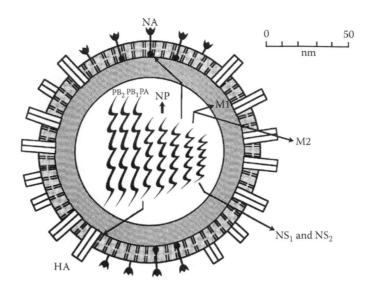

Influenza virus.

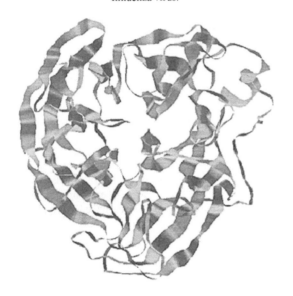

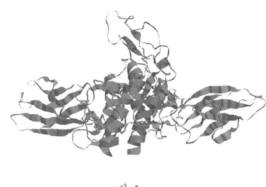

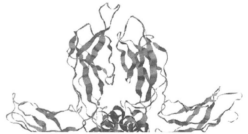

Influenza B/LEE/40 neuraminidase (sialidase).

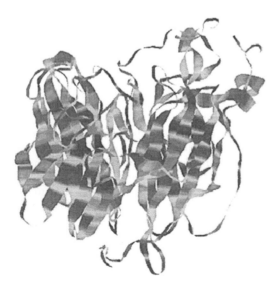

Influenza A subtype N2 neuraminidase (sialidase). A/Tokyo/3/67.

the NA are in a central cavity encircled by two antigenic sites. Influenza A viruses undergo variability that includes antigenic drift, which yields variants of contemporary epidemic strains that are sufficiently different to avoid neutralization by antibody. The more extensive antigenic shift may be a consequence of dual infection with human and animal influenza A viruses. This can lead to the development of a novel pandemic strain for which humans have no preexisting antibodies. CD8+ virus-immune cytotoxic T lymphocytes can clear influenza A virus from infected lungs. It is necessary for the effector lymphocyte to come into direct contact with the virus-infected target cell. Immune CD4+ T lymphocytes are involved in lung consolidation in influenza pneumonia and have a significant role in clearance of the virus. CD4+ T cells facilitate antibody production. They also facilitate the generation of "helper cytokines" such as interleukin-4 (IL4) and IL5 that promote clonal expansion and differentiation of

B cells into antibody-secreting plasma cells. Influenza A virus infection primes the host for a secondary CD8+ T lymphocyte response to other influenza A viruses. Influenza-immune CD4+ helper T cells are specific for viral peptides presented in the context of self major histocompatibility complex (MHC) class II glycoproteins.

influenza virus vaccine
Purified and inactivated immunizing preparation made from viruses grown in eggs. It cannot lead to infection. For example, it might contain H1N1 and H3N2 type A strains and one type B strain. These are the strains considered most likely to cause influenza in the United States. Whole- and split-virus preparations are available; children tolerate the split-virus preparation better than the whole-virus vaccine. The vaccine is a polyvalent immunizing preparation that contains inactivated antigenic variants of the influenza virus (types A and B) individually or combined for annual use. It protects against epidemic disease and the morbidity and mortality induced by influenza virus, especially in the aged and chronically ill. The vaccine is reconstituted each year to protect against the strains of influenza virus present in the population. For active immunization against specific strains of influenza virus. Highly recommended for all individuals over the age of 6 months who, because of age or underlying medical conditions, are at increased risk of complications from influenza. Healthcare workers and others in close contact with high risk people should be vaccinated. Fluvirin is not indicated in children below 4 years of age. FluMist is indicated for healthy children and adolescents (5 to 17 years of age) and healthy adults (18 to 49 years of age). Influenza A viruses are classified into subtypes based on their surface antigens designated hemagglutinin (H) and neuraminidase (N). Immunity against these surface antigens, especially the hemagglutinin, diminishes the likelihood of infection and severity of disease if infection occurs. Influenza vaccines are standardized to contain hemagglutinins of strains, typically two type A and one type B, representing the influenza viruses postulated to circulate in the United States in the upcoming influenza season. The vaccine is prepared from highly purified egg-grown viruses made from noninfectious (inactivated) preparations. Subvirion and purified surface antigen preparations are also available. Since the vaccine viruses are initially in embryonated hens' eggs, the vaccine may contain minute quantities of residual egg protein. The trivalent influenza vaccine prepared for the 2006–2007 season contained A/New Caledonia/20/99 (H1N1), A/Wisconsin/67/2005 (H3N2), and B/Malaysia/2506/2004 antigens. These viruses were used because they were postulated to be representative of the influenza viruses likely to circulate in the United States during the 2006–2007 influenza season. Influenza vaccine is available in a split-virus preparation that causes diminished febrile reactions. Thus, the split-virus vaccines are recommended for use in children younger than 13 years of age. Split-virus vaccines may also be referred to as subvirion or purified surface antigen vaccines.

inhibin α (R1), mouse
Anti-inhibin α is an antibody against a peptide hormone that has demonstrated utility in differentiation between adrenal cortical tumors and renal cell carcinoma. Sex cord stromal tumors of the ovary and trophoblastic tumors also demonstrate cytoplasmic positivity with this antibody.

inhibition test
(1) Blocking an established serological test such as agglutination or precipitation through the addition of an antigen for which the antibody in the test system is specific; it shows the specificity of the reactants. (2) Inhibition of an antigen–antibody interaction through the addition of a hapten for which the antibody is specific; refer to hapten inhibition test. (3) Preventing the action of a virus through addition of an antibody specific for the virus.

inhibition zone
Refer to prozone.

initiation
The initial event in carcinogenesis. A cell in which a mutation is not repaired gains an irreversible growth advantage and makes it a target cell for subsequent malignant transformation.

innate or constitutive defense system
Humans are confronted with a host of microorganisms with the potential to induce serious or fatal infections, but nature provided appropriate molecules, cells, and receptors that can protect against these microbes. Many of these defenses are general or nonspecific and do not require previous exposure to the offending pathogen (or closely related organism). These important mechanisms constitute the innate or constitutive defense system. Another important defense system is acquired immunity that can develop after contact with an organism through infection (overt or subclinical).

innate defense system
General or nonspecific system that does not require previous exposure to an offending pathogen (or closely related organism).

innate immune mechanisms against parasites
Whereas parasitic stages isolated from invertebrates may be lysed through activation of the alternate complement pathway, parasites isolated from humans and other vertebrate hosts are often susceptible to complement lysis. This may be attributable to disappearance of surface molecules that activate complement or adherence to the surfaces of decay-accelerating factor (DAF) or other regulatory proteins.

innate immunity
Natural or native immunity present from birth and designed to protect the organism from injury or infection without previous contact with infectious agents. Attributable to physical, chemical, and molecular defenses that prevent contact with antigens in a nonspecific manner. Also mediated by PRM and PRR receptors that identify a selected number of molecular patterns shared by a broad spectrum of pathogenic organisms. Does not involve immunological memory: there is no difference in the kinetics and magnitude of primary and secondary immune responses. It includes such factors as protection by the skin, mucous membranes, lysozyme in tears, stomach acid, and other factors. Phagocytes, natural killer cells, complement, and cytokines represent key participants in natural innate immunity.

innate immunity against intracellular bacteria
Natural or native immunity that is frustrated by the resistance of many intracellular microbes to intracellular dissolution. Thus, the natural immune mechanism of phagocytosis is of little use in controlling infection by intracellular microorganisms. Bacteria of this category may persist in the tissues, leading to chronic infection.

innocent bystander

A cell that is fatally injured during an immune response specific for a different cell type.

innocent bystander hemolysis

Drugs acting as haptens induce immune hemolysis of "innocent" red blood cells. The reaction is drug-specific and involves complement through activation of the alternate complement pathway. The direct antiglobulin (Coombs') test identifies split products that are membrane associated, yet the indirect Coombs' test remains negative.

inoculation

The introduction of an immunogen into an animal to induce immunity, usually to protect against an infectious disease agent.

Inosiplex (isoprinosine)

An immunomodulating agent that increases natural killer cell cytotoxicity as well as T cell and monocyte functional activites. It has produced slight benefits in acquired immune deficiency syndrome (AIDS) patients and has been used in Europe to treat diverse immunodeficiency diseases but is not yet approved for use in the United States.

inositol 1,4,5-triphosphate (IP3)

A signaling molecule in the cytoplasms of lymphocytes activated by an antigen formed by phospholipase C (PLC γ_1)-mediated hydrolysis of plasma membranes. Phospholipid PIP_2. The principal function of IP_3 is to induce the release of intracellular Ca^{2+} from membrane-bound compartments such as the endoplasmic reticulum (ER).

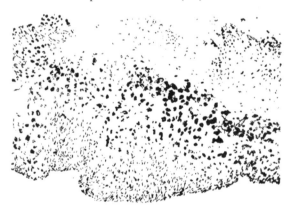

In situ hybridization.

in situ hybridization

A technique to identify specific DNA or RNA segments in cells or tissues, viral plaques, or colonies of microorganisms. DNA in cells or tissue fixed on glass slides must be denatured with formamide before hybridization with a radiolabeled or biotinylated DNA or RNA probe that is complementary to the tissue mRNA sought. Proof that the probe has hybridized to its complementary strand in the tissue or cell under study must be by autoradiography or enzyme-labeled probes, depending on the technique used.

in situ transcription

A method in which mRNA acts as a template for complementary DNA for reverse transcription in tissues that have been fixed.

insect resistance (immunity)

Toll receptors in insects induce the formation of antimicrobial proteins in response to molecular motifs present on

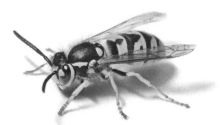

Insect.

the insect pathogen surfaces and fungal polysaccharides. Infection of higher insects leads to the rapid production of antimicrobial peptides after activation of transcription factors that link to promoter sequence configurations homologous to regulatory features of the acute phase response in animals. *Drosophila* have toll molecules that serve as receptors for PAMPs that activate NFκB. A loss of function toll mutation renders these flies susceptible to infection by fungi. Antimicrobial peptides synthesized by insects include cyclic peptides, including anti-Gram-positive defensins (4kDa) and drosomycin, a 5-kDa antifungal agent. Infection-induced linear peptides include cecropins that induce lethal injury of microbial membranes by producing ion channels. Other linear peptides include anti-Gram-negative glycine and proline-rich polypeptides. Integrins in insects may be related to complement receptor CR3.

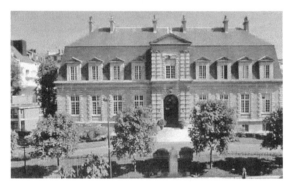

Institut Paris Pasteur.

Institut Pasteur, Paris

Famous research center founded by Louis Pasteur, and the site of many discoveries in immunology and microbiology, including the AIDS virus for which the Nobel Prize in Medicine was awarded in 2008.

instructional model

A theory of antibody diversity postulating that antigen serves as a template for the antibody, which assumes a complementary shape.

instructive theory

A hypothesis that postulates acquisition of antibody specificity after contact with a specific antigen. According to one template theory of antibody formation, it is necessary for an antigen to be present during the process of antibody synthesis. According to the refolding template theory, uncommitted and specific globulins may become refolded upon the antigen, serving as a template for it. The cell released complementary antibodies that rigidly retained their shapes through disulfide bonding. This theory had to be abandoned

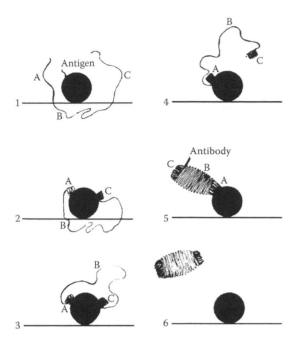

Instructive theory of antibody formation.

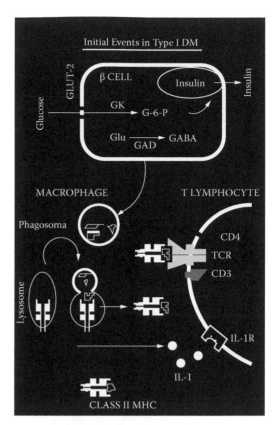

Diabetes mellitus type I.

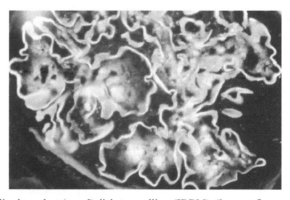

Insulin-dependent (type I) diabetes mellitus (IDDM). (Immunofluorescence of renal glomerulus.)

when it was shown that the specificity of antibodies in all cases is due to the particular arrangement of their primary amino acid sequences. *De novo* synthesis template theories that recognized the necessity for antibodies to be synthesized by amino acids in the proper and predetermined order still had to contend with the serious objection that proteins cannot serve as informational models for the synthesis of proteins. Instructive theories were abandoned when immunologic tolerance was demonstrated and antigen was shown not to be necessary for antibody synthesis. The template theories never explained the anamnestic (memory) immune response. Antibody specificity depends on the variable region amino acid sequence, especially the complementarity-determining or hypervariable regions.

instructive theory of antibody formation
Refer to instructive theory.

insulin-dependent (type I) diabetes mellitus (IDDM)
Juvenile-onset diabetes caused by diminished capacity to produce insulin. Genetic factors play a major role, as the disease is more common in HLA-DR3- and HLA-DR4-positive individuals. Significant autoimmune features include immunoglobulin G (IgG) autoantibodies against glucose transport proteins and anticytoplasmic and antimembrane antibodies directed to antigens in the pancreatic islets of Langerhans; β cells are destroyed, and the pancreatic islets become infiltrated by T lymphocytes and monocytes in the initial period of the disease. Experimental models of IDDM include the NOD mouse and the BB rat.

insulin-like growth factors (IGFs)
Insulin-like growth factors consist of prohormones IGF-I and IGF-II with M_r of 9 and 14 K, respectively. IGF-I is a 7.6-kDa side chain polypeptide hormone that resembles proinsulin structurally. It is formed by the liver and by fibroblasts. IGF-I is the sole effector of growth hormone activity and is a primary growth regulator that is age-dependent. It is expressed in juvenile life but declines after puberty. Circulating IGFs are not free in the plasma but are associated with binding proteins that may have the function of limiting

the bioavailability of circulating IGFs that may be a means of controlling growth factor activity. IGF-II is present mainly in various tissues during the embryonic and fetal stages of mammalian development. It is also present in the circulating plasma in association with binding proteins, reaching its highest level in the fetal circulation and declining following birth. IGF-II is important for growth of the entire organism.

insulin-like growth factor-II (IGF-II)
A fetal growth factor expressed at high levels in many tissues during fetal and early postnatal development but only in the central nervous system thereafter.

insulin receptor antibodies
Antibodies that lead to insulin resistance and may also be associated with acanthosis nigricans and manifestations of autoimmune disease. Insulin receptor antibodies may lead to hypoglycemia possibly associated with autoimmune disease and Hodgkin disease. Selected patients with

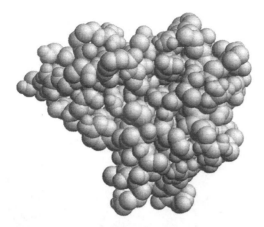

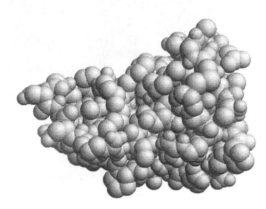

Insulin-like growth factors (IGFs)

insulin-dependent and non-insulin-dependent diabetes mellitus may have insulin receptor antibodies that react at either the site that binds insulin or at some other binding region.

insulin receptor autoantibodies

Autoantibodies that induce type B insulin resistance. This syndrome may be accompanied by acanthosis nigricans and autoimmune disease. Selected patients with insulin-dependent diabetes mellitus (IDDM) and non-insulin-dependent diabetes mellitus have antibodies that react with these insulin receptors at their insulin-binding site or other binding sites. Individuals who have insulin autoantibodies and islet cell antibodies and first-degree relatives of patients with IDDM have a predictive value of 60 to 77% for the development of IDDM within 5 to 10 years.

insulin resistance

Diminished responsiveness to insulin as revealed by its decreased capacity to induce hypoglycemia may or may not have an immunologic basis. The administration of bovine or porcine insulin to humans can lead to antibody production that may contribute to insulin resistance.

insulitis

Lymphocytic or other leukocytic infiltration of the islets of Langerhans in the pancreas, which may accompany the development of diabetes mellitus.

Intal®

Commercial preparation of disodium cromoglycate.

integrase

Retroviral enzyme such as the HIV enzyme that facilitates insertion of viral DNA into the genome of the host cell.

integrin family of leukocyte adhesive proteins

The CD11/CD18 family of molecules.

integrins

A family of cell membrane glycoproteins that are heterodimers comprised of α and β chain subunits and serve as extracellular matrix glycoprotein receptors. They identify the RGD sequence of the β subunit, which consists of the arginine–glycine–aspartic acid tripeptide that occasionally also includes serine. The RGD sequence serves as a receptor recognition signal. Extracellular matrix glycoproteins, for which integrins serve as receptors, include fibronectin, C3, and lymphocyte-function-associated antigen 1 (LFA-1), among other proteins. Differences in the β chain serve as the basis for division of integrins into three categories. Each category has distinctive α chains. The β chain provides specificity. The same 95-kDa β chain is found in one category of integrins that includes LFA-1, p150, p95, and complement receptor 3 (CR3). The same 130-kDa β chain is shared among VLA-1, VLA-2, VLA-3, VLA-4, VLA-5, VLA-6, and integrins found in chickens. A 110-kDa β chain is shared in common by another category that includes the vitronectin receptor and platelet glycoprotein IIb/IIIa. There are four repeats of 40-amino acid residues in the β chain extracellular domains, and there are 45-amino acid residues in the β chain intracellular domains. The principal function of integrins is to link the cytoskeleton to extracellular ligands. They also participate in wound healing, cell migration, killing of target cells, and phagocytosis. Leukocyte adhesion deficiency syndrome occurs when the β subunit of LFA-1 and Mac-1 are missing. VLA proteins facilitate binding of cells to collagen (VLA-1, -2, and -3), laminin (VLA-1, -2, and -6), and fibronectin (VLA-3, -4, and -5). The cell-to-cell contacts formed by integrins are critical for many aspects of the immune response such as antigen presentation, leukocyte-mediated cytotoxicity, and myeloid cell phagocytosis. Integrins comprise an essential part of an adhesion receptor cascade that guides leukocytes from the bloodstream across endothelium and into injured tissues in response to chemotactic signals.

integrins, HGF/SF activation of

Integrins and growth factor receptors can share common signaling pathways. Each type of receptor can impact the signal and ultimate response of the other. An example of a growth factor shown to influence members of the integrin family of cell adhesion receptors is hepatocyte growth factor/scatter factor (HGF/SF), a multifunctional cytokine that promotes mitogenesis, migration, invasion, and morphogenesis. HGF/SF-dependent signaling can modulate integrin function by promoting aggregation and cell adhesion. Morphogenic responses to HGF/SF are dependent on adhesive events. HGF/SF-induced effects occur via signaling of the MET tyrosine kinase receptor, following ligand binding. HGF/SF binding to MET leads to enhanced integrin-mediated B cell and lymphoma cell adhesion. Blocking experiments with monoclonal antibodies directed against integrin subunits indicate that $\alpha_{4\beta1}$ and $\alpha_{5\beta1}$ integrins on hematopoietic progenitor cells are activated by HGF/SF to induce adhesion to fibronectin. The HGF/SF-dependent signal transduction pathway can also induce ligand binding activity in functionally inactive $\alpha_{v\beta3}$ integrins. The effects of HGF/SF highlight the importance of growth factor regulation of integrin function in both normal and tumor cells.

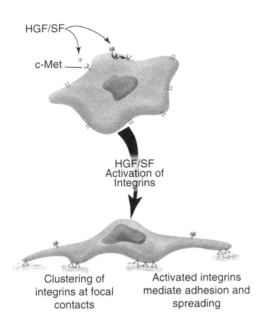

Following binding of HGF/SF, MET receptor signaling can modulate integrin function by promoting aggregation of integrins and adhesion to integrin-specific ligands.

interallelic conversion

Genetic recombination between two alleles of a locus in which a segment of one allele is replaced with a homologous segment from another. Human leukocyte antigen (HLA) class I and HLA class II alleles are formed in this way.

intercalated cell autoantibodies

Autoantibodies against renal tubular (intercalated) cells are detected from time to time by using immunofluorescence with frozen sections of normal human or rabbit kidney. The clinical significance of these antibodies remains to be determined.

intercellular adhesion molecules (ICAMs)

Leukocyte integrin ligands that facilitate the binding of lymphocytes and other leukocytes to various cells such as antigen-presenting cells and endothelial cells.

intercellular adhesion molecule-1 (ICAM-1)

A 90-kDa cellular membrane glycoprotein that occurs in multiple cell types including dendritic and endothelial cells. It is the lymphocyte-function-associated antigen 1 (LFA-1) ligand. The LFA-1 molecules on cytotoxic T lymphocytes (CTLs) interact with ICAM-1 molecules found on CTL target cells. Interferon γ (IFN-γ), tumor necrosis factor (TNF), and interleukin-1 (IL1) can elevate ICAM-1 expression. ICAM-1 is a member of the immunoglobulin gene superfamily of cell adhesion molecules. It plays a major role in the inflammatory response and in T-cell-mediated host responses, serving as a costimulatory molecule on antigen-presenting cells to activate major histocompatibility complex (MHC) class II restricted T cells and on other types of cells in association with MHC class I to activate cytotoxic T cells. On endothelial cells, it facilitates migration of activated leukocytes to sites of injury. It is the cellular receptor for a subgoup of rhinoviruses.

intercellular adhesion molecule-2 (ICAM-2)

A member of the immunoglobulin superfamily of proteins that is important in cellular interactions. It is a cell surface molecule that serves as a ligand for leukocyte integrins. It facilitates lymphocyte binding to antigen-presenting cells or endothelial cells and binds to LFA-1, a T lymphocyte integrin.

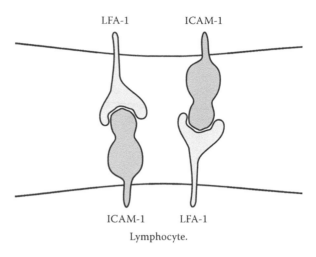

Lymphocyte.

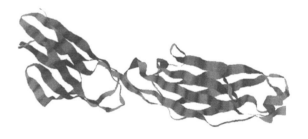

ICAM-2. Ribbon diagram. Resolution 2.2 Å.

intercellular adhesion molecule-3 (ICAM-3)

A leukocyte cell surface molecule that plays a critical role in the interaction of T lymphocytes with antigen-presenting cells. This interaction through union of ICAM-1, ICAM-2, and ICAM-3 with LFA-1 molecules is also facilitated by the interaction of the T cell surface molecule CD2 with LFA-3 present on antigen-presenting cells.

intercrine cytokines

A family composed of a minimum of 8- to 10-kDa cytokines that share 20 to 45% amino acid sequence homology. All are believed to be basic heparin-binding polypeptides with proinflammatory and reparative properties. Their cDNA has conserved, single, open reading frames, 5′ region typical signal sequences, and 3′ untranslated regions that are rich in AP sequences. Human cytokines that include interleukin-8, platelet factor 4, β thromboglobulin, IP-10, and melanoma growth-stimulating factor or GRO comprise a subfamily encoded by genes on chromosome 4. They possess a unique structure. LD78, ACT-2, I-309, RANTES, and macrophage chemotactic and activating factor (MCAF) comprise a second subset and are encoded by genes on chromosome 17 in humans. Human chromosome 4 bears the intercrine α genes, and human chromosome 17 bears the intercrine β genes. Four cysteines are found in the intercrine family. Adjacent cysteines are present in the intercrine β subfamily, which includes huMCAF, huBLD-78, huACT-II, huRANTES, muTCA-III, muJE, muMIP-1α and muMIP-1β. One amino acid separates cysteines of the intercrine α subfamily, which is composed of huPF-4, hubetaTG, huIL-8, ch9E3, huGRO, huIP-10, and muMIP-2. The cysteines are significant for tertiary structure and for intercrine binding to receptors.

interdigitating dendritic cell

An antigen-presenting dendritic cell, different from the follicular dendritic cell, that is major histocompatibility complex (MHC) class II-positive and Fc receptor-negative and is located in lymph node and spleen T cell regions.

interdigitating reticular cells

Refer to dendritic cells.

interfacial test

Refer to ring test.

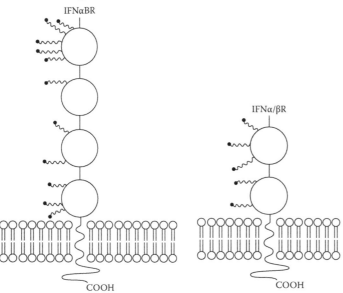

Three-dimensional crystal structure of recombinant murine interferon α. Overall similarity of basic polypeptide chain folding exists among all the interferon α and β molecules from various sources.

interferon α (IFN-α)

It includes at least 13 immunomodulatory, 189-amino acid-residue glycoproteins synthesized by macrophages and B cells that are able to prevent the replication of viruses, are antiproliferative, and are pyrogenic, inducing fever. IFN-α stimulates natural killer (NK) cells and induces expression of major histocompatibility complex (MHC) class I antigens. It also has an immunoregulatory effect through alteration of antibody responsiveness. The 14 genes that encode IFN-α are positioned on the short arm of chromosome 9 in humans. Polyribonucleotides, as well as RNA or DNA viruses, may induce IFN-α secretion. Recombinant IFN-α has been prepared and used in the treatment of hairy cell leukemia, Kaposi's sarcoma, chronic myeloid leukemia, human papilloma virus (HPV)-related lesions, renal cell carcinoma, chronic hepatitis, and selected other conditions. Patients may experience severe flu-like symptoms as long as the drug is administered. They also have malaise, headache, depression, and supraventricular tachycardia and may possibly develop congestive heart failure. Bone marrow suppression has been reported in some patients.

interferon α-2a, recombinant (injection)

An antitumor and antiviral immunomodulator whose mechanism of action is not clearly understood but is believed to be antiproliferative against tumor cells and inhibit virus replication. Its biological activities are species-restricted. *In vivo*, it inhibits the growth of several human tumors grown in immunocompromised (nude) mice. Serum neutralizing activity has been detected in 25% of all patients receiving the drug.

interferon α-2b recombinant (injection)

Interferons are naturally occurring small proteins and glycoproteins, with molecular weights of 15,000 to 27,600 daltons, synthesized and secreted by cells following a viral infection or in response to synthetic or biological inducers. They produce their effect on cells by binding to specific membrane receptors on cell surfaces where they initiate a complex sequence of intracellular events including the induction of certain enzymes, suppression of cell proliferation, immunomodulatory activities such as enhancement of the phagocytic activities of macrophages and augmentation of specific cytotoxicity of lymphocytes for target cells, and inhibition of virus replication in virus-infected cells.

interferon α-n3 (injection)

Binds to the same specific membrane cell surface receptor as interferon α-2b. These receptors are very specific for the binding of human but not mouse interferon, reflecting high species specificity. The binding of interferon to membrane cell surface receptors activates induction of protein synthesis among other effects. This is followed by various cellular responses, including inhibition of virus replication and suppression of cell proliferation. Immunomodulation, including enhanced macrophage phagocytosis, augmentation of lymphocyte cytotoxicity, and enhancement of human leukocyte antigen expression results from exposure to interferon.

interferon β (IFN-β)

An antiviral, 20-kDa protein comprised of 187-amino acid residues. It is produced by fibroblasts and prevents replication of viruses. It has 30% amino acid sequence homology with interferon α. RNA or DNA viruses or polyribonucleotides can induce its secretion. The gene encoding it is located on chromosome 9 in humans.

interferon β-1a

Interferon β-1a is a 166-amino acid glycoprotein synthesized by mammalian cells into which the human interferon β gene has been introduced. Its amino sequence is identical to that of natural human interferon β. Interferon β-1b is a purified protein that has 165 amino acids but does not include the carbohydrate side chains present in the natural material. Interferon β is synthesized by fibroblasts, macrophages, and various other cell types. It has antiviral, antiproliferative, and immunoregulatory properties. Binding to its receptor activates a sequence of intracellular events that leads to expression of multiple interferon-induced gene products and markers.

interferon γ (IFN-γ)

A glycoprotein that is a 21- to 24-kDa homodimer synthesized by activated CD4 Th1 cells, CD8 T cells, and NK cells, causing it to be classified as a lymphokine. IFN-γ has antiproliferative and antiviral properties. It is a powerful activator of mononuclear phagocytes, increasing their ability to destroy intracellular microorganisms and tumor cells. It causes many types of cells to express major histocompatibility complex (MHC) class II molecules and can also increase expression of class I. It facilitates differentiation of both B and T lymphocytes. IFN-γ is a powerful activator of NK cells and also activates neutrophils and vascular endothelial cells.

It is decreased in chronic lymphocytic leukemia, lymphoma, and IgA deficiency, and in patients infected with rubella, Epstein–Barr virus, and cytomegalovirus. Recombinant IFN-γ has been used to treat a variety of conditions, including chronic lymphocytic leukemia, mycosis fungoides, Hodgkin disease, and various other disorders. It has been found effective in decreasing synthesis of collagen by fibroblasts and may have potential in the treatment of connective tissue diseases. Patients receiving it may develop headaches, chills, rash, and even acute renal failure. The one gene that encodes IFN-γ in humans is found on the long arm of chromosome 12. Also termed immune or type II interferon.

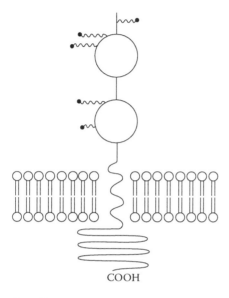

Preliminary three-dimensional structure of human interferon γ (recombinant form). Resolution = 3.5 Å.

interferon γ-1b (injection)

Interferon γ differs from other classes of interferons mainly in its immunomodulatory properties. Whereas α, β, and γ interferons share certain characteristics, interferon γ exerts potent phagocyte-activating effects not produced by other interferon molecules. These effects include the generation of toxic oxygen metabolites within phagocytes *in vitro* that can mediate intracellular killing of selected microorganisms such as *Staphylococcus aureus*, *Toxoplasma gondii*, *Leishmania donovani*, *Listeria monocytogenes*, and *Mycobacterium avium intracellulare*. Among its myriad biological activities are the enhancement of the oxidative metabolism of tissue macrophages and enhancement of antibody-dependent cellular cytotoxicity (ADCC) and natural killer (NK) cell activity. Interferon γ also affects Fc receptor expression on monocytes and major histocompatibility antigen expression. It is produced by antigen-stimulated T lymphocytes and regulates the activity of immune cells, causing it to be classified as a lymphokine of the interleukin type. It interacts with other interleukin molecules such as IL2 within the lymphokine regulatory network. It has been used in chronic granulomatous disease to enhance phagocyte function.

interferon γ (IFN-γ) inducible protein-10 (IP-10)

A chemokine of the α (CXC) family. IP-10 is a gene product following stimulation of cells with IFN-γ. It does not possess the ELR motif that determines the biological significance of a particular α chemokine. IP-10 has angiostatic potential, which is opposite to the angiogenic effects of other ELR-containing α chemokines. This potential renders IP-10 a unique α chemokine family member. Tissue sources include endothelial cells, monocytes, fibroblasts, and keratinocytes. High levels of IP-10 transcripts are present in lymphoid organs. Monocytes, progenitor cells and NK cells serve as a target cells.

interferon γ receptor

A 90-kDa glycoprotein receptor composed of one polypeptide chain. The only cells lacking this receptor are erythrocytes. Interferon γ receptor is encoded by a gene on chromosome 6q in humans.

interferon λ (IFN λ)

This interferon group mediates the induction of antiviral protection in various cell types. It consists of λ1, λ2, and λ3, also known as IL29, IL28A, and IL28B, respectively. IFN-λs share with type I interferons an intracellular signaling pathway that drives expression of a common set of IFN-stimulated genes. IFN-λs initiate many biological activities, including upregulation of class I MHC gene product expression. They mediate their antiviral protection through a class II cytokine receptor complex different from that of type I interferons. Comprised of two receptor proteins designated CRF2-12/IFN/λR1, unique to IFN-λs and CRF2-4/IL10R2, which is shared with IL10, IL22 and IL26 receptors. The IL28 and IL29 IFN-λs are reported to prime dendritic cells to induce proliferation of Foxp3-bearing regulatory T cells. IFN-λ-matured dendritic cells express high levels of class I and class II MHC gene products, but low levels of costimulatory molecules, and specifically induce IL2 dependent proliferation CD4$^+$ CD25$^+$ Foxp3$^+$ T cells with contact-dependent suppressive activity on T cells.

interferon producing cells (IPCs)

Specialized blood cells that resemble lymphocytes and synthesize 100-fold more type I interferon than other types of cells. Refer to plasmacytoid dendritic cells.

interferon regulatory factors (IRFs)

A family of transcription factors that have novel helix–turn–helix DNA-binding motifs. In addition to two structurally related members, IRF-1 and IRF-2, seven additional members have been described. Virally encoded IRFs that may interfere with cellular IRFs have also been identified. These factors play a functional role in the regulation of host defenses such as innate and adaptive immune responses.

interferon response

Alterations in human gene expression in cells subjected to interferon.

interferons (IFNs)

A group of immunoregulatory cytokines synthesized by T lymphocytes, fibroblasts, and other types of cells following stimulation with viruses, antigens, mitogens, double-stranded DNA, or lectins. They facilitate cell resistance to viral infection. Class α and β interferons have antiviral properties. The γ class is known as immune interferon. Interferons α and β share a common receptor, but γ has its own. Interferons have immunomodulatory functions and enhance the abilities of macrophages to destroy tumor cells, viruses, and bacteria. Interferons α and β were formerly classified as type I interferons. They are acid-stable and synthesized mainly by leukocytes and fibroblasts. Interferon γ is acid-labile and is formed mainly by T lymphocytes stimulated by antigen or mitogen. This immune interferon was known as type II in the past. Whereas the ability of interferon to prevent infection of noninfected cells is species-specific, it is not virus-specific. Essentially, all viruses are subject to its inhibitory action. Interferons induce formation of a second inhibitory protein that prevents viral messenger RNA translation. In addition to interferon γ formation by T cells activated with mitogen, natural killer cells also secrete it. Interferons are not viricidal.

interfollicular region

Tissue separating lymphoid follicles situated in a group; it exhibits a predominance of mature T cells encircling high endothelial venules (HEVs).

interleukin (IL)

A general term for numerous cytokines synthesized by leukocytes. Includes multiple secreted proteins that facilitate inflammation exchange among leukocytes and activate signaling that regulates hematopoietic cell growth, differentiation, and function.

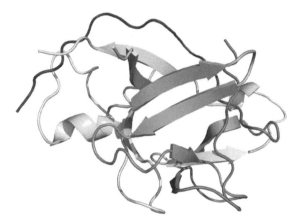

Interleukin-1α.

interleukin-1 (IL1)

The two proteins comprising the IL1 molecule and designated IL1α and IL1β belong to the interleukin-1 superfamily of cytokine molecules. The molecules identified within the IL1 superfamily include IL18 and cytokines encoded by six more genes with structural homology to IL1α, IL1β, or IL1RA. These latter six members are terned IL1F5 through IL1F10. IL1α, IL1β, and IL1RA are now known as IL1F1, IL1F2, and IL1F3. IL33 is an additional member of the IL1 family; it is also known as IL1F11. Macrophages, monocytes and dendritic cells synthesize IL1α and IL1β, which constitute significant parts of the body's inflammatory response to infection. These cytokines elevate adhesion molecule expression on endothelial cells to facilitate transmigration of leukocytes to sites of infection and reset the hypothalamus thermoregulatory center, which causes an elevation in body temperature manifested as fever. Thus, IL1 is an endogenous pyrogen. IL1 also plays a significant role in regulation of hematopoiesis. IL1 is a cytokine synthesized by activated mononuclear phagocytes stimulated by ribopolysaccharide or by interaction with CD4+ T lymphocytes. It is a monokine and a mediator of inflammation, sharing many properties in common with tumor necrosis factors (TNFs). IL1, IL6, and TNF-α induce a variety

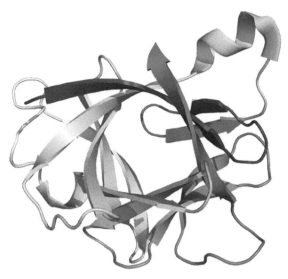

Interleukin-1β.

of inflammatory responses early during infection. IL1 is composed of two principal polypeptides of 17 kDa, each with isoelectric points of 5.0 and 7.0. They are designated IL1α and IL1β, respectively. Genes found on chromosome 2 encode these two molecular species. They have the same biological activities and bind to the same receptors on cell surfaces. Both IL1α and IL1β are derived by proteolytic cleavage of 33-kDa precursor molecules. IL1α acts as a membrane-associated substance, whereas IL1β is found free in the circulation. IL1 receptors are present on numerous cell types. IL1 may activate adenylate cyclase, elevating cAMP levels and then activating protein kinase A, or it may induce nuclear factors that serve as cellular gene transcriptional activators. IL1 may induce synthesis of enzymes that generate prostaglandins, which may in turn induce fever, a well known action of IL1. The actions of IL1 differ according to whether it is produced in lower or higher concentrations. At low concentrations, the effects are mainly immunoregulatory. IL1 acts with polyclonal activators to facilitate CD4+ T lymphocyte proliferation and B lymphocyte growth and differentiation. It stimulates multiple cells to act as immune or inflammatory response effector cells. It also induces further synthesis of itself and of IL6 by mononuclear phagocytes and vascular endothelium. It resembles TNF in inflammatory properties. IL1 secreted in greater amounts produces endocrine effects as it courses through the peripheral blood circulation. For example, it produces fever and promotes the formation of acute phase plasma proteins in the liver. It also induces cachexia. Natural inhibitors of IL1 may be produced by mononuclear phagocytes activated by immune complexes in humans. The inhibitor is biologically inactive and prevents the action of IL1 by binding with its receptor, serving as a competitive inhibitor. Corticosteroids and prostaglandins suppress IL1 secretion. IL1 was formerly called lymphocyte-activating factor (LAF).

interleukin-1 receptor (IL1R)

An 80-kDa receptor found on T lymphocytes, chondrocytes, osteoblasts, and fibroblasts that binds IL1α and IL1β. Helper/inducer CD4+ T lymphocytes are richer in IL1R than suppressor/cytotoxic (CD8+) T cells. IL1R has

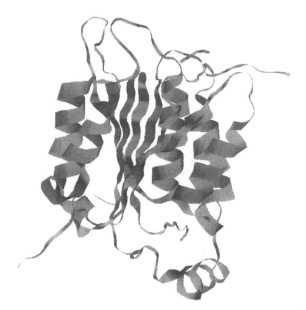

Human IL1β-converting enzyme (x-ray diffraction; resolution = 2.6 Å).

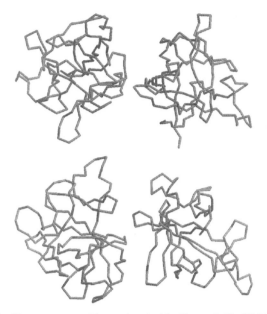

Backbone structure of human interleukin-1β revealed by NMR.

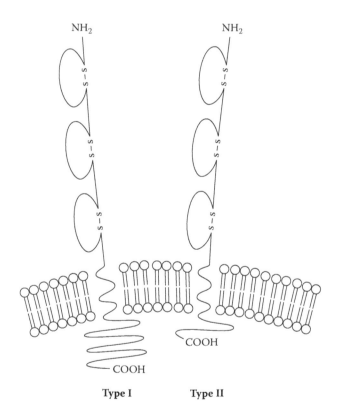

Type I   Type II

Interleukin-1 receptors, types I and II.

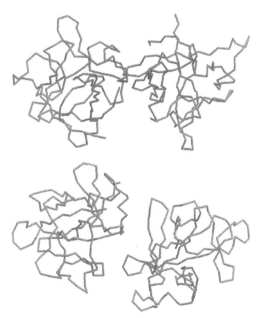

Interleukin-1 receptor antagonist protein (resolution = 3.2 Å).

an extracellular portion that binds ligand and contains all N-linked glycosylation sites. A 217-amino-acid segment, apparently confined to the cytoplasm, may be involved in signal transduction. Further studies of ligand binding have been facilitated through the development of a soluble form of the cloned IL1R molecule that contains the extracellular part but not the transmembrane cytoplasmic region of the molecule. IL1α and IL1β molecules bind with equivalent affinities. It has been claimed that the IL1R has more than one subunit based on the demonstration of bands, such as

a 100-kDa band, in addition to that characteristic of the receptor which is 80 kDa. Recombinant IL1R functions in signal transduction. When the cytoplasmic part of the IL1R is depleted, the molecule does not function. The human T cell IL1R has been cloned and found to be similar to its murine counterpart. Two affinity classes of binding sites for IL1 have been described.

interleukin-1 receptor antagonist protein (IRAP)
    A substance on T lymphocytes and endothelial cells that inhibits IL1 activity.

interleukin-1 receptor deficiency
    CD4⁺ T cells deficient in IL1 receptors in affected individuals fail to undergo mitosis when stimulated and fail to generate IL2. This leads to a lack of immune responsiveness and constitutes a type of combined immunodeficiency. Opportunistic

infections are increased in affected children who have inherited the condition as an autosomal-recessive trait.

interleukin-1 Ra

IL1 receptor antagonist is a soluble protein that interacts with IL1R leading to prevention of signal transduction and prevention of inflammation. Counteracts endotoxic shock.

interleukin-1 receptor antagonist (IL1ra)

An IL1 inhibitor that is structurally homologous to IL1 and is synthesized by mononuclear phagocytes. This biologically inactive molecule blocks IL1 activity by binding to its receptor. Plays a central role in acute and chronic inflammation, both locally and systemically. It is produced primarily by monocytes and macrophages and is synthesized as a precursor that is cleaved by IL1β–converting enzyme (ICE) to mature IL1β plus a prosegment. Some combination of mature IL1β, IL1β precursor, and the prosegment is released by cells.

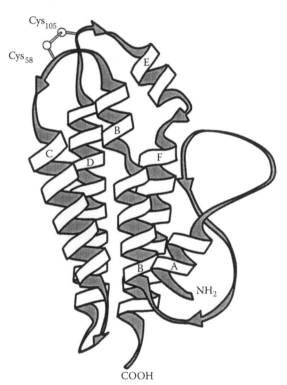

Schematic representation of interleukin-2 (IL-2).

interleukin-2 (IL2)

A 15.5-kDa glycoprotein synthesized by CD4+ T helper lymphocytes; it was formerly called T cell growth factor. Critical to the body's natural defense against microbial infection and discrimination between self and nonself, IL2 is a member of a cytokine family that includes IL4, IL7, IL9, IL15, and IL21. It interacts with a specific IL2 receptor α (CD25), IL2 receptor β (CD122), and a common γ chain (γc) possessed by λ members of this family of cytokines. IL2 binding activates the Ras/MAPK, JAK/Stat and PI 3-kinase/Akt signaling molecules. IL2 is synthesized during an immune response. Antigens binding to the T cell receptor activate IL2 secretion and expression of IL2 receptors (IL2Rs). The binding of IL2 to its receptor activates growth, differentiation, and survival of antigen-

selected cytotoxic T cells through the activation of specific genes. IL2 is needed for the development of T cell immunologic memory. It exerts an autocrine effect, acting on the CD4+ T cells that produce it. Although mainly produced by CD4+ T cells, a small amount is produced by CD8+ T cells. Physiologic amounts of IL2 do not have endocrine effects; it acts on the cells producing it or on those nearby acting as a paracrine growth factor. The main effects of IL2 are on lymphocytes. The amount of IL2 that CD4+ T lymphocytes synthesize is a principal factor in determining the strength of an immune response. It also facilitates formation of other cytokines produced by T lymphocytes, including interferon γ and lymphotoxins. Inadequate IL2 synthesis can lead to antigen-specific T lymphocyte anergy. IL2 interacts with T lymphocytes by reacting with IL2 receptors and also promotes natural killer (NK) cell growth and potentiates the cytolytic action of NK cells through generation of lymphokine-activated killer (LAK) cells. Although NK cells do not have the p55 lower affinity receptor, they do express the high-affinity p70 receptor and thus require high IL2 concentrations for their activation. IL2 is a human B cell growth factor and promotes synthesis of antibody by these cells. However, it does not induce isotype switching. IL2 promotes the improved responsiveness of immature bone marrow cells to other cytokines. In the thymus, it is also necessary for T cell development for the maturation of a unique subset of T cells critical to immunoregulation and called regulatory T cells (T-regs). T-reg cells leaving the thymus inhibit other T cells from recognizing and reacting against self antigens that may lead to autoimmunity. They accomplish this by preventing the responding cells from synthesizing IL2, which is necessary to differentiate between self and nonself. Both IL2 and IL15 aid the synthesis of immunoglobulins by B cells and induce differentiation and proliferation of natural killer cells. The main difference between IL2 and IL15 is in adaptive immune responses. Whereas T-regs prevent self reactivity by T cells, IL15 is requisite for maintaining specific T cell responses through supporting survival of CD8+ memory T cells. The IL2 gene is located on chromosome 4 in humans. Corticosteroids, cyclosporin A, and prostaglandins inhibit IL2 synthesis and secretions. Proleukin® is a commercially available recombinant form of IL2 approved by the FDA to treat tumors such as malignant melanoma and renal cell carcinoma. A number of immunosuppressive drugs used in prevention of organ transplant rejection, such as cyclosporin and tacrolimus, or corticosteroids used in the treatment of autoimmune diseases inhibit IL2 synthesis by antigen-activated T cells. Rapamycin inhibits IL2R signaling.

interleukin-2 receptor (IL2R)

Also known as CD25. IL2R is a structure on the surfaces of T lymphocytes, natural killer cells, and B lymphocytes characterized by the presence of a 55-kDa polypeptide (p55) and a 70-kDa polypeptide (p70) that interact with IL2 molecules at cell surfaces. The p55 polypeptide chain is referred to as Tac antigen, an abbreviation for T activation. The expression of both p55 and p70 permits a cell to bind IL2 securely with a K_d of about 10^{-8}. p55, the low affinity receptor, apparently complexes with p70, the high affinity receptor, to accentuate the affinity of p70 receptor for IL2. This permits increased binding in cells expressing both receptors. In addition, lesser quantities of IL2 than would otherwise be required for stimulation are effective when both receptors are present on cell surfaces. Antibodies against p55 or p70 can block IL2 binding. Powerful antigenic stimulation such as in transplant rejection may lead to the shedding of p55 IL2 receptors into the serum. The gene encoding the p55 chain is located on chromosome 10p14 in humans. IL2, IL1, IL6, IL4, and TNF may induce IL2R expression.

interleukin-2 receptor α subunit (IL2Rα)

The 55-kDa polypeptide subunit of IL2R with a K_d of 10^{-8} M. The α subunit is responsible for increasing the affinity between cytokine and receptor; however, it has no role in signal transduction. It is expressed only on antigen stimulation of T cells, usually within 2 hours. Following long-term T cell activation, the α subunit is shed, making it a potential candidate as a serum marker of strong or prolonged antigen stimulation. The gene encoding IL2Rα is located on chromosome 10p14 in humans.

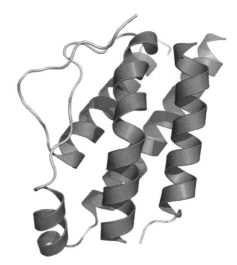

Interleukin-2.

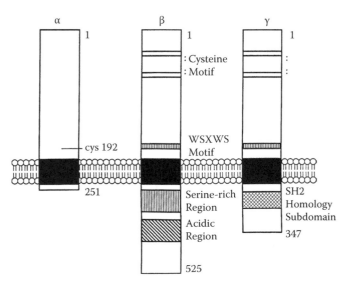

Schematic representation of interleukin-2 receptor αβγ subunit (IR-2Rαβγ.)

interleukin-2 receptor αβγ subunit (ILα2Rβγ)

The complete IL2 receptor consists of two distinct polypeptides: IL2α, induced upon activation, and IL2βγ, present on resting T cells. Upon expression of all three proteins, affinity increases to 10^{-11} M and very low (physiologic) levels of IL2 are capable of stimulating cells. IL2R is found on T lymphocytes, natural killer (NK) cells, and B lymphocytes, although NK cells do not express IL2Rα. IL2, IL1, IL6, IL4, and TNF may induce IL2R expression.

interleukin-2 receptor β subunit (IL2Rβ)

The 70- to 74-kDa subunit of IL2R with a K_d of 10^{-9} M. The β subunit is a member of the cytokine receptor family type I due to its tryptophan–serine–X–tryptophan–serine (WSXWS) domain. It is a constitutive membrane protein coordinately expressed with IL2Rγ.

interleukin-2 receptor βγ subunit (IL2Rβγ)

A heterodimer found on resting T cells. Only T cells expressing IL2R are capable of growth in response to IL2, as this is the portion of the receptor responsible for signal transduction.

interleukin-2 receptor γ subunit (IL2Rγ)

This subunit is also a type I (WSXWS) receptor associated with IL4 and IL7 receptors as well as IL2Rγ. Mutations in the γ subunit have been found in some cases of severe combined immunodefiency syndrome (SCIDS) with X-linked inheritance, resulting in decreased proliferation of B and T cells.

interleukin-3 (IL3)

A 20-kDa lymphokine synthesized by activated CD4+ T helper lymphocytes that acts as a colony-stimulating factor by facilitating proliferation of some hematopoietic cells and promoting proliferation and differentiation of other lymphocytes. It acts by binding to high and low affinity receptors, inducing tyrosine phosphorylation and colony formation of erythroid, myeloid, megakaryocytic, and lymphoid hematopoietic cells. It also facilitates mast cell proliferation, the release of histamine, and T lymphocyte maturation through induction of 20α-hydroxysteroid dehydrogenase. The gene encoding IL3 is situated on the long arm of chromosome 5. The IL3 gene in humans encodes a 152-amino acid long protein, and the naturally occurring form of IL3 is glycosolated. IL3 facilitates natural immune defenses against disease.

interleukin-3 receptor

A low-affinity IL3-binding α subunit (IL3α; CD123) that associates with a β subunit to produce a high affinity IL3 receptor. The IL3α subunit has an N terminal region consisting of 100-amino acid residues, a cytokine receptor domain, and a fibronectin III domain containing the WSXWS motif. The truncated cytoplasmic domain is associated with the inability to signal. The β subunit has two homologous segments in the extracellular region. A cytokine receptor domain followed by a fibronectin domain is present in each segment. The human α chain contains six potential N-linked glycosylation sites, whereas the β chain has three. Tyrosine and serine/threonine phosphorylation of numerous cellular proteins occurs rapidly following union of IL3 with its receptor. The β subunit is requisite for signal transduction.

interleukin-4 (IL4; B cell growth factor)

A 20-kDa cytokine that induces differentiation of naïve helper T (Th0) cells to Th2 cells, subsets of CD4+ helper T lymphocytes, that subsequently become the main producers of the cytokine and may also be synthesized by activated mast cells. Among its numerous biological functions are the stimulation of activated B cell and T cell proliferation and the differentiation of CD4+ T cells into Th2 cells. It is a

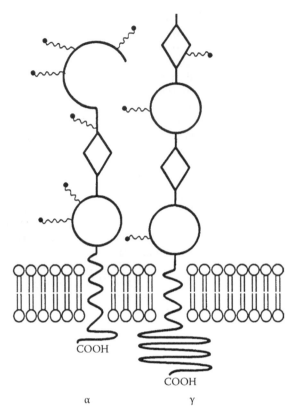

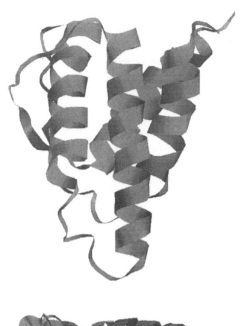

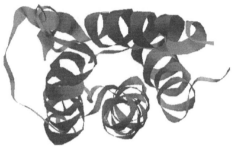

A ribbon diagram of IL-4 that constitutes a theoretical model of human IL-4.

Schematic representation of the interleukin-3 (IL-3) receptor. Schematic representation of the interleukin-6 (IL-6) receptor. IL-6 receptors of high affinity are composed of two subunits that are noncovalently associated. Low-affinity binding of IL-6 to the IL-6Rα chain occurs, but no signal is produced. The gp130 extracellular domain is composed of an IgSF C to set domain at the N-terminus. The cytokine receptor-SF domain and four fibronectin III domains follow. The WSXWS motif is present only in the first of the fibronectin III domains. The human IL-6Rα chain has five potential N-linked glycosylation sites, and the gp130 domain has ten.

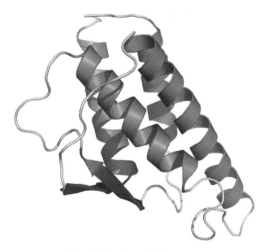

Interleukin-4 crystal structure.

principal regulator of humoral and adaptive immunity. IL4 induces B cell class switching to IgE and upregulates MHC class II production. Most studies of IL4 have been in mice, where it serves as a growth and differentiation factor for B cells and is a switch factor for synthesis of immunoglobulin E (IgE). It also promotes growth of a cloned CD4+ T cell subset. Further properties of murine IL4 include its function as a growth factor for mast cells and activation factor for macrophages. It also causes resting B lymphocytes to enlarge and enhances major histocompatibility complex (MHC) class II molecule expression. IL4 was previously termed B cell growth factor I (BCGF-I) and B cell-stimulating factor 1 (BSF-1). In humans, CD4+ T lymphocytes also produce IL4, but the human variety has not been shown to serve as a B cell or mast cell growth factor. Human IL4 also fails to activate macrophages. Both murine and human IL4s induce switching of B lymphocytes to synthesize IgE; thus IL4 may be significant in allergies. Human IL4 also induces CD23 expression by B lymphocytes and macrophages in humans. It may play some role in cell-mediated immunity. It induces differentiation of T_h2 cells from naïve CD4+ precursor cells, stimulates IgE formation by B cells, and suppresses IFN-γ-dependent macrophage functions.

interleukin-4 receptor (IL4R)

A structure composed of two major complexes, one of which is a 140-kDa single chain that constitutes a high affinity IL4 binding site (IL4Rα). The IL4Rα possesses pairs of cysteine residues and the WSXWS motif present in other members of the hematopoietin receptor superfamily, a classic transmembrane domain, and a 500-amino acid cytoplasmic domain. The IL4 receptor complex also contains other polypeptide chains. Following the binding

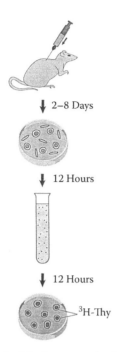

Induction of Interleukin-4 response in short-term culture.

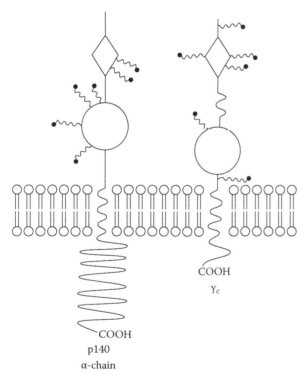

Interleukin-4.

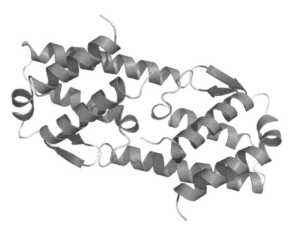

Interleukin-5 crystal structure.

length and murine IL5 is 133-amino acids long. The IL5 gene is located on chromosome 11 in mice and on chromosome 5 in humans. Formerly, it was called T cell-replacing factor or B cell growth factor II. It facilitates B cell growth and differentiation into cells that secrete immunoglobulin A (IgA). It is a costimulator with IL2 and IL4 of B cell growth and differentiation. IL5 also stimulates eosinophil growth and differentiation. It activates mature eosinophils to render them capable of killing helminths. Through IL5, T lymphocytes exert a regulatory effect on inflammation mediated by eosinophils. Because of its action in promoting eosinophil differentiation, it has been called eosinophil differentiation factor (EDF). IL5 can facilitate B cell differentiation into plaque-forming cells of the immunoglobulin M (IgM) and IgG classes. It is associated with various allergic diseases including allergic rhinitis and asthma, in which large numbers of eosinophils are observed in the tissues and sputum. In parasitic diseases, IL5 leads to eosinophilia.

interleukin-5 receptor complex

A structure comprised of an α chain and a β chain, both of which resemble members of the hematopoietin receptor superfamily. The α chain is a 415-amino acid glycoprotein and binds with low affinity to IL5. Even though the β chain does not bind to IL5, it associates with the α chain to form the high-affinity receptor. The β chain is common to IL3 and granulocyte–macrophage colony-stimulating factor (GM-CSF) receptors. The IL5 receptor is a member of the type 1 cytokine receptor family, comprised of a heterodimer containing an α subunit that binds IL5 and confers cytokine receptor specificity and a β subunit that contains the signal transduction domains. Eosinophils, whose principal function is to eliminate antibody bound parasites from the body through release of cytotoxic granule proteins, are the main IL5Rα expressing cells, which permits them to respond to IL5.

interleukin-6 (IL6)

A 26-kDa cytokine produced by vascular endothelial cells, mononuclear phagocytes, fibroblasts, activated T lymphocytes, and various neoplasms such as cardiac myxomas, bladder cancer, and cervical cancer. A cytokine synthesized by T cells and macrophages that is proinflammatory and activates immune responses to trauma, specifically burns amd other tissue injuries resulting in inflammation. It is required for murine resistance against *Streptococcus pneumoniae*. IL6 is produced by muscle, osteoblasts, and tunica

of IL4, the IL2 receptor γ chain associates with the ILRα chain. This complex comprises the type I IL4 receptor. The IL13 low affinity binding chain (IL13Rα) can also associate with IL4Rα. The IL4 receptor containing the IL13Rα is termed type II.

interleukin-5 (IL5; eosinophil differentiation factor)

A 20-kDa cytokine synthesized by some activated CD4⁺ T$_h$2 lymphocytes and activated mast cells. A part of the hematopoietic family, human IL5 is 150-amino acids in

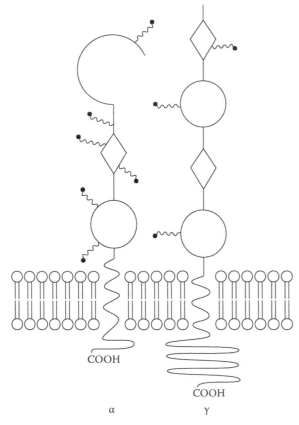

Interleukin-5 receptor complex.

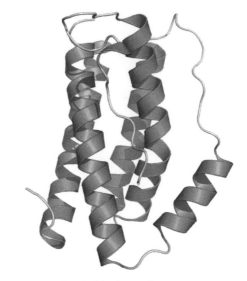

Interleukin-6 crystal structure.

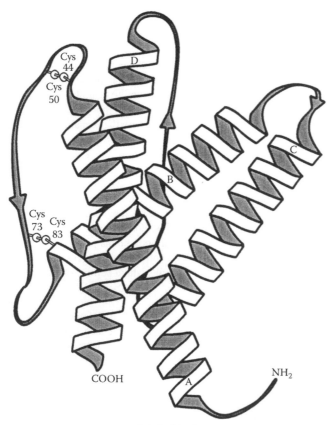

Interleukin-6.

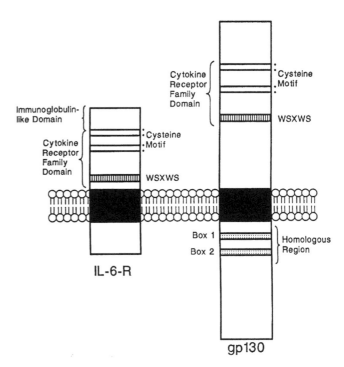

Schematic representation of the IL-6 receptor.

media smooth muscle cells. It is a significant mediator of fever and of the acute phase response. It leads to elevation of body temperature. Pathogen-associated molecular patterns (PAMPs) activate IL6 secretion by macrophages. PAMPs interact with Toll-like receptors of the innate immune system. This leads to intracellular signaling that results in inflammatory cytokine synthesis. It is secreted in response to IL1 or tumor necrosis factor (TNF). Its main actions are on hepatocytes and B cells. Although it acts on many types of cells, a significant function is its ability to cause B lymphocytes to differentiate into cells that synthesize antibodies. IL6 induces hepatocytes to form acute phase proteins that include fibrinogen. It is the main growth factor for activated B lymphocytes late in B cell differentiation. IL6 is a growth factor for plasmacytoma cells that

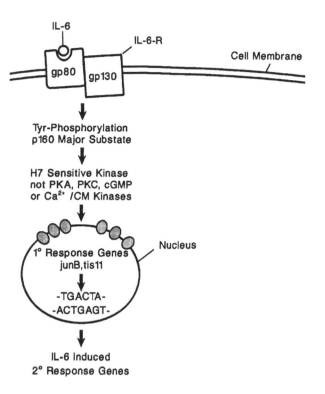

Pathway of IL-6 induction and signaling.

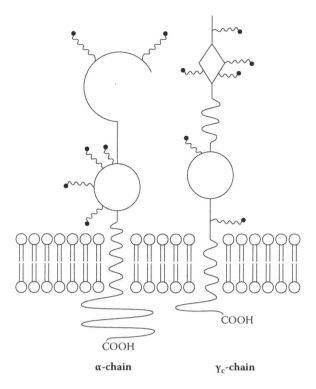

Interleukin-7 receptor.

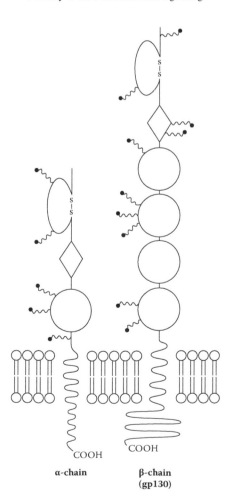

Interleukin-6 receptor.

produce it. IL6 also acts as a costimulator of T lymphocytes and thymocytes. It acts in concert with other cytokines that promote the growth of early bone marrow hematopoietic stem cells. It acts with IL1 to costimulate activation of Th cells. IL6 was formerly termed B cell differentiation factor (BCDF) and B cell-stimulating factor 2 (BSF-2). It has been implicated in the pathogenesis of plaques in psoriasis. With IL1 and TNF-α, IL6 produces a broad spectrum of responses early in infection.

interleukin-6 receptor

A structure composed of 468 amino acids: a 19-amino acid signal peptide, a 339-amino acid extracellular portion, a 28-amino acid transmembrane domain, and an 82-amino acid intracytoplasmic portion. The receptor has six potential N-linked glycosylation sites and 11 cysteine residues. The mature receptor has a molecular weight of 80 kDa and O- and N-glycosylation. The IL6 receptor system is composed of two functional chains, the ligand-binding 80-kDa IL6 receptor and the nonligand-binding gp130. This receptor is expressed on lymphoid as well as nonlymphoid cells. IL6 signals via a cell surface type I cytokine receptor complex comprised of the ligand-binding IL6Rα chain (CD126) and the signal-transducing component gp130 (CD130). Interaction of IL6 with this receptor leads to activation of gp 130 and IL6R proteins to produce a complex, thereby activating the receptor. Such complexes assemble the intracellular regions of gp 130 to activate a signal transduction cascade through such transcription factors as Janus kinases (JAKs) and signal transducers and activators of transcription (STATs).

interleukin-7 (IL7)

Interleukin-7 facilitates lymphoid stem cell differentiation into progenitor B cells. It mainly serves as a T lymphocyte growth factor synthesized by bone marrow stromal cells. It promotes lymphopoiesis, governing stem cell differentiation into early pre-T and -B cells. It is also formed by thymic stroma and promotes the growth and activation of T cells and activates macrophages. It enhances fetal and adult thymocyte proliferation. Thus, IL7 has a significant role for proliferation during selected stages of B cell maturation, T and NK cell survival, development, and homeostasis.

interleukin-8 (IL8; neutrophil-activating protein 1)

A chemokine 8-kDa protein of 72 residues produced by macrophages, epithelial cells, and endothelial cells. Innate immune system Toll-like receptors recognize antigen patterns such as lipopolysaccharides in Gram-negative bacteria. A cascade of biochemical reactions leads to the secretion of IL8, a significant mediator of innate immune system responses. The gene encoding this protein is a member of the CXC chemokine family, which is one of the principal mediators of the inflammatory response. This chemokine is secreted by various cell types and acts as a chemoattractant and also a powerful angiogenic factor. This gene is critical in the pathogenesis of viral-induced bronchiolitis. It and ten other members of the CXC chemokine gene family form a chemokine gene cluster mapped to chromosome 4q. Any innate immune system cells bearing Toll-like receptors can secrete IL8, whose primary function is to recruit neutrophils to phagocytize antigen, which activates the antigen pattern Toll-like receptors. It has a powerful chemotactic effect on T lymphocytes and neutrophils and

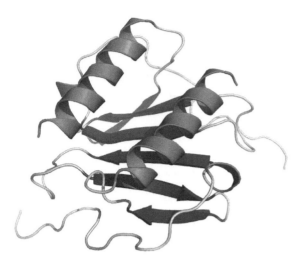

Interleukin-8.

upregulates the binding properties of leukocyte adhesion receptor CD11b/CD18. IL8 is released from macrophages processing antigen and is one of the chemokines designed to signal other immune cells to a site of inflammation. Its ability to attract neutrophils to sites of inflammation makes it also known as neutrophil chemotactic factor. IL8 regulates expression of its own receptor on neutrophils and has antiviral, immunomodulatory, and antiproliferative properties. It prevents adhesion of neutrophils to endothelial cells activated by cytokines, thereby blocking neutrophil-mediated injury. It participates in inflammation and the migration of cells and facilitates neutrophil adherence to endothelial cells through the induction of β_2 integrins by neutrophils. Pregnant females with elevated IL8 levels face increased risk of bearing offspring with schizophrenia. It is the prototypic and most widely investigated chemokine. Its powerful neutrophil chemotactic action makes IL8 a primary regulatory molecule of acute inflammation. High affinity neutralizing anti-IL8 antibodies have been used to reveal the regulatory action of IL8 on neutrophil infiltration into tissues. IL8 also has a second significant effect in promoting angiogenesis. It contains the ELR motif that is crucial to the chemotactic action of several α chemokine family members. Monocytes, macrophages, CD4+, CD8+, and CD45RA+ lymphocytes, among many other cell types

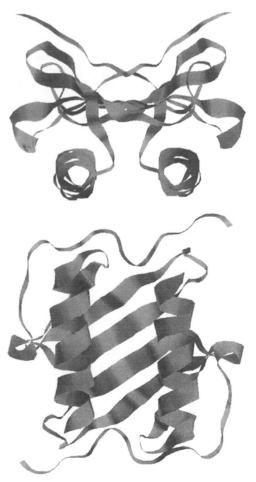

Interleukin-8.

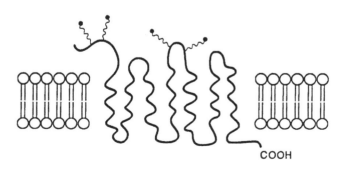

Schematic representation of the interleukin-8 (IL-8) receptor, which may be of either high or low affinity. These receptors are seven transmembrane spanning and are G-protein linked. They belong to the rhodopsin superfamily. Whereas the high-affinity receptor binds IL-8 exclusively, the low affinity receptor also shows specificity for NAP-2 and GRO/MPSA.

serve as tissue sources. Neutrophils, T lymphocytes, basophils, eosinophils, keratinocytes, and HUVEC cells serve as targets. The two types of human IL8 receptors are types A and B consisting of 351 and 360 amino acids, respectively. They belong to a family of G protein-coupled receptors with seven transmembrane domains and have high sequence homologies at the amino acid level. IL8 is also called CXCL8.

interleukin-8 receptor, type A (IL8RA, α)

The high affinity IL8 receptor, class I IL8R belongs to the G protein-coupled receptor family, the chemokine receptor branch of the rhodopsin family. The tissue sources are human neutrophils. Murine IL8 receptor knockout mice develop splenomegaly, enlarged cervical lymph nodes, extramedullary myelopoiesis, and impaired neutrophil acute migration. IL8RA nRNA is present in neutrophils, monocytes, basophils and freshly isolated T cells.

interleukin-8 receptor, type B (IL8RB, β)

A low affinity IL8 receptor, class II, CXCR2, F3R (rabbit). IL8RB mRNA is present in neutrophils, monocytes, basophils, T cells, and primary keratinocytes. It is expressed in the lesional skin of psoriasis patients. G-CSF upregulates IL8RB mRNA expression, whereas IL8 and MGSA downregulate IL8RB surface expression on human neutrophils.

interleukin-9 (IL9; murine growth factor P40; T cell growth factor III)

A cytokine that facilitates the growth of some T helper cell clones but not cytolytic T lymphocyte clones. It is encoded by genes comprised of five exons in a 4-kb segment of DNA in both mice and humans. The gene encoding IL9 is located on chromosomes 5 and 13. This hematopoietic growth factor glycoprotein can be derived from a megakaryoblastic leukemia. Selected human T lymphocyte lines and peripheral lymphocytes activated by mitogen express it. IL9 is related to mast cell growth-enhancing activity both structurally and functionally. In the presence of erythropoietin, IL9 supports erythroid colony formation. In conjunction with IL2, IL3, IL4, and erythropoietin, IL9 may enhance hematopoiesis *in vivo*. It may facilitate bone marrow-derived mast cell growth stimulated by IL3 and fetal thymocyte growth in response to IL2. T_h2 cells preferentially express IL9 following stimulation with concanavalin A (con A) or by antigen presented on syngeneic antigen-presenting cells.

interleukin-9 (IL9)

A cytokine synthesized by T cells and specifically by CD4+ helper cells. It facilitates the growth of some T helper cell clones but not of clones of cytolytic T lymphocytes. It is encoded by genes comprised of 5 exons in the 4-kb segment of DNA in both mice and humans. In the presence of erythropoietin, IL9 supports erythroid colony formation. In conjunction with IL2, IL3, IL4, and erythropoietin, IL9 may enhance hematopoiesis *in vivo*. It may facilitate bone marrow-derived mast cell growth stimulated by IL3 and fetal thymocyte growth in response to IL2. Th2 cells preferentially express IL9 following stimulation with con A or by antigen presented on syngeneic antigen-presenting cells. It is a hematopoietic growth factor glycoprotein derived from a megakaryoblastic leukemia. Selected T lymphocyte lines and peripheral lymphocytes activated by mitogen express it. IL9 is related to mast cell growth-enhancing activity both structurally and functionally. The genes encoding IL9

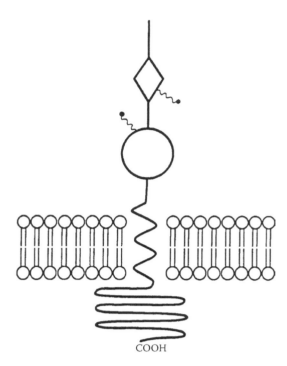

Interleukin-9 receptor. Schematic representation of the interleukin-9 (IL-9) receptor, only one type of which has been found on murine T cell lines. Investigation of the recombinant murine receptor has demonstrated association between the IL-2Rγ chain and the IL-9R. Macrophages, some T cell tumors, and mast cell lines have been shown to express IL-9 receptors.

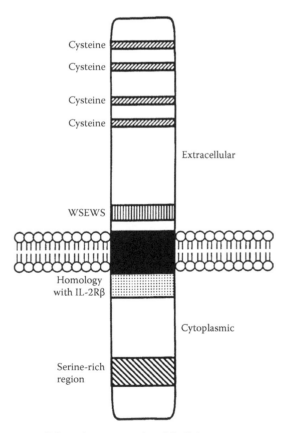

Schematic representation of the Il-9 receptor.

are located on chromosomes 5 and 13. Genes encoding this cytokine are believed to have a role in asthma. Genetic investigations on murine models of asthma show that this cytokine is a determining factor in the pathogenesis of bronchial hyperresponsiveness. The murine IL9 receptor encodes a 469-amino acid polypeptide with two potential N-linked glycosylation sites and six cysteine residues in the extracellular domain. Contemporary research suggests that IL9R is a member of the hematopoietin receptor superfamily.

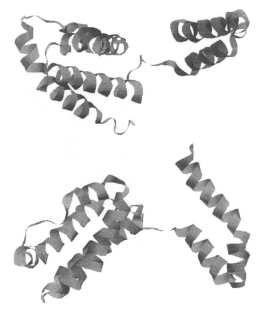

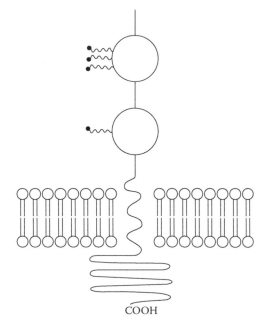

Interleukin-10 receptor.

Interleukin-10.

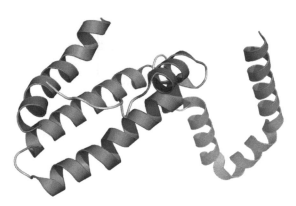

Interleukin-10 crystal structure.

interleukin-10 (IL10)

A multifunctional cytokine synthesized by CD4 Th2 cells that inhibits activation and effector functions of T cells, mononocytes, and macrophages. It has diverse effects on hematopoietic cell types and ultimately terminates inflammatory responses. IL10 regulates growth and/or differentiation of B cells, natural killer (NK) cells, cytotoxic and helper T cells, mast cells, granulocytes, dendritic cells, keratinocytes, and endothelial cells. It plays a key role in differentiation and function of T regulatory cells that are critical in the control of immune responses and tolerance *in vivo*.

interleukin-10 (IL10) cytokine synthesis inhibitory factor

An 18-kDa polypeptide devoid of carbohydrates in humans that acts as a cytokine synthesis inhibitory factor.

It is expressed by CD4+ Th2 and CD8+ T lymphocytes, monocytes and macrophages, activated B lymphocytes, B lymphoma cells, and keratinocytes. It downregulates the expression of Th1 cytokines, MHC class II antigens and costimulatory molecules on macrophages. It enhances B cell survival, proliferation, and antibody synthesis. This cytokine can block NF-κB activity and participates in the regulation of the JAK-STAT signaling pathway. It inhibits some immune responses and facilitates others. It inhibits cytokine synthesis by Th1 cells and blocks antigen presentation and the formation of interferon γ (IFN-γ). It also inhibits the ability of macrophages to present antigen and form IL1, IL6, and TNF-α. It also participates in IgE regulation. Although IL10 suppresses cell-mediated immunity, it stimulates B lymphocytes, IL2, and IL4 T lymphocyte responsiveness *in vitro*, and murine mast cells exposed to IL3 and IL4. IL10 may have potential for suppressing T lymphocyte autoimmunity in multiple sclerosis and type I diabetes mellitus and in facilitating allograft survival. Murine Th2 cells secrete IL10, which suppresses synthesis of cytokines by Th1 cells. Knockout studies in mice suggest that this cytokine functions as an essential immunoregulator in the intestinal tract. Mouse studies also show that IL10 is produced by mast cells, counteracting their inflammatory effects at sites of allergic reactions. In humans, the IL10 gene is located on chromosome 1 and consists of five exons. The IL10 protein is a homodimer. Each subunit is 178 amino acids long. The principal function of IL10 is to inhibit activated macrophages, thereby maintaining homeostatic control of innate and cell-mediated immune reactions.

interleukin-11 (IL11)

A cytokine produced by stromal cells derived from the bone marrows of primates. It activates B cells and megakaryocytes and serves as a growth factor that induces IL6-dependent murine plasmacytoma cells to proliferate. IL11 has several biological actions that include its hematopoietic effect. In humans, the genomic sequence and gene encoding IL11 are composed of five exons and four introns. The gene is located at band 19q13.3–13.4 on the long arm of chromosome 19. It may facilitate plasmacytoma establishment, possibly representing an important role for IL11 in tumorigenesis. In combination with IL3, IL11 can potentiate megakaryocyte growth, producing increased numbers, sizes, and ploidy values. It may be important in the formation of platelets. In the presence of functional T lymphocytes, IL11 can stimulate the production of B cells that secrete immunoglobulin G (IgG). It has a synergistic effect in primitive hematopoietic cell proliferation that is IL3-dependent. IL11 belongs to the IL6 superfamily. It facilitates platelet recovery after chemotherapy-induced thrombocytopenia, induces acute phase proteins, modulates antigen–antibody responses, participates in the regulation of bone cell proliferation and differentiation, and may be used as a therapeutic agent for osteoporosis. Apart from its lymphopoietic, hematopoietic, and osteotrophic properties, it functions in numerous tissues including brain, intestines, and testes. It facilitates growth of selected lymphocytes and in mouse studies has been shown to promote cortical thickness and strength of long bones. The IL11 receptor (IL11R) is composed of at least one ligand-binding subunit (IL11Rα) and a signal transduction subunit (gp130). The murine and human IL11R cDNAs encode 432- and 422-amino acid polypeptides, respectively, with two potential N-linked glycosylation sites and four cysteine residues in the extracellular domain. IL11Rα is believed to be a member of the hematopoietin receptor superfamily. Murine and human IL11Rα have 84% homology at the amino acid level and 85% homology at the nucleotide level.

interleukin-11 receptor (IL11R)

IL11R is composed of at least one ligand-binding subunit (IL11Rα) and a signal transduction subunit (gp130). Murine and human IL11R cDNAs encode 432- and 422-amino acid polypeptides, respectively, with two potential N-linked glycosylation sites and four cysteine residues in the extracellular domain. IL11Rα is believed to be a member of the hematopoietin receptor superfamily. Murine and human IL11Rαs have 84% homology at the amino acid level and 85% homology at the nucleotide level.

interleukin-12 (IL12)

Comprised of a bundle of four α helices, interleukin-12 is a heterodimeric cytokine encoded by two separate genes, IL12A(p35) and IL12B(p40). The active heterodimer and a homodimer of p40 are generated following protein synthesis. The molecule is composed of 35-kDa and 40-kDa chains linked by disulfide bonds. IL12 participates in the differentiation of naïve T cells into Th1 cells that play a significant role in resistance against pathogens. It acts on T cells as a cytotoxic lymphocyte maturation factor (CLMF). As a T cell-stimulating factor, it can activate the growth and function of T cells. It also serves as a natural killer (NK) cell stimulatory factor (NKSF). It induces the synthesis of IFN-γ and tumor necrosis factor-α (TNF-α) from T and NK cells and diminishes IL4-mediated suppression of IFN-γ. IL12 is a growth factor for activated CD4+ and CD8+ T lymphocytes and for NK cells. It facilitates NK cell and LAK cell lytic action exclusive of IL2. It can induce resting peripheral blood mononuclear cells to form IFN-γ in vitro. IL12 may act synergistically with IL2 to increase responses by cytotoxic lymphocytes. T cells that synthesize IL12

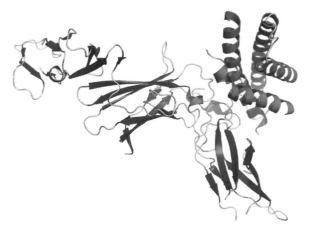

Interleukin-12 crystal structure.

have CD30 coreceptors associated with IL12 activity. IL12 may have potential as a therapeutic agent in the treatment of tumors or infections, especially if used in combination with IL2. IL12 promotes IFN-γ formation by NK cells and T cells, enhances the cytolytic activity of NK cells and CTLs, and facilitates the development of Th2 cells. IL2 and signal transduction of IL12 in NK cells appear to be linked. IL2 induces the expression of two IL12 receptors, IL12Rβ₁ and IL12β₂, maintaining the expression of a critical protein associated with IL12 signaling in NK cells. IL12 reveals an antiangiogenic property by increasing synthesis of IFN-γ, which increases the formation of a chemokine known as inducible protein 10 (IP-10 or CXCL 10) that mediates the antiangiogenic effect. IL12 receptor is designated IL12R. Two receptor chains, IL12Rβ1and IL12Rβ2, have been identified and cloned. Both β1 and β2 chains are members of the cytokine receptor superfamily. They are related to gp130 of the IL6R and to the receptors of LIF and G-CSF. Coexpression of both these receptors confers IL12 responsiveness. Both human- and mouse-activated T cells have IL12 binding sites of high, intermediate, and low affinities. IL12Rβ2 has a key role in IL12 function because it is present on activated T cells and is induced by cytokines that facilitate Th1 cell development and inhibited by those that promote Th2 cell development. Following binding, IL12Rβ2 becomes tyrosine phosphorylated and provides binding sites for kinases, Tyk2 and Jak2, that are significant in activating critical transcription factor proteins such as STAT4 that are involved in IL12 signaling in T cells and NK cells. This is known as the JAK-STAT pathway. IL12 is associated with autoimmunity. Its administration to autoimmune disease patients worsens their condition, possibly associated with its prominent role in the induction of Th1 immune responses. By contrast, administration of anti-IL12 antibodies to mice and studies in IL12 gene knockout mice revealed diminished autoimmune responses.

interleukin 12 receptor (IL12R)

Two receptor chains, IL12Rβ₁ and IL12Rβ₂, have been identified and cloned. Both β₁ and β₂ chains are members of the cytokine receptor superfamily. They are related to gp130 of the IL6R and to receptors of LIF and G-CSF. Coexpression of both these receptors confers IL12 responsiveness. Both human- and mouse-activated T cells have IL12 binding sites of high, intermediate, and low affinities.

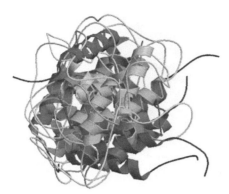

Interleukin-13.

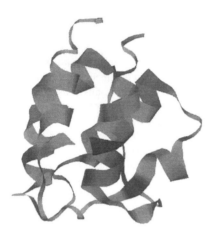

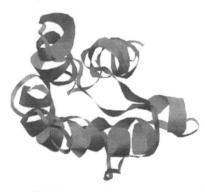

Ribbon diagram of IL-13 that constitutes a theoretical model of human IL-13. This is the first of two alternative structures of IL-13 generated by homology modeling.

interleukin-13 (IL13)

A cytokine synthesized by numerous cell types, especially T helper type 2 (Th2) cells. A significant mediator of allergic inflammation and disease. It exerts effects on immune cells that resemble those of the closely related IL4 cytokine. It is a central mediator of allergic inflammation in numerous tissues. It induces its effects through a multisubunit receptor that includes the α chain of the IL4 receptor (IL4Rα) that is also a constituent of the IL4 receptor and one of two known IL13-specific binding chains. IL13's biological effects are associated with a single transcription factor, signal transducer and activator of transcription 6 (STAT6). The functions of IL13 resemble those of IL4, especially with respect to changes induced on hematopoietic cells. IL13 can induce IgE secretion from activated human B cells. It acts as a molecular bridge linking allergic inflammatory cells to nonimmune cells in contact with them, thereby altering physiologic function. In addition to its role in the induction of airway disease, IL13 also has anti-inflammatory properties. The protein degrading enzymes known as airway matrix metalloproteinases (MMPs) are requisite to induce egression of effete parenchymal inflammatory cells into the airway lumen where they are cleared. IL13 induces these MMPs as a mechanism to protect against excessive allergic inflammation that may lead to asphyxiation. IL13 facilitates the expulsion of offending organisms or their products from parasitized organs. Expulsion of helminths from the mouse gut required IL13 secreted by Th2 cells. The cytokine fosters an environment hostile to the parasite, including enhanced contractions and glycoprotein hypersecretion from gut epithelial cells, leading ultimately to detachment of the organism from the gut wall and its removal. *Schistosoma mansoni* eggs may lodge in various organs and tissues including the gut wall, liver, lung, and central nervous system, leading to the formation of granulomas with the control of IL13. This leads ultimately to organ injury and often significant or fatal disease, not resolution of the infection. IL13 may antagonize Th1 responses required for resolution of intracellular infections, leading to recruitment of aberrantly large numbers of Th2 cells. IL13 inhibits the ability of host immune cells to destroy intracellular pathogens. It mediates many features of allergic lung disease including airway hyperresponsiveness, goblet cell metaplasia, and mucus hypersecretion, all of which contribute to airway obstruction. IL4 also contributes to these changes but is less significant than IL13 in that regard. IL13 induces secretion of chemokines needed for recruitment of allergic effector cells to the lung. STAT6 transgenic mouse investigations reveal the possibility that IL13 signaling occurring only through the airway epithelium is requisite for most of these effects. The high affinity IL13 receptor complex consists of the IL4Rα chain and an IL13-binding protein designated the IL13Rα chain. The IL13 receptor is expressed on B cells, monocytes/macrophages, basophils, mast cells, and endothelial cells but not on T cells. The IL13R complex also acts as a second receptor for IL4. The IL13Rα chain is a specific binding protein for IL13. IL4 can signal through both IL13R and IL4R complexes. Both IL4 and IL13 can mediate their biological actions through the IL13R complex.

interleukin-14 (IL14)

Formerly known as high molecular-weight B cell growth factor (HMW-BCGF), IL14 is a cytokine produced by follicular dendritic cells, germinal center T cells, and some malignant B cells. Normal and malignant B cells, notably germinal center B cells and NHL-B cells, respectively, express receptors for IL14. Its predominant activity is to enhance the proliferation of B cells and induce memory B cell production and maintenance. It also inhibits antibody secretion. It is synthesized principally by T cells and selected malignant B cells. Work with NHL-B cell lines has shown that inhibition of the expression of the IL14 gene results in diminished cell growth and eventual cell death. Also called taxilin. Two distinct transcripts produced from opposite strands of the *il14* locus gene are called IL14α and

IL14β. The *il14* locus is situated near the gene for LCK on chromosome 1 in humans.

interleukin-15 (IL15)

A T cell growth factor synthesized by mononuclear phagocytes and other cells in response to viral infections. It has many of the biological properties of IL2. Its principal function is to stimulate the proliferation of natural killer (NK) cells. IL15 enhances peripheral blood T cell proliferation, and *in vitro* studies demonstrate its ability to induce cytotoxic T cells. IL15 mRNA is expressed by monocyte-enriched peripheral blood cell lines and placental and skeletal muscle tissues. IL15 regulates T cell and NK cell activation and proliferation. This cytokine shares many biological activities with IL2. Both cytokines bind common hematopoietin receptor subunits and may even compete for the same receptor, and thus negatively regulate each other's activities. CD4$^+$ memory cells are shown to be controlled by a balance between this IL15 and IL2. IL15 induces activation of JAKs as well as the phosphorylation and activation of transcription factors STAT3, STAT5, and STAT6. Murine studies suggest that IL15 may elevate expression of apoptosis inhibitor BCL2L1/BCL-x(L), perhaps through the transcription activation activity of STAT6, thereby preventing apoptosis. IL15 may provide survival signals for memory lymphocytes. NK cells fail to develop in transgenic mice in which the IL15 receptor α (IL15Rα) gene has been knocked out. Infectious mononucleosis infection appears to be associated with the loss of IL15R expression by lymphocytes. The IL2 and IL15 receptors also share a common component for successful signal transduction. IL15 receptors are widely expressed. IL15 plays a major role related to NK cell development and cytolytic activity. The receptors for IL15 on T cells contain IL2Rβ, γ$_c$, one unique protein, IL15Rα, and an alternate IL15 receptor designated IL15RX and detected on mast cells. IL15 mediates its action by combination with a heterotrimeric receptor composed of both β and γ$_c$ chains of the IL2R as well as a unique IL15-binding subunit known as IL15α. The IL15Rα chain is requisite for high affinity binding but not signaling by IL15. IL2 and IL15 have the same signaling pathways.

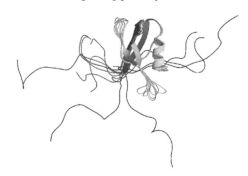

Interleukin-16.

interleukin-16 (IL16)

A 13.2-kDa protein containing 130-amino acid residues. It is also called lymphocyte chemoattractant (LCA). It activates a migratory response in CD4$^+$ T cells and CD4$^+$ monocytes, eosinophils, and dendritic cells. Human IL16 also induces IL2 receptor expression by T lymphocytes. IL16 has been found to suppress T cell proliferation and mixed lymphocyte reactions. IL16 is structurally distinct

from chemokines and in the active form is a homotetramer comprised of four 16-kDa chains. IL16 is produced as a precursor peptide (pro-IL16) that requires processing by an enzyme known as caspase-3 to become active. CD4 is the cell signaling receptor for mature IL16. It is synthesized by CD4$^+$ T cells, mast cells, and eosinophils. Its gene is located on human chromosome 15q26.1. CD4 may be a receptor for IL16. IL16 is chemotactic for resting and activated T cells, eosinophils, and monocytes. It facilitates CD4$^+$ T cell adhesion, expression of IL2Rα (CD25) and HLA-DR, and cytokine synthesis. It suppresses antigen and alloantigen (MLR)-induced lymphocyte proliferation. IL16 does not competitively inhibit HIV–gp120 binding. It is a potent survival factor and counters apoptotic effects of growth-inducing cytokines such as IL2. It has been found in bronchial airway epithelial cells and fluids of asthmatics. It may exacerbate allergic reactions. IL16 is a proinflammatory and immunomodulatory cytokine.

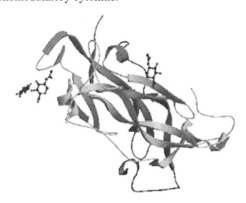

Interleukin-17.

interleukin-17 (IL17)

IL17A belongs to the IL17 family of cytokines. Other family members include IL17B, IL17C, IL17D, IL17E (IL25), and IL17F. All members share similar protein structures with four highly conserved cysteine residues relevant for their three-dimensional shapes, although they exhibit no sequence resemblance to other known cytokines. Amino acids are 62 to 88% conserved between the human and mouse homologs. The IL17 cytokine family has many immune regulatory functions attributable to their induction of numerous immune signaling molecules. IL17 participates in the induction and mediation of proinflammatory responses and is often associated with allergic phenomena. It induces the synthesis of numerous other cytokines including IL6, G-CSF, GM-CSF, IL1β, TGF-β, TNF-α and chemokines including IL8, GRO-α, and MCP-1. It also stimulates the synthesis of prostaglandins such as PGE$_2$ from numerous cell types such as fibroblasts, endothelial cells, epithelial cells, keratinocytes, and macrophages. A feature of IL17 cytokine-mediated responses includes airway remodeling. Chemokine expression may attract neutrophils. IL17 function is critical to the CD4$^+$ T cell subset called T helper 17 (Th17) cells. IL17 family members have been associated with such immune or autoimmune phenomena as asthma, lupus, allograft rejection and antitumor immunity. The human IL17 gene cloned from CD4$^+$ T cells is 1874 base pairs in length. The IL17 family members have a unique pattern of cellular expression. For example, IL17A and IL17F are expressed by activated T cells that are upregulated in inflammatory responses. IL17B is expressed in immune tissues and IL17C is upregulated in inflammation. IL17D is expressed in the nervous system and skeletal muscle tissue. IL17E is expressed at low levels in various peripheral tissues. IL17 was shown to be dependent on IL23. STAT3 and NF-κB signaling are required for IL23-mediated IL17 synthesis. SOCS3 has a significant role in IL17 synthesis. Whether IL17 induction is dependent on IL23 or not, IL23 is important in promoting survival and/or proliferation of IL17-synthesizing T cells. A 155-amino acid protein, IL17A is a disulfide-linked, homodimeric-secreted glycoprotein. The molecular mass is 35 kDa. The homodimer subunits range from 15 to 20 kDa. IL17 is comprised of a single peptide of 23 amino acids followed by a 123-amino acid chain region that is a feature of the IL17 family. It has an *N*-linked glycosylation site. IL17 family members contain four conserved cysteines that form two disulfide bonds. IL17 is dissimilar from all other interleukins, and bears no resemblance to other known proteins or structural domains. Five receptors with unique ligand specificities comprise the IL17 receptor family. IL17R interacts with both IL17A and IL17F and is expressed by vascular endothelial cells, peripheral T cells, B cells, fibroblasts, lung, myelomonocytic cells, and marrow stromal cells. IL17RB interacts with both IL17B and IL17E. Kidney, pancreas, brain, liver, and intestine express IL17RB, whereas prostate, cartilage, kidney, liver, heart, and muscle express IL17RC. Pancreas, brain, and prostate express IL17RE. Identification and characterization of IL12 and IL17 cytokine family members have elucidated a new arm of the adaptive immune response known as Th17 and a significant new player in the Th2 arm. Th17 responses are controlled by IL12 family cytokines, IL23, IL27, IL6, prototype for IL12 cytokines, and innate immune cell products. IL6 is a principal danger signal that switches the proregulatory TGF-β cytokine into a Th17-diverting mediator, making it a principal cytokine in self–nonself discrimination. The discovery of IL17 cytokines and the Th17 pathway has important implications for treating human diseases. IL23- and IL17-targeting treatments should prove highly effective in controlling certain autoinflammatory disorders.

interleukin-18 (IL18)

A proinflammatory cytokine synthesized by macrophages and other cells that belongs to the IL1 cytokine family based on its structure, receptor family, and signal transduction pathways. It functions with IL12 to induce cell-mediated immunity in the defense against intracellular bacteria including *Listeria*, *Shigella*, *Salmonella*, and *Mycobacterium tuberculosis*. As with IL1β, IL18 is synthesized as a precursor requiring caspase-1 for cleavage into an active IL18 molecule. With respect to its capacity to induce synthesis of Th1 cytokines and enhance cell-mediated cytotoxicity, IL18 is related to IL12. It is formed mainly by antigen-presenting cells and is a pleiotropic factor involved in the regulation of both innate and acquired immune responses, playing a key role in autoimmune, inflammatory and infectious diseases. Following stimulation by IL18, NK cells and selected T cells release IF-γ that plays a significant role in activating macrophages and other cells. The combination of IL18 with IL12 inhibits IL4-dependent IgE and IgG1 synthesis and facilitates IgG2a production by B cells. IL18 binding protein (IL18BP) binds specifically with the cytokine to negatively regulate its biological activity. With IL12, IL18 stimulates Th1-mediated immune responses critical for host defense against infection with intracellular microbes through the induction of IFN-γ. IL18 is a potent proinflammatory cytokine, since overproduction of IL12 and IL18 induces severe inflammatory disorders. IL18 enhances IL12-driven Th1 immune responses, but it can also stimulate Th2 immune responses in the absence of IL12.

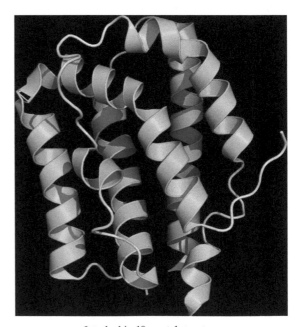

Interleukin-19 crystal structure.

interleukin-19 (IL19)

A novel homolog of IL10, with which it shares 21% amino acid identity and thus belongs to the IL10 family along with IL20, IL22, IL24, IL26, and several virus-encoded cytokines. The expression of IL19mRMA can be induced in monocytes by LPS treatment. GM-CSF can directly induce IL19 gene expression by monocytes. IL19 shares a receptor complex with IL20, indicating that the biological

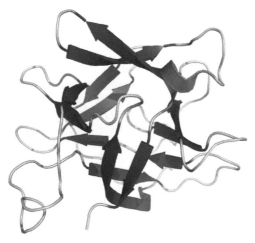

Interleukin-18.

activities of these two cytokines overlap and that both may play important roles in regulating development and proper functioning of the skin. In contrast to IL10, which forms an intercalated dimer, the IL19 molecule is a monomer comprised of seven amphipathic helices designated A through G, creating a unique helical bundle.

interleukin-20 (IL20)

A member of the IL10 cytokine family. Its overexpression in transgenic mice causes neonatal lethality with skin abnormalities that include aberrant epidermal differentiation. It is synthesized by activated keratinocytes and monocytes, and mediates an intracellular signal through two distinct cell surface receptor complexes on keratinocytes and other epithelial cells. Recombinant IL20 protein stimulates a signal transduction pathway through STAT3 in a keratinocyte line. An IL20 receptor was identified as a heterodimer to orphan class II cytokine receptor subunits. Both receptor subunits are expressed in skin and are significantly upregulated in psoriatic skin. IL20 regulates proliferation and differentiation of keratinocytes during inflammation, especially that associated with the skin. It also induces expansion of multi-potential hematopoietic progenitor cells.

interleukin-21 (IL21)

A cytokine most closely related to IL2 and IL15. It exerts powerful regulatory effects on immune system cells including natural-killer (NK) and cytotoxic T cells that can fatally injure virally infected or tumor cells. IL21 activates cell division and/or proliferation of its target cells. Its action on immune system cells is through its cell surface receptor, IL21R, expressed on bone marrow cells and lymphocytes. *In vitro* assays suggest that IL21 plays a role in proliferation and maturation of NK cell populations from the bone marrow and in the proliferation of mature B cell populations, costimulating with anti-CD40 and in the proliferation of T cells, costimulating with anti-CD3.

interleukin-22 (IL22)

A human cytokine distantly related to IL10 and produced by activated T cells. It was previously called IL10-related

T cell-derived inducible factor (IL-TIF). It is a ligand for CRFs 2 through 4 and a member of the class II cytokine receptor family. Human IL-TIF activates the transcription factors STAT1 and STAT3 in selected hepatoma cell lines and upregulates synthesis of acute phase proteins including serum amyloid A, 1-antichymotrypsin, and haptoglobin in HepG2 human hepatoma cells. IL22 signals through the interferon receptor-related proteins CFT2 through 4 and IL22R. IL22 does not bind the IL10 receptor. In contrast to IL10, IL22 does not inhibit the synthesis of proinflammatory cytokines by monocytes in response to lipopolysaccharide (LPS), nor does it affect IL10 function on monocytes. It exerts a modest inhibitory effect on IL4 synthesis by Th2 T cells.

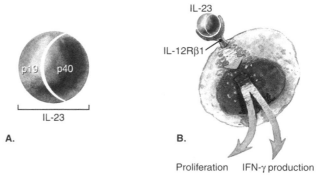

(A) IL-23 is a biologically active cytokine composed of two subunits: p19 and the p40 subunit of IL-12. (B) IL-23 binds specifically to the IL-12Rβ₁ subunit and can stimulate IFN-γ production and proliferation in PHA blast T cells and activated CD45RO (memory) T cells.

interleukin-23 (IL23)

A heterodimeric cytokine comprised of two parts, the p40 subunit of IL12 with a different p19 subunit (the IL23α subunit). It is produced predominantly by macrophages and dendritic cells and shows activity on memory T cells. It may also affect macrophage function directly. It has a significant role in the inflammatory response to infection and promotes upregulation of the MMP9 matrix metalloprotease, increases angiogenesis and diminishes CD8⁺ T cell infiltration. It has been implicated in the development of malignant neoplasms. IL23 along with IL6 and TGF-β1 induces naïve CD4⁺ T cells to differentiate into Th17 cells that are distinct from classical Th1 and Th2 cells. Th17 cells synthesize IL17, a proinflammatory cytokine that promotes T cell priming and stimulates synthesis of proinflammatory molecules that include IL1, IL6, TNF-α, NOS-2, and chemokines leading to inflammation. Knockout mice deficient in p40 or p19 or in one of the IL23 receptor subunits reveal milder symptoms of multiple sclerosis and inflammatory bowel disease, pointing to the significance of IL23 in the inflammatory pathway.

interleukin-24 (IL24)

A member of the IL10 family of cytokines that signals through two heterodimeric receptors: IL20R1/IL20R2 and IL22R1/IL20R2. Based on its role as a tumor suppressing protein, it is also known as melanoma differentiation-associated 7 (mda-7). It controls cell survival and proliferation by initiating rapid activation of the transcription factors designated STAT1 and STAT3. It is synthesized by activated

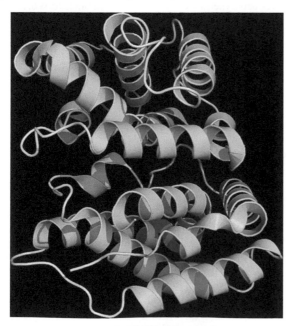

Interleukin-22.

monocytes, macrophages, and Th2 cells. Other sources include melanocytes, breast epithelium, fibroblasts (rat), monocytes, vascular and smooth muscle, NK, B, and naïve T cells. It acts on nonhematopoietic tissues including skin, lung, and reproductive tissues. It has important functions in wound healing, psoriasis, and cancer. It is also involved in megakaryocyte differentiation, induces apoptosis of human breast tumor cells, and induces IL6 and TNF-α formation by monocytes. It shares receptors with IL20 and IL19. The IL24 gene is present on chromosome 1 in humans.

interleukin-25 (IL25)

A member of the IL17 cytokine family secreted by Th2 helper T cells and mast cells. It is also called IL17E. It facilitates the synthesis of other cytokines such as IL4, IL5, and IL13 in numerous tissues that induce the expansion of eosinophils. Lineage-negative cells with high MHC class II levels are targets of IL25. It supports proliferation of lymphocytes, signature Th2 effects: induces serum IgG1 and IgE, increases eosinophil production and inflammation and mediates its effects through the induction of IL4, IL5 and IL13. It is significant in controlling gut immunity and has been implicated in chronic inflammation of the GI tract. The IL25 gene is in a chromosomal region associated with autoimmune diseases of the GI tract, including inflammatory bowel disease, even though it has not been shown to play a role in this disorder. Its receptor is the thymic-shared antigen TSA-1.

interleukin-26 (IL26)

A 171-amino acid protein and member of the IL10 family of cytokines. It was previously called AK155 and is composed of a signal sequence, six helices, and four conserved cysteine residues. It is expressed in selected herpesvirus-transformed T cells but not in primary stimulated T cells. Cell sources include CD4, CD45RO T cells, NK cells, and Th1 cells. It signals through a receptor complex consisting of IL20 receptor 1 and IL10 receptor 2. Signaling through this pathway permits the rapid phosphorylation of transcription factors STAT1 and STAT3, thus enhancing IL10 and IL8 secretion, and facilitates CD54 expression on epithelial cell surfaces. The target of IL26 action is the epithelial cell.

interleukin 27 (IL27)

A heterodimeric cytokine of the IL12 family composed of two subunits, Epstein–Barr virus (EBV)-induced gene 3 (EBI3, also known as IL27B) and IL27-p28 (also termed IL28). Mature dendritic cells serve as sources of IL17. Its targets are NK cells and naïve CD4$^+$ T cells. It induces proliferation of naïve, but not memory, CD4$^+$ T cells and serves as an initial activator of Th1 responses (induces T-bet; downregulates GATA-3). Its effects are listed by its interaction with a specific cell surface receptor complex comprised of IL27R and gp130. The gene symbol of IL27 refers to its IL30 subunit. WSX-1/T cell cytokine receptor (TCCR) and gp130 are receptors for IL27.

interleukin 28 (IL28)

A cytokine that exists in two isoforms: IL28A and IL28B. It has a significant role in immune defense against viruses. The isoforms are members of the type III interferon cytokine family and closely resemble IL29 in amino acid sequence. IL28 genes are positioned near IL29 on chromosome 19 in humans.

interleukin 28A (IL28A)

Also called IFN-λ2, related to IL10 and type I IFNs. Produced by plasmacytoid dendritic cells, induced by virus infection or double-stranded RNA. Most tissues except brain and spinal cord serve as targets. It has antiviral activity, inhibiting replication of the hepatitis B and C viruses; induces oligoadenylate synthetase and MxA; and upregulates class I MHC. It shares a receptor with IL28B and IL29, IL28Rα/IFN-λR1, and IL10Rβ.

interleukin-28B (IL28B)

Also known as IFN-λ3 and related to IL10 and type I IFNs. It is synthesized by plasmacytoid dendritic cells, induced by virus infection of dsRNA. Most tissues except brain and spinal cord serve as targets. It exerts antiviral activity, inhibiting replication of hepatitis B and C viruses; induces oligoadenylate synthetase and MxA; and upregulates class I MHC. It shares a receptor with IL28A and IL29, IL28Rα/IFN-λR1, and IL10Rβ.

interleukin-29 (IL29)

A helical cytokine family member and type III interferon, also called IFN-λ1. Related to IL10 and type I IFNs. Produced by plasmacytoid dendritic cells, induced by virus infection or dsRNA. Most tissues other than brain and spinal cord serve as targets. It has antiviral activity (inhibits replication of hepatitis B and C viruses); induces oligoadenylate synthetase and MxA; and upregulates class I MHC. It has an amino acid sequence similar to those of IL28 and other type III interferons. It plays a significant role in host defense against microorganisms and its gene is highly upregulated in virus infected cells. The IL29 gene is positioned on chromosome 19 in humans. It shares a receptor with IL28A and IL28B, IL28Rα/IFN-λR1, and IL10Rβ.

interleukin-30 (IL30)

A 28-kDa protein that comprises one chain of the heterodimeric cytokine known as IL27. Thus IL30 is also called IL27-p28. The other chain of IL27 is termed an Epstein–Barr-induced gene 3 (EBI3). It is a member of the long chain, four-helix bundle cytokine family; this explains its structural similarity to IL6. IL27 triggers expansion of antigen-specific naïve CD4$^+$ T cells and facilitates development of a Th1 phenotype with expression of interferon-γ. IL27 acts synergistically with IL12 and binds to WSX1. The IL30 gene is designated *IL27* under HGNC rules.

interleukin-31 (IL31)

A cytokine with a four-helix bundle structure, synthesized by type 2 helper T (Th2) cells. It is structurally similar to IL6 cytokines. It signals via a receptor complex comprised of IL31 receptor A (IL31RA) and oncostatin M receptor subunits that are expressed by activated monocytes and unstimulated epithelial cells. IL31 is believed to have a role in skin inflammation.

interleukin-32 (IL32)

A cytokine that induces the secretion of tumor necrosis factor-α (TNF-α) by immune system cells including monocytes and macrophages in addition to chemokines such as IL8 and MIP-2/CXCL2. IL32 induces various cytokines, human TNF-α, and IL8 in THP-1 monocytic cells, as well as mouse TNF-α and MIP-2 in raw macrophages. It activates typical cytokine signal pathways of nuclear factor-κ B (NF-κB) and p38 mitogen-activated protein kinase. Induced in human peripheral lymphocytes after mitogen stimulation, in human epithelial cells by IFN-γ and in NK cells after exposure to IL12 plus IL18, IL32 is believed to play a role in inflammatory and autoimmune diseases.

interleukin-33 (IL33)

An IL1-like cytokine that signals via the IL1 receptor-related protein ST 2 and induces T helper type II-associated cytokines. IL33 also activates NF-κB and MAP kinases. *In vivo*, it induces the expression of IL4, IL5, and IL13 and leads to severe pathological changes in mucosal organs.

interleukin-34 (IL34; FPT025)

A 242-amino acid cytokine secreted with signal peptide. It has no sequence homology to known cytokines or other genes. Human primary monocytes are target cells of this cytokine. It activates ERK1/2 phosphorylation in monocytic THP-1 in the Th1 cell line. IL34 is expressed in human spleen, skin, brain, and other tissues. It promoted formation of myeloid lineage colonies (CFU-M) in a human bone marrow formation assay, and enhanced proliferation of cells with myeloid cell surface markers from human monocytes. IL34 functions as a novel ligand of the CSF-1 receptor and participates in the regulation of myeloid lineage differentiation, proliferation, and survival.

intermediate filaments

Lineage-specific 7- to 11-nm diameter intracellular filaments observed by electron microscopy. They are intermediate in size between actin microfilaments (6-nm diameters) and microtubules (25-nm diameters). They are detected in cell and tissue preparations by monoclonal antibodies specific for the filaments and are identified by the immunoperoxidase method. The detection of various types of intermediate filaments in tumors is of great assistance in determining the histogenetic origins of many types of neoplasms.

intermolecular epitope spreading

A phenomenon in which the immune response is first directed against a single antigenic molecular epitope and then responds to epitopes on different proteins.

internal image

According to the Jerne network theory, antibodies are produced against the antibodies induced by an external antigen. Some of the antiantibodies produced will bear idiotopes that precisely fit the paratope or antigen-binding site of the original antibody against the external antigen. Because the antibody bears close structural similarity to the epitope on the antigen molecule that was originally administered, it serves as the internal image of the antigen and thus acquired the name.

international unit of immunological activity

The use of an international reference standard of a biological preparation of antiserum or antigen of a precise weight and strength. The potencies or strengths of biological preparations such as antitoxins, vaccines, and test antigens derived from microbial products and antibody preparations may be compared against such standards.

interstitial dendritic cells

Dendritic cells found in most organs such as heart, lungs, liver, kidney, and gastrointestinal tract.

interstitial fluid

Fluid present in the spaces between cells of an organ or tissue.

interstitial nephritis

Inflammation characterized by mononuclear cell (lymphocytic) infiltrate in the interstitia surrounding renal tubules following autoantibody reaction with tubular basement membranes in the kidneys. Other etiologies include analgesic abuse.

intervening sequence

Refer to intron.

intestinal cryptopatches

Tiny areas of lymphoid tissue in the lamina propria of the small intestinal crypts that represent sites of extrathymic lymphopoiesis.

intestinal follicles

Lymphoid follicles present in the lamina propria of the intestine as Peyer's patches, in the appendix, or scattered individually. A follicle consists of a germinal center comprised of B cells and follicular dendritic cells covered by a dome of dendritic cells, macrophages, CD4+ T cells, regulatory T cells, and mature B cells. Follicles are encircled by CD4+ Th and CD8+ T cells.

intestinal lymphangiectasia

Escape of immunoglobulins and other proteins and lymphocytes into the intestinal tract as a consequence of lymphatic dilation in the intestinal villi. The loss of immunoglobulin leads to secondary immunodeficiency. In addition to primary intestinal telangiectasia, obstruction of lymphatic drainage of the intestine produced by a lymphoma represents a secondary type.

intimin

A bacterial membrane protein expressed on enteropathogenic *Escherichia coli* that can bind to both $\alpha_{4\beta1}$ and $\alpha_{4\beta7}$ integrins.

intolerance

Adverse reactivity following administration of normal doses of a drug.

intrabody

Intracellular antibody that binds the key targets to inhibit tumor growth. It is postulated that this may be accomplished by gene therapy. Intrabodies can be expressed within mammalian cells in precise locations by modifying intrabody genes (in scFv or Fab format) with sequence-encoding classical intracellular trafficking signals.

intracellular antigen

Endogenous antigen.

intracellular bacterium

A bacterium that survives or replicates in the endosomes of cells. Cell-mediated immunity is the main defense against these intracellular microorganisms.

intracellular cytokine staining

The use of fluorescent-labeled anticytokine antibodies to stain permeabilized cells that synthesize the cytokine in question.

intracellular immunization

Interference with wild-type virus replication by a dominant, negative, mutant, viral gene. The action has been suggested to be of possible use in protecting cells against HIV-1 infection because of the easy accessibility of CD4+ cells. By using *tat*, *gag*, and *rev* mutant genes and a mutant CD4 cell that bears the KDEL sequence, HIV envelope protein transport to the cell surfaces is inhibited.

intracellular pathogens

Microorganisms, including viruses and bacteria, that grow within cells.

intracellular signaling pathway

The mechanism whereby ligand binding to its cell surface receptor ultimately activates new gene expression patterns in the cell nucleus. Interaction between ligand and receptor activates a sequence of interactions among proteins, including enzymes and adaptors, leading to activation of transcription factors with access to the nucleus where they change transcription patterns of genes governing cellular proliferation, differentiation, and effector functions.

intraepidermal lymphocytes

Primarily CD8⁺ T cells within the epidermis. Murine intraepidermal lymphocytes express mainly the γδ receptor. It is believed that these cells have a more restricted repertoire of antigen receptors than those homing to extracutaneous sites. Most skin-associated lymphocytes are found in the dermis, with only about 2% in the epidermis. Intraepidermal lymphocytes express CLA-1, which may play a role in homing.

intraepithelial lymphocytes (IELs)

Lymphocytes present in the intestinal epithelium or other specialized epithelial layer. αβ and γδ lymphocytes resident in the intestinal epithelium or specialized layer tend to congregate in the epithelium as intestinal IELs, and iIELs, and in superior layers of the skin as dendritic epidermal T cells. Intraepithelial NK cells may also be present.

intraepithelial pocket

An invagination within the follicle-associated epithelium produced by infolding of an M cell basolateral surface. Comprises CD4⁺ memory T cell subpopulations, naïve B cells, dendritic cells, and macrophages. Enables interaction with antigens conveyed through M cells by transcytosis.

intraepithelial T lymphocytes

T lymphocytes present in the epidermis and in the mucosal epithelial layer. They characteristically manifest a limited diversity of antigen receptors. They may identify glycolipids from microbes, associated with nonpolymorphic major histocompatibility complex (MHC) class I-like molecules. They can function as effector cells of innate immunity and facilitate host defense by secreting cytokines, activating phagocytes, and destroying infected cells.

intramolecular epitope spreading

A mechanism whereby the immune response is first directed against epitopes in one area of an antigenic molecule and then responds to additional, non-crossreactive epitopes on the same molecule.

intrathecal chemotherapy

The administration of a chemotherapeutic drug beneath the spinal cord's protective sheath.

intravenous immune globulin (IVIG)

An immunoglobulin preparation comprised principally of immunoglobulin G (IgG) derived from the blood plasma of about 1000 donors. This preparation may be effective against hepatitis A and B, cytomegalovirus, rubella, varicella zoster, tetanus, and various other agents. IVIG is administered to children with common variable immunodeficiency, X-linked agammaglobulinemia, and other defects of the antibody limb of the immune system. Although acquired immune deficiency syndrome (AIDS) is a CD4⁺ T cell defect, IVIG may help to protect against microbial infection in HIV-I-infected children. It may also be effective in autoimmune or idiopathic thrombocytopenia, autoimmune neutropenia, or Kawasaki's disease. IVIG may induce anaphylactic reactions and fever, headaches, muscle aches, and cardiovascular effects on blood pressure and heart rate.

intrinsic affinity

Synonym for intrinsic association constant.

intrinsic apoptotic pathway

A means whereby mammalian cell apoptosis is initiated by inducing alterations in the mitochondrial membrane leading to the release of cytochrome c, which interacts with caspase-9 and Apaf-1 in the apoptosome, which activates the caspase-3 cascade.

intrinsic association constant

The association constant that describes univalent ligand binding to a special site on a protein macromolecule if all sites of this type are identical and noninteracting when found on the same molecule. Equilibrium dialysis and other techniques that determine bound and free ligand concentration evaluate the intrinsic association constant.

intrinsic asthma

Nonallergic or idiopathic asthma that usually occurs first during adulthood and follows a respiratory infection. Patients experience chronic or recurrent obstruction of bronchi associated with exposure to pollen or other allergens. This is in marked contrast to patients with extrinsic (allergic) asthma mediated by immune (IgE) mechanisms in the bronchi. Intrinsic asthma patients have negative skin tests to ordinary allergens when the IgE contents of their sera are normal. They manifest eosinophilia. There is no family history of atopic diseases.

intrinsic factor

A glycoprotein produced by parietal cells of the gastric mucosa required for vitamin B₁₂ absorption. A lack of intrinsic factor leads to vitamin B₁₂ deficiency and pernicious anemia.

intrinsic factor antibodies

Antibodies found in three fourths of pernicious anemia patients that are specific for either the binding site (type I or blocking antibodies) or some other intrinsic factor antigenic determinant (type II antibodies).

intron

Structural gene segment not transcribed into RNA. Introns have no known function and are believed to be derived from "junk" DNA.

inulin

A homopolysaccharide of d-fructose found in selected plants such as dahlias. Although it is used to measure renal clearance, soluble inulin is known to activate the alternative complement pathway.

Inv

Former designation for human κ light polypeptide chain allotype; allotypic epitopes in the immunoglobulin κ light chain constant region. Km replaced Inv.

Inv allotype

Early terminology for Km allotype; Km is now the preferred nomenclature.

Inv allotypic determinant

Refer to Km allotypic determinant.

Inv marker

Refer to Km allotypic determinant.

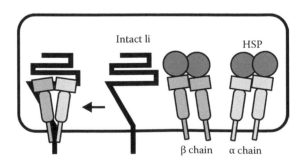

Invariant chain promotes assembly of class II heterodimers from free chains.

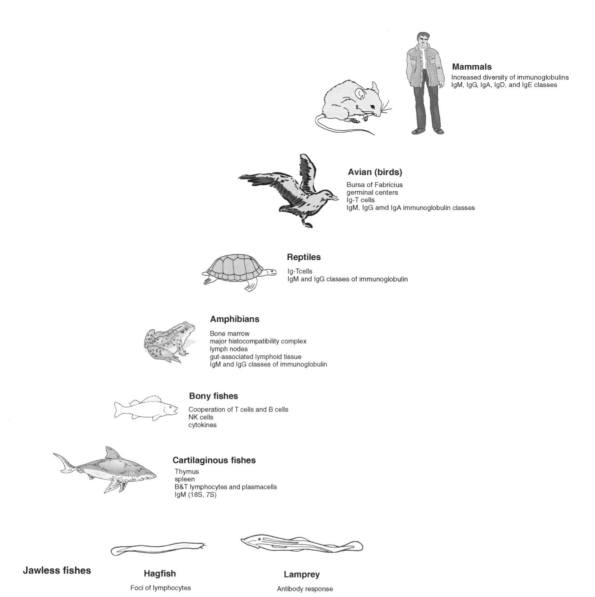

VERTEBRATES

Mammals
Increased diversity of immunoglobulins
IgM, IgG, IgA, IgD, and IgE classes

Avian (birds)
Bursa of Fabricius
germinal centers
Ig-T cells
IgM, IgG amd IgA immunoglobulin classes

Reptiles
Ig-Tcells
IgM and IgG classes of immunoglobulin

Amphibians
Bone marrow
major histocompatibility complex
lymph nodes
gut-associated lymphoid tissue
IgM and IgG classes of immunoglobulin

Bony fishes
Cooperation of T cells and B cells
NK cells
cytokines

Cartilaginous fishes
Thymus
spleen
B&T lymphocytes and plasmacells
IgM (18S, 7S)

Jawless fishes

Hagfish
Foci of lymphocytes

Lamprey
Antibody response

INVERTEBRATES

Coelomate

Multicellular

Unicellular

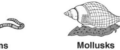

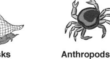

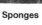

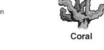

Worms
Specialized cells
opsonins
lysins
agglutinins

Mollusks
Lack of graft rejection

Anthropods
Alternative
complement pathway

Tunicates
Stem cells
MHC
lymphocytes

Echinoderms
Phagocytic cells
memory of graft rejection
cytokines
agglutinins

Self recognition
Specific aggregation

Sponges

Recognition of nonself
graft rejection

Coral

Phagocytosis

Protozoa

Enzymes

Bacteria

Evolution of immunity.

invariant (Ii) chain

A nonpolymorphic, 31-kDa glycoprotein that associates with class II histocompatibility molecules in the endoplasmic reticulum. It inhibits the linking of endogenous peptides with the class II molecule, conveying it to appropriate intracellular compartments. Truncation of the invariant chain stimulates a second signal that may function in the *trans*-Golgi network prior to the conveyance of major histocompatibility complex (MHC) class II molecules to cell surfaces. It directs the MHC class II molecules to endosomes where Ii is degraded, permitting MHC class II molecules to bind peptides in the endosomes. The Ii chain stabilizes the class II molecule before it acquires an antigenic peptide.

invasin

A membrane protein derived from *Yersina pseudotuberculosis* that binds to $\alpha_{4\beta1}$ integrins and has the capacity to induce T cell costimulatory signals.

invasive pathogen

A pathogenic microorganism that successfully gains access to the body even though defense mechanisms are intact.

invasive tumor

A neoplasm capable of accessing and obliterating healthy architectures of adjacent organs.

inversional joining

An event that takes place during V(D)J recombination when the two gene segments to be united are in the opposite transcriptional orientation.

invertebrate immunity

Invertebrates have various mechanisms to recognize and respond to nonself substances even though they lack lymphoid immune systems. They possess both cellular and humoral components that mediate immune-like responses. Invertebrate internal defense responses include phagocytosis, encapsulation, and nodule formation. The molecular recognition and effector mechanisms among species are diverse. Some of the factors involved include α_2 macroglobulins, C-reactive proteins, antibacterial peptides, serine proteinases and proteinase inhibitors, C-type lectins and complement-related factors, glucan-binding proteins, and some antibacterial peptides. Alloaggressive responses have been observed in noncolonial invertebrates. Invertebrates form certain members of the immunoglobulin superfamily such as adhesion molecules and receptors for tyrosine kinases. Within the immunoglobulin superfamily, only hemolin, a protein isolated from lepidopterans, is induced following bacterial challenge. Hemolin has four immunoglobulin-like domains whose primary structures more closely resemble cell adhesion molecules than immunoglobulins. With respect to invertebrate effector molecules, antibacterial peptides are classified into several families that include lysozymes, cecropins, sapecins or insect defensins, and attacin-like and proline-rich antibacterial peptides. Invertebrates have cascades of endogenous serine proteinases that are important in defense. Cytokine-like activity, possibly mediated by factors equivalent to IL1 and IL6, has been recognized. Receptors have also been identified on phagocytic cells. Thus, invertebrate cytokine-like factors may play a role in the regulation of nonspecific responses to tissue injury and infection. Opioid peptides, opiate alkaloids, and other neuropeptides may modulate chemotaxis and cell adhesion.

invertebrates

Animals without backbones.

inverted repeat

Complementary sequence segments on a single strand of DNA. A palindrome when the halves of an inverted repeat are placed side by side.

in vitro ("in glass")

Investigations with living cells or cellular components performed outside the bodies of intact organisms. The investigations are performed in tissue culture plates or test tubes.

in vivo ("in life")

Investigations performed in intact living organisms.

ion exchange chromatography

A method that permits the separation of proteins in a solution, taking advantage of their net charge differences. It involves the electrostatic binding of proteins onto a charged resin suspended in a buffer and packed into a column. Because serum protein charges vary, binding to or elution from the column is possible by gradually increasing or decreasing the salt concentration (with or without changes in pH). This affects the types of proteins binding to the resin. With buffers of low molarity and pH >6.5, the immunoglobulin G (IgG) in solution is not adsorbed on the column and passes through with the first buffer volume.

ionic bonds

Electrostatic bonds.

$$-NH_3 \quad OOC-$$

Electrostatic forces.

ionic (or Coulombic) forces

Forces resulting from the interactions of oppositely charged ionic groups on antigen and antibody molecules. Based on Coulomb's equation:

$$F = \frac{Q^+Q^-}{\varepsilon r^2}$$

where ε is the dielectric constant of the medium, Q^+ and Q^- are the positive and negative charges in electrostatic units, respectively, and r is the distance between the centers of the charged sites, the Coulombic force of attraction is inversely proportional to the square of the distances between antigen and antibody.

IP-10

Interferon γ (IFN-γ)-inducible protein 10. A chemokine of the α (CXC) family. IP-10 is a gene product following stimulation of cells within IFN-γ. It does not posses the ELR motif that determines the biological significance of a particular α chemokine. IP-10 has an angiostatic potential, which is opposite to the angiogenic effect of other ELR-containing α chemokines. This potential renders IP-10 a unique α chemokine family member. Tissue sources include endothelial cells, monocytes, fibroblasts, and keratinocytes. High levels of IP-10 transcripts are present in lymphoid organs. Monocytes, progenitor cells, and natural killer cells serve as targets.

IPEX

Abbreviation for immunodysregulation, polyendocrinopathy, enteropathy X-linked (IPEX) syndrome.

Ir genes

Immune response (Ir) genes. Major histocompatibility complex (MHC) class II genes that control immune responses are found in the Ir region. These genes govern the ability of an animal to respond immunologically to any particular antigen. Ir genes encode polymorphic MHC molecules that bind peptides needed for T cell activation and are also necessary for helper T cell-dependent B cell antibody responsiveness to protein antigens.

iridovirus immunity

Insect immunity against this virus consists mainly of cellular responses including phagocytosis, encapsulation, nodule formation, and coagulation to recognize foreignness. Attacin, cecropins, lysozyme, and phenol oxidase occur in various dipteran and lepidopteran species. These inducible agents may play a toxic role in the defense mechanism. Only nonspecific immunity not associated with antigen antibody reactions or complement or interferon occurs.

iron and immunity

Iron has two effects on immune function. Micronutrients such as iron are redistributed in the body during infection. Dietary iron deficiency produces iron deficiency anemia and decreases immunocompetence. Both iron deficiency and iron excess compromise the immune system.

irradiation chimera

An animal or human whose lymphoid and myeloid tissues have been destroyed by lethal irradiation and successfully repopulated with donor bone marrow cells that are genetically different.

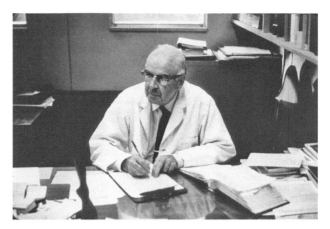

M.R. Irwin.

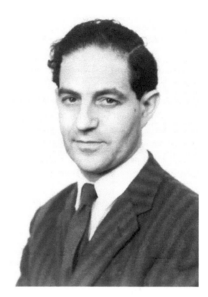

Alick Isaacs.

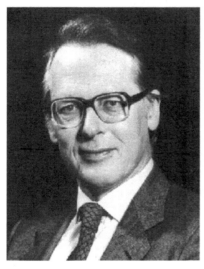

J. Irvine.

Irvine, J.

British authority on autoimmune diseases.

Irwin, M.R.

A professor at the University of Wisconsin, Madison, who first used the term *immunogenetics* in 1933 to describe an uncertain association between immunology and genetics.

Isaacs, Alick

An investigator who, with Jean Lindenmann, discovered a substance they named *interferon*. They were studying the phenomenon of viral interference, i.e., the resistance shown by cells infected by one virus to simultaneous infection by another. In their experiments, chick cells infected with influenza viruses were resistant to infection with other viruses.

ischemia

Deficient blood supply to a tissue as a consequence of vascular obstruction.

ISCOMs

Immune stimulatory complexes of antigen bound in a matrix of lipid that serves as an adjuvant and facilitates

uptake of antigen into the cytoplasm of a cell following plasma membrane–lipid fusion. One example is a vaccine composed of a pathogen antigen combined with cholesterol, phospholipid, and saponin to yield a soccer ball-shaped configuration bearing a strong negative charge. Frequently, the vaccine antigen is amphipathic protein.

Ishizaka, Kimishige (1925–) and Terako

Discovered immunoglobulin E (IgE) and contributed to elucidation of its function.

islet cell autoantibodies (ICAs)

Autoantibodies specific for the β cells of the pancreatic islets. They are found in 80% of newly diagnosed cases of insulin-dependent diabetes mellitus (IDDM) by indirect immunofluorescence on frozen sections of human pancreas. Individuals with high titers of persistent ICAs are more likely to have IDDM than those with fluctuating ICAs. Half of relatives with a single positive ICA assay and 60 to 80% of relatives with both ICA and insulin autoantibodies (IAAs) will develop IDDM within 10 years. Strong persistently positive ICAs (>40 JDF-U) are the best predictors of subsequent onset of IDDM, especially if insulin secretion is greatly diminished. ICAs are found in 31% of women who develop gestational diabetes mellitus.

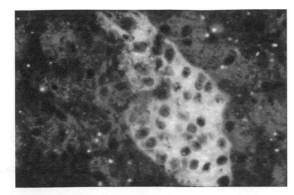

Islet cell autoantibodies

islet cell transplantation

An experimental method aimed at treatment of type I diabetes mellitus. The technique has been successful in rats, but less so in humans. It requires sufficient functioning islets (from a minimum of two cadaveric donors) that have been purified, cultured, and shown to produce insulin. The islet cells are administered into the portal vein. The liver serves as the host organ in the recipient, who is treated with FK506 or other immunosuppressant drugs.

islets of Langerhans

Groups of endocrine cells within the exocrine pancreas that consist of α cells that secrete glucagon, β cells that secrete insulin, and δ cells that secrete somatostatin.

isoagglutinin

An alloantibody present in some individuals of a species; isoagglutinin is capable of agglutinating cells of other members of the same species.

isoallergens

Allergenic determinants with similar size, amino acid composition, peptide fingerprint, and other characteristics. They are present as a group but each one can individually to sensitize a susceptible subject. They are molecular variants of the same allergen.

isoallotypic determinant (nonmarker)

An antigenic determinant present as an allelic variant on one immunoglobulin class or subclass heavy chain that occurs on every molecule of a different immunoglobulin class or subclass heavy chain.

isoantibody

An antibody specific for an antigen present in other members of the species in which it occurs; thus, it is an antibody against an isoantigen. Also called alloantibody.

isoantigen

An antigen found in a member of a species that induces an immune response if injected into a genetically dissimilar member of the same species. These antigens carry identical determinants in a given individual. Isoantigens of two individuals may or may not have identical determinants. In the latter case, they are allogeneic with respect to each other and are called alloantigens. Because the individual red blood cell antigens have the same molecular structures and are identical in different individuals, they were in the past called isoantigens. This is a descriptive term only and should not be used, because two individuals may be allogeneic by virtue of the assortment of the antigens present on their red blood cells. An isoantigen is an antigen of an isograft.

isoelectric focusing (IEF)

An electrophoretic method to fractionate amphoteric molecules, especially proteins, according to their distribution in a pH gradient in an electric field created across the gradient. Molecular distribution is according to isoelectric pH values. The anode repels positively charged proteins and the cathode repels negatively charged proteins. Thus, each protein migrates in the pH gradient and bands at a position where the gradient pH is equivalent to the isoelectric pH of the protein. A chromatographic column is used to prepare a pH gradient by the electrolysis of amphoteric substances.

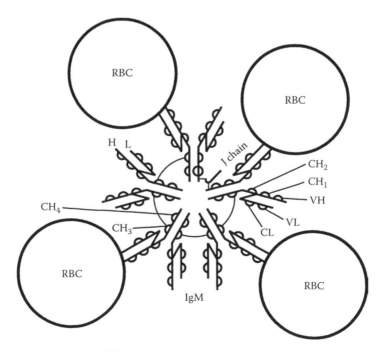

Agglutination of human RBCs by the natural isohemagglutinins in serum (antibodies of IgM class).

A density gradient or a gel is used to stabilize the pH gradient. Proteins or peptides focus into distinct bands at the parts of the gradient that are equivalent to their isoelectric points. Isoelectric focusing permits the separation of protein substances on the basis of their isoelectric characteristics. Thus, it can be used to define heterogeneous antibodies and also to purify homogeneous immunoglobulins from heterogeneous pools of antibody.

isoelectric point (pI)

The pH at which a molecule has no charge—the number of positive and negative charges is equal. At isoelectric pH, a molecule does not migrate in an electric field. The solubility of most substances is minimal at their isoelectric points.

isoforms

Different versions of a protein encoded by alleles of a gene or by different but closely related genes.

isogeneic (isogenic)

Implying genetic identity, e.g., identical twins. Although used as a synonym for syngeneic when referring to a genetic relationship between members of an inbred strain (of mice), the inbred animals never show the absolute dentity (identical genotypes) observed in identical twins.

isograft

A tissue transplant from a donor to an isogeneic recipient. Grafts exchanged between members of an inbred strain of laboratory animals such as mice are syngeneic rather than isogeneic.

isohemagglutinins

Naturally occurring immunoglobulin M (IgM) antibodies in some members of a species that recognize erythrocyte isoantigens on the surfaces of red blood cells from other members of the same species. In the ABO blood group system, the anti-A antibodies in the sera of group B individuals and the anti-B antibodies in the sera of group A individuals are examples of isohemagglutinins. They may be formed as a result of immunization by bacteria in the gastrointestinal and respiratory tracts.

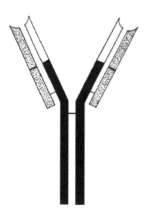

IgG showing the isotype, designated in black, is determined by the heavy chain.

isoimmunization

An immune response induced in the recipient of a blood transfusion in which the donor red blood cells express isoantigens not present in the recipient. The term also refers to maternal immunization by fetal red blood cells bearing isoantigens the mother does not possess.

isoleukoagglutinins

Antibodies in the sera of multiparous females and patients receiving multiple blood transfusions that recognize surface isoantigens of leukocytes and lead to their agglutination.

isologous

Derived from the same species; also called isogeneic or syngeneic.

isophile antibody

An antibody induced by and specifically reactive with erythrocytes but not reactive with other species' red blood cells. These antibodies are against antigens of red blood cells unique to the species from which they were derived.

isophile antigen

Antigen that is species-specific; often refers to erythrocyte antigens.

isoproterenol

Its chemical name is dl-β-[3,4-dihydroxyphenyl]-α-isopropylaminoethanol; a β-adrenergic amine used to treat patients with asthma. It relaxes the bronchial smooth muscle constriction that occurs in asthmatics.

isoschizomer

One of several restriction endonucleases derived from different organisms that identify the same DNA base sequence for cleavage but do not always cleave DNA at the same location in the sequence. Target sequence methylation affects the actions of isoschizomers that are valuable in investigations of DNA methylation.

isotope

An isotypic determinant or epitope of an isotype.

isotopic (radionuclide) labeling

The introduction of a radioactive isotope into a molecule via external labeling through tagging molecules with ^{125}I or another appropriate isotope or by internal labeling in which ^{14}C- or ^{3}H-labeled amino acids are added to tissue culture, allowing cells to incorporate the isotope. Once labeled, molecules can be easily traced and their fate monitored by measuring radioactivity.

isotypes

Antigens that determine the class or subclass of heavy chains or the type and subtype of light chains of immunoglobulin molecules, based on the amino sequences of their constant regions. Mice and humans have five different Ig heavy chain constant regions, $C\mu$, $C\delta$, $C\alpha$, $C\gamma$, and $C\epsilon$, that define the five antibody isotypes IgM, IgD, IgA, IgG and IgE, respectively. Every normal member of a species expresses each isotype. Immunoglobulin subtypes are found in all normal individuals. Among the immunoglobulin classes, immunoglobulin G (IgG) and IgA have subclasses designated by Arabic numerals. They are distinguished according to domain number and size and also the number of intrachain and interchain disulfide bonds in the constant region. The four isotypes of IgG are designated IgG_1, IgG_2, IgG_3, and IgG_4. The two IgA isotypes are designated IgA_1 and IgA_2. Each of the μ, δ, and ϵ heavy chains and the κ and λ light chains has one isotype. Immunoglobulin isotypes are responsible for the biological effector functions of an antibody molecule. IgM, IgG, IgD, IgA, and IgE that differ in heavy chain constant regions constitute antibody classes or isotypes. Light chain isotypes are defined by either a κ light chain constant region ($C\kappa$) or one of several λ light chain constant regions ($C\lambda$).

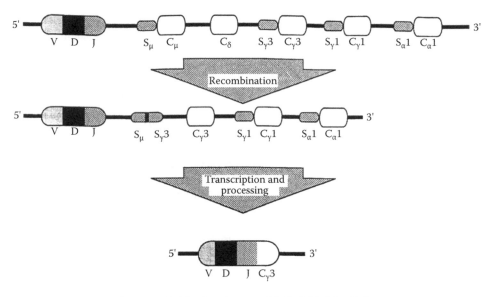

Isotype switching from immunoglobulin M (IgM) to IgG.

isotype switching

The mechanism whereby a cell changes from synthesizing a heavy polypeptide chain of one isotype to that of another, as from μ chain to γ chain formation in B cells that received switch signals from T cells. Refer also to switch region and switch site. Antigenic specificity remains the same during isotype switching that involves joining a rearranged *VDJ* gene unit to a different heavy chain constant region gene.

isotypic determinant

Immunoglobulin epitope present in all normal individuals of a species. Isotypic determinants of immunoglobulin heavy and light chains determine immunoglobulin class and subclass and light-chain type.

isotypic exclusion

The use by a B cell or antibody of one light polypeptide chain isotype, κ or λ.

isotypic specificities

Species-specific variability of antibody (human, mouse, rabbit, etc.). Examples of isotypes include IgG, IgM, and κ light chains.

isotypic variation

Differences among antigens found in members of a species such as the epitopes that differentiate immunoglobulin classes and subclasses and light chain types among immunoglobulin chains.

ITAM

Abbreviation for immunoreceptor tyrosine-based activation motif.

ITIM

Abbreviation for immunoreceptor tyrosine-based inhibition motif.

ITIM/ITAM immunoreceptors

ITAMs (immunoreceptor tyrosine-based activation motif; consensus sequence $YxxI/Lx_{6-12}YxxII/L$) and ITIMs (immunoreceptor tyrosine-based inhibition motif; $S/I/V/LxYxxI/V/L$) are phosphorylation motifs found in a large number of receptors or adaptor proteins. Phosphorylated ITAMs serve as docking sites for tandem SH2 domains of Syk family kinases, whereas phosphorylated ITIMs recruit tyrosine phosphatases. Signaling through ITAM-bearing receptors usually results in cell activation, while engagement of ITIM-bearing receptors is usually inhibitory. Most of these receptors are involved in tumor development and regulation of the immune system, although they also function in tissues such as bone and brain.

ITP

Abbreviation for idiopathic thrombocytopenic purpura.

IVIG

Abbreviation for intravenous immunoglobulin.

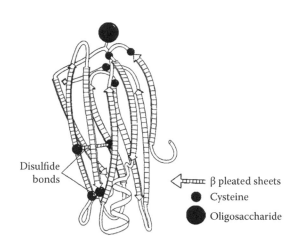

Disulfide bonds

⇦ β pleated sheets
● Cysteine
⬤ Oligosaccharide

Structure of J chain that occurs in secretory IgA and IgM molecules and facilitates polymerization.

J (joining) chain

A 17.6-kDa polypeptide chain present in polymeric immunoglobulins, including IgM and IgA. A diminutive acidic polypeptide that can bind to tail pieces of α and μ Ig heavy chains, stabilizing polymeric IgA or IgM molecules. It links four-chain immunoglobulin monomers to produce the polymeric immunoglobulin structure. J chains are produced in plasma cells and incorporated into IgM or IgA molecules prior to their secretion. Incorporation of the J chain appears essential for transcytosis of these immunoglobulin molecules to external secretions. The J chain comprises 2 to 4% of an IgM pentamer or a secretory IgA dimer. Tryptophan is absent from both mouse and human J chains. J chains are composed of 137-amino-acid residues and a single, complex, N-linked oligosaccharide on asparagine. Human J chain contains three forms of the oligosaccharide that differ in sialic acid content. The J chain is fastened through disulfide bonds to penultimate cysteine residues of μ or α heavy chains. The human J chain gene is located on chromosome 4q21, whereas the mouse J chain gene is located on chromosome 5.

J exon

A DNA sequence that encodes part of the third hypervariable region of a light or heavy chain located near the 5' ends of the κ, λ, and γ constant region genes. An intron separates the J exon from them. The J exon should not be confused with the J chain. The H constant region gene is associated with several J exons. The V region gene is translocated to a site just 5' to one of the J exons during stem cell differentiation to a lymphocyte.

J gene segment

DNA sequence that codes for the carboxyl terminal 12 to 21 residues of T lymphocyte receptor or immunoglobulin polypeptide chain variable regions. Through gene rearrangement, a J gene segment unites either a V or D gene segment to intron 5' of the C gene segment.

J region

The variable part of a polypeptide chain consisting of a T lymphocyte receptor or immunoglobulin that a J gene segment encodes. The J region of an immunoglobulin light chain is composed of the third hypervariable region carboxyl terminal (1 or 2 residues) and the fourth framework region (12 or 13 residues). The J region of an immunoglobulin heavy chain is composed of the third hypervariable region carboxyl terminal portion and the fourth framework region (15 to 20 residues). The J region of the heavy chain is slightly longer than that of the light chain. The variable region carboxyl terminal portion represents the J region of the T cell receptor.

JAK-3 SCID

Severe combined immune deficiency (SCID) attributable to JAK-3 deficiency. Immunophenotypic and functional analysis of circulating lymphoid cells permits classification of SCID into distinct subgroups. Neither immunological nor clinical features can distinguish between X-linked and (AR) T–B+ SCID. Cytokine receptors that utilize the common γ chain always associate with the intracellular tyrosine kinase designated JAK-3. The major cytokine receptor transducing subunit binds to another JAK kinase, JAK-1. Markedly reduced expression of JAK-3 protein due to mutations in the JAK-3 gene in unrelated infants with T–B+ SCID reveals the critical role of JAK for lymphoid development and function. Fewer than 10 SCID patients in the United States are characterized by defective expression of JAK-3; the incidence has been greater in Europeans.

JAK–STAT signaling pathway

A signaling mechanism induced by the binding of cytokine to type I and type II cytokine receptors. Sequential activation of receptor-associated Janus kinase (JAK) tyrosine kinases, JAK-mediated tyrosine phosphorylation of cytokine receptor cytoplasmic tails, docking of signal transducers and activators of transcription (STATs) to phosphorylated receptor chains, JAK-mediated tyrosine phosphorylation of the associated STATs, dimerization and nuclear translocation of the STATs, and binding STAT to regulatory regions of target genes leading to transcriptional activation of those genes all occur.

Janus kinases (JAKs)

Nonreceptor tyrosine kinases that transduce activating signals from cytokine receptors with which they associate and phorphorylate STAT transcription factors. Tyrosine kinases that associate with cytoplasmic tails of various cytokine receptors such as receptors for IL2, IL4, IFN-γ, and IL12, among others. They are activated by the aggregation of cytokine receptors. JAKs phosphorylate cytokine receptors that facilitate the binding of STATs. This is followed by phosphorylation and activation of the STATs by JAKs. JAKs associate selectively with different cytokine receptors. STATs in the cytosol transfer to the nucleus following phosphorylation where they activate various genes. The four known JAKs are JAK-1, JAK-2, JAK-3, and TYK-2.

Japanese encephalitis virus vaccine

Intended for protection against Japanese encephalitis, a mosquito-borne arboviral flavivirus infection that is a prominent cause of viral encephalitis in Asia. United States travelers and military personnel should receive three-dose vaccinations. Neutralizing antibody has been shown to be produced in fewer than 80% of vaccinated individuals after two doses of the vaccine and antibody levels decline substantially in most persons vaccinated within 6 months. In another study, two regiments of three doses induced neutralizing antibodies 2 months and 6 months after initiation of vaccination. Vaccination on days 0, 7, and 30 led to higher antibody responses than vaccination on days 0, 7, and 14. The full duration of protection is unknown.

Jarisch–Herxheimer reaction

A systemic reaction associated with fever, lymphadenopathy, skin rash, and headaches that follows the injection of penicillin into patients with syphilis. It is apparently produced by the release of significant quantities of toxic or antigenic substances from multiple *Treponema pallidum* microorganisms.

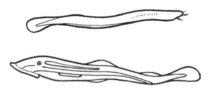

California hagfish and lamprey.

jawless fishes (cyclostomes, e.g., hagfish and lampreys)

The lowest vertebrate investigated, the California hagfish, does not manifest true lymphocytes and adaptive T and B cell responses. This species has no thymus, an erythropoietic spleen or lymphocyte-like cells in the circulation and γ M macroglobulin. The hagfish responds to hemocyanin if its body temperature is maintained at 20°C, but true immunoglobulins are not synthesized.

Jenner, Edward (1749–1823)

Jenner studied medicine under John Hunter and for most of his career was a country doctor in Berkeley in southern England. It was common knowledge that an eruptive skin disease of cattle (cowpox) and a similar disease in horses called grease conferred immunity to smallpox on those who cared for the animals and caught infections from them, and Jenner carefully observed and recorded 23 cases. The results of his experiments were published, establishing his claim of initiating the technique of vaccination. He vaccinated James Phipps, an 8-year old boy. The vaccination contained matter taken from the arm of Sarah Nelmes, a milkmaid who suffered from cowpox.

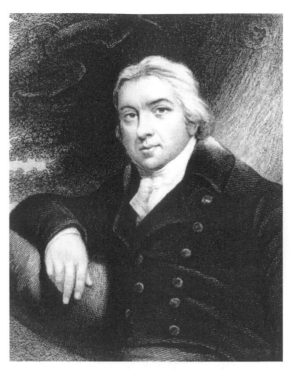

Edward Jenner (1749–1823) is often called the founder of immunology based on his contribution of the first reliable method for conferring lasting immunity to a major contagious disease.

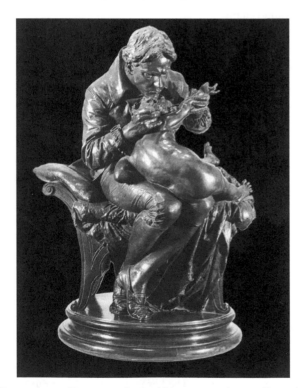

Bronze statue of Jenner vaccinating his own son against smallpox with cowpox lymph.

After the infection subsided, Jenner inoculated the child with smallpox and found that the inoculation had no effect. His results led to widespread adoption of vaccination in England and elsewhere, leading ultimately to the eradication of smallpox.

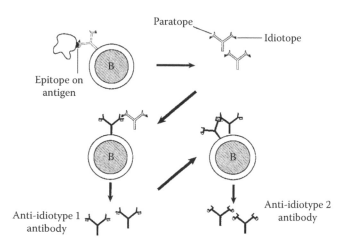

Jerne network theory.

Jerne network theory

Niels Jerne's hypothesis that antibodies produced in response to a specific antigen would induce a second group of antibodies that in turn would downregulate the original antibody-producing cells. The second antigen (Ab-2) would recognize epitopes of the antibody-binding region of antibody 1. These would be anti-idiotypic antibodies that would also be reactive with the antigen-binding regions of T cell receptors for which they were specific. Thus, a network of antiantibodies would produce a homeostatic effect on the immune response to a particular antigen. This theory was subsequently proven and confirmed by numerous investigators.

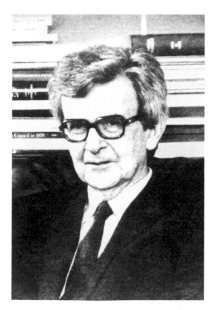

Niels Kaj Jerne.

Jerne, Niels Kaj (1911–1994)

Immunologist born in London and educated at Leiden and Copenhagen who shared the Nobel Prize in 1984 with Kohler and Millstein for his contributions to immune system theory. These include his selective theory of antibody formation, the functional network of interacting antibodies and lymphocytes, and distinction of self from nonself by T lymphocytes. He studied antibody synthesis and avidity, perfected the hemolytic plaque assay, developed the natural selection theory of antibody formation, and formulated the idiotypic network theory. He was the director of the Paul Ehrlich Institute in Frankfurt-am-Main, 1966, and director of the Basel Institute for Immunology, 1969.

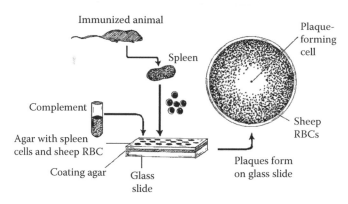

Jerne plaque assay.

Jerne plaque assay

Refer to hemolytic plaque assay.

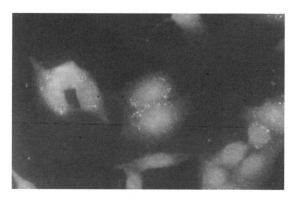

Jo-1 autoantibodies.

Jo-1 autoantibodies

Thirty percent of adult patients with myositis (including polymyositis, dermatomyositis, and combination syndromes) form autoantibodies against the Jo-1 antigen (histidyl-tRNA synthetase). These antibodies against Jo-1 occur in approximately 60% of patients with both myositis and interstitial lung disease. Jo-1 antibodies are most often found in addition to other aminoacyl synthetases in individuals with antisynthetase syndrome, which is marked by acute onset, steroid-responsive myositis with interstitial lung disease, fever, symmetrical arthritis, Raynaud's phenomenon, and mechanic's hands. Jo-1 autoantibodies in patients with idiopathic polymyositis are usually associated with severe relapse and poor prognosis.

Jo-1 syndrome

A clinical condition in which anti-Jo-1 antigen (histidyl-tRNA synthetase) antibodies are produced. Arthritis, myositis, and interstitial lung disease, may be present. One quarter of myositis patients may manifest anti-Jo-1 antibodies.

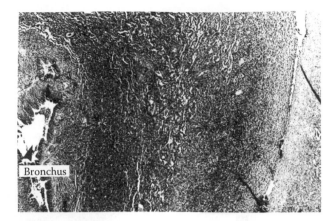

Job's syndrome with bronchogenic abscess.

Job's syndrome
Recurring cold staphylococcal abscesses or infections by other agents. Eczema, elevated levels of immunoglobulin E (IgE) in the serum, and phagocytic dysfunction are associated with glutathione reductase and glucose-6-phosphatase deficiencies. The syndrome has an autosomal-recessive mode of inheritance.

johnin
An extract from culture medium in which *Mycobacterium johnei* is growing. It can be used in a skin test of cattle for the diagnosis of Johne's disease. Its preparation parallels the extraction of the purified protein derivative (PPD) used in the tuberculin test.

joining (J) gene segment
A type of gene segment in immunoglobulin and T-cell receptor genes that is rearranged to render functional variable region exons.

Jones criteria
Signs and symptoms used in the diagnosis of acute rheumatic fever.

Jones–Mote hypersensitivity
Delayed (type IV) hypersensitivity involving prominent basophil infiltration of the skin immediately beneath the epidermis. It can be induced by the intradermal injection of a soluble antigen such as ovalbumin incorporated into Freund's incomplete adjuvant. Swelling of the skin reaches a maximum 7 to 10 days following induction and vanishes when antibody is formed. Histologically, basophils predominate, but lymphocytes and mononuclear cells are also present. Jones–Mote hypersensitivity is greatly influenced by lymphocytes that are sensitive to cyclophosphamide (suppressor lymphocytes).

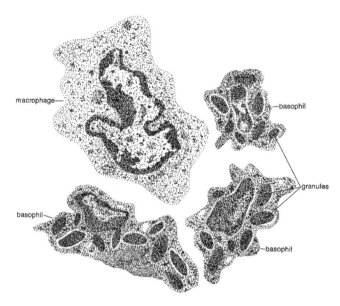

Cutaneous basophil hypersensitivity.

Jones–Mote reaction
Delayed-type hypersensitivity to protein antigens associated with basophil infiltration, which gives the reaction

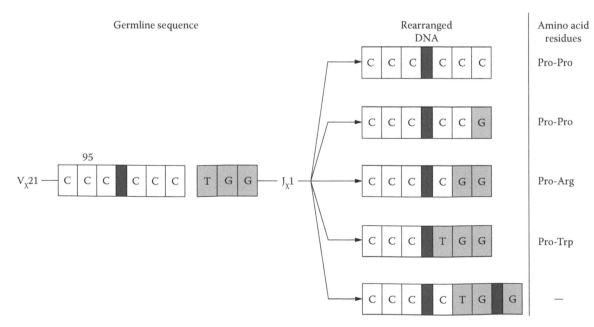

Junctional diversity.

the additional name of *cutaneous basophil hypersensitivity*. Compared to the other forms of delayed-type hypersensitivity, it is relatively weak and appears on challenge several days following sensitization, with minute quantities of protein antigens in aqueous medium or in incomplete Freund's adjuvant. No necrosis is produced. Jones–Mote hypersensitivity can be produced in laboratory animals such as guinea pigs appropriately exposed to protein antigens in aqueous media or in incomplete Freund's adjuvant. It can be passively transferred by T lymphocytes.

jugular bodies

Nodules ventral to external jugular veins that contain lobules of lymphoid cells separated by sinusoids paved with phagocytic cells. Jugular bodies filter the blood but are not a part of the lymphoid system. They may be found in selected amphibian species.

junctional diversity

Amino acid sequence variation in immunoglobulin and T cell receptor polypeptides that arises during V(D)J gene rearrangement in the immunoglobulin or T cell receptor loci with the addition of nucleotides into the junctions between gene segments. When gene segments join imprecisely, the amino acid sequence may vary and affect variable region expression, which can alter codons at gene segment junctions. These include the V–J junction of the genes encoding immunoglobulin κ and λ light chains and the V–D, D–J, and D–D junctions of genes encoding immunoglobulin heavy chains or the genes encoding T cell receptor β and δ chains.

juvenile onset diabetes

Synonym for type I insulin-dependent diabetes mellitus.

juvenile rheumatoid arthritis

Juvenile rheumatoid arthritis is the diagnosis when a child has inflammation in one or more joints that persists for a minimum of 3 months with no other explanation. The condition may be associated with uveitis, pericarditis, rheumatoid nodules, fever, and rash; however, rheumatoid factor (RF) is found in the serum in fewer than 10% of these patients. Subgroups include (1) polyarticular disease divided into group 1, which is HLA-DR4-associated, and group 2, which is HLA-DR5- and DR8-associated; (2) systemic Still's disease with hepatosplenomegaly, enlarged lymph nodes, pericardial inflammation, rash, and fever; and (3) pauciarticular disease, in which one to nine joints are affected and which is associated with uveitis and anti-DNA antibodies, principally in young women.

J

K

K antigens

Surface epitopes of Gram-negative microorganisms. They are either proteins (fimbriae) or acid polysaccharides found on the surfaces of *Klebsiella* and *Escherichia coli* microorganisms. K antigens are exterior to somatic O antigens. They are labile to heat and crossreact with the capsules of other microorganisms such as *Hemophilus influenzae*, *Streptococcus pneumoniae*, and *Neisseria meningitidis*. K antigens may be linked to virulent strains of microorganisms that induce urinary tract infections. Anti-K antibodies are only weakly protective.

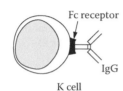

Schematic representation of a K (NK) cell.

K (killer) cell

Name originally given to null cells that were first recognized as non-B non-T lymphocytes. They were described to have lymphocyte-like morphology but functional characteristics different from those of B and T cells. Killer cells are now called natural killer (NK) cells. One type of immune response in which they are involved is antibody-dependent cell-mediated cytotoxicity (ADCC) in which they kill target cells coated with immunoglobulin G (IgG) antibodies. A K cell is an Fc-bearing killer cell that has an effector function in mediating antibody-dependent, cell-mediated cytotoxicity. An IgG antibody molecule binds through its Fc region to the Fc receptor of the K cell. Following contact with a target cell bearing antigenic determinants on its surface for which the Fab regions of the antibody molecule attached to the K cell are specific, the lymphocyte-like K cell releases lymphokines that destroy the target. This represents a type of immune effector function in which cells and antibody participate. Other cells that mediate antibody-dependent cell-mediated cytotoxicity include cytotoxic T cells, neutrophils, and macrophages.

K region

The K region and the D region relate to major histocompatibility complex (MHC) class I segments in the murine genome.

K562 cells

A chronic myelogenous leukemia cell line that serves as a target cell in a ^{51}Cr release assay of natural killer (NK) cells. Following incubation of NK cells with ^{51}Cr-labeled target K562 cells, the amount of chromium released into the supernatant is measured and the cytotoxicity is determined by use of a formula.

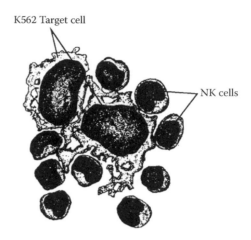

Schematic representation of a K562 target cell bound to natural killer (NK) cells.

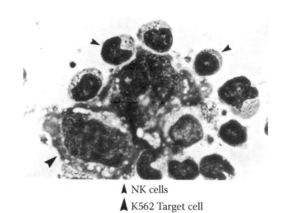

K562 target cell (large arrow) bound to natural killer (NK) cells (small arrows).

Kabat, Elvin Abraham (1914–)

American immunochemist; with Tiselius, he was the first to separate immunoglobulins electrophoretically. He also demonstrated that γ globulins can be distinguished as 7S or 19S. Other contributions include research on antibodies to carbohydrates, antibody combining sites, and the discovery of immunoglobulin chain variable regions. He received the National Medal of Science. (Refer to *Experimental Immunochemistry* [with Mayer], 1948; *Blood Group Substances: Their Chemistry and Immunochemistry*, 1956; *Structural Concepts in Immunology and Immunochemistry*, 1968.)

Kabat Wu plot

Refer to Wu Kabat plot.

K

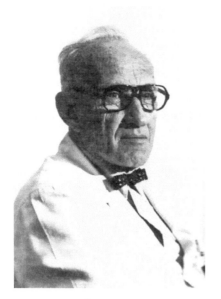

Elvin Abraham Kabat.

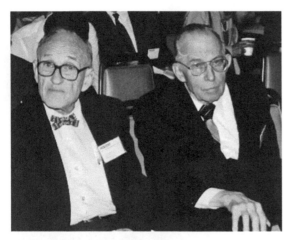

Elvin A. Kabat (left) of Columbia University and Merrill W. Chase of Rockefeller University at the 75th Annual Meeting of the American Association of Immunologists in Las Vegas, Nevada, 1988.

kallidin

Refer to kinins.

kallikrein

An enzyme that splits kininogens to generate bradykinin, which has an effect on pain receptors and smooth muscle and exerts a chemotactic effect on neutrophils. Bradykinin is a nonapeptide that induces vasodilation and increases capillary permeability. Kallikreins, also known as kininogenases, are present in both plasma and tissues and also in glandular secretions such as saliva, pancreatic juice, tears, and urine, among others. Trypsin, pepsin, proteases of snake venoms, and bacterial products are also able to hydrolyze kininogens, but the substrate specificity and potency of kallikreins are greater. Plasma and tissue kallikreins are physically and immunologically different. It is not known whether plasma contains more than one form of kallikrein.

kallikrein inhibitors

Natural inhibitors of kallikreins belong to the group of natural inhibitors of proteolysis. They also inhibit other proteolytic enzymes, but each has its own preference for one protease or another. Apronitin, also known by its registered name of Trasylol™, is particularly active on tissue kallikreins.

kallikrein–kinin system

Vasopressive peptides that control blood pressure through maintenance of regional blood flow and the excretion of water and electrolytes. Kallikrein causes the release of renin and the synthesis of kinins that interact with the immune system, increase urinary sodium excretion, and act as powerful vasodilators.

Kaposi's sarcoma

A malignant neoplasm that may consist of a discrete intradermal nodule with vascular channels lined by atypical endothelial cells and extravasated erythrocytes with deposits of hemosiderin. This vascular tumor, seen largely in elderly patients of Mediterranean and Jewish heritage, is now recognized in a more aggressive form as one of the presentations of AIDS. Whereas classical Kaposi's sarcoma is on the lower limbs and is only very slowly progressive, the more aggressive form seen in AIDS involves discrete vascular tumors scattered widely over the body. This tumor is associated with infection by Kaposi's-sarcoma-associated herpesvirus (human herpesvirus 8).

κ (kappa)

Designation for one of the two types of immunoglobulin light chains; the other designation is λ.

κ–λ exclusion

Means whereby the generation of a functional κ light chain from the Igk locus on one chromosome prevents futher V(D)J rearrangement at the other Igk allele, and also blocks V(D)J rearrangement of either Igl allele.

κ chain

One of two types of light polypeptide chains present in immunoglobulin molecules of humans and other species. κ Light chains are found in approximately 60% of human immunoglobulin, whereas λ light chains are present in approximately 40%. A single immunoglobulin molecule contains either κ or λ light chains, not one of each.

κ light chain deficiency

A rare condition in which point mutations in the Cκ gene at chromosome 2p11 cause an absence of κ light chains in the serum and generate B lymphocytes whose surfaces are bereft of κ light chains.

karyotype

The number and shape of chromosomes within a cell. A karyotype may be characteristic for a particular species.

Kawasaki's disease

Mucocutaneous lymph node syndrome that occurs in children under 5 years of age. The incubation period may be 1 to 2 weeks. It is an acute febrile disease characterized by erythema of the conjunctiva and oral cavity, skin rash, and swollen (especially cervical) lymph nodes. It occurs mostly in Japan, although some cases have been reported in the United States. Cardiac lesions such as coronary artery aneurysms may be found in 70% of the patients. Coronary arteritis causes death in 1 to 2% of patients. Necrosis and inflammation of the vessel wall are present. The etiology is unknown, but it has been suggested to be infection by a retrovirus. Considered to be an autoimmune disease. Associated immunoregulatory disorders include T and B lymphocyte activation, circulating immune complexes, and autoantibodies cytolytic for endothelial cells activated by cytokines.

Kell Blood Group System

Phenotype	K	K	Reactions with Anti-				Phenotype Frequency	
			Kpᵃ	Kpᵇ	Jsᵃ	Jsᵇ	Caucasian	African American
K+k–	+	0					0.2	Rare
K+k+	+	+					8.8	2
K–k+	0	+					91	98
Kp (a+b–)			+	0			Rare	0
Kp (a+b+)			+	+			2.3	Rare
Kp (a–b+)			0	+			97.7	100
Js (a+b–)					+	0	0	1
Js (a+b+)					+	+	Rare	19
Js (a–b+)					0	+	100	80
K₀	0	0	0	0	0	0	Very rare	Very rare

Kell blood group system

Antibody specific for the K (KELI) antigen that induces hemolytic disease of the newborn, described in 1946. Nine percent of Caucasians and 2% of African-Americans have the *K* gene that encodes this antigen. Subsequently, the *K* allele was identified. Anti-k (KEL2) antibodies reacted with the erythrocytes of more than 99% of the random population. Kell system antigens are present only in relatively low density on erythrocyte membranes. The strong immunogenicity of the K antigen leads to the presence of anti-K antibodies in sera of transfused patients. Anti-K antibodies cause hemolytic transfusion reactions of both immediate and delayed varieties. Ninety percent of donors are K–, thus considerably simplifying the task of finding compatible blood for patients with anti-K.

keratin layer

External structure of skin that protects the body from microorganisms and resists penetrating stimuli. It is comprised of keratin protein filaments synthesized by keratinocytes.

keratinocyte growth factor (KGF)

A 19-kDa protein composed of 163-amino acid residues that binds heparin and facilitates the growth of keratinocytes and other epithelial cells that comprise 95% of the epidermis.

keratinocytes

Squamous epithelial cells of the epidermis that are produced in waves. They are joined together by desmosomes and synthesize keratin. Their constant upward migration permits skin regeneration. The keratin layer is a consequence of the orchestrated death of a wave of keratinocytes. In the lower epidermis, these cells secrete proinflammatory cytokines and complement components.

keratoconjunctivitis sicca

A condition characterized by hyperemia of the conjunctiva, lachrymal deficiency, corneal epithelium thickening, itching and burning of the eye, and often reduced visual acuity.

kernicterus

Deposition in the skin (leading to yellowish discoloration) and in the central nervous system of erythrocyte breakdown products in the blood of infants with erythroblastosis fetalis. It may lead to neurologic dysfunction.

ketokonazole

An antifungal drug used to treat chronic mucocutaneous candidiasis.

keyhole limpet hemocyanin (KLH)

A traditional antigen widely used as a carrier in studies on immune responsiveness to haptens. This respiratory pigment containing copper is found in mollusks and crustaceans. It is usually immunogenic in vertebrate animals.

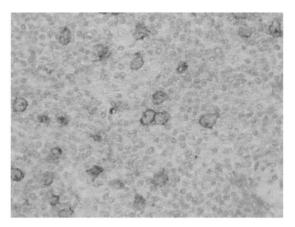

CD30—Hodgkin lymphoma.

Ki-1 (CD30 antigen)

A marker of Reed–Sternberg cells found in Hodgkin disease of the mixed cellularity, nodular sclerosing, and lymphocyte-depleted types and in selected cases of large cell non-Hodgkin lymphomas.

Ki-67 or Ki-780

Nuclear antigens expressed by both normal and neoplastic proliferating cells demonstrable by immunoperoxidase staining. A relatively high percentage of positive cells in a neoplasm implies an unfavorable prognosis.

Ki autoantibodies

Autoantibodies specific for a 3-kDa nonhistone nuclear protein from rabbit thymus present in 19 to 21% of systemic lupus erythematosus (SLE) patients by enzyme immunoassay (EIA) and 8% by DD. They are present in smaller quantities in mixed connective tissue disease, systemic sclerosis, and rheumatoid arthritis. At present, this autoantibody is

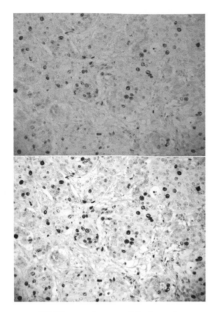

Ki-67—carcinoma of the breast.

not clinically useful. The Ki protein contains an antigenic determinant that is homologous to the Sv40 large T antigen nuclear localization signal.

Kidd Blood Group System

Phenotype	Reactions with Anti-		Phenotype Frequency	
	Jk^a	Jk^b	Caucasian	African American
Jk (a+b−)	+	0	28	57
Kj (a+b+)	0	+	49	34
Jk (a−b+)	+	+	23	9
Jk (a−b−)	0	0	Very rare	Very rare

Kidd blood group system

The anti-Jk^a antibodies originally detected in the serum of a woman giving birth to a baby with hemolytic disease of the newborn (HDN). The anti-Jk^b antibodies were discovered in the serum of a patient following a transfusion reaction. Although Kidd system antibodies sometimes lead to HDN, the disease is not usually severe; however, the antibodies are problematic and cause severe hemolytic transfusion reactions, especially of the delayed type. These occur when antibodies developing quickly in a booster response to antigens on transfused erythrocytes destroy red cells in the circulation. As shown in the table, four phenotypes are revealed by the reactions of anti-Jk^a and anti-Jk^b antibodies. A dominant inhibitor gene (In[Jk]) may encode a null phenotype. Jk3 is believed to be present on both Jk(a$^+$) and Jk(b$^+$) red cells. Anti-Jk3 is frequently induced by red blood cell stimulation.

killed vaccine

An immunizing preparation composed of viral or bacterial microorganisms that are dead but retain their antigenicity, making them capable of inducing a protective immune response with the formation of antibodies and/or stimulation of cell-mediated immunity. Inactivation is by irradiation, chemical treatment, or heat. Killed vaccines do not induce even mild cases of the disease that are sometimes observed with attenuated (greatly weakened but still living) vaccines. Although the first killed vaccines contained intact dead microorganisms, some modern preparations contain subunits or parts of microorganisms to be used for immunization. Killed microorganisms may be combined with toxoids, as in the case of the DPT (diphtheria–pertussis–tetanus) preparations administered to children.

killed virus vaccines

Immunogen preparation containing virons deliberately killed by heat, chemicals, or radiation.

killer activatory receptors (KARs)

Natural killer (NK) cell or cytotoxic T cell surface receptors that can activate killing by these cell types.

killer cell (K cell)

A large granular lymphocyte bearing Fc receptors on its surface for immunoglobulin G (IgG), which makes it capable of mediating antibody-dependent, cell-mediated cytotoxicity. Complement is not involved in the reaction. Antibody may attach through its Fab regions to target cell epitopes and link to the killer cell through attachment of its Fc region to the Fc receptor of the K cell, thereby facilitating cytolysis of the target by the killer cell, or an IgG antibody may first link via its Fc region to the Fc receptor on the killer cell surface and direct the K cell to its target. Cytolysis is induced by insertion of perforin polymer in the target cell membrane in a manner that resembles the insertion of C9 polymers in a cell membrane in complement-mediated lysis. Perforin is showered on the target cell membrane following release from the K cell.

killer cell immunoglobulin-like receptors (ICIRs)

Molecular configurations on NK cells that interact with MHC class I molecules and transmit either activating or inhibitory signals to natural killer (NK) cells. NK cell receptors that bind to MHC class I molecules and transmit either activating or inhibitory signals to the T cell.

killer inhibitory receptors (KIRs)

Natural killer (NK) cell receptors that recognize self major histocompatibility complex (MHC) class I molecules and transmit inhibitory signals that block activation of NK cell cytolytic processes. These receptors prevent NK cells from killing normal host cells expressing MHC class I molecules but allow lysis of virus-infected cells for which MHC class I expression has been suppressed. The inhibitory receptors fall into several classes that include immunoglobulin superfamily members, heterodimers of CD94 and selectin, and Ly49. These receptors possess cytoplasmic tails bearing immunoreceptor tyrosine inhibition motifs (ITIMs) that participate in initiating inhibitory signal pathways.

killer T cell

A T lymphocyte that mediates a lethal effect on a target cell expressing a foreign antigen bound to major histocompatibility complex (MHC) molecules on target cell surfaces. A synonym for a cytotoxic T cell.

kilobase (kb)

One thousand DNA or RNA base pairs.

kinetochore autoantibodies

Autoantibodies specific for the mitotic spindle apparatus; also known as centromere autoantibodies. They have been found in the cutaneous form of systemic sclerosis,

Raynaud's phenomenon, and primary biliary cirrhosis patients with features of systemic sclerosis.

kininases

An enzyme in the blood that degrades kinins to inactive peptides. Inactivation occurs when any of the eight bonds in the kinin are cleaved. Plasma contains two kininases. Kininase I, or carboxy peptidase N, cleaves the C terminal arginines of kinins and of anaphylatoxins. It differs from pancreatic carboxy peptidase B with respect to molecular weight, subunit structure, carbohydrate content, antigenic properties, substrate specificity, and inhibition pattern. The purified enzyme has a molecular weight of 280 kDa. The site of synthesis of carboxy peptidase N is believed to be the liver. Kininase II, a peptidyl dipeptidase, cleaves the C terminal Phe–Args of kinins and also liberates angiotensin II from angiotensin I. (Angiotensin is another vasoactive substance.) The vascular endothelia of both lung and peripheral vascular beds are rich in this enzyme. Peptidyl dipeptidase is also present outside the circulatory system and has different functions at these sites. Other enzymes with kininase activity are present in the spleen and kidney (cathepsin) and the endothelial cells of the gastrointestinal tract.

kininogens

The precursors of kinins, kininogens are glycoproteins synthesized in the liver. Plasma kininogens comprise two, possibly three, classes of compounds with species variation: (1) Low molecular weight kininogens (LMKs) are acidic proteins with molecular weights of about 57 kDa and are susceptible to conversion into kinins by kininogen-converting enzymes (kallikreins) of tissue origin. Forms I and II represent the main plasma kininogens. (2) High molecular weight kininogens (HMKs) are α glycoproteins with molecular weights of 97 kDa that may be converted into kinins both by plasma and tissue kallikreins. HMKs exist in forms a and b that differ both in enzyme sensitivity and generated kinin.

kinins

A family of straight chain polypeptides generated by enzymatic hydrolysis of plasma α_2 globulin precursors, collectively called kininogens. They exert potent vasomotor effects, causing vasodilatation of most vessels in the body but vasoconstriction of the pulmonary bed. They also cause smooth muscle contraction and pain and increase vascular permeability and promote the diapedesis of leukocytes. Peptide kinins are released during inflammatory responses.

Kissmeyer-Nielsen, F.

Danish immunologist who sponsored the Sixth Histocompatibility or Transplantation Workshop in 1975. Six HLA-D alleles were described and the HLA-C locus was demonstrated at the workshop.

Kitasato, Shibasaburo (1892–1931)

Co-discoverer, with Emil von Behring, of antitoxin antibodies.

Klebsiella immunity

Most healthy adults have high levels of natural resistance against *Klebsiella pneumoniae*. The organism classically induces lung infection, leading to a massive confluent lobar consolidation with polymorphonuclear leukocytes, edema, and abscess formation with extensive cavity formation. Type-specific antibodies to the carbohydrate capsule are critical to recovery. These antibodies that appear within 2 weeks following infection serve as opsonins to facilitate the killing of this microorganism by phagocytes. Immunity

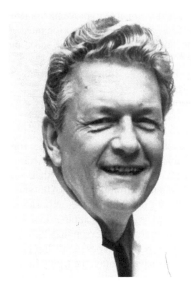

F. Kissmeyer-Nielsen.

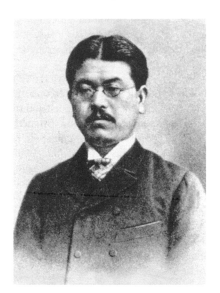

Shibasaburo Kitasato.

to *K. pneumoniae* is long lasting. This microorganism is believed to play a part in the development of ankylosing spondylitis (AS) because AS patients develop high levels of serum immunoglobulin A (IgA) against the microbe. AS is associated with HLA-B27 antigen. The mechanism has been claimed to be (1) molecular mimicry, in which antibody against this antigen will bind to self-antigenic determinants, leading to destructive immunity, or (2) that *Klebsiella* plasmids may encode the formation of a bacterial modifying factor that reacts with HLA-B27, rendering it susceptible to immune attack. The main virulence factor of the microbe is the capsule that helps it resist phagocytosis. Despite reports of several enterotoxins, the main pathologic effect is associated with the production of an endotoxin. The extracellular toxic complex (ETC) contains endotoxin, capsule, and protein and is lethal when injected into mice; it leads to pathologic changes that resemble those produced in *K. pneumoniae* lobar pneumonia in humans. Vaccines are aimed at developing antibodies against capsule polysaccharides that are able to prevent experimental *K. pneumoniae* sepsis. An effective vaccine must contain capsular polysaccharides from 25 different serotypes.

KLH

Abbreviation for keyhole limpet hemocyanin.

Km (formerly Inv)

The designation for the κ light chain allotype genetic markers.

Km allotypes

The three Km allotypes described in human immunoglobulin κ light chains are designated Km1, Km1,2, and Km3. They are encoded by alleles of the gene that codes for the human κ light chain constant regions. Allotype differences are based on the amino acid residues at positions 153 and 191 that are in proximity to one another in a folded immunoglobulin Cκ domain. One person may have a maximum of two of the three Km allotypes on his light chains. To fully express Km determinants, the heavy immunoglobulin chains should be present, probably to maintain appropriate three-dimensional configuration.

knock-in transgene

A transgene with a specific mutation flanked by sequences that are homologous to the endogenous locus, thereby ensuring that the transgene integrates in its natural position.

knockout gene

Generation of a mutant organism in which the function of a particular gene is completely eliminated (a null allele). To successfully "knock out" a gene, cloned and sequenced genomic DNA and a suitable embryonic (ES) cell line are necessary. A sequence insertion targeting approach may be used. The advantage of an insertion vector is that the frequency of integration is ninefold higher than with an equal length replacement-type vector. Homologous recombination techniques can be used to achieve targeted disruption of one or more genes in mice. Knockout mice deprived of functional genes that encode cytokines, cell-surface receptors, signaling molecules, and transcription factors are critical for contemporary immunologic research.

knockout, genetic

A technique to introduce precise genetic lesions into the mouse genome to cause gene disruption and generate an animal model with a specific genetic defect. Specific defects may be introduced into any murine gene by permitting investigation of this alteration *in vivo*. Technological advances that made this possible include homologous recombination to introduce defined changes into the murine genome and the reintroduction of genetically altered embryonic stem cells into the murine germline to produce mutant mouse strains.

knockout mouse

A transgenic mouse in which a mutant allele or disrupted form of a gene replaces a normal gene, leading to the mouse's failure to produce a functional gene product. Much has been learned about the roles of cytokines, cell surface receptors, signaling molecules, and transcription factors in the immune system through experiments on knockout mice.

Koch, Heinrich Hermann Robert (1843–1910)

German bacteriologist awarded the Nobel Prize in 1905 for his work on tuberculosis. Koch made many contributions to the field of bacteriology. Along with his postulates for proof of etiology, Koch instituted strict isolation and culture methods. He studied the life cycle of anthrax and discovered

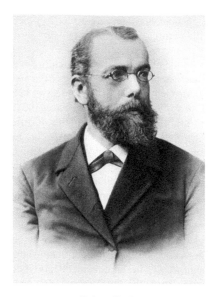

Robert Koch.

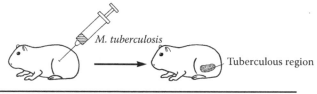

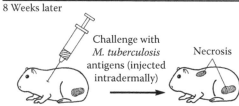

Koch phenomenon.

both *Vibrio cholerae* and the tubercle bacillus. The Koch phenomenon and Koch–Weeks bacillus both bear his name.

Koch phenomenon

Delayed hypersensitivity reaction in the skin of a guinea pig after it has been infected with *Mycobacterium tuberculosis*. Robert Koch described the phenomenon in 1891 following the injection of living or dead *M. tuberculosis* microorganisms into guinea pigs previously infected with the same microbes. He observed severe necrotic reactions at the sites of inoculation that occasionally became generalized and induced death. The injection of killed *M. tuberculosis* microorganisms into healthy guinea pigs caused no ill effects. This is a demonstration of cell-mediated immunity and is the basis for the tuberculin test.

Köhler, Georges J.F. (1946–1995)

German immunologist who shared the Nobel Prize in 1984 with Cesar Milstein for their work in the production of monoclonal antibodies by hybridizing mutant myeloma cells with antibody-producing B cells (hybridoma technique). Monoclonal antibodies have broad applications in both basic and clinical research and in diagnostic assays.

Koprowski, Hilary (1916–)

In the 1960s, Koprowski and Marin Kaplan developed a superior rabies vaccine from virus grown in human embryonic cell cultures. It had the advantage of requiring fewer

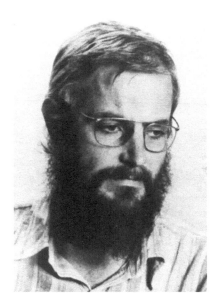

Georges J.F. Köhler.

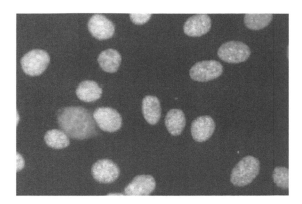

Ku antibodies.

Japanese patients in contrast to systemic lupus erythematosus (SLE) and overlap syndromes in Americans. These antibodies are also present in selected patients with mixed connective tissue disease, scleroderma, polymyositis, Graves' disease, and primary pulmonary hypertension, making them nondiagnostic for any specific autoimmune disease. The Ku autoantigen is a heterodimeric nucleolar protein composed of 70-kDa and 80- to 86-kDa subunits which, in association with a 350-kDa catalytic subunit, constitute the DNA-binding component of a DNA-dependent protein kinase involved in double-stranded DNA repair and V(D)J recombination. Ku autoantibodies are of unknown pathogenicity and clinical significance.

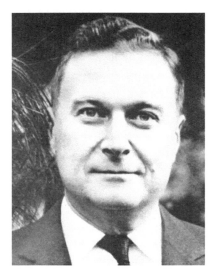

Hilary Koprowski.

injections than the Pasteur treatment and eliminated the possibility of allergy to duck embryo antigens.

Ku

An antigen present in a particle comprised of two noncovalently linked 70- and 80-kDa proteins that bind DNA. Nuclear factor IV (NF IV) and Ku antigen are the same. Anti-Ku antibodies recognize conformational epitopes.

Ku antibodies

Antibodies detectable in 15 to 50% of individuals with Sjögren's syndrome, systemic lupus erythematosus (SLE), mixed connective tissue disease, and scleroderma. They are found in 5 to 15% of myositis patients in the United States.

Ku antigen

A 70- to 80-kDa DNA-binding protein that is the target of autoantibodies in a few Japanese myositis patients manifesting the overlap syndrome.

Ku autoantibodies

Autoantibodies against the Ku epitope that reveal a strong association with systemic autoimmunity in

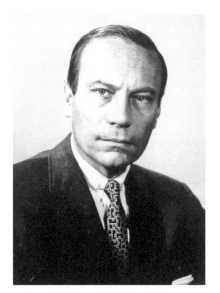

Henry George Kunkel.

Kunkel, Henry George (1916–1983)

American physician and immunologist whose work focused on immunoglobulins; he characterized myeloma proteins as immunoglobulins and rheumatoid factor as an autoantibody. He also discovered IgA and contributed to immunoglobulin structure and genetics. Kunkel received the Lasker Award and the Gairdner Award. A graduate of Johns Hopkins Medical School, he served as a professor of medicine at the Rockefeller Institute for Medical Research.

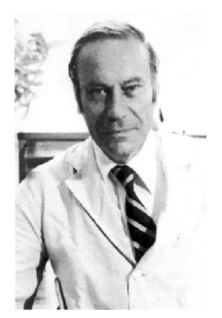

Henry George Kunkel.

Kupffer's cell

A liver macrophage that has become fixed as a mononuclear phagocytic cell in the liver sinusoids. It is an integral part of the mononuclear phagocyte (reticuloendothelial) system. Monocytes become attached to the interior surfaces of liver sinusoids, where they develop into macrophages. They have CR1 and CR2 receptors, surface Fc receptors, and major histocompatibility complex (MHC) class II molecules. They are actively phagocytic and remove foreign substances from the blood as it flows through the liver. Under certain disease conditions, they may phagocytize erythrocytes, leading to the deposition of hemosiderin particles derived from hemoglobulin breakdown products.

kuru

A slow virus disease of some native tribes of Guinea that practice cannibalism. Transmission is through skin lesions of individuals preparing infected brains for consumption. The virus accumulates in brain cell membranes.

Kveim reaction (historical)

A skin reaction for the diagnosis of sarcoidosis in which ground lymph node tissue of a known sarcoidosis patient is suspended in physiological salt solution and inoculated intracutaneously into a suspected sarcoidosis patient. A positive reaction, on histopathologic examination of an injection-site biopsy 1 month to 6 weeks after inoculation, reveals a nodular epithelioid cell granuloma-like reaction. A positive Kveim test confirms the diagnosis of sarcoidosis. The danger of possibly transmitting hepatitis, AIDS, and other viruses precludes the use of this reaction.

L

L₊ dose (historical)

The smallest amount of toxin that, when mixed with one unit of antitoxin and injected subcutaneously into a 250-g guinea pig, will kill the animal within 4 days. This is the unit used for standardization of antitoxin.

L2C leukemia

A B cell neoplasm of guinea pigs that is transplantable.

L3T4

A CD4 marker on mouse lymphocytes that signifies the T helper/inducer cell. It is detectable by specific monoclonal antibodies and is equivalent to the CD4⁺ lymphocyte in humans.

L3T4⁺ T lymphocytes

Murine CD4⁺ T cells.

lactalbumin

A breast epithelial cell protein demonstrable by immunoperoxidase staining found in approximately one half to two thirds of breast carcinomas for which it is relatively specific. More than 50% of metastatic breast tumors and some salivary gland and skin appendage tumors stain positively for lactalbumin.

lacteals

Minute lymphatics that drain intestinal villi.

lactoferrin

A protein that combines with iron and competes for it with microorganisms. This represents a nonantibody humoral substance that contributes to natural defenses against infection. It is present in polymorphonuclear neutrophil granules and in milk. By combining with iron molecules, it deprives bacterial cells of this needed substance.

lactoperoxidase

An enzyme present in milk and saliva that may be inhibitory to a number of microorganisms and serves as a nonantibody humoral substance that contributes to nonspecific immunity. Its mechanism of action resembles that of myeloperoxidase.

LAF (lymphocyte-activating factor)

Refer to interleukin-1.

LAG-3

A natural killer (NK) cell activation molecule whose structure is closely related to CD4. It is a type I integral membrane protein and a member of the immunoglobulin (Ig) superfamily with an Ig V-region-like domain and three Ig C2-region-like domains. Its gene colocalizes with but is distinct from the CD4 gene on mouse chromosome 6. LAG-3 is expressed on activated T and NK cells but not on resting lymphocytes. It may be a coreceptor for a putative activation receptor.

LAK cells

Lymphokine-activated killer cells.

LAM-1 (leukocyte adhesion molecule 1)

A homing protein found on membranes that combines with target cell-specific glycoconjugates. It helps regulate migration of leukocytes through lymphocyte binding to high endothelial venules and neutrophil adherence to endothelium at inflammatory sites.

λ (lambda)

One of the two light polypeptide chain types found in immunoglobulin (Ig) molecules.

λ (lambda) chain

One of the two light polypeptide chain types found in immunoglobulin (Ig) molecules. The κ light chain is the other. Each immunoglobulin molecule contains two λ or two κ light chains. The ratio of κ to λ light chains differs among species. Approximately 60% of IgG molecules in humans are κ and 40% are λ.

λ cloning vector

A genetically engineered λ phage that can accept foreign DNA and act as a vector in recombinant DNA studies. Phage DNA is cleaved with restriction endonucleases, and foreign DNA is inserted. An insertion vector has a single site where phage DNA is cleaved and foreign DNA inserted. A substitution or replacement vector has two sites that span a DNA segment that can be excised and replaced with foreign DNA.

λ5

Refer to pre-B cell receptor.

λ5 B cell development

Refer to VpreB protein.

lamin antibodies

Antibodies present in the sera of chronic autoimmune disease patients manifesting hepatitis, leukocytoclastic angiitis or brain vasculitis, cytopenia, and circulating anticoagulant or cardiolipin antibodies. The antibodies form a rim-type antinuclear staining pattern in immunofluorescence assays. A minority of systemic lupus erythematosus (SLE) patients develop antibodies to lamin.

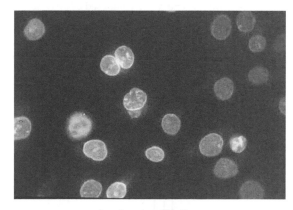

Lamin autoantibodies.

lamin autoantibodies

Autoantibodies against lamin, a nuclear antigen. They are found in selected patients with autoimmune and inflammatory diseases. Incomplete Freund's adjuvant (IFA) is the method of choice for their detection. Lamin autoantibodies occur in selected patients with chronic autoimmune disease marked by delta hepatitis, cytopenia with circulating anticoagulants or cardiolipin antibodies, and cutaneous leukocytoclastic angiitis. They may occur naturally, may be cross-reacting, or may be formed in response to antigen. They have no known clinical significance.

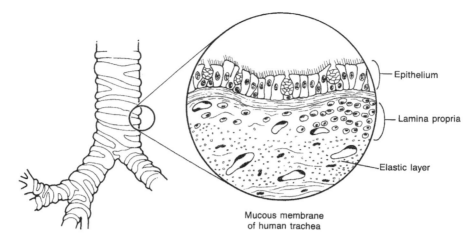

Lamina propria.

lamina propria

The thin connective tissue layer that supports the epithelium of the gastrointestinal tract. The epithelium and lamina propria form the mucous membrane. The lamina propria may be the site of immunologic reactivity in the gastrointestinal tract, representing an area where lymphocytes, plasma cells, and mast cells congregate.

laminin

A relatively large (820-kDa) basement membrane glycoprotein composed of three polypeptide subunits. It belongs to the integrin receptor family, which includes a 400-kDa α heavy chain and two 200-kDa light chains designated β_1 and β_2. By electron microscopy the molecule is arranged in the form of a cross. The domain structures of the α and β chains resemble one another. There are six primary domains. Domains I and II have repeat sequences forming α helices. Domains III and V are composed of cysteine-rich repeating sequences. The globular regions are composed of domains IV and VI. An additional short cysteine-rich α domain is located between the I and II domains in the β_1 chain. A relatively large globular segment is linked to the C terminal of domain I, designated the "foot" in the α chain. Five "toes" on the foot contain repeat sequences. Laminins have biological functions and characteristics that include facilitation of cellular adhesion and linkage to other basement membrane constituents such as collagen type IV, heparan, and glycosaminoglycans. Laminins also facilitate neurite regeneration, an activity associated with the foot of the molecule. Each form of laminin represents different gene products, although they possess a high degree of homology. S laminin describes a form found only in synaptic and nonmuscle basal lamina. Its is a single 190-kDa polypeptide (in reduced form) and its weight is >1000 kDa in the nonreduced form. It is associated with the development or stabilization of synapses and is homologous to the β_1 chain of laminin. Laminin facilitates cell attachment and migration, plays a role in differentiation and metastasis, and is produced by macrophages, endothelial cells, epithelial cells, and Schwann cells.

laminin receptor

A membrane protein composed of two disulfide bond-linked subunits, one relatively large and one relatively small. Its function appears to be the attachment of cells. It may share structural similarities with fibronectin and vitronectin, both of which are also integrins.

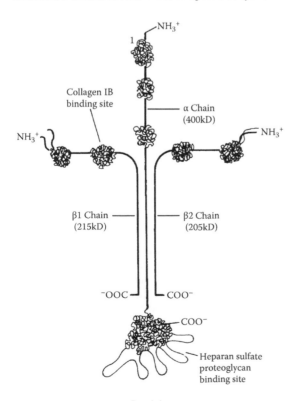

Laminin.

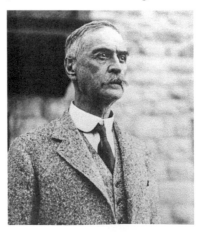

Karl Landsteiner.

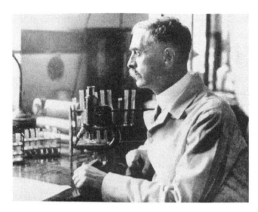

Karl Landsteiner in his laboratory.

LAMP 1 and LAMP 2

Lysosome-associated membrane proteins that are complex molecular structures involved in maintaining lysosomal membrane integrity in cytotoxic lymphocytes and in platelets. LAMP 1 is designated CD107a; LAMP 2 is designated CD107b.

Lancefield precipitation test

A ring precipitation test developed by Rebecca Lancefield to classify streptococci according to their group-specific polysaccharides. The polysaccharide antigen is derived by treatment of cultures of the microorganisms with HCl, formimide, or a *Streptomyces albus* enzyme. Antiserum is first placed into a serological tube, followed by layering the polysaccharide antigen over it. A positive reaction is indicated by precipitation at the interface.

Landsteiner, Karl (1868–1943)

Discoverer of the ABO and other blood group systems including MN and the Rh factor. Landsteiner developed

---

Landsteiner, Zur Kenntnis der antifermentativen etc. Wirkungen des Blutserums. 357

Nachdruck verboten.

Zur Kenntnis der antifermentativen, lytischen und agglutinierenden Wirkungen des Blutserums und der Lymphe.

[Aus dem pathol.-anat. Univ.-Institute des Prof. Weichselbaum in Wien.]

Von Dr. **Karl Landsteiner** in Wien.

I. Zur Serumdiagnostik der Fermente.

Durch die Arbeiten von Fermi[1], Pernossi[1], Hammarsten, Hahn[2], Röden[3], Hildebrandt[4] und Morgenroth[5] wurde festgestellt, daß dem Blutserum die Fähigkeit zukomme, die Wirkung mancher Fermente aufzuheben. Fermi und Hahn führten ihre Untersuchungen an verdauenden Fermenten aus, Röden und Morgenroth am Labenzym.

Die Hoffnung, dieses eigentümliche Verhalten des Serums zur Untersuchung der Fermente benutzen zu können, ist leicht begreiflich, und es hat Morgenroth[6] Versuche in Aussicht gestellt, die mit Hilfe der Einwirkung von Serum beweisen, daß im Lab verschiedene wirksame Gruppen vorhanden sind. In anderer Weise versuchte v. Dungern[7] die antifermentativen Serumwirkungen zu verwerten, indem er Tiere mit verschiedenen Mikrobien immunisierte und zeigte, daß das resultierende Serum spezifisch gegen die Fermente der eingeführten Bakterien wirke. Es handelt sich in diesen Versuchen also um eine Art von Serodiagnostik von Bakterien auf dem Umwege über ihre Fermente. Wie es scheint, ist eine praktische Verwertung dieses Verhaltens bis jetzt nicht erzielt worden.

Versuche, die ich anstellte, gingen darauf aus, das Serum als Hilfsmittel zur Unterscheidung solcher tierischen Fermente zu benutzen, die auf anderem Wege keine Differenzen erkennen lassen. Ich wählte das tryptische Ferment als Objekt der Untersuchung. Dabei ging ich von der Vermutung aus, daß die gleich benannten Fermente verschiedener Tierspecies ebenso jeder Art eigentümlich sein könnten wie die wirksamen Serumstoffe, die Hämoglobine und gewisse andere Bestandteile der roten Blutkörperchen und tierischen Zellen überhaupt.

Die Erkenntnis der gesetzmäßigen Besonderheit sehr ähnlicher, zunächst nicht unterscheidbarer Stoffe bei den verschiedenen Species gelang bisher zum Teil durch chemische Untersuchung, namentlich durch die Serumreaktionen, andererseits führten physiologische und morphologische Ueberlegungen zu ähnlichen Schlüssen. So hat erst vor kurzem Rabl[8] auf Grund der Erfahrungen bei Transplantationsversuchen und seiner Untersuchungen über den Bau der Linse des Auges auf die Konstanz der Unterschiede homologer Strukturen bei den verschiedenen Tierspecies hingewiesen.

1) Zeitschr. f. Hyg. Bd. XVIII. u. a. a. O.
2) Berl. klin. Wochenschr. 1897. p. 499.
3) Cit. nach Hahn.
4) Virch. Arch. Bd. CXXXI.
5) Centralbl. f. Bakt. etc. Bd. XXVI. No. 11, 12.
6) l. c.
7) Ref. Münch med. Wochenschr. 1898. p. 1040.
8) 71. Versamml. deutscher Naturforscher.

Title page of Karl Landsteiner's article describing the human blood groups.

artificial haptens to investigate antibody specificity and received the Nobel Prize in Medicine or Physiology in 1930 for discovery of the human blood groups. He was born in Vienna in 1868. He attended the University of Vienna and graduated in 1891 as a medical doctor. He maintained a strong interest in chemistry and took special instruction under Emil Fischer and Eugen von Bamberger. In 1896, he became an assistant at the Institute of Hygiene directed by Max von Grüber and was introduced to immunology and serology that occupied his research interests for the remainder of his career. He also conducted research in pathology. He coauthored nine papers with Donath, including a report on paroxysmal hemoglobinuria. Landsteiner was appointed a research assistant at the Vienna Pathological Institute in 1898. He remained there until 1908 when he became chief of pathology at the Royal Imperial Wilhelminen Hospital in Vienna and adjunct professor on the Medical Faculty of the University of Vienna. After World War I, Austria was chaotic and experienced inflation and fuel and food shortages. Landsteiner left for the Hague in The Netherlands in 1919, where he accepted a position at the Catholic Hospital. He was lured to the Rockefeller Institute for Medical Research in New York in 1923 at the invitation of its director, Dr. Simon Flexner. He became an American citizen in 1929 and died in New York on 26 June 1943. He discovered the human blood groups in 1900 when he found that the sera of some individuals could cause the agglutination of red cells from others. This led him to characterize red blood cells according to their antigens, leading subsequently to a description of the ABO blood groups. The development of citrates as anticoagulants in 1914 by Richard Lewisohn and Landsteiner's blood grouping system led to the widespread use of blood transfusion. In 1927, Landsteiner and Phillip Levine discovered the M and N blood group antigens that are not of significance in transfusion since human blood serum does not contain isoagglutinins (antibodies) against them, differentiating MN from the ABO groups. In 1940 Landsteiner, Levine, and Weiner discovered the Rh blood group system when they found that antibodies raised in rabbits and guinea pigs immunized with blood from a rhesus monkey agglutinated the red blood cells of many humans (termed Rh positive). Those not possessing this blood factor were termed Rh negative. The Rh factor was shown to be important in hemolytic disease of the newborn. Landsteiner investigated poliomyelitis between 1908 and 1922. He discovered that a rhesus monkey became paralyzed following the injection of brain and spinal cord from a polio victim. After finding no bacteria in the monkey's nervous system, Landsteiner concluded that a virus was the causative agent. He perfected a technique to diagnose poliomyelitis. He discovered that an extract of ox hearts could replace the antigen derived from livers of babies with congenital syphilis for use in the Wassermann test for syphilis. Landsteiner continued his serology and immunology work at the Rockefeller Institute. He examined the effects of position on attached radicals. He discovered that immunochemical specificity was altered by the *ortho, meta*, or *para* position on aromatic rings of stereoisomers; position was more important than the nature of the radical. Landsteiner further showed that partial antigens (called haptens) were unable to elicit antibody formation, but could react with those formed in response to a complete antigen comprising a hapten bound to a carrier molecule. He demonstrated carrier- and hapten-specific

antibodies. His extensive investigations on immunochemical specificity were summarized in his book titled *Die Specifizität der serologischen Reactionen* published in 1933. The English translation was published in 1936, and a revised edition titled *The Specificity of Serological Reactions* appeared after his death in 1945. Landsteiner found that haptens could combine with pre-existing antibodies to produce allergic desensitization. His work laid a foundation for much of modern immunology, including the construction of synthetic vaccines.

Landsteiner's rule (historical)

In 1900, Karl Landsteiner discovered that human red blood cells could be separated into four groups based on their antigenic characteristics. The groups were designated O, A, B, and AB. He found naturally occurring isohemagglutinins in the sera of individuals specific for the (ABO) blood group antigen which they did not possess (i.e., anti-A and anti-B isohemagglutinin in group O subjects, anti-B in group A individuals, anti-A in group B persons, and neither anti-A nor anti-B in individuals of group AB). This principle became known as Landsteiner's rule.

lane

The path of migration of a molecule of interest from a well or point of application in gel electrophoresis. A substance is propelled within the confines of this path or corridor by an electric current that induces migration and separation of the molecules into bands according to size.

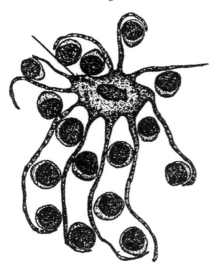

Langerhans cell.

Langerhans cells

Phagocytic- and dendritic-appearing accessory cells interspersed between cells of the upper layer of the epidermis. They function as antigen-presenting cells and produce cytokines that attract lymphocytes to the skin. They can be visualized by gold chloride impregnation of unfixed sections and show dendritic processes but no intercellular bridges. By electron microscopy, they lack tonofibrils or desmosomes, have indented nuclei, and contain tennis racket-shaped Birbeck granules (relatively small, round to rectangular vacuoles that measure 10 nm). Following their formation from stem cells in the bone marrow, Langerhans cells migrate to the epidermis and then to the lymph nodes, where they are described as dendritic cells based upon their thin cytoplasmic processes that course between adjacent cells. Langerhans cells express both class I and class II histocompatibility antigens, as well as C3b receptors and IgG Fc receptors on their surfaces. They function as antigen-presenting cells. Epidermal Langerhans cells express complement receptors 1 and 3, Fcγ receptors, and fluctuating quantities of CD1. They are important in the development of delayed-type hypersensitivity through the uptake of antigen in the skin and its transport to the lymph nodes. Dendritic cells do not express Fcγ receptors or CD1. Langerhans cells in the lymph nodes are found in the deep cortex. Veiled cells in the lymph are indistinguishable from Langerhans cells.

lapinized vaccine
A preparation used for immunization that is attenuated by passage through rabbits until its original virulence has been lost.

LAR
Refer to local acquired resistance.

large granular lymphocytes (LGLs)
Refer to natural killer cells.

large lymphocyte
A 12-μm or greater diameter lymphocyte.

large pre-B cells
Immature B cells with surface pre-B cell receptors that are deleted on transition to small pre-B cells, which undergo light chain gene rearrangement.

large pyroninophilic blast cell
Cells that stain positively with methyl green pyronin stain. They are found in thymus-dependent areas of lymph nodes and other peripheral lymphoid tissues.

LAT
Refer to linker of activation in T cells.

late onset immune deficiency
A disease of unknown cause associated with gastric carcinoma, pernicious anemia, atrophic gastric autoimmunity, and several other conditions.

late phase reaction (LPR)
An inflammatory response that begins approximately 5 to 8 hours after exposure to antigen in immunoglobulin E (IgE)-mediated allergic diseases. Leukocytes, attracted to the allergen site by early phase reaction mediators, produce cytokines, enzymes, and inflammatory mediators that cause further injury. Eosinophils are the predominant NANT cell type. Inflammation is accompanied by pruritus and minor cellular infiltration. Asthmatic patients may produce delayed or secondary responses following antigenic challenge involving the release of histamines from neutrophils. This induces secondary degranulation of mast cells and basophils which stimulates bronchiole hyperreactivity. Whereas prostaglandin and then PGD_2 are produced in the primary response, they are not formed in the late phase reaction. Cold air, ozone, viruses, and other irritants may induce the late phase reaction. This condition may be treated with β-adrenergic aerosols; it is resistant to treatment with antihistamine. Repeated episodes of late phase reactivity can produce tissue injury.

late pro-B cell
Refer to pro-B cell.

latency
A condition in which viruses enter a cell but do not replicate. Once reactivated, the virus may replicate and cause disease.

latent allotype
The detection of an unexpected allotype in an animal's genetic constitution. This allotype is expressed as a temporary replacement of the nominal heterozygous allotype of the animal. It has been described among rabbit immunoglobulin allotypes. Whereas an F_1 rabbit would be expected to synthesize α_1 or α_2 heavy chain allotypes if one parent were homozygous for α_1 and its other parent homozygous for α_2, the F_1 rabbit might under certain circumstances of stimulation produce immunoglobulin molecules of the α_3 (latent) allotype.

latent infection
The long-term presence of a pathogenic microorganism that remains uninfectious and fails to produce clinical symptoms. A consequence of viral genome integration into host cell DNA or altered expression of viral genes.

latex allergy
Hypersensitivity to natural latex, the milky sap from the rubber tree *Hevea brasiliensis*. The symptoms range from hand dermatitis to life-threatening anaphylaxis. Three percent of the general population shows sensitivity to latex and 2 to 25% of healthcare workers manifest this type of hypersensitivity; 9% of nurses have natural latex-specific immunoglobulin E (IgE) antibodies. Patients with increased frequency of operations have increased prevalence of the allergy (29%). The number of operations and total serum IgE are the most important factors in predicting latex allergy. Natural latex-specific IgE is detectable by RAST, enzyme immunoassay (EIA), flow cytometry, and electrochemiluminescence. Patients with latex allergy show increased frequency of allergy to foods such as avocado, potato, banana, tomato, chestnut, and kiwi.

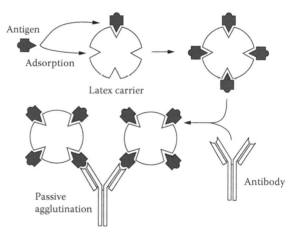

Latex fixation test.

latex fixation test
A technique in which latex particles are used as passive carriers of soluble antigens adsorbed to their surfaces. Antibodies specific for the adsorbed antigen then cause agglutination of the coated latex particles. This technique is widely used and is the basis of a rheumatoid arthritis (RA) test in which pooled human immunoglobulin G (IgG) molecules are coated on the surfaces of latex particles that are then agglutinated by anti-immunoglobulin antibodies in the sera of rheumatoid arthritis patients.

latex particles
Inert particles of defined size that serve as carriers of antigens or antibodies in latex agglutination immunoassays. An example is the rheumatoid arthritis (RA) test in which latex particles are coated with pooled human IgG that serves as the antigen. The coated particles are

agglutinated by rheumatoid factor (anti-immunoglobulin antibody) that may be detected in the serum of a patient with rheumatoid arthritis.

LATS (long-acting thyroid stimulator)
See long-acting thyroid stimulator.

LATS protector
An antibody found in Graves' disease patients that inhibits LATS neutralization *in vitro*. It forms the basis for a LATS protector assay in which sera from patients with Graves' disease are tested for the ability to "protect" a known LATS serum from neutralization by binding to human thyroid antigen.

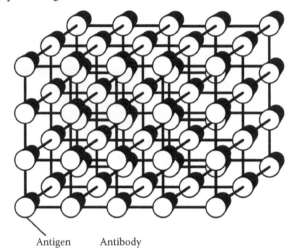

Antigen   Antibody

Antigen–antibody lattice formation.

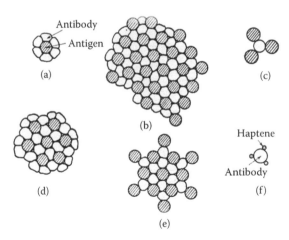

Marrack's proposal of a lattice network theory of antigen–antibody interaction.

lattice theory
The concept that soluble antigen and antibody combine in a precipitation reaction to produce an interconnecting structure of molecules. This structure has been likened to a crisscross pattern of wooden strips fastened together to reveal a series of diamond-shaped structures. Lattice formation requires interaction of bivalent antibodies with multivalent antigens to produce a connecting linkage of many molecules that constitute a complex whose density becomes sufficient to settle out of solution. The more epitopes recognized by the antibody molecules present, the more extensive the complex formation.

Laurell crossed immunoelectrophoresis
Refer to crossed immunoelectrophoresis.

Laurell rocket test
A method to quantify protein antigens by rapid immuno-electrophoresis. Antiserum is incorporated in agarose, into which wells are cut and protein antigen samples are distributed. The application of an electric current at 90° angles to the antigen row drives antigen into the agar. Dual lines of immune precipitate emanate from each well and merge to form a point where no more antigen is present, producing a structure that resembles a rocket. The amount of antigen can be determined by measuring the rocket length from the well to the point of precipitate. This length is proportional to the total amount of antigen in the preparation.

LAV
Lymphadenopathy-associated virus. Refer to HIV-1.

Lawrence, Henry Sherwood (1916–2004)
American immunologist. While studying type IV hypersensitivity and contact dermatitis, he discovered transfer factor. (See *Cellular and Humoral Aspects of Delayed Hypersensitivity*, 1959.)

lazy leukocyte syndrome
A disease of unknown cause in which patients experience increased incidence of pyogenic infections such as abscess formation, pneumonia, and gingivitis. The disease is linked to defective neutrophil chemotaxis in combination with neutropenia. Random locomotion of neutrophils is diminished and abnormal, demonstrated by the vertical migration of leukocytes in capillary tubes. The exodus of neutrophils from the bone marrow is also impaired.

LCA (leukocyte common antigen)
See leukocyte common antigen.

LCAM
Leukocyte cell adhesion molecule.

L cell conditioned medium
A powerful growth factor for macrophages, termed macrophage colony-stimulating factor (M-CSF), present in L cell cultures.

L chain
A 22-kDa polypeptide chain found in all immunoglobulin molecules. The two types are designated κ and λ. Each four-chain immunoglobulin monomer contains two κ or two λ light chains. The two types of light chains never occur in one molecule under natural conditions. Refer to light chain.

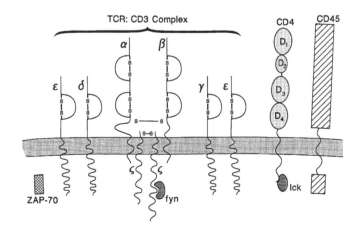

Structure of TCR/CD3 complex showing the lck, fyn, and ZAP phosphotyrosine kinases.

L

lck, fyn, ZAP (phosphotyrosine kinases in T cells)

The phosphotyrosine kinases (PTKs) associated with early signal transduction in T cell activation. *Lck* is a *src*-type PTK found on T cells in physical association with CD4 and CD8 cytoplasmic regions. Deficiency of *lck* results in decreased stimulation of T cells and decreased T cell growth. *Fyn* is also a *src* PTK; it is found on hematopoietic cells. Increased *fyn* results in enhanced T cell activation, but a deficiency of *fyn* has not been shown to decrease T cell growth. A *fyn* deficiency inhibits T cell activation in only some T cell subsets. *ZAP*, or ζ-associated protein kinase, is like the *syk* PTK in B cells. It is found only on T cells and natural killer (NK) cells. Activity of the enzyme is dependent on association of *ZAP* with the ζ chain following T cell receptor (TCR) activation.

LCM

Refer to lymphocytic choriomeningitis.

LD$_{50}$

The dose of a substance, such as a bacterial toxin or microbial suspension, that leads to the death of 50% of a group of test animals within a certain period following administration. The measurement is employed to evaluate toxicity or virulence and the protective qualities of vaccines administered to experimental animals.

LDCF (lymphocyte-derived chemotactic factor)

Lymphokines that are chemotactic factors, especially for mononuclear phagocytes.

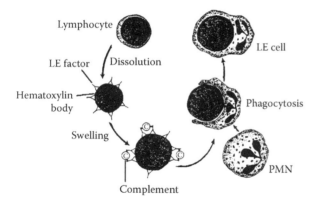

Formation of a lupus erythematosus (LE) cell.

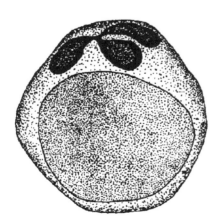

Lupus erythematosus (LE) cell.

LE cell

A neutrophil (polymorphonuclear neutrophil, or PMN) in the peripheral blood or synovia of lupus erythematosus (LE) patients produced when the PMNs phagocytize with Wright's stain, a reddish-purple staining homogeneous lymphocyte nucleus coated with antinuclear antibody. In addition to LE, these cells are seen also in scleroderma, drug-induced lupus erythematosus, and lupoid hepatitis.

LE cell "prep"

Glass beads are added to heparinized blood samples, causing the release of nuclei from some blood cells that become coated with antinuclear antibody present in the serum. These opsonized nuclei are then phagocytized by polymorphonuclear neutrophils to produce lupus erythematosus (LE) cells. The LE cells produce homogeneous chromatin that imparts a glassy appearance to the phagocytized nuclear material.

LE cell test

A no-longer-used diagnostic test that detects antinuclear antibodies in the sera of systemic lupus erythematosus (SLE) patients. Antinuclear antibodies in the serum react with nascent lymphocyte nuclei and serve as opsonins, enhancing phagocytosis of the nucleus–antibody complex by polymorphonuclear neutrophils. Thus, the so-called LE cell is represented by the appearance of a polymorphonuclear neutrophil with its own nucleus displaced to the periphery by an ingested lymphocyte nucleus that appears as a homogeneous mass and is coated with antinuclear antibody. These cells develop following incubation of blood containing the appropriate antibody for 1 hour at 37°C. This early diagnostic test for the presence of antinuclear antibody in SLE has been replaced by a more sophisticated test. LE cells are also present in other connective tissue diseases in addition to SLE.

LE factor

Antinuclear antibodies present in the blood sera of systemic lupus erythematosus patients. LE factor facilitates LE cell formation.

leader peptide

A 20-amino acid sequence situated at the N termini of free heavy and light polypeptide chains and absent in secreted immunoglobulins. Once the light and heavy polypeptide chains reach the cisternal space of the endoplasmic reticulum, the peptide is split from the polypeptide chains. It is thought to facilitate vectorial release of the chains and their secretions.

leader sequence

Refer to leader peptide.

leading front technique

A method to assay chemotaxis or cell migration that evaluates differences in the migration of stimulated and nonstimulated cells.

lectin

A glycoprotein that binds to specific sugars and oligosaccharides and links to glycoproteins or glycolipids on cell surfaces. They can be extracted from plants, seeds, and other sources. They are able to agglutinate cells such as erythrocytes through recognition of specific oligosaccharides and occasionally react with a specific monosaccharide. Many lectins also function as mitogens and induce lymphocyte transformation, during which a small resting lymphocyte becomes a large blast cell that may undergo mitosis. Well known mitogens used in experimental immunology include phytohemagglutinin, pokeweed mitogen, and concanavalin A.

lectin-like receptors

Macrophage and monocyte surface structures that bind sugar residues. The ability of these receptors to anchor polysaccharides and glycoproteins facilitates attachment during phagocytosis of microorganisms. Steroid hormones elevate the number of these cell surface receptors.

lectin pathway of complement activation

A complement-activation pathway, not involving antibody, that is initiated by the binding of microbial polysaccharide to circulating lectins such as the plasma mannose-binding lectin (MBL) which structurally resembles C1q. Similar to C1q, it activates the C1r–C1s enzyme complex or another serine esterase, termed mannose-binding protein-associated serine esterase. Involves MASP1/2, MAp19 and C4, C2, and C3 cleavage and activation. Beginning with C4 cleavage, the lectin pathway is the same as the classical pathway.

Lederberg, Joshua (1925–2008)

American biochemist who made a significant contribution to immunology with his work on the clonal selection theory of antibody formation. He received a Nobel Prize in 1958 (with Beadle and Tatum) for his research on genetic recombination and organization of genetic material in bacteria.

LEF-1

Lymphoid enhancer factor 1 (LEF-1) is a cell-type-specific transcription factor and member of the family of high motility group (HMG) domain proteins that recognizes a specific nucleotide sequence in the T cell receptor (TCR) α enhancer. The function of LEF-1 is dependent, in part, on the HMG domain, which induces a sharp bend in the DNA helix, and on an activation domain, which stimulates transcription only in the specific context of other enhancer-binding proteins.

leflunomide

A prodrug of an inhibitor of pyrimidine synthesis. An isoxazole immunomodulatory agent that blocks dihydroorotate dehydrogenase, an enzyme involved in *de novo* pyrimidine synthesis that has antiproliferative effects. Leflunomide has an anti-inflammatory effect. Its active metabolite has a long half-life of several weeks. It is approved only for treatment of rheumatoid arthritis but may have future potential in combination with mycophenolate mofetil in the treatment of selected autoimmune and inflammatory skin disorders, as well as in combating allograft rejection for solid organ transplants. Toxicities include some risk of liver injury, renal impairment and teratogenic effects.

Legionella immunity

Immunity against *Legionella pneumophila*, a facultative intracellular pathogen that induces Legionnaires' disease in humans, depends on cellular immune mechanisms, including the release of IFN-γ. T$_H$1 CD4$^+$ T cells play a significant role in the development of acquired immunity in mice. Acquired immunity to *Legionella pneumophila* is believed to be a consequence of both humoral and cellular immune responses that facilitate enhanced uptake of the microorganisms by activated mononuclear phagocytic cells.

Leishmania

An obligate intracellular protozoan parasite with an affinity for infecting macrophages. It produces chronic inflammatory disease of numerous tissues. In mice, Th1 responses to *Leishmania major,* including IFN-γ-synthesis, control

infection. By contrast, Th2 responses to IL4 synthesis result in disseminated lethal disease.

leishmaniasis

A parasitic human infection that can lead to the development of various disease conditions ranging from cutaneous lesions to fatal visceral infection. Mouse models of infection have yielded much information on mechanisms of susceptibility and resistance to this infection, rendering experimental leishmaniasis. This is a fine model system to evaluate T cell subset polarization and its relationship to pathogenesis. These intracellular protozoan parasites affect 12 million people worldwide. *Leishmania major* and *L. tropica* may cause cutaneous leishmaniasis; *L. baraziliensas* causes mucocutaneous leishmaniasis; and *L. donovini and L. infantum* induce visceral leishmaniasis to produce the clinical disease known as kala-azar (black disease), dum dum fever, or ponos. This disease follows the spread of the parasite from a skin lesion to tissue macrophages in the liver, spleen, and bone marrow. Patients develop fever, malaise, weight loss, coughing, and diarrhea, anemia, darkening skin, and hepatosplenomegaly. Immunity depends on polarization of CD4$^+$ Th cell subsets. In a Th2 response to infection, interleukin-4 (IL4) and IL10 correlate with disease susceptibility, whereas a murine Th1 response is associated with production of interferon γ (IFN-γ) and IL2, which lead to resolution of lesions in animals that remain refractory to further challenge.

lenalidomide (oral)

An immunomodulatory and antiangiogenic agent, whose mechanism of action remains to be fully determined. It blocks the secretion of proinflammatory cytokines and increases the secretion of anti-inflammatory cytokines from peripheral blood mononuclear cells. It inhibits the expression of cyclooxygenase-2 (COX-2) but not COX-1 *in vitro*.

lens-induced uveitis

An inflammatory reaction in the eye related to sensitization or toxicity to lens material. It also includes inflammation that occurs following dislocation and breakdown of the lens. The lens contains very strong organ-specific antigen that can stimulate the formation of autoantibodies. Lens antigens are normally sequestered and do not induce antibody responses until exposed to the immune system of the host. The principal lens antigen is α crystallin. Evidence that lens-induced uveitis is an immunological disease is based mainly on animal studies, in which its potent immunogenic properties and capacity to produce autoimmune disease have been revealed. The condition is treated by surgically removing the lens or its remnants soon after diagnosis.

lentiviruses

A group of slow retroviruses that have long incubation periods and take years to manifest. Human immunodeficiency virus (HIV) is included in this group.

LEP (low egg passage)

A type of vaccine for rabies that has been employed for the immunization of dogs and cats.

Lepow, Irwin

Lepow and Louis Pillemer were instrumental in describing the alternative pathway of complement activation.

lepra cells

Foamy macrophages that contain clusters of *Mycobacterium leprae* microorganisms that are not degraded because cell-mediated immunity has been lost.

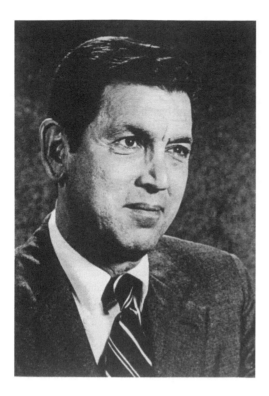

Irwin H. Lepow.

These cells are found in lepromatous leprosy but are not observed in tuberculoid leprosy.

lepromatous leprosy

A chronic granulomatous disease induced by *Mycobacterium leprae*. The condition is contagious and is also known as Hansen's disease. A second form known as tuberculoid leprosy is a more benign and stable form. Both forms infect the peripheral nervous system.

lepromin

A heat-inactivated extract of skin nodules laden with *Mycobacterium leprae*. It is used as a skin test antigen, which, upon intradermal injection, induces formation of a nodular granuloma within 2 to 4 weeks in patients with tuberculoid leprosy but not in those with lepromatous leprosy who are anergic. The development of a positive test signifies the presence of cell-mediated immunity against *M. leprae*.

lepromin test

A tuberculin-type skin test in which a *Mycobacterium leprae* suspension of microorganisms is used as the test material. This delayed-type (type IV) hypersensitivity reaction is negative in lepromatous leprosy but positive in tuberculoid leprosy as well as in normal subjects. The reaction may occur early and peak at 24 to 48 hours (described as a Fernandez reaction), or it may occur late at approximately 4 weeks (referred to as a Mitsuda reaction). Although not useful in diagnosis, this test has been used in the past to classify leprosy and to give some idea of prognosis.

leptin

Endothelial cells express OB-Rβ, the leptin receptor. In addition, leptin, the anti-obesity hormone, is an endothelial cell mitogen and chemoattractant that induces angiogenesis in a cornea implant model.

Leptospira immunity

Newly isolated leptospires evade the host immune system by not reacting with specific antibody, which permits their multiplication. On entering the host, they also evade the host immune system by their sequestration in renal tubules, uterine lumen, eye, or brain. The humoral immune response is marked by production of immunoglobulin M (IgM), which together with complement and phagocytic cells begins to clear leptospires from the host. This is followed by the production of opsonizing and neutralizing IgG. Cell-mediated immunity to *Leptospira* infection is only low grade. Vaccines for use in animals consist of chemically inactivated whole *Leptospira* cultures, which have proven to be somewhat effective. The immunity induced is serovar-specific. These antibodies do not afford protection. Virulent leptospires are better immunogens than are avirulent organisms. It is significant that antigens located on the outer envelope maintain their natural configuration. Both IgM and IgG are induced following parenteral administration of a vaccine, as the IgM is a more efficient agglutinating and neutralizing antibody for leptospires than is IgG.

Lesch–Nyhan syndrome

A deficiency of hypoxanthine-guanine phosphoribosyl transferase that leads to neurological dysfunction and B cell immunodeficiency.

LESTR

Leukocyte-derived 7-transmembrane domain receptor. LESTR is a member of the G protein-coupled receptor family, the chemokine receptor branch of the rhodopsin family. Tissue sources include the human blood monocyte cDNA library and human fetal spleen. It is expressed on monocytes, neutrophils, lymphocytes, and phytohemagglutinin (PHA)-activated T cell blasts. CHO and COS cells transfected with LESTR fail to bind IL8, NAP-2, GRO-α, MCP-1, MCP-3, MIP-1α, and RANTES. Also called fusin and CXCR4.

lethal dose

An amount of a toxin, virus, or other material that produces death in all members of the species receiving it within a specified period of time following administration.

lethal hit

The induction of irreversible injury to a target cell following binding with a cytotoxic T lymphocyte. Exocytosis, cytotoxic lymphocyte granules, polymerization of perforin in target cell membranes, and the passage of calcium ions and granzymes (apoptosis-inducing enzymes) into the cytoplasm of the target cell are observed.

Letterer–Siwe disease

A macrophage lineage tumor (histiocytosis X) that may appear in the skin, lymph nodes, and spleen.

Leu-CAM

Leukocyte cell adhesion molecules.

Leu-M1

A granulocyte-associated antigen. Immunoperoxidase staining detects this marker on myeloid cells but not on B or T cells, monocytes, erythrocytes, or platelets. It can be detected in Hodgkin cells and Reed–Sternberg cells.

leukapheresis

A method that removes circulating leukocytes from the blood of healthy individuals for transfusion to recipients with decreased immunity or who are leukopenic. Leukapheresis is also used in leukemia patients who have too many white cells. The procedure leads to temporary

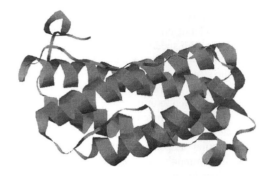

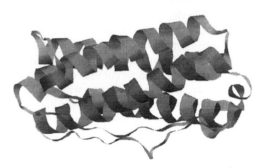

Leukemia inhibitory factor. Resolution = 2.0 Å.

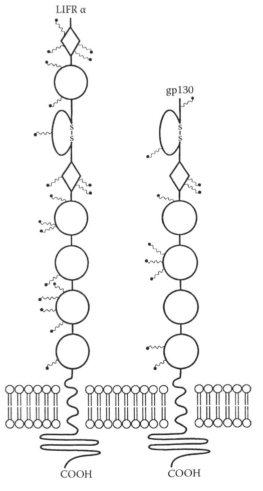

Leukemia inhibitory factor.

relief of symptoms attributable to hyperleukocytosis. Conditioning of a donor with cytokines to mobilize hematopoietic stem cells from the bone marrow into the peripheral blood may be employed to enrich the donor leukocyte preparation for hematopoietic stem cells.

leukemia

Clonal expansion of lymphohematopoietic cells. Acute leukemias are characterized by elevated numbers of immature lymphohematopoietic cells (blasts) in the blood and/or bone marrow. By contrast, chronic leukemias are marked by a neoplastic population of mature-appearing cells. With increasing age, the incidence of acute and chronic myeloid leukemias and of chronic lymphoid leukemias is increased. By contrast, acute lymphoblastic leukemia occurs more frequently among children, reaching a sharp age peak at 3 to 4 years of age. Leukemia cell biology classification has been dramatically advanced through immunological characterization of normal and leukemic hematopoietic cells, the demonstration of immunoglobulin and T cell receptor gene rearrangement, and the molecular elucidation of genetic abnormalities associated with leukemogenesis.

leukemia inhibitory factor (LIF)

A lymphoid factor that facilitates maintenance of embryonic stem cells through suppression of spontaneous generation. It also induces mitogenesis of selected cell lines, stimulation of bone remodeling, facilitation of megakaryocyte formation *in vivo,* and suppression of cellular differentiation in culture. The recombinant form is a 20-kDa protein comprised of 180-amino acid residues. This cytokine has pleiotropic activities. LIF is a member of the interleukin-6 (IL6) family of cytokines which includes oncostatin m, ciliary neurotrophic factor (CNTF), IL11, IL6, and cardiotrophin-1. The receptors for these cytokines consist of a cytokine-specific ligand-binding chain in the shared gp130 transducer chain. Two signal-transducing pathways downstream of gp130 include the Janus kinase (JAK)/signal transducer and activator of transcription (STAT) and the Ras/mitogen-activated protein kinase (MAPK) pathway. LIF can induce the same acute-phase proteins as IL6. It is released at local injury sites where monocytes and polymorphic nuclear cells are recruited. LIF can induce stimulation of proliferation of cancer cells. It also modulates tumor cell capacity to adhere to matrix components.

leukemia viruses

Leukemia is a neoplasm of hematopoietic cells. It may have a viral etiology in humans to produce adult T cell leukemia as well as in mice, cats, cattle, and birds. The leukemia-inducing viruses are members of the Oncovirinae subfamily of the Retroviridae family. Additional retroviruses comprise the lentiviruses, a subfamily of pathogenic slow viruses that include the human immunodeficiency virus (HIV) and the spumaviruses and formiviruses that induce persistent infections unaccompanied by clinical disease. Oncoviruses infect target cells and cause their transformation to produce infected cells with tumor-producing potential. Viral carcinogenesis involves (1) overexpression of a viral *onc* gene; (2) protooncogene (c-*onc*) capture in a retroviral vector and the occurrence of mutations in the captured gene that render it highly oncogenic (v-*onc*); (3) inclusion of two cooperation v-*onc*s in the same provirus; (4) viral protein and activation of a c-*onc* cooperation; and (5) reorganization of cellular transcription processes by a viral transactivation protein.

leukoagglutinin

An antibody or other substance that induces the aggregation or agglutination of white blood cells into clumps.

leukocidin

A cytolytic bacterial toxin produced especially by staphylococci. It is toxic principally for polymorphonuclear leukocytes and to a lesser extent for monocytes. It contains F and S components that combine with cell membranes, causing altered permeability. Less than toxic doses interfere with locomotion of polymorphonuclear neutrophils (PMNs).

leukocyte

White blood cell. The principal types of leukocytes in the peripheral blood of humans include polymorphonuclear neutrophils, eosinophils and basophils (granulocytes), and lymphocytes and monocytes.

leukocyte activation

The first step in activation is adhesion through surface receptors on cells. Stimulus recognition is also mediated through membrane-bound receptors. An inducible endothelial–leukocyte adhesion molecule that provides a mechanism for leukocyte–vessel wall adhesion has been described. Surface-adherent leukocytes undergo a large prolonged respiratory burst. NADPH oxidase, which utilizes hexose monophosphate shunt-generated NADPH, catalyzes the respiratory burst. Both Ca^{2+} and protein kinase C play key roles in the activation pathway. Complement receptor 3 (CR3) facilitates the ability of phagocytes to bind and ingest opsonized particles. Molecules found to be powerful stimulators of polymorphonuclear neutrophil (PMN) activity include recombinant interferon-γ (IFN-γ), granulocyte–macrophage colony-stimulating factor (GM-CSF), tumor necrosis factor (TNF), and lymphotoxin.

leukocyte adhesion deficiency (LAD)

Recurrent bacteremia with staphylococci or *Pseudomonas* linked to defects in the leukocyte adhesion molecules known as integrins, which mainly alters the ability of leukocytes to reach extracellular pathogens at sites of infection, thereby preventing their effective eradication. These include the CD11/CD18 family of molecules. CD18 β chain gene mutations lead to a lack of complement receptors CR3 and CR4 to produce a congenital disease marked by recurring pyogenic infections. Deficiency of p150,95, leukocyte-function-associated antigen 1 (LFA-1), and complement receptor 3 (CR3) membrane proteins leads to diminished adhesion properties and mobility of phagocytes and lymphocytes. All three of these molecules share a flaw in the synthesis of the 95-kDa β chain subunit. The defect in mobility is manifested as altered chemotaxis, defective random migration, and faulty spreading. Particles coated with C3 are not phagocytized and therefore fail to activate a respiratory burst. The CR3 and p150,95 deficiencies account for the defective phagocytic activity. The T cells of patients with LAD fail to respond normally to antigen or mitogen stimulation and are also unable to provide helper function for B cells producing immunoglobulin. They are ineffective in fatally injuring target cells, and they do not produce the lymphokine interferon-γ (IFN-γ). LFA-1 deficiency accounts for the defective responses of these T lymphocytes and all natural killer (NK) cells that also have impaired ability to fatally injure target cells. Clinically, the principal manifestations are consequences of defective phagocyte function rather than of defective T lymphocyte function. Patients may have recurrent severe infections, defective inflammatory responses, abscesses, gingivitis, and periodontitis. LAD has two forms; those with the severe deficiency do not express the three α and four β chain complexes, whereas those with moderate deficiency express 2.5 to 6% of these complexes. The two human LAD syndromes thus far recognized include LAD I, in which the integrin family is defective, and LAD II, in which sialyl Lewis^X, the ligand for selectins, is absent. LAD has an autosomal-recessive mode of inheritance; LAD I is attributable to mutations in the gene that encodes the CD18 protein which is part of the β_2 integrins, whereas mutations in the gene that encodes an enzyme needed for the synthesis of leukocyte ligands for endothelial selectins causes LAD II.

leukocyte adhesion molecule-1

A homing protein found on membranes that combines with target-cell-specific glycoconjugates. It helps regulate migration of leukocytes through lymphocytes binding to high endothelial venules and neutrophil adherence to endothelium at inflammatory sites.

leukocyte adhesion molecules (LAMs)

Facilitators of vascular endothelium aggregation, chemotaxis, cytotoxicity, binding of iC3b-coated particles, lymphocyte proliferation, and phagocytosis. The three main families of LAMs include the selectins, integrins, and immunoglobulin superfamily. Leukocyte adhesion deficiencies are partial or complete inherited deficiencies of cell surface expression of CD18 and CD11a–c. These deficiencies prevent granulocytes from migrating to extravascular sites of inflammation, leading to recurrent infections and possibly death.

leukocyte adhesion protein

A membrane-associated dimeric glycoprotein composed of a unique α subunit and a shared 95-kDa β subunit involved in cell-to-cell interactions. This protein group includes lymphocyte function-associated antigen 1 (LFA-1) found on lymphocytes, neutrophils, and monocytes; membrane attack complex 1 (MAC-1) found on neutrophils, eosinophils, natural killer (NK) cells, and monocytes; and p150,95, which is common to all leukocytes.

leukocyte chemotaxis inhibitors

Humoral factors that inhibit the chemotaxis of leukocytes. They play a role in the regulation of inflammatory responses of both immune and nonimmune origin.

leukocyte common antigen (LCA, CD45)

A family of high molecular weight glycoproteins (180 to 220 kDa) densely expressed on lymphoid and myeloid cells, including lymphocytes, monocytes, and granulocytes. Expression of LCA on leukocytes but not on other cells makes LCA a valuable marker in immunophenotyping of tumors to determine histogenetic origin. LCA antigen function is unknown, but it has a high carbohydrate content and is believed to be associated with the cytoskeleton. LCA molecules are heterogeneous and appear on T and B lymphocytes and selected other hematopoietic cells. Some LCA epitopes are present in all LCA molecules, while others are confined to B lymphocyte LCA; still other epitopes are associated with B cell, CD8$^+$ T cell, and most CD4$^+$ T cell LCA molecules. About 30 exons are present in the gene that encodes LCA molecules; it is designated as CD45.

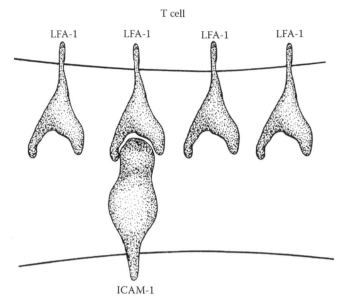

Adhesion to artificial membranes.

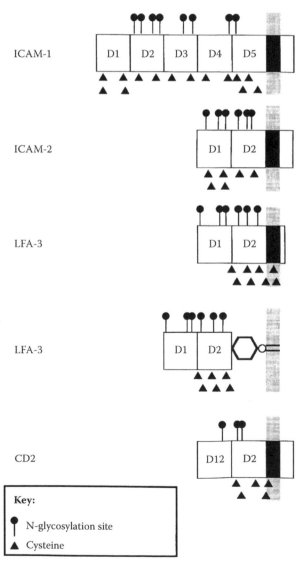

Immunoglobulin superfamily adhesion receptors.

leukocyte culture

In the past, mononuclear blood cells have been cultured *in vitro* in a medium containing serum to support growth; however, culture of cells to be used for patient reinfusion must be grown in a medium that is free of serum, endotoxin, and antibiotics. Tissue culture vessels for the large-scale expansion of leukocytes include polystyrene flasks that can be stacked on top of one another in an incubator; gas-permeable cell-culture bags (30 of which contain 1500 mL of cell culture each) that may be placed in an incubator; tissue-culture bioreactors that include the hollow-fiber cell culture bioreactors; and the rotary cell culture system, both of which provide a three-dimensional growth environment. Clinical applications of leukocyte culture include (1) generation of lymphokine-activated killer (LAK) cells and tumor-infiltrating lymphocytes (TILs) for adoptive immunotherapy; (2) CD34⁺ cell culture and *in vitro* generation of hematopoietic precursors for bone marrow reconstitution; and (3) culture of dendritic cells for use in active immunization.

leukocyte-function-associated antigens (LFAs)

Cell adhesion molecules that include LFA-1, a β_2 integrin; LFA-2, an immunoglobulin superfamily member; and LFA-3, an immunoglobulin superfamily member now designated CD58. LFA-1 facilitates T cell adhesion to endothelial cells and antigen-presenting cells.

leukocyte groups

Leukocytes may be grouped according to their surface antigens such as major histocompatibility complex (MHC) class I and class II histocompatibility antigens. These surface antigens may be detected by several techniques including the microlymphotoxicity assay and DNA typing.

leukocyte inhibitory factor (LIF)

A lymphokine that prevents polymorphonuclear leukocyte migration. T lymphocytes activated *in vitro* may produce this lymphokine, which can interfere with the migration of polymorphonuclear neutrophils from a capillary tube, as observed in a special chamber devised for a laboratory demonstration. Serine esterase inhibitors inhibit LIF activity, although they do not have this effect on macrophage migration inhibitory factor (MIF). This inhibitor is released by normal lymphocytes stimulated with the concanavalin A lectin or by sensitized lymphocytes challenged with the specific antigen. LIF is a 65- to 70-kDa protein.

leukocyte integrins

Refer to leukocyte-function-associated antigens.

leukocyte migration inhibitory factor

Refer to leukocyte inhibitory factor.

leukocyte sialoglycoprotein

Refer to LGSP.

leukocyte transfer

Refer to adoptive transfer.

leukocytoclastic vasculitis

A type of vasculitis with karyorrhexis of inflammatory cell nuclei. Fragments of neutrophil nuclei and immune complexes are deposited in vessels. Direct immunofluorescence reveals IgM, C3, and fibrin in vessel walls. Nuclear dust, necrotic debris, and fibrin staining of the postcapillary venules are present. Leukocytoclastic vasculitis represents a type of allergic cutaneous arteriolitis or necrotizing angiitis. It is seen in a variety of diseases, including Henoch–Schönlein purpura, rheumatoid arthritis, polyarteritis nodosa, and Wegener's granulomatosis, and other diseases.

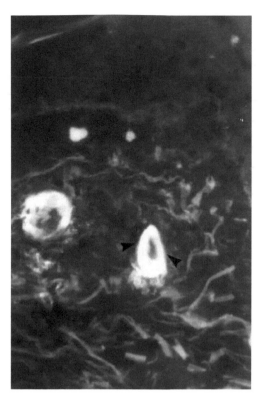

Leukocytoclastic vasculitis.

leukocytosis

An above-normal increase of peripheral blood leukocytes as reflected by a total white blood cell count >11,000/mm of blood. This occurs frequently with acute infection.

leukopenia

A below-normal reduction of the number of white blood cells in the peripheral blood.

leukophysin (LKP)

An RNA helicase A-related molecule identified in cytotoxic T cell granules and vesicles. It is a 28-kDa protein of cytotoxic T lymphocytes and U937 monocytic cells located in the membranes of high density granules and lighter cytoplasmic granules or vesicles. Based on the expression of the C terminal LKP epitope, vesicular structures and granules detected in cytotoxic T lymphocytes (CTLs) are distinct from classical granzyme-containing cytolytic granules.

leukotaxis

Chemotaxis of leukocytes.

leukotriene

An arachidonic acid product generated during an anaphylactic reaction. May include lipid mediators of inflammation and type 1 hypersensitivity. Synthesized following degradation and conversion to arachidonic acid of phospholipids in macrophage, monocytes, neutrophils, and mast cell membranes. Leukotriene formation follows arachidonic acid metabolism via the lipoxygenase pathway. In the past, leukotrienes were referred to as slow-reacting substances of anaphylaxis (SRS-A). These lipid inflammatory mediators are produced by the lipoxygenase pathway in various types

Arachidonic acid

12-HPETE

12-HETE

5-HPETE

5-HETE

Leukotriene A_4

Leukotriene B_4

S-Cys-Gly-Glu

Leukotriene C_4

S-Cys-Gly

Leukotriene D_4

S-Cys

Leukotriene E_4

Lipoxygenase pathway or arachidonic acid metabolism that participates in mediation of type I hypersensitivity reactions.

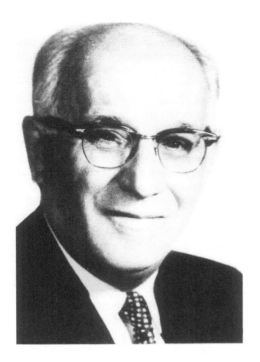

Philip Levine.

of cells. Most cells synthesize plentiful amounts of leukotriene C (LTC) and its breakdown products, LTD and LTE, which bind to smooth muscle cell receptors to produce prolonged bronchoconstriction. Leukotrienes play a significant role in the pathogenesis of bronchial asthma. The former SRS-A term covered the collective actions of LTD and LTE. Refer also to arachidonic acid (AA) and leukotrienes.

levamisole

An antihelminthic drug used extensively in domestic animals and birds that was found to also produce immunostimulant effects. It may potentiate or restore the functions of T lymphocytes and other leukocytes. It increases the magnitude of delayed-type hypersensitivity or T-cell-medicated immunity in humans. It has some efficacy in the treatment of rheumatoid arthritis and induces severe agranular cytosis, which requires discontinuation of use. It also potentiates the action of fluorouracil in adjuvant therapy of colorectal cancer.

Levine, Philip

Russian–American immunohematologist. With Landsteiner, he conducted pioneering research on blood group antigens, including discovery of the MNP system. His work contributed much to transfusion medicine and transplantation immunobiology.

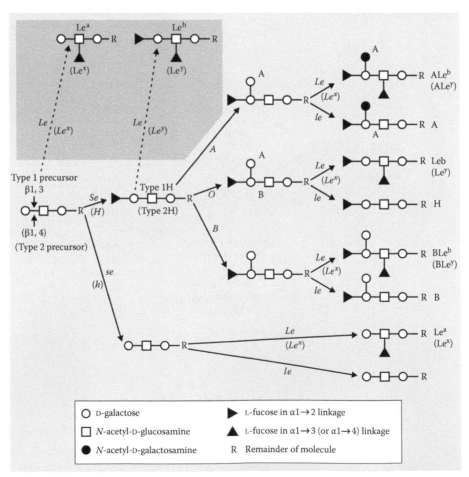

Biosynthetic pathways of ABH, Lewis, and XY antigens derived from type I and type II core chains. Genes controlling steps in the pathway are shown in italics. Types I and II precursors differ in the nature of the linkage between the nonreducing terminal galactolose and *N*-acetylglucosamine: β 1–3 in type I and β 1–4 in type II. Type II structures and the genes that act on them are shown in parentheses. Dashed lines show how Le^a and (Le^x)Le^d(Le^y), produced from the precursor and H structures, respectively, are not substrates for the H, Se, or ABO transferases and remain unconverted.

Lewis Blood Group System

Genotype	Secretor Status	Phenotype
(a) Le, H, se	Nonsecretor	Lea+b–
(b) Le, H, Se	Secretor	Lea–b+
(a) le, H, se	Nonsecretor	Lea–b–
(a) le, H, Se	Secretor	Lea–b–

Lewis blood group system

An erythrocyte antigen system that differs from other red cell groups in that the antigen is present in soluble form in blood and saliva. Lewis antigens are adsorbed from the plasma onto red cell membranes. The Lewis phenotype expressed is based on whether the individual is a secretor or nonsecretor of the Lewis gene product. Expression of the Lewis phenotype is dependent also on the ABO phenotype. Chemically, Lewis antigens are carbohydrates. Lewis secretors face increased likelihood of urinary tract infections induced by *Escherichia coli* and other microbes because of the linkage of carbohydrate residues of glycolipids and glycoproteins on urothelial cells.

Lewis^x/sialyl-Lewis^x: CD15/CD15S

The blood-group-related antigen Lewis^x (Le^x) and related oligosaccharide sequences on glycoproteins and glycolipids serve as ligands for selectins, the leukocyte–endothelium adhesion molecules critical to the early stages of leukocyte recruitment in inflammation. Le^x and sialyl-Lewis^x are human granulocyte and monocyte markers designated CD15 and CD15s, respectively. Monocytes express mainly the sialyl-Le^x. Sialic acid masks the expression of Le^x antigen. Le^x and sialyl-Le^x are tumor-associated antigens. The oligosaccharides may be inappropriately expressed on tumor cells but are established as distinctive markers of myeloid cells in human peripheral blood. Le^x- and Le^a-related sequences serve as ligands for carbohydrate-binding receptors, the selectins. All three selectins bind to sialyl-Le^x-related sequences when they are exhibited in the clustered state on protein or lipid. E-selectin also binds the asialo-Le^x sequence, but less avidly.

L$_f$ dose (historical)

The flocculating unit of diphtheria toxin; the amount of toxin that flocculates most rapidly with one unit of antitoxin in a series of mixtures containing constant amounts of toxin and varying amounts of antitoxin. This unit must be calculated.

L$_f$ flocculating unit (historical)

The flocculating unit of diphtheria toxin; the amount of toxin that flocculates most rapidly with one unit of antitoxin in a series of mixtures containing constant amounts of toxin and varying amounts of antitoxin. Historically, a unit of antitoxin was considered as the least quantity that would neutralize 100 minimal lethal doses of toxin administered to a guinea pig. Modern usage relates antitoxic activity to an international standard antitoxin.

LFA-1, LFA-2, LFA-3

Refer to leukocyte-function-associated antigens.

LFA-1 deficiency

An immunodeficiency caused by a defect in lymphocyte function-associated antigen, a 95-kDa β chain linked to CD11a that ds natural killer (NK) cell binding, T helper cell reactivity, and cytotoxic-T-cell-mediated killing.

This deficiency is associated with pyogenic mucocutaneous infections, pneumonia, diminished respiratory burst, and abnormal cell adherence in chemotaxis, causing poor wound healing among other features.

LFA-2

A T cell antigen that is the receptor molecule for sheep red cells, also known as the T11 antigen and leukocyte-function-associated antigen 2 (LFA-2). The molecule has a weight of 50 kDa. The antigen also seems to be involved in cell adherence, probably binding LFA-3 as its ligand.

LFA-3

A 60-kDa polypeptide chain expressed on the surfaces of B cells, T cells, monocytes, granulocytes, platelets, fibroblasts, and endothelial cells of vessels. It is the ligand for CD2 and is encoded by genes on chromosome 1 in humans.

LGLs (large granular lymphocyte or null cells)

These lymphocytes do not express B and T cell markers, but have Fc receptors for immunoglobulin G (IgG) on their surfaces. They comprise approximately 3.5% of lymphocytes and originate in the bone marrow. LGLs include natural killer (NK) cells (70%) and killer cells that mediate antibody-dependent cell-mediated cytotoxicity (ADCC).

LGSP (leukocyte sialoglycoprotein)

A richly glycosylated protein present on thymocytes and T lymphocytes. B lymphocytes are devoid of LGSP.

Liacopoulos phenomenon (nonspecific tolerance)

The daily administration of 0.5 to 1.0 g of bovine γ globulin and bovine serum albumin to guinea pigs for at least 8 days suppresses their immune responses to these antigens. If an unrelated antigen is injected and continued for several days thereafter, the response to the unrelated antigen is reduced. This phenomenon has been demonstrated for circulating antibody, delayed hypersensitivity, and graft-vs.-host reaction. It describes the induction of nonspecific immunosuppression for one antigen by the administration of relatively large quantities of an unrelated antigen.

liberated CR1

A truncated complement receptor 1 (CR1) without transmembrane and intracytoplasmic domains that may help limit the size of myocardial infarcts by diminishing complement activation. Liberated CR1 may also play a therapeutic role in other types of ischemia, burns, autoimmunity, and inflammation because it is a natural inhibitor of complement activation.

lichenification

Profound hyperkeratosis or skin thickening produced by chronic inflammation.

LICOS

The ligand for ICOS, a CD28-related protein induced on activated T cells that can enhance T cell responses. LICOS is formed on activated dendritic cells, B cells, and monocytes.

Li–Fraumeni syndrome

Inherited susceptibility to selected tumors, usually attributable to germline mutations of p53.

ligand

A molecule that binds or forms a complex with another molecule such as a cell surface receptor.

light chain

A 22-kDa polypeptide chain found in all immunoglobulin molecules. Each four-chain immunoglobulin monomer contains two identical light polypeptide chains joined to two like heavy chains by disulfide bonds. The two types of light

L

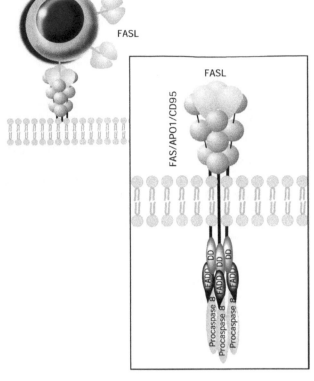

Fas Is a member of the tumor necrosis factor (TNF) receptor superfamily and contains a cytoplasmic death domain (DD) required for Induction of apoptosis. *Fas* ligand (*Fas*L)-Induced receptor trimerization aggregates the DD of *Fas* and recruites the adaptor protein FADD and procaspase 8. Following activation of caspase 8, the DD-Induced complex can trigger subsequent events of apoptosis.

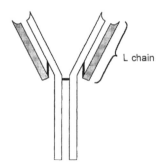

Ligh polypeptide chains of immunoglobulins that are fastened to heavy chains through disulfide bonds and are found in all classes of immunoglobulin.

chains are designated κ and λ. An individual immunoglobulin molecule possesses two light chains that are κ or λ, but never a combination of both. The types of light polypeptide chains occur in all five immunoglobulin classes. Each light chain has an N terminal V region that constitutes part of the antigen-binding site of the antibody molecule. The C region or constant terminal reveals no variation except for the Km and Oz allotype markers in humans.

light chain deficiencies

The ratio of κ to λ light chains may be altered in individuals with immunodeficiencies. κ Chain deficiency has been associated with respiratory infections, megaloblastic anemia, and diarrhea. It has also been associated with

achlorhydria and pernicious anemia and has even been seen in cases of malabsorption, diabetes, and cystic fibrosis. T cell function in all these cases was within normal limits, with only defective B cell immunity observed. Abnormal κ and λ light-chain ratios are secondary findings in certain diseases; they may also act as primary etiologic agents.

light chain disease

A paraproteinemia also known as Bence–Jones myeloma that comprises one fifth of all myelomas. Excess monoclonal light chains are produced. These are linked to renal amyloidosis and renal failure as a consequence of blockage of tubules by certain Bence–Jones proteins. Four fifths of patients have monoclonal light chains in the blood circulation, and 60% have diminished γ globulin and lytic lesions of the bone. The λ type is usually more severe than the κ type. Patients with light chain disease experience a worse course than patients with IgA or IgG myelomas.

light chain subtype

The subdivision of a type of light polypeptide chain based on its primary or antigenic structure that appears in all members of a species. Subtype differences distinguish light chains that share a common type. These relatively minor structural differences are located in the light chain constant region. Oz+, Oz−, Kern+, and Kern− markers represent subtypes of λ light chains in humans.

light chain type

The classification of immunoglobulin light chains based on their primary or antigenic structures. Two types of light chain have been described and are designated κ and λ. Two κ chains or two λ chains, never one of each, are present in each monomeric immunoglobulin subunit of vertebrate species.

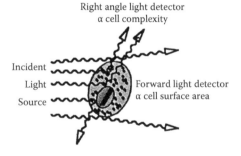

Forward scatter—diffracted light

▼ Related to cell surface area

▼ Detected along axis of incident light in the forward direction

Side Scatter—reflected and refracted light

▼ Related to cell granularity and complexity

▼ Detected at 90° to the laser beam

Properties of forward scatter light and side scatter light are measured by observing how light disperses when a laser hits a cell.

light scatter

Light dispersion in any direction that may be useful for studying cells by flow cytometry. A cell passing through a laser beam absorbs and scatters light. Fluorochrome staining of cells permits absorbed light to be emitted as fluorescence. Forward angle light scatter permits identification of a cell in flow and determination of its size. If higher angle light scatter is added, certain specific cell populations may also be identified. Light scatter measured at 90° to the laser beam and

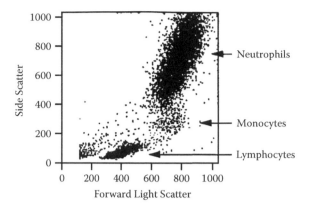

Each dot represents data from one cell. The bigger the cell, the larger the FSC signal and the farther to the right the dot will appear on the *x*-axis. The more complex or granular the cell, the larger the SCC signal and the higher it will appear on the *y*-axis. It is possible to discern lymphocytes, monocytes, and neutrophils in this plot.

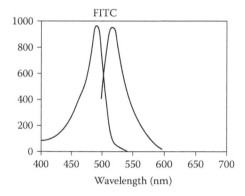

The absorption and emission spectra for the FITC fluorochrome are shown. The peak absorption is around 488 nm and the peak emission is around 530 nm.

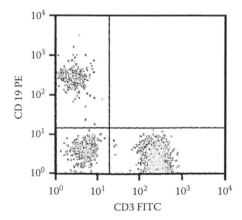

FITC-positive cells fall in the lower right quadrant and PE-positive cells fall in the upper left quadrant. Cells that are positive for both FITC and PE are in the upper right quadrant.

flow stream yields data on cell granularity or fine structure. Light scatter depends on such factors as cell size and shape, cell orientation in flow, cellular internal structure, laser beam shape and wavelength, and angle of light collection.

light zone

A region of a germinal center in secondary lymphoid tissue containing centrocytes that do not divide but interact with follicular dendritic cells. A site of isotype switching where B cells in which immunoglobulin genes have undergone somatic hypermutation are negatively selected to facilitate peripheral B cell tolerance or selected for affinity maturation, i.e., increased affinity for antigen.

limiting dilution

A method of preparing aliquots that contain single cells through dilution to a point where each aliquot contains only one cell. The apportionment of cells by this method follows the Poissonian distribution that yields 37% of aliquots without cells and 63% with one or more cells. This technique may be used to estimate the frequency of a certain cell in a population. For example, it may be employed to approximate the frequency of helper T lymphocytes, cytotoxic T lymphocytes, or B lymphocytes in a lymphoid cell suspension or to isolate cells for cloning in the production of monoclonal antibodies.

lineage infidelity

Cells that undergo neoplastic transformation may express molecules on their surfaces that are alien to their lineage.

linear determinant

Antigenic determinant produced by adjacent amino acid residues in the covalent sequence in proteins. Linear determinants of six amino acids interact with specific antibodies. Occasionally, they may appear on the surface of a native folded protein, but they are more commonly unavailable in the native configuration and become available only for interaction with antibody upon denaturation of the protein.

linear epitope

Antigenic determinant of a protein molecule recognized by an antibody that consists of a linear sequence of amino acids within the protein's primary structure.

linear staining

The interaction of IgG and possibly C3 on peripheral capillary loops of renal glomeruli in antiglomerular basement membrane diseases such as Goodpasture's syndrome. The use of fluorescein-labeled goat or rabbit antiimmunoglobulin preparations permits this smooth, thin, delicate, ribbon-like staining pattern to be recognized by immunofluorescence microscopy. This pattern is in sharp contrast to the lumpy, bumpy patterns of immunofluorescence staining seen in immune complex diseases.

linkage analysis

The use of simple tandem repeat sequences or microsatellites to screen an entire genome for linkage with a trait and identify non-MHC loci linked with disease.

linkage disequilibrium

The appearance of human leukocyte antigen (HLA) genes on the same chromosome with greater frequency than would be expected by chance. This has been demonstrated by detailed studies of populations and families, employing outbred groups in which numerous different haplotypes are present. With respect to the HLA-A, -B, and -C loci, a possible explanation for linkage disequilibrium is that the genes have not had sufficient time to reach equilibrium; however, this possibility is remote for HLA-A, -B, and -D linkage disequilibrium. Natural selection has been suggested to maintain linkage disequilibrium that is advantageous. If products of two histocompatibility loci play a role in the immune response and appear on the same chromosome, they may reinforce one another and represent an advantageous association. An example of linkage

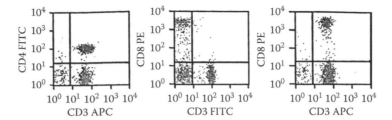

Three bivariate plots displaying stained lymphocytes. CD3⁺ cells are stained with APC, CD4⁺ cells are stained with FITC, and CD8⁺ cells are stained with PE.

Structure

Bound to DNA

DNA content can be quantified by the use of propidium iodide (PI) fluorescent dye. The dye intercalates between the base pairs to stain double-stranded nucleic acids. The amount of DNA that PI binds is proportional to the DNA content.

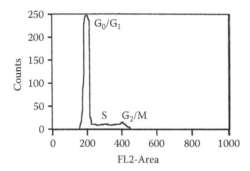

Staining DNA with PI and analyzing the sample by flow cytometry permits the percentage of cells in each phase of the cell cycle to be determined.

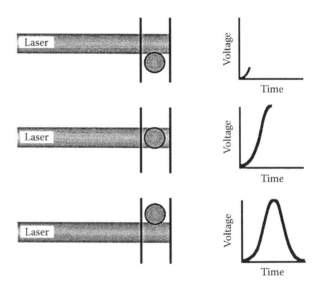

A pulse is created when a particle enters the laser beam and starts to scatter light. The highest point of the pulse occurs when the particle is in the center of the beam and the maximum amount of scatter is achieved. As the particle leaves the laser, the pulse returns to baseline.

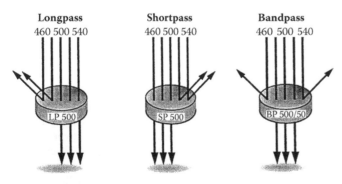

The specificity of an optical detector for a particular fluorescent dye is optimized by placing a filter in front of the detector that allows a narrow range of wavelengths to pass through the filter.

disequilibrium in the HLA system of humans is the occurrence on the same chromosome of HLA-A3 and HLA-B7 in the Caucasian American population.

linked recognition

The need for helper T cells and B cells participating in the antibody response to a thymus-dependent antigen to interact with different epitopes linked physically in the same antigen. Epitopes that B cells and helper T cells recognize must be linked physically for the helper T cell to activate the B cell, which constitutes linked recognition. The need for hapten and carrier to be linked physically rather than merely mixed together to stimulate a secondary response to the hapten.

L

List-Mode Data

	FSC	SSC	FL1	FL2
Event 1	30	60	638	840
Event 2	100	160	245	85
Event 3	300	650	160	720

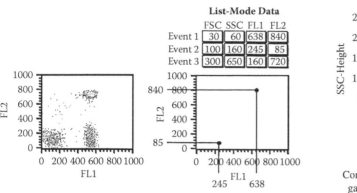

Useful information can be obtained with a dot plot by determining the percentage for each population.

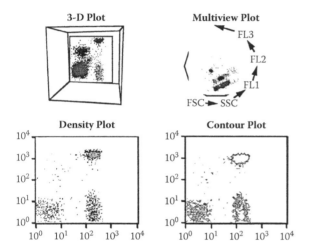

The different plots can be used to clearly display and analyze populations of interest.

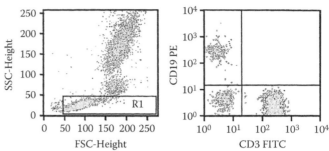

Conventional method for identifying lymphocyte subsets is light scatter gating. The lymphocytes are gated, markers are set using a two-color isotype control, then subsequent immunofluorescence analyses of the remaining files are completed.

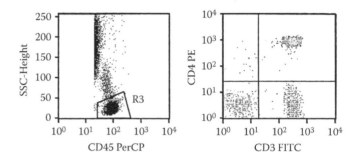

Unlike traditional methods of light scatter gating in which lymphocyte gate purity and recovery are concerns, TriTEST allows the CD45+ lymphocyte population to be gated, providing unambiguous identification.

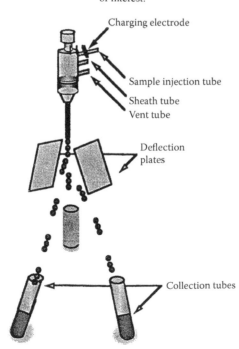

Particles can be isolated by charging them after they are passed through a laser. Depending on the charge, the particular will travel to the left or right sort tube, repelled by or attracted toward the charge plate. All noncharged particles travel to waste.

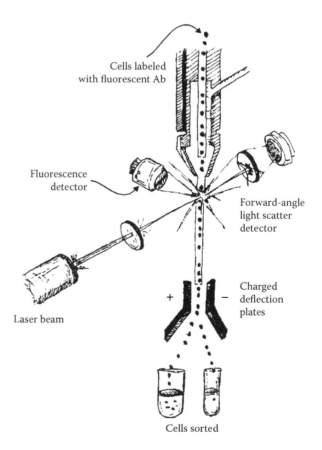

Light scatter.

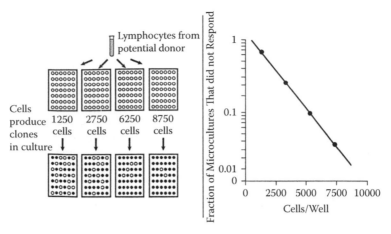

Limiting dilution.

linked suppression

Mechanism whereby peripheral tolerance to one antigen extends to other antigens nearby within the same host. Dependent on regulatory T cells.

linker of activation in T cells (LAT)

An adaptor cytoplasmic protein with several tyrosines that are phosphorylated by ZAP-70, a tyrosine kinase. It associates with membrane lipid rafts and coordinates downstream signaling events in T lymphocyte activation.

lipid raft

A plasma membrane subdomain rich in cholesterol and glycosphingolipid in which cellular activation molecules are concentrated. Proteins in an activated T cell requisite for T cell receptor signaling interact with the rafts and produce a large stable immunosome that attracts and activates more molecular signals. The rafts and signaling molecules act with the T cell receptors' cytoplasmic regions to transduce T cell receptor signaling to the nucleus.

lipopolysaccharide (LPS)

Refer to endotoxin. Refer to LPS.

liposome

A spherical lipid vesicle comprised of 5-nm phospholipid bilayers that enclose one or several aqueous units. These microspheres can be produced by dispersing phospholipid mixtures with or without sterols in aqueous solution. The liposomes produced consist of concentric phospholipid bilayers and thus represent ideal models of cell membranes into which antigens may be embedded to induce an immune response. They also have been used to deliver drugs. They may or may not fuse with cell membranes, and other problems surround their use, e.g., whether they will leave the circulatory system or be phagocytized by reticuloendothelial cells. Liposomes may act as immunologic adjuvants when antigens are incorporated into them. Liposomes serving as biological membrane models have also been used in studies on complement-mediated lysis. They may serve as vehicles for vaccine delivery if the vaccine antigen is incorporated in the aqueous solution.

lipoxygenase pathway

Enzymatic metabolism of arachidonic acid derived from the cell membrane which is the source of leukotrienes.

liquefactive degeneration

Dermal–epidermal interface liquefaction induced by immune mechanisms. This process engages basal cells,

leading to coalescing subepidermal vesicles in such skin diseases as dermatitis herpetiformis, erythema multiforme, fixed drug reaction, lichen planus, lupus erythematosus, and many other conditions.

lissamine rhodamine (RB200)

A fluorochrome that produces orange fluorescence. Interaction with phosphorus pentachloride yields a reactive sulfonyl chloride useful for labeling protein molecules to be used in immunofluorescence staining.

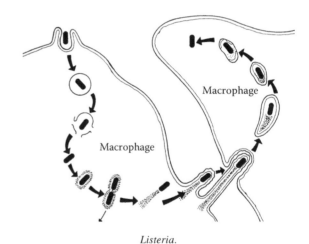

Listeria.

Listeria

A genus of small Gram-positive motile bacilli that have palisade growth patterns. The best known is *L. monocytogenes*, which has a special affinity for monocytes and macrophages, in which it takes up residence. It may be transmitted in contaminated milk and cheese. Approximately one third of the cases occur in pregnant females, resulting in transplacental infection that may induce abortion or stillbirth. Infected infants may develop septicemia, vomiting, diarrhea, cardiorespiratory distress, and meningoencephalitis. Individuals with defective immune reactivity may develop endocarditis, meningoencephalitis, peritonitis, or other infectious processes. Treatment is with ampicillin, erythromycin, gentamycin, or chloramphenicol.

Listeria **immunity**

Immune responsiveness to *Listeria* has been investigated mostly in mouse models. The microorganism may be found in macrophages and also in hepatocytes of infected hosts. Natural immunity in mice is controlled by the Lr1 locus on chromosome II. Mice resistant to *Listeria* respond to the inoculated microorganisms with large numbers of inflammatory phagocytes. Neutrophils and mononuclear phagocytes kill *L. monocytogenes in vitro* although resident macrophages are less effective. Oxygen-dependent and -independent bactericidal mechanisms facilitate destruction of *Listeria*. Multiple cell types and mediators are involved in resistance. T-cell-mediated immunity is significant but is not the only factor in resistance to listeriosis. Neutrophils are also significant to resistance. Other cells implicated include granulocytes, natural killer (NK) cells, and cytotoxic T cells. Infection with the microorganism is followed by the expression of several cytokines that include IFN-γ, IL1β, TNF-α, and GM-CSF, among others. The two cytokines most critical for resistance to listeriosis are IFN-γ and TNF-α. IFN-γ (Th1) is necessary for resistance but IL4 and IL10 (Th2) hinder resistance. Recombinant cytokines that can increase resistance to *L. monocytogenes* infection include IFN-γ, TNF-α, IL1β, and IL12. Experimental animals injected with sublethal doses of viable *Listeria* develop resistance to rechallenge for a few months followed by decreased resistance. Killed microorganisms failed to provide effective immunity.

Listeria monocytogenes

Specific immune responses can be mounted against intracellular bacteria and fungi. Some bacteria reproduce inside cells of a host. For example, mycobacteria and *Listeria monocytogenes* are organisms of high pathogenicity that survive in phagocytic cells such as macrophages where they resist dissolution. Within macrophages, they are not exposed to specific antibody. In addition to mycobacteria and *Listeria* species, a number of fungi are also intracellular pathogens.

live attenuated measles (rubeola) virus vaccine

An immunizing preparation that contains live measles virus strains. It is the preferred form except in patients with lymphoma, leukemia, and other generalized malignancies; radiation therapy; pregnancy; active tuberculosis; egg sensitivity; prolonged drug treatment that suppresses the immune response, such as corticosteroids or antimetabolites; or administration of γ globulin, blood, or plasma. Immune globulin should be administered to persons in these groups immediately following exposure.

live attenuated vaccine

An immunizing preparation consisting of microorganisms whose disease-producing capacity has been weakened deliberately so that they may be used as immunizing agents. Response to a live attenuated vaccine more closely resembles a natural infection than does the immune response stimulated by killed vaccines. The microorganisms in live vaccines continue to divide, which increases the dose of immunogen. Microorganisms in killed vaccines do not reproduce and the amount of injected immunogen remains unchanged. Thus, in general, the protective immunity conferred by responses to live attenuated vaccines is superior to that conferred by killed vaccines. Examples of live attenuated vaccines include those that protect against measles, mumps, polio, and rubella.

live attenuated viral vaccines

An immunizing preparation comprised of live viruses in which the accumulation of mutations interferes with their reproduction in human cells and their ability to cause disease.

live measles and mumps virus vaccine

A standardized immunizing preparation containing attenuated measles and mumps viruses.

live measles and rubella virus vaccine

A standardized immunizing preparation that contains attenuated measles and rubella viruses.

live measles virus vaccine

A standardized attenuated virus immunizing preparation used to protect against measles.

live oral poliovirus (Sabin) vaccine

An immunizing preparation prepared from three types of live attenuated polioviruses. An advisory panel to the Centers for Disease Control and Prevention recommended in 1999 that its routine use be discontinued. It contains a weakened live virus linked to eight to ten cases of polio each year. Now that the polio epidemic has been eliminated in the United States, this risk is no longer acceptable.

live rubella virus vaccine

An attenuated virus immunizing preparation employed to protect against rubella (German measles). All nonpregnant susceptible women of childbearing age should receive this vaccine to prevent fetal infection and congenital rubella syndrome (possible fetal death, prematurity, impaired hearing, cataracts, mental retardation, and other serious consequences).

live vaccine

An immunogen for protective immunization that contains an attenuated strain of the causative agent, an attenuated strain of a related microorganism that cross protects against the pathogen of interest, or the introduction of a disease agent through an avenue other than its normal portal of entry or in combination with an antiserum.

liver cytosol autoantibodies

Autoantibodies against liver cystolic antigen type I (LC1) are present in 20% of patients who are liver–kidney microsome 1 (LKM-1) autoantibody positive, in less than 1% of subjects infected with chronic hepatitis C virus, and in some patients with autoimmune hepatitis (AIH).

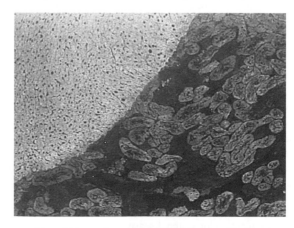

Liver–kidney microsome 1 (LKM-1) autoantibodies.

liver–kidney microsomal antibodies

Antibodies present in a subset of antinuclear antibody (ANA)-negative individuals who have autoimmune chronic active hepatitis. By immunofluorescence, these antibodies can be shown to interact with hepatocyte and proximal renal tubule cell cytoplasm. The antibodies are not demonstrable in the sera of non-A, non-B chronic active hepatitis patients.

liver–kidney microsome 1 (LKM-1) autoantibodies

Autoantibodies associated with autoimmune hepatitis type II. Their principal feature is the exclusive staining of the P3 portions of the proximal renal tubules. Sixty-seven percent of patients with this disease have antibodies to liver cytosol type I (anti-LC-1). Cytochrome P-450 2D6 is the major antigen for LKM-1 autoantibodies, which are specific for cytoplasmic constituents of hepatocytes and proximal renal tubule cells. They are present in selected patients with antinuclear antibody (ANA)-negative autoimmune chronic active hepatitis (CAH) (HBsAg negative). They are not found in CAH non-A, non-B. LKM-1-autoantibody-positive CAH type II is the most frequent autoimmune liver disease in children, who have a relatively poor prognosis. LKM-1 autoantibodies are not believed to be pathogenic in autoimmune CAH of children. They show specificity for cytochrome P-450. LKM-2 autoantibodies are present in tienilic acid (Ticrynafen)-induced hepatitis. LKM-3 autoantibodies are present in 10% of chronic delta virus hepatitis cases. The LKM-1 antigen is cytochrome P-450IID6. The LKM-2 antigen is cytochrome P-450IIC8/9/10.

liver–kidney microsome 2 (LKM-2) autoantibodies

Antibodies associated only with drug-induced hepatitis caused by tienilic acid and not an autoimmune hepatitis. These antibodies are specific for cytochrome P-450-2 C9.

liver–kidney microsome 3 (LKM-3) autoantibodies

An autoantibody that detects a protein band of 55 kDa in approximately 10% of patients with autoimmune chronic hepatitis type II.

liver membrane (LM) antibodies

Antibodies specific for the 26-kDa LM protein target antigen in the sera of 70% of autoimmune chronic active hepatitis patients who are HBsAg-negative. These antibodies are demonstrable by immunofluorescence, and they may also be demonstrated in patients with primary biliary cirrhosis, chronic hepatitis B, alcoholic liver disease, and sometimes Sjögren's syndrome. Lupoid autoimmune chronic active hepatitis patients may develop antibodies against liver membrane and also against smooth muscle and nuclear constituents. Liver membrane antibodies are not useful for diagnosis or prognosis.

liver membrane autoantibodies

A heterogeneous group of autoantibodies that include liver-specific membrane lipoprotein (LSMP) autoantibodies linked to chronic autoimmune hepatitis (AIH). They lack disease specificity but are useful prognostically for treatment withdrawal. Characteristic autoantibodies usually aid in the diagnosis of autoimmune hepatitis. Persistence or reappearance of liver-specific protein antibodies in chronic AIH patients in remission during treatment withdrawal may signify reactivation of the disease.

LM autoantibodies

Antimicrosomal antibodies that react exclusively with liver tissue have been found in drug-induced hepatitis caused by dihydralazine. They interact with cytochrome P-450-1A2. LM antibodies against cytochrome P-450-1A2 in non-drug-induced autoimmune liver disease suggest that the liver

disease may be a manifestation of autoimmune polyendocrine syndrome type II (APS-1).

LMP-2 and LMP-7

Catalytic subunits of the organelles (proteasomes) that degrade cytosolic proteins into peptides in the major histocompatibility complex (MHC) class I pathway of antigen presentation. MHC genes encode these two subunits that are upregulated by INF-γ and are especially significant in the generation of MHC class I-binding peptides.

LMP genes

Two genes located in the major histocompatibility complex (MHC) class II regions in humans and mice that code for proteasome subunits. They are closely associated with the two *TAP* genes.

L$_0$ dose (historical)

The largest amount of toxin that, when mixed with one unit of antitoxin and injected subcutaneously into a 250-g guinea pig, produces no toxic reaction.

local acquired resistance

Metabolic changes in plant cells that result in the deposition or cross linking of lipoproteins and other locally acquired resistance molecules to strengthen plant cell walls and isolate a pathogenic microorganism. Antimicrobial peptides and plant regulatory peptides that activate pathogenesis-related proteins are induced.

local anaphylaxis

A relatively common type I immediate hypersensitivity reaction. Local anaphylaxis is mediated by immunoglobulin E (IgE) cross linked by allergen molecules at the surfaces of mast cells that then release histamines and other pharmacological mediators that produce signs and symptoms. The reaction occurs in a particular target organ such as the gastrointestinal tract, skin, or nasal mucosa. Hay fever and asthma represent examples.

local immunity

Immunologic reactivity confined principally to a particular anatomic site such as the respiratory or gastrointestinal tract. Local antibodies and lymphoid cells present in the area may mediate a specific immunologic effect. For example, secretory IgA produced in the gut may react to food or other ingested antigens.

loci

Plural of locus.

locus

The precise location of a gene on a chromosome or other marker; the DNA at that position. The use of *locus* is sometimes restricted to regions of DNA that are expressed.

locus accessibility

The extent to which the chromatin architecture of a specific antigen receptor gene permits it to be a substrate for the recombinase complex. Controlled by enhancers.

London forces

Forces that contribute somewhat to the stabilization of the antigen–antibody complex resulting from attraction of oscillating dipoles of atoms and molecules moving their electrons from one side to another. Dispersion forces occur only when the two molecules are very close together and decrease with the sixth power of the distance between interaction groups.

long-acting thyroid stimulator (LATS)

An immunoglobulin G (IgG) autoantibody that mimics the action of thyroid-stimulating hormone in its effect on

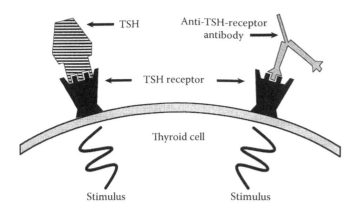

Third form of type II hypersensitivity in which long-acting thyroid stimulator (LATS), an immunoglobulin G (IgG) antibody specific for the thyroid-stimulating hormone (TSH) receptor, leads to continuous stimulation of thyroid parenchyma cells, leading to hyperthyroidism. The IgG antibody mimics the action of TSH.

the thyroid. Most patients with Graves' disease (hyperthyroidism) produce LATS. This IgG autoantibody reacts with the receptors on thyroid cells that respond to thyroid-stimulating hormone. Thus, the antibody–receptor interaction produces the same biological consequence as hormone interaction with the receptor. This represents a stimulatory type of hypersensitivity and is classified in the Gell and Coombs classification as a form of type II hypersensitivity.

long homologous repeat

Refer to consensus sequence of C3/C4-binding proteins.

long-lived lymphocyte

Small lymphocyte derived principally from the thymus that survives for months to years without dividing, unlike short-lived lymphocytes.

long-term nonprogressors (LTNPs)

Persons infected with HIV whose virus loads remain controlled without the administration of antiretroviral drugs.

long terminal repeat (LTR)

In retroviruses, the repeated sequence at the 5′ and 3′ terminals of the provirus. The 5′ LTR of HIV possesses an active promoter that facilitates transcription and regulatory sites that govern transcription following signals from host cells or viral proteins. Sequences in the 3′ LTR govern cleavage of the primary transcript and poly-a tail addition.

low dose tolerance

Antigen-specific immunosuppression induced by the administration of antigen in a suboptimal dose. Low dose tolerance is achieved easily in the neonatal period when the lymphoid cells are not sufficiently mature to mount an antibody or cell-mediated immune response. This renders helper T lymphocytes tolerant, thereby inhibiting them from signaling B lymphocytes to respond to immunogenic challenge. Although no precise inducing dose of antigen can be defined, usually in low dose tolerance 10^{-8} mol antigen per kg body weight is effective. Low dose tolerance is relatively long lasting. Also called low zone tolerance.

low responder mice

Inbred mouse strains that produce poor immune responses to selected antigens in comparison to responses by other inbred mouse strains. This is associated with the low responder's lack of appropriate *Ir* genes. Low

responsiveness is governed by major histocompatibility complex (MHC) class II genes.

low zone tolerance

Specific antigen-induced immunosuppression resulting from the repeated administration of a minute dose of immunogen over a long time. Refer to low dose tolerance.

lower invertebrates

Coelenterates, including corals and jellyfish; platyhelminths (flatworms), nematodes (roundworms), and nemertines (ribbonworms).

LPAM-1

A combination of α4 and β7 integrin chains that mediate the binding of lymphocytes to the high endothelial venules of Peyer's patches in mice. The addressin for LPAM-1 is MadCAM-1.

L-phenylalanine mustard

A nitrogen mustard employed for therapy of multiple myeloma patients.

L-plastin (LPL)

A 65-kDa actin-bundling protein, also called fimbrin, that is expressed in leukocytes, embryonic endoderm, and transformed cells. LPL localizes to phagocytic cups, phagosomes, and podosomes in phagocytes but its role is unclear. It is believed to be important in the formation and stabilization of F-actin filaments during phagocytosis.

LPR

Abbreviation for late-phase reaction.

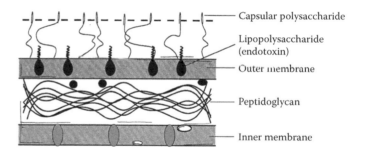

Cross-section of Gram-negative bacterial cell wall.

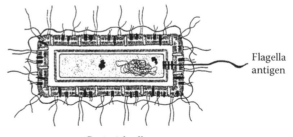

Lipopolysaccharide (LPS).

LPS

Abbreviation for lipopolysaccharide. LPS may serve as an endotoxin; is a constituent of Gram-negative bacterial cell walls associated with endotoxin; and may lead to endotoxin shock.

LPS-binding protein (LBP)

A substance that can bind a bacterial lipopolysaccharide (LPS) molecule; this enables it to interact with CD14, an LPS:LBP-binding protein, on macrophages and selected other cells.

L$_r$ dose (historical)

The least amount of toxin that, after combination with one unit of antitoxin, will produce a minimal skin lesion when injected intracutaneously into a guinea pig.

L-selectin

An adhesion molecule of the selectin family found on lymphocytes; it is responsible for the homing of lymphocytes to lymph node high endothelial venules where it binds to CD34 and GlyCAM-1. It induces the migration of naïve lymphocytes into secondary lymphoid tissues. L-selectin is also found on neutrophils, where it acts to bind the cells to activated endothelium early in the inflammatory process. Also called CD62L.

LSGP (leukocyte sialoglycoprotein)

A richly glycosylated protein present on thymocytes and T lymphocytes. B lymphocytes are devoid of leukocyte sialoglycoprotein.

LT

Abbreviation for lymphotoxin.

LTα

A mediator of killing by cytolytic T cells, helper/killer T cells, natural killer cells, and lymphokine-activated killer cells.

lung autoantibodies

Autoantibodies to lung have been described in the sera of patients with farmer's lung. Cytotoxic autoantibodies against lung tissue have been reported in sarcoidosis and extrinsic asthma but are not well defined. Antibasement membrane antibodies specific for lung and kidney antigens are recognized in Goodpasture's syndrome.

lupoid hepatitis

Autoimmune hepatitis usually found in young females who may produce antinuclear, antimitochondria, and antismooth muscle antibodies. Fifteen percent of these patients may show lupus erythematosus (LE) cells in the blood. This form of hepatitis has the histologic appearance of chronic active hepatitis, which generally responds well to corticosteroids.

lupus anticoagulant (LAC)

Immunoglobulin G (IgG) or IgM antibody that develops in lupus erythematosus (LE) patients, in certain individuals with neoplasia or drug reactions, in some normal persons, and in some AIDS patients who have active opportunistic infections. These antibodies are specific for phospholipoproteins or phospholipid constituents of coagulation factors. *In vitro,* these antibodies inhibit coagulation dependent upon phospholipids. Members of a family of acquired circulating anticoagulants, lupus anticoagulants are immunoglobulins that lead to prolonged coagulation screening tests that include activated partial thromboplastin time (APTT) and prothrombin time (PT). LAC shows species specificity for a prothrombin–anionic phospholipid neoepitope in primary antiphospholipid syndrome (PAPS). LAC assays may be useful for predicting thrombosis.

lupus erythematosus (LE)

A connective tissue disease associated with the development of autoantibodies against DNA, RNA, and nucleoproteins. It is believed to be due to hyperactivity of the B cell limb of the immune response. Clinical manifestations include skin lesions (including the so-called butterfly rash on the cheeks and across the bridge of the nose) that are light sensitive. Patients may develop vasculitis, arthritis, and glomerulonephritis. When the disease is confined to the skin, it is referred to as discoid LE or cutaneous LE. Approximately 75% of patients with lupus have renal involvement.

lupus erythematosus (LE) and pregnancy

Pregnant patients with lupus erythematosus may experience fetal wasting caused by thromboses. Spontaneous abortion together with anticardiolipin antibody and anti-Rh antibodies may be linked to fertility failure and death of the fetus.

lupus erythematosus (LE), drug-induced

Certain drugs such as procainamide, hydralazine, d-penicillamine, phenytoin, isoniazid, and ergot substances may produce a condition resembling lupus in patients who receive them. Most cases develop

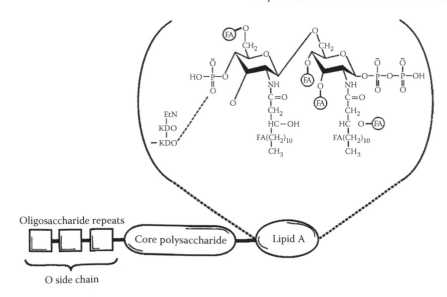

Lipopolysaccharide or endotoxin.

antinuclear and antihistone antibodies; about a third develop clinical signs and symptoms of lupus such as arthralgia, serositis, and fever. These cases do not usually develop the renal and CNS lesions seen in classic lupus. Nonacetylated metabolites accumulate in many patients, who are described as slow acetylators. The nonacetylated metabolites act as haptens by combining with macromolecules. This may lead to an autoimmune response due to metabolic abnormality.

lupus inhibitor

Refer to lupus anticoagulant.

lupus nephritis

Renal involvement in cases of systemic lupus erythematosus (SLE) that can be classified into five histologic patterns according to morphologic criteria developed by the World Health Organization: (1) normal by light electron and immunofluorescent microscopy (class I); (2) mesangial lupus glomerulonephritis (class II); (3) focal proliferative glomerulonephritis (class III); (4) diffuse proliferative glomerulonephritis (class IV); and (5) membranous glomerulonephritis (class V). None of these patterns is specific for lupus.

Lutheran Blood Group

Phenotype	Reactions with Anti-		Phenotype
	Lu^a	Lu^b	Frequency
Lu (a+b−)	+	0	0.15
Lu (a+b+)	+	+	7.5
Lu (a−b+)	0	+	92.35
Lu (a−b−)	0	0	Very rare

Lutheran blood group

Human erythrocyte epitopes recognized by alloantibodies against Lu^a and Lu^b products. Antibodies developed against Lutheran antigens during pregnancy may induce hemolytic disease of the newborn.

Lw antibody

An antibody initially believed to be anti-Rh specific and subsequently shown to be directed against a separate red cell antigen closely linked to the Rh gene family. Its inheritance is separate from that of the Rh group. Lw is the designation given to recognize the research of Landsteiner and Wiener on the rhesus system. The rare anti-Lw antibody reacts with Rh$^+$ or Rh$^-$ erythrocytes and is nonreactive with Rh$_{null}$ red cells.

Ly antigen

A murine lymphocyte alloantigen expressed to different degrees on mouse T and B lymphocytes and thymocytes. Also referred to as Lyt antigen.

Ly1 B cell

A murine B lymphocyte that expresses CD5 (Ly1) epitope on its surface. This cell population is increased in inbred strains of mice such as the New Zealand strain that are susceptible to autoimmune diseases.

Ly6

Glycosylphosphatidylinositol (GPI)-linked murine cell surface alloantigens found most often on T and B cells but also on nonlymphoid tissues such as brain, kidney, and heart. Monoclonal antibodies to these antigens indicate T cell receptor (TCR) dependence.

Lyb

A murine B lymphocyte surface alloantigen.

Lyb-3 antigen

Mature murine B cells express a surface marker designated Lyb-3. It is a single, membrane-bound, 68-kDa polypeptide. On sodium dodecyl sulfate polyacrylamide gel electrophoresis (SDS-PAGE), it appears distinct from the SIg chains δ and μ. It does not contain disulfide bridges. The gene coding for Lyb-3 appears X-linked and recessive, and mutant mice lacking Lyb-3 antigens are known. Lyb-3 is involved in the cooperation of T and B cells in response to thymus-dependent antigens and seems to be manifested particularly when the amount of antigen used for immunization is suboptimal. The number of cells carrying Lyb-3 increases with age.

Lyme disease

A condition named after the town of Lyme, Connecticut, where an epidemic of juvenile rheumatoid arthritis (Still's disease) was found to be due to *Borrelia burgdorferi*. It is the most frequent zoonosis in the United States, with concentration along the eastern coast. Insect vectors include the deer tick (*Ixodes dammini*), white-footed mouse tick (*I. pacificus*), wood tick (*I. ricinus*), and lone star tick (*Amblyomma americanum*). Deer and field mice are the hosts. In stage I, a rash termed erythema chronicum migrans occurs. The rash begins as a single reddish papule and plaque that expands to as much as 20 cm. This is accompanied by induration at the periphery, with central clearing that may persist for months to years. The vessels contain IgM and C3 deposits. Stage II is the cardiovascular stage that may be accompanied by pericarditis, myocarditis, transient atrial ventricular block, and ventricular dysfunction. Neurological symptoms also ensue and include Bell's palsy, meningoencephalitis, optic atrophy, and polyneuritis. Stage III is characterized by migratory polyarthritis. The diagnosis requires the demonstration of IgG antibodies against the causative agent by western immunoblotting. Lyme disease is treated with tetracycline, penicillin, and erythromycin antibiotics.

lymph

The fluid that circulates in the lymphatic system vessels. Its composition resembles that of tissue fluids, although lymph contains less protein than plasma. Lymph in the mesentery contains fat, and lymph draining the intestine and liver often possesses more protein than does other lymph. The principal cell type in lymph is the small lymphocyte, with only rare large lymphocytes, monocytes, and macrophages. Occasional red cells and eosinophils are present. Coagulation factors are also present in lymph.

lymphadenitis

Lymph node inflammation often caused by microbial (bacterial or viral) infection.

lymphadenoid goiter

Refer to Hashimoto's thyroiditis.

lymphadenopathy

Lymph node enlargement due to any of several causes. Lymphadenopathies are reactive processes in lymph nodes arising from various exogenous and endogenous stimulants. Possible etiologies include microorganisms, autoimmune diseases, immunodeficiencies, foreign bodies, tumors, and medical procedures. The term *lymphadenitis* is reserved for lymph node enlargement caused by microorganisms; *Lymphadenopathy* applies to all other etiologies of lymph node enlargement. Lymphadenopathies are classified as (1) reactive, (2) those associated with clinical syndromes, (3) vascular lymphadenopathies, (4) foreign body lymphadenopathies, and (5) lymph node inclusions. Variability of germinal center size, no invasion of the capsule or fat, confinement of mitotic activity to germinal centers, and localization in the cortex and nonhomogenous follicle distribution are observed in benign lymphadenopathy.

lymphatic system

Network of lymphoid channels that transports lymph, a tissue fluid derived from the blood. It collects extracellular fluid from the periphery and channels it via the thoracic duct to the blood circulation. Lymph nodes at the intersections of lymphatic vessels trap and retain antigens from the lymph. Situated at lymphatic vessel intersections are lymph nodes, Peyer's patches, and other organized lymphoid structures except the spleen, which communicates directly with the blood. The main functions of the lymphatic system include the concentration of antigen from various body locations into a few lymphoid organs. The circulation of lymphocytes through lymphoid organs permits antigen to interact with antigen-specific cells and to carry antibody and immune effector cells to the blood circulation and tissue.

lymphatic vessels

Thinly walled channels through which lymph and cells of the lymphatic system move through secondary lymphoid tissues, such as lymph nodes, except for the spleen, to the thoracic duct that joins the blood circulation.

lymphatics

Vessels that transport the interstitial fluid called lymph to lymph nodes and away from them, directing it to the thoracic duct, from which it reenters the blood stream.

lymph gland

More correctly referred to as lymph node.

lymph node

A relatively small (0.5 cm) secondary lymphoid organ that serves as a major site of immune reactivity. It is surrounded by a capsule and contains lymphocytes, macrophages, and dendritic cells in a loose reticulum environment. Lymph enters this organ from afferent lymphatics at the periphery, percolates through the node until it reaches the efferent lymphatics, exits at the hilus, and circulates to central lymph nodes and finally to the thoracic duct. The lymph node is divided into a cortex and medulla. The superficial cortex contains B lymphocytes in follicles, and the deep cortex is composed of T lymphocytes. Differentiation of the specific cells continues in these areas and is driven by antigen and thymic hormones. Conversion of B cells into plasma cells occurs chiefly in the medullary region, where enclosed lymphocytes are protected from undesirable influences by a macrophage sleeve. The postcapillary venules from which lymphocytes exit the lymph node are also located in the medullary region. Macrophages and follicular dendritic cells interact with antigen molecules that are transported via lymph to the lymph nodes. Reticulum cells form medullary cords and sinuses in the central region. T lymphocytes percolate through the lymph nodes and enter from the blood at the postcapillary venules of the deep cortex. They then enter the medullary sinuses and pass from the node through

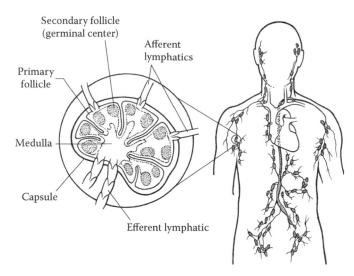

Lymph node.

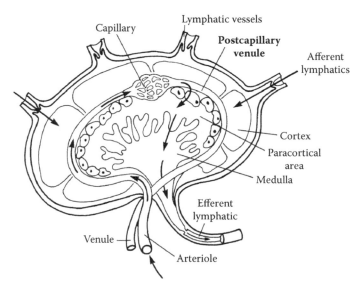

Lymph node.

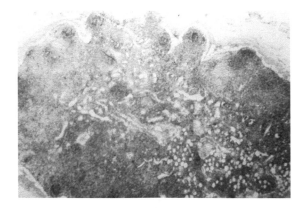

Lymph node (low power).

the efferent lymphatics. T cells that interact with antigens are detained in lymph nodes, which may be sites of major immunologic reactivity. A lymph node is divided into B and T lymphocyte regions. Individuals with B cell or T cell immunodeficiencies may reveal an absence of one or the other lymphocyte type in the areas of the lymph node

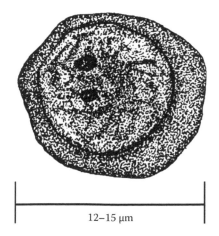

Subcapsular sinus lymph node.

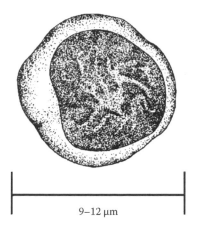

9–12 μm

Lymphocyte.

normally occupied by that cell population. The lymph
node acts as a filter and may be an important site for
phagocytosis and the initiation of immune responses.

lymphoblast

A relatively large cell of lymphocyte lineage that bears
a nucleus with fine chromatin and basophilic nucleoli.
Induced within 18 to 24 hours following engagement of resting lymphocytes' TCRs or BCRs. They frequently form following antigenic or mitogenic challenge of lymphoid cells,
which leads to enlargement and division to produce effector
lymphocytes that are active in immune reactions. They
divide rapidly and differentiate into memory and effector
lymphocytes. The Epstein–Barr virus (EBV) is commonly
used to transform B cells into B lymphoblasts in tissue
culture to establish B lymphoblast cell lines. Lymphoblasts
have increased rates of synthesis of RNA and protein.

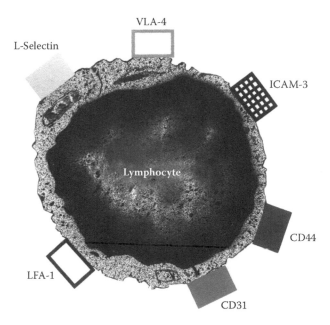

Lymphocyte.

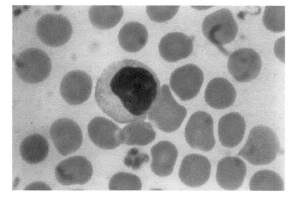

Lymphocyte in peripheral blood.

12–15 μm

Lymphoblast.

lymphoblastic leukemia

A malignancy that is a consequence of T or B precursor
cell transformation.

lymphocyte

A round cell that measures 7 to 12 μm and contains a round
to ovoid nucleus that may be indented. The chromatin is
densely packed and stains dark blue with Romanowsky
stain. Small lymphocytes contain a thin rim of robin's egg
blue cytoplasm, and a few azurophilic granules may be
present. Large lymphocytes have more cytoplasm and a
similar nucleus. Electron microscopy reveals villi that cover

most of the cell surface. Lymphocytes are divided into the
two principal groups of B and T lymphocytes that can be
distinguished phenotypically by their cell surface receptors,
BCRs and TCRs respectively. They are distinguished not
by morphology but by the expression of distinctive surface
molecules that have precise roles in immune reaction. In

L

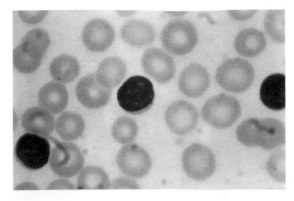

Small lymphocyte in peripheral blood.

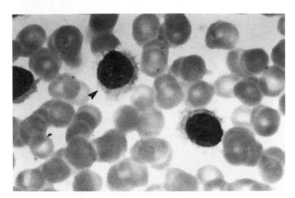

Lymphocytes in peripheral blood.

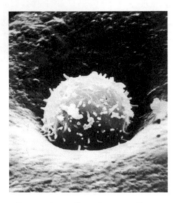

Lymphocyte (scanning electron microscope).

addition, natural killer cells, which are large granular lymphocytes, comprise a small percentage of the lymphocyte population. Lymphocytes express variable cell surface receptors for antigen.

lymphocyte-activating factor (LAF)

Refer to interleukin-1.

lymphocyte activation

The stimulation of lymphocytes *in vitro* by an antigen or mitogen that renders them metabolically active. Activated lymphocytes may undergo transformation or blastogenesis. Follows binding of numerous copies of a specific epitope to a resting lymphocyte's TCR or BCR, resulting in formation of a lymphoblast that undergoes proliferation. Costimulation and cytokines are also necessary to activate naïve cells. There is triggering of multiple genes leading the progeny cells to undergo alterations that result in memory and effector lymphocytes.

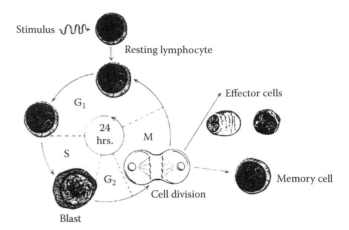

Lymphocyte activation.

lymphocyte activation threshold

The number of receptors for antigen required to be aggregated and activated, together with costimulatory signals, to produce a proliferative signal.

lymphocyte anergy

The failure of clones of T or B lymphocytes to react to antigen; may represent a mechanism to maintain immunologic tolerance to self. Antigen stimulation of a lymphocyte without costimulation leads to tolerance. Unresponsiveness may stem from a failure of T lymphocytes to proliferate on rechallenge with antigen presented by professional antigen-presenting cells. Occupancy of the T cell receptor by peptide–MHC complexes leads to anergy. IL2 and selected other cytokines are inhibited in anergic T cell clones. Anergy appears to be a growth arrest condition designed to diminish proliferation in the T cell immune response. Also called clonal anergy.

lymphocyte antigen receptor complex

Immunoglobulin α (Igα) and Igβ function in B lymphocytes as CD3 and proteins do in T cells. Requisite for signal transduction are immunoreceptor tyrosine-based activation motifs (ITAMs) in the cytoplasmic domains of Igα and Igβ. Cross linking of the B cell receptor complex by antigen leads to increased cell size and cytoplasmic ribonucleic acid with increased biosynthetic organelles including ribosomes as resting cells enter the G_1 stage in the cell cycle. Class II molecules and B7-2 and B7-1 costimulators show increased expression. B cells stimulated by antigen are then able to activate helper T cells. Expression of receptors for T cell cytokines increases, thereby facilitating the ability of antigen-specific B cells to receive T cell help. The effect of B cell receptor complex signaling on proliferation and differentiation depends in part on the type of antigen. Following activation as a result of combination with antigen, cell proliferation and differentiation are facilitated by interaction with helper T lymphocytes. Helper T cells must recognize antigen, and there must be interaction between protein antigen-specific B cells and T lymphocytes for antibody to be formed. When B cells, acting as antigen-presenting cells, interact with helper T lymphocytes that are specific for the peptide presented, numerous ligand-receptor interactions facilitate transmission of signals to B cells required to generate a humoral immune response. Among these are B7 molecules:CD28 and CD40:CD40 ligand interactions. Cytokines play important heavy chain isotype and provide amplification mechanisms through argumentation of B lymphocyte proliferation and differentiation. Germinal centers are the sites of synthesis of antibodies of high affinity and of memory B cells.

lymphocyte antigen stimulation test

An assay for the *in vitro* assessment of impaired cell-mediated immunity. It is useful to evaluate patients with genetic or acquired immunodeficiencies, bacterial and viral infections, cancers, autoimmune disorders, transplantation-related disorders, antisperm antbodies, and previous exposures to a variety of antigens, allergens, pathogens, metals, and chemicals. Lymphocyte antigen stimulation is assayed by [³H]-thymidine uptake or a flow cytometric assay (based on expression of the activation antigen CD69) with [³H]-thymidine incorporation. Antigen-stimulated culture supernatants can be assessed for cytokine production by enzyme immunoassay (EIA).

lymphocyte chemokine (BLC)

A CSC chemokine that induces B lymphocytes and activated T cells to enter peripheral lymphoid tissue follicles by binding to the CXCR5 receptor.

lymphocyte chemotaxis

Lymphocytes comprise a heterogeneous motile cell population. Both T and B cells recirculate continuously between the blood and the lymphoid tissues. This recirculating cell population consists of naïve small lymphocytes that are not in the cell cycle. Once lymphocytes recognize antigen, their migration behavior changes. They enter the cell cycle and exit the recirculatory pool. An adhesion phenotype changes with loss of L-selectin and loss of affinity for the high endothelial venule (HEV) cells of lymphoid tissue. They increase expression and activity of various other adhesion molecules which prevents them from attaching to the endothelium at sites of inflammation, to cluster around antigen-presenting cells, and to interact with target cells for cytotoxicity. Rather than continuing to monitor the environment for antigen, the lymphocyte changes to a cell that mediates effector functions. Interleukin-2 (IL2) and IL15 are both excellent chemotactic factors for activated T lymphocytes. IL16 is also a T cell attractant with selective activity for CD4⁺. Several chemokines including both α and β types exert activity. B and T cells respond better to attractants following their activation. Natural killer (NK) cells activated with IL2 can respond to chemoattractants, including several chemokines such as MIP-1α, MCP-1, RANTES, and IL8.

lymphocyte-defined (LD) antigens

Histocompatibility antigens on mammalian cells that induce reactivity in a mixed-lymphocyte culture (MLC) or mixed-lymphocyte reaction.

lymphocyte determinant

Target cell epitopes identified by lymphocytes rather than antibodies from a specifically immunized host.

lymphocyte-function-associated antigen-1 (LFA-1)

A leukocyte integrin that facilitates lymphocyte adhesion to endothelial cells and antigen-presenting cells. A glycoprotein comprised of a 180-kDa α chain and a 95-kDa β chain expressed on lymphocyte and phagocytic cell membranes. The ligand of LFA-1 is the intercellular adhesion molecule 1 (ICAM-1). It facilitates natural killer (NK) cell and cytotoxic T cell interaction with target cells. Complement receptor 3

Adhesion to Artificial Membranes

T cell

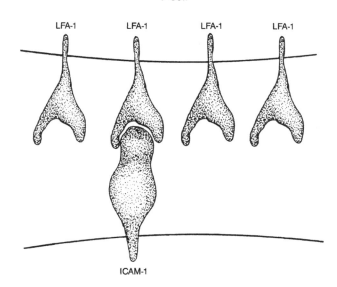

Lymphocyte-function-associated antigen 1 (LFA-1).

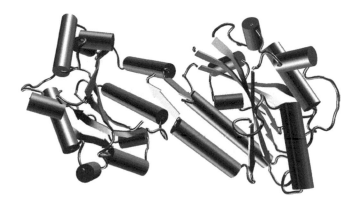

Lymphocyte-function-associated antigen-1 (LFA-1) I domain.

and p150,95 share the same specificity of the 769-amino acid residue β chain found in LFA-1. A gene on chromosome 16 encodes the α chain and a gene on chromosome 21 encodes the β chain. This leukocyte integrin (β₂) adhesion molecule plays a critical role in adhesion of leukocytes to each other and to other cells and microbial recognition by phagocytes. LFA-1 binds not only ICAM-1 but also ICAM-2 or ICAM-3. LFA-1-dependent cell adhesion is also temperature-, magnesium-, and cytoskeleton-dependent. LFA-1 induces costimulatory signals believed to be significant in leukocyte function. LFA-1 function is critical to most aspects of the immune response. Refer to CD11a and CD18.

lymphocyte-function-associated antigen-2 (LFA-2)

Refer to CD2.

lymphocyte-function-associated antigen-3 (LFA-3)

An immunoglobulin superfamily cell adhesion molecule found on antigen-presenting cells, among others, that facilitates their adhesion to T cells. A 60-kDa polypeptide chain expressed on the surfaces of B cells, T cells, monocytes, granulocytes, platelets, fibroblasts, and endothelial cells of vessels. LFA-3 is the ligand for CD2 and is encoded by genes on chromosome 1 in humans. LFA-3 or CD58 is expressed as a transmembrane- or lipid-linked cell surface protein. The transmembrane form consists of a 188-amino acid extracellular region, a 23-amino acid transmembrane hydrophobic region, and a 12-amino acid intracellular hydrophilic region ending in the C terminus. LFA-3 expression by antigen-presenting cells that include dendritic cells, macrophages, and B lymphocytes points to a possible role in regulating the immune response.

lymphocyte homing

The directed migration of circulating lymphocyte subsets to specific tissue locations. The action is regulated by adhesion molecules (homing receptors), such as addressins, expressed on specific tissues in different vascular beds. Selected T cells that home specifically to intestinal lymphoid tissues such as Peyer's patches are directed by binding of VLA-4 integrin on their surfaces to MadCAM addressin on the endothelia of Peyer's patches.

lymphocyte immune globulin (injection)

Indicated for the management of allograft rejection in renal allotransplant recipients. When administered with conventional therapy at the time of rejection, it increases the frequency of resolution of acute rejection episodes. May be used also in conjunction with other immunosuppressive therapy to delay the onset of the first rejection episode. Indicated also for the treatment of moderate to severe aplastic anemia patients who are unsuitable for bone marrow transplantation. Unlabeled uses include its use as an immunosuppressant in liver, bone marrow, heart, and other organ transplants, treatment of multiple sclerosis, myasthenia gravis, pure red cell aplasia, and scleroderma even though efficacy is not fully established.

lymphocyte maturation

The development of pluripotent bone marrow precursor cells into T or B lymphocytes that express antigen receptors present in peripheral lymphoid tissue. B cell maturation takes place in the bone marrow, and T cell maturation is governed by the thymus.

lymphocyte mitogen stimulation test

An assay used for the *in vitro* assessment of cell-mediated immunity in patients with immunodeficiency, autoimmunity, infectious diseases, cancers, and chemical-induced hypersensitivity reactions. Healthy human lymphocytes have receptors for mitogens such as the plant lectin known as concanavalin A (Con A), pokeweed mitogen (PWM), *Staphylococcus* protein A, and chemicals. Lymphocytes respond to these mitogens, which stimulate large numbers of lymphocytes, without prior sensitization. In contrast to antigens, mitogens do not require a sensitized host. Mitogens may stimulate both B and T cells, and the inability of lymphocytes to respond to mitogens suggests impaired cell-mediated or humoral immunity.

lymphocyte precursors

Hematopoietic stem cell-derived immature cells in the bone marrow or thymus that develop into lymphocytes, such as pro-B, pre-B, pro-T, pre-T, and immature B and T cells.

lymphocyte receptor repertoire

All of the highly variable antigen receptors of B and T lymphocytes.

lymphocyte recirculation

Lymphocyte migration through the lymphatic system from the tissues into the blood, from which they return to the tissues by extravasation. Refer to lymphocyte trafficking.

lymphocyte specificity

The restricted and unique epitopes a lymphocyte may be able to bind based on its expression of only one type of randomly generated antigen receptor gene.

lymphocyte tolerization

Inducing a lymphocyte to become anergic. In B cells, it may follow B cell receptor engagement without T cell help or result from receptor blockade. Tolerization of T cells may be a consequence of lymphocyte interaction with immature dendritic cells, modulated dendritic cells, or regulatory T cells. Tolerization may be a consequence of insufficient costimulation and/or intracellular suppressor signaling.

lymphocyte toxicity assay

A test to evaluate adverse reactions to drugs, especially anticonvulsants. Incubation with liver microsomes is believed to metabolize the drug to the *in vivo* metabolite that kills lymphocytes from sensitized patients but not from controls. Lymphocytes derived from nonreactive individuals do not show significant lymphocyte toxicity.

lymphocyte trafficking

A process that is critical for interaction of the lymphocyte surface antigen receptor with epitopes. Lymphocytes continuously migrate from the blood into lymphoid and nonlymphoid organs and back again to the blood by way of the lymphatics and venules. Lymphocytes remain in the blood circulation for approximately 30 minutes on each passage. Lymphocytes in the blood circulation are exchanged approximately 48 times per day, and about 5×10^{11} lymphocytes leave the circulation each day. Lymphocyte migration is regulated during entry, transit, and exit. Because only a few immunocompetent lymphocytes are specific for each antigen, lymphocyte trafficking increases the probability of interaction between the lymphocyte and the epitope for which it is specific. Several adhesion molecules participate in receptor–ligand interactions involved in the entry of lymphocytes into lymphoid organs through endothelial venules. Refer also to lymphocytes, circulating (or recirculating).

lymphocyte transfer reaction

Refer to normal lymphocyte transfer reaction.

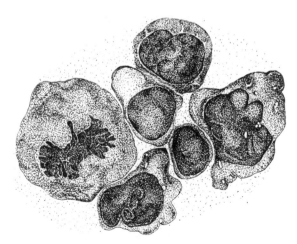

Lymphocyte transformation.

lymphocyte transformation

An alteration in the morphology of a lymphocyte induced by an antigen, mitogen, or virus interacting with a small, resting lymphocyte. The transformed cell increases in size and amount of cytoplasm. Nucleoli develop in the nucleus, which stains lighter as the cell becomes a blast. Epstein–Barr virus transforms B cells, and the human T cell leukemia virus transforms T cells. The lymphocyte transformation test involves activation of lymphocytes with mitogens, antigen, superantigens, and antibodies to components of cell membranes. This leads to their synthesis of proteins that include immunoglobulins, cytokines, and growth factors. The activated lymphocyte enters the cell cycle, synthesizes DNA, replicates, and undergoes metabolic and morphologic changes. Phytohemagglutinin (PHA) and concanavalin A (con A), superantigens, anti-CD3 mitogens, and antigens presented by antigen-presenting cells activate T lymphocytes. Anti-immunoglobulin, bacterial lypopolysaccharides, and staphylococcal protein A activate B lymphocytes. The lymphocyte transformation assay is a broadly used *in vitro* test to evaluate lymphocyte function.

lymphocytes, circulating (or recirculating)

The lymphocytes present in the systemic circulation represent a mixture of cells derived from different sources: (1) B and T cells exiting from bone marrow and thymus on their way to seed the peripheral lymphoid organs; (2) lymphocytes exiting the lymph nodes via lymphatics, collected by the thoracic duct, and discharged into the superior vena cava; and (3) lymphocytes derived from direct discharge into the vascular sinuses of the spleen. About 70% of cells in the circulating pool are recirculating, that is, they undergo a cycle during which they exit the systemic circulation to return back to lymphoid follicles, lymph nodes, and spleen and start the cycle again. The cells in the recirculating pool are mostly long-lived mature T cells. About 30% of the lymphocytes of the intravascular pool do not recirculate. They comprise mostly short-lived immature T cells that live their lifespans intravascularly or are activated and exit the intravascular space. The exit of lymphocytes into the spleen occurs by direct discharge from the blood vessels. In lymph nodes and lymphoid follicles, the exit of lymphocytes occurs through specialized structures called postcapillary venules. These differ from other venules in that they have tall endothelial coverings. The exiting lymphocytes percolate through the endothelial cells, a mechanism whose significance is not known. A number of agents such as cortisone or *Bordetella pertussis* bacteria increase the extravascular exit of lymphocytes and prevent their return to circulation. The lymphocytes travel back and forth between the blood and lymph. They attach to and pass through the high endothelial cells of the postcapillary venules of lymph nodes or the marginal sinuses of the spleen. Within 24 to 48 hours they return via the lymphatics to the thoracic duct, where they then reenter the blood.

lymphocytic choriomeningitis (LCM)

A murine viral disease that produces inflammatory brain lesions in affected mice as a result of delayed-type hypersensitivity to viral antigens on brain cells infected with the LCM virus. This infectious agent, classified as an arenavirus, is endemic in the mouse population and occasionally occurs in humans. Only adult mice that become infected develop the lesions; those infected *in utero* are rendered immunologically tolerant to the viral antigens and fail to develop disease. An adult with an intact immune system exposed to LCM virus becomes immune or succumbs to the

acute infection, which is associated with lymphadenopathy, splenomegaly, and T lymphocyte perivascular infiltration of the viscera, especially the brain. A chronic carrier state can be induced in neonatal mice or those with impaired immune systems through infection with the virus. Although carriers generate significant quantities of antiviral antibodies, the infection persists, and virus–antibody immune complexes become deposited in the renal glomeruli, walls of arteries, liver, lungs, and heart. The passive transfer of cytotoxic T lymphocytes from an immune animal to a carrier results in specific reactivity against LCM viral epitopes on cell membranes in the brain and meninges, which leads to profound inflammation and death. Transmission of this disease is via the excrement of rodents and is seen especially in winter when rodents enter dwellings. Fever, headache, flu-like symptoms, and lymphocytosis in the cerebrospinal fluid are present, as may be associated leukopenia and thrombocytopenia. This disease must be distinguished from infectious mononucleosis, herpes zoster, and enterovirus infection.

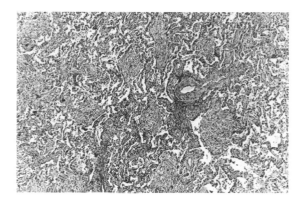

Lymphocytic interstitial pneumonia (LIP) with organization.

lymphocytic interstitial pneumonia (LIP)

A diffuse pulmonary disease of middle-aged females who may also have Sjögren's disease, hypergammaglobulinemia, or hypogammaglobulinemia. They develop shortness of breath, and reticulonodular infiltrates appear on chest films. Mature lymphocytes and plasma cells appear in the nodular interstitial changes in alveolar and interlobular septae with perivascular accumulation of round cells. LIP may resemble lymphoma based on the monotonous accumulation of small lymphocytes, and patients may ultimately develop end-stage lung disease or lymphoma.

lymphocytic leukemia

A malignancy in which abnormal proliferation of transformed T or B cells manifests a mature peripheral cell phenotype.

lymphocytopenic center

Refer to germinal center.

lymphocytosis

An elevated number of peripheral blood lymphocytes.

lymphocytotoxic autoantibodies

A heterogeneous group of autoantibodies including (1) those that occur naturally and in selected diseases, are of the immunoglobulin M (IgM) isotype, and are cold-reactive at temperatures near 15°C; (2) lymphocytotoxic autoantibodies associated with infections such as mumps, herpes, mycoplasma, chronic parasitic infections, and autoimmune diseases such as systemic lupus erythematosus (SLE) and rheumatoid arthritis (RA). The sera of most SLE patients react with CD45 on mitogen-stimulated T lymphocytes; some interact with T cell receptor and β_2 microglobulin, and selected B cell antigens. Alloantibodies against lymphocytes usually result from immunization, blood transfusion, transplantation, and pregnancy. IgG alloantibodies are warm-reactive (at 37°C or room temperature). Major histocompatibility complex (MHC) class I and class II antigens on lymphocyte surfaces are the targets of lymphocyte autoantibodies. The microlymphocytotoxicity test is the method of choice for lymphocytotoxic autoantibody detection.

lymphocytotoxin

Refer to lymphotoxin.

lymphocytotrophic

Possessing a special attraction or affinity for lymphocytes. Examples include the attraction of the Epstein–Barr virus for B lymphocytes and the affinity of human immunodeficiency virus (HIV) for helper/ inducer (CD4) T lymphocytes.

lymphogranuloma venereum (LGV)

A sexually transmitted disease induced by *Chlamydia trachomatis* that is divided into L_1, L_2, and L_3 immunotypes. It is rare in the United States but endemic in Africa, Asia, and South America. Clinically, patients develop papule ulcers that heal spontaneously at the inoculation site. This is followed by development of inguinal and perirectal lymphadenopathy, as well as skin sloughing, hemorrhagic proctocolitis, purulent draining, fever, headache, myalgia, aseptic meningitis, arthralgia, conjunctivitis, hepatitis, and erythema nodosum. Various antibody assays used in the diagnosis of LGV include complement fixation, with a titer >1:32, and immunofluorescence. The Frei test, which consists of the intracutaneous inoculation of a crude antigen into the forearm, is also used and can be read after 72 hours. It is considered positive if the area of induration exceeds 6 mm.

lymphoid

Tissues such as lymph nodes, thymus, and spleen that contain large populations of lymphocytes.

lymphoid cell

A cell of the lymphoid system. The classic lymphoid cell is the lymphocyte. A cell that arises from a common lymphoid progenitor, including T and B lymphocytes, NK cells, and NKT cells.

lymphoid cell series

(1) Cell lineages whose members morphologically resemble lymphocytes, their progenitors, and their progeny.
(2) Organized tissues of the body in which the predominant cell type is the lymphocyte or cells of the lymphoid cell lineage. These include the lymph nodes, thymus, spleen, and gut-associated lymphoid tissue, among others.

lymphoid enhancer factor-1(LEF-1)

A cell-type specific transcription factor and member of the family of high motility group (HMG) domain proteins that recognizes a specific nucleotide sequence in the T cell receptor (TCR) α enhancer. The function of LEF-1 is dependent in part on the HMG domain that induces a sharp bend in the DNA helix and on an activation domain that stimulates transcription only in the specific context of other enhancer-binding proteins.

lymphoid follicles

Organized aggregates of lymphocytes. Refer to the lymphoid nodules.

lymphoid lineage

Lymphocytes of all varieties and the bone marrow cells that are their precursors.

lymphoid nodules (or follicles)

Aggregates of lymphoid cells present in the loose connective tissue supporting the respiratory and digestive membranes. They are also present in the spleen and may develop beneath any mucous membrane as a result of antigenic stimulation. They are poorly defined at birth. Characteristic lymphoid nodules are round and nonencapsulated. They may occur as isolated structures or may be confluent, such as in the tonsils, pharynx, and nasopharynx. In the tongue and pharynx, they form a characteristic structure referred to as Waldeyer's ring. In the terminal ileum, they form oblong areas called Peyer's patches. The lymphoid nodules contain B and T cells and macrophages. Plasma cells in submucosal sites synthesize immunoglobulin A (IgA), which is released in secretions.

lymphoid organs

Organized lymphoid tissues in which numerous lymphocytes interact with nonlymphoid stroma. The thymus and bone marrow are the primary lymphoid organs where lymphocytes are formed. The principal secondary lymphoid tissues where adaptive immune responses are initiated include the lymph nodes, spleen, and mucosa-associated lymphoid tissues, including the tonsils, Peyer's patches, and appendix.

lymphoid patches

Unencapsulated clusters of lymphoid follicles.

lymphoid progenitor cell

A cell belonging to the lymphoid lineage, such as a bone marrow stem cell that gives rise to all lymphocytes.

lymphoid system

The lymphoid organs and the lymphatic vessels.

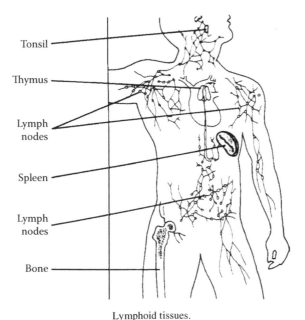

Lymphoid tissues.

lymphoid tissues

Lymphocyte-containing tissues that include the lymph nodes, spleen, thymus, Peyer's patches, tonsils, bursa of

Fabricius in birds, and other lymphoid organs for which the predominant cell type is the lymphocyte.

lymphokine

A nonimmunoglobulin polypeptide substance, i.e., a cytokine synthesized mainly by T lymphocytes that affects the function of other cells. It may enhance or suppress an immune response. Lymphokines may facilitate cell proliferation, growth, and differentiation, and they may act on gene transcription to regulate cell function. Lymphokines exert paracrine or autocrine effects. Many lymphokines have now been described. Well known examples include interleukin-2 (IL2), IL3, migration inhibitory factor (MIF), and interferon-γ (IFN-γ). The term *cytokine* includes lymphokines and soluble products produced by lymphocytes, as well as monokines and soluble products produced by monocytes. Lymphokines are more frequently known as cytokines formed by lymphocytes, soluble protein mediators of immune responses.

lymphokine-activated killer (LAK) cells

Lymphoid cells derived from normal or tumor patients cultured in medium with recombinant interleukin-2 (IL2) become capable of lysing natural killer (NK)-resistant tumor cells as revealed by ^{51}Cr-release cytotoxicity assays. These cells are also known as lymphokine-activated killer cells. Most LAK activity is derived from NK cells. The large granular lymphocytes (LGLs) contain all LAK precursor activity and all active NK cells. In accord with the phenotype of precursor cells, LAK effector cells are also granular lymphocytes expressing markers associated with human NK cells. The asialo $G_{1+}m$ population, known to be expressed by murine NK cells, contains most LAK precursor activity. Essentially all LAK activity resides in the LGL population in rats. LAK cell and IL2 immunotherapy has been employed in human cancer patients with a variety of histological tumor types when conventional therapy has been unsuccessful. Approximately one fourth of LAK- and IL2-treated patients manifested significant responses, and some individuals experienced complete remissions. Serious side effects include fluid retention and pulmonary edema attributable to the administration of IL2.

lymphoma

A malignant neoplasm of lymphoid cells. Hodgkin disease, non-Hodgkin lymphoma, and Burkitt's lymphoma are examples. Lymphomas or lymphocyte tumors grow in lymphoid or other tissues but fail to enter the blood in large numbers. The numerous types of lymphomas are characterized by various classes of transformed lymphoid cells. Lymphomas often manifest the phenotype of the normal lymphocytes from which they arose.

lymphoma belt

An area across central Africa on both sides of the Equator where an increased incidence of Epstein–Barr virus (EBV)-induced Burkitt's lymphoma occurs. Burkitt's lymphoma is a relatively common childhood cancer in Uganda.

lymphomatoid granulomatosis

Vasculitis in the lung of unknown etiology with an ominous prognosis. Atypical lymphocytes and plasma cells extensively infiltrate the pulmonary vasculature. Many of these lymphocytes undergo mitosis. The lungs may develop cavities, and occasionally the nervous system, skin, and kidneys may be sites of nodular vasculitis.

lymphomatosis

Numerous lymphomas occurring in different parts of the body, such as those occurring in Hodgkin disease.

lymphopenia

A decrease below normal in the number of lymphocytes in the peripheral blood.

lymphopoiesis

The differentiation of hematopoietic stem cells into common lymphoid progenitors and ultimately into lymphocytes.

lymphoreticular

A system composed of lymphocytes, monocytes–macrophages, and the stromal elements that support them. The thymus, lymph nodes, spleen, tonsils, bone marrow, Peyer's patches, and avian bursa of Fabricius comprise the lymphoreticular tissues.

lymphorrhages

Accumulations of lymphocytes in inflamed muscle in selected muscle diseases such as myasthenia gravis.

lymphotactin (Ltn)

A member of the γ or C family of chemokines. Human lymphotactin (Ltn) resembles some β chemokines but is lacking the first and third cysteine residues characteristic of the α and β chemokines. Ltn is chemotactic for lymphocytes but not monocytes and employs a unique receptor. An ATAC cDNA clone derived from human T cell activation genes encodes a protein 73.8% identical to mouse lymphotactin. Tissue sources include thymocytes and activated T cells. T lymphocytes are the target cells.

lymphotoxin (LT)

A T lymphocyte lymphokine produced by some CD4$^+$ T cells; it is a heterodimeric glycoprotein comprised of 5- and 15-kDa protein fragments. Lymphotoxin is inhibitory to the growth of tumors *in vitro* and *in vivo,* and it also blocks chemical-, carcinogen-, and ultraviolet light-induced transformation of cells. Lymphotoxin has cytolytic or cytostatic properties for tumor cells that are sensitive to it. Approximately three quarters of the amino acid sequences of human and mouse lymphotoxins are identical. Human lymphotoxin has 205-amino acid residues and the mouse variety has 202-amino acid residues. Lymphotoxin does not produce membrane pores in its target cells, such as those produced by perforin or complement, but it is taken into cells after it is bound to their surfaces and subsequently interferes with metabolism. Lymphotoxin is also called tumor necrosis factor β (TNF-β). This T cell cytokine is homologous to and binds to the same receptors as TNF. It is proinflammatory, activating both endothelial cells and neutrophils. It is necessary for normal lymphoid organ development. A surface form on T cells is mainly a heterotrimer of one LTα subunit with two LTβ molecules (LTα$_{1β2}$). LTα and LTβ are related to TNF-α, sharing sequence and structural characteristics in addition to a tight genetic linkage. TNFα, LTα, and LTα$_{1β2}$ all bind to TNF receptor family molecules.

lysins

Factors such as antibodies and complement or microbial toxins that induce cell lysis. For an antibody to demonstrate this capacity, it must be able to fix complement.

lysis

Disruption of cells due to interruption of their membrane integrity. This may be accomplished nonspecifically, as with hypotonic salt solution, or via interactions of surface membrane epitopes with specific antibody and complement or with cytotoxic T lymphocytes.

L

lysogeny

The condition in which a viral genome (provirus) is associated with the genome of the host in such a manner that the genes of the virus remain unexpressed.

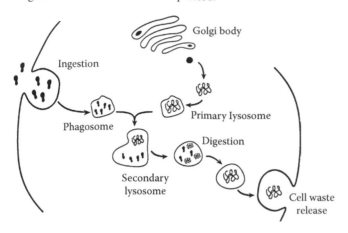

Lysosome.

Factor	Function	Source
Lysozyme	Catalyzes hydrolysis of cell wall mucopeptide	Tears, saliva, nasal secretions, body fluids, lysosomal granules
Lactoferrin, transferrin	Binds iron and competes with microorganisms for it	Specific granules of PMNs
Lactoperoxidase	May be inhibitory to many microorganisms	Milk and saliva
Beta-lysin	Effective mainly against gram-positive bacteria	Thrombocytes, normal serum
Chemotactic factors	Induce reorientation and directed migration of PMNs, monocytes, and other cells	Bacterial substances and products of cell injury and denatured proteins
Properdin	Activates complement in the absence of antibody-antigen complex	Normal plasma
Interferons	Act as immunomodulators to increase the activities of macrophages	Leukocytes, fibroblasts, natural killer cells, T cells
Defensins	Block cell transport activities	Polymorphonuclear granules

Nonspecific humoral defense mechanisms.

lysosome

A cytoplasmic organelle enclosed by a membrane that contains multiple hydrolytic enzymes including ribonuclease, deoxyribonuclease, phosphatase, glycosidase, collagenase, arylsulfatase, and cathepsins. Lysosomes occur in numerous cells but are especially prominent in neutrophils and macrophages. The enzymes are critical for intracellular digestion. Lysosomes participate in antigen processing by the major histocompatibility complex (MHC) class II pathway. Refer also to phagosome and phagocytosis.

lysozyme (muraminidase)

A cationic, low molecular weight enzyme found in egg white, tears, nasal secretions, body fluids, lysosomal granules, on skin, and in lesser amounts in serum that leads to hydrolysis of the β-1,4 glycosidic bond that joins N-acetylmuramic acid with N-acetylglucosamine in bacterial cell wall mucopeptides. This causes osmotic lysis of bacterial cells. Lysozyme is effective principally against Gram-positive cocci. It may facilitate the effects of antibodies and complement on Gram-negative microorganisms. This substance, which is found widely among vertebrates, invertebrates, plants, and bacteria, has been sequenced and its three-dimensional structure determined. It is widely distributed in such normal cells as histiocytes, and leukocytes including neutrophil granules, and monocytes. By immunoperoxidase staining, this marker identifies histiocytes and neoplasms associated with them.

lysozyme (muramidase) antibody

An antibody specific for lysozyme (muramidase) in a variety of cells that include histiocytes, myeloid cells, renal tubular cells, salivary acinar cells, reactive histiocytes in granulomatous conditions, and histiocytic neoplasms. It may be useful in the identification of histiocytic neoplasms and myeloid and monocytic leukemias.

Lyt antigens

Murine T cell surface alloantigens that distinguish T lymphocyte subpopulations designated as helper (Lyt1) and suppressor (Lyt2 and Lyt3) antigens. Corresponding epitopes on B cells are termed Ly.

Lyt1, Lyt2, and Lyt3

A category of murine T lymphocyte surface antigens subdivided into helper T cells (Lyt1) and suppressor T cells (Lyt2 and Lyt3).

lytic granules

Perforin and granzyme-containing intracellular storage granules of cytotoxic T cells and natural killer (NK) cells. They are characteristic of armude effector cytotoxic cells.

M

M13 bacteriophage

An *Escherichia coli* bacteriophage that contains single-stranded, circular DNA. It is male-specific and infects *E. coli* by linking to the F pili on bacterial cell surfaces. Viral DNA becomes double-stranded after entering a host cell and replicates quickly. M13 bacteriophage has been popular as a cloning vector because of the ease of obtaining single- or double-stranded DNA with it. Double-stranded DNA isolated from bacterial cells can be employed to prepare recombinants *in vitro*. Single-stranded DNA from phage can be employed as a template for DNA sequencing. Due to the filamentous structure of M13, it can house variable quantities of DNA.

mAb

Abbreviation for monoclonal antibody.

MAC

(1) Abbreviation for membrane attack complex of the complement system. (2) *Mycobacterium avium* complex, a systemic infection that regularly affects subjects with AIDS, up to 66% of whom still have peripheral blood CD4$^+$ T lymphocytes. Infection with this complex is a clear indication of immunosuppression. MAC is successfully treated with clarithromycin.

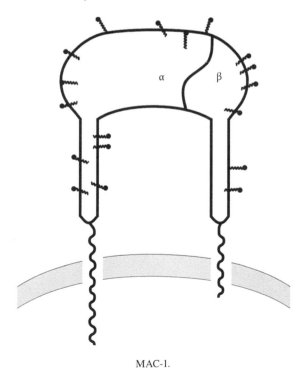

MAC-1.

MAC-1

A monoclonal antibody specific for macrophages.

Mackay, Ian

Widely known for his investigations of autoimmunity and autoimmune diseases, especially autoimmune liver disease.

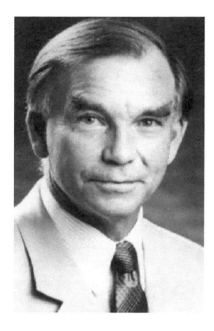

Ian Mackay.

He described lupoid hepatitis, believed to result from autoimmunization. He and Noel R. Rose are the authors of multiple editions of a famous textbook about autoimmune diseases.

macroglobulin

A relatively high molecular weight serum protein. Macroglobulins have a sedimentation coefficient of 18 to 20 S and high carbohydrate content. Each type of macroglobulin belongs to a particular immunoglobulin (Ig) class and is more homogeneous than the Igs resulting from immune responses. Elevated levels appear on electrophoresis as sharp peaks in the migration area of the corresponding Ig class. Macroglobulins are monoclonal in origin and restricted to one κ or λ light chain type. The level of macroglobulins increases significantly in lymphocytic and plasmolytic disorders such as multiple myeloma or leukemia. It also increases in some collagen diseases, reticulosis, chronic infectious states, and carcinoma. The 820- and 900-kDa IgM molecules are both α_2 macroglobulins.

macroglobulinemia

The presence of greater than normal levels of macroglobulins in the blood.

macroglobulinemia of Waldenström

A condition usually of older men in which monoclonal immunoglobulin M (IgM) is detected in the serum and elevated numbers of lymphoid cells and plasmacytoid lymphocytes expressing cytoplasmic IgM are found in the bone marrow; however, these subjects do not exhibit the osteolytic lesions observed in multiple myeloma. Due to the high molecular weight of the IgM and increased levels of this immunoglobulin, blood viscosity increases, leading

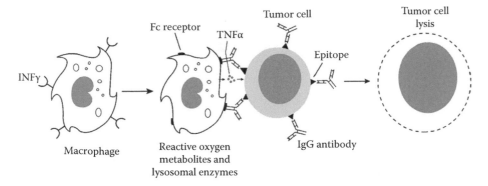

Macrophage-mediated tumor cell lysis proceeds by several mechanisms. Activated macrophages express Fcγ receptors that anchor IgG molecules attached to tumor cells but not normal cells, resulting in the release of lysosomal enzymes and reactive oxygen metabolites and leading to tumor cell lysis. Another mechanism of macrophage-mediated lysis includes the release of tumor necrosis factor α (TNF-α) that may unite with its high affinity receptors on tumor cell surfaces, resulting in lysis, or exert its effects on small blood vessels and capillaries of vascularized tumors, leading to hemorrhagic necrosis, producing a localized Shwartzman-like reaction.

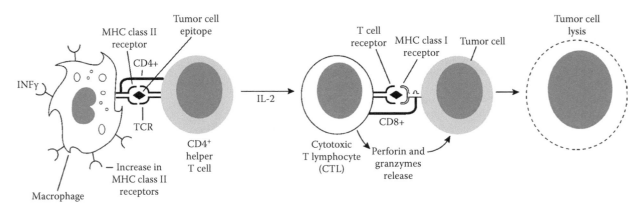

Macrophage-mediated tumor immunity.

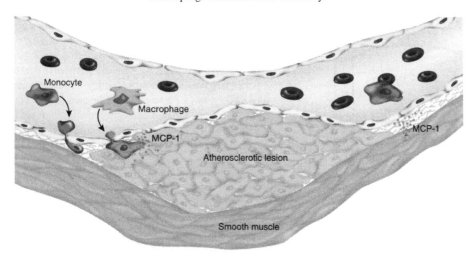

MCP-1 released by smooth muscle and endothelial cells promotes the recruitment of monocytes and macrophages to the subendothelial cell layer. Deposition of lipids within these monocytes and macrophages then leads to development of atherosclerotic lesions.

to circulatory embarrassment. Patients often develop skin hemorrhages, anemia, and neurological problems. This condition is considered less severe than multiple myeloma.

macrophage

A large mononuclear phagocytic cell found in many tissues. It is derived from monocytes in the blood and is active in innate immunity and early phases of nonadaptive host defense. It acts as a professional antigen-presenting cell and

an effector cell in both humoral and cell-mediated immunity. Interferon-γ (IFN-γ) activates macrophages to increase their capacity to kill intracellular microorganisms. IFN-γ activated and primed macrophages can engage in both antigen presentation and costimulation. A combination of IFN-γ and bacterial endotoxin may cause an activated macrophage to become hyperactivated, i.e., become a triggered cytolytic macrophage possessing increased activity against pathogens

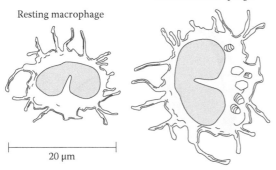

Cell differentiation factors	Alpha interferon
CSF	Plasma proteins
Cytotoxic factors	Coagulation factors
TNFα	Oxygen metabolites H_2O_2 Superoxide anion
Cachectin	Arachidonic acid metabolites Prostaglandins Thromboxanes Leukotrienes
Hydrolytic enzymes Collagenase Lipase Phosphatase	Complement components C1 to C5 Properdin Factors B, D, I, H
Endogenous pyrogen IL-1	

Secreted products of macrophages that have a protective effect on the body.

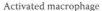

Resting macrophage   Activated macrophage

20 µm

Macrophage.

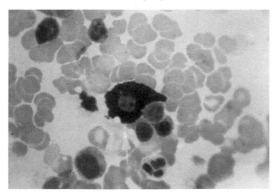

Macrophage-histiocyte in bone marrow.

and the ability to kill tumor cells. Macrophages are known by different names according to the tissue in which they are found such as the microglia of the central nervous system, Kupffer cells of the liver, alveolar macrophages of the lung, and osteoclasts in the bone.

macrophage-activating factor (MAF)

A lymphokine such as interferon-γ (IFN-γ) that accentuates the ability of macrophages to kill microbes and tumor cells; a lymphokine that enhances the phagocytic activity of a macrophage and bactericidal and tumoricidal properties.

macrophage activation

Multiple processes are involved in stimulation of macrophages including increases in size and number of cytoplasmic granules and a spread of membrane ruffling. Functional alterations include elevated metabolism and transport of amino acids and glucose, increased enzymatic activity, and an elevation in the number of prostaglandins, cyclic guanosine monophosphate (cGMP), plasminogen activator, intracellular calcium ions, phagocytosis, and pinocytosis and ability to lyse bacteria and tumor cells.

macrophage chemotactic and activating factor (MCAF or MCP-1)

A chemoattractant and activator of macrophages produced by fibroblasts, monocytes, and endothelial cells as a result of exogenous stimuli and endogenous cytokines such as tumor necrosis factor (TNF), interleukin-1 (IL1), and PDGF. It also has a role in activating monocytes to release an enzyme that is cytostatic for some tumor cells. MCAF also plays a role in endothelial leukocyte adhesion molecule 1 (ELAM-1) and CD11a and b surface expression in monocytes and is a potent degranulator of basophils. MCP-1 is a member of the chemokine β family and has a CC (cysteine–cysteine) amino acid sequence. It is chemotactic toward monocytes *in vivo* and *in vitro*, and activates monocytes. It shares 21% amino acid sequence homology with IL8. The 76-amino-acid mature form is derived from a 99-amino acid precursor. The MCP-1 receptor (CCR2A CCR2B) is a seven-transmembrane spanning G protein-coupled molecule of 39 kDa with homology to other cyokine receptors. Various normal and malignant cell types synthesize MCP-1, which can induce chemotaxis, enzyme release, and increased β_2-integrin cell adhesion molecule expression in monocytes and facilitate monocyte cytostatic activity against tumor cells activated by oxidized low density lipoprotein (LDL).

macrophage chemotactic factors (MCFs)

Cytokines that act with macrophages to facilitate migration. The group includes interleukins and interferons.

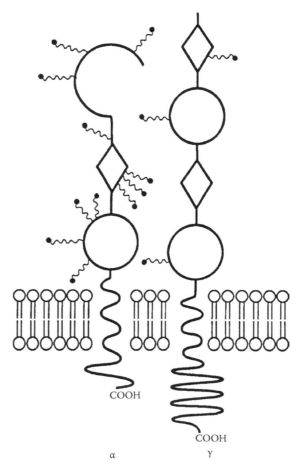

COOH

COOH

α   γ

Macrophage colony-stimulating factor (M-CSF).

M

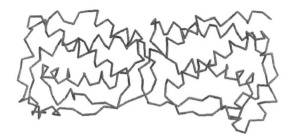

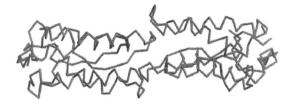

Human macrophage colony-stimulating factor (M-CSF).
Resolution = 2.5 Å.

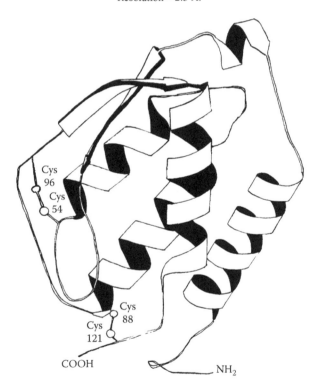

Three-dimensional structure of dimeric human recombinant macrophage
colony-stimulating factor (M-CSF; α form, soluble). Resolution = 2.5 Å.

macrophage colony-stimulating factor (M-CSF)

Facilitates growth, differentiation, and survival and serves as
an activating mechanism for macrophages and their precursors. It is derived from numerous sources such as lymphocytes, monocytes, endothelial cells, fibroblasts, epithelial
cells, osteoblasts, and myoblasts. X-ray crystallography of
recombinant CSF reveals a structure in which four α helices
are placed end to end in two bundles. Human and mouse
M-CSF share 82% homology in the N terminal 227 amino
acids of the mature sequence; there is only 47% homology
in the remainder of the molecular structure. M-CSF derived
from humans and from mice was formerly called colony-
stimulating factor 1 (CSF-1). M-CSF is homodimeric and is

secreted as an 80- to 100-kDa glycoprotein or a 130- to 160-
kDa chondroitin sulfate proteoglycan, or it is expressed as
a biologically active, cell surface membrane, 68- to 86-kDa
glycoprotein. Both forms are present in the blood circulation. The cell surface participates in local regulation, but the
proteoglycan form may be sequestered to specific sites. The
CSF-1 receptor mediates the effects of CSF-1. This receptor
is expressed on osteoclasts and tissue macrophages, their
precursors, embryonic cells, decidual cells, and trophoblasts.
Circulating CSF-1 is postulated to be derived from endothelial cells that line small blood vessels.

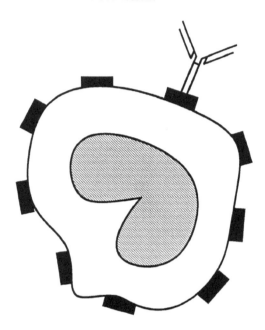

Macrophage cytophilic antibody.

macrophage cytophilic antibody

A cytophilic antibody that becomes anchored to the Fc
receptors on macrophage surfaces. It can be demonstrated
by the immunocytoadherence test.

macrophage functional assays

Tests of macrophage function. (1) Chemotaxis, in which
macrophages are placed in one end of a Boyden chamber
and a chemoattractant is added to the other end; macrophage migration toward the chemoattractant is assayed.
(2) Lysis, in which macrophages acting against radiolabeled
tumor cells or bacterial cells in suspension can be measured
after suitable incubation by measuring the radioactivity of
the supernatant. (3) Phagocytosis, in which the radioactivity
of macrophages that have ingested a radiolabeled target can
be assayed.

macrophage immunity

Cellular immunity.

macrophage inflammatory peptide 2 (MIP-2)

Interleukin-8 (IL8) type II receptor competitor and
chemoattractant also involved in hematopoietic colony
formation as a costimulator. It also degranulates murine
neutrophils. The inflammatory activities of MIP-2 are very
similar to those of IL8.

macrophage inflammatory protein 1α (MIP-1α)

A chemokine of the β (CC) family and endogenous fever-
inducing substance that binds heparin and is resistant to
cyclooxygenase inhibition. Macrophages stimulated by

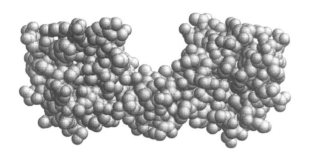

MIP-1α (NMR).

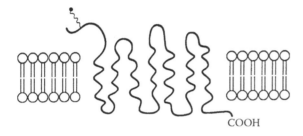

COOH

Macrophage inflammatory protein 1α.

endotoxin may secrete this protein, termed MIP-1, which differs from tumor necrosis factor (TNF), interleukin-1 (IL1), and other endogenous pyrogens because its action is not associated with prostaglandin synthesis. It appears indistinguishable from hematopoietic stem cell inhibitor and may function in growth regulation of hematopoietic cells. It has a broad spectrum of biological activities that include prostaglandin-independent pyrogenic activity, possible participation in wound healing, monocyte chemotaxis, and suppression of immature bone marrow stem and progenitor cells. Significantly, MIP-1α has an HIV-suppressive effect. Tissue sources include fibroblasts, monocytes, lymphocytes, neutrophils, eosinophils, smooth muscle cells, mast cells, platelets, and bone marrow stromal cells, among other cell types. T lymphocytes, basophils, hematopoietic precursor cells, monocytes, eosinophils, neutrophils, mast cells, natural killer (NK) cells, and dendritic cells, among other types, are target cells.

macrophage inflammatory protein 1β(MIP-1β)

A chemokine of the β (CC) family. It shares 70% homology with MIP-1α. Although the two molecules resemble one another structurally, they are significantly different in functions. Unlike MIP-1α, MIP-1β does not activate neutrophils. Unlike MIP-1α, which inhibits early hematopoietic progenitor growth, MIP-1β potentiates it. Both MIP-1α and MIP-1β exert synergistic HIV-suppressive effects. Tissue sources include monocytes, fibroblasts, T lymphocytes, B lymphocytes, neutrophils, smooth muscle cells, mast cells, and selected tumor cell lines. Monocytes, T lymphocytes, hematopoietic precursor cells and basophils are target cells.

macrophage inflammatory protein-2 (MIP-2)

A chemokine of the α (CXC) family. The MIP-2 class is comprised of MIP-2α, also called GRO-β gene product, and MIP-2β, the GRO-γ gene product. MIP-2 has a role in anti-GBM antibody-induced glomerulonephritis in mice. Anti-MIP-2 antibody injection 30 minutes before anti-GBM antibody effectively decreases neutrophil influx and PAS positive deposits containing fibrin. Tissue sources include mast cells, cardiac myocytes, mesangial cells, alveolar macrophages, epidermal cells, and nasal and bronchial epithelium. Neutrophils, basophils, and epithelial cells are the target cells.

macrophage migration inhibitory factor

Migration inhibitory factor.

	No antigen	Ovalbumin	Toxoid
Normal cells	A	B	C
Ovalbumin–sensitive cells	D	E	F
Toxoid–sensitive cells	G	H	I

Macrophage migration test.

M

macrophage migration test

An *in vitro* assay of cell-mediated immunity. Macrophages and lymphocytes to be tested are placed into segments of capillary tubes about the size of microhematocrit tubes and incubated in tissue culture medium containing the soluble antigen of interest, with maintenance of appropriate controls incubated in the same medium not containing the antigen. Lymphocytes from an animal or human sensitized to the antigen release a lymphokine called migration inhibitory factor (MIF) that blocks migration of macrophages from the end of the tube where the cells form an aggregated mass. The macrophages in the control preparation (which does not contain antigen) will migrate out of the tube into a fan-like pattern.

macrophage–monocyte chemotaxis

Macrophages and monocytes are strongly adherent cells and have a rate of locomotion slower than that of neutrophils. They mount a chemotactic response to microorganisms, formyl–Met–Leu–Phe, C5a, C5a des Arg, leukotriene B_4, platelet-activating factor, thrombin, and elastin. Tumors in humans and animals may produce an inhibitor that causes monocytes or macrophages to migrate poorly in chemotaxis assays.

macrophage–monocyte inhibitory factor (MIF)

A substance synthesized by T lymphocytes in response to immunogenic challenge that inhibits the migration of macrophages. MIF is a 25-kDa lymphokine. Its mechanism of action is by elevating intracellular cAMP, polymerizing microtubules and stopping macrophage migration. MIF may increase the adhesive properties of macrophages, thereby inhibiting their migration. The two types of the protein MIF include one of 65 kDa with a pI of 3 to 4 and another of 25 kDa with a pI of approximately 5.

macrophages

Mononuclear phagocytic cells derived from monocytes in the blood that were produced by stem cells in the bone marrow. These intensely phagocytic cells have a powerful although nonspecific role in immune defense. They contain lysosomes and exert microbicidal action against microbes they ingest. They also have effective tumoricidal activity. They may take up and degrade both protein and polysaccharide antigens and present them to T lymphocytes in the context of major histocompatibility complex (MHC) class II molecules. They interact with both T and B lymphocytes in immune reactions. They are frequently found in areas of epithelium, mesothelium, and blood vessels. Macrophages have been called adherent cells as they readily adhere to and spread on glass and plastic and manifest chemotaxis. They have receptors for Fc and C3b on their surfaces, stain positively for nonspecific esterase and peroxidase, and are Ia antigen-positive when acting as accessory cells that present antigen to CD4+ lymphocytes in the generation of an immune response. Monocytes that may differentiate into macrophages when they migrate into the tissues comprise 3 to 5% of leukocytes in the peripheral blood. Tissue-bound macrophages may be found in the lung alveoli, as microglial cells in the central nervous system, as Kupffer's cells in the liver, as Langerhans' cells in the skin, and as histiocytes in connective tissues, as well as macrophages in lymph nodes and peritoneum. Multiple substances are secreted by macrophages including complement components C1 through C5, factors B and D, properdin, C3b inactivators, and β-1H. They also produce monokines such as interleukin-1 (IL1), acid hydrolase, proteases, lipases, and numerous other substances.

macropinocytosis

Antigen uptake through engulfment by a cell of extracellular fluid droplets containing soluble macromolecules and creating macropinosomes that join the endocytic pathway. Referred to also as cell drinking.

macropinosome

A structure produced by invagination of a plasma cell membrane to produce a vesicle containing an extracellular fluid droplet. Refer to macropinocytosis.

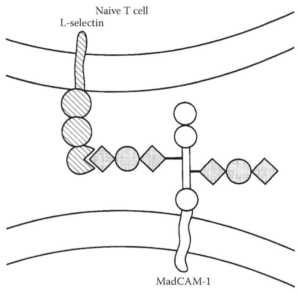

MadCAM-1.

MadCAM-1

Mucosal addressin cell adhesion molecule-1; an addressin in Peyer's patches of mice. This three-immunoglobulin domain structure with a polypeptide backbone binds the $\alpha_{4\beta7}$ integrin. The lymphocyte surface proteins L-selectin and VLA-4 recognize MadCAM-1. MadCAM-1 facilitates access of lymphocytes to the mucosal lymphoid tissues, as in the gastrointestinal tract.

Madsen, Thorvald

Danish bacteriologist who, with Svante Arrhenius, a colleague of Paul Ehrlich, formed an opinion that the reaction of antibody and antigen was a reversible equilibrium between the substances as when a weak acid and weak base are combined according to the ordinary law of mass action.

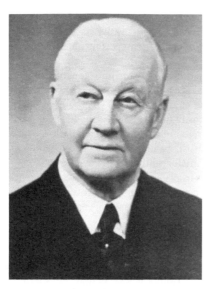

Thorvald Madsen.

MAF

Macrophage-activating factor.

MAGE-1

Melanoma antigen 1 gene derived from a malignant melanoma cell line in humans. It codes for an epitope recognized by a cytotoxic T lymphocyte clone specific for melanoma. This clone was isolated from a patient bearing melanoma.

MAGE-1 protein

A protein found on one half of all melanomas and one fourth of all breast carcinomas but not expressed on the majority of normal tissues. Even though MAGE-1 has not been shown to induce tumor rejection, cytotoxic T lymphocytes in patients with melanoma manifest specific memory for MAGE-1 protein.

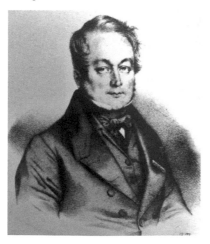

François Magendie.

Magendie, François (1783–1855)

French physician who in 1837 noted the violent death of rabbits following repeated injections of egg albumin and published his findings in 1839. This was the first observation of anaphylaxis in rabbits.

magic bullet

A term coined by Paul Ehrlich in 1900 to describe the affinity of a drug for a particular target. He developed 606 (salvarsan), an arsenical preparation, to treat syphilis. In immunology, the term describes a substance that may be directed to a target by a specific antibody and injure the target after it arrives. Monoclonal antibodies have been linked to toxins such as diphtheria toxin or ricin, as well as to cytokines, for use as magic bullets.

MAIDS

Abbreviation for (1) murine acquired immunodeficiency syndrome, and (2) monoclonal anti-idiotypic antibodies.

MAIS complex

Mycobacterium avium/intracellulare/scrofulaceum. Three species of mycobacteria that express the same antigens and lipids on their surfaces and exhibit the same biochemical reactions, antibiotic susceptibility, and pigment formation. They frequently occur together clinically. MAIS complex is relatively rare; it occurs in 5 to 8% of AIDS patients when their CD4+ T lymphocyte levels diminish to fewer than 100 cells per cubic millimeter of blood. Affected patients have persistent diarrhea, night sweats and fever, abdominal pain, anemia, and extrahepatic obstruction. Ciproflozacin, clofazimine, ethambutol, rifampicin, rifabutin, clarithromycin, and azithromycin have been used in treatment.

major basic protein (MBP)

A 10- to 15-kDa protein present in eosinophilic granules that is released when eosinophils are activated. It causes mast cell degranulation. It has an isoelectric point that exceeds pH 10, thus the inclusion of *basic* in its name. MBP induces injury to the bronchial epithelium and is linked to asthma. When inoculated intracutaneously, it can induce a wheal-and-flare response. It induces tissue injury in allergic and inflammatory diseases.

major histocompatibility complex (MHC)

A locus on a chromosome composed of multiple genes encoding histocompatibility antigens that are cell-surface glycoproteins. MHC genes encode both class I and class II MHC antigens. These antigens play critical roles in interactions among immune system cells, such as class II antigen participation in antigen presentation by macrophages to CD4+ lymphocytes and the participation of MHC class I antigens in cytotoxicity mediated by CD8+ T lymphocytes against target cells such as those infected by viruses, as well as various other immune reactions. MHC genes are very polymorphic and also encode a third category of class III molecules that include complement proteins C2, C4, and factor B; P-450 cytochrome 21-hydroxylase; tumor necrosis factor; and lymphotoxin. The MHC locus is designated HLA in humans, H2 in mice, B in chickens, DLA in dogs, GPLA in guinea pigs, and RT1 in rats. The mouse and human MHC loci are the most widely studied. When organs are transplanted across major MHC locus differences between donor and recipient, graft rejection is prompt.

major histocompatibility complex class II deficiency (MHC II deficiency)

A condition characterized by the lack of MHC class II expression. It leads to a severe defect in both cellular and humoral immune responses to foreign antigens and is consequently characterized by an extreme susceptibility to viral, bacterial, fungal, and protozoal infections, primarily of the respiratory and gastrointestinal tracts. Severe malabsorption with failure to thrive ensues, often leading to death in early childhood. Also called bare lymphocyte syndrome type II.

major histocompatibility complex (MHC) molecule

MHC locus-encoded heterodimeric membrane proteins used by T lymphocytes to recognize antigen. They are divided into two structural types designated class I and class II. Most nucleated cells of the body express MHC class I molecules, which bind peptides derived from cytosolic proteins and are recognized by CD8$^+$ T lymphocytes. The distribution of MHC class II molecules is more restricted, confined mostly to professional antigen-presenting cells that bind peptides from enocytosed proteins recognized by CD4$^+$ T cells.

major histocompatibility complex restriction

Refer to MHC restriction.

major histocompatibility system

Refer to major histocompatibility complex.

Makari test

A no-longer-recommended assay that consisted of preparing an extract from a patient's tumor, incubating it with the patient's serum, and inoculating it into the skin, where it would induce an immediate skin reaction.

malaria

A disease induced by protozoan parasites (*Plasmodium* species) with a complex life cycle in a mosquito and a vertebrate host. Four species are responsible for human malaria. Numerous immunogenic proteins are formed at each morphologically distinct stage in the life cycle. The asexual stage in the blood stream causes the disease. The parasite employs various mechanisms to evade a protective immune response; however, immunity against the parasite and the disease eventually develops from repeated exposure. Malaria vaccine development is in progress.

malaria vaccine

Although no vaccine is presently effective against malaria, several candidates are under investigation including an immunogenic but nonpathogenic *Plasmodium* sporozoite attenuated by radiation. Circumsporoite (CS) proteins combined with sporozoite surface protein 2 (SSP-2) are immunogenic. Murine studies have shown the development of transmission-blocking antibodies following immunization with vaccinia into which the *P. falciparum* surface 25-kDa protein designated Pfs25 has been inserted. Attempts have

been made to increase natural antibodies against CS protein to prevent the prehepatoinvasive stage. The high mutability of *P. falciparum* makes prospects for an effective vaccine dim.

malignant

Leading to death, e.g., a malignant neoplasm.

malignant conversion

Stage IV of carcinogenesis. The progressive accumulation of mutations in neoplastic cells rendering it a malignant tumor with total lack of growth regulation. The tumor may become invasive and metastatic.

malignant transformation

Alterations in a cell render it neoplastic. A neoplasm characterized by uncontrolled growth, invasive properties, and metastatic potential. Left untreated, it can lead to death of the host.

malignolipin (historical)

A substance claimed to be specific for cancer and detectable in blood early in the course of the disease. This concept is no longer considered valid. Malignolipin is comprised of fatty acids, phosphoric acid choline, and spermine. When injected into experimental animals, it can produce profound anemia, leukopoiesis, and cachexia.

MALT

Refer to mucosa-associated lymphoid tissue.

mammals

Compared with lower forms, mammals develop additional immunoglobulin classes, e.g., IgD, IgG, and subclasses. They also manifest increased diversity of major histocompatibility complex (MHC) antigens. Three distinct recognition systems are recognized in mammals. These include antibody, on B cells only, the T cell receptor, on T lymphocytes only, and on a spectrum of cells (MHC), all of whose genes evolved from a common ancestor. The close similarity of murine and human immune systems has

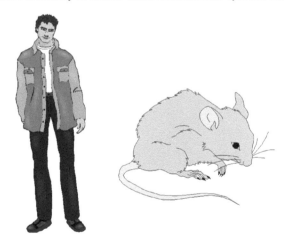

Mammals (man and mouse).

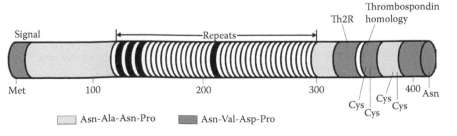

Circumsporate protein of malaria.

greatly facilitated elucidation of human immunity through inbred and transgenic mouse research. Whereas rats have powerful natural immunity, other mammals such as whales and Syrian hamsters manifest little MHC polymorphism.

Mancini test

Single radial diffusion test.

mannan-binding protein (Man-BP)

A substance that induces carbohydrate-mediated activation of complement, in contrast to complement activation mediated by immune complexes which is initiated by C1q. For example, the inability to opsonize *Saccharomyces cerevisiae* may be attributable to Man-BP deficiency. Alveolar macrophage mannose receptors facilitate ingestion of *Pneumocystis carinii.*

mannose-binding lectin (MBL)

A plasma protein also known as collectin binds mannose residues on bacterial cell walls, thereby acting as an opsonin to facilitate phagocytosis of the bacterium by macrophages. A surface receptor for C1q on macrophage surfaces also binds MBL and facilitates phagocytosis of the opsonized microorganisms. Union with the mannose-binding lectin activates lectin-mediated complement activation. Also called mannose-binding protein (MBP) and mannan-binding lectin.

mannose-binding protein pathway

Refer to lectin-mediated pathway.

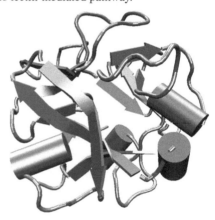

Mannose-receptor complexed with acetylgalactosamine-4-sulfate.

mannose receptor

A lectin or carbohydrate-binding receptor on macrophages that binds mannose and fucose residues on cell wall microorganisms, thereby facilitating their phagocytosis.

mantle

A dense zone of lymphocytes that encircles a germinal center.

mantle zone

The rim of a B lymphocyte that encircles lymphoid follicles. The function and role of mantle zone lymphocytes remain to be determined.

mantle zone lymphoma

A type of follicular lymphoma of intermediate grade. Small lymphocyte proliferation in the mantle zone encircling benign germinal centers, splenomegaly, and generalized lymphadenopathy are present. Histopathologically, B cells vary in size from small to relatively large blasts containing clumped chromatin. Immunoglobulin M (IgM) is usually present.

Mantoux test

A type of tuberculin reaction in which an intradermal injection of tuberculin tests for cell-mediated immunity. A positive test signifies delayed (type IV) hypersensitivity to

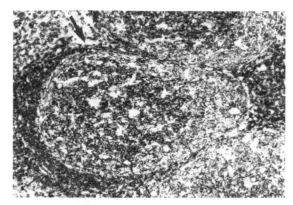

Mantle zone.

Mycobacterium tuberculosis, which indicates previous or current infection with this microorganism.

MAPK

Abbreviation for mitogen-activated protein kinase. Refer also to Ras/MAPK signaling pathway.

Marek's disease

A lymphoproliferative disease of chickens induced by a herpesvirus. Demyelination may occur as a consequence of autoimmune lymphocyte reactivity.

marginal zone

Exterior layer of lymphoid follicles of the spleen where T and B lymphocytes are loosely arranged encircling the periarterial lymphatic sheath. When antigens are injected intravenously, macrophages in this area actively phagocytize them. Marginal zone macrophages are especially adept at trapping polysaccharide antigens on their surfaces, where they may persist for long periods and be recognized by specific B cells or conveyed into follicles.

marginal zone B cells

A B cell subset present in the marginal zone that encircles splenic lymphoid follicles. It plays a significant role during the early adaptive immune response to immunogens, principally Ti antigens. They are precursors of abbreviated life span plasma cells in the spleen but not memory cells.

margination

The adherence of leukocytes in the peripheral blood to the endothelia of vessel walls. Adherence to post-capillary venule endothelium occurs in three phases: selectin-mediated binding, integrin-mediated activation, and arrest and flattening that are activation-dependent. Approximately 50% of polymorphonuclear neutrophils marginate at one time. Margination of leukocytes occurs during inflammation, followed by their migration out of the vessels.

Marrack, John Richardson (1899–1976)

British physician who served as a professor of chemical pathology at Cambridge and at London Hospital. He hypothesized that antibodies are bivalent, labeled antibodies with colored dyes, and proposed a lattice theory of antigen–antibody complex formation in fundamental physicochemical studies.

marsupial immunity

Opossums have been studied as representatives of the marsupialia. At birth, the pouch neonates are immunologically incompetent and antigenically inexperienced; they must develop immune competence without delay. This is facilitated by a rapidly developing thymus in a cervical location. Whereas some species may pass maternal antibodies across

M

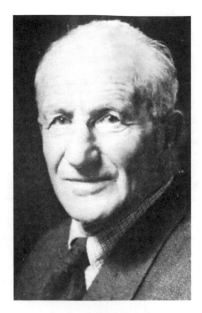

John Richardson Marrack.

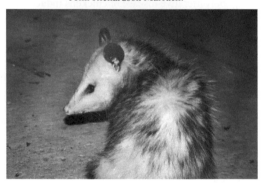

Marsupial.

the placenta, most of the transfer of maternal antibodies begins with suckling and continues until the young leave the pouch, at which time immune competence is fully developed. Adult marsupials possess lymphoid organs that participate in both humoral and cellular immune responses. Some data suggest that the humoral immune response may be initially sluggish and that selective immune responses may be refractory to certain cytokines.

MART-1 (M2-7C10), mouse
A melanocyte differentiation antigen present in melanocytes of normal skin and retina, nevi and in more than 85% of melanomas. This antibody is very useful in establishing the diagnosis of metastatic melanoma. Also known as melan A.

mass vaccination
Immunization with vaccines during an outbreak of a communicable disease in an effort to prevent an epidemic. For example, mass vaccinations may be carried out in schools and hospitals during meningitis or hepatitis epidemics.

mast cell activation
Mast cells may be activated immunologically through cross linking by antigen of surface immunoglobulin E (IgE) attached to FcεRI. They may be activated also by anti-IgE antibody, C5a, substance P, or local trauma.

mast cell–eosinophil axis
Interactions between mast cells and eosinophils during inflammatory reactions recognized as immediate hypersensitivity.

This involves the attraction of eosinophils and their activation by mast-cell-derived ECF-A along with a dampening effect exerted by eosinophils upon mast cells. The released mediators influence the reactions in the microenvironment. When the causative agent is a parasite, the antiparasitic cytotoxic mechanisms of eosinophils reinforce the defense. The other effector cells attracted to the involved sites join forces in the defense activities. The inhibitory effects of eosinophils upon mast cells are exerted through a number of enzymes that inactivate or destroy some of the mast-cell-derived mediators. Intact granules released from mast cells in the microenvironment are phagocytized by eosinophils and can be demonstrated in these cells by metachromatic staining. This represents an important detoxification mechanism, as even intact granules have been shown to exert proteolytic activity.

mast cell growth factor 1
Synonym for interleukin-3 (IL3).

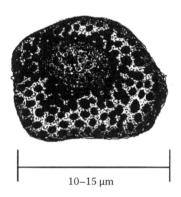

10–15 μm

Mast cell.

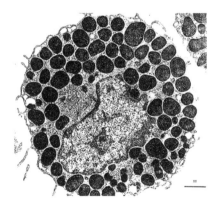

Mast cell.

mast cell growth factor 2
Synonym for interleukin-4 (IL4).

mast cells
A normal component of connective tissue that plays an important role in immediate (type I) hypersensitivity and inflammatory reactions by secreting a large variety of chemical mediators from storage sites in their granules upon stimulation. Mast cells possess high-affinity Fcε receptors (Fcε RI) that bind free IgE. Their locations at mucosal and cutaneous surfaces and about venules in deeper tissues is related to this role. They can be identified easily by their characteristic granules that stain metachromatically. The sizes and shapes of mast cells vary in diameter (10 to 30 μm). In adventitia of

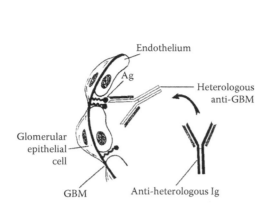

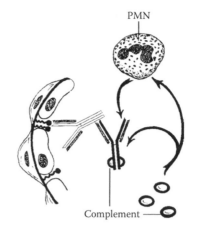

Masugi nephritis.

large vessels, mast cells are elongated. In loose connective tissue, they are round or oval; their shape in fibrous connective tissue may be angular. On their surfaces, they have Fc receptors for immunoglobulin E (IgE). Cross linking by either antigen for which the IgE Fab regions are specific or by anti-IgE or antireceptor antibody leads to degranulation with the release of pharmacological mediators of immediate hypersensitivity from their storage sites in the mast cell granules. Leukotrienes, prostaglandins, and platelet-activating factor are also produced and released following Fcε receptor cross linking. Mast cell granules are approximately 0.5 μm in diameter and are electron-dense. They contain many biologically active compounds, of which the most important are heparin, histamine, serotonin, and a variety of enzymes. Histamine is stored in the granule as a complex with heparin or serotonin. Mast cells also contain proteolytic enzymes such as plasmin and hydroxylase, β glucuronidase, phosphatase, and a high uronidase inhibitor, to mention only the most important. Zinc, iron, and calcium are also found. Some substances released from mast cells are not stored in a preformed state but are synthesized following mast cell activation. These represent secondary mediators as opposed to preformed primary mediators. Mast cell degranulation involves adenylate cyclase activation with rapid synthesis of cyclic AMP, protein kinase activation, phospholipid methylation, and serine esterase activation. Mast cells of the gastrointestinal and respiratory tracts that contain chondroitin sulfate produce leukotriene C_4, whereas connective tissue mast cells that contain heparin produce prostaglandin D_2.

mast cell tryptase

A serine protease present in secretory granules of mast cells and released with histamine during mast cell activation. Serum tryptase is a clinical indicator of diseases of mast cell activation such as systemic anaphylaxis or mastocytosis. Tryptase is a better *in vitro* marker of anaphylaxis than histamine because it has a slower release and is more stable. The half-life of tryptase is 90 minutes. It takes at least 15 minutes to reach detectable concentrations. The best time to measure tryptase is 1 to 2 hours but not more than 6 hours after the reaction. In anaphylaxis, both α and β tryptase are elevated. Most studies indicate that tryptase is increased in postmortem blood following severe anaphylaxis and is a reliable postmortem indicator of fatal anaphylaxis.

Masugi nephritis

Experimental model of human antiglomerular basement membrane (anti-GBM) nephritis. The disease is induced by the injection of rabbit antirat glomerular basement membrane antibody into rats. The antiserum for passive transfer is raised in rabbits immunized with rat kidney basement

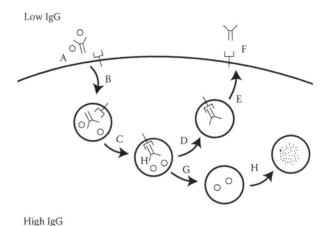

Mechanism of γ globulin protection from catabolism. IgG (γ) and plasma prteins (o) (A) are internalized into endosomes of endothelium (B) without prior binding. In the low pH (H^+) of the endosome (C), binding of IgG is promoted (D, E, F). IgG retained by receptor recycles to the cell surface and dissociates in the neutral pH of the extracellular fluid, returning to circulation (G, H). Unbound proteins are shunted to the lysosomes for degradation. With "low IgG," receptor efficiently "rescues" IgG from catabolism. With "high IgG," receptor is saturated and excess IgG passes to catabolism for a net acceleration of IgG catabolism.

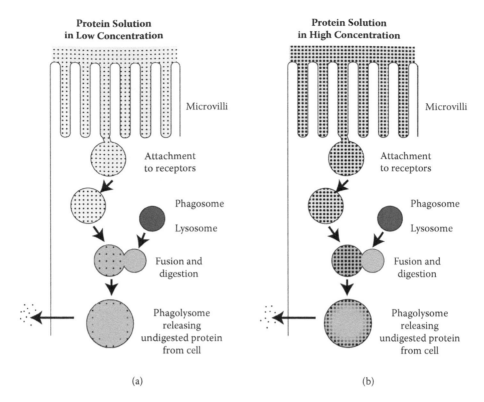

Maternal antibodies.

membranes. The passively administered antibodies become bound to the glomerular basement membrane, fix complement, and induce glomerular basement membrane injury with increased permeability. Neutrophils and monocytes may infiltrate the area. Masugi nephritis is an experimental model of Goodpasture's syndrome in humans. Also called nephrotoxic nephritis.

maternal antibodies

Maternal immunoglobulins are passed to offspring both *in utero* and in the neonatal period. In humans, immunoglobulin G (IgG) is transferred by way of the placenta as early as the 38th day of gestation. Transfer remains stable until the 17th week and then increases until term. Only the IgG class of antibodies crosses the placenta. The SC portion of the immunoglobulin is bound to specific placental membrane receptors of the Scγ type III variety (CD16) that possess binding sites for the Foc region of IgG in addition to epitopes that can be recognized by the antigen-binding site of IgG. The receptors have low affinity for aggregated or complex IgG, with the strongest affinity for IgG$_1$ and IgG$_3$, less for IgG$_4$, and least for IgG$_2$; they have no affinity for IgM and IgA. The receptors are concentrated on syncytiotrophoblasts that make direct contact with the mother's circulation. Human colostrum and fresh breast milk contain numerous specific and nonspecific host resistance factors. Secretory IgA is present in these fluids, with the highest concentration in colostrom that peaks during the first 34 days postpartum. Breast-fed children receive 0.5 g of secretory IgA per day. Human milk also contains IgG and IgM, as well as secretory IgA but in lower concentrations. Factors other than immunoglobulins that protect against infections include lactoferrin that acts as a bacteriostatic agent depriving microbes of iron. Lysozyme is also present in milk. Breast milk also contains macrophages, T and B

cells, neutrophils, epithelial cells, and immunomodulators. Diseases caused by maternal antibodies are listed individually. Refer also to Brambell receptor.

maternal immunity

Passive immunity conferred on the neonate by its mother. This is accomplished prepartum by active immunoglobulin transport across the placenta from the maternal to the fetal circulation in primate animals including humans. Other species such as ungulates transfer immunity from mother to young via antibodies in the colostrum, as the intestine can pass immunoglobulin molecules across its surface in the early neonatal period. The egg yolk of avian species is the mechanism through which immunity is passed from mother to young.

maternal immunoglobulins

Refer to maternal antibodies.

maternal imprinting

Alteration of the maternal allele chromatin of a gene in a subject to render it more likely to be expressed than the paternal allele. Concerns the relationship between a disease-related allele and the incidence of the disease.

matrix (HIV)

Provides the scaffolding that the viral envelope enfolds.

matrix metalloproteinases (MMPs)

A family of zinc-containing endoproteinases that adjust specific components of extracellular matrix, thereby contributing to matrix equilibrium and structural integrity. They are grouped in three categories: (1) interstitial collagenases, (2) stromelysins, and (3) gelatinases. Dysregulation of MMP synthesis and activation is believed to contribute to tissue injury in inflammatory and neoplastic diseases. Macrophages, T lymphocytes, eosinophils, and neutrophils all produce MMPs with cell-specific patterns. MMPs from macrophages contribute to the degradation, removal, and remodeling of connective tissues. The gelatinase-type MMPs synthesized by T lymphocytes mainly facilitate T cell migration. MMPs facilitate shedding of L-selectin, an adhesion receptor, from the leukocyte surface.

maturation of affinity

During the course of immunization with a particular antigen, the antibodies formed show a progressive increase in affinity.

mature B cells

B lymphocytes that expresses immunoglobulin M (IgM) and IgD and are functionally capable of responding to antigen. These cells constitute the final step in B cell maturation of the bone marrow and reside in peripheral lymphoid organs.

mature dendritic cells

Antigen-presenting cells of secondary lymphoid tissues that bear costimulatory molecules among other cell surface molecules that render them capable of presenting antigen to naïve T cells that become activated.

mature T cells

Classified on the basis of their surface markers, such as CD4 and CD8. CD4$^+$ T lymphocytes recognize antigens in the context of MHC class II histocompatibility molecules, whereas CD8$^+$ T lymphocytes recognize antigen in the context of MHC class I molecules. CD4$^+$ T cells participate in the afferent limb of the immune response to exogenous antigen via antigen-presenting cells. This stimulates the synthesis of interleukin-2 (IL2), which activates CD8$^+$ T cells, natural killer (NK) cells, and B cells, thereby orchestrating an immune response to the antigen. Thus these cells are called helper T lymphocytes. They also mediate delayed-type hypersensitivity reactions. CD8$^+$ T lymphocytes include cytotoxic and suppressor cell populations. They react to endogenous antigen and often express their effector function through a cytotoxic mechanism (e.g., against a virus-infected cell). Other molecules on mature T cells in humans include the E rosette receptor CD2 molecule, the T cell receptor, the pan T cell marker (CD3), and transferrin receptor.

Matzinger danger theory

A concept that abandons the idea of self–nonself discrimination as the basic immunologic metaphor. Matzinger proposes that the function of the immune system is to protect the individual from "danger." His concept requires a discriminating event to mark the entry of potentially dangerous material into the system. This is associated with the activity of antigen-presenting cells, which at rest are unable to provide a source of signal 2, which expresses the S phenotype. A dangerous event converts this cell to the S$^+$ state that provides costimulatory activity, signal 2 for the initiation of the T cell response, and subsequent T-cell-dependent immune phenomena.

Mayer, Manfred

A student of Michael Heidelberger and later a professor at Johns Hopkins University Medical School in Baltimore, Mayer was an authority on the molecular aspects of complement activity, especially its role in hemolysis.

MBP

Acronym for (1) myelin basic protein or (2) major basic protein.

MBSA

Acronym for methylated bovine serum albumin.

McCleod phenotype

Human erythrocytes without Kell or Cellano antigens. These red cells lack Kx, a precursor in the biosynthetic

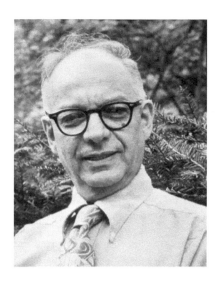

Manfred M. Mayer.

pathway of the Kell blood group system. Kx is encoded by a gene on the X chromosome termed *X1k* and is normally found on granulocytes and fibroblasts. Red cells lacking Kx exhibit decreased survival and diminished permeability to water and are acanthocytic morphologically with spikes on their surfaces. They also show decreased expression of Kell system antigens. This group of erythrocyte abnormalities is termed the McCleod phenotype. Subjects with McCleod erythrocytes have a neuromuscular system abnormality characterized by elevated serum levels of creatine phosphokinase (CPK). Older individuals may have disordered muscular functions. The *X1k* gene maps to the short arm of the X chromosome, where it is linked to the chronic granulomatous disease gene.

M cell

A gastrointestinal tract epithelial cell, with an intraepithelial pocket that trayscytoses antigens from a lumen such as the gastrointestinal tract across the epithelium to its basolateral surface. The M cell conveys microorganisms and macromolecular substances from the gut lumen to Peyer's patches. M cells do not possess glycocalyx and brush borders that enable antigen capture. M cells are non-antigen-presenting cells found in the epithelial layers of Peyer's patches that nevertheless may have an important role in antigen delivery. They have relatively large surfaces with microfolds that attach to microorganisms and macromolecular surfaces. The M cell cytoplasmic processes extend to CD4$^+$ T cells underneath them. Materials attached to microvilli are conveyed to coated pits and moved to the basolateral surface, which has pronounced invaginations rich in leukocytes and mononuclear phagocytes. Thus, materials gaining access by way of M cells come into contact with lymphoid cells as they reach the basolateral surface. This is believed to facilitate induction of immune responsiveness. M signifies membranous or microfold cells.

Mcg isotypic determinant

A human immunoglobulin λ chain epitope that occurs on a number of every person's λ light polypeptide chains in immunoglobulin molecules. The Mcg isotypic determinant is characterized by asparagine at position 112, threonine at position 114, and lysine at position 163.

M component

A spike or defined peak observed on electrophoresis of serum proteins which suggests monoclonal proliferation of mature B lymphocytes synthesizing immunoglobulin G (IgG), IgA, or IgM. M component can be seen in such diseases as multiple myeloma, heavy chain disease, and Waldenström's macroglobulinemia.

MCP-1 (monocyte chemoattractant protein 1)

A prototypic chemokine of the β (CC) family that was first isolated as a product of the immediate early gene, *JE,* induced by PDGF. Cloning of the human homolog of *JE* reveals an encoded protein identical to an authentic chemokine MCP-1, which is believed to be one of the most significant chemokines in chronic inflammatory diseases controlled by mononuclear leukocytes. Tissue sources include fibroblasts, monocytes, macrophages, mouse spleen lymphocytes, and endothelial cells, among others. Target cells include monocytes, hematopoietic precursors, T lymphocytes, basophils, eosinophils, mast cells, natural killer (NK) cells, and dendritic cells.

MCP-1 in atherosclerosis

Chemokines are involved in the pathogenesis of atherosclerosis by promoting directed migration of inflammatory cells. Monocyte chemoattractant protein-1 (MCP-1), a CC chemokine, has been detected in atherosclerotic lesions by anti-MCP-1 antibody detection and *in situ* hybridization. MCP-1 mRNA expression has been found in endothelial cells, macrophages and vascular smooth muscle cells in atherosclerotic arteries of patients undergoing bypass revascularization. MCP-1 functions in the development of atherosclerosis by recruiting monocytes into the subendothelial cell layer. MCP-1 is critical for the initiation and development of atherosclerotic lesions. During the progression of atherosclerosis, low density lipoprotein (LDL) accumulates within macrophages and monocytes present in the intimal layer. Deposition of lipids within these cells leads to the formation and eventual enlargement of atherosclerotic lesions. Studies suggest a noncholesterol-mediated effect of MCP-1 in the development of atherosclerotic lesions. MCP-1 plays a crucial role in initiating atherosclerosis by recruiting macrophages and monocytes to vessel walls.

MCP-2 (monocyte chemoattractant protein 2)

A chemokine of the β (CC) family. It is a variant of MCP-1, but is independent and has several distinct biological properties that include eosinophil and basophil activation. The principal differences between MCP-1 and MCP-2 appear in the N terminal molecular region. Tissue sources include fibroblasts, peripheral blood mononuclear cells, leteal cells, and osteosarcoma cell line MG 63. Target cells include T lymphocytes, monocytes, eosinophils, basophils, and natural killer (NK) cells.

MCP-3 (monocyte chemoattractant protein 3)

A chemokine of the β (CC) family that has very different binding characteristics and actions from MCP-1. MCP-3 binds to unique monocyte receptors shared by MCP-1. In contrast to MCP-1, MCP-3 is chemotactic to eosinophils and more potent toward basophils. It is the only β chemokine that fails to form dimers at elevated concentrations. Tissue sources include fibroblasts, platelets, mast cells, monocytes, and osteosarcoma MG-63. Target cells include monocytes, T cells, basophils, eosinophils, activated natural killer (NK) cells, dendritic cells, and neutrophils.

M-CSF (macrophage colony-stimulating factor)

Facilitates growth, differentiation, and survival and serves as an activating mechanism for macrophages and their precursors. It is derived from numerous sources such as lymphocytes, monocytes, endothelial cells, fibroblasts, epithelial cells, osteoblasts, and myoblasts. X-ray crystallography of recombinant CSF reveals a structure in which four α helices are placed end to end in two bundles. Human and mouse M-CSF share 82% homology in the N terminal 227 amino acids of the mature sequence, but there is only 47% homology in the remainder of the molecular structure. M-CSF derived from humans and from mice has been previously termed colony-stimulating factor 1 (CSF-1).

MCTD

Acronym for mixed-connective tissue disease.

MDP

Muramyl dipeptide.

measles vaccine

An attenuated virus vaccine administered as a single injection to children at 2 years of age or between 1 and 10 years old. Contraindications include a history of allergy or convulsions. Puppies may be protected against canine distemper in the neonatal period by the administration of attenuated measles virus which represents a heterologous vaccine. Passive immunity from the mother precludes early immunization of puppies with live canine distemper vaccine.

measles virus vaccine (live, injection)

Measles, a common childhood disease, is induced by a paramyxovirus. It can be associated with serious complications, including pneumonia, encephalitis, and even death. Subjects first vaccinated with measles virus vaccine at 12 months of age or older require revaccination with measles, mumps, and rubella virus vaccine (live) before entering elementary school. Revaccination may induce seroconversion. The Advisory Committee on Immunization Practices advises that the first dose of measles–mumps–rubella vaccine be administered at 12 to 15 months of age and that the second dose be given at 4 to 6 years of age.

measles–mumps–rubella virus vaccine (live, injection)

For simultaneous vaccination in individuals at least 12 months of age. These subjects should be revaccinated prior to admission to elementary school. Vaccination of persons exposed to natural measles may afford protection if the vaccine is administered within 72 hours of exposure. If given a few days prior to exposure, greater protection is possible.

mechanical barrier

The papilloma virus and a few other infection agents may penetrate the skin but most microorganisms are excluded by it. Free fatty acids from sebaceous glands and lactic acid present in perspiration together with an acid pH of 5 to 6 and the dryness of the skin are unfavorable to microorganisms. *Staphylococcus aureus* may colonize hair follicles and sweat glands to produce furuncles, carbuncles, and abscesses. *Pseudomonas aeruginosa* may infect skin injured by burns. Injury to the gastric mucosa by irradiation or cytotoxic drugs may culminate in infection by the normal flora of the intestine.

Medawar, Peter Brian (1915–1987)

British transplantation biologist. Earned a PhD in 1935 at Oxford, where he served as a lecturer in zoology. He later became a professor of zoology at Birmingham (1947) and at University College, London (1951). He was named

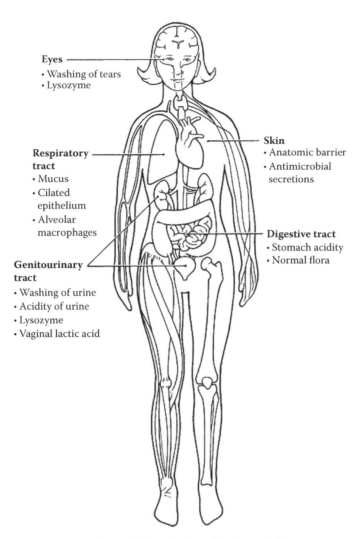

Eyes
• Washing of tears
• Lysozyme

Respiratory tract
• Mucus
• Cilated epithelium
• Alveolar macrophages

Genitourinary tract
• Washing of urine
• Acidity of urine
• Lysozyme
• Vaginal lactic acid

Skin
• Anatomic barrier
• Antimicrobial secretions

Digestive tract
• Stomach acidity
• Normal flora

External defense barriers of the human body.

Intact skin

Mucus
  Motion of cilia
  Coughing/sneezing

Cell shedding
Flushing of microbes by tears, saliva, urine, perspiration, other body fluids
Emesis and diarrhea aid microbial elimination

Mechanical barriers against infection.

director of the Medical Research Council in 1962 and of the Clinical Research Center at Northwick Park in 1971. With Billingham and Brent, he made seminal discoveries in transplantation and immunobiology and described immunological tolerance and its importance for tissue transplantation. He shared the 1960 Nobel Prize in Medicine or Physiology with Sir MacFarlane Burnett.

mediastinal mass

A structure situated in proximity to the heart and thymus that lies between the sternum and the vertebral column.

Mediterranean lymphoma

Refer to immunoproliferative small intestinal disease (IPSID).

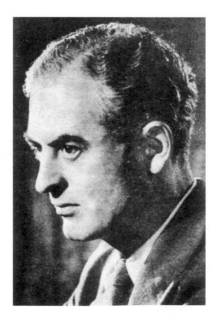

Peter Brian Medawar.

medulla

The innermost or central region of an organ. The central area of a thymic lobe is the thymic medulla, which is rich in antigen-presenting cells derived from the bone marrow and medullary epithelial cells. Macrophages and plasma cells are rich in the lymph node medulla through which lymph passes en route to the efferent lymphatics.

medullary cord

A region of the lymph node medulla composed of macrophages and plasma cells that lies between the lymphatic sinusoids.

medullary sinus

Potential cavities in the lymph node medulla that receive lymph prior to its entering efferent lymphatics.

medullary thymic epithelial cells (mTECs)

Refer to thymic epithelial cells.

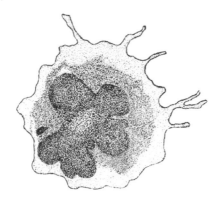

Megakaryocyte.

megakaryocyte

Relatively large bone marrow giant cells of myeloid lineage that are multinucleate and from which blood platelets are derived by the breaking up of membrane-bound cytoplasm to produce thrombocytes.

MEL-14

A selectin on the surfaces of lymphocytes significant in lymphocyte interaction with endothelial cells of peripheral lymph nodes. Selectins are important for adhesion despite shear forces associated with circulating blood. MEL-14 is lost from the surfaces of both granulocytes and T lymphocytes following their activation. It combines with phosphorylated oligosaccharides.

MEL-14 antibody

A gp90 receptor that permits lymphocyte binding to peripheral lymph node high endothelial venules. Immature double-negative thymocytes comprise cells that vary from high to low in MEL-14 content. The gp90 MEL-14 epitope is a glycoprotein on murine lymph node lymphocyte surfaces. MEL-14 antibody prevents these lymphocytes from binding to postcapillary venules. The gp90 MEL-14 is apparently a lymphocyte homing receptor that directs these cells to lymph nodes in preference to lymphoid tissue associated with the gut.

melanization reaction

Refer to ProPO system.

melanocyte

A melanin pigment-producing cell of the skin.

melanoma

Malignant tumors of melanocytes in the skin.

melanoma antigen-1 gene

See MAGE-1.

melanoma-associated antigens (MAAs)

Antigens associated with the aggressive, malignant, and metastatic tumors arising from melanocytes or melanocyte-associated nevus cells. Monoclonal antibodies have identified more than 40 MAAs. They are classified as major histocompatibility complex (MHC) molecules, cation binding proteins, growth factor receptors, gangliosides, high molecular weight extracellular matrix-binding molecules, and nevomelanocyte differentiation antigens. Some of the antigens are expressed on normal cells; others are expressed on tumor cells. Melanoma patient blood sera often contain anti-MAA antibodies that are regrettably not protective. Monoclonal antibodies against MAAs aid studies on the biology of tumor progression, immunodiagnosis, and immunotherapy trials.

melanoma growth stimulatory activity

See MGSA.

melanosome

A melanocyte organelle linked to the endocytic pathway that is charged with synthesis of pigment proteins.

$$HOOC-\underset{\underset{NH_2}{|}}{CH}-CH_2-\bigcirc-N\underset{CH_2-CH_2-Cl}{\overset{CH_2-CH_2-Cl}{<}}$$

Structure of melphalan (l-phenylalanine mustard).

melphalan (l-phenylalanine mustard)

Nitrogen mustard used to treat multiple myeloma patients.

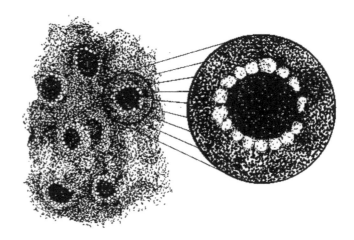

Membrane perforations resulting from membrane attack complex (MAC) action.

membrane attack complex (MAC)

Five terminal proteins (C5, C6, C7, C8, and C9) associate into a membrane attack complex (MAC) on a target cell membrane to mediate injury. Initiation of MAC assembly begins with C5 cleavage into C5a and C5b fragments. A (C5b678)$_1$(C9)$_n$ complex then forms either on natural membranes or, in their absence, in combination with such plasma inhibitors as lipoproteins, antithrombin III, and S protein. C9 and C8 α proteins resemble each other structurally and also in sequence homologies. Both bind

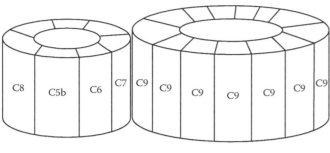

MAC.

calcium and furnish domains that bind lipid, enabling MAC to attach to membranes. Mechanisms proposed for complement-mediated cytolysis include extrinsic protein channel incorporation into the plasma membrane or membrane deformation and destruction. Central regions of C6, C7, C8α, C8β, and C9 have been postulated to contain amphiphilic structures that may be membrane anchors. A single C9 molecule per C5b678 leads to erythrocyte lysis. Gram-negative bacteria that have both outer and inner membranes resist complement action by lengthening the O-antigen chain at the outer membrane or heightening surface carbohydrate content, which interferes with MAC binding. MAC assembly and insertion into the outer membrane are requisite for lysis of bacteria. Nucleated cells may rid their surfaces of MAC through endocytosis or exocytosis. Platelets have provided much data concerning sublytic actions of C5b–9 proteins. Control proteins acting at different levels may inhibit killing of homologous cells mediated by MAC. Besides C8-binding protein or homologous restriction factor (HRF) found on human erythrocyte membranes, the functionally similar but smaller

phosphatidyl inositol glycan (PIG)-tailed membrane protein harnesses complement-induced cell lysis. Sublytic actions of MAC may be of greater consequence for host cells than its cytotoxic effects.

membrane attack unit

Lytic unit exclusive of the recognition and activation units. C5b binds to cell membranes, followed by the successive interaction of single molecules of C6, C7, and C8 with the membrane-bound C5b. Finally, further interaction with several C9 molecules finishes the formation of the lytic unit through noncovalent interactions without enzymatic alteration. Formation of a membrane attack unit or membrane attack complex (MAC) leads to a cell membrane lesion that permits loss of K$^+$ and ingress of Na$^+$ and water, leading to hypotonic lysis of cells.

membrane-bound immunoglobulin (mIg)

An immunoglobulin molecule on the surface that possesses a transmembrane region and extended C terminal region and lacks a tail piece. It is the antigen-binding structure of the B cell receptor.

membrane cofactor protein (MCP)

A type I transmembrane regulatory protein of the complement system that is a cofactor for the factor-I-mediated proteolytic cleavage and inactivation of C3b and C4b deposited on self tissue. MCP protects the cell on which it is located rather than neighboring cells. It also serves as the measles virus receptor and participates in the adherence of *Streptococcus pyogenes* (group A streptococcus) to endothelial cells. It is a member of a group of structurally, functionally, and genetically related proteins called regulators of complement activation (RCAs). They include decay-accelerating factor DAF (CD55), complement receptors 1

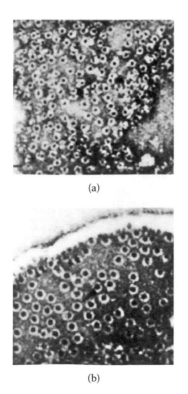

(a)

(b)

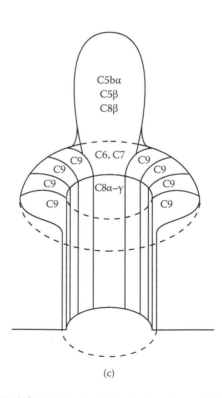

(c)

Perforations in cell membrane (a) and (b) induced by complement (poly C9 tubular complexes). (c) Model of membrane attack complex (MAC) subunit arrangement.

and 2, and factor H and C4-binding protein in plasma. MCP is also called CD46.

membrane cofactor of proteolysis (MCP or CD46)

A host cell membrane protein that functions in association with factor I to cleave C3b to its inactive derivative iC3b, thereby blocking formation of convertase.

membrane complement receptors

Receptors are expressed on blood cells and tissue macrophages of humans. They include Clq-R (Clq receptor), CR1 (C3b/C4b receptor; CD35), CR2 (C3d/Epstein–Barr virus [EBV] receptor; CD21), CR3 (iC3b receptor; CD11b/CD18), CR4 (C3bi receptor; CD11c/CD18), CR5 (C3dg-dimer receptor), fH-R (factor H receptor), C5a-R (C5a receptor), and C3a/C4a–R (C3a/C4a receptor). Ligands for C receptors generated by the classic or alternate pathway include fluid phase activation peptides of C3, C4, and C5 designated C3a, C4a, and C5a that are anaphylatoxins that interact with C3a/C4a–R or C5a–R and participate in inflammation. Other ligands for C receptors include soluble or particulate complement proteins deposited on immune complexes. Fixed C4 and C3 fragments (C4b, C3b, C3bi, C3dg, and C3d), Clq, and a factor H constitute these ligands. These receptors play a major role in facilitating improved recognition of pathogenic substances. They aid the elimination of bacteria and soluble immune complexes. Neutrophils, monocytes, and macrophages express C3 receptors on their surface. Neutrophils and erythrocytes express immune adherence receptors (CR1s) on their surfaces. Four other receptors for C3 are designated CR2, CR3, CR4, and CR5. Additional receptors for complement components other than C3 and C3a are termed Clq receptor, C5a-R (C5a receptor), C3a-R (C3a receptor), and fH-R (factor H receptor).

membrane immunofluorescence

The reaction of a fluorochrome-labeled antibody with surface receptors of viable cells. This reaction of fluorescent antibody with surface antigens rather than internal antigens is the basis for many immunologic assays such as labeling of lymphocytes with such reagents for immunophenotyping by flow cytometry, patching, and capping and to detect changes in surface antigens through antigenic variation.

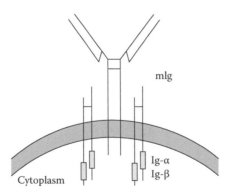

Membrane immunoglobulin.

membrane immunoglobulin

Cell surface immunoglobulin that serves as an antigen receptor. Virgin B cells contain surface membrane IgM and IgD molecules. Following activation by antigen, the B cells differentiate into plasma cells that secrete IgM molecules. Whereas membrane-bound IgM is a four-polypeptide chain monomer,

the secreted IgM is a pentameric molecule containing five four-chain unit monomers and one J chain. Other immunoglobulin classes have membrane and secreted types. IgG and IgA membrane immunoglobulins probably serve as memory B cell antigen receptors. The segment of the immunoglobulin introduced into the cell membrane is a hydrophobic heavy chain region in the vicinity of the carboxyl terminus. Within a particular isotype, the heavy chain is of greater length in the membrane form than in the secreted molecule. This greater length is at the carboxyl terminal end of the membrane form. Separate mRNA molecules from one gene encode the membrane and secreted forms of heavy chain.

membrane nibbling

Process whereby a dendritic cell acquires part of the membrane of an intact living whole cell.

membranoproliferative glomerulonephritis (MPGN)

A nephropathy in which the glomerular basement membrane is altered and glomerular cells proliferate, especially in mesangial areas, leading to the synonymous mesangiocapillary GN. Patients may present with hematuria and/or proteinuria. In type I MPGN, IgG-, Clq-, C4-, and C3-containing subendothelial electron-dense deposits are present in approximately 66% of cases, as revealed by immunofluorescence and electron microscopy. Conventional light microscopy reveals splitting of basement membranes. In type II MPGN, also called dense deposit disease, the lamina densa of the glomerular basement membrane appears as an electron-dense ribbon, on either side of which C3 can be detected by immunofluorescence. Complement is fixed only by the alternate pathway. Type II patients have C3 nephritic factor (C3NeF) in their sera which facilitates stabilization of alternate C3 convertase, thereby promoting C3 degradation and hypocomplementemia. Half of these patients develop chronic renal failure over a 10-year period.

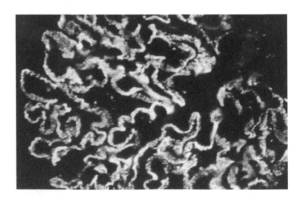

Types of glomerulonephritis.

membranous glomerulonephritis

A disease induced by deposition of electron-dense, immune (Ag–Ab) deposits in the glomerular basement membrane in a subepithelial location. This leads to progressive thickening of glomerular membranes. Most cases are idiopathic, but membranous glomerulonephritis may follow development of other diseases such as systemic lupus erythematosus (SLE), lung or colon carcinoma, and exposure to gold, mercury, penicillamine, or captopril. It can also be a sequela of certain infections (e.g., hepatitis B) or metabolic disorders (e.g., diabetes mellitus). Clinically, it is a principal cause of nephrotic syndrome in adults. The subepithelial immune deposits are shown by immunofluorescence to contain both immunoglobulins and complement. Proteinuria persists in 70 to 90% of cases, and half of the patients develop renal insufficiency over a period of years. A less severe course appears in 10 to 30% of cases.

memory

The capacity of the adaptive immune system to respond more rapidly, more effectively, and with greater magnitude to a second (or subsequent) exposure to an immunogen compared to its response to the primary exposure. Refer to immunological memory.

memory B cells

Long-lived antigen-specific B cells generated during exposure of naïve B lymphocytes to antigen in a primary immune response. Subsequent exposure to the antigen for which they are specific leads to reactivation and differentiation into plasma cells as a secondary or subsequent immune response.

memory cells

Immunocompetent T and B lymphocytes generated during a primary immune response. They have the ability to mount an accentuated response to antigen, compared with that of virgin immunocompetent cells, because of their previous exposure to the antigen through immunization or infection. Activated memory cells yield effector cells more rapidly and with less costimulation than naïve lymphocytes. Homing and chemokine receptors of memory cells direct them to sites where they were first exposed to antigen. Memory cells are responsible for immunological memory and protective immunity.

memory lymphocytes

Lymphocytes of the B or T type that respond rapidly with an enhanced memory or recall response to second or subsequent exposure to an antigen to which they were primed previously. Antigen stimulation of naïve lymphocytes leads to the production of memory B and T cells that persist in a functionally dormant state years following antigen elimination.

memory response

Refer to immunological memory.

memory T cells

Long-lived antigen-specific T lymphocytes that are activated in secondary and subsequent immune responses to antigen and respond in an immediate and exaggerated manner to induce a heightened immune response to a specific antigen.

meningococcal D (Groups A,C,Y, and W-135)polysaccharide diphtheria toxoid conjugate vaccine

Bactericidal anticapsular meningococcal antibodies are associated with protection from invasive meningococci. Meningococcal polysaccharide diphtheria toxoid conjugate vaccine induces synthesis of bactericidal antibodies specific for the capsular polysaccharides of serogroups A, C, Y, and W-135. Immunogenicity and clinical efficacy of serogroups A and C meningococcal vaccines are well established. The serogroup A polysaccharide induces antibodies in children as young as 3 months of age, although a response comparable with that among adults is not achieved until 3 to 5 years of age; the serogroup C component is weakly immunogenic in recipients who are younger than 18 to 24 months of age. The serogroups A and C vaccines have clinical efficacies of 85 to 100% in older children and adults and are used to control epidemics. Serogroups Y and W-135 polysaccharides

are safe and immunogenic in adults and in children above 2 years of age. In the first 3 years following a single dose of vaccine, the measurable levels of antibodies against groups A and C polysaccharides decrease significantly. This decrease in antibody occurs more rapidly in infants and younger children than in adults. Vaccine-induced clinical protection probably persists in school children and adults for at least 3 years.

meningococcal vaccine

An immunizing preparation that contains bacterial polysaccharides from certain types of meningococci. Meningococcal polysaccharide vaccines A, C, Y, and W-135 are available for preventing diseases induced by those serogroups. There is no vaccine for meningococcal serogroup B.

2-Mercaptoethanol agglutination test.

2-mercaptoethanol agglutination test

A simple test to determine whether an agglutinating antibody is of the immunoglobulin M (IgM) class. If treatment of an antibody preparation such as a serum sample with 2-mercaptoethanol can abolish the ability of the serum to agglutinate cells, then agglutination was due to IgM antibody. Agglutination induced by IgG antibody is unaffected by 2-mercaptoethanol treatment and is just as effective after the treatment as it was before. Dithiothreitol (DTT) produces the same effect as 2-mercaptoethanol in this test.

Structure of 6-mercaptopurine (6-MP).

6-mercaptopurine (6-MP)

A powerful immunosuppressive drug used prior to the introduction of cyclosporine in organ transplantation. It is also an effective chemotherapeutic agent for the treatment of acute leukemia of childhood and other neoplastic conditions. 6-MP is a purine analog in which a thiol group replaces the 6-hydroxyl group. Hypoxanthine–guanine phosphoribosyl transferase (HGPRT) transforms 6-MP to 6-thioinosine-5′-phosphate. This reaction product blocks various critical purine metabolic reactions. 6-MP is also incorporated into DNA as thioguanine.

mercury and immunity

Mercury does not have any known physiologic function in humans. This highly toxic metal affects enzyme function and calcium ion channels. It is especially toxic for the kidneys and the central nervous system and may affect

M

the reproductive system. It has been postulated to have a carcinogenic effect. Mercury is allergenic, affects immuno-globulin synthesis, and induces multispecific antibodies and autoimmune reactions. Mercuric chloride serves as a poly-clonal activator of both B and T lymphocytes. Mercury's immunological effects are under genetic influence.

mesangial phagocytes

Renal macrophages.

metaproterenol (dl-β-[3,5-dihydroxyphenyl]-α-isopropylamino-ethanol)

A β-adrenergic amine that induces smooth muscle relaxation, especially in the bronchi, and is used to treat asthma.

metastases

Secondary tumors that arise from daughter cells released by spread from a primary tumor to other anatomical sites.

metastasis

The transfer of disease from one organ or part to another not directly connected with it. For example, malignant tumors may seed anatomical sites distant from the site of origin of the primary tumor, leading to the establishment of secondary tumors.

metatype autoantibodies

Anti-immunoglobulin antibodies that recognize an anti-body-liganded active site but are not specific for the ligand or idiotype alone. Metatype antibody interactions with anti-metatype–metatype immunoglobulins serve as models for T cell receptor and antigen–MHC complex interactions that could be considered as metatype immunoglobulins and liganded antibody, respectively.

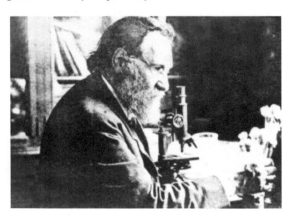

Elie (Ilya) Metchnikoff.

Metchnikoff, Elie (1845–1916)

Elie (Ilya) Metchnikoff (also spelled Mechnikov) was born in Avanovska, Ukraine. He showed an interest in natural sciences from childhood and completed his 4-year university studies in 2 years at the University of Kharkov, graduating in 1864. He received a Ph.D. degree at the University of Odessa. He studied with several researchers in Germany and Italy and began publishing original observations at

a young age. He returned to Russia in 1867 as professor of zoology and comparative anatomy at the University of Odessa. He was plagued with eye trouble and depression, and lost his young wife to tuberculosis despite his devoted efforts to save her life. His second marriage to a neighbor was happy and the world is indebted to her for writing his biography. Metchnikoff was not temperamentally suited to teaching and left to pursue private studies in Messina. He first studied phagocytes, examining the transparent larvae of starfish. He observed that cells surrounded and engulfed foreign particles introduced into the larvae. He also discovered that special amoeba-like cells surrounded bacteria introduced into starfish larvae and fungal spores introduced into water fleas (*Daphnia*) and engulfed them. He observed the digestive powers of the mesodermal cells in starfish larvae and connected the process with the cause of immunity against infectious disease. He returned to Odessa and continued studies of parasite infection of *Daphnia*, from which he built a theory of cellular immunity involving phagocytosis. He was appointed director of the Bacteriological Institute in Odessa. He was unhappy in that position and visited the Hygiene Institute of Robert Koch, who showed no interest in his research. When Metchnikoff visited Pasteur in Paris, he was invited to remain, and spent the rest of his life at Institut Pasteur. He found that many white blood cells or leukocytes are phagocytic, defending the body against acute infection by engulfing invading microorganisms. After discovering the role of phagocytes in host defense, he devoted much of his later career to elaborating and championing his cellular theory of immunity. He attracted a number of students including Jules Bordet and published many papers, a series of *Lectures on the Comparative Pathology of Inflammation* and a thorough and balanced review of the entire field of comparative and human immunity titled *L'immunité dans les maladies infectieuses*. He was a colorful and influential personality. He shared the Nobel Prize in Medicine or Physiology for 1908 with Paul Ehrlich for his work in immunology and made many more contributions to immunity and bacteriology. Metchnikoff became interested in longevity and aging in his later years, and advocated the consumption of yogurt. He believed that lactic acid-producing bacteria in the gut prolonged life span.

methotrexate (N-[p-{(2,4-diamino-6-pteridinyl-methyl) methylamino} benzoyl] glutamic acid)

A drug that blocks synthesis of DNA and thymidine in addition to its well known use as a chemotherapeutic agent against neoplasia. It blocks dihydrofolate reductase, the enzyme required for folic acid conversion to tetrahydrofolate. Methotrexate has been used to treat cancer, psoriasis, rheumatoid arthritis, polymyositis, Reiter's syndrome, graft-vs.-host disease, and steroid-dependent bronchial asthma. It inhibits both humoral and cell-mediated immune responses. Its major toxicity is hepatic fibrosis, which is dose-related. It may also produce hypersensitivity pneumonitis and

Structure of methotrexate.

megaloblastic anemia. It interferes with the binding of IL1β to its receptor and may function as an anticytokine.

methyl green pyronin stain

A stain used in histology or histopathology that renders DNA green and RNA red. It is widely used to demonstrate plasma cells and lymphoblasts that contain multiple ribosomes containing RNA in their cytoplasm.

metronidazole

The drug of choice to treat intestinal and extraintestinal amebiasis and neurogenital trichomoniasis and an alternative drug for the treatment of *Giardia lamblia*, *Balantidium coli*, and *Blastocystis hominis* infections.

MGSA (melanoma growth-stimulating activity)

MGSA is a chemokine of the α (CXC) family. It is a mitogenic polypeptide secreted by human melanoma cells. The MGSA/GRO-α gene product has powerful chemotactic, growth regulatory, and transforming functions. Its many tissue sources include monocytes, neutrophils, bronchoalveolar macrophages, and endothelial cells, among other cell types. Neutrophils, lymphocytes, monocytes, and epidermal melanocytes are target cells.

MGUS

Refer to monoclonal gammopathy of undetermined significance.

MHC

Abbreviation for major histocompatibility complex.

MHC-I antigen presentation

Proteins in the cytosol, such as those derived from viruses, may be processed through the class I MHC route of antigen presentation. The multiprotein complex in the cytoplasm known as the proteasome effect involves proteolytic degradation of proteins in the cytoplasm to yield many of the peptides presented by class I MHC molecules. TAP molecules transport peptides from the cytoplasm to the endoplasmic reticulum where they interact with and bind to class I MHC dimeric molecules. Once the class I MHC molecules have become stabilized through peptide binding, the complex leaves the endoplasmic reticulum, entering the Golgi apparatus en route to cell surfaces. Thus, mechanisms are provided through MHC-restricted antigen presentation to guarantee that peptides derived from extracellular microbial proteins can be presented by class II MHC molecules to CD4$^+$ helper T cells and that peptides derived from intracellular microbes can be presented by class I MHC molecules to CD8$^+$ cytotoxic T lymphocytes. The generation of microbial peptides produced through antigen processing to combine with self MHC molecules is critical to the development of an appropriate immune response.

MHC class I deficiency

A type of severe combined immunodeficiency in which MHC class I molecules are not expressed on lymphocyte membranes. The trait has an autosomal-recessive mode of inheritance.

MHC class I molecules

Major histocompatibility complex polymorphic glycoproteins that present cytosol-generated peptides to CD8$^+$ T lymphocytes. They are heterodimers comprised of a class I heavy chain associated with β$_2$ microglobulin.

MHC class IB molecules

Molecules encoded by the major histocompatibility complex that are less polymorphic than the MHC class I and class II molecules and which present a restricted set of antigens.

MHC class Ib and IIb

MHC proteins that are nonclassical and have restricted polymorphism. The majority do not participate in antigen presentation. Genes at the Q, T, and M loci in mice and genes at the HLA-X, -E, -J, -G and -F and HFE loci in humans encode class Ib proteins. Murine P locus genes and human DM and DO loci genes encode class IIb proteins.

MHC class I proteins

Heterodimeric proteins on cell surfaces comprised of a polymorphic transmembrane MHC class Iα chain noncovalently united with an invariant β$_2$ microglobulin (β$_{2m}$) chain. Murine genes in the K and D loci and human genes in the HLA-A, -B, and -C loci encode the MHC class I α chain, whereas the β$_{2m}$ is encoded independent of the MHC. These molecules unite with 8 to 10 endogenous amino acid peptides that they present to CD4$^+$ T cells. Nearly all nucleated cells of the body express them.

MHC class II molecules

Major histocompatibility complex molecules that present peptides formed in intracellular vesicles to CD4$^+$ T cells. Structurally they are heterodimers of class IIα and class IIβ chains.

MHC class II compartment (MIIC)

A cellular site where MHC class II molecules concentrate, interact with HLA-DM, and bind antigenic peptides prior to migrating to the cell surface.

MHC class II deficiency

A type of combined immunodeficiency in which lymphocytes and monocytes fail to express MHC class II molecules on their surfaces. The cells also have diminished expression of MHC class I antigens. The condition, which appears principally in North African children, has an autosomal-recessive mode of inheritance. Patients are able to synthesize the class I invariant chain β$_2$ microglobulin. Whereas the numbers of B cells and T lymphocytes in the circulating blood are normal, patients have agammaglobulinemia and diminished cell-mediated immunity. Malabsorption in the gastrointestinal tract and diarrhea are commonly associated with this deficiency.

MHC class II proteins

Heterodimeric proteins on cell surfaces comprised of polymorphic MHC class IIα and class IIβ chains. Genes at the A and E murine loci and by DP, DQ, and DR loci genes in humans encode the α and β chains. These proteins unite with 13 to 18 exogenous amino acid peptides that are then presented to CD4$^+$ T cells. Antigen-presenting cells express them.

MHC class II region

Region composed of three subregions designated DR, DQ, and DP. Multiple genetic loci are present in each subregion. DN (previously DZ) and DO subregions are composed of a single genetic locus. Each class II HLA molecule includes one α chain and one β chain that constitute a heterodimer. Genes within each subregion encode the α and β chains of a particular class II molecule. Class II genes that encode α chains are designated A; class II genes that encode β chains are designated B. A number is used following A or B if a particular subregion contains two or more A or B genes.

MHC class II transactivator (CIITA)

A protein that activates major histocompatibility complex (MHC) class II gene transcription. The gene that encodes this molecule is one of several defective genes in bare

M

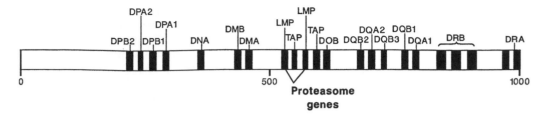

Major histocompatibility complex (MHC) class II.

lymphocyte syndrome, which is characterized by a lack of MHC class II molecules on all cells.

MHC class III proteins

Murine S region genes and human MHC class III region genes that encode these numerous proteins that participate in immune response functions comprise this group that includes complement; heat shock proteins; TNF; and LT.

MHC congenic mice

Mice that differ only at the major histocompatibility complex.

MHC disease associations

Refer to HLA disease association.

MHC functions

Major histocompatibility complex class I molecules were originally identified as strong histocompatibility antigens. MHC class II glycoproteins were first described as immune response (Ir) gene products. MHC class I and class II molecules have a central immunological function of focusing CD8+ and CD4+ T lymphocytes, respectively, to the surfaces of appropriate lymphocytes. The principal role of MHC in immunity is to alert T cells to alterations in the surface integrity of other cells so that they may be dealt with in a manner appropriate for maintenance of the interior milieu. MHC class I and class II molecules define self to the immune system. They represent a self surveillance complex.

MHC-like proteins

Molecules with a structural and functional resemblance to MHC proteins that are nonpolymorphic, including CD1 molecules, and are encoded independent of the MHC region.

MHC genes

Major histocompatibility complex genes. Genes that encode the major (as opposed to minor) histocompatibility antigens expressed on cell membranes. MHC genes in mice are located at the H-2 locus on chromosome 17, whereas the MHC genes in humans are located at the HLA locus on the short arm of chromosome 6.

MHC haplotype

The set of genes in a haploid genome inherited from one parent. Children of parents designated ab and cd will probably be ac, ad, bc, or bd haplotypes.

MHC molecules

Major histocompatibility complex (MHC)-encoded glycoproteins that are highly polymorphic. They complex

with immunogenic peptides for antigen presentation to T lymphocytes. The two classes are designated MHC class I and MHC class II, each of which has a different role in the immune response. Also termed major histocompatibility antigens, they serve as the principal alloantigens that are the targets of rejection in tissue and organ transplantation.

MHC mutant mice

Mice that are mutant at one or more loci.

MHC peptide-binding specificity

The highly polymorphic membrane glycoprotein major histocompatibility complex (MHC) molecules bind peptide fragments of proteins and display them for recognition by T lymphocytes. Their *raison d'etre* is to present self antigens in the thymus for tolerance induction and foreign antigens in the periphery for immune responsiveness. The organism distinguishes self from nonself through MHC peptide recognition by T cells.

MHC–peptide tetramers

A molecular complex fastened together by fluorescent streptavidin which possesses four binding sites for biotin. The complex is attached to the tail of the MHC molecule. This makes its possible to stain specific T lymphocytes in any species.

MHC recombinant mice

Mice that have crossovers within the MHC.

MHC restriction

The recognition of antigen in the context of class I or class II molecules by the T cell receptor for antigen. In the afferent limb of the immune response, the presentation of antigen at the surface of a macrophage, dendritic cell, or other antigen-presenting cell to CD4+ T lymphocytes must be in the context of MHC class II molecules for the CD4+ lymphocyte to recognize the antigen and proliferate in response to it. By contrast, cytotoxic (CD8+) T lymphocytes recognize foreign antigens such as viral antigens on infected target cells only in the context of class I MHC molecules. Once this recognition system is in place, the cytotoxic T cell can fatally injure the target cell through release of perforin and granzyme molecules that penetrate the target cell surfaces. T cells recognize a firm peptide antigen only in the context of a specific allelic form of an MHC molecule to which it is bound.

Major histocompatibility complex (MHC) class II.

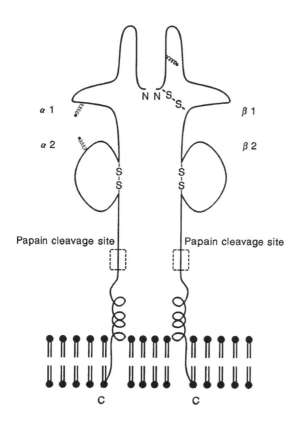

Class II MHC molecules are glycoprotein histocompatibility antigens that play a critical role in immune system cellular interactions. Each class II MHC molecule is comprised of a 32- to 34-kDa α chain and a 29- to 32-kDa β chain, each of which possesses N-linked oligosaccharide groups, amino termini that are extracellular, and carboxyl termini that are intracellular. Approximately 70% of both α and β chains are extracellular.

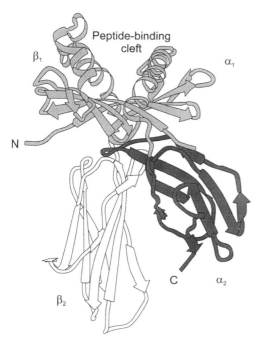

Major histocompatibility complex (MHC) class II molecular structure.

MHD

Minimal hemolytic dose; the amount of complement used in a complement fixation test. MHD is also an abbreviation for minimal hemagglutinating dose of a virus, as in a hemagglutination inhibition test.

MICA, MICB

Human MHC class I chain-related genes located within the HLA class I region of chromosome 6 encode MHC class I chain-related A and B. MIC proteins are markers of "stress" in the epithelia, and act as ligands for cells expressing a common activatory NK cell receptor (NKG2D). Heat or other environmental stress, virus infection, or tumor regenesis may lead to upregulation of these human stress ligands. These molecules combine with the NK activatory receptor, NKG2D, and to VγlVδ1 T cell receptors. In mice, the corresponding Rae-1 and H60 molecules also combine with NKG2D. Refer to NK activatory receptors and γδ T cell receptors.

MIC molecules

Major histocompatibility complex (MHC) class-I-like molecules expressed in the gastrointestinal tract during stress. Genes within the class I region of the human MHC encode these molecules.

microchimerism

The establishment in a transplant recipient of passenger donor hematopoietic cells that accompanied the solid organ transplant.

microenvironment

An organized local interaction among cells that provides an interactive, dynamic, structural, or functional compartmentalization. The microenvironment may facilitate or regulate cell and molecular interactions through biologically active molecules. Microenvironments may exert their influence at the organ, tissue, cellular, or molecular levels. In the immune system, they include the thymic cortex and the thymic medulla, which are distinct; a microenvironment of lymphoid nodules; and a microenvironment of B cells in a lymphoid follicle, among others.

microfilaments

Cellular organelles that comprise a network of fibers of about 60 Å in diameter present beneath the membranes of round cells, occupying protrusions of the cells, or extending down microprojections such as microvilli. They are found as highly organized and prominent bundles of filaments concentrated in regions of surface activity during motile processes or endocytosis. Microfilaments consist mainly of actin, a globular 42-kDa protein. In media of appropriate ionic strength, actin polymerizes in a double array to form the microfilaments that are critical for cell movement, phagocytosis, fusion of phagosomes and lysosomes, and other important functions of cells belonging to the immune and other systems.

microfold cells

Refer to M cells.

microglia

Non-neural brain cells derived from a macrophage-like precursor. They are migratory and have phagocytic function.

microglial cell

Phagocytic cell in the central nervous system that is a bone marrow-derived perivascular cell of the mononuclear phagocyte system. In the central nervous system, it may act as an antigen-presenting cell, functioning in a major histocompatibility complex (MHC) class-II-restricted manner.

microglobulin

Refer to β2 microglobulin. A globulin molecule or its fragment with a molecular weight of 40 kDa or less.

Short Arm of Chromosome 6

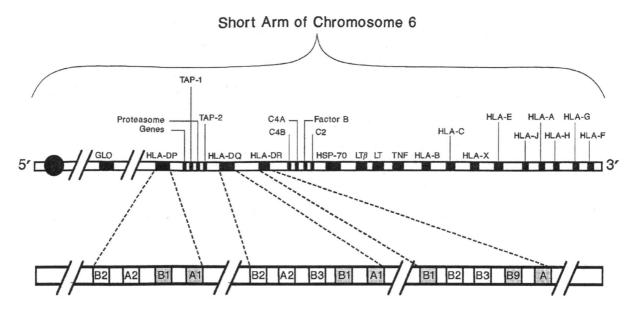

Major histocompatibility complex (MHC) genes encode the major histocompatibility antigens that are expressed on cell membranes. MHC genes in the mouse are located at the H-2 locus on chromosome 17, and MHC genes in humans are located at the HLA locus on the short arm of chromosome 6.

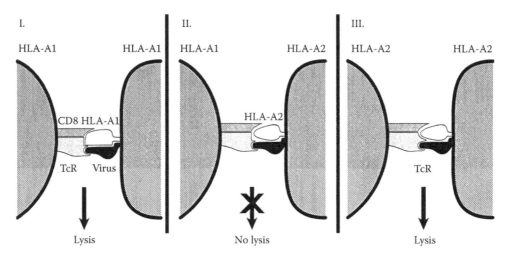

Major histocompatibility (MHC) restriction.

Bence–Jones proteins in the serum or urine are examples. β_2 microglobulin that is a constituent of major histocompatibility complex (MHC) class I molecules is another example.

microinjection

A technique for introducing a solution of DNA into a pronuclear cell or blastocyst using a fine microcapillary pipet.

microlymphocytotoxicity

A widely used technique for human leukocyte antigen (HLA) tissue typing. Lymphocytes are separated from heparinized blood samples by layering over Ficoll-Hypaque, centrifuging and removing lymphocytes from the interface or by using beads. After appropriate washing, these purified lymphocyte preparations are counted, and aliquots are dispensed into microtiter plate wells containing predispensed quantities of antibody. When used for human histocompatibility HLA testing, antisera in the wells are specific for known HLA antigenic specificities. After incubation of the cells and antisera, rabbit complement is added, and the plates are again incubated. The extent of cytotoxicity induced is determined by incubating the cells with Trypan blue, which enters dead cells and stains them blue, while leaving live cells unstained. The plates are read with an inverted phase contrast microscope. A scoring system from 0 to 8 (8 implies >80% of target cells killed) indicates cytotoxicity. Most of the sera used to date are multispecific because they were obtained from multiparous females who were sensitized during pregnancy by HLA antigens determined by their spouses. Monoclonal antibodies are used with increasing frequency in tissue typing. This technique is useful to identify HLA-A, HLA-B, and HLA-C antigens. When purified B cell preparations and specific antibodies against B cell antigens are employed, HLA-DR and HLA-DQ antigens can be identified.

microorganisms

Microscopic life forms that are mostly unicellular, with the exception of selected fungi. The term may apply to bacteria, yeast and other fungi, and protozoa, all of which have been implicated in human diseases.

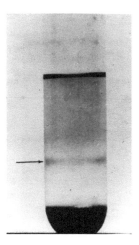

The separation of lymphocytes from peripheral blood by centrifugation using Ficoll-Hypaque.

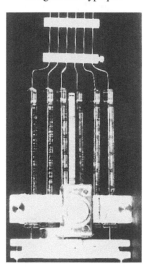

A Hamilton syringe that is used to dispense lymphocytes into Terasaki plates for tissue typing.

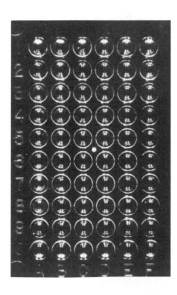

A Terasaki plate consisting of depressions in a plastic plate that contains pre-dispensed antibodies to HLA antigens of various specificities and into which are placed patient lymphocytes and rabbit complement for tissue typing.

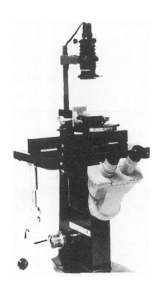

An inverted light microscope used to read Terasaki plates to determine tissue type.

microtiter technique

Refer to Takatsy method.

microtubules

These organelles are hollow, cylindrical fibers about 240 Å in diameter, radiating from the centers of eukaryotic cells, including lymphocytes, phagocytes, and mast cells, in all directions toward plasma membranes. Mitotic spindles are composed of microtubules. They form a sturdy cytoskeleton. They originate from centrioles, structures occupying the concavities of nuclei. Microtubules provide orientation of gross membrane activities, associate directly or indirectly with granules to enable their contact and fusion with endocytic vesicles, and direct reorganization of cell membranes. Although not critical for the cell movement of chemotaxis, they are needed for "fine tuning" of cell locomotion. Their major component is tubulin, a dimeric protein.

mid-piece (historical)

A term used by investigators in the early 1900s to refer to components of complement present in the serum euglobulin fraction that actually contains the entire C1 and selected other complement components, but no C2 component.

Miescher, Peter (1923–)

Swiss physician, authority on autoimmune diseases, and prolific author of research articles about them.

MIF

Macrophage–monocyte migration inhibitory factor. A substance synthesized by T lymphocytes in response to immunogenic challenge that inhibits the migration of macrophages. MIF is a 25-kDa lymphokine. Its mechanism of action is by elevating intracellular cAMP, polymerizing microtubules, and stopping macrophage migration. MIF may increase the adhesive properties of macrophages, thereby inhibiting their migration. The two types of protein MIF include one of 65 kDa with a pI of 3 to 4 and another of 25 kDa with a pI of approximately 5.

mIg

Abbreviation for membrane-bound immunoglobulin.

MIG

Monokine induced by interferon-γ (IFN-γ) is a chemokine of the α (CXC) family. It is derived from a cDNA library from

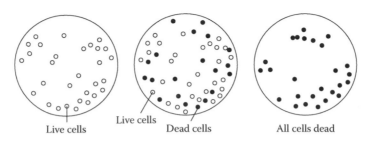

Microlymphocytotoxicity.

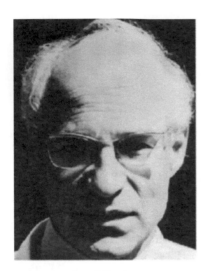

Peter Miescher.

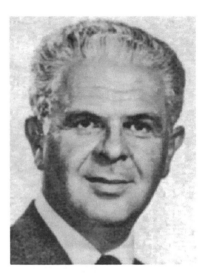

Felix Milgrom.

lymphokine-activated macrophages. IFN-γ can induce macrophages to express the *MIG* gene. Tissue sources include lymphokine-activated macrophages, IFN-γ-treated human peripheral blood monocytes, and IFN-γ-treated human monocytic cell line THP-1. Target cells include human tumor-infiltrating lymphocytes (TILs) and monocytes.

MiHA

Refer to minor histocompatibility antigens.

MIICs

MHC class compartments or class II vesicles. These specialized late endosomal spaces comprise a segment of the exogenous (endocytic) antigen processing pathway. Endolysosomal MHC-CLIP complexes enter MIICs where CLIP exchange and peptide loading occur.

Mikulicz's syndrome

Lymphocytic inflammation in the parotid gland. This condition represents a type of Sjögren's syndrome.

Milgrom, Felix (1919–2007)

Polish-American investigator who worked at the University of Buffalo in New York State. He and Ernest Witebsky described anti-immunoglobulin antibodies. They immunized rabbits with aggregated autologous globulin and discovered that the rabbits produced antibodies with greater reactivity for human globulin than for rabbit globulin.

Miller, J.F.A.P. (1931–)

Proved the role of the thymus in immunity while investigating Gross' leukemia in neonatal mice.

Miller–Fisher syndrome (MFS)

A variant of Guillain–Barré syndrome (GBS) that has a subacute onset and follows infectious illnesses of which

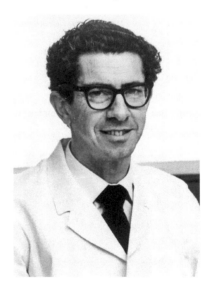

J.F.A.P. Miller.

Campylobacter jejuni infection is the most common. Fewer than 5% of GBS cases have MFS. Clinically, MFS presents as ophthalmoplegia, ataxia, and areflexia. The extremity and trunk muscles exhibit little or no weakness. The spinal fluid protein is seldom increased, and nerve conduction studies are usually normal. Most MFS patients have circulating polyclonal antibodies to GQb1 ganglioside, a minor ganglioside component of both the central and peripheral nervous systems. These antibodies are highest initially and fall with recovery.

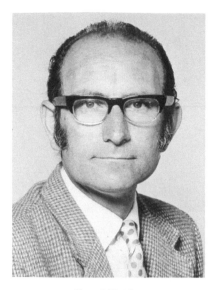

Cesar Milstein.

Milstein, Cesar (1927–)
Argentinian-born immunologist who worked in the United Kingdom. He shared the 1984 Nobel Prize with G.F. Köhler for their production of monoclonal antibodies by hybridizing mutant myeloma cells with antibody-producing B cells (hybridoma technique). Their method revolutionized immunological research.

minimal hemagglutinating dose (MHD)
In the hemagglutination inhibition test for antiviral antibodies, the MHD is the least amount of hemagglutinating virus that will completely agglutinate the red cells in a single volume of a standard suspension.

minimal hemolytic dose (MHD)
The smallest amount of complement that can completely lyse a defined volume of a standardized suspension of red blood cells sensitized with antibody.

minimum lethal dose (MLD)
The dose of a substance or agent that kills 100% of the population tested.

mini pigs
A strain of diminutive pigs designed specifically to serve as organ and tissue donors for human xenografts. Their organ sizes are equivalent to those of humans.

minisatellite
DNA regions comprised of tandem repeats of DNA short sequences.

minor blood group antigens
Non-ABO erythrocyte antigens, such as Duffy, Kell, and Kidd groups. Delayed mild transfusion reactions may occur in subjects alloimmunized against these antigens.

minor H peptides
Donor minor histocompatibility antigen peptides that antigen-presenting cells display to recipient T cells.

minor histocompatibility antigens (MiHAs)
Molecules expressed on cell surfaces that are encoded by minor histocompatibility loci, not the major locus. They represent weak transplantation antigens by comparison with the major histocompatibility antigens, but they are multiple and their cumulative effect may contribute considerably to organ or tissue graft rejection. Graft rejection based on a minor histocompatibility difference between donor and recipient requires several weeks compared to the 7 to 10 days required for a major histocompatibility difference. Minor histocompatibility antigens may be difficult to identify by serological methods. The epitopes occur in a small number of different allelic forms in the population. Allogeneic MiHA donor peptides are recognized as nonself by recipient T cells in a transplant situation.

minor histocompatibility locus
A chromosomal site of genes encoding minor histocompatibility antigens that stimulate immune responses against grafts containing these antigens.

minor histocompatibility peptides
H antigens. Among minor antigens thus far identified are H-3 antigens, male-specific H-Y antigen, β_2 microglobulin, and others that have not yet been firmly established.

minor lymphocyte-stimulating (Mls) determinants
Characterized by their activation of a marked primary mixed lymphocyte reaction (MLR) between lymphocytes of mice sharing an identical major histocompatibility complex (MHC) haplotype. MHC class II molecules on various cell surfaces present Mls epitopes to naïve T lymphocytes that mount a significant response. V–β-specific monoclonal antibodies have facilitated the definition of Mls epitopes. Mls determinants activate T lymphocytes expressing selected β specificities. Refer also to Mls antigens.

minor lymphocyte-stimulating genes
See *Mls* genes.

minor lymphocyte-stimulating (Mls) loci
Refer to Mls antigens.

minor transplantation antigens
Refer to minor histocompatibility antigens.

MIP-1 (macrophage inflammatory protein 1)
See macrophage inflammatory protein.

MIP-1α (macrophage inflammatory protein 1α)
A chemokine of the β (CC) family. It exhibits a broad spectrum of biological activities that include prostaglandin-independent pyrogenic activity, possible participation in wound healing, monocyte chemotaxis, and suppression of immature bone marrow stem and progenitor cells. Significantly, MIP-1α has an HIV-suppressive effect. Tissue sources include fibroblasts, monocytes, lymphocytes, neutrophils, eosinophils, smooth muscle cells, mast cells, platelets, and bone marrow stromal cells, among other cell types. T lymphocytes, basophils, hematopoietic precursor cells, monocytes, eosinophils, neutrophils, mast cells, natural killer (NK) cells, and dendritic cells, among many other types, are target cells.

MIP-1α receptor
A seven-membrane-spanning structure. There is 32% homology between the receptor for MIP-1α and those for IL8. A calcium flux occurs when MIP-1α binds to its receptor. Murine T cells, macrophages, and eosinophils have been shown to express a receptor for MIP-1α. The human MIP-1α receptor has one potential *N*-linked glycosylation site. The gene for the MIP-1α receptors in humans is found on chromosome 3p21.

MIP-1β (macrophage inflammatory protein 1β)
A chemokine of the β (CC) family, sharing 70% homology with MIP-1α. Although both molecules resemble one another structurally, they differ significantly in function. Unlike MIP-1α, MIP-1β does not activate neutrophils. Unlike MIP-1α, which inhibits early hematopoietic progenitor growth, MIP-1β potentiates it. Both MIP-1α and

M

MIP-1β exert synergistic HIV-suppressive effects. Tissue sources include monocytes, fibroblasts, T lymphocytes, B lymphocytes, neutrophils, smooth muscle cells, mast cells, and selected tumor cell lines. Monocytes, T lymphocytes, hematopoietic precursor cells, and basophils are target cells.

MIP-2 (macrophage inflammatory protein 2)

A chemokine of the α (CXC) family. The MIP-2 class is comprised of MIP-2α, also termed GRO-β gene product, and MIP-2β, the GRO-γ gene product. MIP-2 has a role in anti-GBM antibody-induced glomerulonephritis in mice. Anti-MIP-2 antibody injection 30 minutes before anti-GBM antibody effectively decreases neutrophil influx and PAS-positive deposits containing fibrin. Tissue sources include mast cells, cardiac myocytes, mesangial cells, alveolar macrophages, epidermal cells, human nasal, and bronchial epithelium. Neutrophils, basophils, and epithelial cells are the target cells.

MIRL (membrane inhibitor of reactive lysis)

Inhibitor of membrane attack complexes on self tissue. Also known as CD59.

missing self hypothesis

The hypothesis that interaction of NK cells with cells failing to express self MHC class I antigens on their surfaces leads to T cell activation. Examples include neoplastic cells; virus-infected cells; and allogeneic cells.

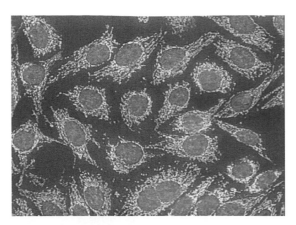

Mitochondrial autoantibodies.

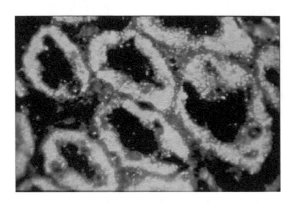

Mitochondrial antibody (mouse kidney, 500× magnification).

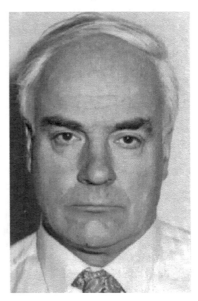

N.A. Mitcheson.

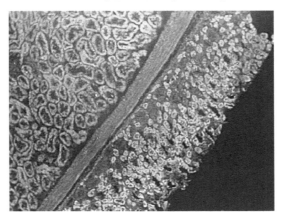

Mitochondrial autoantibodies (mouse kidney and stomach).

Mitcheson, N.A. (1928–)

British investigator who demonstrated the role of helper T cells in immunoregulation.

mitochondria

Cytoplasmic organelles in aerobic eukaryotic cells where respiration, electron transport, oxidative phosphorylation, and citric acid cycle reactions occur. Mitochondria possess DNA and ribosomes.

mitochondrial antibodies

Immunoglobulin G (IgG) antibodies present in 90 to 95% of primary biliary cirrhosis (PBC) patients. These antibodies, which are of doubtful pathogenic significance, are specific for the pyruvate dehydrogenase enzyme complex E2 component situated at the inner mitochondrial membrane (M2). They are also specific for another E2-associated protein. Other antimitochondrial antibodies include the M1

antibodies of syphilis, the M3 antibodies found in pseudo-lupus, the M5 antibodies in collagen diseases, the M6 antibodies in hepatitis induced by iproniazid, the M7 antibodies associated with myocarditis and cardiomyopathy, the M8 antibodies that may be markers for prognosis, and the M9 antibodies that serve as markers for beginning primary biliary cirrhosis. Mitochondrial antibody titer may be an indicator of primary biliary cirrhosis progression. A patient with a titer of 1 to 40 or more should be suspected of having primary biliary cirrhosis, whether symptoms are present or absent and even if alkaline phosphatase is normal.

mitochondrial autoantibodies (MAs)

Immunoglobulin G (IgG) autoantibodies specific for the E2 component (lipoate acetytransferase) of the pyruvate dehydrogenase enzyme complex located at the inner mitochondrial membrane (M2) as well as against another protein in E2 preparations. They are present in 90 to 95% of patients with primary biliary cirrhosis (PBC); however, they are not believed to be pathogenic. MAs that do not react with M2 are found in other conditions, such as M1 autoantibodies in syphilis, M3 autoantibodies in pseudolupus, M5 autoantibodies in poorly defined collagen diseases, M6 autoantibodies in iproniazid-induced hepatitis, M7 autoantibodies in cardiomyopathy and myocarditis, and M8 autoantibodies that serve as indicators of early PBC. The titer of MAs in PBC correlates with disease progression; a titer of 1 to 40 or greater suggests PBC in the absence of symptoms and in the presence of a normal alkaline phosphatase. Nuclear autoantibody (ANA) patterns in PBC include (1) multiple nuclear dots ANA (MND–ANA) present in 10 to 15% of PBC and mainly associated with sicca syndrome; and (2) membrane-associated ANA (MANA) present in 25 to 50% of PBC.

mitogen

A substance often derived from plants that nonspecifically stimulates DNA synthesis and induces blast transformation and cell division by mitosis. The mitogen-binding sites on lymphocytes are distinct from the antigen-binding sites of B cell receptors and T cell receptors. Lectins, representing plant-derived mitogens or phytomitogens, have been widely used in both experimental and clinical immunology to evaluate T and B lymphocyte function *in vitro*. Phytohemagglutinin (PHA) is principally a human and mouse T cell mitogen, as is concanavalin A (con A). By contrast, lipopolysaccharide (LPS) induces B lymphocyte transformation in mice, but not in humans. Staphylococcal protein A is the mitogen used to induce human B lymphocyte transformation. Pokeweed mitogen (PWM) transforms B cells of both humans and mice, as well as their T cells.

mitogen-activated protein (MAP) kinase cascade

Enzymes that become phosphorylated and activated when cells are stimulated by various ligands, leading to new gene expression by phosphorylating critical transcription factors. The inactive form of the Ras protein initiates this signal transduction cascade that includes sequential activation of three serine/threonine kinases, including MAP kinase, which phosphorylates and activates other enzymes or transcription factors. When antigen binds to the T cell receptor, MAP kinase pathway is one of the signal pathways activated.

mitogen-activated protein (MAP) kinases

Kinases that become phosphorylated and activated following cell stimulation by various ligands and induce new gene expression by phosphorylating key transcription factors.

mitogenic factor

A substance that induces cell division and proliferation of cells, such as phytohemagglutinin (PHA), which induces proliferation of lymphocytes. Many substances may serve as mitogenic factors.

mitotic spindle apparatus autoantibodies

Antibodies present in the sera of individuals with various autoimmune diseases that include rheumatoid arthritis, Sjögren's syndrome, Hashimoto's thyroiditis, and localized scleroderma, respiratory infection, dilated cardiomyopathy, and melanoma. The clinical usefulness of autoantibodies to the mitotic spindle apparatus protein is unknown.

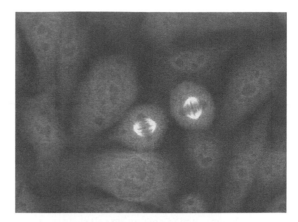

Mitotic spindle apparatus autoantibodies.

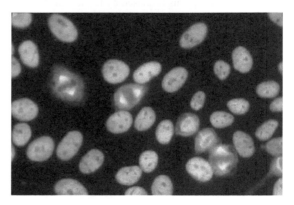

Mitotic spindle apparatus autoantibodies.

Mitsuda reaction

A graduated response to an intracutaneous inoculation of lepromin, a substance used in the lepromin test. A nodule representing a subcutaneous granulomatous reaction to lepromin occurs 2 to 4 weeks after inoculation and is maximal at 4 weeks; it indicates granulomatous sensitization in a leprosy patient. Although not a diagnostic test, it can distinguish tuberculoid from lepromatous leprosy in that this test is positive in tuberculoid leprosy and in normal adult controls but negative in lepromatous leprosy patients.

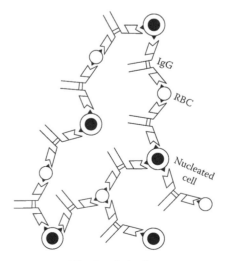

Mixed agglutination.

mixed agglutination

Aggregation (agglutination) produced when morphologically dissimilar cells that share a common antigen are reacted with antibody specific for this epitope. The technique is useful in demonstrating antigens on cells that by virtue of their size or irregular shape are not suitable for study by conventional agglutination tests. It is convenient to use an indicator, such as a red cell, that possesses the antigen sought. Thus, the demonstration of mixed agglutination in which the indicator cells are linked to the other cell type suspected of possessing the common antigen constitutes a positive test.

mixed antiglobulin reaction

A test to demonstrate antibodies adsorbed to cell surfaces. The addition of antiglobulin-coated red cells to a suspension of cells suspected of containing cell surface antibodies results in formation of erythrocyte–test cell aggregates if the test is positive. This is caused by linkage of the antiglobulin to the immunoglobulin on the surfaces of test cells.

mixed chimerism

In a non-myeloablative conditioned hematopoietic cell transplant recipient who has received a donor cell infusion, the recipient's surviving hematopoietic stem cells coexist with donor hematopoietic stem cells and yield cells of the myeloid and lymphoid lineages.

mixed connective tissue disease (MCTD)

A connective tissue disease that shares characteristics in common with systemic lupus erythematosus (SLE), rheumatoid arthritis (RA), and dermatomyositis. Under immunofluorescence, a speckled nuclear pattern attributable to antinuclear antibody in the circulation is revealed. The titers of antinuclear antibodies specific for nuclear ribonucleoproteins are high. Treatment with corticosteroids is very effective. Also called Sharp syndrome or overlap syndrome.

mixed hemadsorption

The demonstration of antiviral antibody by the mixed antiglobulin reaction.

mixed leukocyte reaction (MLR)

Refer to mixed lymphocyte reaction.

mixed lymphocyte culture (MLC)

The combination of lymphocytes from two members of a species in culture where they are maintained and incubated for 3 to 5 days. Lymphoblasts are formed as a consequence

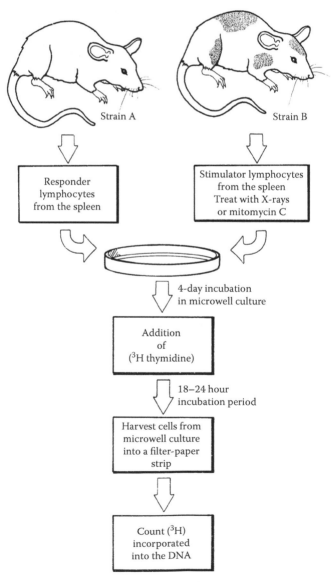

Mixed lymphocyte reaction (MLR).

of histoincompatibility between the two individuals donating the lymphocytes. The lymphocyte antigens of these genetically dissimilar subjects stimulate DNA synthesis by each other which is measured by tritiated thymidine uptake assayed in a scintillation counter. Refer to mixed lymphocyte reaction (MLR).

mixed lymphocyte reaction (MLR)

Lymphocytes from a potential donor and recipient are combined in tissue culture. Each of these lymphoid cells has the ability to respond by proliferating following stimulation by antigens of the other cells. In the one-way reaction, the donor cells are treated with mitomycin or irradiation to render them incapable of proliferation. Thus, the donor antigens stimulate the untreated responder cells. Antigenic specificities of the stimulator cells absent in the responder cells lead to blastogenesis of the responder lymphocytes and a subsequent increase in the synthesis of DNA and cell division. This process is followed by introduction of a measured amount of tritiated thymidine, which is incorporated into the newly synthesized DNA. In the two-way MLR, lymphoid cells from two individuals are incubated together and total proliferation is measured. The mixed lymphocyte reaction usually measures a proliferative response and not an effector cell killing response. The test is important in bone marrow and organ transplantation to evaluate the degree of histoincompatibility between donor and recipient. Both CD4+ and Cd8+ T lymphocytes proliferate and secrete cytokines in the MLR. Also called mixed lymphocyte culture.

mixed vaccine

A preparation intended for protective immunization that contains antigens of more than one pathogenic microorganism. Thus, it induces immunity against those disease agents whose antigens are represented in the vaccine. It may also be called a polyvalent vaccine.

MK-571

A powerful synthetic antagonist of leukotriene D_4 receptor that prevents bronchoconstriction induced by exercise in patients with asthma.

MLC

Acronym for mixed lymphocyte culture.

MLD (minimum lethal dose)

That dose of a substance or agent that will kill 100% of the population tested. Ehrlich defined MLD as the least amount of a toxin that will kill a 250-g guinea pig within 4 days after subcutaneous injection.

MLNS (mucocutaneous lymph node syndrome)

Refer to Kawasaki's disease.

Mls antigens

Minor lymphocyte-stimulating antigens; cell surface molecules originally observed on mouse cells that stimulate previously unsensitized T lymphocytes. They occur in two stimulatory forms designated Mls*a* and Mls*c*. The Vβ chain of the T cell receptor is encoded by the *Mls* genes. The anti-Mls response is linked to T lymphocyte receptor Vβ expression. The anti-Mls responses also link to intrathymic contact of CD8+ T lymphocytes and are critical in the induction of immunologic tolerance. As the immune system matures, clones of autoreactive T lymphocytes expressing the T cell receptor Vβ chain are deleted.

***Mls* genes**

Minor lymphocyte-stimulating genes. Mouse mammary tumor retroviruses code for *Mls* genes. The proteins formed

serve as superantigens that are powerful inducers of CD4+ T lymphocyte proliferation in mixed lymphocyte cultures.

M macroglobulin

An IgM paraprotein that occurs in Waldenström's macroglobulinemia.

MMR vaccine

Measles–mumps–rubella vaccine. A live attenuated virus vaccine given at 15 months of age or earlier. A booster injection is given later. The vaccine is effective in stimulating protective immunity in most cases. It may prove ineffective in children younger than 15 months of age if they still have transferred antibodies from their mothers. This vaccine should not be given to pregnant women, immunodeficient individuals undergoing immunosuppressive therapy, or patients with acute febrile disease.

MNS Blood Group System

Reactions		Phenotype Frequency		
Anti-M	Anti-N	Phenotype	Caucasian	African American
+	0	M+N–	28	26
+	+	M+N+	50	45
0	+	M–N+	22	30
Anti-s	Anti-s			
+	0	S+s–	11	3
+	+	S+s+	43	28
0	+	S–s+	45	69
0	0	S–s–	0	<1

MNS blood group system

Human erythrocyte glycophorin epitopes. The four distinct sialoglycoproteins (SGPs) on red cell membranes include α-SGP (glycophorin A, MN), β-SGP (glycophorin C), γ-SGP (glycophorin D), and δ-SGP (glycophorin B). MN antigens are present on α-SGP and δ-SGP. M and N antigens are present on α-SGP, with approximately 500,000 copies detectable on each erythrocyte. This is a 31-kDa structure composed of 131 amino acids, with about 60% of the total weight attributable to carbohydrate. This transmembrane molecule has a carboxyl terminus that stretches into the cytoplasm of the erythrocyte with a 23-amino acid hydrophobic segment embedded in the lipid bilayer. The amino terminal segment extends to the extracellular compartment. Blood group antigen activity is in the external segment. In α-SGP with M antigen activity, the first amino acid is serine and the fifth is glycine. When it carries N antigen activity, leucine and glutamic acid replace serine and glycine at positions 1 and 5, respectively. The Ss antigens are encoded by allelic genes at a locus closely linked to the MN locus. The U antigen is also considered a part of the MNSs system. Whereas anti-M and anti-N antibodies may occur without red cell stimulation, antibodies against Ss and U antigens generally follow erythrocyte stimulation. The MN and Ss alleles positioned on chromosome 4 are linked. Antigens of the MNSs system may provoke the formation of antibodies that can mediate hemolytic disease of the newborn.

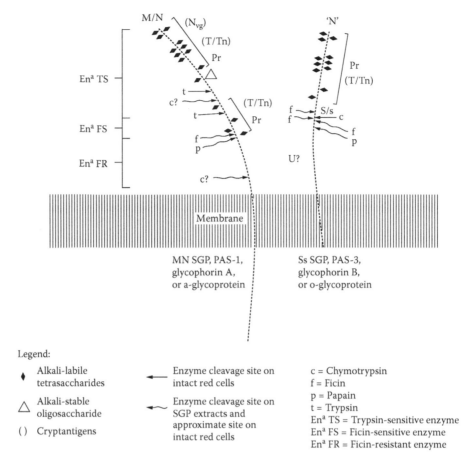

Legend:

♦	Alkali-labile tetrasaccharides	← Enzyme cleavage site on intact red cells
△	Alkali-stable oligosaccharide	↜ Enzyme cleavage site on SGP extracts and approximate site on intact red cells
( )	Cryptantigens	

c = Chymotrypsin
f = Ficin
p = Papain
t = Trypsin
En^a TS = Trypsin-sensitive enzyme
En^a FS = Ficin-sensitive enzyme
En^a FR = Ficin-resistant enzyme

Membrane glycoproteins and glycosphingolipids that carry blood group antigens.

Mo1

An adhesive glycoprotein present on neutrophils and monocytes. It is also called Leu-CAM, which is an iC3b receptor and thus helps mediate monocyte functions that are complement-dependent.

modulated dendritic cell

A dendritic cell (DC) that induces anergy rather than activation of naïve T cells, and/or propagation of T_{reg} cells. Interaction of DCs with T suppressor cells *in vitro* or culture in the presence of low GM-CSF, high IL10 or TGF-β, or the presence of aspirin, corticosteroids, or cyclosporine A that interferes with NF-κβ signaling may lead to modulation. Referred to also as a tolerized or tolerogenic DC.

modulation

Refer to antigenic modulation.

mofetumomab

A mouse monoclonal antibody labeled with ^{99m}Tc used as a diagnostic aid to ascertain the extent of disease and stage of patients with small cell lung cancers. It unites with 40-kD antigen present on numerous tumor cell types and also on selected normal cells.

moesin

During chemokine-induced lymphocyte polarization, the moesin cytoskeletal protein is important for the redistribution of adhesion molecules to the cellular uropod.

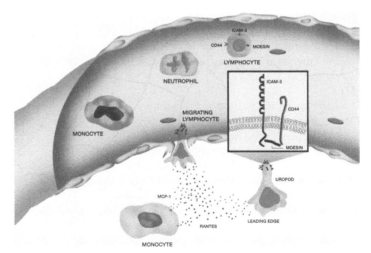

Moesin.

molecular (DNA) typing (sequence-specific priming or SSP)

A method that employs a primer with a single mismatch in the 3′ end that cannot be employed efficiently to extend a DNA strand because the enzyme Taq polymerase, during the PCR reaction, and especially in the first PCR cycles which are very critical, does not manifest 3′-5′ proofreading endonuclease activity to remove the mismatched nucleotide. If primer pairs are designed to have perfectly matched 3′ ends with only a single allele or a single group of alleles and the PCR reaction is initiated under stringent conditions, a

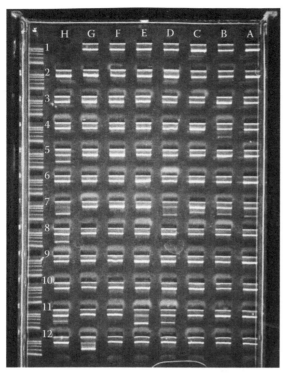

Example of high resolution DRBI typing using sequence-specific primer methodology. Far left column shows molecular weight ladder of known base pairs for base pair sizing.

perfectly matched primer pair results in an amplification product, whereas a mismatch at the 3′ end primer pair will not provide an amplification product. A positive result, i.e., amplification, defines the specificity of the DNA sample. The PCR amplification step provides the basis for identifying polymorphism. The postamplification processing of the sample consists only of a simple agarose gel electrophoresis to detect the presence or absence of amplified product. DNA amplified fragments are visualized by ethidium bromide staining and exposure to UV light. A separate technique detects amplified product by color fluorescence. The primer pairs are selected in such a manner that each allele should have a unique reactivity pattern with the panel of primer pairs employed. Appropriate controls must be maintained.

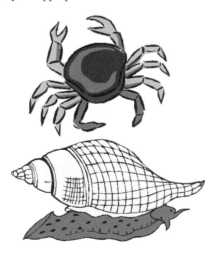

Mollusks and arthropods.

molecular hybridization probe

A molecule of nucleic acid labeled with a radionuclide or fluorochrome that can reveal the presence of complementary nucleic acid through molecular hybridization such as *in situ.*

molecular mimicry

The sharing of antigenic determinants or epitopes between cells of an immunocompetent host and a microorganism may lead to pathologic sequelae if antibodies produced against the microorganism combine with antigens of self and lead to immunologic injury. Ankylosing spondylitis and rheumatic fever are examples. Immunologic cross reactivity between a viral antigen and a self antigen or between a bacterial antigen such as streptococcal M protein and human myocardial sarcolemmal membranes may lead to tissue injury. Cross reactive epitopes involving molecular mimicry may be sequential (common amino acid determinants between host and pathogen) or conformational (cross reactivity to chemical moieties such as glycans, phosphates, or sulfates that reveal a specific tertiary configuration and electrostatic potential). Rothbard epitopes, which are common cognate T cell epitopes, may also induce cross reactive T lymphocyte responses. Molecular mimicry may also be observed in the idiotype network in which anti-Id antibodies can generate a mirror image of the original antigen.

mollusks and arthropods

Mollusks and arthropods fail to manifest graft rejection even though they possess significant humoral factors including what may be the most primitive alternative complement pathway components that may provide resistance to selected parasites.

Moloney test

Diphtheria toxoid is injected intradermally, and the skin response is observed to determine whether the subject is hypersensitive to diphtheria prophylactic substances.

monoclonal

Derived from a single clone.

monoclonal antibody (mAb)

Monoclonal antibodies are synthesized by a single clone of B lymphocytes or plasma cells and have identical structure and antigen specificity. The first to be observed were produced by malignant plasma cells in patients with multiple myeloma and associated gammopathies. The identical copies of the antibody molecules produced contain only one class of heavy chain and one type of light chain. Kohler and Millstein in the mid-1970s developed B lymphocyte hybridomas by fusing an antibody-producing B lymphocyte with a mutant myeloma cell that was not secreting antibody. The B lymphocyte product provided the specificity, whereas the myeloma cell conferred immortality on the hybridoma clone. Today monoclonal antibodies (mAbs) are produced in large quantities against a plethora of antigens for use in diagnosis and sometimes treatment. mAbs are homogeneous and widely employed in immunoassays, single antigen identification in mixtures, delineation of cell surface molecules, and assays of hormones and drugs in serum, among other uses. Since the responses to some immunogens are inadequate in mice, monoclonal antibodies have also been generated using rabbit cells. Monoclonal antibodies have been radioactively labeled and used to detect tumor metastases, to differentiate subtypes of tumors with monoclonal antibodies against membrane antigens or intermediate filaments, to identify microbes in body fluids, and for circulating hormone assays. mAbs may be used to

M

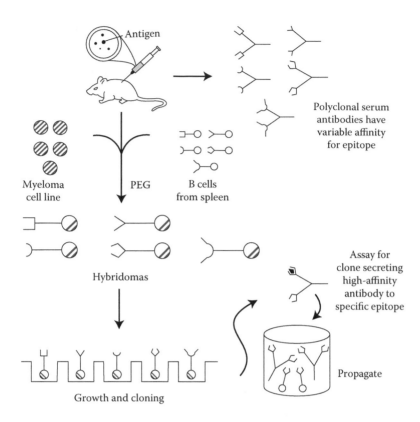

direct immunotoxins or radioisotopes to tumor targets with potential for tumor therapy.

monoclonal antibody HECA-452

An antibody that recognizes cutaneous lymphocyte antigen.

monoclonal antibody (MAb) therapy

Treatment with monoclonal antibodies to suppress immune function, kill target cells, or treat specific inflammatory diseases. MAbs demonstrate highly specific binding to precise cellular or molecular targets. Because MAbs are derived from mouse cells, they have the potential to induce allergic reactions in recipients. They have multiple uses in health care. For example, Edrecolomab® is used to treat solid tumors, Enlimomab® is used to treat organ transplant rejection, Infliximab® is used to treat Crohn's disease and rheumatoid arthritis, OKT3® is used to treat organ transplant rejection, Palivizumab® is used for respiratory syncytial virus, Rituxamab® is used to treat leukemias and lymphomas, Rhumabvegf® is used to treat solid tumors, and Transtuzumab® is used to treat metastatic breast cancer.

monoclonal anti-insulin antibody

An antibody used for the immunohistochemical localization of the polypeptide hormone insulin that is the most reliable means to accurately characterize the functional repertoire of islet cell tumors. Islet cell neoplasms of the pancreas appear as solitary or multiple circumscribed lesions that contrast sharply with the neighboring pancreatic parenchyma. These tumors are grouped on the basis of their predominant secretory hormones. This monoclonal antibody is used for the specific and qualitative localization of insulin in routinely fixed paraffin-embedded or frozen tissue sections.

monoclonal gammopathy

A pathologic state characterized by a monoclonal immunoglobulin (M component) in serum. Examples include multiple myeloma, benign monoclonal gammopathy, and Waldenström's macroglobulinemia.

monoclonal gammopathy of undetermined significance (MGUS)

Benign monoclonal gammopathy. A condition in which the serum contains an M component, serum albumin is less than 2 g/dL, and no Bence–Jones protein is present in the urine. There are no osteolytic lesions, and plasma cells comprise less than 5% of bone marrow constituents. Of these patients, 20 to 40% ultimately develop monoclonal malignancies. When monoclonal spikes exceed 2 g/dL, other immunoglobulins decrease, and no Bence–Jones protein appears in the urine, a condition that is usually malignant. One to two percent of myelomas are nonsecretory monoclonal gammopathies. More than half of the patients with elevated monoclonal IgM have monoclonal gammopathy of undetermined significance (MGUS), with other cases evolving into Waldenström's macroglobulinemia and a few progressing to lymphoma or chronic lymphocytic leukemia.

monoclonal immunoglobulin

A protein formed by an expanding clone of antibody-synthesizing cells in the body of a patient with a tumor or a benign condition. A classic example is multiple myeloma or Waldenström's macroglobulinemia, in which an expanded clone of cells producing a homogeneous and uniform immunoglobulin product can be demonstrated. A number of tumors may stimulate monoclonal immunoglobulin synthesis. These include adenocarcinoma and carcinoma of the

M

Therapeutic Monoclonal Antibodies

Antibody Name	Target Antigen	Conditions Treated and/or Prevented
Abciximab (ReoPro)	Glycoprotein II_b and III_a receptor	Complications of coronary angioplasty
ABX-CBL	CD147	GVHD
ABX-EGF	EGFR	EGF-dependent human tumor
ABX-IL8	IL8	Rheumatoid arthritis, psoriasis
AcuTect		Diagnosis of acute venous thrombosis
Adalimumab (Humira)	TNF	Rheumatoid arthritis
AFP-Scan	AFP	Detection of liver and germ cell cancers
Alemtuzumab (Campath)	CD52	B cell chronic lymphocytic leukemia, multiple sclerosis, kidney transplant rejection
Apolizumab (Remitogen)	1D10 antigen	B cell non-Hodgkin lymphoma, solid tumors
Arcitumomab (CEA-Scan), technetium 99m labeled	Carcinoembryonic antigen	Detection and location of recurrent and metastatic colorectal cancer
Anti-CD11a hu1 124	CD11a	Psoriasis
Basiliximab (Simulect)	CD25 (IL2 receptor)	Allograft rejection
Bectumomab		Non-Hodgkin lymphoma
Bevacizumab (Avastin)	VEGF	Metastatic renal carcinoma
Capromab Pendetide (Prostascint), indium 111 labeled	Prostate membrane-specific antigen	Radioimmunoscintigraphy for prostate cancer
Cetuximab	EGFR	Head and neck, breast, pancreatic, colorectal cancers
CEACide	Carcinoembryonic antigen	
Daclizumab (Zenapax)	CD25 (IL2 receptor)	Allograft rejection
Edrecolomab (Panorex)	17-1A cell surface antigen	Colorectal cancer
Efalizumab (Xanelim)	CD11a	Rheumatoid arthritis
Enlimomab	CD54 (ICAM-1)	Organ transplant rejection
Epratuzumab (LymphoCide)	CD22	Non-Hodgkin lymphoma
Gemtuzumab ozogamicin (Mylotarg)	CD33 calicheamicin	Acute myeloid leukemia
Hu23F2G (LeukArrest)	CD11/18 (leukointegrin)	Ischemic stroke
Hu1124	CD11a	Psoriasis
Ibritumomab tiuxetan (Zevalin)	CD20	B cell non-Hodgkin lymphoma
Igovomab (Indimacis 125)	Tumor-associated antigen CA125	Detection of ovarian adenocarcinoma
Imciromab pentetate (Myoscint)	Human cardiac myosin	Myocardial infarction imaging
IMC-C225 (Erbitux)	EGFR	EGF-dependent human tumor
Infliximab (Remicade)	TNF-α	Crohn's disease, rheumatoid arthritis
Inolimomab	IL2 receptor	Organ transplant rejection
LDP-01	β2 integrin	Stroke, kidney transplant rejection
LDP-02	α4β7 Integrin receptor	Crohn's disease, ulcerative colitis
LeuTech 99cTc-anti-CD15 anti-granulocyte antibody	CD15	Imaging infection sites
Lerdelimumab	TGFb2	Glaucoma, cataract
Lym-1, yttrium 90 labeled	HLA-DR	Non-Hodgkin lymphoma
Lymphoscan	CD22	Detection of B cell non-Hodgkin lymphoma
MAK-195F	TNFα	Hyperinflammatory response in sepsis syndrome
MDX-33	CD64	Idiopathic thrombocytopenic purpura
MCX-H210	Bispecific HER2 x CD64	Breast, colorectal, kidney, ovarian, and prostate cancers
MDX-447	Bispecific EGFR x CD64	Head, neck, and renal cancers
Mitumomab (BEC2)	GD3 idiotypic	Small cell lung cancer, melanoma

(*Continued*)

M

Therapeutic Monoclonal Antibodies

Antibody Name	Target Antigen	Conditions Treated and/or Prevented
Muromonab (Orthoclone OKT3)	CD3	Allograft rejection
Natalizumab (Antegren)	α-4 Integrin (VLA-4)	Multiple sclerosis, Crohn's disease
Nebacumab (Centoxin)	Bacterial endotoxins	Gram-negative bacteria sepsis
Nofetumomab (Verluma)	Carcinoma-associated antigen	Detection of small cell lung cancer
OctreoScan, indium 111 labeled	Somatostatin receptor	Immunoscintigraphic localization of primary and metastatic neuroendocrine tumors containing somatostatin receptors
Olizuma, rhuMAb-E25	Ig-E	Allergic asthma, allergic rhinitis
Oncolym (131Lym-1), iodine 131 labeled	HLA-DA	B cell non-Hodgkin lymphoma
Omalizumab (Xolari)	IgE	Allergic asthma, allergic rhinitis
Oregovomab (OvaRex)	Tumor-associated antigen CA125	Ovarian cancer
Orthoclone OKT4A	CD4	CD4-mediated autoimmune diseases, allograft rejection
Palivizumab (Synagis)	Antigenic site of F protein of respiratory syncytial virus	Respiratory syncytial virus infection
Pexelizumab (5G1.1-SC)	Complement C5	AMI, UA, CPB, PTCA
Priliximab	CD4	Crohn's disease, multiple sclerosis
Regavirumab	Cytomegalovirus	Acute CMV disease
Rituximab (Rituxan)	CD20	Non-Hodgkin lymphoma
Satumomab pendetide (OncoScint CR/OV)	Tumor-associated glycoprotein-72	Detection of colorectal and ovarian cancers
Sevirumab (Protovir)	Cytomegalovirus	Prevention of CMV infection in bone marrow transplant patients
Siplizumab (MEDI-507)	CD2	Acute GVHD, psoriatic arthritis
Smart M195	CD33	Acute myeloid leukemia, myelodysplastic syndrome
Sulesomab (LeukoScan), technetium 99m labeled	Surface granulocyte nonspecific cross-reacting antigen	Detection of osteomyelitis, acute atypical appendicitis
Tecnemab K1 (withdrawn from market)	High molecular weight melanoma-associated antigen	Diagnosis of cutaneous melanoma lesions
Tositumomab (Bexxar), iodine 131 attached	B cell surface protein	Non-Hodgkin lymphoma
Trastuzumab (Herceptin)	Her2/neu	Her2-positive metastatic breast cancer
Visilizumab (Nuvion, Smart, anti-CD3)	CD3	GVHD, ulcerative colitis
Vitaxin	αvβ3 Integrin	Solid tumors
Votumumab (Humaspect)	Cytokeratin tumor-associated antigen	Detection of carcinoma of colon and rectum
YM-337	GPIIb/IIIa	Prevention of platelet aggregation
Zolimomab	CD5, ricin, A chain toxin	GVHD

AFP = α α fetoprotein.

AMI = acute myocardial infarction.

CPB = cardiopulmonary bypass.

EGFR = epidermal growth factor receptor.

GPIIb/IIIa = glycoprotein IIbIIIa.

GVHD = graft-vs-host disease.

HLA = human leukocyte antigen.

ICAM-1 = intercellular adhesion molecule-1.

IL-2 = interleukin-2.

IL-8 = interleukin-8.

PTCA = percutaneous transluminal coronary angioplasty.

TGFb2 = transforming growth factor b2.

TNF-α = tumor necrosis factor α.

UA = unstable angina.

VEGF = vascular endothelial growth factor.

VLA-4 = very late antigen-4.

Monoclonal Antibodies

Drug Name	Active Ingredient
Avastin	Bevacizumab
Campath	Alemtuzumab
Cea-Scan	Arcitumomab
Erbitux	Cetuximab
Hemabate	Carboprost tromethamine
Herceptin	Trastuzumab
Humira	Adalimumab
Lucentis	Ranibizumab
Mylotarg	Gemtuzumab ozogamicin
Myoscint	Imciromab pentetate
Prostascint	Capromab pendetide
Raptiva	Efalizumab
Remicade	Infliximab
Reopro	Abciximab
Rituxan	Rituximab
Simulect	Basiliximab
Soliris	Eculizumab
Synagis	Palivizumab
Tysabri	Natalizumab
Vectibix	Panitumumab

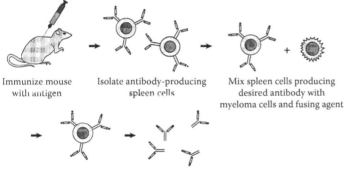

Immunize mouse with antigen   Isolate antibody-producing spleen cells   Mix spleen cells producing desired antibody with myeloma cells and fusing agent

Select and culture immortalized fused spleen/myeloma cells producing desired antibody   Purify antibody from hybridoma culture medium

Development of a hybridoma for monoclonal antibody production.

cervix, liver, and bladder, Kaposi's sarcoma, and angiosarcoma. Selected infections may also evoke monoclonal immunoglobulin responses, e.g., viral hepatitis, tuberculosis, and schistosomiasis. Other conditions that stimulate this response include thalassemia, autoimmune hemolytic anemia, autoimmune diseases such as scleroderma and pemphigus vulgaris, and various other conditions.

monoclonal immunoglobulin deposition disease (MIDD)
A condition in which monotypic light or heavy chains are deposited in tissues. The deposits may be fibrillar or nonfibrillar. The AL type of amyloidosis, characterized by light chains and amyloid P component, represents an example of fibrillar deposits, whereas light chain or light and heavy chain diseases represent nonfibrillar deposits. Patients may develop azotemia, albuminuria, hypogammaglobulinemia, cardiomyopathy, or nephropathy. Some may develop multiple myeloma or another plasma cell neoplasm. Another variety of MIDD is amyloid H, which is composed of V_H, D_D, J_H, and C_H3 domains.

monoclonal protein
A protein synthesized by a clone of identical cells derived from a single cell.

monocyte
Mononuclear phagocytic blood cell derived from promonocytes in the bone marrow. Following a relatively brief residence in the blood, i.e., approximately one day, they migrate into the tissues and serous cavities and are transformed into macrophages. They are less mature than macrophages, as suggested by fewer surface receptors, cytoplasmic organelles, and enzymes than the latter. Monocytes are larger than polymorphonuclear leukocytes, are actively phagocytic, and constitute 2 to 10% of the total white blood cell count in humans. Monocytes in the blood circulation have diameters of 15 to 25 μm and a grayish-blue cytoplasm that contains lysosomes with enzymes such as acid phosphatase, arginase cachetepsin, collagenase, deoxyribonuclease, lipase, glucosidase, and plasminogen activator. The cell has a reniform nucleus with delicate lace-like chromatin. Monocytes have surface receptors such as the Fc receptor for immunoglobulin G (IgG) and a receptor for CR3. They are actively phagocytic and play a significant role in antigen processing. Monocyte numbers are elevated in both benign and malignant conditions. Certain infections stimulate reactive types of monocytosis such as in tuberculosis, brucellosis, HIV-1 infection, and malaria.

monocyte chemoattractant protein (MCP-1)
A prototypic chemokine of the β (CC) family first isolated as a product of the immediate early gene, *JE,* induced by PDGF. Cloning of the human homolog of *JE* reveals an encoded protein identical to authentic chemokine MCP-1, which is believed to be one of the most significant chemokines in chronic inflammatory diseases controlled by mononuclear leukocytes. Tissue sources include fibroblasts, monocytes, macrophages, mouse spleen lymphocytes, and endothelial cells, among others. Target cells include monocytes, hematopoietic precursors, T lymphocytes, basophils, eosinophils, mast cells, NK cells, and dendritic cells.

monocyte chemoattractant protein-2 (MCP-2)
Refer to MCP-2.

monocyte chemoattractant protein-3 (MCP-3)
Refer to MCP-3.

monocyte colony-stimulating factor (M-CSF)
A cytokine that induces the production of monocytes from bone marrow precursor cells. It is synthesized by T lymphocytes, macrophages, endothelial cells, and stromal fibroblasts.

monocyte-derived neutrophil chemotactic factor
Refer to interleukin-8 (IL8).

monocyte–phagocytic system
A system of cells that provides nonspecific immunity and is dependent on the activity of the monocyte–macrophage lineage cells that are especially prominent in the spleen.

monogamous bivalency
The binding of a bivalent antibody molecule such as IgG with two identical antigenic determinants or epitopes on the same antigen molecule, in contrast to each Fab region of the IgG molecule uniting with an identical antigenic determinant on two separate antigen molecule. For this monogamous binding to take place, the epitopes must be positioned on the surface of the antigen molecule in such a manner that the binding of one Fab region to an epitope can position the remaining Fab of the IgG molecule

Therapeutic Monoclonal Antibodies and Their Potential Clinical Uses

Monoclonal Antibody	Condition Treated or Prevented
Abciximab (c7E3 Fab), specific for platelet glycoprotein 11b-111a receptors	Adjunct to percutaneous coronary intervention to prevent cardiac ischemic complications
Alemtuzumab (Campath-1H), anti CD52	B cell chronic lymphocytic leukemia
Antimyosin MAb (Octreoscan®), indium 111 labeled	Cardiac scintigraphy
Anti-CD66 (a,b,c,e) MAb (Basiliximab), rhenium 188 labeled	Conditioning for stem cell transplantation
Basiliximab	Acute organ rejection
Bectumomab	B cell lymphomas and leukemias
Capromab pendetide (indium 111 labeled)	Immunoscintigraphy
Daclizumab	Acute organ rejection
Edobacomab	Gram-negative bacterial endotoxins
Endrecolomab	Solid tumors (e.g., colorectal carcinoma)
Enlimomab (anti-ICAM-1)	Organ transplant rejection
Felvizumab	Respiratory syncytial virus
Gemtuzumab ozogamicin (Mylotarg®), anti-CD33	Acute myeloid leukemia
Ibritumomab tiuxetan, anti-CD20, yttrium 90 labeled	Non-Hodgkin B cell lymphoma
Infliximab (anti-TNFα)	Crohn's disease; rheumatoid arthritis
Inolimomab (anti-IL2 receptor)	Organ transplant rejection
Iodine 131 Tositumomab	Non-Hodgkin B cell lymphomas
Muromonab-CD3	Acute allograft rejection
Nebacumab (Centoxin®)	Anti-Gram-negative bacterial endotoxins
OKT3 (anti-CD3)	Organ transplant rejection
Olizumab (anti-IgE)	Allergic asthma; allergic rhinitis
Omalizumab (anti-IgE)	Allergic asthma; allergic rhinitis
Omalizumab (anti-IgE)	Allergic asthma; allergic rhinitis
Palivizumab	Respiratory syncytial virus
Priliximab (anti-CD4)	Heart transplant rejection; mycosis fungoides
RhuMAbVEGF	Solid tumors
Rituximab (anti-CD20)	CD20+ non-Hodgkin B cell lymphoma
Satumomab pendetide (indium labeled)	Diagnostic imaging; immunoscintigraphy
Tc-99m anti-CD15 (Acutect®), antineutrophil	Imaging agent for diagnosis of infection
Transtuzumab (anti-p185-HER2)	Metastatic breast cancer
Votumumab, Tc-99m radiolabeled	Cancer imaging agent
Zolimomab aritox (anti-CD5–ricin A chain toxin)	Graft-vs.-host disease

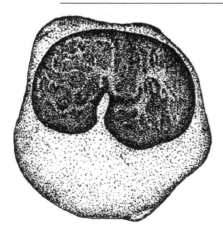

16–22 μm.

Monocyte.

for easy interaction with an adjacent identical epitope. Interaction of this type represents high affinity of binding, which lends a stability to the antigen–antibody complex. The combination of one IgM molecule to multiple epitopes on a single molecule of antigen would represent monogamous multivalency.

monogamous multivalency

Refer to monogamous bivalency.

monokine

A cytokine produced by monocytes. Any one of a group of biologically active factors secreted by monocytes and macrophages that have a regulatory effect on the functions of other cells such as lymphocytes. Examples include interleukin-1 (IL1) and tumor necrosis factor (TNF).

monomers

(1) Subunits of an immunoglobulin molecule; two heavy and two light chains that comprise the four polypeptide chains of a typical IgG molecule. (2) Also used to refer to a basic four-chain monomer or monomeric unit of an immunoglobulin molecule. In contrast to one monomeric

M

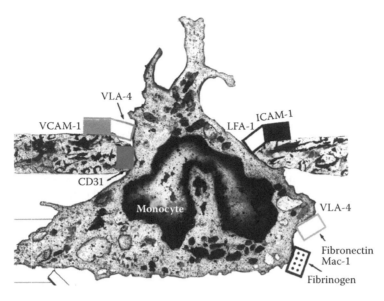

Monocyte.

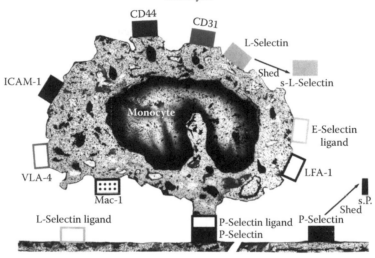

Monocyte.

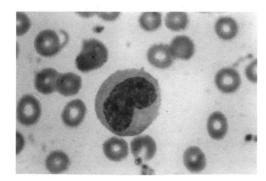

Monocyte in peripheral blood.

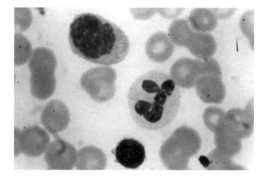

Monocyte, lymphocyte, and polymorphonuclear neutrophil.

immunoglobulin unit for IgG, IgM possesses five that are linked by disulfide bonds.

monomorphic

Existing only in one form. In genetics, refers to a gene with only one allele.

monomorphic population

A group exhibiting only one trait with potential for variable expression, attributable to fixation with one allelic form of the gene encoding that trait. Only a single nucleotide sequence (one allele) is present in a population for a monomorphic gene.

mononuclear cell

Leukocytes with single, round nuclei such as lymphocytes and macrophages, in contrast to polymorphonuclear leukocytes; thus, the term refers to the mononuclear phagocytic system or to lymphocytes.

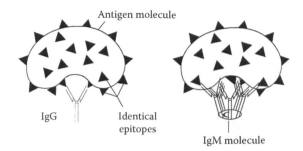

Monogamous bivalency and monogamous multivalency.

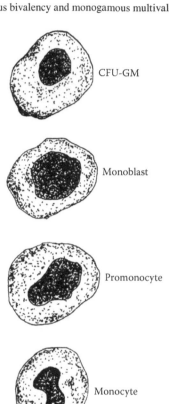

CFU-GM

Monoblast

Promonocyte

Monocyte

Tissue macrophage

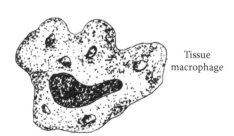

Mononuclear phagocyte system.

mononuclear phagocyte

Refer to mononuclear phagocyte system.

mononuclear phagocyte system

Mononuclear cells with pronounced phagocytic ability that are distributed extensively in lymphoid and other organs. *Mononuclear phagocyte system* should replace the previous *reticuloendothelial system* term to describe this group of cells. Mononuclear phagocytes originate from stem cells in the bone marrow that first differentiate into monocytes

that appear in the blood for approximately 24 hours or more with final differentiation into macrophages in the tissues. Macrophages usually occupy perivascular areas. Liver macrophages are termed Kupffer's cells; those in the lung are alveolar macrophages. The microglia represent macrophages of the central nervous system. Histiocytes represent macrophages of connective tissue. Tissue stem cells are monocytes that wander from the blood into the tissues and may differentiate into macrophages. Mononuclear phagocytes have a variety of surface receptors that enable them to bind carbohydrates or such protein molecules as C3 via complement receptor 1 and complement receptor 3, and IgG and IgE through Fcγ and Fcε receptors. The surface expression of MHC class II molecules enables both monocytes and macrophages to serve as antigen-presenting cells to CD4+ T lymphocytes. Mononuclear phagocytes secrete a rich array of molecular substances with various functions: interleukin-1; tumor necrosis factor α; interleukin-6; C2, C3, C4, and factor B complement proteins; prostaglandins; leukotrienes; and other substances.

monospecific antiserum

An antiserum against only a single antigen or epitope.

monovalent

Univalent; a combining power of one.

monovalent antiserum

A monospecific antiserum.

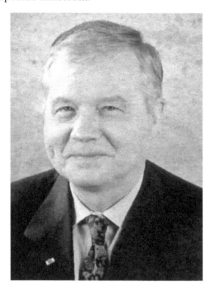

Luc Montagnier.

Montagnier, Luc

First to isolate the human immunodeficiency virus that causes acquired immune deficiency syndrome (AIDS) with his colleagues F. Barre-Sanoussi and J. C. Chermann at Institut Pasteur in Paris. They isolated the virus in early 1983 from a culture of activated T lymphocytes derived from a lymph node biopsy of a homosexual patient with lymphadenopathy. Montagnier is credited with the original isolation. Another investigator, Robert Gallo of the United States NIH, successfully propagated the virus in cell culture and developed critically needed diagnostic tests. Both groups made major contributions to AIDS biology. Montagnier received the Nobel Prize in Physiology or Medicine in 2008, together with Francoise Barre-Sinoussi for discovery of the AIDS virus.

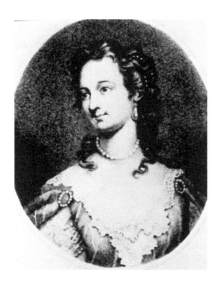

Lady Mary Wortley Montagu.

Montagu, Lady Mary Wortley (1689–1762)

Often credited as the first to introduce inoculation as a means of preventing smallpox in England in 1722. After observing the practice in Turkey, where her husband was posted as Ambassador to the Turkish court, she had both her young son and daughter inoculated and interested the Prince and Princess of Wales in the practice. Accounts of inoculation against smallpox are found in her *Letters*, 1977. Robert Halsband authored her biography, *The Life of Lady Mary Wortley Montagu* (Clarendon Press, Oxford, 1956).

Montenegro test

A diagnostic assay for South American leishmaniasis induced by *Leishmania brasiliensis*. The intracutaneous injection of a polysaccharide antigen derived from the causative agent induces a delayed hypersensitivity response.

Mooren's ulcer

A chronic progressive marginal corneal degeneration of unknown cause. It has an increased incidence in older persons and is associated with marked pain and ceaseless melting of the peripheral cornea. Autoimmune phenomena and collagenolytic enzymes have been considered in the pathogenesis of this condition. Circulating antibodies to human corneal epithelium and serum antibodies to a bovine corneal antigen (CO-Ag) have been demonstrated. Immunoglobulins and complement component patterns discovered in the affected epithelia and stroma were not found in normal controls. It remains to be determined whether these immunology phenomena lead to corneal inflammation or are consequences of it.

Moro test

A variant of the tuberculin test in which tuberculin is incorporated into an ointment that is applied to the skin to permit the tuberculin to enter the body by inunction.

moth-eaten mouse

A C57Bl/6J mouse strain mutant designated me/me. These animals are especially prone to develop autoimmune and infectious diseases. They have a mutation of the gene encoding SHP-1, a phosphatase that normally acts as a negative regulator of B cell receptor signaling and exhibit areas of hair loss. Immunologically, they develop polyclonal hypergammaglobulinemia, defective cell-mediated

immunity, and a type of autoimmune disease in which immune deposits are found in the kidneys.

MOTT (mycobacteria other than *Mycobacterium tuberculosis*)

An acronym for mycobacteria other than those that induce tuberculosis. Their recognition is increasing.

MOTT cell

A type of plasma cell containing refractile eosinophilic inclusion bodies that resemble Russell bodies. The cells are associated with African sleeping sickness and are demonstrable in periarteriolar cuffs in the brains of patients in late stages of African trypanosomiasis.

mouse hepatitis virus (MHV)

A DNA virus that causes murine hepatitis and encephalitis. MHV infects oligodendrocytes and leads to demyelination without the presence of immune system cells.

mouse immunoglobulin antibodies

Forty percent of human subjects may harbor heteroantibodies that include human antimouse antibodies (HAMAs). HAMAs in serum may induce falsely elevated results in immunoassays that involve mouse antibodies. This may present a problem for organ transplant patients who receive mouse monoclonal antibodies such as anti-CD3, anti-CD4, and anti-IL2R treatments.

mouse inbred strains

Refer to inbred strain.

M protein

(1) Monoclonal immunoglobulin or immunoglobulin components such as myeloma proteins. The M protein represents 3 to 10% of total serum proteins and the level remains constant throughout life or decreases with age. (2) Group Aβ hemolytic streptococcal type-specific cell surface antigens such as streptococcal M protein.

MRL-lpr/lpr mice

A mouse strain genetically prone to developing lupus erythematosus (LE)-like disease spontaneously. Its congenic subline is MRL-+/+. The lymphoproliferation (*lpr*) gene in the former strain is associated with development of autoimmune disease (i.e., murine lupus). This natural mouse mutant has a Fas mutation. Although the MRL-+/+ mice are not normal immunologically, they develop autoimmune disease only late in life and without lymphadenopathy. MRL-lpr/lpr mice differ from New Zealand mice mainly in the development of striking lymphadenopathy in both males and females of the MRL-lpr/lpr strain between 8 and 16 weeks of age with a 100-fold increase in lymph node weight. Many Thy-1+, Ly-1+, Ly-2- and L3T4- lymphocytes that express and rearrange α and β genes of the T cell receptor but fail to rearrange immunoglobulin genes are present in the lymph nodes. Multiple antinuclear antibodies, including anti-Sm, are among serological features of murine lupus in the MRL-lpr/lpr mouse model. These are associated with the development of immune complexes that mediate glomerulonephritis. Although the *lpr* gene is clearly significant in the pathogenesis of autoimmunity, the development of anti-DNA and anti-Sm even in low titers and late in life in the MRL-+/+ congenic line points to the role of factors other than the *lpr* gene in the development of autoimmunity in this strain.

MS

Abbreviation for multiple sclerosis.

μ chain

The IgM heavy polypeptide chain. Membrane μ chain is designated μ$_m$. Secreted μ chain is designated μ$_s$.

M

µ heavy chain disease

A type of myelomatosis in which aberrant monoclonal immunoglobulin µ chains are present in serum but not in urine, and Bence–Jones proteins are present in urine. Although very rare, this condition may be associated with chronic lymphocytic leukemia or reticulum cell sarcoma. Vacuolated plasma cells have been demonstrated in the bone marrow and are very suggestive of the diagnosis of µ heavy chain disease. The µ chains produced by bone marrow plasma cells have deletions in the variable regions and involve the C_H1 domain but have a normal sequences in the C_H2 domain. Light chains synthesized by these patients are not incorporated into molecular IgM; therefore, these individuals demonstrate distinct failures in the assembly of immunoglobulin molecules. Heavy and light chains have different electrophoretic motilities, which becomes an important observation in establishing a diagnosis of µ heavy chain disease by electrophoresis.

mucin

Heavily glycosated serine- and threonine-rich proteins that serve as ligands for selectins.

mucocutaneous candidiasis

Cellular immunodeficiency is associated with this chronic *Candida* infection of the skin, mucous membranes, nails, and hair, with about 50% of patients manifesting endocrine abnormalities. Cell-mediated immunity to *Candida* antigens alone is absent or suppressed. The individual manifests anergy following the injection of *Candida* antigen into the skin. Immunity to other infectious agents, including other fungi, bacteria, and viruses, is not impaired. The B cell limb of the immune response, even to *Candida* antigens, does not appear to be affected. The antibody response to *Candida* and other antigens is within normal limits. The relative numbers of both T and B lymphocytes are normal, and immunoglobulins are at normal or elevated levels. Four clinical patterns have been described. The most severe is known as early chronic mucocutaneous candidiasis with granuloma and hyperkeratotic scales on the nails or face. This condition has associated endocrinopathy in about 50% of the cases. The second type is late-onset chronic mucocutaneous candidiasis, which involves the oral cavity or occasionally the nails. The third form is transmitted as an autosomal-recessive trait and is usually not associated with endocrine abnormalities. It is a mild to moderately severe disorder. The fourth form is known as juvenile familial polyendocrinopathy with candidiasis, which may be associated with hypoparathyroidism with or without Addison's disease. Those individuals in whom endocrinopathy is associated with mucocutaneous candidiasis may demonstrate autoantibodies against the endocrine tissue involved. In addition to the immunologic abnormalities described above, there is diminished formation of lymphokines (e.g., macrophage migration inhibitory factor, or MIF) directed against *Candida* antigens. Recommended treatment includes antimycotic agents and immunologic intervention designed to improve resistance of the host.

mucocutaneous lymph node syndrome

Refer to Kawasaki's disease.

mucosa

The mucus-secreting epithelial layers that cover the exterior surfaces of the respiratory, gastrointestinal, and urogenital

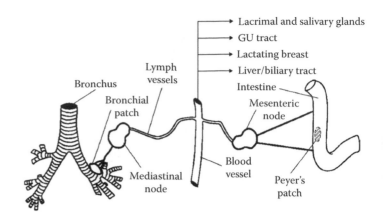

Cell traffic.

tracts. The conjunctiva of the eye and the mammary glands also belong to this classification.

mucosa homing

The selective return of immunologically reactive lymphoid cells that originated in mucosal follicles, migrated to other anatomical locations, and then returned to their site of origin in mucosal areas.

mucosa-associated lymphoid tissue (MALT)

Extranodal lymphoid tissue associated with the mucosa at various anatomical sites including the skin (SALT), bronchus (BALT), gut (GALT), nasal-associated lymphoid tissue (NALT), breast, and uterine cervix. MALTs provide localized or regional immune defense, as they are in immediate contact with foreign antigenic substances, thereby differing from the lymphoid tissues associated with lymph nodes, spleen, and thymus. Secretory or exocrine immunoglobulin A (IgA) is associated with the MALT system of immunity. The lymphoid tissues comprising MALT include intraepithelial lymphocytes, principally T lymphocytes together with B cells beneath the mucosal epithelia and in the lamina propria.

mucosal immune system

Aggregates of lymphoid tissues or lymphocytes near mucosal surfaces of the respiratory, gastrointestinal, and urogenital tracts that protect against microorganisms gaining access to the body through mucosal surfaces. The mucosal immune system is comprised of mucosa-associated lymphoid tissues that consist of lymphocyte and accessory cell aggregates in the epithelia and lamina propria of mucosal surfaces. There is local synthesis of secretory IgA and T cell immunity at these sites. Research in this field is so extensive that the Society for Mucosal Immunology was established to represent interests in this area.

mucosal immunity

Refer to mucosal immune system.

mucosal lymphoid follicles

These structures include Peyer's patches in the small intestine and pharyngeal tonsils. The appendix and other areas of the gastrointestinal tract and respiratory tract contain similar aggregates of lymphoid cells. Germinal centers at the centers of lymphoid follicles have an abundance of B cells. CD4+ T cells are present in interfollicular regions of Peyer's patches. One half to three quarters of the lymphocytes in murine Peyer's patches are B cells,

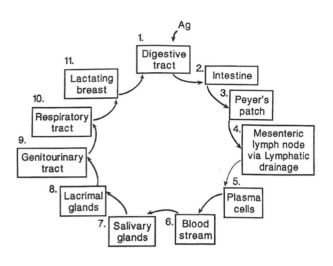

Secretory immune system.

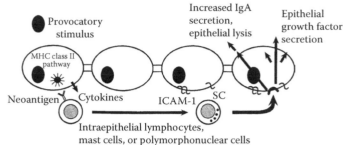

Common mucosal inflammatory pathway.

whereas 10 to 30% are T lymphocytes. M cells overlying Peyer's patches are membranous (M) cells devoid of microvilli, are pinocytic, and convey macromolecules to subepithelial tissues from the lumen of the intestine. Although M cells are believed to transport antigens to Peyer's patches, they do not act as antigen-presenting cells. Lymphoid cells in the blood migrate to the gut mucosa. The α_4-associated β_7 integrin is critical for endothelial binding of lymphocytes in the intestine and migration of cell into the mucosa.

mucosal tolerance
The hypothesis that continuous exposure of an individual to a modest quantity of a specific antigen through a mucosal route renders tolerance to that antigen systemically. As a consequence, there is abrogation of the immune response to that same antigen administered later by a nonmucosal route. Refer to oral tolerance.

mucous adhesive
Viscous liquid on the luminal surfaces of mucosal cells. Secretory antibodies and antimicrobial molecules are present in this secretion, which is a constituent of mucosal immunity. It is produced by multiple internal epithelia.

mucous membranes
Refer to mucosa.

Müller-Eberhard, Hans J. (1927–1998)
Investigator at the Scripps Research Institute in La Jolla, California. He was an authority on complement research and was instrumental in demonstrating the immunobiology of the late acting complement components in immune lysis.

multicatalytic proteinase autoantibodies
Of patients with systemic lupus erythematosus (SLE), 35% manifest autoantibodies to multicatalytic proteinases (proteasomes), macromolecular structures comprised of at least 14 subunits involved in the intracellular degradation of proteins. They are not usually found in myositis, scleroderma, or Sjögren's syndrome.

multilocus probes (MLPs)
Probes used to identify multiple related sequences distributed throughout each person's genome. Multilocus probes may reveal as many as 20 separate alleles. Because of this

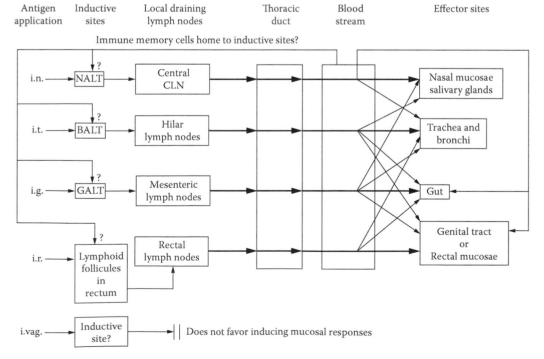

Compartmentalized common mucosal immune system.

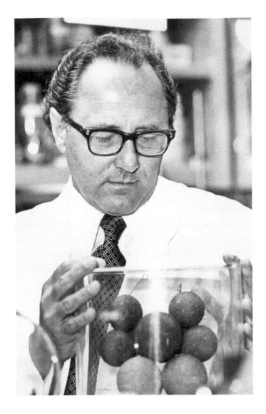

Hans J. Müller-Eberhard.

multiplicity of alleles, the possibility that two unrelated persons share the same pattern is remote (i.e., about 1 in 30 billion). There is, however, a problem in deciphering the multibanded arrangement of minisatellite restriction fragment length polymorphisms (RFLPs), as it is difficult to ascertain which bands are allelic. Mutation rates of minisatellite HVRs remain to be demonstrated but are recognized occasionally. Used in resolving cases of disputed parentage.

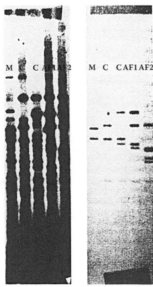

| M C CAF1AF2 | M C CAF1AF2 |

Multilocus probes   Single locus probes

multiple autoimmune disorder (MAD)

In type I MAD, a patient must manifest a minimum of two of the diseases designated Addison's disease, mucocutaneous candidiasis, or hypoparathyroidism. Type II MAD is known as Schmidt syndrome; patients manifest at least two conditions from a category that includes autoimmune thyroid disease, Addison's disease, mucocutaneous candidiasis, and insulin-dependent diabetes mellitus, with or without hypopituitarism.

multiple emulsion adjuvant

Water-in-oil-in-water emulsion adjuvant.

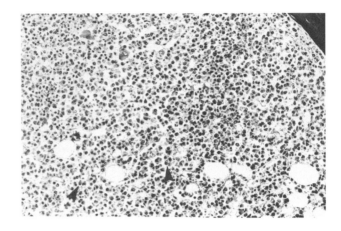

Multiple myeloma. Bone marrow plasma cell myeloma.

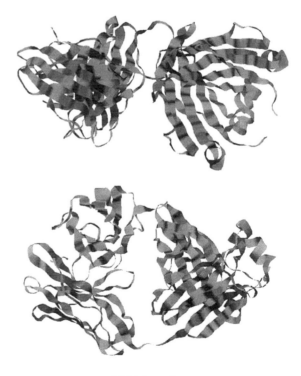

Multiple myeloma.

multiple myeloma

A plasmacytoma or plasma cell neoplasm associated with the production of a paraprotein that appears in the serum. The neoplastic plasma cells usually synthesize and secrete monoclonal, highly homogenous immunoglobulins. Serum electrophoresis reveals a narrow monoclonal band in 98 to 99% of patients. IgG paraimmunoglobulin manifests in 80% of myeloma patients, while 15% of the patients manifest monoclonal IgA. A few cases of the IgD and IgE types have been described. Homogeneous light chain dimers identical to the corresponding light chain portions of immunoglobulin in the blood appear in the urine. These light chain dimers in the urine are called Bence–Jones proteins. The segments of light polypeptide chains do not represent degradation products of immunoglobulin, as they are synthesized separately from it. The disease affects 3 in 100,000 persons, usually men over 50 years of age. Patients develop anemia, anorexia, and weakness. The tumor infiltrates the bone marrow cavities, ultimately leading to erosion of the bone cortex. This may take years. Osteolytic lesions are the hallmarks of multiple myeloma. The long bones, ribs, vertebrae, and skull manifest diffuse osteoporosis, which leads to the appearance of punched-out areas and pathologic fractions. Tumor invasion of the marrow, erosion of the cortex, and osteoclast-activating substances produce the bone lesions. Lung or renal infections may also occur. Hypogammaglobulinemia results from decreased functioning of normal plasma cells and leads to diminished antibody to combat infections. The malignant plasma cells produce an excess of nonsense paraimmunoglobulin which does not protect against infection. There is also defective phagocytic activity. Patients may have altered B cell function and increased susceptibility to pyogenic infections. Some patients may develop myeloma kidney, signified by proteinuria, followed by oliguria, kidney failure, and possibly death.

Zone Electrophoresis
Patterns of Cerebrospinal Fluid

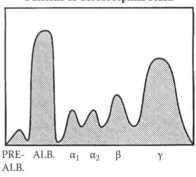

PRE-   ALB. α_1 α_2 β γ
ALB.

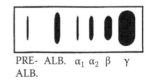

PRE- ALB. α_1 α_2 β γ
ALB.

Multiple sclerosis (100× concentrate).

multiple sclerosis (MS)

A demyelinating nervous system disease of unknown cause. It is most frequent in young adult females and has an incidence of 1 in 2500 individuals in the United States. MS shows a disease association with HLA-A3, B7, and Dw2 haplotypes. Patients express multiple neurological symptoms that are worse at some times than others, together with inhibition of nerve impulse transmission.

They have paresthesias, muscle weakness, visual and gait disturbances, ataxia, and hyperactive tendon reflexes. Lymphocytes and macrophages infiltrate into the nervous system which facilitates demyelination. Autoimmune mechanisms mediated by T cells, which constitute the majority of infiltrating lymphocytes, are involved. At least 20 viruses have been suggested to play a role in the etiology of MS. Infected oligodendrocytes are destroyed by the immune mechanism, and "innocent bystander" demyelination may also occur. Antibodies against HTLV-I GAG (p24) protein have been identified in the cerebrospinal fluid of MS patients. HTLV-I gene sequences have been identified in monocytes of MS patients. An oligoclonal increase in cerebrospinal fluid IgG occurs in 90% of MS patients. Inflammation, demyelination, and glial scarring are observed. Paraventricular, frontal, and temporal areas of the brain are first involved, followed by regions of the brain stem, optic tracts, and white matter of the cortex with patchy lesions of the spinal cord. Attempts at treatment have included COP-1, a polypeptide mixture that resembles myelin basic protein, and numerous other agents.

multiplicity

The presence in the genome of numerous independent genes that encode proteins that have the same function.

multivalent

Antibody or antigen molecules with a combining power greater than two.

multivalent antiserum

An immune serum preparation containing antibodies specific for more than two antigens. *Multivalent* means possessing more than two binding sites.

multivalent vaccine

Refer to polyvalent vaccine.

mumps vaccine

A live attenuated immunizing preparation employed to prevent mumps. It should be administered under the same guidelines and restrictions that apply to live attenuated measles virus vaccine.

mumps virus vaccine (live, injection)

For immunization of individuals over 12 months of age. Not recommended for infants younger than 12 months because of the possible presence of maternal mumps-neutralizing antibodies that may interfere with the immune response. Mumps is a common childhood disease induced by a paramyxovirus that may lead to such serious complications as aseptic meningitis, deafness, orchitis, and even death. As proven in clinical trials, the vaccine is highly immunogenic and well tolerated. A single injection can induce mumps-neutralizing antibodies in 95% of susceptible children and 93% of susceptible adults. Even though the antibody level is relatively lower than that following natural infection, it is protective and of long duration. A few (1 to 5%) individuals receiving the vaccine may fail to seroconvert following primary immunization. Protective efficacy of mumps vaccine has been established in controlled field trials. Seroconversion has been shown to parallel protection from the disease. Antibodies appearing following vaccination may be assayed by neutralization, hemagglutination inhibition, or ELISA techniques. Antibodies are often detectable 11 to 13 days after primary vaccination. Children vaccinated at or after 12 months of age should be revaccinated

M

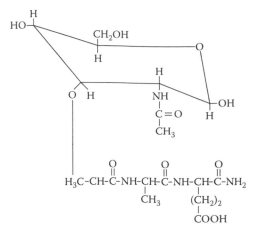

N-acetylmuramyl-L-alanyl-D-isoglutamine

Muramyl dipeptide (MDP).

with measles–mumps–rubella virus vaccine before admission to elementary school.

muramyl dipeptide (MDP)
N-Acetyl-muramyl-l-alanyl-d-isoglutamine; the active compound responsible for the immunologic adjuvant properties of complete Freund's adjuvant. It is an extract of the peptidoglycans of cell walls of mycobacteria in complete Freund's adjuvant that has the immunopotentiating property of inducing delayed-type hypersensitivity and boosting antibody responses. It induces fever and lyses blood platelets and may produce a temporary leukopenia; however, purified derivatives without adverse side effects have been prepared for use as immunologic adjuvants and may prove useful for use in human vaccines.

muromonab CD3 (injection)
A murine monoclonal antibody specific for CD3 antigen of human T cells used as an immunosuppressant. For intravenous administration only. It is biochemically purified IgG2a immunoglobulin that counteracts allograft rejection, possibly by blocking T cell function that plays a principal role in acute allograft rejection. It interacts with and inhibits the functioning of CD3 molecules in human T cell surface membranes associated with antigen recognition structures of T cells and is critical for signal transduction. It inhibits all known

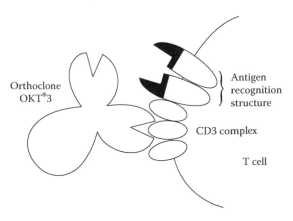

Orthocone OKT®3 blocks T cell effect or function involved in renal allograft rejection.

T cell functions and interacts with most peripheral T cells in blood and body tissues. Following cessation of therapy, T cell function returns to normal within approximately 1 week. Within minutes following administration, the number of circulating $CD2^+$, $CD3^+$, $CD4^+$, and $CD8^+$ T cells decreases precipitously. T cell activation leads to the release of numerous cytokines and/or lymphokines believed to be responsible for many of the acute clinical effects that follow muromonab CD3 therapy. Antibodies have been detected. The mean time of appearance of IgG antibodies is 20 days.

mutagen
A chemical, radiation or other agent that can induce a mutation.

mutant
A mutation in a gene, protein, or cell.

mutation
A structural change in a gene that leads to a sudden and stable alteration in the genotype of a cell, virus, or organism. It is a heritable change in the genome of a cell, virus, or organism apart from that induced through the incorporation of "foreign" DNA. It represents an alteration in the base sequence of DNA. Germ cell mutations may be inherited by future generations, whereas somatic cell mutations are inherited only by the progeny of cells produced through mitotic division. A point mutation is an alteration in a single base pair. Mutations in chromosomes may be expressed as translocation, deletion, inversion, or duplication.

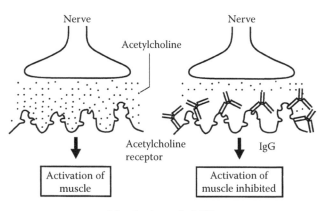

Myasthenia gravis (MG).

myasthenia gravis (MG)
An autoantibody-mediated autoimmune disease. Antibodies specific for the nicotinic acetylcholine receptor (AChR) of skeletal muscle react with the postsynaptic membranes at neuromuscular junctions and diminish the number of functional receptors. Patients develop muscular weakness and some voluntary muscle fatigue. The severe muscle weakness may interfere with breathing if respiratory muscles are affected. Thus, MG is a receptor disease mediated by antibodies. The nicotinic AChR is the autoantigen. Contemporary research hopes to identify epitopes on the autoantigens that interact with B and T cells in an autoimmune response. AChR is a four-subunit transmembrane protein. Most autoantibodies in humans are against the main immunogenic regions (MIRs). Antibodies against the MIRs cross link AChR molecules, leading to their internalization and lysosomal degradation followed by a decreased number of postsynaptic membrane AChRs. Humans with MG

and animals immunized against AChR develop circulating antibodies and clinical manifestations of MG. A subgroup of patients have seronegative MG; they resemble classic MG patients clinically but have no anti-AChR antibodies in their circulation. Because the IgG anti-AChR autoantibodies cross the placenta from mother to fetus, newborns of mothers with this disease may also manifest signs and symptoms. Neonatal MG establishes the antibody-mediated autoimmune nature of the disease. The thymus of an MG patient may reveal lymphofollicular hyperplasia (70%) or thymoma (10%). Anti-AChR-synthesizing B cells and T helper lymphocytes may be found in hyperplastic follicles. These are often encircled by myoid cells that express AChR. Interdigitating follicular dendritic cells closely associated with myoid cells have been suggested to present AChR autoantigen to autoreactive T helper lymphocytes. Anti-idiotypic antibodies have been used to suppress or enhance experimental autoimmune myasthenia gravis (EAMG), depending on the antibody concentration employed. Conjugate immunotoxins to anti-Id antibodies have been able to suppress autoimmunity to AChR. Both thymectomy and anticholinesterase drugs have proven useful in treatment.

myc

An oncogene designated v-*myc* when isolated from an avian myelocytomatosis retrovirus and c-*myc* when referring to the cellular homolog. Two others designated N-L-*myc* have been cloned. *myc* Genes are activated by overexpression by upregulation caused by transcriptional regulatory signal mutations in the first intron or by gene amplification. Normal tissues contain c-*myc*. When c-*myc* is in its normal position on chromosome 8, it remains transcriptionally silent, but when it is translocated, as in Burkitt's lymphoma, it may become activated. The protooncogene c-*myc* is amplified in early carcinoma of the uterine cervix and lung and in promyelocytic leukemia.

mycobacteria immunity

Immunity to tuberculosis is highly complex and involves cell-mediated mechanisms. The host immune response to tuberculosis is inappropriate, leading to tissue injury through immune mechanisms rather than elimination of the invading microorganism. In mice, immunity depends upon TNF-α, a Th1 cytokine pattern, and MHC class II. Mouse murine macrophages activated by IFN-γ inhibit proliferation of *M. tuberculosis*. β_2 microglobulin is requisite for immunity to mycobacteria which may point to the participation of CD8$^+$ MHC class I restrictor cytotoxic T cells. γδ T cell receptors identify mycobacterial antigens such as heat-shock proteins. These cell types secrete IFN-γ and are cytotoxic and classified as a type I response. A type II response renders mice more susceptible to tuberculosis. Immunity in humans is also associated with a Th1 type of response associated with macrophage activation and cytotoxic removal of infected cells. Human tuberculosis patients form specific IgE and IgG$_4$ antibodies, both of which are IL4-dependent. IL10 levels may also be increased. A Th2 response is associated with progressive disease in humans. *M. tuberculosis* can cause release of TNF-α from primed macrophages. This cytokine is requisite for protection but also has a role in immunopathology. Patients with tuberculosis develop necrotic lesions believed to help wall off established infections. The TNF-α toxicity in a mycobacterial lesion depends on whether the T cell response is Th1 or Th2. Necrosis is not produced when TNF-α is injected into a Th1 inflammatory site, but marked tissue injury results when it is injected into a Th1/Th2-mediated site. Infection by *M. leprae* is weakly associated with MHC haplotypes. It appears to determine the type of disease that will develop instead of susceptibility. In tuberculoid leprosy, both *in vivo* and *in vitro* equivalents of T cell-mediated responsiveness such as skin test reactivity in lymphoproliferation in response to antigens of *M. leprae* are intact. Th1 cytokines are produced in these lesions. Unless treated, they will develop into lepromatous leprosy in which the Th1 response is impaired. In leprosy, immunity probably requires macrophage activation and cytotoxic T cells activated by the Th1 response. In lepromatous leprosy, T cell-mediated immunity is depressed *in vivo* and *in vitro*. Numerous macrophages packed with bacilli are present in the lesions, but no response occurs. There is a continuous heavy antigen load and lack of a T cell-mediated response to the microorganism. The T cells express a Th2 cytokine pattern.

mycobacterial adjuvants

Substances used to enhance both humoral and cellular immune responses to antigen. Killed, dried mycobacteria, including *Mycobacterium tuberculosis* among other strains, are ground and suspended in lightweight mineral oil. With the aid of an emulsifying agent such as arlacel A, added antigen in aqueous medium is incorporated to produce a water-in-oil emulsion used for immunization. The mycobacteria are especially effective in stimulating cell-mediated immunity to the antigen. The administration of this adjuvant without antigen may induce adjuvant arthritis in rats. Incorporation of normal tissues such as thyroid or adrenal into Freund's complete adjuvant may induce autoimmune disease if reinoculated into the animal of origin or other members of the strain with the same genetic background.

mycobacterial peptidoglycolipid

A constituent of the wax D fraction of *Mycobacterium tuberculosis* var. hominis that contains the component associated with such mycobacterial adjuvants as Freund's adjuvant. Under electron microscopy, the peptidoglycolipid exhibits a homogeneous, intertwined filamentous structure.

Mycobacterium

A genus of aerobic bacteria including *Mycobacterium tuberculosis* that can survive within phagocytic cells and produce disease. Cell-mediated immunity is the principal host defense mechanism against mycobacteria.

Structure of mycophenolate mofetil.

mycophenolate mofetil

A semisynthetic derivative of mycophenolic acid isolated from the mold *Penicillum glaucum*. An immunosuppressive agent used to prolong survival of allogeneic transplants including kidney, heart, liver, intestine, limb, small bowel, pancreatic islets, and bone marrow. This immunosuppressive drug induces reversible antiproliferative effects specifically on lymphocytes but does not induce renal, hepatic, and neurologic toxicity. Its action is based on the requirement for adequate amounts of guanosine and deoxyguanosine nucleotides for lymphocytes to proliferate following antigenic stimulation. Thus, an agent that reversibly inhibits the final steps in purine synthesis, leading to a depletion of guanosine and deoxyguanosine nucleotides, may induce effective immunosuppression. Mycophenolate mofetil was found to produce these effects. It is the morpholinoethyl ester of mycophenolic acid. *In vivo*, it is hydrolyzed to the active form, mycophenolic acid glucuronide, which is biologically inactive and excreted in the urine. Mycophenolate blocks proliferation of peripheral blood mononuclear cells of humans to both B and T cell mitogens. It also blocks antibody formation as evidenced by inhibition of a recall response by human cells challenged with tetanus toxoid. Its ability to block glycosylation of adhesion molecules that facilitate leukocyte attachment to endothelial cells and target cells probably diminishes recruitment of lymphocytes and monocytes to sites of rejection or chronic inflammation. It does not affect neutrophil chemotaxis, microbicidal activity, or superoxide production. *In vivo*, mycophenolate prevents cytotoxic T cell generation and rejection of allogeneic cells. It inhibits antibody formation in a dose-dependent manner and effectively prevents allograft rejection in animal models, especially when used in conjunction with cyclosporine. Mycophenolate mofetil is effective in the treatment of refractory rejection in solid organ transplant recipients and in combination with prednisone as an alternative to cyclosporine or tacrolimus. It is also used for therapy of steroid-refractory graft-vs.-host disease in hematopoietic stem cell transplant patients. It is used with tacrolimus to prevent graft-vs.-host disease, and has been suggested for use in autoimmune disorders including lupus nephritis and rheumatoid arthritis. Toxicities include gastrointestinal disturbances, headache, hypertension, and reversible myelosuppression (principally neutropenia). It is used to reverse acute rejection in canine renal and rat cardiac allograft models. It inhibited proliferative arteriopathy in experimental models of aortic and heart allografts in rats and in primate cardiac xenografts. It inhibits immunologically mediated inflammatory responses in animal models and inhibits tumor development and prolongs survival in murine tumor transplant models. It is absorbed rapidly following oral administration and hydrolyzed to form mycophenolic acid, the active metabolite. Mycophenolic acid is a potent, selective, uncompetitive, and reversible inhibitor of inosine monophosphate dehydrogenase and, therefore, inhibits the *de novo* pathway of guanosine nucleotide synthesis without incorporation into DNA. Since T and B cells depend for their proliferation on *de novo* synthesis of purines unlike other cell types that can utilize salvage pathways, mycophenolic acid has potent cytostatic effects on lymphocytes. It inhibits proliferative responses of T and B lymphocytes to both mitogenic and allospecific stimulation. It also suppresses antibody formation by B cells and inhibits the glycosylation of lymphocyte and monocyte glycoproteins involved in intercellular adhesion to endothelial cells; it may inhibit leucocyte recruitment to sites of inflammation and graft rejection.

Mycoplasma–AIDS link

A mechanism postulated by Luc Montagnier for AIDS development. HIV-1 virus binds to cells first activated by *Mycoplasma* infection.

mycoplasma immunity

High-titer cold agglutinin autoantibodies against sialo-oligosaccharide of the Ii antigen type are sometimes found during *Mycoplasma pneumoniae* infections. The first line of defense against these microorganisms is phagocytosis, yet mycoplasmas can survive neutrophil phagocytosis if specific antibodies are not present. Secretory IgA is significant in preventing localized colonization, but systemic antibodies protect from primary infection and secondary spread from localized colonization. Mycoplasmas can evade the humoral immune response by undergoing antigenic variation of surface antigens. T cells also appear to play a role in immunity to mycoplasma that should be further investigated.

mycoses

Diseases produced by fungus infection.

mycosis fungoides

A chronic disorder involving the lymphoreticular system. The skin appears scaly and exhibits eczematous areas that are erythematous, with infiltration by lichenified plaques. Finally, ulcers and neoplasms of the internal organs and lymph nodes develop. Cells in skin lesions reveal markers that identify them as T lymphocytes. This disease usually appears after 50 years of age and is more frequent in males than females and in blacks than Caucasians. The number of null cells in the blood circulation increases, with a simultaneous decrease in the numbers of B and T lymphocytes. T cell immunity is diminished both *in vitro* and *in vivo,* as revealed by diminished lymphocyte unresponsiveness to mitogens and by a poor response and skin test. Immunoglobulin A and E levels may be elevated in the serum. A type of cutaneous T cell non-Hodgkin lymphoma.

myelin-associated glycoprotein (MAG) autoantibodies

Autoantibodies against the glycoprotein constituent of myelin that are found in the periaxonal region, Schmidt–Lanterman incisures, lateral loops, and outer mesaxon of the myelin sheath; belong to the immunoglobulin superfamily; and act as adhesion molecules that facilitate myelination. MAG autoantibodies recognize the *N*-linked L1 and J1 carbohydrate moiety, which is also found on PO and P2 glycoproteins, sulfate-3-glucuronyl paragloboside (SGPG), and sulfate-3-glucuronyl lactosaminyl paragloboside (SGLPG) glycolipids of peripheral nerves, neural cell adhesion molecules, and Li and J1 of lymphocytes and human natural killer cells. MAG autoantibodies are present in half of polyneuropathy patients with monoclonal gammopathy, which may be associated with other lymphoid proliferative diseases. T lymphocyte responses to MAG have been found in multiple sclerosis.

myelin autoantibodies

The detection of autoantibodies to myelin used previously to screen for autoantibodies in idiopathic and paraproteinemic neuropathy patients leads to inconsistent results due to imprecise myelin preparations leading to poor clinical specificity. Autoantibodies against myelin in Guillain–Barré syndrome (GBS) and sensory polyneuropathy with monoclonal gammopathy of unknown significance involve autoantibodies against glycolipids, including sulfatide, Forssman antigen, galactosyl–cerebroside (Gal–Cer) and gangliosides.

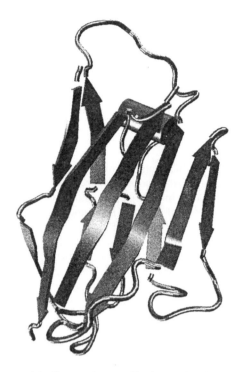

Myelin membrane adhesion molecule.

myelin basic protein (MBP)

A principal constituent of the myelin lipoprotein that first appears during late embryogenesis. It is a 19-kDa protein that is increased in multiple sclerosis patients who may generate T lymphocyte reactivity against MBP. T lymphocytes with the Vβ-17 variant of the T cell receptor are especially prone to react to MBP.

myelin basic protein (MBP) antibodies

Antibodies against myelin proteins have been investigated for their possible role in the demyelination that accompanies multiple sclerosis, acute idiopathic optic neuritis, Guillain–Barré syndrome, chronic relapsing polyradiculoneuritis, carcinomatous polyneuropathy, and subacute sclerosing panencephalitis. Antibodies against myelin basic protein are well known to play a role in experimental allergic encephalomyelitis in laboratory animals, but the role they play in patients with multiple sclerosis and other neurological diseases has yet to be established. MBP autoantibody titers are closely correlated with exacerbations and relapses in MS and are present in 75% of MS patients and 89% of optic neuritis subjects. They have also been detected in 64% of HIV-associated neurological syndrome cases, in 58% of autistic children, in 30% of Japanese encephalitis cases, and in 30% of patients with subacute sclerosing panencephalitis (SSPE). Humoral and cellular immune responses participate in inflammatory demyelination.

myeloablative conditioning

A type of therapy required prior to bone marrow transplantation in which a patient's hematopoietic cells in the bone marrow are eliminated through the use of aggressive chemotherapy and total body irradiation, causing depletion of immune system cells from both the peripheral blood and the secondary lymphoid tissues. This therapy is used before hematopoietic cell transplantation and bone marrow transplantation.

myeloblast

A myeloid lineage immature hematopoietic cell produced by and present in the bone marrow but not usually found in the peripheral blood. It leads to the formation of granulocyte precursors and possesses nongranular basophilic cytoplasm.

myelodysplastic syndromes (MDS)

Category of hematopoietic disorders characterized by increased infection, anemia, and hemorrhage. The disorders

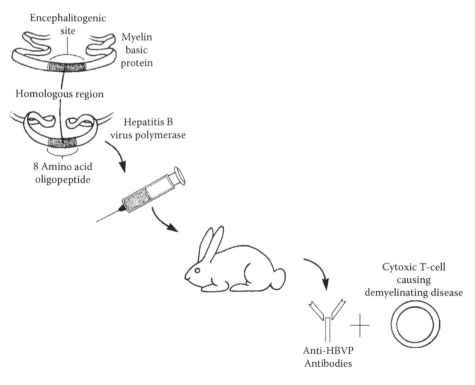

Myelin basic protein (MBP).

M

develop as a consequence of ineffective hematopoiesis marked by abnormal myeloid, erythroid, and megakaryocytic precursors and may develop into acute myeloid leukemia (AML).

myelogenous leukemia

A myeloid lineage cell malignancy.

myeloid antigen

A surface epitope of myeloid leukocytes. Examples include CD13, CD14, and CD33. A poor prognosis is indicated when the leukocytes of a patient with acute lymphocytic leukemia express myeloid antigens. Their expression is a better indicator of decreased survival than are other features of the disease.

myeloid cells

Cells that arise from common myeloid progenitors, comprising erythrocytes, neutrophils, monocyte/macrophages, eosinophils, basophils, and megakaryocytes.

myeloid cell series

An immature bone marrow cell (myeloblast) that is a precursor of the polymorphonuclear leukocyte series. This 18-μm diameter cell has a relatively large nucleus with finely distributed chromatin and two conspicuous nucleoli. The cytoplasm is basophilic when stained. During maturation, the cytoplasm becomes populated with large azurophilic primary granules, representing the promyelocyte stage. Later, the specific or secondary granules appear, representing the myelocyte stage. The nucleoli vanish as the nuclear chromatin forms dense aggregates. The chromatin in the nucleus condenses, and the cells no longer divide at this metamyelocyte stage. The nucleus assumes a sausage-like configuration known as a band. This subsequently develops into a three-lobed polymorphonuclear leukocyte that subsequently becomes a neutrophil, eosinophil, or basophil of the myeloid cell group. All three types of myeloid cells are present in normal peripheral blood.

myeloid lineage

A bone marrow-derived subset of cells, including granulocytes, monocytes, and macrophages.

myeloid progenitors

Bone marrow stem cells that lead to the formation of granulocytes, monocytes, and macrophages.

myeloma

A plasma cell dyscrasia characterized by highly malignant plasma cells in solid masses or dispersed as clones in the bone marrow. A plasmacytoma represents proliferation of a neoplastic plasma cell clone in bone marrow with the production of a monoclonal immunoglobulin paraprotein in addition to Bence–Jones proteins (free Ig light chains). Besides myeloma in humans, an experimental variety can be induced in certain inbred mouse strains such as BALB/c by intraperitoneal injection of mineral oil.

myeloma, IgD

A myeloma in which the monoclonal immunoglobulin is IgD. It constitutes 1 to 2% of myelomas and usually occurs in older males. Lymphadenopathy and hepatosplenomegaly are present. Approximately one half of the cases develop dissemination beyond the bones. Patients develop osteolysis, hypercalcemia, anemia, azotemia, aberrant plasma cells, and plasma blasts.

myeloma protein

The immunoglobulin synthesized in excess in patients with multiple myeloma (plasmacytoma). Myeloma proteins are products of proliferating plasma cells of a malignant clone. The heavy and light chains are usually assembled to produce the homogeneous monoclonal paraimmunoglobulin, but if the synthesis of light chains is exclusive or exceeds that of heavy chains, a Bence–Jones protein may appear in addition to the paraimmunoglobulin or it may occur alone. A myeloma protein may be a whole molecule of monoclonal immunoglobulin or part of the molecule synthesized by malignant plasma cells.

myelomatosis

A condition in which bone marrow plasma cells undergo malignant transformation and produce excessive homogeneous monoclonal immunoglobulin molecules that represent a paraprotein of a specific immunoglobulin isotype such as IgG or IgA. IgD and IgE myelomas also occur. Serum electrophoresis reveals a clearly demarcated band. Isoelectric focusing shows a classic monoclonal banding pattern. Some patients also have Bence–Jones protein in their urine. Patients are often males past 50 years of age and commonly present with spontaneous bone fracture or anemia due to replacement of bone marrow.

myeloperoxidase

An enzyme present in the azurophil granules of neutrophilic leukocytes that catalyzes peroxidation of many microorganisms. Myeloperoxidase, in conjunction with hydrogen peroxidase and halide, has a bactericidal effect.

myeloperoxidase (MPO) deficiency

A lack of 116-kDa myeloperoxidase in both neutrophils and monocytes. This enzyme is located in the primary granules of neutrophils. It possesses a heme ring that imparts a dark green tint to the molecule. MPO deficiency has an autosomal-recessive mode of inheritance. Affected patients have a mild version of chronic granulomatous disease. *Candida albicans* infections are frequent in this condition.

myelopoiesis

The generation of descendant myeloid lineage cells from hematopoietic stem cells differentiating into common myeloid progenitors in the bone marrow.

myeloproliferative diseases (MPD)

Chronic hematopoietic neoplasms of myeloid lineage cells, including chronic myelogenous leukemia (CML), polycythemia vera, essential thrombocythemia, and myelofibrosis.

myocardial antibodies

Antibodies against myocardium that have been demonstrated in two thirds of coronary artery bypass patients and in Dressler syndrome. Patients with acute rheumatic fever often manifest myocardial antibodies reactive with sarcolemmal, myofibrillar, or intermyofibrillar targets. Dilated cardiomyopathy patients and patients with systemic hypertension/autoimmune polyendocrinopathy may develop autoantibodies against myocardium.

myocardial autoantibodies (MyAs)

Myocardial autoantibody titers increase in approximately two thirds of coronary artery bypass patients, but this is not necessarily related to postcardiotomy syndrome. MyAs with sarcolemmal, intermyofibrillar patterns are demonstrable in most acute rheumatic fever patients. Their molecular mimicry is believed to have a role in pathogenesis. The sera of patients with idiopathic dilated cardiomyopathy react with the adenine nuclear translocator protein, a mitochondrial branched chain α-ketoacid dehydrogenase, cardiac β adrenoreceptor protein, and heat-shock protein (HSP)-60. The autoantigen in Dressler syndrome has not yet been identified.

myogenin (F5D, mouse)

Anti-myogenin monoclonal antibody labels the nuclei of myoblasts in developing muscle tissue, and is expressed in tumor cell nuclei of rhabdomyosarcoma. Positive nuclear staining may occur in Wilm's tumor and some myopathies.

myoglobin

Oxygen-storing muscle protein that serves as a marker of muscle neoplasms, demonstrable by immunoperoxidase staining for surgical pathologic diagnosis.

myoglobin antibody

A reagent that stains normal striated muscle and striated muscle containing tumor. Using immunohistochemical procedures on formalin-fixed, paraffin-embedded tissues, this antibody stains human skeletal and cardiac muscle.

myoid cell

A cell present in the neonatal thymus of humans and other species. It contains skeletal myofibrils.

myositis-associated autoantibodies

Antibodies to the nucleolar antigen PM-Scl are found in patients with features of scleroderma and polymyositis/dermatomyositis. This antibody is specific for a complex of nucleolar proteins. The principal antigen having a molecular mass of 100 kDa is found mainly in Caucasians with overlap syndrome. Antibodies against the Ku antigen are found in a few Japanese patients with overlap syndrome. The Ku antibody is specific for 70- and 80-kDa DNA-binding proteins. Anti-Ku autoantibodies are also found in systemic lupus erythematosus (SLE), dermatomyositis, scleroderma, thyroid disease, and Sjögren's syndrome. Other autoantibodies found in inflammatory myopathies include anti-U_1 RNP, which helps define mixed connective tissue disease (MCTD); high titers of anti-RNP may also be found in inflammatory muscle disease. Autoantibodies against SSA (Ro), antithyroid microsome antibodies, and rheumatoid factor have also been found in myositis syndromes.

myositis-specific autoantibodies

Many patients with idiopathic inflammatory myopathies (IIMs) generate autoantibodies against aminoacyl-transfer (tRNA) synthetases (myositis-specific antibodies) that represent a group of cellular enzymes that catalyze binding of one amino acid to their tRNA. Autoantibodies against eight of these synthetases have been found in IIMs. Jo-1 antibodies specific for histidyl-tRNA synthetase are most common (found in 20 to 30% of IIMs). Aminoacyl-tRNA synthetase autoantibodies are closely associated with interstitial lung disease, arthritis, and Raynaud's phenomenon. Other myositis-specific autoantibodies include those that react with signal recognition particles (SRPs) in acute onset severe myalgic IIM, Mi-2 antibodies reactive with 235- to 240-kDa nuclear antigen in 15 to 25% of dermatomyositis patients, anti-elongation factor Iα autoantibodies, and RNA-reactive autoantibodies.

M

N

N addition

Appending nucleotides by terminal deoxynucleotidyl transferase during D–J joining or V to-D–J joining.

naïve

B and T lymphocytes that have not been exposed to antigen. Also called unprimed or virgin lymphocytes.

naïve B cell

A mature lymphocyte that has exited the bone marrow but has not yet come into contact with the antigen for which it is specific.

naïve lymphocyte

Mature T or B lymphocytes that have never been exposed to antigen and are not derived from antigen-stimulated mature lymphocytes. Exposure of naïve lymphocytes to antigen leads to their differentiation into effector lymphocytes such as antibody-secreting B cells or helper T cells and cytolytic T lymphocytes (CTLs). Lymphocytes that migrate from the central lymphoid organs are naïve (e.g., naïve T cells from the thymus and naïve B cells from the bone marrow). The surface markers and recirculation patterns of naïve lymphocytes differ from those of lymphocytes activated previously. Also termed unprimed or virgin lymphocytes.

naïve T cell

A mature T lymphocyte that has exited the thymus but has not yet come into contact with the antigen for which it is specific.

naked DNA vaccine

An immunizing preparation composed of an isolated DNA plasmid that encodes the vaccine antigen. Following introduction into the host body, the plasmid becomes incorporated into the host cells that form pathogen protein.

NALT

Abbreviation for nasopharynx-associated lymphoid tissue. Refer also to MALT.

NANBH

The principal cause of transfusion-related hepatitis. Risk factors include intravenous drug abuse (42%), unknown risk factors (40%), sexual contact (6%), blood transfusion (6%), household contact (3%), and health professional occupations (2%). Of the 150,000 cases per year in the United States, 30 to 50% become chronic carriers, and one fifth develop cirrhosis. Parental NANBH is usually hepatitis C, and enteric NANBH is usually hepatitis E.

NAP

Neutrophil alkaline phosphatase.

NAP-1

Neutrophil attractant or activation protein-1. Refer to interleukin-8 (IL8).

NAP-2 (neutrophil activating protein 2)

A chemokine of the α (CXC) family. NAP-2 is a proteolytic fragment of platelet basic protein (PBP) corresponding to amino acids 25 to 94. CTAP-III and LA-PF4 or β-TG released from activated platelets are inactive NAP-2 precursors. Leukocytes and leukocyte-derived proteases convert the inactive precursors into NAP-2 by proteolytic cleavage at the N terminus. Platelets represent the tissue source.

naprosyn

A nonsteroidal anti-inflammatory drug (NSAID).

naproxen (2-naphthaleneacetic acid, 6-methoxy-α-methyl)

An anti-inflammatory drug used in the treatment of arthritis, especially rheumatoid arthritis of children and adults, as well as ankylosing spondylitis.

nasopharyngeal-associated lymphoreticular tissue (NALT)

Tissue that includes the palatine and nasopharyngeal tonsils (adenoids) that are mostly covered by squamous epithelium. The palatine tonsils usually contain 10 to 20 crypts that increase their surface area. The deeper regions of these crypts contain M cells that may take up encountered antigens. The tonsils contain all major classes of antigen-presenting cells, including dendritic and Langerhans' cells, macrophages, class I-positive B cells, and antigen-retaining follicular dendritic cells in B cell germinal centers. Approximately one half of tonsillar cells are B lymphocytes situated mainly in follicles containing germinal centers. Immunoglobulin G (IgG) blasts are predominant in germinal centers; plasma cells, in the parafollicular area. Approximately 40% of tonsillar cells are T cells, and more than 98% express the αβ TCR. Higher CD4:CD8 ratios are found in tonsils compared with peripheral blood. The tonsils reveal not only features of mucosal inductive sites but also characteristics of effector sites with high numbers of plasma cells. The role of tonsils in host mucosal immunity following intranasal immunization remains to be determined. NALT also includes diffuse aggregates of lymphocytes in the upper respiratory epithelium.

native immunity

Genetically determined host responsiveness that prevents healthy humans from becoming infected under normal circumstances by selected microorganisms that usually infect animals. This may be altered in the case of profound immunosuppression of humans, as in the case of acquired immune deficiency syndrome (AIDS), in which humans become infected with microorganisms such as *Mycobacterium avium intracellulare*.

natural antibody

Polyreactive antibodies (principally IgM antibodies) found in the serum of an individual who has no known previous contact with that antigen such as by previous immunization or infection with a microorganism containing the antigen. The anti-A and anti-B antibodies related to the ABO blood group system are natural antibodies. Natural antibodies may be consequences of exposure to cross reacting antigens (e.g., ABO blood group antibodies resulting from exposure to bacterial antigens in the gut). Also refers to immunoglobulin M (IgM) antibodies produced by B-1 (CD5⁺) cells specific for microorganisms found in the environment and gastrointestinal tract. The two kinds of natural antibodies in blood sera are (1) specific, antigen-induced antibodies, the synthesis of which depends on external antigenic stimuli and corresponds to acquired specificities; and (2) a type that expresses broad specificity, is genetically determined, and does not depend on a specific antigenic stimulus. Both kinds of natural antibodies of the IgM, IgG, and IgA isotypes specific for many antigens are present in normal sera of humans and other animals. Natural antibodies have a variety of biological functions ranging from physiological to pathological effects. They comprise a component of innate immunity.

natural antiviral immunity

Occurs when virus-infected host cells synthesize type I interferon. This blocks virus replication. Natural killer (NK) cells that are not MHC-restricted provide early antiviral effects following infection. Type I interferon accentuates their action. Both complement and phagocytosis play significant roles in removal of extracellular viruses.

natural autoantibodies

Polyreactive antibodies of low affinity synthesized by CD5+ B cells that compose 10 to 25% of circulating B lymphocytes in normal individuals, 27 to 52% in those with rheumatoid arthritis, and less than 25% in patients with systemic lupus erythematosus (SLE). Natural autoantibodies may appear in first-degree relatives of autoimmune disease patients and in older individuals. They may be predictive of disease in healthy subjects. They are often present in patients with bacterial, viral, or parasitic infections and may have a protective effect. In contrast to natural antibodies, autoantibodies may increase in disease and lead to tissue injury. The blood group isohemagglutins are also considered natural antibodies even though they are believed to be of heterogenetic immune origin as a consequence of stimulation by microbial antigens.

natural cytotoxicity

NK cell cytotoxicity of target cells mediated by perforin and granzyme.

natural cytotoxicity receptors (NCRs)

Activating NK cell receptors that belong to the immunoglobulin family.

natural fluorescence

Autofluorescence.

natural immunity

Innate immune mechanisms that do not depend upon previous exposure to an antigen. Among the factors that contribute to natural resistance are the skin, mucous membranes, and other barriers to infection; lysozyme in tears and other antibacterial molecules; and natural killer (NK) cells.

natural interferon-producing cells (NIPCs)

Refer to interferon-producing cells.

natural killer (NK) cells

Lymphoid cells that recognize nonself molecular configurations with broad specificity. They attack and destroy tumor cells and certain virus-infected cells. They constitute an important part of the natural immune system, do not require prior contact with antigen, and are not major histocompatibility complex (MHC)-restricted by MHC antigens. NK cells are lymphoid cells of the natural immune system that express cytotoxicity against various nucleated cells including tumor cells and virus-infected cells. NK cells, killer (K) cells, and antibody-dependent, cell-mediated cytotoxicity (ADCC) cells induce lysis through the action of antibody. Immunologic

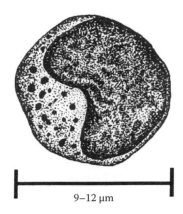

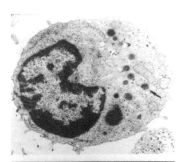

9–12 μm

Natural killer (NK) cell schematic representation.

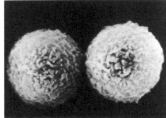

Natural killer (NK) cell schematic representation, transmission and scanning electron microscopy (SEM) of human large granular lymphocyte.

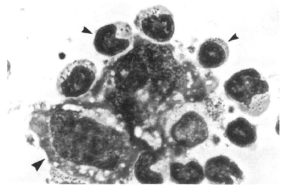

▲ NK cells

▲ K562 Target cell

NK cells.

memory is not involved, as previous contact with the antigen is not necessary for NK cell activity. The NK cell is approximately 15 μm in diameter and has a kidney-shaped nucleus with several, often three, large cytoplasmic granules. The cells are also called large granular lymphocytes (LGLs). In addition to their ability to kill selected tumor cells and some virus-infected cells, they also participate in ADCC by

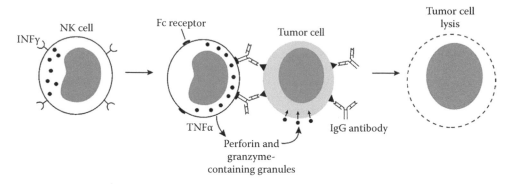

NK-cell-mediated killing of tumor cells by antibody-dependent cell-mediated cytotoxicity.

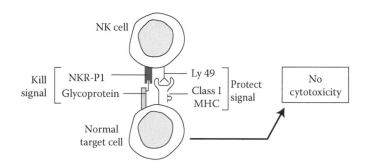

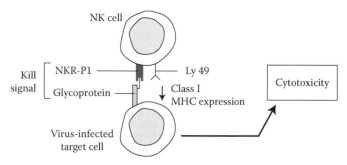

Natural killer (NK) cell cytotoxicity.

anchoring antibody to the cell surface through an Fcγ receptor; thus, they are able to destroy antibody-coated nucleated cells. NK cells are believed to represent a significant part of the natural immune defense against spontaneously developing neoplastic cells and against infection by viruses. NK cell activity is measured by a ^{51}Cr release assay employing the K562 erythroleukemia cell line as a target. NK cells secrete IFN-γ and fail to express antigen receptors such as immunoglobulin receptors or T cell receptors. Cell surface stimulatory receptors and inhibitory receptors that recognize self MHC molecules regulate their activation. NK cells become activated if a target cell that expresses ligands that bind to NK activating receptors does not express MHC class I molecules to interact with NK inhibitory receptors. NK cells are sentinels of natural innate immunity.

natural killer gene complex (NKC)
NK inhibitory/activatory receptor genes, including Ly-49, CD95, CD69, NKG2, and NKRP1 (NK1.1) molecules. This gene cluster is located on chromosome 6 in mice and on chromosome 12 in humans.

natural killer T (NKT) cells
Lymphoid cells that manifest characteristics of both T cells and NK cells. NKT cells bear semi-invariant TCRs that recognize glycolipids or lipid antigens presented in the context of CD1d molecules. Following activation, NKT cells rapidly secrete Th0 cytokines that facilitate activation and differentiation of both B and T cells. Similar to NK cells, NKT cells may also induce cytolysis of target cells.

natural passive immunity
The transfer of immunoglobulin G (IgG) antibodies across the placenta from mother to child.

natural resistance
Refer to natural immunity.

natural suppressor cells
Lymphocytes that demonstrate nonspecific inhibition of some immune responses. They have been found following total irradiation and in neonatal animals. They may share a common lineage and function with NK cells.

naturally acquired immunity

Immunity that develops as a consequence of unplanned and coincidental contact with an antigen, as contrasted with immunity acquired through deliberate immunization.

NCR

Refer to natural cytotoxicity receptor.

necrosis

Cell or tissue death caused by chemical or physical injury as opposed to apoptosis (biologically programmed cell death). Necrosis leaves extensive cellular debris that must be removed by phagocytes; apoptosis does not. "Danger signal" mediators that initiate inflammation may be released from necrotic cells.

necrotaxis

The attraction of leukocytes to dead or injured cells and tissues.

Nef (HIV)

A multifunctional protein in an HIV-infected cell that forces internalization of certain MHC class I, class II, and CD4 molecules mediated by clathrin, disturbs the proton pump needed for endosome acidification, activates intracellular signaling pathways to induce infected cells to promote viral DNA synthesis, upregulates FasL, activates caspase-3, and downregulates survival signaling.

negative induction apoptosis

Negative induction of apoptosis by loss of suppressor activity involves the mitochondria. Release of cytochrome c from the mitochondria into the cytosol serves as a trigger to activate caspases. Permeability of the mitochondrial outer membrane is essential to initiation of apoptosis through this pathway. Proteins belonging to the Bcl-2 family appear to regulate the membrane permeability to ions and possibly to cytochrome c as well. Although these proteins can form channels in membranes, the molecular mechanisms by which they regulate mitochondrial permeability and the solutes released are less clear. The Bcl-2 family is composed of a large group of anti-apoptosis members that when overexpressed prevent apoptosis and pro-apoptosis members that when overexpressed induce apoptosis. The balance between the anti- and pro-apoptotic Bcl-2 family members may be critical to determining whether a cell undergoes apoptosis. Thus, the suppressor activity of the anti-apoptotic Bcl-2 family appears to be negated by the pro-apoptotic members. Many members of the pro-apoptotic Bcl-2 family are present in cells at levels sufficient to induce apoptosis. However, these members do not induce apoptosis because their activity is maintained in a latent form. Bax is present in the cytosols of live cells. After an appropriate signal, Bax undergoes a conformational change and moves to the mitochondrial membrane where it causes release of mitochondrial cytochrome c into the cytosol. BID is also present in the cytosols of live cells. After cleavage by caspase-8, it moves to the mitochondria where it causes release of cytochrome c, possibly by altering the conformation of Bax. Similarly, BAK appears to undergo a conformational change that converts it from an inactive to an active state. Thus, understanding the molecular mechanisms responsible for regulating the Bcl-2 family activities creates the potential for pharmaceutical intervention to control apoptosis. The viability of many cells is dependent on a constant or intermittent supply of cytokines or growth factors. In the absence of an apoptosis-suppressing cytokine, cells may undergo apoptosis. BAD is a pro-apoptotic member of the Bcl-2 family and is sequestered in the cytosol when cytokines are present. Cytokine binding can activate PI3 kinase, which phosporylates Akt/PKB, which in turn phosphorylates BAD. Phosphorylated BAD is sequestered in the cytosol by the 14-3-3 protein. Removal of the cytokine turns the kinase pathway off, the phosphorylation state of BAD shifts to the dephosphorylated form, and dephosphorylated BAD causes release of cytochrome c from the mitochondria.

negative phase

The decrease in antibody titer immediately following injection of a second or booster dose of antigen to an animal previously given a primary injection of the same antigen. Following this initial drop of preformed antibody in the circulation, there is a rapid and pronounced rise in antibody titer, representing immunologic memory.

negative selection

The process whereby thymocytes that recognize self antigens in the context of self major histocompatibility complex (MHC) undergo clonal deletion (apoptosis) or clonal anergy (inactivation). The resulting cell population is self MHC-restricted and self antigen-tolerant (refer to positive selection). Developing thymocytes in the thymus, whose TCRs show high affinity/avidity for self-peptide complexed to self MHC presented by thymic epithelial cells, undergo apoptosis. Negative selection of NK T cells also occurs in the thymus. Autoreactive B cells undergo a similar process in the bone marrow. Autoreactive B cells, whose BCRs have high affinity/avidity for self antigens present on bone marrow stromal cells, are induced to undergo apoptosis.

NEHJ pathway

Refer to non-homologous end-joining pathway.

Neisser–Wechsberg phenomenon

The deviation of complement by antibody. Although complement does not react with antigen alone, it demonstrates weak affinity for unreacted antibody.

***Neisseria* immunity**

Even though patients with gonococcal infection develop increased levels of serum and mucosal antibody of immunoglobulin G (IgG) and IgA classes reactive with gonococcal surface antigens, they are subject to repeated episodes of urogenital infections; thus, natural infection does not confer protective immunity. The surface antigens may be antigenically heterogeneous or this phenomenon may be attributable to the brevity of the mucosal antibody response and the lack of activity of serum antibody in the mucosal infection. Attachment and colonization of the mucosa with gonococci during their encounter with polymorphonuclear neutrophils (PMNs) play important roles. Protective immunity against meningococcal infection is associated with complement-dependent, bactericidal serum antibodies specific for capsular polysaccharide. Cell-mediated immunity does not appear to have a significant role. There is no successful gonococcal vaccine. Polysaccharide vaccines to protect against *N. meningitidis* of serogroups A and C induce protective bactericidal antibodies. The current vaccine contains polysaccharide from serogroups A, C, Y, and W-135. Polysaccharide A and C vaccine is conjugated to tetanus toxoid or another protein carrier to enhance immunogenicity in young children. Polysaccharide vaccines may not induce protection in serogroup B meningococcal disease. Protection against these strains may be linked to antibody specific for outer membrane proteins that can be used to induce immunity.

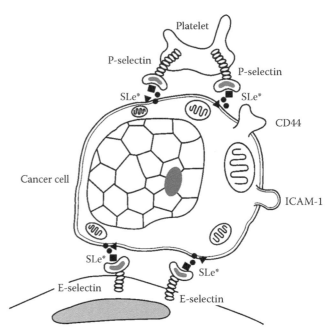

Nelfinavir mesylate (Viracept). A powerful HIV-1 protease inhibitor, effective orally, used together with HIV reverse transcriptase inhibitors to treat HIV infection.

N-formyl peptide receptor (FPR)

A member of the G protein coupled receptor family, the chemokine receptor branch of the rhodopsin family. Tissue sources include HL-60 cells differentiated with Bt2 cAMP. Undifferentiated HL-60 cells transfected with FPR bound FMLP with two affinities. COS7 cells transfected with FPR bound FMLPK-Pep12 with low and high affinity. The receptor is expressed in neutrophils. Dibutyryl cAMP includes FPR transcription in HL-60 cells.

neoantigen

Modification of proteins by phosphorylation or specific proteolysis may change their covalent architecture to yield new antigenic determinants or epitopes termed neoantigens; a neoantigen is also an epitope newly expressed on cells during development or in neoplasia. Neoantigens include tumor-associated antigens. New antigenic determinants may also emerge when a protein changes conformation or when a molecule is split, exposing previously unexpressed epitopes. A neoantigen may be produced by the union of a xenobiotic with a self protein.

neonatal Fc receptor (FcRn)

An Fc receptor is specific for immunoglobulin G (IgG) that facilitates the transport of maternal IgG across the placenta and the neonatal intestinal epithelium. FcRn is similar to a class I molecule. An adult variety of this receptor protects plasma IgG antibodies from catabolism.

neonatal immunity

Resistance in the newborn attributable to maternal circulating antibodies that reached the fetus via the placenta or maternal secretory antibodies translated to the newborn in breast milk. The quality and quantity of both humoral and cellular immune responses of neonates differ from those of adults. These differences may be a consequence of the lower incidence and decreased function of immunocompetent cells, such as B cells, T cells, and antigen-presenting cells early in ontogeny. Restriction of T and B cell function early in ontogeny compared with function in the adult may be due partially to limitations in the diversity of antigen-specific repertoires. Differences in responses to various types of activation by neonatal and adult lymphocytes also affect immunity. A type of passive immunization.

neonatal thymectomy syndrome

Refer to wasting disease.

neonatal tolerance

The concept that immunologic tolerance to an antigen is established more easily in neonates than in mature animals. Attributable to functional immaturity and decreased numbers of neonatal T and B lymphocytes, dendritic cells, macrophages, and follicular dendritic cells, as well as modified patterns of lymphocyte recirculation.

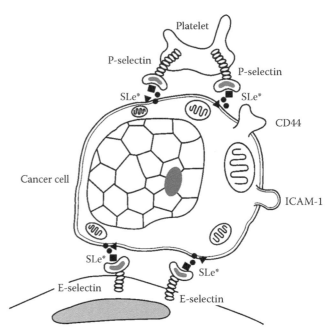

Tumor cell attached through E-selectin molecules to endothelial cell surface.

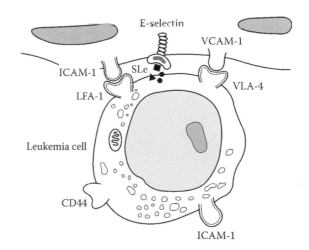

Leukemia cell attached to endothelial cell surface via adhesion molecules.

neoplasm

Any new and abnormal growth that may be a benign or malignant tumor.

neopterin

A guanosine triphosphate metabolite synthesized by macrophages following their stimulation by interferon-γ (IFN-γ) from activated T lymphocytes. Neopterin levels in both serum and urine of patients infected with HIV-1 rise as the infection progresses. The increase in neopterin along with

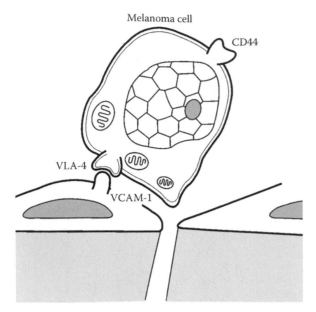

Melanoma cell attached to endothelial cell surface through VLA-4–VCAM-1 interaction.

diminishing CD4 lymphocyte levels reflects the progression of HIV-1 infection to clinical AIDS.

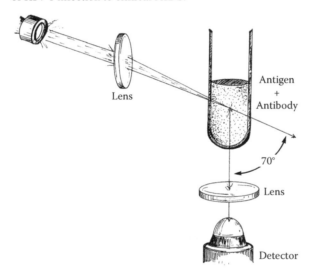

Nephelometry.

nephelometry

A technique to assay proteins and other biological materials through the formation of a precipitate of antigen and homologous antibody. The assay depends on the turbidity or cloudiness of a suspension and is based on determination of the degree to which light is scattered when a helium–neon laser beam is directed through the suspension. The antigen concentration is ascertained using a standard curve devised from the light scatter produced by solutions of known antigen concentration. This method is used by many clinical immunology laboratories for the quantification of complement components and immunoglobulins in patients' sera or other body fluids.

nephritic factor

C3 nephritic factor (C3NeF) is found in the sera of patients with type II membranoproliferative glomerulonephritis (i.e., dense-deposit disease). This factor can activate the alternate complement pathway; it is an immunoglobulin that interacts with alternate complement pathway C3 convertase and stabilizes it. Thus, it activates the pathway and leads to the generation of biologically active complement fragments. C3NeF is an autoantibody against alternate pathway C3 convertase. Membranoproliferative glomerulonephritis patients have a genetic predisposition to develop the disease. The excessive C3 consumption leads to hypocomplementemia.

nephritic factor autoantibodies

The most frequently encountered of the four types of autoantibodies reactive with the complement system in membranoproliferative glomerulonephritis (MPGN) are antibodies to a neoepitope on the Bb moiety of C3bBb (properdin-independent C3NeF). These autoantibodies are designated C3NeF (or as Nfa, NFII, or C3bBb stabilizing factor). They belong to the immunoglobulin G (IgG) or IgM class and are found in type II (dense-deposit) MPGN. They have also been found in partial lipodystrophy (PLD), post-streptococcal glomerulonephritis, systemic lupus erythematosus, idiopathic rapidly progressive glomerulonephritis, and rarely in MPGN types I and III. The sera of patients with MPGN contain anti-idiotypic antibodies. C3NeF (Nfa) interaction with inhomologous antigen induces prolonged *in vitro* C3bBb C3-cleaving activity half-life and decreased serum C3 concentrations. The presence of these antibodies is used to distinguish types of MPGN and monitor treatment.

nephritic syndrome

A clinical complex of acute onset characterized by hematuria with red cell and hemoglobin casts in the urine, oliguria, azotemia, and hypertension. There may be limited proteinuria. Inflammatory reactions within glomeruli cause injury to capillary walls which permits the release of erythrocytes into the urine. Acute diffuse proliferative glomerulonephritis is an example of a primary glomerular disease associated with acute nephritic syndrome.

nephrotic syndrome

A clinical complex that consists of massive proteinuria with the loss of greater than 3.5 g of protein per day, generalized edema, hypoalbuminemia (i.e., <3 g/dL), hyperlipidemia, and lipiduria. Nephrotic syndrome in children often follows lipoid nephrosis; in adults it is frequently associated with membranous glomerulopathy. Both are primary glomerular diseases.

network hypothesis

Niels Jerne's theory that anti-idiotypic antibodies form in response to the antigen-binding regions of antibody molecules or of lymphocyte surface receptors. These in turn elicit anti-anti-idiotypic antibodies, etc. Each new immune response stimulated in this network interrupts the finely tuned immune network balance as anti-idiotype antibodies are produced, eventually downregulating the response and bringing it back to homeostasis.

network theory

A hypothesis proposed by Niels Jerne that explains immunoregulation through a network of idiotype–anti-idiotype reactions involving T cell receptors and the antigen-binding (paratope) regions of antibody molecules. Exposure to antigens interrupts the delicate balance of the idiotype–anti-idiotype network, leading to the increased synthesis of some idiotypes and the corresponding anti-idiotypes, modulating the response. Anti-idiotypes occur following immunization against selected antigens and may prevent the response to

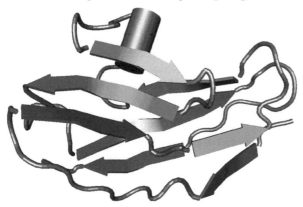

Jerne network theory.

the antigen. Selected anti-idiotypic antibodies have binding sites similar to the immunizing epitopes known as internal images of the epitopes. Other anti-idiotypic antibodies are directed to idiotopes of the antigen-binding region and are not internal images. Anti-idiotypic antibodies with internal images may be substituted for an antigen, leading to specific antigen-binding antibodies. These are the bases for so-called idiotypic vaccines in which an individual is never exposed to the infecting agent. Anti-idiotypes may also block T cell receptors for the corresponding antigen.

Neural cell adhesion molecule L1 (NCAM-L1).

neural cell adhesion molecule L1 (NCAM-L1)

Member of the immunoglobulin gene superfamily. Although originally identified in the nervous system, NCAM-L1 is also expressed in hematopoietic and epithelial cells. It may function in cell–cell and cell–matrix interactions. It can support homophilic NCAM-L1–NCAM-L1 and integrin cell binding and bind with high affinity to the neural proteoglycan neurocan. NCAM-L1 promotes neurite outgrowth by functioning in neurite extension.

neuraminidase

An enzyme that cleaves the glycosidic bond between neuraminic acid and other sugars. Neuraminic acid is a critical constituent of multiple cell-surface glycoproteins and confers a negative charge on the cells. Cells treated with neuraminidase agglutinate more readily than do normal cells because of the diminished Coulombic forces between them. Cells treated with neuraminidase activate the alternate complement pathway. Neuraminidase is produced by myxoviruses, paramyxoviruses, and such bacteria as *Clostridium perfringens* and *Vibrio cholerae*. Neuraminidase and hemagglutinin are found on the spikes of the influenza virus.

neurofilament

A marker, demonstrable by immunoperoxidase staining, for neural-derived tumors and selected endocrine neoplasms with neural differentiation.

neurofilament (2F11), mouse antibody

Neurofilament antibody stains an antigen localized in a number of neural, neuroendocrine, and endocrine tumors. Neuromas, ganglioneuromas, gangliogliomas, ganglion-euroblastomas, and neuroblastomas stain positively for neurofilament. Neurofilament is also present in paragangliomas and adrenal and extraadrenal pheochromocytomas. Carcinoids, neuroendocrine carcinomas of the skin, and oat cell carcinomas of the lung also express neurofilament.

neuroleukin

A cytokine synthesized in the brain and in T lymphocytes as a 56-kDa protein that shares sequence homology with the gp120 of HIV-1 and with phosphohexose isomerase. Thus, the ability of the gp120 of the AIDS virus to compete with neuroleukin for the neuroleukin receptor may be associated with AIDS dementia.

neurological autoimmune diseases

Disorders that can alter function of the nerve–muscle junction. Nerve–muscle junction disorders include myasthenia gravis and Lambert–Eaton syndrome. Guillain-Barré syndrome is an example of a peripheral nerve disorder. Multiple sclerosis and post-infectious vaccination encephalomyelitis are examples of central nervous system disorders.

neuromuscular junction autoimmunity

The three autoantibody-mediated disorders of the neuromuscular junction include: (1) myasthenia gravis (MG), a disorder in which antibodies lead to loss of muscle acetylcholine receptors (AChRs)—a disease that satisfies all Witebsky's criteria for antibody-mediated autoimmune diseases listed elsewhere in this volume; (2) the Lambert–Eaton myasthenic syndrome (LEMS), an antibody-mediated presynaptic disease in which the target is the nerve terminal voltage-gated calcium channel that meets two of Witebsky's criteria; and (3) acquired neuromyotonia (Isaacs' syndrome), a disorder induced by autoantibodies against voltage-gated potassium channels in peripheral motor nerves, resulting in increased excitability and continuous muscle fiber activity that satisfies two of Witebsky's criteria.

neuronal antibodies

Antibodies present in the cerebrospinal fluids of approximately three fourths of patients who have systemic lupus erythematosus (SLE) with neuropsychiatric manifestations; 11% of SLE patients who do not manifest neuropsychiatric disease also develop neuronal antibodies. Neuronal antibodies are identified by their interactions with human neuroblastoma cell lines. The presence of neuronal antibodies generally indicates central nervous system (CNS) SLE. The lack of neuronal antibodies in the serum and cerebrospinal fluid mitigates against CNS involvement in SLE patients.

neuronal autoantibodies

Autoantibodies that react with neuroblastoma cell surface antigens present in 75% of SLE cases with neuropsychiatric

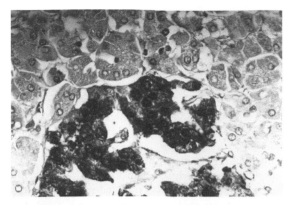

Neuron-specific enolase (immunoperoxidase stain).

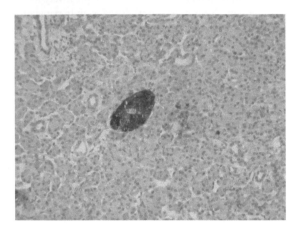

Neuron-specific enolase (NSE)—pancreas.

manifestations, in Raynaud's phenomenon, and in antiphospholipid syndromes. They may be detected by flow cytometry, but their clinical usefulness remains to be determined.

neuron-specific enolase (NSE)
An enzyme of neurons and neuroendocrine cells and their derived tumors (e.g., oat cell carcinoma of lung) demonstrable by immunoperoxidase staining. NSE also occurs in some neoplasms not derived from neurons or endocrine cells.

neuron-specific enolase (NSE) antibody
A murine monoclonal antibody directed against γ-γ enolase present on most human neurons, normal and neoplastic neuroendocrine cells, and some megakarocytes. This reagent may be used to aid in the identification of cells of neural or neuroendocrine lineage. The antibody is intended for qualitative staining in sections of formalin-fixed, paraffin-embedded tissue. Anti-NSE antibody specifically binds to the γ-γ enolase located in the cytoplasms of normal and neoplastic neuroendocrine cells. Unexpected antigen expression or loss of expression may occur, especially neoplasms. Occasionally stromal elements surrounding heavily stained tissue and/or cells will show immunoreactivity. The clinical interpretation of staining or its absence must be complemented by morphological studies and evaluation of proper controls.

neuropeptides
Substances that associate the nervous system with the inflammatory response. Neuropeptides serve as inflammatory mediators released from neurons in response to local tissue injury. They include substance P, vasoactive intestinal peptide, somatostatin, and calcitonin-gene-related peptide.

Multiple immunomodulatory activities have been attributed to these substances.

neuropilin
A cell surface protein that is a receptor for the collapsin/semaphorin family of neuronal guidance proteins.

neurotoxin
An exotoxin that can interfere with the conduction of a nerve impulse or block transmission at the synapse by linking to a voltage-gated Na^{2+} channel protein. *Corynebacterium diphtheriae*, *Clostridium tetani*, *C. botulinum*, and *Shigella dysenteriae* produce neurotoxins. Conotoxin is an example of another neurotoxin.

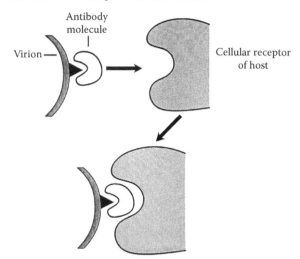

Neutralizing antibody molecules.

neutralization
The inactivation of a microbial product such as a toxin by antibody or counteraction of the infectivity of a microorganism, especially the neutralization of viruses. Antibody binding to viral antigen physically blocks its binding to and infecting a host cell.

neutralization test
An assay based on the ability of antibody to inactivate the biological effects of an antigen or of a microorganism expressing it. Neutralization applies especially to inactivation of virus infectivity or of the biological activity of a microbial toxin.

neutralizing antibody
Refer to neutralization and neutralization test.

neutropenia
A diminished number of polymorphonuclear neutrophilic leukocytes in the peripheral blood circulation.

neutrophil activating factor 1
Interleukin-8 (IL8).

neutrophil activating peptide 2 (NAP-2)
A 75-amino acid chemokine produced by the proteolysis of β-thromboglobulin (β-TG) by neutrophil cathepsin-G. It can activate neutrophils and monocytes by binding to their interleukin-8 (IL8) type B receptors. NAP-2 has about 60% amino acid sequence similarity with platelet factor 4 (PF-4). It is believed to augment inflammation by cooperative interactions between platelets and neutrophils. Autoantibodies against NAP-2 and IL8 have been identified in heparin-associated thrombocytopenia, but their clinical significance remains to be determined.

neutrophil activating protein 1 (NAP-1)

Former term for interleukin-8 (IL8).

neutrophil activating protein 2 (NAP-2)

A chemokine of the α (CXC) family, NAP-2 is a proteolytic fragment of PBP corresponding to amino acids 25 through 94. CTAP-III and LA-PF4 or β-TG released from activated platelets are inactive NAP-2 precursors. Leukocytes and leukocyte-derived proteases convert the inactive precursors into NAP-2 by proteolytic cleavage at the N terminus.

neutrophil attracting peptide 2 (NAP-2)

Chemoattractant of neutrophils to sites of platelet aggregation. NAP-2 competes weakly with interleukin-8 (IL8) for the IL8 type II receptor. However, because it can be found at much higher concentrations than IL8 at platelet aggregation sites, NAP-2 is considered an active participant in the inflammatory process.

neutrophil chemotaxis

Refer to chemotaxis and chemotactic factors.

neutrophil cytoplasmic antibodies

Autoantibodies specific for myeloid-specific lysosomal enzymes. Antineutrophil cytoplasmic antibodies (ANCAs) are of two types. The cANCA variety stains the cytoplasm where it reacts with α granule proteinase-3 (PR-3). By contrast, pANCA stains the perinuclear zone through its reaction with myeloperoxidase (MPO). Of patients with Wegener's granulomatosis with generalized active disease, 84 to 100% develop cANCA, although fewer individuals with the limited form of Wegener's granulomatosis develop these antibodies. Organ involvement cannot be predicted from the identification of cANCA or pANCA antibodies. pANCA antibodies reactive with MPO may be found in patients with certain vasculitides including Churg–Strauss syndrome, polyarteritis nodosa, microscopic polyarteritis, and polyangiitis. A pANCA staining pattern unrelated to antibodies against PR-3 or MPO has been described in inflammatory bowel disease (IBD); 59 to 84% of ulcerative colitis patients and 65 to 84% of primary sclerosing cholangitis patients are positive for pANCA. By contrast, only 10 to 20% of patients with Crohn's disease are positive for it. These antibodies are classified as neutrophil nuclear antibodies (ANAs). Hep-2 cells are used to differentiate granulocyte-specific ANAs from ANAs that are not tissue-specific.

neutrophil leukocyte

A peripheral blood polymorphonuclear leukocyte derived from the myeloid lineage. Neutrophils comprise 40 to 75% of the total white blood count, numbering 2500 to 7500 cells per cubic millimeter. They are phagocytic and have multilobed nuclei and azurophilic and specific granules that appear lilac following staining with Wright's or Giemsa stains. They may be attracted to a local site by such chemotactic factors as C5a. They are the principal cells of acute inflammation and actively phagocytize invading microorganisms. Besides serving as the first line of cellular defense in infection, they participate in such reactions as the uptake of antigen–antibody complexes in the Arthus reaction. The neutrophil leukocyte expresses Fc receptors and can participate in antibody-dependent cell-mediated cytoxicity. It has the capacity to phagocytize microorganisms and digest them enzymatically.

neutrophil microbicidal assay

A test that assesses the capacity of polymorphonuclear neutrophil leukocytes to kill intracellular bacteria.

neutrophil nicotinamide adenine dinucleotide phosphate oxidase

Refer to chronic granulomatous disease.

neutrophilia

Significantly elevated numbers of neutrophils in the blood circulation.

neutrophils

Leukocytes. Also called polymorphonuclear cells (PMNs).

Newcastle disease

Follicular conjunctivitis induced by an avian paramyxovirus that blocks the oxidative burst in phagocytes. Cytokines that produce fever are formed. Recovery occurs in approximately 1 to 2 weeks. In birds, the agent induces pneumoencephalitis, which is fatal.

Newcastle disease vaccine

(1) An inactivated virus raised in chick embryos that is incorporated into aluminum hydroxide gel adjuvant. (2) A live virus grown in chick embryos and attenuated in a graded manner. Strains with medium virulence are administered parenterally; less virulent strains are given to birds in drinking water as aerosols.

New Zealand black (NZB) mice

An inbred strain of mice that serve as animal models of autoimmune hemolytic anemia. They develop antinuclear

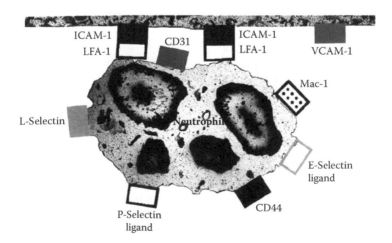

Neutrophil leukocyte.

antibodies in low titer and have defective T lymphocytes, defects in DNA repair, and B cells that are spontaneously activated.

New Zealand white (NZW) mice

An inbred strain of white mice that, when mated with the NZB strain (that develops autoimmunity), produces an F_1 generation of NZB/NZW mice that represent animal models of autoimmune disease and especially of a lupus erythematosus (LE)-like condition.

Nezelof's syndrome

Hypoplasia of the thymus leading to a failure of the T lymphocyte compartment with no T cells and no T cell function. By contrast, B lymphocyte function remains intact. Thus, this syndrome is classified as a T lymphocyte immunodeficiency.

NFAT (nuclear factor of activated T cells)

A transcription factor activated as a consequence of T cell receptor signaling. It acts as a complex of the NFAT protein with the dimer of Fos and Jun proteins called AP-1.

NFc (nephritic factor of classical pathway)

Binds to a neoantigen of the C4b2a complex and is associated with low C4 and C3 concentrations. It is found in patients with membranoproliferative glomerulonephritis (MPGN) type I, acute post-infectious glomerulonephritis, systemic lupus erythematosus (SLE), and chronic glomerulonephritis.

NFid3 nuclear factor KB

A transcription factor that facilitates immune system gene expression.

N-formylmethionine

An amino acid that initiates all bacterial proteins but no mammalian proteins other than those produced within mitochondria. It alerts the innate immune system to infection of the host. Neutrophils express specific receptors for N-formylmethionine-containing peptides. These receptors mediate neutrophil activation.

NF-κB

A group of heterodimeric transcription factors comprised of two chains of 50 and 65 kDa. Activation follows engagement of BCR, TCR, and multiple cytokine/growth factor receptors. Under physiologic conditions, NFκB is found in the cytosol, where it is bound to a chain termed $I_\kappa B$, an inhibitor of NF-κB transcription. Engagement of the receptor induces intracellular signaling that activates the IKK kinase, which phosphorylates IκB, inducing its degradation. Entrance of NF-κB into the nucleus and binding to κB DNA binding motif induces new gene transcription.

NFt (C3bBb-P stabilizing factor)

An autoantibody to alternate pathway C3 convertase present in patients with membranoproliferative glomerulonephritis (MPGN) types 1 and 3. Ft activity in these patients is inversely correlated with serum C3 concentrations.

NHEJ pathway

Refer to nonhomologous end joining pathway.

nick translation

A technique used to make a radioactive probe of a DNA segment. Nick translation signifies the movement of a nick (i.e., single-stranded break in the double-stranded helix) along a duplex DNA molecule.

NIP (4-hydroxy,5-iodo,3-nitrophenylacetyl)

Used as a hapten in experimental immunology.

NIPC

Refer to interferon-producing cell.

nitric oxide (NO)

A biological molecule with multiple effects, including an important role in intracellular signaling and functioning in macrophages as a powerful microbicidal agent against ingested microorganisms. Also acts as a neurotransmitter and an agent that maintains hemodynamic stability. Its role in human host defense has been controversial. Nitrite has been generated in human macrophage cultures in response to tumor necrosis factor α (TNF-α) and granulocyte–macrophage colony-stimulating factor (GM-CSF), together with avirulent mycobacterial strains. High levels of nitric oxide synthesis have been shown in response to a select group of stimuli. Interferes with the citric acid cycle and microbial enzymes that contain iron or sulfur atoms. Inhibits virus replication.

nitric oxide (NO) and reactive oxygen species (ROS)

Reactive oxygen species (ROS) break down to form or generate free radicals. Cells possess elaborate systems to scavenge free radicals. When free radicals exceed the capacity of these systems, however, cells die. Cell death induced by free radicals has characteristics of both apoptosis and necrosis. The most compelling observation that cell death resulting from free radicals is related to the apoptotic process is found at the level of the mitochondria. The antiapoptotic Bcl-2 protein inhibits cell death in response to free radicals. The mechanisms involved are not fully understood. Radical-induced cell death may involve the mitochondrial permeability transition pore. Bcl-2 has been observed to be located near the pore in the mitochondrial membrane. Nitric oxide (NO) is produced by iNOS, eNOS, and nNOS. It is a biological signaling molecule that elicits numerous biochemical responses. Reports suggest that NO may affect key proteins or signaling pathways involved in apoptosis. Based on the rapidly expanding roles for signaling through the generation of NO, NO may exert important influences on apoptosis.

nitric oxide synthetase

An enzyme or family of enzymes that synthesizes the vasoactive and microbicidal nitric oxide from l-arginine. The activation of macrophages by microorganisms or cytokines can induce a form of this enzyme.

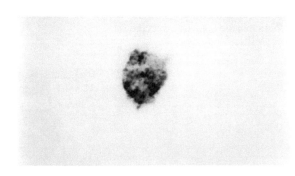

Nitroblue tetrazolium (NBT) test.

nitroblue tetrazolium (NBT) test

An assay that evaluates the hexose monophosphate shunt in phagocytic cells. The soluble yellow NBT dye is taken up by neutrophils and monocytes during phagocytosis. In normal neutrophils, NBT is reduced by enzymes to insoluble, dark blue formazan crystals within cells. Neutrophils from patients with chronic granulomatous disease are unable to reduce NBT. The ability to reduce NBT to the insoluble formazan crystals depends on the generation of superoxide in the neutrophil tested.

Nijmegen breakage syndrome (NBS)

A primary immunodeficiency including variable hypogammaglobulinemia and CID. Ionizing radiation of patient cells reveals significant levels of chromosomal defects. Induced by mutations in the gene that encodes nibrin, a protein associated with the NHEJ pathway of DNA repair.

NK1.1

A natural killer (NK) cell alloantigen identified in selected inbred mouse strains such as C57BL/6 mice.

NK1.1 CD4 T cells

A minor T cell subset that expresses the NK1.1 marker, a molecule usually present on natural killer cells. NK1.1 T lymphocytes also express α:β T cell receptors of limited diversity and coreceptor molecule CD4 or no coreceptor. They are present in abundance in the liver and synthesize cytokines soon after stimulation.

NK1-T cell

A lymphocyte that shares certain characteristics with T cells such as T cell receptors in addition to those of natural killer cells.

NK activatory receptors

ITAM-bearing receptors which, when engaged with inhibitory receptor interaction, lead to natural cytotoxicity and cytotoxic cytokine secretion by NK cells causing deaths of target cells bereft of self MHC class I molecules. The group includes NCR, KAR, NKG2D, -C and –E and Ly-49D, -H, -P and –W.

NK cell lectin-like receptors

One of the two principal structural classes of NK cell activating and inhibitory receptors.

NK cells

Refer to natural killer cells.

NK inhibitory receptors

ITIM-bearing receptors that, when engaged by self-MHC class I molecules on a target, dampen the effects of NK activatory receptor engagement, thereby inhibiting destruction of target cells. Includes KIRs; Ly-49A, -B, -C, -E, -F, -G, Ly-49I: NKG2A and –B; and IL-T2.

NK/T precursor

Common lymphoid progenitor derived predecessor capable of differentiating into T or NK cells but not B cells.

NKT

Refer to natural killer T cells.

NKT cell

A lymphoid cell that is intermediate between T lymphocytes and natural killer (NK) cells with respect to morphology and granule content. Lymphoid cells may be CD4⁻8⁻ or CD4⁺8⁻ weakly expressed α:β T cell receptors (TCRs) with an invariant α chain and highly restricted β chain specificity. They have a powerful capacity to synthesize interleukin-4 (IL4). Many of these TCRs recognize antigens presented by the nonclassical major histocompatibility complex (MHC)-like CD1 molecule. Their surface NK1.1 receptors are lectin-like and are believed to recognize microbial carbohydrates.

NK tolerance

Fostered during NK cell development through selection of only NK clones bearing NK inhibitory receptors that are capable of recognizing self-MHC and sending a strong

enough signal to overcome NK activatory receptory signaling induced by host cells.

N-linked oligosaccharide

An oligosaccharide covalently linked to asparagine residues in protein molecules. N-linked oligosaccharide manifests a branched core structure composed of two N-acetylglucosamine residues and three mannose residues. The three types differ on the basis of their exterior branches: (1) high-mannose oligosaccharide reveals two to six additional mannose residues linked to the polysaccharide core; (2) complex oligosaccharide composed of two to five terminal branches that consist of N-acetylglucosamine, galactose, often N-acetylneuraminic acid, and occasionally fucose or another sugar; and (3) hybrid molecules that reveal characteristics of high mannose and complex oligosaccharides.

N nucleotides

Nontemplated nucleotides that terminal deoxynucleotidyl transferase (TdT) adds to the 3′ cut ends of V, D, and J coding segments during rearrangement. They are added to junctions between V, D, and J gene segments in immunoglobulin or T cell receptor genes during lymphocyte development. When as many as 20 of these nucleotides are added, the diversity of the antibody and T cell receptor repertoires is expanded.

Nocardia immunity

Infection by microorganisms of this genus usually begins as a pulmonary infection that may be localized or disseminated. Nocardia species have complex antigenic structures. Immunocompromised patients face increased likelihood of developing nocardial infections. Defects in the mononuclear phagocyte system increase host susceptibility. The microorganisms grow in monocytes and macrophages. T cells of mice immunized against whole cells of Nocardia species become immunologically reactive against the microorganism and kill it directly. T cell-deficient athymic mice show increased susceptibility to nocardial infection, but B cell-deficient mice do not. Thus, T cells rather than B cells are critical for host immunity against nocardial infection. No effective vaccine against Nocardia is currently available.

NOD (nonobese diabetic) mouse

A mutant mouse strain that spontaneously develops type I insulin-dependent diabetes mellitus, an autoimmune disease; the strain exhibits an autosomal-recessive pattern of inheritance for the NOD mutation. Lymphocytes infiltrate NOD mouse islets of Langerhans in the pancreas and kill β cells. Humans with insulin-dependent diabetes mellitus have defects in the HLA-DQ parts of the major histocompatibility complex (MHC) class II region. There is also a defect in the class II IA region of murine MHC class II. A major DNA segment is missing from the NOD mouse MHC IE region. When the IE segment is inserted or the IA defect is corrected in these mice, disease progression is halted. This strain represents a significant animal model for human type I diabetes mellitus.

NOD proteins

Nucleotide-binding oligomerization domain proteins. Cytoplasmic pattern recognition molecules capable of detecting intracellular pathogen products. Related structurally to Toll-like receptors. NOD protein engagement leads to expression of pro-inflammatory cytokines.

NON mouse

The normal control mouse for use in studies involving the NOD mouse strain that spontaneously develops type I (insulin-dependent) diabetes mellitus. The two strains differ only in genes associated with the development of diabetes. Nonobese normal mouse.

non-A non-B hepatitis

Refer to hepatitis, non-A and non-B.

non-classical Hodgkin lymphoma

Nodular lymphocyte-predominant Hodgkin lymphoma that comprises 5% of all Hodgkin lymphomas. The neoplastic cells are CD30-, CD15-, CD19+, and CD20+ popcorn cells.

non-Hodgkin lymphoma (NHL)

All lymphoid neoplasms without the characteristics of Hodgkin disease constitute non-Hodgkin lymphomas. They are monoclonal lymphoid neoplasms that are very heterogeneous morphologically, antigenically, and with respect to kinetic phenotypes. They also differ greatly in clinical expression. They are divided into low, intermediate, and high grade. Low grade lymphomas are treated conservatively. Intermediate and high grade lymphomas are aggressive and are appropriately treated. T lymphocyte, B lymphocyte, and NULL cell lymphomas make up the NHL group. Tumor derived from a transformed peripheral B cell or occasionally a transformed peripheral T cell. A heterogeneous group of neoplasms that include precursor B lymphoblastic leukemia/lymphoma, mantle cell lymphoma, B cell chronic lymphocytic leukemia, follicular lymphoma, mucosa-associated lymphoid tissue lymphoma, diffuse large cell lymphoma, Burkitt's lymphoma, precursor T lymphoblastic leukemia/lymphoma, adult T cell leukemia/lymphoma, mycosis fungoides, Sezary syndrome, anaplastic large cell lymphomas, angio-immunoblastic T cell lymphoma, and peripheral T cell lymphoma (unspecified.)

nonadherent cell

A cell that fails to stick to a surface such as a culture flask. A lymphocyte is an example. Conversely, macrophages readily adhere to the glass surfaces of tissue culture flasks.

noncovalent forces

Include hydrogen bonding, ionic or Coulombic bonding, Van der Waals interactions, hydrophobic bonding, and steric repulsion forces that are extremely sensitive to distances between interacting groups. Although charged on antigen–antibody binding, these forces may play a very important role in determining the stability of the antigen–antibody complex. The literature differs on the issue of whether charged antigens elicit antibodies of reciprocal charge effect per se or if the effect is exerted by the microenvironment of the antigen and antibody molecules and not so much by the net of the molecules as a whole.

noncytopathic virus

A virus that appropriates cellular functions and reproduction without injuring the host cell.

nondeletional tolerance

The development of donor-specific tolerance without a discernible change in anti-donor reactivity *in vitro*. Nondeletional tolerance develops to antigen-presenting cell (APC)-depleted islet or thyroid allografts.

nonhomologous end-joining (NEHJ) pathway

A DNA repair pathway possessed by all cells that repairs double-stranded DNA breaks without the requirement for DNA sequence homology between the ends to be joined. The DNA ends are merely ligated back together. Some of the proteins that participate in V(D)J recombination are involved.

nonimmunologic classic pathway activators

Selected microorganisms such as *Escherichia coli* and low-virulence *Salmonella* strains and certain viruses such as parainfluenza react with C1q and lead to C1 activation without antibody which represents classic pathway activation that facilitates defense mechanisms. Various other substances such as myelin basic protein, denatured bacterial endotoxin, heparin, and urate crystal surfaces may also directly activate the classic complement pathway.

nonmyeloablative conditioning

A diminished level of chemotherapy that induces only partial depletion of the bone marrow as part of the conditioning process prior to transplantation.

nonobese normal mice (NON mice)

Normal control mice for use in studies involving the nonobese diabetic (NOD) mouse strain that spontaneously develops type I (insulin-dependent) diabetes mellitus. The two strains differ only in genes associated with the development of diabetes.

nonprecipitating antibodies

The addition of antigen in increments to an optimal amount of antibody precipitates only ~78% of the amount of antibody that would be precipitated by one-step addition to the antigen. This demonstrates the presence of both precipitating and nonprecipitating antibodies. Although the nonprecipitating variety cannot produce formation of insoluble antigen–antibody complexes, they can be assimilated into precipitates that correspond to their specificity. Rather than being univalent as was once believed, they may merely have a relatively low affinity for the homologous antigen. Monogamous bivalency, which describes the combination of high affinity antibody with two antigenic determinants on the same antigen particle, represents an alternative explanation for the failure of these molecules to precipitate with their homologous antigen. The formation of nonprecipitating antibodies, which usually represents 10 to 15% of the antibody population produced, is dependent upon such variables as heterogeneity of the antigen, characteristics of the antibody, and animal species. The equivalence zone is narrower with native proteins of 40 to 60 kDa and their homologous antibodies than with polysaccharide antigens or aggregated denatured proteins and their specific antibodies. The equivalence zone with synthetic polypeptide antigens varies with the individual compound used. The solubility of antibody–antigen complexes and the nature of the antigen are related to these variations at the equivalence zone. The extent of precipitation is dependent upon characteristics of both the antigen and antibody. At the equivalence zone, not all antigen and antibody molecules are present in the complexes. For example, rabbit anti-BSA (bovine serum albumin) precipitates only 46% of BSA at equivalence.

nonproductive rearrangement

Rearrangements in which gene segments are joined out of phase, leading to failure to preserve the triplet-reading frame for translation. Nonproductive rearrangements of gene segments encoding T and B cell receptors lead to failure to encode a protein because the coding sequences are in the wrong translational reading frame.

nonresponder

An animal that fails to generate an immune response following antigenic challenge. This may be genetically based, as in strain 13 guinea pigs that reveal unresponsiveness to selected antigens based upon genetic factors. Failure of an individual to generate an immune response to immunogenic challenge to which other members of the same species mount a strong immune response is attributable to failure of expression of an MHC allele capable of presenting an immunogenic peptide from the foreign protein immunogen.

nonsecretor

An individual whose body secretions such as gastric juice, saliva, tears, and ovarian cyst mucin do not contain ABO blood group substances. Nonsecretors comprise approximately one fifth of the population and are homozygous for the *se* gene.

nonsequential epitopes

Antigenic determinants that are widely separated in the primary sequence of the polypeptide chain but are near one another in the tertiary structure of the molecule.

nonspecific esterase (α naphthyl acetate esterase)

An enzyme of mononuclear phagocytes and lymphocytes demonstrable by cytochemical staining, which reveals diffuse granular staining of the cytoplasm of mononuclear phagocytes that may help to identify them. Some human T cells are positive for nonspecific esterase but appear as one or several small localized dots within T cells.

nonspecific fluorescence

Fluorescence emission that does not reflect antigen–antibody interaction and may confuse interpretation of immunofluorescence tests. Free fluorochrome or fluorochrome tagging of proteins other than antibody such as serum albumin, α globulin, or β globulin may contribute to nonspecific fluorescence. Nonspecific staining is accounted for in appropriate controls.

| Natural killer (NK) cells |
| Antibody-dependent cytotoxic cells
  K cells
  NK cells |
| Lymphokine-activated killer (LAK) cells |
| Tumor-infiltrating lymphocytes (TILS) |

Lymphoid cells participating in nonspecific immunity.

nonspecific immunity

Mechanisms such as phagocytosis that nonspecifically remove invading microorganisms along with the chemical and physical barriers to infection such as acid in the stomach and the skin, respectively. Other nonspecific protective factors include lysozyme, β lysin, and interferon. Nonspecific or natural immunity does not depend on immunologic memory. Natural killer cells represent an important part of the natural immune cell system. Phagocytosis of invading microorganisms by polymorphonuclear neutrophils and monocytes represents another important aspect of nonspecific immunity.

nonspecific suppression

A state induced by soluble molecules released from cells, in a nonantigen-specific manner, that downmodulate immune function such as cytokines, nitric oxide, and prostaglandins. Nonspecific suppressive cell populations such as natural suppressor (NS) cells may induce suppression through soluble mediators. Nonspecific suppressive mechanisms would be of interest for tolerance induction if they could be induced temporarily during a critical period when an alloreactive was present.

nonspecific T cell suppressor factor

A CD8+ suppressor T lymphocyte-soluble substance that nonspecifically suppresses the immune response.

nonspecific T lymphocyte helper factor

A soluble factor released by CD4+ helper T lymphocytes that nonspecifically activates other lymphocytes.

nonsquamous keratin (NSK)

A marker, demonstrable by immunoperoxidase staining, that is found in glandular epithelium and adenocarcinomas, but not in stratified squamous epithelium.

nonsterile immunity

Refer to premunition.

nonsteroidal antiinflammatory drugs (NSAIDs)

A group of drugs used to treat rheumatoid arthritis, gouty arthritis, ankylosing spondylitis, and osteoarthritis. The drugs are weak organic acids. They block prostaglandin synthesis by inhibiting cyclooxygenase and lipooxygenase. They also interrupt membrane-bound reactions such as NADPH oxidase in neutrophils, monocyte phospholipase C, and processes regulated by G proteins. They exert a number of other possible activities such as diminished generation of free radicals and superoxides that may alter intracellular cAMP levels, diminishing vasoactive mediator release from granulocytes, basophils, and mast cells. NSAIDs include salicylates and similar drugs that are used to treat rheumatic disease through their capacity to suppress the signs and symptoms of inflammation. These drugs also exert antipyretic and analgesic effects. Their anti-inflammatory properties make them most useful in the management of disorders in which pain is related to the intensity of the inflammatory process. NSAIDs used for special indications include indomethacin and ketorolac. Gastric irritation caused by some of the original NSAIDs led to the introduction of newer nonsteroidal antiinflammatory drugs that include phenylbutazone and a host of other compounds for use and treatment of such conditions as rheumatoid arthritis and osteoarthritis.

nontissue-specific antigen

An antigen that is not confined to a single organ but is distributed in more than one normal tissue or organ, e.g., nuclear antigen.

normal cellular antigen (class of TAA)

Overexpression of a normal macromolecule on tumor cells frequently induced by gene amplification. Refer to tumor-associated antigen.

normal flora

Refer to commensal microorganisms.

normal lymphocyte transfer reaction

The intracutaneous injection of an individual with peripheral blood lymphocytes from a genetically dissimilar allogeneic member of the same species leads to the development of a local erythematous reaction that becomes most pronounced after 48 hours. The size of the reaction has been claimed to qualitatively indicate histocompatibility or histoincompatibility between a donor and recipient. This test is not used in clinical practice.

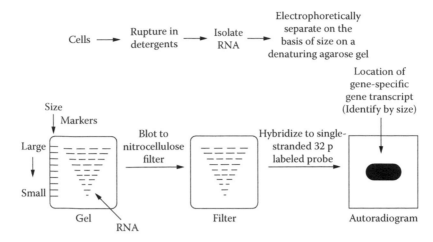

Northern blotting.

northern blotting

A method to identify specific mRNA molecules. Following denaturation of RNA in a particular preparation with formaldehyde to cause the molecule to unfold and become linear, the material is separated by size through gel electrophoresis and blotted onto a natural cellulose or nylon membrane. This preparation is then exposed to a solution of labeled DNA probe of complementary sequence for hybridization, followed by autoradiography. Northern blotting corresponds to a similar method used for DNA fragments which is known as southern blotting.

Norvir®

A peptidomimetic inhibitor of both human immunodeficiency virus 1 (HIV-1) and HIV-2 proteases. It is FDA-approved for the treatment of HIV. The mechanism of action includes inhibition of HIV protease, rendering the enzyme incapable of processing the *gag–pol* polyprotein precursor that leads to production of noninfectious immature HIV particles. Ritonavir is the active component.

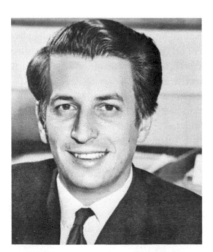

Gustav Joseph Victor Nossal.

Nossal, Gustav Joseph Victor (1931–)

Australian immunologist whose seminal works concentrated on antibodies and their formation. He is director emeritus of the Walter and Eliza Hall Institute of Medical Research in Melbourne. (Refer to *Antibodies and Immunity,* 1969; *Antigens, Lymphoid Cells and the Immune Response* [with Ada] 1971.)

notch 1

A molecule that determines cell fate by regulating transcription through direct associated nuclear transcription factors. It facilitates T cell development at the expense of B cell development, DN to DP thymocyte transition, and Th1 differentiation at the disadvantage of Th2 differentiation.

NP (4-hydroxy,3-nitrophenylacetyl)

A hapten used in experimental immunology that exhibits limited cross reactivity with NIP (4-hydroxy,5-iodo, 3-nitrophenylacetyl).

N region

A brief segment of the variable region of an immunoglobulin molecule or T cell receptor chain that is not encoded by germline genes, but instead by brief nucleotide (N) insertions at recombinational junctions. These N nucleotides may be present both 3′ and 5′ to the D gene segment of the rearranged immunoglobulin heavy chain, as well as at the V–J, V–D–J, and D–D junctions of the variable region genes of the T lymphocyte receptor.

N region diversification

In junction diversity, the addition at random of nucleotides that are not present in the genomic sequence at V–D, D–J, and V–J junctions. Terminal deoxynucleotidyl transferase (TdT) catalyzes N region diversification, which takes place in TCR α and β genes and in immunoglobulin (Ig) heavy chain genes but not in Ig light chain genes.

NSAID (nonsteroidal antiinflammatory drug)

Used in the treatment of arthritis.

N terminus

The amino end of a polypeptide chain bearing a free amino–NH$_2$ group.

nuclear dust (leukocytoclasis)

Extensive basophilic granular material representing karyolytic nuclear debris that accompanies areas of inflammation and necrosis, as in leukocytoclastic vasculitis.

nuclear factor of activated T cells (NFAT)

A transcription factor that is a complex of a protein called NFATc, as it is held in the cytosol by serine/threonine phosphorylation, and the Fos/Jun dimer termed AP-1. It migrates from the cytosol to the nucleus following cleavage of the phosphate residues by calcineurin, a serine/threonine protein phosphatase.

nuclear matrix protein

A marker expressed preferentially by malignant cells rather than by normal cells; demonstrated by immunoperoxidase staining.

nuclear matrix proteins (NMPs)

Substances that organize nuclear chromatin. They are associated with DNA replication, RNA synthesis, and hormone receptor binding. Antibodies against NMPs react with nuclear mitotic apparatus protein. Thus, much of the nuclear matrix is devoted to formation of the mitotic apparatus (MA). NMPs participate in cellular events that result in programmed cell death (apoptosis).

nucleolar autoantibodies

Antibodies associated with systemic sclerosis (SSc) include autoantibodies to nucleolar 7-2 RNA, present in only a small percentage of patients with SSc; RNA polymerase I, found in 4% of patients with SSc; the fibrillarin component of U3 RNP, found in 6% of patients with SSc; and PM-Scl autoantibodies, found in 3% of polymyositis–scleroderma overlap syndrome cases. Nucleolar autoantibodies have also been observed in chronic graft-vs.-host disease following bone marrow transplantation. Indirect immunofluorescence is used to demonstrate nucleolar staining patterns that include speckled or punctuate (RNA polymerase I specificity), homogeneous (PM-Scl specificity), and clumpy (U3 RNP specificity). Hep-2 cells are useful as a substrate to detect nucleolar autoantibodies.

nucleoside phosphorylase

An enzyme that is only seldom decreased in immunodeficiency patients. It catalyzes inosine conversion into hypoxanthine.

nucleotide excision pathway (NER)

A DNA repair pathway with participation by products of the XPA-XPG genes capable of excising nucleotides injured by UV irradiation.

nude mouse

A strain of hairless mouse that has a congenital absence of the thymus and of T lymphocyte function. An autosomal-recessive mutation that inhibits hair follicle development and prevents or greatly diminishes thymus development. The mice are hairless and lack T cells and serve as highly effective animal models to investigate the immunologic consequences of the absence of a thymus. The mice fail to develop cell-mediated (T-lymphocyte-mediated) immunity, are unable to reject allografts, and cannot synthesize antibodies against the majority of antigens. Their B lymphocytes and natural killer cells are normal even though T lymphocytes are missing. Also called nu/nu mice. Valuable in the investigation of graft-vs.-host disease. Partial model for DiGeorge syndrome in humans.

null cell

A lymphocyte that does not manifest any markers of T or B cells, including cluster of differentiation (CD) antigens or surface immunoglobulins. Approximately 20% of peripheral lymphocytes are null cells. They play a role in antibody-dependent cell-mediated cytotoxicity (ADCC) and may be the principal cells in certain malignancies such as acute lymphocytic leukemia of children. The three types of null cells include (1) undifferentiated stem cells that may mature into T or B lymphocytes, (2) cells with labile immunoglobulin G (IgG) and high affinity Fc receptors that are resistant to trypsin, and (3) large granular lymphocytes that constitute natural killer (NK) and killer (K) cells.

null cell compartment

Null cells constitute 37% of the bone marrow lymphocytes (i.e., they do not have any markers characteristic of B or T cell lineage). They may differentiate into B or T cells upon appropriate induction, the mechanism of which is unknown. Some null cells differentiate into killer (K) cells by developing Fc and complement receptors. Natural killer (NK) cells are also present in this cell population. Null, K, and NK cells, like committed lymphocytes, also migrate to the peripheral lymphoid organs such as spleen and lymph nodes, or the thymus, but they represent only a very small fraction of the total cells present there. At all locations, the null cells are part of the rapidly renewed pool of immature cells with short lifespans (5 to 6 days). The null cells committed to T cell lineage migrate to the thymus to continue their differentiation.

null phenotype

The failure to express protein because the gene that encodes it is either defective or absent on both inherited haplotypes. Most of these involve erythrocytes, but they are quite rare.

nurse cell

Refer to thymus.

nutrition and immunity

The most frequent cause of immunodeficiency worldwide is malnutrition. Protein energy malnutrition has an adverse effect on immunity, increases the frequency of opportunistic infections, and leads to lymphoid tissue atrophy with reduction in size of the thymus, depletion of lymphoid cells in thymus-dependent areas of lymph nodes, and a loss of lymphoid cells around small vessels in the spleen. It leads to delayed hypersensitivity responses in the skin to both new and recall antigens. The helper/suppressor ratio is significantly decreased, and lymphocyte proliferation and synthesis of DNA are diminished. Serum antibody responses are usually unaffected. Phagocytosis is affected as a consequence of decreased complement, component C3, factor B, and total hemolytic activity. Ingestion by phagocytes is intact. Metabolic destruction of microorganisms is decreased, as is synthesis of various cytokines, including interleukin-2 (IL2) and interferon-γ (IFN-γ). Deficiency of pyridoxine, folic acid, vitamin A, vitamin C, and vitamin E leads to impaired cell-mediated immunity and diminished antibody responses. Vitamin B_6 deficiency leads to decreased lymphocyte stimulation responses to mitogens. A moderate increase in vitamin A enhances immune responses. Zinc deficiency leads to lymphoid atrophy, decreased cutaneous delayed hypersensitivity responses and allograft rejection, and diminished thymic hormone activity. Iron deficiency, the most common nutritional problem worldwide, leads to impaired lymphocyte proliferation in response to mitogens and antigens and a low response to tetanus toxoid and herpes simplex antigens. Copper-deficient animals have fewer antibody-forming cells compared to healthy controls. Dietary deficiencies of selected amino acids diminish antibody responses but in other states an amino acid imbalance may enhance selected antibody responses, perhaps reflecting alterations in suppressor cells.

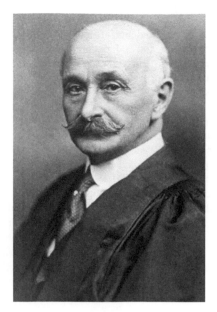

George H.F. Nuttall.

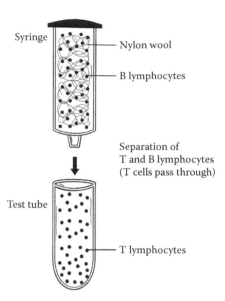

Nylon wool.

Nuttall, George H.F. (1862–1937)

Author of a landmark publication titled *Blood Immunity and Blood Relationship*. He was an early pioneer in comparative immunology.

nylon wool

A material used to fractionate T and B cells from a mixture based on the tendency for B cells to adhere to nylon wool, while T cells pass through it. B cells are then eluted from the column. Tissue typing laboratories previously used this technique to isolate B lymphocytes for major histocompatibility complex (MHC) class II (B cell) typing. Magnetic beads have replaced nylon wool for lymphocyte T and B cell separation.

NZB/NZW F$_1$ hybrid mice

A mouse strain genetically prone to develop lupus erythematosus (LE)-like disease spontaneously. This was the first murine lupus model and was developed from the NZB/B$_1$ mouse model of autoimmune hemolytic anemia mated with the NZW mouse, which develops a positive Coombs' test, antinuclear antibodies, and glomerulonephritis. This F$_1$ hybrid develops various antinuclear autoantibodies and forms immune complexes that subsequently induce glomerulonephritis and shorten life spans due to renal disease. Hemolytic anemia is minimal in the F$_1$ strain compared to the NZB parent. NZB mice show greater lymphoid hyperplasia than do the F$_1$ hybrids, yet the latter show features that are remarkably similar to those observed in human lupus, such as major sex differences.

O

O125 (ovarian celomic)

Nonmucinous ovarian tumor antigen demonstrable with homologous antibody by immunoperoxidase staining. Selected mesotheliomas express this antigen as well.

OA

Abbreviation for ovalbumin.

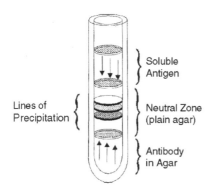

Oakley–Fulthorpe test.

Oakley–Fulthorpe test

Double-diffusion type of precipitation test performed by incorporating antibody into agar placed in a tube followed by a layer of plain agar. A solution of antigen is placed on top of the plain agar, and precipitation occurs where antigen and antibody meet in the plain agar layer.

O antigen

(1) A lipopolysaccharide–protein antigen of enteric microorganisms used for their serological classification. O antigens of the *Proteus* species serve as the basis for the Weil–Felix reaction used to classify *Rickettsia*. O antigens of *Shigella* permit their subdivision into 40 serotypes. The exterior oligosaccharide repeating unit side chain is responsible for specificity and is joined to lipid A to form lipopolysaccharide and to lipid B. The O antigen is the most variable part of the lipopolysaccharide molecule. (2) In the ABO blood group system, O antigen is an oligosaccharide precursor form of A and B antigens: a fucose-galactose-*N*-acetylglucosamine-glucose.

O blood group

One of the groups described by Landsteiner in the ABO blood group system. Refer to ABO blood group system.

O phage antibody library

Cloned antibody variable region gene sequences that may be expressed as Fab or svFv fusion proteins with bacteriophage coat proteins. They may be exhibited on phage surfaces. The phage particle contains the gene encoding a monoclonal recombinant antibody and can be selected from the library by binding of the phage to specific antigen.

occupational allergy

Allergy induced by the type of work in which an individual is engaged.

Oct-2

A protein formed early in the development of B lymphocytes that has a role in immunoglobulin heavy chain transcription.

OKT monoclonal antibodies

Commercially available preparations used to enumerate human T cells according to their surface antigens to determine the immunophenotype. OKT designations have been replaced by CD designations.

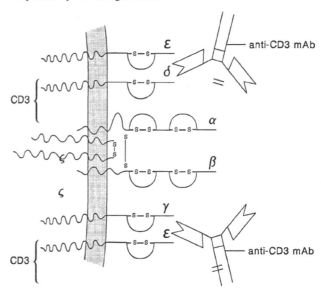

Anti-CD3 monoclonal antibody interaction with CD3 at the T cell surface. Specifically reacts with the T3-Antigen recognition structure of human T cells

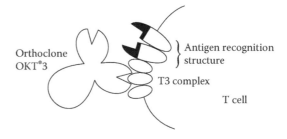

Orthoclone OKT®3 blocks T cell effector function involved in renal allograft rejection

OKT®3 bound to CD3 complex of a T cell.

OKT®3 (Orthoclone OKT®3)

A commercial mouse monoclonal antibody against the CD3 T cell surface marker. It may be used therapeutically to diminish T cell reactivity in organ allotransplant recipients experiencing rejection episodes. OKT3 may act in concert with the complement system to induce T cell lysis or it may act as an opsonin, rendering T cells susceptible to phagocytosis.

OKT4

Refer to CD4.

OKT8

Refer to CD8.

old tuberculin (OT)

A broth culture, heat-concentrated filtrate of medium in which *Mycobacterium tuberculosis* microorganisms are grown. Robert Koch developed it for use in tuberculin skin tests nearly a century ago.

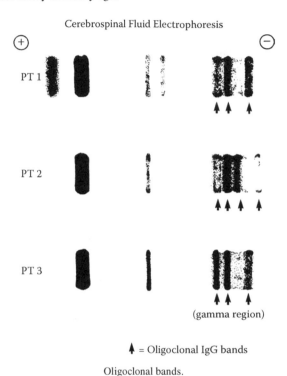

Cerebrospinal Fluid Electrophoresis

(gamma region)

⬆ = Oligoclonal IgG bands

Oligoclonal bands.

oligoclonal bands

When the cerebrospinal fluids of some multiple sclerosis patients are electrophoresed in agarose gel, immunoglobulins with restricted electrophoretic mobility may appear as multiple distinct bands in the γ region. Although nonspecific, 90 to 95% of multiple sclerosis patients show this banding. The bands may appear in selected other central nervous system diseases such as herpetic encephalitis, bacterial or viral meningitis, carcinomatosis, toxoplasmosis, neurosyphilis, progressive multifocal leukoencephalopathy, and subacute sclerosing panencephalitis, and may appear briefly during the course of Guillain-Barré disease, lupus erythematosus vasculitis, spinal cord compression, diabetes, and amyotrophic lateral sclerosis.

oligoclonal response

An immune response characterized by only a few separate clones of immunocompetent cells responding to yield a small number of immunoglobulin bands in agarose gel electrophoresis.

oligomorphic

Genes that possess only a relatively small number of different alleles in the population.

oligosaccharide determinant

An epitope or antigenic determinant of a polysaccharide hapten that consists of relatively few (two to seven) pentoses, hexoses, or heptoses united by glycoside linkages.

Omenn's syndrome

A severe immunodeficiency characterized by the development soon after birth of a generalized erythroderma desquamation, failure to thrive, protracted diarrhea, hepatosplenomegaly, hypereosinophilia, and markedly elevated serum immunoglobulin E (IgE) levels. It has been observed in association with neonatal minimal-change nephritic syndrome. Circulating and tissue-infiltrating activated T lymphocytes that do not respond normally to mitogens or antigen *in vitro* are increased. These T cells are both oligoclonal and polyclonal. Circulating B cells are not found, and the only hypogammaglobulinemia is for IgE. Superficial lymph node architecture is grossly abnormal due to a proliferation of interdigitating, S-100, protein-positive, nonphagocytic reticulum cells and a depletion of B lymphocytes. This is believed to be a Th2-mediated condition, even though the fundamental defect has not been discovered. This form of severe combined immunodeficiency is induced by amino acid substitution mutations in the RAG genes that significantly diminish the activity of the corresponding proteins to 1 to 25% of normal. The condition is fatal in the first 5 months of life unless corrected by bone marrow transplantation following chemoablation.

Onchocerca volvulus immunity

This filarial parasite that can induce dermal and ocular complications contains antigens that induce antigen-specific immunoglobulin G (IgG), IgM, IgE, and IgA antibodies in addition to polyclonal stimulation. Humoral immunity develops early in chimpanzees, but the exact role of antibodies in protection remains to be determined. Antibodies against microfilariae facilitate adherence of granulocytes *in vitro*, and eosinophils and neutrophils mediate antibody-dependent killing. Massive eosinophil degranulation may lead to tissue injury. Infected subjects develop elevated IgE that may worsen ocular lesions by contributing to acute inflammation. Much of the IgE antibody is *O. volvulus* antigen-specific. Immune complexes may also contribute to acute inflammation. Cell-mediated immunity is downregulated to antigens that are specific and nonspecific for the infectious agent. Onchocerciasis is marked by predominant Th2 cytokine responses in subjects with ocular pathologies, whereas a Th1 response is associated with immunity. Thus, the host immune response is significant in both pathology and protection in onchocerciasis. The HLA-D allele influences the pathogenesis of *O. volvulus* infection. Ocular pathology is the most serious result, affecting both anterior and posterior segments of the eye. Protection against onchocerciasis has been directed to vector control, but development of a protective vaccine would be a better solution. Larval antigens are the best targets for a prophylactic vaccine.

oncofetal antigens

Markers or epitopes present in fetal tissues during development and not present or found only in minute quantities in adult tissues. These cell-coded antigens may reappear in certain neoplasms of adults due to derepression of the gene responsible for their formation. Examples include carcinoembryonic antigen (CEA) found in the liver, intestine, and pancreas of the fetus and also in both malignant and benign gastrointestinal conditions. It is still useful to detect the recurrence of adenocarcinoma of the colon based on demonstration of CEA in the patient's serum; α-fetoprotein

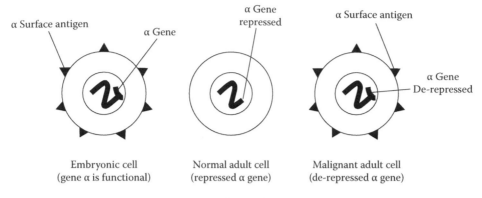

Oncofetal antigen.

(AFP) is demonstrable in approximately 70% of hepatocellular carcinomas.

oncogene

A gene linked to carcinogenesis when deregulated. Such genes may encode positive regulators of cell growth. They may be activated by mutation or retroviral integration. They are involved in the control of cell growth and when defective in structure or expression can lead to abnormal cell proliferation resulting in tumor generation. Genes with the capacity to induce neoplastic transformation of cells, they are derived from normal genes (proto-oncogenes) or from oncogenic RNA (oncorna) viruses. Their protein products are critical for the regulation of gene expression and growth signal transduction. Translocation, gene amplification, and point mutation may lead to neoplastic transformation of proto-oncogenes. Oncogenes may be revealed through the use of viruses that induce tumors in animals or by derivation of tumor-causing genes from cancer cells. The human genome has more than 20 proto-oncogenes and cellular oncogenes. An oncogene alone cannot produce cancer. It must be accompanied by malignant transformation involving multiple genetic steps. Oncogenes encode four types of proteins, including growth factors, receptors, intracellular transducers, and nuclear transcription factors.

oncogenesis

The process by which tumors develop.

oncogene theory

A concept of carcinogenesis that assigns tumor development to latent retroviral gene activation through irradiation or carcinogens. These retroviral genes are considered to be normal constituents of cells. Following activation, these oncogenes are presumed to govern the neoplasm through synthesized hormones and even the possible construction of a complete oncogenic virus. This concept states that all cells may potentially become malignant.

oncogenic virus

Any virus, whether DNA or RNA, that can induce malignant transformation of cells. An example of a DNA virus is human papillomavirus. Retroviruses are RNA viruses.

oncomouse

Commercially developed transgenic mice into which human genes have been introduced to make the mice more susceptible to neoplasia. Transgenic mice are used for both medical and pharmaceutical research.

one gene, one enzyme theory (historical)

An early hypothesis that proposed that one gene encodes one enzyme or other protein. Although basically true, it is now known that one gene encodes a single polypeptide chain, and it is necessary to splice out mRNA introns composed of junk DNA before mRNA can be translated into a protein.

one-hit theory

A concept related to complement activation that states that only a single site of preparation is necessary for red cell lysis during complement-antibody-mediated injury to a cell membrane.

one-turn recombination signal sequence

Immunoglobulin gene recombination signal sequence separated by an intervening sequence of 12 base pairs.

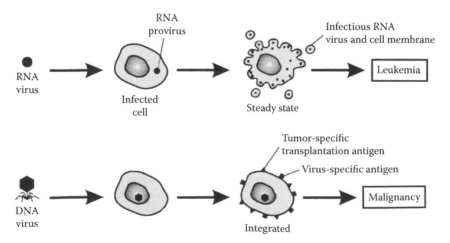

Oncogenic virus.

ontogeny

The development of an individual organism from conception to maturity.

open reading frame (ORF)

A length of RNA or DNA that encodes a protein and may signal the identification of a protein not described previously. An ORF begins with a start codon, ends at a stop codon, and lacks a termination codon.

opisthorchiasis (clonorchiasis) immunity

Antibodies synthesized in patients with opisthorchiasis (or chlonorchiasis) react with the various developmental stages of the parasites. Stage-specific and cross reactive common antigens have been detected and identified. Immunoglobulin G (IgG) is the predominant class of antibodies in serum, but IgE has also been detected to a lesser degree. The bile contains secretory IgA as the principal immunoglobulin. The parasite antigens manifest IgE-potentiating activity. Although high antibody titers are achieved in infected patients, their protective ability is doubtful. Some investigations have suggested that complement-fixing antibodies may play a role but *Opisthorchis* may be able to activate complement by way of the alternative pathway leading to lymphocyte killing. Cell-mediated immunity also occurs following natural infection or immunization with the parasite antigen. The role of T cells remains to be determined. Primary infection does not appear to protect against reinfection by the same parasite. Thus, there appears to be a lack of protective acquired immunity. The liver flukes survive in the biliary system that may serve as a type of immunologically privileged site. These parasites can shed their surface teguments following injury by immune mechanism, representing yet another mechanism to evade host defenses.

opportunistic infection

An infection produced by microorganisms that are usually of relatively low virulence but become more aggressive in subjects with altered or defective cell-mediated immunity. Susceptible individuals include individuals with acquired immune deficiency (AIDS) and severe combined immunodeficiency (SCID) and organ transplant recipients. Typical microorganisms producing opportunistic infections include *Pneumocystis carinii, Candida albicans, Mycobacterium avium intracellulare, Cryptosporidium, Toxoplasma*, cytomegalovirus, and herpesvirus.

opportunistic pathogen

A microorganism that produces disease only in persons whose immune defense mechanisms are compromised as in AIDS.

opsonin

A substance that binds to bacteria, erythrocytes, or other particles to increase their susceptibility to phagocytosis. A host protein that coats a pathogenic microorganism or macromolecule to make it bind more readily to phagocyte receptors, thereby enhancing phagocytosis. Opsonins include antibodies such as IgG_3, IgG_1, and IgG_2 that are specific for epitopes on particle surfaces. Following interaction, the Fc region of the antibody becomes anchored to Fc receptors on phagocyte surfaces, thereby facilitating phagocytosis of the particles. In contrast to these so-called heat-stable antibody opsonins are the heat-labile products of complement activation such as C3b or C3bi that are linked to particles by transacylation with the C3 thiolester. C3b combines with complement receptor 1 and C3bi combines

with complement receptor 3 on phagocytic cells. Besides immunoglobulins of the mentioned isotypes and complement proteins, other opsonic complement intermediates include iC3b and C4b. Opsonins facilitate phagocytosis of particulate antigens by neutrophils or macrophages. Other substances that act as opsonins include the basement membrane constituent known as fibronectin.

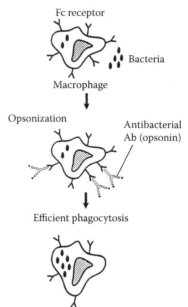

Opsonization.

opsonization

Facilitation of the phagocytosis of microorganisms or other particles such as erythrocytes through the coating of their surfaces with immune or nonimmune opsonins. The enhanced phagocytosis of a pathogenic microorganism or macromolecule is attributable to the linkage of molecules that interact with phagocyte cell surface receptors. Antibodies such as immunoglobulin G (IgG) molecules and complement fragments may opsonize extracellular bacteria or other microorganisms, rendering them susceptible to destruction by neutrophils and macrophages through phagocytosis.

opsonophagocytosis

Antibodies and/or complement, mainly C3, serve as opsonins by binding to epitopes on microorganisms and increasing their susceptibility to phagocytosis by polymorphonuclear leukocytes, especially neutrophils. Serum bactericidal activity and phagocytic killing are two principal mechanisms in host defense against bacteria. Opsonic antimicrobial antibodies are critical for optimal functioning of phagocytes in the uptake and containment of bacteria.

oral immunology

Saliva rinses the oral cavity and also contains numerous molecules such as lysozyme and secretory immunoglobulin A (IgA) that serve as parts of the mucosal immune system to help protect the oral cavity. Polymorphonuclear leukocytes are important in protection of gingival tissues and ultimately the periodontium. In addition to secretory IgA, the systemic vascular humoral immune response is significant in oral immunity. The relative contribution of Th1 and Th2 cells in an immune response to plaque bacterial pathogens is

Oral tolerance.

significant in periodontal disease. Individuals with immunodeficiencies often have increased mucosal infections by opportunistic microorganisms such as by *Candida albicans*. Immunopathologic mechanisms that involve types II, III, and IV hypersensitivity may be involved in the development and progression of chronic periodontitis. Vaccines may be used in the future to prevent or control dental caries and periodontal diseases. Oral or intranasal routes of vaccine administration may prove useful to protect against oral infections.

oral tolerance

Antigen-induced specific suppression of humoral and cell-mediated immunity to an antigen following oral administration of that antigen as a consequence of anergy of antigen-specific T lymphocytes or the formation of immunosuppressive cytokines such as transforming growth factor β (TGF-β). Oral tolerance may inhibit immune responses against food antigens and bacteria in the intestine. Proteins passing through the gastrointestinal tract induce antigen-specific hyporesponsiveness. Oral tolerance is believed to have evolved to permit the gut-associated immune system to be exposed to external proteins without becoming sensitized. If proteins such as ovalbumin or myelin basic protein (MBP) are fed to animals that are then immunized, the immune response against the fed antigen, but not against the control antigen, is subsequently diminished. Based on the quantity of antigen fed, orally administered antigen may induce regulatory cells that suppress the antigen-specific response (low doses) or inhibit antigen-specific T cells by induction of clonal anergy (high doses). Antigens passing through the gastrointestinal tract preferentially induce T helper (Th2)-type T cells that secrete interleukin-4 (IL4), IL10, and TGF-β.

oral unresponsiveness

The selective ability of the mucosal immune system to react immunologically against antigens of food and intestinal microorganisms even though it responds vigorously to pathogenic microorganisms.

organ bank

A site where selected tissues for transplantation, such as acellular bone fragments, corneas, and bone marrow, may be stored for relatively long periods until needed. Several hospitals often share such a facility. Organs such as kidneys, liver, heart, lung, and pancreatic islets must be transplanted within 48 to 72 hours and are not suitable for storage in an organ bank.

organ brokerage

The selling of an organ such as a kidney from a living related donor to the transplant recipient is practiced in certain parts of the world but is considered unethical and is illegal in the United states because it violates the National Organ Transplant Act (Public Law 98-507, 3 USC).

organ-specific antigen

An antigen that is unique to a particular organ even though it may be found in more than one species.

organ-specific autoimmune diseases

Autoimmune reactivity against specific organs, such as the thyroid in Hashimoto's thyroiditis, leads to cell and tissue damage to specific organs. By contrast, systemic lupus erythematosus (SLE) affects a wide variety of tissues and organs of the body.

organ specific autoimmunity

An autoimmune response directed against a specific anatomical site.

organism-specific antibody index (OSAI)

The ratio of organism-specific immunoglobulin G (IgG) to total IgG in cerebrospinal fluid (CSF) compared to the ratio of organism-specific IgG in serum to total serum IgG. This is illustrated in the following formula: an index >1 signifying a greater quantity of organism-specific immunoglobulin in CSF than in the blood serum implies that organism-specific IgG is being synthesized in the intra-blood–brain barrier (IBBB) and suggests that the specific organism of interest is producing an infection of the central nervous system. Similar indices can be calculated for IgM and IgA antibody classes.

original antigenic sin

When an individual is exposed to an antigen that is similar but not identical to an antigen to which he was previously exposed by infection or immunization, the immune response to the second exposure is still directed against the first antigen. This was first noticed in influenza virus infection. Due to antigenic drift and shift in influenza virus, reinfection with an antigenically altered strain generates a secondary immune response specific for the virus strain that produced an earlier infection. The antibody response against a second infection with influenza is restricted to epitopes that the second strain shares with the first strain that infected the host. Other highly immunogenic epitopes on second and subsequent viruses are ignored. B cell clones activated by an original antigen are reactivated in response to a new cross reactive antigen that possesses novel B cell epitopes in addition to T cell epitopes present on the original antigen.

Orthoclone OKT®3

A commercial antibody against the T cell surface marker CD3. It may be used therapeutically to diminish T cell reactivity in organ allotransplant recipients experiencing

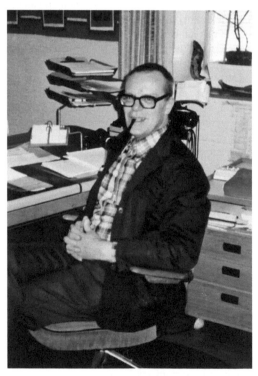

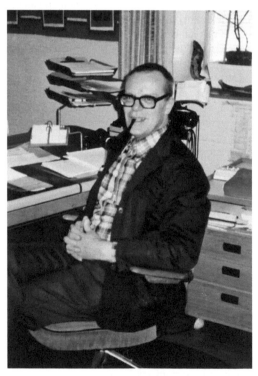
Orthotopic graft.

Oseltamivir.

rejection episodes. It may act in concert with the complement system to induce T cell lysis or act as an opsonin, rendering T cells susceptible to phagocytosis. Rarely, recirculating T lymphocytes are removed in patients experiencing rejection crisis by thoracic duct drainage or extracorporeal irradiation of the blood. Plasma exchange is useful for temporary reduction in circulating antibody levels in selective diseases, such as hemolytic disease of the newborn, myasthenia gravis, or Goodpasture's syndrome. Immunosuppressive drugs act on all of the T and B cell maturation processes.

orthotopic

An organ or tissue transplant at a site usually occupied by that organ or tissue.

orthotopic graft

An organ or tissue transplant placed in the location usually occupied by that particular organ or tissue.

oseltamivir (Tamiflu®)

A powerful inhibitor of the neuraminidase enzyme of influenza viruses A and B. Neuraminidase leads to cleavage of sialic acid residues on newly formed virions and is critical to the release and spread of progeny viruses. On contact with oseltamivir, influenza virions aggregate on host cell surfaces, which limits the extent of infection within the mucosal secretions and diminishes viral infectivity. This drug is indicated in the prophylaxis of influenza and for the treatment of uncomplicated acute illness due to influenza in patients 1 year and older who have manifested symptoms for no more than 2 days. H5N1 influenza virus strains are usually sensitive to the drug, but no clinical data of efficacy are available. Drugs in this category diminish the duration of influenza-related symptoms if administered within 48 hours of onset. Clinical efficacy is 60 to 70%. Symptoms including myalgia, fever, and headache diminished if treatment started within 48 hours. Therapy is more effective

if begun within 30 hours of symptom onset. Oseltamivir exerts no adverse effect on cellular immune responses to influenza virus infection *in vivo*. Its only clinical side effect is mild gastrointestinal distress. Oseltamivir is an ethyl ester prodrug that undergoes ester hydrolysis when converted to the active form of oseltamivir carboxylate. The drug has a potent antiviral effect *in vitro* also against H9N2 strains and recombinant viruses composed of the 1918 NA or both the 1918 HA and 1918 NA in tissue cultures and mouse studies, suggesting that it may be effective against a re-emergent 1918-like virus.

osteoclast

A macrophage-like cell present in bone that is responsible for bone resorption.

osteoclast-activating factor (OAF)

A lymphokine produced by antigen-activated lymphocytes that promotes bone resorption through activation of osteoclasts. Besides lymphotoxin produced by T cells, interleukin-1 (IL1), tumor necrosis factor (TNF), and prostaglandins synthesized by macrophages also have OAF activity. OAFs may be responsible for the bone resorption observed in multiple myeloma and T cell neoplasms.

OT (historical)

Old tuberculin.

Orjan Thomas Gunnersson Ouchterlony.

Ouchterlony, Orjan Thomas Gunnersson (1914–2004)

Swedish bacteriologist who developed the antibody detection test that bears his name. Two-dimensional double diffusion with subsequent precipitation patterns is the basis of the assay. (Refer to *Handbook of Immunodiffusion and Immunoelectrophoresis,* 1968.)

Ouchterlony test

A double diffusion in a gel type precipitation test. Antigen and antibody solutions are placed in separate wells cut into an agar plate prepared with electrolyte. As the antigen

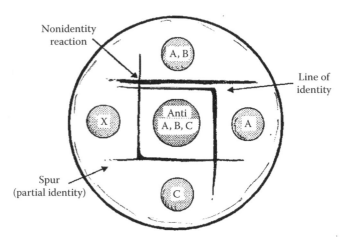

Ouchterlony test.

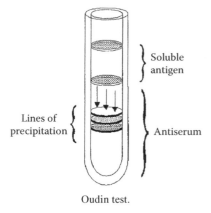

Oudin test.

and antibody diffuse through the gel medium, a line of precipitation forms at the point of contact between antigen and antibody. Results are expressed as a reaction of identity, reaction of partial identity, or reaction of nonidentity (refer to those entries for further details).

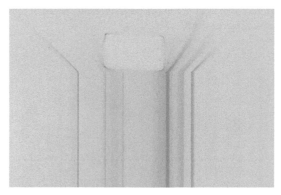

Gel precipitation using Ouchterlony technique.

Oudin, Jacques (1908–1986)

French immunologist who was director of analytical immunology at Institut Pasteur in Paris. His accomplishments include discovery of idiotypy and the agar single-diffusion-method antigen–antibody assay.

Oudin test

A type of precipitation in gel that involves single diffusion. Antiserum, incorporated into agar, is placed in a narrow test tube and overlaid with an antigen solution that diffuses into the agar to yield precipitation rings. Also called single radial diffusion test. A band of precipitation forms at the equivalence point.

outbreeding

Mating of subjects who show greater genetic differences between themselves than randomly chosen individuals of a population. This process encourages genetic diversity, in contrast to inbreeding and random breeding.

ovalbumin (OA)

A protein derived from avian egg albumin (egg white) used extensively as an antigen in experimental immunology.

ovary antibodies (OAs)

Antibodies present in 15 to 50% of premature ovarian failure patients in whom ovarian function failed after puberty but prior to 40 years of age. These individuals have elevated levels of gonadotropins in serum but diminished serum estradiol levels. Premature ovarian failure is associated with an increased incidence of autoimmune disease, especially of the thyroid. Patients also develop autoantibodies of both the organ-specific and nonorgan-specific types. They are often HLA-DR3 positive and have elevated CD4/CD8 ratios. Ovarian antibodies are specific for steroid cells, which causes them to cross react with steroid-synthesizing cells in the placenta, adrenals, and testes.

ovary autoantibodies

Autoantibodies to adrenal glands, ovary, placenta, and testes are known as steroid cell autoantibodies. Adrenal gland steroid autoantibodies commonly react with ovary and testes antigens. Most females with Addison's disease and amenorrhea with autoimmune gonadal failure develop

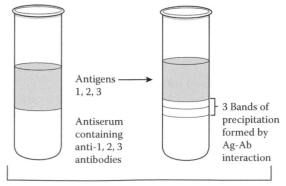

Single diffusion in one dimension

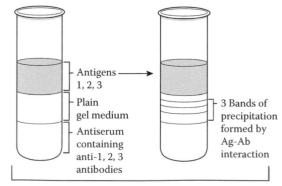

Double diffusion in one dimension

Oudin test.

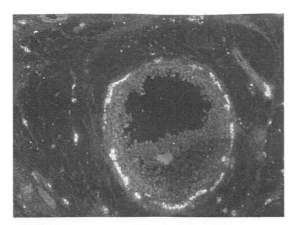

Ovary autoantibodies.

steroid cell autoantibodies. These autoantibodies occur in 78% of patients with premature ovarian failure and Addison's disease.

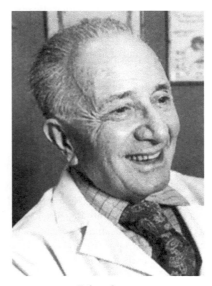

Zoltan Ovary.

Ovary, Zoltan

Investigator at New York University who perfected passive cutaneous anaphylaxis (PCA). The PCA test will always be associated with his name.

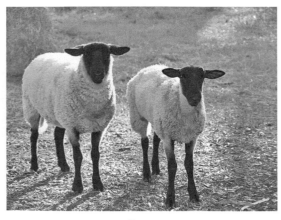

Sheep.

ovine immune system

Sheep are valuable for investigation of the physiology of the immune system. A technique termed lymphatic cannulation of single lymph nodes in sheep offers a powerful tool to analyze immune cell populations within various immunological microenvironments. The cannulated lymph node maintains intact vascular and neurological connections. Cannulation of the efferent lymphatic permits monitoring of immunological events in a single lymph node. Numerous studies have been conducted on ovine cellular and molecular markers of lymphocyte populations, their subsets, and receptors. Major histocompatibility complex (MHC) class I and class II genes and proteins, immunoglobulins, and cytokines have been described. The ileal Peyer's patches in the intestine serve as primary lymphoid organs for B cell lymphopoiesis. Serum immunoglobulin G (IgG) is higher in sheep than in humans. The three principal T cell subsets in sheep include the majority of CD4+ or CD8+ T cells that express the αβ T cell receptor together with adhesion molecules. The double negative CD4−/CD8− T cell subset contains the γδ T cell subset, which is a measured subpopulation in ruminants. Both MHC class I and class II molecules are products of the MHC region in sheep. The afferent lymph of sheep is a physiological source of antigen-presenting dendritic cells.

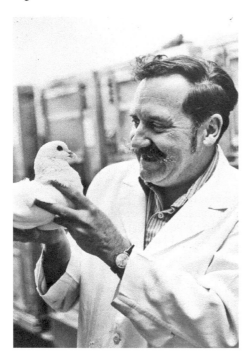

Ray D. Owen.

Owen, Ray David (1915–)

American geneticist who described erythrocyte mosaicism in dizygotic cattle twins. His discovery of reciprocal erythrocyte tolerance contributed to the concept of immunologic tolerance. The observation that cattle twins that shared a common fetal circulation were chimeras and could not reject transplants of each other's tissues later in life. Provided the groundwork for Burnett's ideas about tolerance and Medawar's work in transplantation.

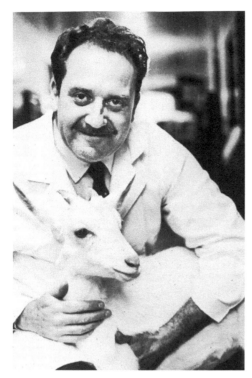

Dr. Owen at work.

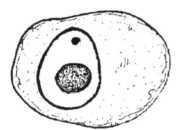

Owl eye appearance.

owl eye appearance

Inclusions found by light microscopy in cytomegalovirus (CMV) infection. CMV-infected epithelial cells are enlarged and exhibit prominent eosinophilic intranuclear inclusions that are half the size of the nucleus and are encircled by a clear halo.

oxazolone (4-ethoxymethylene-2-phenyloxazol-5-one)

A substance used in experimental immunology to induce contact hypersensitivity in laboratory animals.

oxidized low density lipoprotein (ox-LDL) autoantibodies

Autoantibodies against ox-LDL represent good markers of LDL oxidation. Ox-LDL is immunogenic and leads to increased immunoglobulin G (IgG) but not IgM or IgA ox-LDL antibodies with carotid atherosclerosis. Ox-LDL antibodies are also characterized as antiphospholipid antibodies, whereas most antibodies against ox-LDL are specific for apolipoprotein B epitopes, the major lipoprotein of LDL. A considerable number are reactive against peroxidized phospholipid.

oxygen-dependent killing

Activated by a powerful oxidative burst that culminates in the formation of hydrogen peroxide and other antimicrobial substances. In addition to this oxygen-dependent killing mechanism, phagocytized intracellular microbes may be the targets of toxic substances released from granules into phagosomes, leading to microbial cell death by an oxygen-independent mechanism. For oxygen-dependent killing of microbes, membranes of specific granules and phagosomes fuse, permitting interaction of NADPH oxidase with cytochrome. With the aid of quinone, this combination reduces oxygen to superoxide anion O_2. In the presence of a superoxide dismutase catalyst, superoxidase ion is converted to hydrogen peroxide. The clinical relevance of this process is illustrated by chronic granulomatous disease (CGD) in children who fail to form superoxide anions and have diminished cytochrome b, even though phagocytosis is normal. They have impaired ability to oxidize NADPH and destroy bacteria through

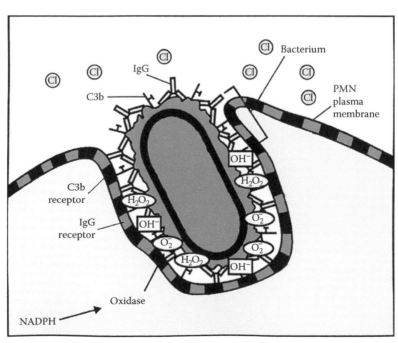

Formation of bactericide and hydrogen peroxide catalyzed by NADPH oxidase.

O

the oxidative pathway. The oxidative mechanism kills microbes through a complex process. Hydrogen peroxide together with myeloperoxidase transforms chloride ions into hypochlorous ions that kill microorganisms. Azurophil granule fusion releases myeloperoxidase to phagolysosomes. Some microorganisms such as pneumococci form hydrogen peroxide.

oxygen-independent killing

Following adherence of opsonized microbes to neutrophil plasma membranes, lysozyme and lactoferrin are discharged from specific granules into phagosomes with which they have fused. Antimicrobial cationic proteins reach phagosomes from azurophil granules. These proteins kill Gram-negative microbes by interrupting their cell membrane integrity. They are far less effective against Gram-positive microorganisms.

Oz isotypic determinant

Oz represents an isotypic marker. λ Light chains of human immunoglobulin that are Oz$^+$ contain lysine at position 190, whereas those that are Oz$^-$ contain arginine at this position. A fraction of each person's λ light chains expresses Oz$^-$ determinants.

P

P

Abbreviation for properdin. Also called factor P.

P1^{A1} antibodies

These antibodies, specific for the P1^{A1} antigen, are responsible for three fourths of the cases of neonatal alloimmune thrombocytopenic purpura and post-transfusion purpura. Anti-P1^{A1} antibodies prevent clot retraction and platelet aggregation.

P1 kinase

A serine/threonine kinase activated by interferons α and β. It prevents translation by phosphorylating eIF2, the eukaryotic protein synthesis initiation factor. This facilitates inhibition of viral replication.

p24 antigen

A human immunodeficiency virus type 1 (HIV-1), 24-kDa core antigen that is the earliest indicator of infection with HIV-1. It is demonstrable days to weeks prior to seroconversion to antibody synthesis against HIV-1. Testing for the p24 antigen does not reveal anti-HIV-1 seronegative persons or those with unapparent infections who wish to donate blood.

p53

The tumor suppressor gene that is most frequently mutated in human neoplasms. It acts as a sentinel of genomic stability. It prompts arrest of the cell cycle to permit repair of DNA or facilitates apoptosis of cells in which injuries cannot be repaired.

P-80

An assay of an antiserum's ability to precipitate antigen. This test yields data equivalent to that obtained by the quantitative precipitation reaction. A constant quantity of radioisotope-labeled antigen is added to doubling dilutions of antiserum in a row of tubes. The end point is the tube in the zone of antigen excess in which precipitation of 80% of the antigen occurs.

P addition

Appending of nucleotides from cleaved hairpin loops produced by the junction of V–D or D–J gene segments during rearrangements of immunoglobulin or T cell receptor (TCR) genes.

PAF

Abbreviation for platelet-activating factor.

PAFR

Platelet-activating factor receptor is a member of the G protein-coupled receptor family, the chemokine receptor branch of the rhodopsin family. Tissue sources include the HL-60 granulocyte cDNA library. The classic ligand of PAFR is the proinflammatory lipid PAF. COS-7 cells expressing PAFR possess a single high affinity binding site for PAF. Transcript 1 is ubiquitous and is expressed on peripheral leukocytes; transcript 2 is expressed in placenta, heart, and lung.

palindrome

A DNA segment with a dyad symmetrical structure. When read from 5′ to 3′, it reveals an equivalent sequence whether read forward or backward or from left or right. The base sequence in one strand is identical to the sequence in the second strand.

panagglutination

Aggregation of cells with multiple antigenic specificities by certain blood sera, such as agglutination of normal red blood cells by a particular serum sample. It may also refer to an antibody that identifies an antigenic specificity held in common by a group of cells bearing a common antigenic specificity even though they differ in other antigenic specificities. Contamination of sera or cells to be typed can result in aggregation of all the cells, leading to false-positive results as in blood grouping or cross matching procedures.

PAMPs

Abbreviation for pathogen-associated molecular patterns.

pancreatic islet cell hormones

Immunoperoxidase staining of islet cell adenomas with antibodies to insulin, glucagon, somatostatin, and gastrin facilitates definition of their clinical phenotype.

pancreatic transplantation

A treatment for diabetes. A complete pancreas or a large segment of it obtained from a cadaver may be transplanted along with kidneys into the same diabetic patient. It is important for the patient to be clinically stable and to have as close a tissue (HLA antigen) match as possible. Graft survival is 50 to 80% at 1 year.

pandemic

A worldwide eruption of an infectious disease.

pan-keratin antibodies

A "cocktail" of antibodies reactive with high molecular weight cytokeratin and low molecular weight keratin (AE1/AE3). By immunoperoxidase staining, these antibodies identify most epithelial cells and their derived neoplasms, regardless of the site of origin or level of differentiation.

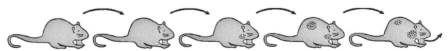

Rat   Diabetic rat   Freshly isolated Lewis islet cells inoculated into thymus, along with antilymphocyte serum   Islet cells transplanted under renal capsule in animals with sustained intrathymic transplant and normal blood glucose   Thymus removed. Rate still has normal blood glucose due to functional transplant of islet cells under renal capsule.

Protocol for pancreas transplant.

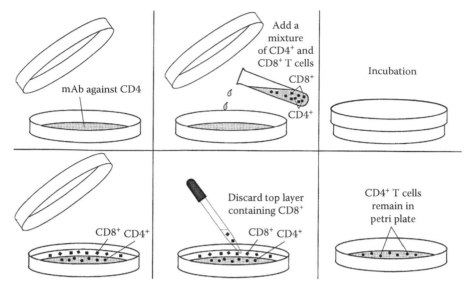

Panning technique.

panel reactive antibody (PRA) test

A laboratory method designed to identify the level of sensitization to potential donors in recipients awaiting organ transplants. The recipient's serum is screened for antibodies reactive with panels of pooled cells that express a wide spectrum of MHC molecules. PRA represents the percentage of subjects in the panel with cells that interact with the patient's antibodies. The test is employed to detect preformed alloantibodies in a recipient that could lead to hyperacute rejection of tissue from selected allogeneic donors.

Paneth cells

Narrow, pyramidal, or columnar epithelial cells, with round or oval nuclei near their bases, present in the fundi of the crypts of Lieberkühn. They manifest large secretory granules that may contain peptidase and produce antimicrobial proteins.

panning

A technique to isolate lymphocyte subsets through the use of petri plates coated with monoclonal antibodies specific for lymphocyte surface markers; thus, only lymphocytes bearing the marker sought bind to the petri plate surface.

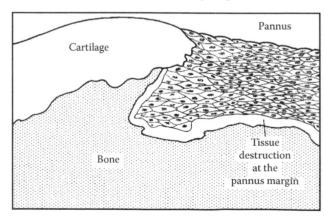

Pannus.

pannus

Granulation tissue reaction that is chronic and progressive and produces joint erosion in patients with rheumatoid arthritis. It is a structure that develops in synovial membranes during the chronic proliferative and destructive

phase of rheumatoid arthritis. It is a membrane of granulation tissue induced by immune complexes deposited in the synovial membranes. They stimulate macrophages to release interleukin-1, fibroblast-activating factor, prostaglandins, substance P, and platelet-derived growth factor which leads to extensive injury to chondro-osseous tissues. The articular surface of the joint is covered by this synovitis. Edema, swelling, and erythema in the joints are present, in addition to palisades of histiocytes. This entire process can fill the joint space, leading to demineralization and cystic resorption.

pan-T cell markers

Surface epitopes found on all normal T lymphocytes. These include the 50-kDa CD2 molecule that is the sheep erythrocyte rosette marker found exclusively on T lymphocytes, the 41-kDa CD7 molecule, CD1 present on peripheral T lymphocytes and cortical thymocytes, the mature T lymphocyte marker CD3, and CD5.

P Antigen

| | Reactions with Anti- | | | | Phenotype Frequency | |
Phenotype	P_1	P	P^k	PP_1P^k	Caucasian	African American
P_1	+	+	0	+	79	94
P_2	0	+	0	+	21	6
P	0	0	0	0	Very rare	
P_1^k	+	0	+	+	Very rare	
P_2^k	0	0	+	+	Very rare	

P antigen

An ABH-blood group-related antigen found on erythrocyte surfaces and composed of three sugars (galactose, N-isoacetyl-galactosamine, and N-acetyl-glucosamine). The P antigens are designated P_1, P_2, P^k, and P. P_2 subjects rarely produce anti-P_1 antibody, which may lead to hemolysis in clinical situations. Paroxysmal cold hemagglutinaria patients develop a biphasic autoanti-P antibody that fixes complement in the cold and lyses red blood cells at 37°C.

palivizumab (injection)

A monoclonal antibody used for the prevention of serious lower respiratory tract disease induced by respiratory syncytial virus (RSV) in pediatric patients at high risk for RSV disease. Manifests neutralizing and fusion-inhibitory activity against RSV, as revealed by RSV replication in laboratory studies. Palivizumab neutralized a panel of 57 clinical RSV isolates.

PAP (peroxidase–antiperoxidase) technique

A method for immunoperoxidase staining of tissue to identify antigens with antibodies that employs unlabeled antibodies and a PAP reagent. The same PAP complex may be used for dozens of different unlabeled antibody specificities. If the primary antibody against the antigen sought is made in rabbits, then tissue sections treated with this reagent are exposed to sheep antirabbit immunoglobulin followed by the PAP complex. For human primary

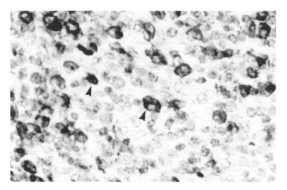

Plasma cells decorated with antibody.

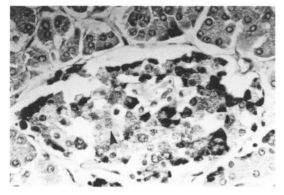

Chromogranin.

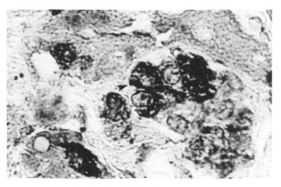

Prolactin staining in pituitary.

Development in chromogenic hydrogen donor and hydrogen peroxide. (The reaction product is seen as a reddish brown or brown granular deposit depending upon the chromogenic hydrogen donor used.)

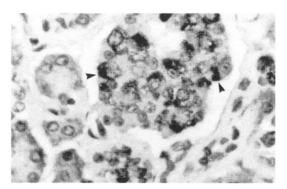

Insulin in β cells.

antibody, an additional step must link the human antibody to the rabbit sandwich technique. Paraffin-embedded tissue sections are first treated with xylene; after deparaffinization, they are exposed to hydrogen peroxide to destroy the endogenous peroxidase. Sections are next incubated with normal sheep serum to suppress nonspecific binding of immunoglobulin to tissue collagen. Primary rabbit antibody against the antigen to be identified is combined with the tissue section. Unbound primary antibody is removed by rinsing the sections that are then covered with sheep antibody against rabbit immunoglobulin. This linking antibody will combine with any primary rabbit antibody in

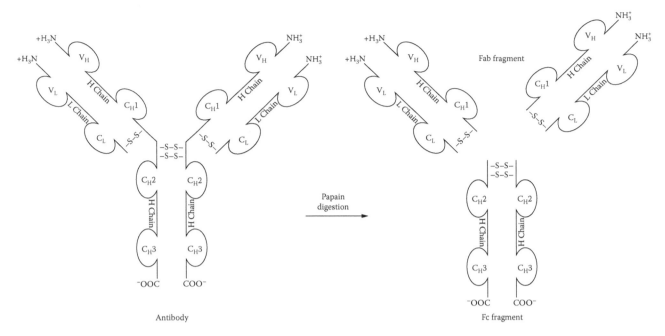

Papain digestion of IgG yielding two Fab and one Fc fragments.

the tissue. It is added in excess, which results in one of its antigen-binding sites remaining free. After washing, the PAP is placed in the section, and the rabbit antibody part of this complex will be bound to the free antigen-binding site of the linking antibody. The unbound PAP complex is then washed away by rinsing. A substrate of hydrogen peroxide and aminoethyl-carbazole (AEC) is placed on the tissue section, leading to formation of a visible color reaction product that can be seen by light microscopy. Peroxidase is localized only at sites where the PAP is bound via linking antibody and primary antibody to antigen molecules, permitting the antigen to be identified as an area

of reddish-brown pigment. Tissues may be counterstained with hematoxylin.

papain

A proteolytic enzyme extracted from *Carica papaya* used to digest each immunoglobulin (IgG) molecule into two Fab fragments and one crystallizable Fc fragment. This aids efforts to reveal the molecular structure of immunoglobulins. Papain cleaves the IgG molecule on the opposite side of the central disulfide bond from pepsin, which cleaves the molecule to the C terminus side, leading to the formation of one bivalent F(ab')$_2$ fragment in contrast to the univalent Fab fragments. The Fc fragment of papain digestion has

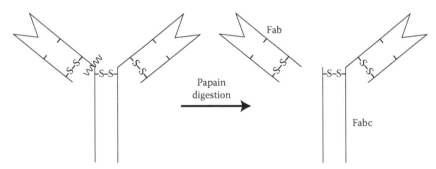

The Fab fragment is comprised of one light chain and the variable and C$_H$1 regions of a heavy chain. They are united by disulfide bonds and have a single binding site for antigen. The heavy chain part of a Fab fragment is referred to as Fd. Further digestion with papain yields and Fc'.

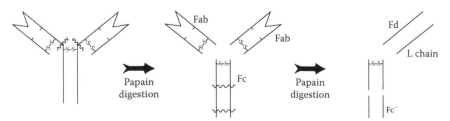

A Fab fragment is comprised of one light chain and the variable and CH1 regions of a heavy chain united by a disulfide bond, with a single binding site for antigen. The heavy chain part of a Fab fragment is referred to as Fd. Further digestion with papain yields an Fc'.

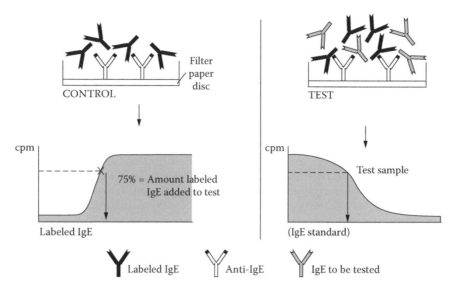

Paper radioimmunosorbent test (PRIST).

no antigen-binding capacity, although it does have complement-fixing functions and attaches immunoglobulin molecules to Fc receptors on cell membranes. The enzyme has also been used to render red blood cell surfaces susceptible to agglutination by incomplete antibody.

papain hydrolysis

Cleavage of immunoglobulin G (IgG) molecules into two Fab fragments and one Fc fragment. When the immunoglobulin is exposed to papain with cysteine present, papain cleaves a histidyl–threonine peptide bond of the heavy chain.

paper radioimmunosorbent test (PRIST)

A technique to assay serum immunoglobulin E (IgE) levels. It resembles the radioimmunoabsorbent test except that filter paper discs impregnated with anti-human IgE are used in place of Sephadex® discs.

papillomavirus immunity

Papillomaviruses induce skin and mucosa neoplasia. Humans infected with this virus develop antibodies that react with papillomavirus capsid proteins. Cervical cancer patients frequently form antibodies against the E7 proteins of HPV 16 and HPV 18. Patient sera have also demonstrated antibodies against E2, E6, and E7 proteins. Chronic infection in immunologically competent hosts points to the possibility that the viral antigens may not be recognized by the immune system. Human papillomavirus (HPV) disease occurs in immunosuppressed transplant patients and in patients with acquired immune deficiency syndrome (AIDS). Thus, cell-mediated immunity is significant for the control of HPV infection. Natural killer (NK) cells are significant in the cellular response to HPV infection. NK cell activity is decreased in patients with HPV-induced neoplasia. Decreased numbers of the potent antigen-presenting cells known as Langerhans' cells occur in HPV precancerous lesions. Viral antigens are presented to T lymphocytes via major histocompatibility complex (MHC) class I molecules that are downregulated in HPV-induced cervical lesions. The papillomavirus evades the immune system through downregulation of MHC class I molecules and Langerhans cells and diminished susceptibility to NK cells. Vaccines have been developed in animal models, especially

cattle. Therapeutic vaccines for subjects already infected with these viruses hold promise.

papovavirus

Minute tumor viruses that are icosahedral and contain double-stranded DNA. Included in the group are SV40 and polyomavirus that may cause malignant and benign tumors. Permissive or nonpermissive infections occur with papovavirus. Following permissive infection of monkey cells, papovavirus replicates, leading to lysis. T antigens—early papovavirus proteins that occur in nonpermissive rodent cells—can lead to transformation of the cells that is not reversible if the viral genome is integrated into the host genome. It is reversible if the cell can eliminate the viral genome.

parabiotic intoxication

The result of a surgical union of allogeneic adult animals. The course of immune reactivity can be modified to take a single direction by uniting parental and F_1 animals. A hybrid recognizes parental cells as its own and does not mount an immune response against them, but alloantigens of F_1 hybrid cells stimulate the parental cells, leading to graft-vs.-host disease.

para-Bombay phenotype

A variant Bombay phenotype of the ABO blood group system. Individuals expressing it have Se secretor genes that encode synthesis of blood groups A and B that are detectable in secretions. However, these subjects do not produce A and B erythrocytes as the H gene is absent. By comparison, Bombay phenotype individuals do not have the H gene or the enzyme it produces (fucosyl transferase) and do not have A or B blood group substances on their erythrocytes or in their secretions.

paracortex

A T lymphocyte, thymus-dependent area beneath and between lymph node cortex follicles.

paracrine

Local effects of a hormone acting on cells in its immediate vicinity.

paracrine factor

A molecule that produces its effect on cells in close proximity to those that synthesize the factor. Powerful cytokine molecules act in this way.

paradoxical reaction

Deaths of experimental animals from anaphylaxis when administered a second injection of an antigen to which they had been previously immunized. Early workers administering repeated injections of tetanus toxoid observed the phenomenon. This term is no longer in use.

paraendocrine syndromes

Clinical signs and symptoms induced by hormones synthesized by neoplasms.

paraimmunoglobulins

(1) The physical characteristics of some immunoglobulins present in a variety of pathologic conditions and in others of unknown etiology. (2) The secretory products of neoplastic lymphocytes. One form, the M protein of macroglobulin, is present in the normal serum, but increased levels may result in increased serum viscosity with sluggish blood flow and development of thrombi or central nervous system lesions. Increased levels of M protein are considered paraimmunoglobulinopathies.

parainfluenza virus (PIV) immunity

Immunity against parainfluenza virus infection (manifested clinically as croup, upper respiratory infections, and pharyngitis) is exhibited as an increase in immunoglobulin G (IgG) antibodies to PIV in 93, 81, and 80% of PIV type 1, 2, and 3 infections, respectively. IgM antibodies occur in 40 to 90% of cases. There are common cross reactions of IgG antibodies to PIV 1 and 3 but not of antibodies to PIV 2 and PIV 1 and 3. Cross reactions are less frequent with IgM antibodies. Enzyme immunoassay (EIA) is more sensitive than complement fixation but is of lower specificity because of cross reactions of PIV with mumps virus. Type-specific PIV antigens are found in 94 to 100% of culture-positive nasopharyngeal aspirates.

paralysis

The masking of an immune response by the presence of excessive quantities of antigen. This finding mimics acquired immunologic tolerance and is considered a false tolerance state.

paralyzed TCRs

T cell receptors that have united with but cannot release an antagonist ligand. Also called spoiled TCRs.

paramyxovirus immunity

Both serum antibody and cell-mediated immunity are induced by infection with human paramyxoviruses that cause such common childhood diseases as measles, mumps, and respiratory tract infections. Both limbs of the immune response are important for recovery from disease, although their relative significance varies with the virus of this group. Secretory antibody is important in some of them, such as respiratory infections, but it is only partially protective. Almost all of the virus-encoded proteins induce serum antibody detectable after infection. Antibodies specific for M protein and F protein are usually of low titer. Even though antinucleocapsid antibody is often present in high titer, the only neutralizing antibodies are those specific for the attachment protein and the fusion protein and are thus protective. Antibodies against either F or HN proteins are protective, but the greatest protection is induced when both antigens are used for immunization. The cell-mediated immune response to paramyxoviruses remains to be defined. These viruses may evade the host immune response and nonspecifically suppress cell-mediated immunity through infection of monocytes and macrophages as observed in measles infection. They also evade host immunity by establishing a persistent infection. Measles, mumps, Newcastle disease, canine distemper, and rhinderpest virus vaccines are presently available. These are all live attenuated virus vaccines.

paraneoplastic autoantibodies

Autoantibodies that cross react with tumor and normal tissue in the same patient. Examples are Yo antibodies against cerebellar Purkinje cells that occur in paraneoplastic cerebellar degeneration, neuronal nuclear (Hu) antibodies in paraneoplastic subacute sensory neuronapathy and sensory neuropathies, antikeratinocyte polypeptides in paraneoplastic pemphigus, antibodies against voltage-gated calcium channels in Lambert–Eaton syndrome, antibodies against retina in retinopathy associated with cancer, and antibodies against myenteric and submucosal plexuses in pseudo-obstruction of the intestine.

paraneoplastic autoimmune syndromes

Paraneoplastic syndromes affect specific organ systems and are induced by tumors but are caused by remote effects of neoplasms and not by direct infiltration or tumor metastases. Neoplasms may induce perturbations of the immune system with injurious effects on various organ systems such as the central nervous system, eyes, and skin. Tumor–immune system interaction induces tissue injury in distant organs by various mechanisms such as autoantibody-induced tissue injury.

paraneoplastic pemphigus

A rare autoimmune condition that may occasionally be seen in lymphoproliferative disorders. It is caused by autoantibodies against desmoplakin I, bullous pemphigoid antigen, and other epithelial antigens. Clinically, erosion of the oropharynx and vermilion border is observed along with pseudomembranous conjunctivitis and erythema of the upper trunk skin.

paraneoplastic syndrome

Clinical symptoms attributable to the indirect action of a malignant neoplasm on remote organs or tissues.

paraprotein

Homogeneous, monoclonal immunoglobulin molecules synthesized by an expanding clone of plasma cells, as observed in patients with plasma cell dyscrasias such as multiple myeloma or Waldenström's macroglobulinemia. The homogeneity of the paraprotein is reflected by all molecules belonging to the same immunoglobulin class and subclass as well as the same light chain type. On electrophoresis, a serum paraprotein appears as a distinct band. This is a consequence of a biologic event such as neoplastic transformation rather than antigenic stimulation.

paraproteinemias

Malignant diseases in which proliferation of a single clone of plasma cells produces monoclonal immunoglobulin. These are commonly grouped as paraproteinemias that may be manifested in several forms. Diseases associated with paraproteinemias include multiple myeloma, Waldenström's macroglobulinemia, cryoglobulinemia, plasmacytoma of soft tissues, amyloidosis, heavy chain disease, lymphomas, leukemias, sarcomas, gastrointestinal disorders associated with tumors, chronic infections, and some endocrine disorders.

parasite immunity

The cytokine network is critical in parasitic infection. Contemporary research is attempting to untangle this complex network to develop appropriate mechanisms to combat infections. Partial success has been achieved in attempting to control the direction of an immune response by incorporating cytokines into a vaccine against leishmaniasis. Interleukin-12 (IL12) has been used to prevent granuloma formation in schistosomiasis. A fine balance must be maintained between ensuring protection and reducing the possibilities of counterprotection. The primary concern in parasitic infections is not to determine whether an immune response occurs but whether the interaction between parasite and host will lead to protection or pathological changes or a combination. It is necessary to determine which antigens induce protection, how this protection may be induced artificially, what causes the pathological changes, and how they may be countered. No commercially available vaccines against any human parasitic diseases exist, and only a few against parasites of veterinary importance are available.

parasites

Organisms that derive sustenance from living hosts such as worms and protozoa. Eukaryotic organisms with several chromosomes in a nucleus surrounded by a membrane. Includes single-celled protozoa and multicellular helminth worms that range in size from a few micrometers to several meters.

parathyroid hormone autoantibodies

Autoantibodies to parathyroid hormone have been observed in unexplained hypocalcemia and hypoparathyroidism associated with normal or increased concentrations of immunoreactive parathyroid hormone.

paratope

The antigen-binding site of an antibody molecule, the variable (V) domain, or T cell receptor that binds to an epitope on an antigen. It is the variable or Fv region of an antibody molecule and the site for interaction with an epitope of an antigen molecule. It is complementary for the epitope for which it is specific. A paratope is the portion of an antibody molecule where the hypervariable regions are located. There is less than 10% variability in the light and heavy chain amino acid positions in the variable regions. There is a 20 to 60% variability in amino acid sequence in the so-called "hot spots" located at light chain amino acid positions 29 to 34, 49 to 52, and 91 to 95 and at heavy chain positions 30 to 34, 51 to 63, 84 to 90, and 101 to 110. Great specificity is associated with this variability and is the basis of an idiotype. This variability permits recognition of multiple antigenic determinants.

parenteral

Administration or injection of a substance into the animal body by any route except the alimentary tract.

parietal cell antibodies

Antibodies present in 50 to 100% of patients with pernicious anemia (PA) and in 2% of normal individuals. Their frequency increases with aging and in subjects with insulin-dependent diabetes mellitus. The frequency of parietal cell antibodies diminishes with disease duration in pernicious anemia. Parietal cell autoantibodies in pernicious anemia and in autoimmune gastritis recognize the α and β subunits of the gastric proton pump (H^+/K^+ ATPase) that are the principal target antigens. Parietal cell antibodies react with the α and β subunits of the gastric proton pump and inhibit the acid-producing H^+/K^+ adenosine triphosphatase of the

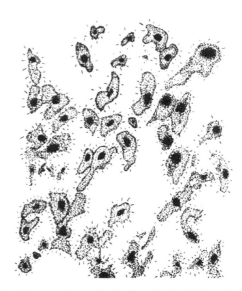

Pernicious anemia; parietal cell antibody (FITC-labeled).

gastric mucosa. Parietal cell antibodies relate to type A gastritis, for which fundal mucosal atrophy, achlorhydria, development of pernicious anemia, and autoimmune endocrine disease are characteristic.

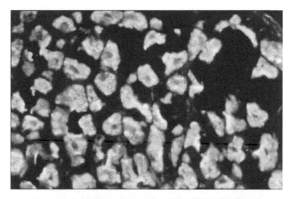

Gastric parietal cell autoantibody.

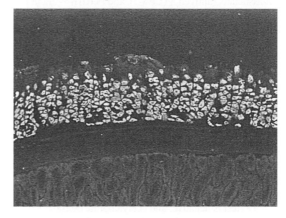

Autoantibody: gastric parietal cell + kidney.

parietal cell autoantibodies (PCAs)

Autoantibodies specific for the α and β subunits of the gastric H^+/K^+-ATPase (gastric proton pump) that secretes acid into the stomach lumen and is expressed specifically in gastric parietal cells. Although parietal cell antibodies can occur in 5% of healthy subjects, they occur in high frequency in pernicious anemia. They are related to type A gastritis, for which

P

atrophy of the fundal mucosa, achlororhydria, tendency to evolve into pernicious anemia, and association with autoimmune endocrine disease are characteristic. PCAs can be detected by incomplete Freund's adjuvant (IFA) as reticular cytoplasmic staining using mouse stomach frozen sections. PCAs have been found in 100% of patients with primary biliary cirrhosis, in three fourths of cases of autoimmune hepatitis, and in 29% of patients with chronic liver disease.

paroxysmal cold hemoglobinuria (PCH)

A rare type of disease that accounts for 10% of cold autoimmune hemolytic anemias. It may be a primary idiopathic disease or secondary to syphilis or viral infection and is characterized by the passage of hemoglobin in the urine after exposure to cold. In addition to passing dark brown urine, a patient may experience chills, fever, and pain in the back, legs, or abdomen. The disease is associated with a hemolysin termed the Donath–Landsteiner antibody, a polyclonal immunoglobulin G (IgG) antibody. It sensitizes red blood cells in the cold, complement attaches to the erythrocyte surface, and hemolysis occurs on warming to 37°C. The specificity of the antibody is for the P antigen of red blood cells.

paroxysmal nocturnal hemoglobinuria (PNH)

A rare form of hemolytic anemia in which the red blood cells, neutrophils, and platelets manifest strikingly increased sensitivity to complement lysis. An acquired membrane defect secondary to a mutation that affects myeloid stem cells. The mutant *PIGA* gene is requisite for the synthesis of a precise intramembranous glycolipid anchor called phosphatidyl inositol glycan (PIG), a component of diverse membrane-associated proteins. This membrane anchor is necessary for the expression of PIG-tailed proteins on cell surfaces. The affected proteins include some that limit the spontaneous activation of complement at the cell surface. Thus, PIG-deficient precursors give rise to red cells that are especially sensitive to the lytic action of complement. The hemolysis is nocturnal as the blood becomes acidic during sleep because of CO_2 retention and an acid pH may facilitate hemolysis. PNH red blood cell membranes are deficient in decay-accelerating factor (DAF), leukocyte-function-associated antigen 3 (LFA-3), and FcRIII. Without DAF, which protects the cell membranes from complement lysis by classic pathway C5 convertase and decreases membrane attack complex formation, the erythrocytes and lymphocytes are highly susceptible to lysis by complement. Interaction of these PNH erythrocytes with activated complement results in excessive C3b binding, which leads to the formation of more C3b through the alternate complement pathway by way of factors B and D. Intravascular hemolysis follows activation of C5 convertase in the C5–C9 membrane attack complex (MAC). The blood platelets and myelocytes in affected subjects are also DAF-deficient and are readily lysed by complement. Leukopenia, thrombocytopenia, iron deficiency, and diminished leukocyte alkaline phosphatase are observed. The Coombs' test is negative, and acetylcholine esterase activity in the red cell membrane is very low. No antibody participating in this process has been found in either the serum or on the erythrocytes. The disease is suggested by episodes of intravascular hemolysis, iron deficiency, and hemosiderin in the urine. It is confirmed by hemolysis in acid medium, termed the HAM test.

partial agonist

Refer to altered peptide ligands.

partial identity

Refer to reaction of partial identity.

parvovirus

A minute icosahedral virus composed of single-stranded DNA that may replicate in previously uninfected host cells or in those already infected with adenovirus.

parvovirus immunity

Specific immunoglobulin M (IgM) followed by IgG antibodies that occur in the second week of exposure can effectively clear parvovirus infection. Parvovirus B19 targets the erythroid bone marrow cells. Antibodies that develop following first exposure to the virus are specific mainly for VP2 epitopes. This is followed by antibodies that are specific for VP1 epitopes. VP1-unique region linear epitopes are critical to induce effective neutralizing antibodies. IgG antibodies persist for life. Immunodeficient individuals who cannot develop adequate antibody responses may develop persistent parvovirus infection. VP1-specific antibodies are crucial for the control of parvovirus B19 infection. Commercial immunoglobulin preparations contain parvovirus B19 neutralizing antibody and are useful for the treatment of persistent parvovirus infection. Antibody synthesis in immunocompetent subjects prevents clinical manifestations as a consequence of direct viral cytotoxicity. Immunodeficient patients who have impaired capacity to synthesize neutralizing antibodies develop severe anemia as a result of suppressed erythropoiesis by the virus. Empty parvovirus capsids enriched for VP1 epitopes induce protective antibody responses. A recombinant form has shown promise in clinical trials.

PAS

(1) Abbreviation for periodic acid Schiff stain for polysaccharides. This technique identifies mucopolysaccharide, glycogen, and sialic acid among other chemicals containing 1,2-diol groups. (2) Abbreviation for para-aminosalicylic acid, used in the treatment of tuberculosis.

passive agglutination

The aggregation of particles with soluble antigens adsorbed to their surfaces by a homologous antibody. The soluble antigen may be linked to the particle surface through covalent bonds rather than by mere adsorption. Red blood cells, latex, bentonite, or collodion particles may be used as carriers for antigen molecules adsorbed to their surfaces. When a red blood cell is used as a carrier particle, its surface has to be altered to facilitate maximal adsorption of the antigen to its surface. Several techniques are employed to accomplish this. One is the tanned red blood cell technique, which involves treating the cells with a tannic acid solution that alters their surfaces in a manner favoring the adsorption of added soluble antigen. A second method is the treatment of red cell preparations with other chemicals such as *bis*-diazotized benzidine. With this passive agglutination technique, even relatively minute quantities of soluble antigens may be detected by the homologous antibody-agglutinating carrier cells on which they are adsorbed. Because red blood cells are the most commonly employed particles, the technique is referred to as passive hemagglutination. Latex particles are used in the rheumatoid arthritis (RA) test, in which pooled immunoglobulin G (IgG) molecules are adsorbed to latex particles and reacted with the sera of patients with rheumatoid arthritis that contain rheumatoid factor (IgM anti-IgG antibody) to produce agglutination. Polysaccharide antigens will stick to red blood cells without treatment. When proteins are used, however, covalent linkages are required.

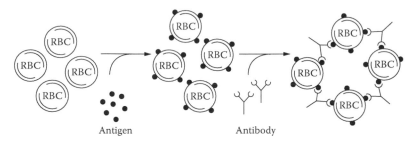

Passive agglutination test.

passive agglutination test

An assay to recognize antibodies against soluble antigens that are attached to erythrocytes, latex, or other particles by adsorption or chemical linkage. In the presence of antibodies specific for the antigen, aggregation of the passenger particles occurs. Examples of this technique include the rheumatoid arthritis (RA) latex agglutination test, the tanned red cell technique, the bentonite flocculation test, and the *bis*-diazotized benzidine test.

passive anaphylaxis

An anaphylactic reaction in an animal that has been administered an antigen after it has been conditioned by an inoculation of antibodies derived from an animal immunized against the antigen of interest.

passive Arthus reaction

An inflammatory vasculitis produced in experimental animals by the passive intravenous injection of significant amounts of precipitating immunoglobulin G (IgG) antibody, followed by the intracutaneous or subcutaneous injection of the homologous antigen for which the antibodies are specific. This permits microprecipitates to occur in the intercellular spaces between the intravascular precipitating antibody and antigen in the extravascular space. This is followed by interaction with complement, attraction of polymorphonuclear leukocytes, and an inflammatory response as described under Arthus reaction.

passive cutaneous anaphylaxis (PCA)

A skin test that involves the *in vivo* passive transfer of homocytotropic antibodies mediating type I immediate hypersensitivity (e.g., IgE in human) from a sensitized to a previously nonsensitized individual by intradermally injecting the antibodies that become anchored to mast cells through their Fc receptors. This is followed hours or even days later by intravenous injection of antigen mixed with a dye such as Evans blue. Cross linking of the cell-fixed (e.g., IgE) antibody receptors by the injected antigen induces a type I immediate hypersensitivity reaction in which histamine and other pharmacological mediators of immediate hypersensitivity are released. Vascular permeability factors act on the vessels to permit plasma and dye to leak into the extravascular space, forming a blue area that can be measured with calipers. In humans, this is called the Prausnitz–Küstner (PK) reaction.

passive hemagglutination

Aggregation by antibodies of erythrocytes bearing adsorbed or covalently bound soluble antigen on their surfaces.

passive hemolysis

The lysis of erythrocytes used as carriers for soluble antigens bound to their surfaces. Following interaction with antibody, complement induces cell lysis. In passive hemolysis, the antigen is not a part of the cell surface structure but is only attached to it.

passive immunity

A form of acquired immunity induced by the transfer of immune serum containing specific antibodies or transfer of sensitized lymphoid cells from an immune to a nonimmune recipient host. Examples of passive immunity are the transfer of immunoglobulin G (IgG) antibodies across the

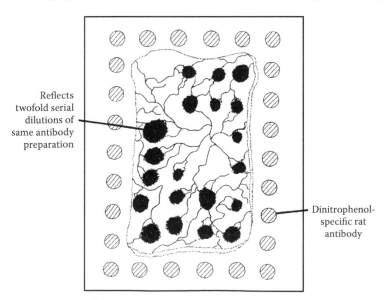

Reflects twofold serial dilutions of same antibody preparation

Dinitrophenol-specific rat antibody

Passive cutaneous anaphylaxis in rats in response to dinitrophenol-specific rat reagin antibody. The diminished size of areas of increased capillary permeability is a consequence of twofold serial dilutions of the antibody.

P

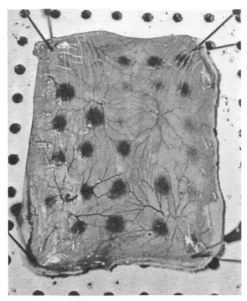

Passive cutaneous anaphylaxis in rats to dinitrophenol-specific rat reagin antibody. The diminished size of areas of increased capillary permeability is a consequence of two-fold serial dilutions of the antibody.

placenta from mother to young or the ingestion of colostrum containing antibodies by an infant. Antitoxins generated to protect against diphtheria or tetanus toxins represent a second example of passive humoral immunity, as used in the past. The transfer of specifically sensitized lymphoid cells from an immune to a previously nonimmune recipient is termed adoptive immunization. The passive transfer of antibodies in immune serum can be used for the temporary protection of individuals exposed to certain infectious disease agents who may be injected with hyperimmune globulin. No immunological memory is established.

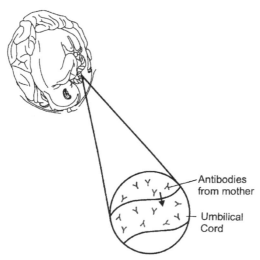

Antibodies from mother

Umbilical Cord

Passive immunization.

passive immunization

The transfer of a specific antibody or sensitized lymphoid cells from an immune to a previously nonimmune recipient host. Unlike active immunity that may be of relatively long duration, passive immunity is relatively brief, lasting only until the injected immunoglobulin or lymphoid cells have disappeared. Examples of passive immunization include

(1) the administration of γ globulin to immunodeficient individuals, and (2) the transfer of immunity from mother to young (i.e., antibodies across the placenta or the ingestion of colostrum containing antibodies). The sources of passively administered antibodies may be human blood donors, immunized humans or other animals, or hybridoma cell lines. No immunological memory is established.

passive sensitization

The transfer of antibodies or primed lymphocytes from a donor previously exposed to antigen to a normal recipient for the purpose of conveying hypersensitivity from a sensitized to a nonsensitized individual. The Prausnitz–Küstner reaction is an example.

passive systemic anaphylaxis

Rendering a normal, previously unsensitized animal susceptible to anaphylaxis by a passive injection, often intravenously, of homocytotrophic antibody derived from a sensitized animal, followed by antigen administration. Anaphylactic shock occurs soon after the passively transferred antibody and antigen interact *in vivo,* releasing the mediators of immediate hypersensitivity from mast cells of the host.

passive transfer

The transfer of immunity or hypersensitivity from an immune or sensitized animal to a previously nonimmune or unsensitized (and preferably syngeneic) recipient animal by serum containing specific antibodies or by specifically immune lymphoid cells. The transfer of immunity by lymphoid cells is referred to as adoptive immunization. Humoral immunity and antibody-mediated hypersensitivity reactions are transferred with serum, whereas delayed-type hypersensitivity, including contact hypersensitivity, is transferred with lymphoid cells. Passive transfer was used to help delineate which immune and hypersensitivity reactions were mediated by cells and which were mediated by serum.

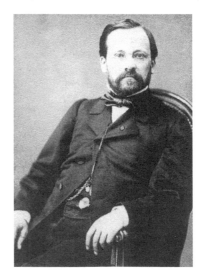

Louis Pasteur.

Pasteur, Louis (1822–1895)

French researcher, the "Father of Immunology," and one of the most productive scientists of modern times. Pasteur's contributions included the crystallization of *L-* and *O*-tartaric acid, disproving the theory of spontaneous generation; studies of disease in wine, beer, and silkworms; and the use of attenuated bacteria and viruses for vaccination against anthrax, fowl cholera, and rabies. He successfully immunized sheep and cattle

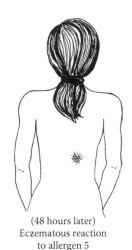

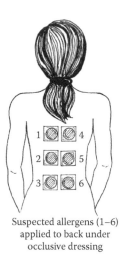

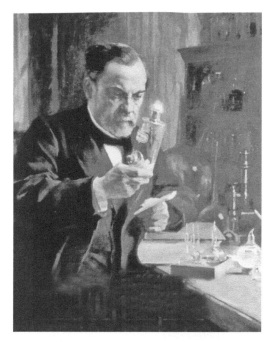

Suspected allergens (1–6)
applied to back under
occlusive dressing

(48 hours later)
Eczematous reaction
to allergen 5

Patch test.

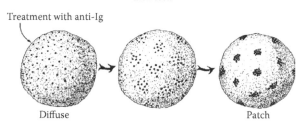

Patching.

Louis Pasteur at work in his laboratory (Edelfeldt painting).

against anthrax, terming the technique *vaccination* in honor of Jenner. He produced a vaccine for rabies by drying the spinal cords of rabbits and using the material to prepare a series of 14 injections of increasing virulence. The life of a child named Joseph Meister was saved by this treatment. (See *Les Maladies des Uers a Soie*, 1865; *Etudes sur le Vin*, 1966; *Etudes sur la Bierre*, 1876; *Oeuvres*, 1922–1939).

Pasteurella immunity

Immunity against *Pasteurella multocida* is mainly humoral antibody-mediated, yet cell-mediated immune responses also occur. Naturally acquired immunity to this organism can develop in unvaccinated cattle and water buffalo even though the organism is surrounded by a capsule that contributes to its virulence. Antibody, acting as opsonin, can render these microorganisms readily susceptible to phagocytosis by monocytes, macrophages, and polymorphonuclear neutrophils. Protein toxins from certain strains can induce the formation of neutralizing antitoxins, but purified proteins have not been shown to induce protective immunity. Cattle, buffalo, and poultry vaccinated with bacterins (formalin-killed organisms in a water-in-oil emulsion) form antibodies against lipopolysaccharide (LPS). Anti-LPS antibodies are also associated with naturally acquired immunity. Not only bacterins but also live attenuated vaccines have been employed to control *P. multocida* infections.

patching

The accumulation of membrane receptor proteins cross linked by antibodies or lectins on a lymphocyte surface prior to capping. The antigen–antibody complexes are internalized following capping, permitting antigen processing and presentation in the context of major histocompatibility complex (MHC) molecules. Membrane protein redistribution into patches is passive and does not require energy. The process depends on the lateral diffusion of membrane constituents in the plane of the membrane.

patch test

An assay to determine the cause of skin allergy, especially contact allergic (type IV) hypersensitivity. A small square of cotton, linen, or paper impregnated with the suspected allergen is applied to the skin for 24 to 48 hours. The test is read by examining the site 1 to 2 days after applying the patch. The development of redness (erythema), edema, and formation of vesicles constitutes a positive test. The impregnation of tuberculin into a patch was used by Vollmer for a modified tuberculin test. Multiple chemicals, toxins, and other allergens may induce allergic contact dermatitis in exposed members of the population.

paternity testing

Tests performed to ascertain the biological (genetic) parentage of a child. In the past, they included erythrocyte enzymes, red blood cell antigens, human leukocyte antigens, immunoglobulin allotypes, nonimmunoglobulin serum proteins, and more recently DNA "fingerprinting" (typing). The demonstration of a genetic marker in a child that is not present in the father or the mother or in cases where no paternal antigens are present in the child is enough evidence for direct exclusion of paternity. Another case of direct exclusion of paternity is when a child fails to express a gene found in both the mother and putative father. A child expressing a gene that only a male can transmit and which the putative father does not express is evidence for indirect exclusion of paternity. When a child is homozygous for a marker not present in the mother or putative father or if the parent is homozygous for a marker not found in the child, then paternity can be excluded as an indirect exclusion. Also called identity testing.

pathogen

An agent such as a microorganism that can produce disease through infection of a host.

pathogen-associated molecular pattern (PAMP)

Repetitive motifs of molecules such as lipopolysaccharide, peptidoglycan, lipoteichoic acids, and mannans that are broadly expressed by microbial pathogens not found on host tissues. Ligands for pattern recognition molecules (PRMs). The pattern-recognition receptors (PRRs) of the immune system use PAMPs to differentiate between pathogen antigens and self antigens.

pathogenesis-related (PR) proteins

Products of plant cells manifesting local acquired resistance. These substances include chitinases, P1,3 glucanases, peroxidases, RNases, proteases and enzyme inhibitors. These PR proteins break down pathogen constituents to yield small degradation products that initiate further plant responses.

pathogenicity

The capacity of a microorganism to induce disease. Factors that contribute to pathogenicity include toxin production, activation of host inflammatory responses, and perturbation of host cell metabolism.

pathologic autoantibodies

Autoantibodies generated against self antigens that induce cell and tissue injury following interaction with the cells bearing epitopes for which they are specific. Many autoantibodies are physiologic, representing an epiphenomenon during autoimmune stimulation, whereas others contribute to the pathogenesis of tissue injury. Autoantibodies that lead to red blood cell destruction in autoimmune hemolytic anemia represent pathogenic autoantibodies, whereas rheumatoid factors such as IgM anti-IgG autoantibodies have no proven pathogenic role in rheumatoid arthritis.

pathology

The study of disease.

pattern recognition molecules (PRMs)

Protein molecules that identify pathogen-associated molecular patterns. They may be soluble or membrane-bound. Collectins, including MBL, acute phase proteins, NOD proteins, and natural antibodies comprise the soluble PRMs. Those that are membrane-bound are termed pattern recognition receptors (PRRs).

pattern recognition receptors (PRRs)

Receptors that bind to pathogen-associated molecular patterns (PAMPs). Natural or innate immune system receptors that recognize molecular patterns comprising frequently encountered structures produced by microorganisms. These receptors enhance natural immune responses against microbes. CD14 receptors on macrophages that bind bacterial endotoxin to activate macrophages and the mannose receptor on phagocytes that bind microbial glycoproteins or glycolipids are examples of PRRs. These plasma membrane or endocytic vesicle membrane-bound pattern recognition molecules have a broad distribution pattern. Toll-like receptors, NK activatory receptors, $\gamma\delta$ T cell receptors, and the NKT semi-invariant TCR also belong to this category of molecules. Binding of PRRs leads to proinflammatory cytokine expression.

Paul–Bunnell test

An assay for heterophile antibodies in patients with infectious mononucleosis. It is a hemagglutination test in which patient serum induces sheep red blood cell agglutination. Absorption of the serum with guinea pig kidney tissue removes antibody to the Forssman antigen but does not remove the sheep red blood cell agglutinin that can be absorbed with ox cells. This hemagglutinin is distinct from antibodies against the causative agent of infectious mononucleosis (i.e., the Epstein–Barr virus).

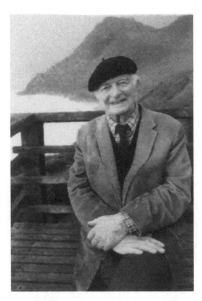

Linus Pauling.

Pauling, Linus (1901–1994)

Nobel Laureate in chemistry and proponent of the template theory of antibody formation that was championed by immunochemists.

Pax-5 gene

DNA that encodes B cell-specific activator protein (BSAP) required as a transcription factor for B lymphocyte development.

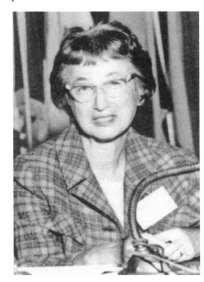

Rose Payne.

Payne, Rose (1909–1999)

A pioneer in human histocompatibility.

PBC

Abbreviation for primary biliary cirrhosis.

PCA

Abbreviation for passive cutaneous anaphylaxis.

PCH

Abbreviation for paroxysmal cold hemoglobinuria.

PCNA

Proliferating cell nuclear antigen (PCNA), which is a 29-kDa protein present mainly in dividing cells. Also called cyclin.

PCP

Abbreviation for *Pneumocystis carinii* pneumonia.

PCR

Abbreviation for polymerase chain reaction.

PDGF

Abbreviation for platelet-derived growth factor.

PECAM (CD31)

An immunoglobulin-like molecule present on leukocytes and at endothelial cell junctions. The molecules participate in leukocyte–endothelial cell interactions, as during an inflammatory response. See also platelet endothelial cell adhesion molecule-1 (PECAM-1; CD31).

pediatric AIDS

Acquired immunodeficiency syndrome (AIDS) in infants who are infected vertically (i.e., from mother to young through intrauterine or intrapartum infection). These infants show symptoms usually between 3 weeks and 2 years of age. They develop lymphadenopathy, fever, increased numbers of B lymphocytes in the peripheral blood, thrombocytopenia, and increased levels of IgG, IgM, and IgD in the serum. They may develop lymphoid interstitial pneumonia, chronic otitis media encephalopathy, recurrent bacterial infections, and *Candida* esophagitis. Epstein–Barr virus infection may produce interstitial pneumonia and salivary gland inflammation. The infants may also have blood-borne infections with such microorganisms as *Hemophilus influenzae* or pneumococci. The adult age patterns of opportunistic infections and Kaposi's sarcoma are rarely seen in HIV-1-infected infants. These children have a 50% 5-year mortality.

PEG (polyethylene glycol)

(1) A synthetic, inert molecule with a long chain structure that masks recognition of certain proteins by the immune system when attached to them. For example, PEG has been linked to adenosine deaminase (ADA), the absence of which may induce severe combined immunodeficiency. This PEG attachment permits extended survival of ADA in the body. (2) PEG is also used to promote cell fusion in hybridoma technology, in which an antibody-secreting cell and a mutant myeloma cell are fused to yield a hybridoma that is immortal and continues to produce a monoclonal antibody product.

pegademase bovine

A modified enzyme used for enzyme replacement treatment of severe combined immunodeficiency disease (SCID) associated with adenosine deaminase deficiency. It is a conjugate of multiple strands of monomethoxy polyethylene glycol (PEG) covalently linked to the adenosine deaminase (ADA) enzyme. It replaces the deficient enzyme, which when absent leads to the accumulation of metabolites toxic to lymphocytes. This treatment corrects metabolic abnormalities, leading to improvement in immune function and decreased frequency of opportunistic infections. The lag time between correction of the metabolic abnormality and improved immune function may vary from a few weeks to as long as 6 months. SCID associated with ADA deficiency is rare, inherited, and frequently fatal. Without ADA, purine substrates adenosine and 2′-deoxyadenosine concentrations increase, leading to metabolic abnormalities that are toxic to lymphocytes. Bone marrow transplantation can cure the immune deficiency.

peginterferon α-2a

Interferons bind to specific receptors on cell surfaces, leading to intracellular signaling via a complex cascade of protein–protein interactions, leading to rapid activation of gene transcription. Genes stimulated by interferon modulate many biological effects, including the inhibition of viral replication in infected cells, inhibition of cell proliferation, and immunomodulation. Peginterferon α-2a stimulates prodution of effector proteins such as serum neopterin and 2′,5′-oligoadenylate synthetase.

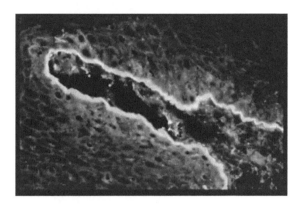

Pemphigoid (primate esophagus).

pemphigoid

A blistering disease of the skin in which bullae form at the dermal–epidermal junction, in contrast to the intra-epidermal bullae of pemphigus vulgaris. Autoantibodies develop against the dermal basement membrane. By using fluorochrome-labeled goat or rabbit antihuman IgG, linear fluorescence can be demonstrated at the bases of subepidermal bullae by immunofluorescence microscopy. Dermal basement membrane IgG autoantibodies can also be demonstrated in serum. This disease occurs principally in elderly individuals. C3 linear fluorescence at the dermal–epidermal junction is often demonstrable as well.

pemphigus erythematosus (Senear–Usher syndrome)

A clinical condition with immunopathologic characteristics of both pemphigus and lupus erythematosus. Skin lesions may appear on the seborrheic regions of the head and upper trunk, as seen in pemphigus foliaceus; however, immune deposits are also demonstrable at the dermal–epidermal junction and in skin biopsy specimens obtained from areas exposed to sunlight, reminiscent of lupus erythematosus. Light microscopic examination may reveal an intraepidermal bulla of the type seen in pemphigus foliaceus. Facial skin lesions may even include the "butterfly rash" seen in lupus. Immunofluorescence staining may reveal intercellular IgG and C3 in a "chickenwire" pattern in the epidermis with concomitant granular immune deposits containing immunoglobulins and complement at the dermal–epidermal junction. The serum may reveal both antinuclear antibodies and pemphigus antibodies. Pemphigus erythematosus has been reported in patients with neoplasms of internal organs and in drug addicts, among other conditions. Indirect immunofluorescence using serum with both antibodies may reveal simultaneous staining for intercellular antibodies and peripheral (rim) nuclear fluorescence in the same specimen of monkey esophagus used as a substrate.

pemphigus foliaceus

A type of pemphigus characterized by subcorneal blisters and anti-dsg1 autoantibodies. Patients develop fragile blisters that rupture early, leaving areas of denuded skin. One

P

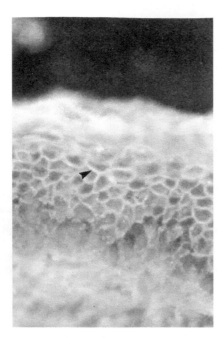

Pemphigus vulgaris; "chickenwire" staining antibody to intercellular antigen.

form of the disease affects individuals of all ethnic backgrounds, whereas a second is endemic to certain regions of Brazil and is known as *fogo selvagem*. This disease rarely involves mucosal surfaces. Histologic studies reveal acantholysis in the subcorneal layers of the epidermis.

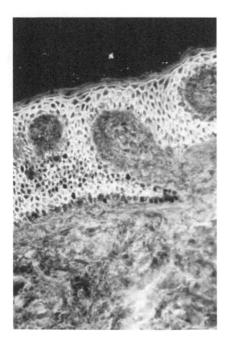

Pemphigus vulgaris.

pemphigus vulgaris

A blistering lesion of the skin and mucous membranes produced by autoantibodies, usually IgG or IgA, that interact with desmogleins requisite for adhesion between epithelial cells. This autoimmune disease has a type II hypersensitivity mechanism. The bullae develop on normal-appearing skin and rupture easily. The blisters are prominent on both

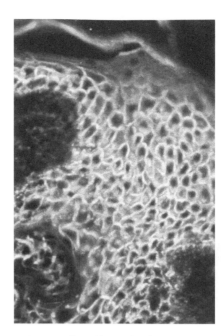

Pemphigus vulgaris.

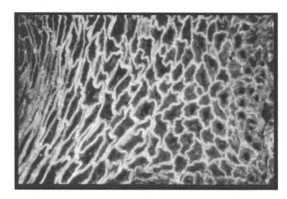

Pemphigus vulgaris.

the oral mucosa and anal/genital mucous membranes. The disorder may have an insidious onset, appearing in middle-aged individuals, and it tends to be chronic. It may be associated with autoimmune diseases, thymoma, and myasthenia gravis. Certain drugs may induce a pemphigus-like condition. By light microscopy, intraepidermal bullae are present; suprabasal epidermal acantholysis with only mild inflammatory reactivity is observed in early pemphigus. Suprabasal unilocular bullae develop, as do autoantibodies to intercellular substance with activation of classic pathway-mediated immunologic injury. Acantholysis results as the epidermal cells become disengaged from one another as the bulla develops. Epidermal proteases activated by autoantibodies may actually cause the loss of intercellular bridges. Immunofluorescence staining reveals IgG, Clq, and C3 in the intercellular substance between epidermal cells. In patients with pemphigus vulgaris, 80 to 90% have circulating pemphigus antibodies. Their titer usually correlates positively with clinical manifestations. Corticosteroids and immunosuppressive therapy, as well as plasmapheresis, have been used with some success.

P

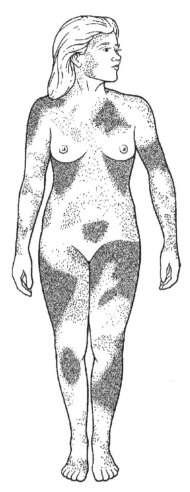

Penicillin hypersensitivity.

penicillin hypersensitivity

Allergic reactions to penicillin or its degradation products such as penicillinic acid may be antibody- or cell-mediated. Penicillin derivatives may act as haptens by conjugating to tissue proteins to yield penicilloyl derivatives. These conjugates may induce antibody-mediated hypersensitivity manifested as an anaphylactic reaction when a patient is subsequently exposed to penicillin, or it may be manifested as a serum sickness-type reaction with fever, urticaria, and joint pains. Penicillin hypersensitivity may also be manifested as hemolytic anemia, in which the penicillin derivatives become conjugated to red blood cells, or as allergic contact dermatitis, especially in pharmacists or nurses who come into contact with penicillin on a regular basis. Whereas a patch test using material impregnated with penicillin may be applied to the skin to detect cell-mediated (delayed-type, type IV) hypersensitivity, individuals who have developed anaphylactic hypersensitivity with IgE antibodies specific for penicilloyl–protein conjugates may be identified by injecting penicilloyl polylysine into their skin. The development of a wheal-and-flare response signifies the presence of IgE antibodies that mediate anaphylactic reactivity in humans.

pentadecacatechol

The chemical constituent of the leaves of poison ivy plants that induces cell-mediated immunity associated with hypersensitivity to poison ivy.

pentamidine isoethionate

A substance useful in the treatment of *Pneumocystis carinii* pneumonia in AIDS patients who failed to respond to trimethoprimsulfamethoxazole therapy. It is administered by aerosol and has diminished *P. carinii* pneumonia by 65%. Adverse effects include azotemia, arrhythmia, hypotension, diabetes mellitus, pancreatitis, and severe hypoglycemia.

pentraxin family

A category of glycoproteins in the blood that have cyclic pentameric symmetric structures. They include C-reactive protein, serum amyloid P, and complement C1.

pentraxins

A family of acute phase plasma proteins composed of five identical globular subunits. Included in this group are C-reactive protein and serum amyloid protein.

pepsin

A proteolytic enzyme used to hydrolyze immunoglobulin molecules into $F(ab')_2$ fragments plus small peptides.

pepsin digestion

A proteolytic enzyme used to cleave immunoglobulin molecules into $F(ab')_2$ fragments together with fragments of small peptides that represent what remains of the Fc fragment. Each immunoglobulin molecule yields only

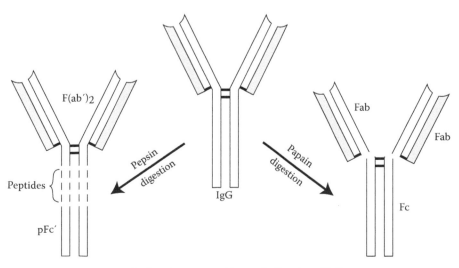

Pepsin digestion compared to papain digestion of IgG.

one F(ab')₂ fragment, which is bivalent and may manifest many of the same antibody characteristics as intact IgG molecules, such as antitoxic activity in neutralizing bacterial toxins. Cleaving the Fc region from an IgG molecule deprives it of its ability to fix complement and bind to Fc receptors on cell surfaces. Pepsin digestion is useful in diminishing the immunogenicity of antitoxins. It converts them to F(ab')₂ fragments that retain antitoxin activity.

pepsinogen antibodies

Antibodies against pepsinogen, which is produced by chief cells and mucous neck cells. Autoantibodies against pepsinogen develop in patients with autoimmune atrophic gastritis with pernicious anemia. Three fourths of patients with peptic ulcers have pepsinogen antibodies. Autoantibodies are present in half of patients with pernicious anemia and a quarter of patients with active duodenal ulcer.

peptide-binding cleft

Part of a major histocompatibility molecule that binds peptides for display to T lymphocytes. Paired α helices on a floor of an eight-stranded β-pleated sheet comprise the cleft. Situated in and around this cleft are polymorphic residues that are the amino acids that differ among various MHC alleles.

peptide-binding motif

The assemblage of anchor residues of an MHC isoform that are common to the peptide amino acid sequences that interact with the isoform.

peptide interception

A possible cross presentation mechanism. An MHC class II compartment holding exogenous peptides combines with a vesicle-harboring MHC class I recycling from the cell surface. A reduced pH in the MHC class II compartment causes release of the endogenous peptide from the recycling MHC class I molecule groove and permits loading of an exogenous MHC class II compartment peptide, independent of TAP, onto MHC class I.

peptide map

A fingerprint of peptides in two dimensions prepared by digestion of a protein with an enzyme such as pepsin. Thin layer chromatography in one direction and electrophoresis in the other direction at pH 6.5 yield the fingerprint pattern.

peptide regurgitation

A possible mechanism of cross presentation. Following internalization of extracellular proteins and processing into peptides within dendritic cell endosomes, the peptides are set free or "regurgitated" back into the extracellular environment. The extracellular exogenous peptide may negotiate an exchange of peptides at the cell surface without intracellular processing. The exogenous peptide displaces MHC-associated peptides displayed on the surface.

peptidergic endothelium-derived contrasting factor (EDCF)

A unique 21-amino acid peptide with two intrachain disulfide bonds. It is homologous to surafotoxin S6b. Also called endothelin (ET). Four isoforms of ET and two ET receptor subtypes have been described.

peptide T

A small HIV-1 envelope polypeptide initially believed to have potential in treating AIDS, but later withdrawn.

peptide vaccine

An immunizing preparation comprised of a small antigenic peptide capable of generating an immune response.

peptidoglycan layer

Humans have innate immunity against extracellular bacteria. Neutrophil (PMN), monocyte, and tissue macrophage phagocytosis leads to rapid microbicidal action against ingested microbes from the extracellular environment. The capacity of a microorganism to resist phagocytosis and digestion in phagocytic cells is a principal feature of its virulence. Complement activation represents a significant mechanism for ridding the body of invading microorganisms. A peptidoglycan layer in the cell walls of Gram-positive bacteria and lipopolysaccharide (LPS) in the cell walls of Gram-negative bacteria are able to activate the alternative pathway of complement without antibody. Also associated with LPS are flagellar antigen and somatic antigen.

peptidoglycolipid

A part of the wax D fraction extracted from mycobacteria that contains the adjuvant principle in Freund's adjuvant.

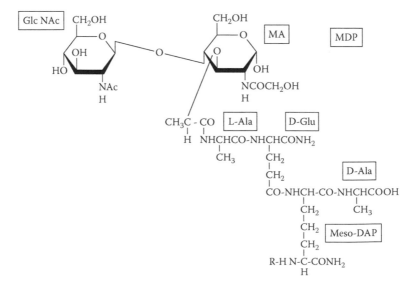

Peptidoglycan (murein).

Percoll®

A density-gradient centrifugation medium used to isolate certain cell populations such as natural killer (NK) cells. It is a colloidal suspension.

perforin

Perforin from cytolytic T lymphocyte and natural killer (NK) cell granules produces target cell lysis. Perforin isolation and sequence determination through cDNA cloning made possible studies on perforin structure and function. Perforin is a 70-kDa glycoprotein. Granules containing perforin mediate lysis in a medium with calcium. A transmembrane polyperforin tubular channel is formed in the lipid bilayer of the membrane. Released perforin inserts into the membranes of target cells to produce 5- to 20-nm, doughnut-shaped, polymeric structures that serve as stable conduits for intracellular ions to escape to the outside extracellular environment, promoting cell death. Both murine and human perforin cDNAs have been cloned and sequenced. They share 67% homology, and each is 534 amino acids long. Perforin and C9 molecules appear to be related in a number of aspects. This is confirmed by sequence comparison, functional studies, and morphologic and immunologic comparisons. Whereas lysis of host cells by complement is carefully regulated, cytotoxic T lymphocytes lyse virus-infected host cells. Decay-accelerating factor (DAF) and homologous restriction factor (HRF) guard host cells against lysis by complement. By contrast, perforin is able to mediate lysis without such control factors. Using perforin cDNA as the hybridization probe, mRNA levels have been assayed for perforin expression. Thus far, all cytotoxic T lymphocytes have been shown to express the perforin message. Perforin expression is an *in vitro* phenomenon, but perforin expression has been shown *in vivo*. This was based upon cytotoxic CD8⁺ T cells containing perforin mRNA. Refer also to perforin–granzyme-mediated cytotoxicity.

perforin–granzyme-mediated cytotoxicity

A means whereby proteases (granzymes) and a pore-forming protein (perforin) fatally injure target cells when these enzymes are released by degranulation from cytotoxic T lymphocytes, NK cells, or NKT cells. Following the uptake of these molecules by the target cells, perforin aids the release of granzyme from endosomes of target cells. Presynthesized perforin and granzyme are held in the cytoplasmic granules of the cells.

periarteriolar lymphoid sheath (PALS)

The thymus-dependent region in the splenic white pulp populated mainly by T cells. Lymphocyte cuffing of these small arterioles of the spleen adjacent to lymphoid follicles is observed. Two thirds of the PALS T cells are CD4⁺ and one third are CD8⁺. During humoral immune responses against protein antigens, B cells are activated at the PALS and follicle interfaces and then migrate into the follicles to produce germinal centers. In addition to mature T cells and some B cells, PALS also contain plasma cells, macrophages, and interdigitating dendritic cells.

periarteritis nodosa

A synonym for polyarteritis nodosa.

perinuclear antibodies

Antibodies against perinuclear granules in buccal mucosal cells in humans. They are present in about 78% of patients with classical rheumatoid arthritis (RA) and in 40% of patients with RA who are IgM rheumatoid factor (RF)-negative. The presence of perinuclear antibodies portends a poor prognosis in the RF-negative group. Perinuclear antibodies may also be found in selected other rheumatic diseases and are often present in subjects infected with Epstein–Barr virus. They are also demonstrable in approximately one fourth of patients with primary biliary cirrhosis.

perinuclear factor (profillagrin) autoantibodies

Autoantibodies against perinuclear granules of human buccal mucosal cells, They are positive in 78% of patients with classical rheumatoid arthritis (RA) and in 40% of patients with RA who are IgM rheumatoid factor (RF)-negative. The presence of these antibodies in RF-negative individuals signals a poor prognosis. They are present in much higher titers in RA patients than in individuals with other rheumatic diseases. The principal target antigen is profillagrin, an insoluble protein rich in histidine.

peripheral blood mononuclear cells

Lymphocytes and monocytes in the peripheral blood that may be isolated by Ficoll-Hypaque density centrifugation.

peripheral lymphoid organs

Lymphoid organs that are not required for ontogeny of the immune response. They include the lymph nodes, spleen, tonsils, and mucosal-associated lymphoid tissues in which immune responses are induced, in contrast to the thymus, a central lymphoid organ in which lymphocytes develop.

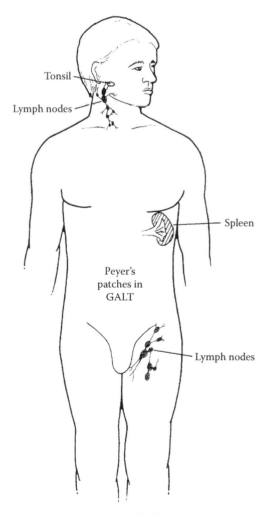

Peripheral lymphoid organs.

P

peripheral lymphoid tissues

Refer to secondary lymphoid tissues.

peripheral tolerance

Suppression of the function or deletion of self-reactive lymphocytes that escaped destruction during the development of central tolerance. Mediated by a variety of means acting outside the thymus and bone marrow. Among these are peripheral clonal deletion, anergization, clonal exhaustion, immunological ignorance, immune privilege, immunosuppressive cytokines, immune deviation, and regulatory T cells. Inhibition of expression of the immune response. The cells delivering the response are functionally impaired but not defective. Peripheral tolerance affects the efferent limb of the immune response, which is concerned with the generation of effector cells. Peripheral tolerance is acquired by mature lymphocytes in peripheral tissues. It is induced by recognition of antigens without sufficient levels of costimulators required for lymphocyte activation or by persistent and repeated stimulation by these self antigens (refer to immunologic tolerance). Mechanisms that interfere with maturation or stimulation of lymphocytes with the potential for reacting with self include self tolerance, which is acquired and not inherited. Lymphocytes reactive with self may be inhibited from responding to self or inactivated upon combination with self antigens. Self tolerance may involve both central and peripheral tolerance. In central tolerance, immature lymphocytes capable of reacting with self encounter self antigen, producing tolerance instead of activation. By contrast, peripheral tolerance involves the interaction of mature self-reactive lymphocytes with self antigens in peripheral tissues under conditions that promote tolerance instead of activation. Clonal deletion and clonal anergy are also principal mechanisms of tolerance in clones of lymphocytes reactive with self antigens.

peripheral-type benzodiazepine receptor (PBR)

An 18-kDa protein found in most steroidogenic tissues. It is found in the outer mitochondrial membrane in association with a 34-kDa, voltage-dependent anion channel (VDAC) protein. PBR is thought to be part of the mitochondrial permeability transition pore and to be involved in apoptosis.

peripolesis

A gathering of cells of one type around another kind of cell, such as the accumulation of lymphocytes around macrophages. This facilitates cell-to-cell interaction in the induction of an immune response.

peritoneal exudate cells (PECs)

Inflammatory cells resident in the peritoneum of experimental animals following the interperitoneal injection of an inflammatory agent such as glycogen, peptone, or paraffin oil. The cell population varies with time after inoculation. The first cells to appear are polymorphonuclear neutrophilic leukocytes, found several hours following injection. These are followed by lymphocytes and, within 72 hours, by macrophages. The desired population of cells such as macrophages may be harvested by peritoneal lavage with an appropriate tissue culture medium.

permeability factors

Refer to vascular permeability factors.

permeability-increasing factor

A lymphokine that enhances the permeability of vessels.

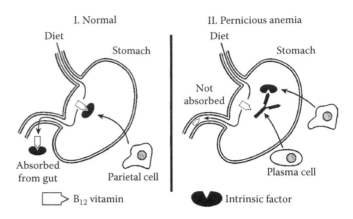

Pernicious anemia.

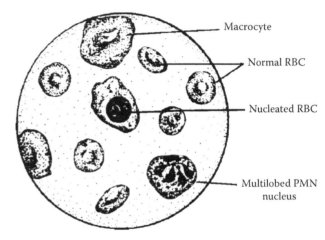

Macrocytic anemia.

pernicious anemia (PA)

An autoimmune disease characterized by the development of atrophic gastritis, achlorhydria, decreased synthesis of intrinsic factor, and malabsorption of vitamin B_{12}. Patients present with megaloblastic anemia caused by the vitamin B_{12} deficiency. The majority of pernicious anemia patients develop antiparietal cell antibodies, and at least half of them also develop antibodies against intrinsic factor, which is necessary for the absorption of B_{12}. The antiparietal cell antibodies are against a microsomal antigen found in gastric parietal cells. Intrinsic factor is a 60-kDa substance that links to vitamin B_{12} and aids its uptake in the small intestine. PA may be a complication of common variable immunodeficiency or may be associated with autoimmune thyroiditis. PA is caused principally by injury to the stomach mediated by T lymphocytes. Patients may manifest megaloblastic anemia, deficiency of vitamin B_{12}, and increased gastrin in serum.

peroxidase–antiperoxidase (PAP)

A technique that employs unlabeled antibodies and a PAP reagent and has proven highly successful for the demonstration of antigens in paraffin-embedded tissues as an aid in surgical pathologic diagnosis. Tissue sections preserved in paraffin are first treated with xylene, and after deparaffinization are exposed to hydrogen peroxide solution that destroys the endogenous peroxidase activity in tissue. The sections are next incubated with normal swine serum, which suppresses nonspecific binding of immunoglobulin molecules to tissues containing collagen. Thereafter, the primary rabbit antibody against the antigen to be identified is reacted with the tissue section. Unbound primary antibody is removed by rinsing the sections that are then covered with swine antibody against rabbit immunoglobulin. This so-called linking antibody will combine with any primary rabbit antibody in the tissue. It is added in excess. As a result, one of its antigen-binding sites remains free. After washing, the PAP is placed on the section, and the antibody portion of this complex raised in rabbits will be bound to the free antigen-binding site of the linking antibody on the sections. The inbound PAP complex is then washed away by rinsing. To read the sections microscopically it is necessary to add a substrate of hydrogen peroxide and aminoethylcarbazole (AEC) that permits formation of a visible product that may be detected with a light microscope. The AEC is oxidized to produce a reddish-brown pigment that is not water-soluble. Peroxidase catalyzes the reaction. Because peroxidase occurs only at sites where the PAP is bound via linking antibody and primary antibody to antigen molecules, the antigen is identified by the reddish-brown pigment. The tissue section can then be counterstained with hematoxylin or other suitable dye, covered with mounting medium and cover slips, and read by conventional light microscopy. The PAP technique has been replaced, in part, by the avidin–biotin complex (ABC) technique.

persistent generalized lymphadenopathy (PGL)

A clinical stage of HIV infection.

persistent infection

The prolonged existence of a pathogenic microorganism in the host body, which may be throughout life. Infections of this type may be latent or induced chronic diseases.

pertussis adjuvant

Killed *Bordetella pertussis* microorganisms mixed with antigen to enhance antibody production. Pertussis adjuvant particularly facilitates immunoglobulin E (IgE) synthesis in rats and other animals. When used as a component in the triple vaccine (diphtheria–pertussis–tetanus [DPT]) preparation used for childhood immunization, the killed *B. pertussis* microorganisms stimulate antibodies that protect against whooping cough and also facilitate antibody synthesis against both the diphtheria and tetanus toxoid preparations, thereby serving as an immunologic adjuvant.

Pertussis Vaccine

Problem	Risk of Occurrence After	
	Vaccination	Disease
Seizure	1:1750	1:25–1:50
Encephalitis	1:100,000	1:1000–1:4000
Severe brain damage	1:310,000	1:2000–1:8000
Death	1:1,000,000	1:200–1:1000

pertussis vaccine

A preparation used for prophylactic immunization against whooping cough in children. It consists of virulent *Bordetella pertussis* microorganisms killed by treatment with formalin. It is administered in conjunction with diphtheria toxoid and tetanus toxoid as a so-called triple

vaccine. In addition to stimulating protective immunity against pertussis, the killed *B. pertussis* microorganisms act as an adjuvant and facilitate antibody production against the diphtheria and tetanus toxoid components in vaccine. Rarely does a hypersensitivity reaction occur. To reduce the toxic effects of the vaccine, an acellular product is now in use.

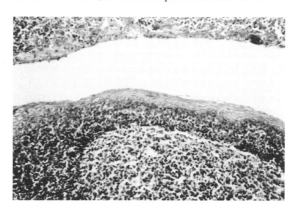

Mucosa of ileum with Peyer's patch.

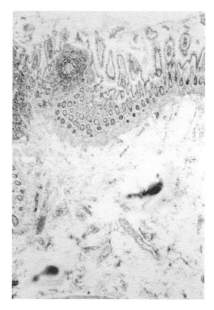

Peyer's patch.

Peyer's patches

Secondary gut-associated lymphoid tissue in the small intestinal wall, particularly the ileum. Sites where immune responses to ingested antigens may be induced. They are composed of lymphocytes, plasma cells, germinal centers, and thymus-dependent areas.

PF-4 (platelet factor 4)

Platelet factor 4 is a chemokine of the α (CXC) family. It is a heat-stable, heparin-binding protein stored with fibronectin, fibrinogen, thrombospondin, von Willebrand factor, and β-thromboglobulin (β-TG) in the α granules of platelets. PF-4 is secreted from stimulated and aggregated platelets. It is a megakaryocyte differentiation marker and a negative autocrine regulator of human megakaryocytopoiesis. A related protein called low affinity platelet factor 4 (LAPF-4) shares 50% homology with PF-4 but, unlike PF-4, is an active mitogenic and chemotactic agent that fails to bind heparin. PF4 interacts with a carrier molecule, a 53-kDa proteoglycan, *in vivo*.

Platelets and megakaryocytes represent the tissue source. Fibroblasts, platelets, adrenal microvascular pericytes, mast cells, basophils, and megakaryocytes are the target cells. PF4 levels increase during cardiopulmonary bypass surgery, in arterial thrombosis, following surgery, in acute myocardial infarction, during acute infections, and during inflammation.

pFc′ fragment

A fragment of pepsin digestion of immunoglobulin G (IgG) or the Fc fragment that yields low molecular weight peptides and a pFc′ fragment that is still capable of binding to an Fc receptor on a macrophage or monocyte. It is a 27-kDa dimer without a covalent bond composed of two C_H3 domains, the carboxyl terminal 116-amino acid residues of each chain. Unlike the Fc′ fragment, it has the basic N terminal and C terminal peptides of this immunoglobulin domain.

PFC (plaque-forming cell)

An *in vitro* technique in which antibody-synthesizing cells derived from the spleen of an animal immunized with a specific antigen produce antibodies that lyse red blood cells coated with the corresponding antigen in the presence of complement in a gel medium. The reaction bears some resemblance to β hemolysis produced by streptococci on a blood agar plate. When examined microscopically, a single antibody-producing cell can be detected in the center of the plaque-forming unit.

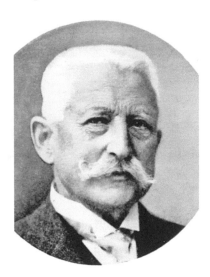

Richard Pfeiffer.

Pfeiffer, Richard (1858–1945)

Pfeiffer was a colleague of Robert Koch in Berlin. He observed that *Vibrio cholerae* organisms were lysed in the peritoneum of immunized guinea pigs and showed the same process *in vitro*. This became known as Pfeiffer's phenomenon.

Pfeiffer's phenomenon

The rapid lysis of *Vibrio cholerae* microorganisms injected into the peritoneal cavities of guinea pigs immunized against them. The microorganisms are first rendered nonmotile, followed by complement-induced lysis in the presence of antibody. Immune bacteriolysis *in vivo* involving *Vibrio cholera* became known as Pfeiffer's phenomenon.

PFU

Abbreviation for plaque-forming unit. An assay of plaques that develop in hemolytic plaque assays and related techniques.

PHA

Abbreviation for phytohemagglutinin. PHA is principally a T lymphocyte mitogen, producing a greater stimulatory effect on CD4+ helper/inducer T lymphocytes than on CD8 suppressor/cytotoxic T cells. It has a weaker mitogenic effect on B lymphocytes.

phacoanaphylactic endophthalmitis

Introduction of lens protein into the circulation following an acute injury of the eye involving the lens may result in chronic inflammation of the lens as a consequence of autoimmunity to lens protein.

phacoanaphylaxis

Hypersensitivity to lens protein of the eye following an injury that introduces lens protein, normally a sequestered antigen, into the circulation. The immune system does not recognize it as self and responds to it as it would any other foreign antigen.

phage display

A technique that permits expression of the humoral immune system *in vitro* by phage display technology and antibody engineering. Large libraries of antibody fragments are displayed on the surfaces of bacteriophage particles. Phages expressing desirable antibody specificity must be selected and expanded. Favorable mutations in the genes encoding a selected antibody specificity must be selected. Antibody fragments are selected from large libraries constructed from B cells or assembled *in vitro* from the genetic elements encoding antibodies. This technique is rapid and unaffected by the immunogenicity of the target antigen. Selection procedures permit the isolation of antibodies specific for membrane molecules and epitopes. Antibody fragments can be tailored to have the desired avidity, pharmacokinetic properties, and biological effector functions. Monoclonal antibodies prepared from phage display libraries formed from human V regions constitute a molecule especially amenable for immunotherapy in humans.

phage antibody library

Cloned antibody variable region gene sequences that may be expressed as Fab or svFv fusion proteins with bacteriophage coat proteins. They can be exhibited on phage surfaces. The phage particle contains the gene encoding a monoclonal recombinant antibody and can be selected from the library by binding of the phage to specific antigen.

phage display library

Antibody-like phage produced by cloning immunoglobulin V region genes and filamentous phage which results in their expressing antigen-binding domains on their surfaces. Antigen-binding phage can be replicated in bacteria and used like antibodies. This method can be employed to develop antibodies of any specificity.

phage neutralization assay

A laboratory test in which bacteriophage is combined with antibodies specific for it to diminish its capacity to infect a host bacterium. This neutralization of infectivity may be quantified by showing the decreased numbers of plaques produced when the phage that has been incubated with specific antibody is plated on appropriate bacteria. The technique is sensitive and can demonstrate even weak antibody activity.

phagocyte

A cell capable of phagocytosis, for example, mononuclear phagocytes and polymorphonuclear neutrophils that ingest

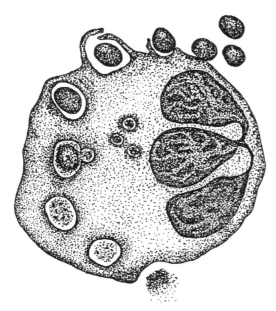

Schematic representation of phagocytosis.

and frequently digest particles such as bacteria, blood cells, and carbon particles, among other particulate substances. Neutrophils and macrophages are the main phagocytic cells in mammals.

phagocyte disorders

Conditions characterized by recurrent bacterial infections that may involve the skin, respiratory tract, and lymph nodes. Evaluation of phagocytosis should include tests of motility, chemotaxis, adhesion, intracellular killing (respiratory burst), enzyme testing, and examination of a peripheral blood smear. Phagocyte disorders include chronic granulomatous disease, myeloperoxidase deficiency, Job's syndrome (hyperimmunoglobulin E syndrome), Chédiak–Higashi syndrome, and leukocyte adhesion deficiency, together with less common disorders.

phagocytic cell function deficiencies

Patients with this group of disorders frequently show increased susceptibility to bacterial infections but are generally able to successfully combat infections by viruses and protozoa. Phagocytic dysfunction can be considered as an extrinsic or intrinsic defect. Extrinsic factors include diminished opsonins that result from deficiencies in antibodies and complement, immunosuppressive drugs or agents that reduce phagocytic cell numbers, corticosteroids that alter phagocytic cell function, and autoantibodies

against neutrophil antigens that diminish the number of polymorphonuclear neutrophils (PMNs) in the blood circulation. Complement deficiencies or inadequate complement components may interfere with neutrophil chemotaxis to account for other extrinsic defects. By contrast, intrinsic defects affect the ability of phagocytic cells to kill bacteria. This is related to deficiencies of certain metabolic enzymes associated with the intracellular digestion of bacterial cells. Among the disorders are chronic granulomatous disease, myeloperoxidase deficiency, and defective glucose-6-phosphate-dehydrogenase.

phagocytic cells

Polymorphonuclear neutrophils, eosinophils, and macrophages (monomuclear phagocytes) that play a critical role in defending a host against microbial infection. Polymorphonuclear neutrophils and occasionally eosinophils appear first in areas of acute inflammation followed later by macrophages. Chemotactic factors including N-formyl–methionyl–leucyl–phenylalanine (f-Met-Leu-Phe) are released by actively multiplying bacteria. This is a powerful attractant for PMNs whose membranes have specific receptors for it. Different types of infectious agents may stimulate different types of cellular responses. When particles larger than 1 μm become attached and engulfed by a cell, the process is known as phagocytosis. Various factors present in the serum and known as opsonins coat microorganisms and other particles and make them more delectable to phagocyte cells. These include nonspecific substances such as complement component C3b and specific antibodies located in the IgG or IgG3 fractions. Capsules enable microorganisms such as pneumococci and *Hemophilus* to resist phagocytosis.

phagocytic dysfunction

An altered ability of macrophages, neutrophils, and other phagocytic cells to ingest microorganisms or to digest them following ingestion. This represents a type of immunodeficiency involving phagocytic function.

phagocytic index (PI)

An *in vivo* measurement of the ability of the mononuclear phagocyte system to remove foreign particles. It may be represented by the rate at which injected carbon particles are cleared from the blood. The PI is increased in graft-vs.-host disease.

phagocytosis

The uptake of particulate materials such as bacteria by endocytosis. Particle ligands unite with numerous receptors on the surfaces of phagocytes in a "zippering" effect and cause

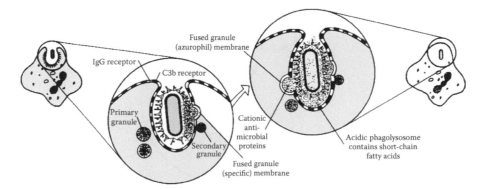

Steps of phagocytic endocytosis.

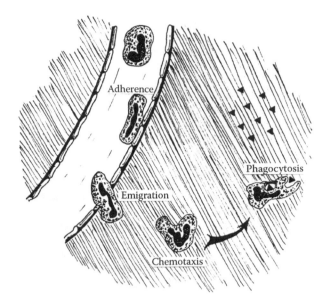

Phagocytosis

polymerization of actin, invagination of plasma membranes, and sequestration of the particle into an intracellular vesicle called a phagosome. Microbes taken up in this manner are killed by reactive oxygen intermediates and reactive nitrogen intermediate species inside the phagosome, which joins the endocytic processing pathway where it matures incrementally to generate a phagolysosome. An important clearance mechanism for the removal and disposition of foreign agents and particles or damaged cells. Macrophages, monocytes, and polymorphonuclear cells are phagocytic. In special circumstances, other cells such as fibroblasts may show phagocytic properties; these are called facultative

phagocytes. Phagocytosis may involve nonimmunologic or immunologic mechanisms. Nonimmunologic phagocytosis refers to the ingestion of inert particles such as latex or other materials modified by chemical treatment or coated with protein. Damaged cells are also phagocytized by nonimmunologic mechanisms. They may become coated with immunoglobulin or other proteins that facilitate their recognition. Phagocytosis of microorganisms involves several steps: attachment, internalization, and digestion. After attachment, the particle is engulfed within a membrane fragment and a phagocytic vacuole is formed. The vacuole fuses with the primary lysosome to form the phagolysosome, in which the lysosomal enzymes are discharged and the enclosed material is digested. Remnants of indigestible material can be recognized subsequently as residual bodies. Polymorphonuclear neutrophils (PMNs), eosinophils, and macrophages play an important role in defending the host against microbial infection. PMNs and occasional eosinophils appear first in response to acute inflammation, followed later by macrophages. Chemotactic factors are released by actively multiplying microbes. These factors are powerful attractants for phagocytic cells that have specific membrane receptors for them. Certain pyogenic bacteria may be destroyed soon after phagocytosis as a result of oxidative reactions; however, certain intracellular microorganisms such as *Mycobacteria* or *Listeria* are not killed merely by ingestion and may remain viable unless adequate cell-mediated immunity is induced by interferon-γ activation of macrophages. Phagocytic dysfunction may be due to extrinsic or intrinsic defects. The extrinsic variety encompasses opsonin deficiencies secondary to antibody or complement factor deficiencies, suppression of phagocytic cell numbers by immunosuppressive agents, corticosteroid-induced interference with phagocytic

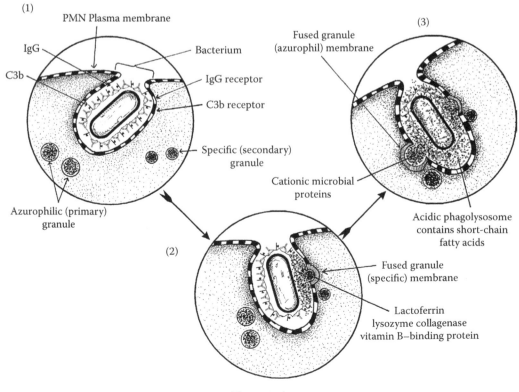

Phagocytosis.

Phenylbutazone.

function, neutropenia, or abnormal neutrophil chemotaxis. Intrinsic phagocytic dysfunction is related to deficiencies in enzymatic killing of engulfed microorganisms. Examples of the intrinsic disorders include chronic granulomatous disease, myeloperoxidase deficiency, and glucose-6-phosphate dehydrogenase deficiency. Consequences of phagocytic dysfunction include increased susceptibility to bacterial infections but not to viral or protozoal infections. Selected phagocytic function disorders may be associated with severe fungal infections. Severe bacterial infections associated with phagocytic dysfunction range from mild skin infections to fatal systemic infections.

phagolysosome
A cytoplasmic vesicle with a limiting membrane produced by the fusion of a phagosome with a lysosome. Substances within a phagolysosome are digested by hydrolysis.

phagosome
A phagocytic membrane-limited vesicle in a phagocyte that contains phagocytized material that is digested by lysosomal enzymes that enter the vesicle after fusion with lysosomes in the cytoplasm.

pharyngeal pouch
Embryonic structure in the neck that provides the thymus, parathyroids, and other tissues with epithelial cells.

pharyngeal pouch syndrome
Thymic hypoplasia.

pharyngeal tonsils
Lymphoid follicles found in the roof and posterior wall of the nasopharynx. They are similar to Peyer's patches in the small intestine. Mucosal lymphoid follicles are rich in IgA-producing B cells that may be found in germinal centers.

(Phe,G)AL
A poly-l-lysine backbone to which side chains of phenylalanine and glutamic acid short polymers are linked by alanine residues.

phenotype
Observable feature of a cell or organism that results from interaction between the genotype and the environment. A phenotype represents genetically encoded characteristics that are expressed. The term may also refer to a group of organisms with the same physical appearance and the same detectable characteristics.

phenylbutazone (4-butyl-1,2-diphenyl-3,5-pyrazolidenedione)
A drug that prevents synthesis of prostaglandin and serves as a powerful anti-inflammatory agent. It is used in therapy of rheumatoid arthritis and ankylosing spondylitis.

Philadelphia chromosome
Abbreviated chromosome 22 as a consequence of the T(9;22)(q34;q11) reciprocal translocation leading to fusion of the *Bcr* gene on chromosome 22 with the *abl* gene on chromosome 9. The *Bcr-abl* fusion gene encodes a chimeric protein that possesses constitutive Abl tyrosine kinase activity as a consequence of abnormal regulation and oligomerization capacity conferred by the Bcr moiety. Present in CML and in selected ALL patients.

***Phoma* species**
Aeroallergenic fungi that can induce hypersensitivity pneumonitis (HP); one type is known as shower curtain disease.

phorbol ester(s)
Esters of phorbol alcohol (4,9,12-β,13,20-pentahydroxy-1,6-tigliadien-3-one) found in croton oil and myristic acid. Phorbol myristate acetate (PMA), which is of interest to immunologists, is a phorbol ester called 12-*O*-tetradecanoylphorbol-13-acetate (TPA). It is a powerful tumor promoter that also exerts pleiotropic effects on cells in culture, such as stimulation of macromolecular

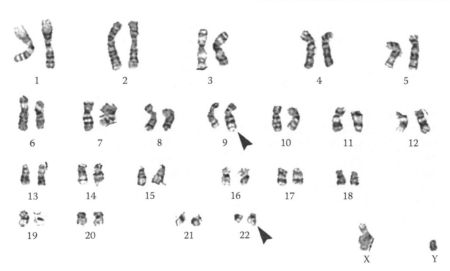

Philadelphia chromosome.

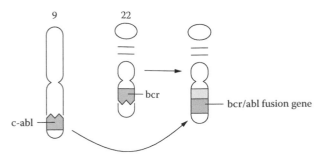

Philadelpia chromosome.

Phorbol 12,13-dibutyrate
(PDBu)

Structure of phorbol ester.

synthesis and cell proliferation, induction of prostaglandin formation, alteration in the morphology and
permeability of cells, and disappearance of surface
fibronectin. PMA also acts on leukocytes. It links to and
stimulates protein kinase C. This leads to threonine and
serine residue phosphorylation in the transmembrane
protein cytoplasmic domains such as in the CD2 and
CD3 molecules. These events enhance interleukin-2
(IL2) receptor expression on T cells and facilitate their
proliferation in the presence of IL1 as well as TPA. Mast
cells, polymorphonuclear leukocytes, and platelets may
all degranulate in the presence of TPA.

phosphatase
An enzyme that deletes phosphate groups from protein
amino acid residue side chains. Lymphocyte protein phosphatases control signal transduction and transcription factor
activity. Protein phosphatases may show specificity for
phosphotyrosine residues or phosphoserine and phospho-
threonine residues.

phosphatidylinositol bisphosphate (PIP$_2$)
A membrane-associated phospholipid cleaved by a phospholipase C-γ to yield the signaling molecules discylglyc-
erol and inositol triphosphate.

phosphocholine antibodies
Antibodies synthesized during some bacterial infections
especially by streptococcus (S) but also by *Mycoplasma*,
Proteus, *Trichinella*, and *Neisseria* in addition to
helminthic parasites. CD5$^+$ B cells form IgM antibodies that
have a limited idiotype spectrum and V$_H$/V$_L$ gene usage and
provide protective immunity from infection. These antibodies cross-react with phosphotidylcholine, pneumococci,
dsDNA, and sphingomyelin. Phosphocholine antibody
affinity diminishes with age.

phospholipase C-γ
A principal enzyme in signal transduction. It is activated
by protein tyrosine kinases that are activated by receptor
ligation. Activated phospholipase C-γ cleaves inositol phospholipid into inositol triphosphate (IP$_3$) and diacylglycerol
(DAG).

phospholipase Cγ (PLC-γ)
An enzyme that participates in signal transduction involved
in T and B cell activation. It cleaves phosphatidylinositol
bisphosphate (PIP$_2$) into diacylglycerol (DAG) and inositol
triphosphate (IP$_3$), initiating activation of two principal
signaling pathways.

phospholipid autoantibodies
Autoantibodies that include those specific for cardiolipin,
phosphatidylserine, and lupus present in individuals with
antiphospholipid antibody syndrome and systemic lupus
erythematosus, drug-induced disorders, and infectious and
neurological diseases. Phospholipid autoantibodies, primary
markers for antiphospholipid antibody syndrome, are linked
to increased risk of thrombosis, thrombocytopenia, and
recurrent abortion.

photoallergy
An anaphylactoid reaction induced by exposing an individual to light.

photoimmunology
The investigation of the effects of photons on the immune
system. The effects are initiated in the skin from the
interaction of ultraviolet radiation with immune cells.
Ultraviolet-induced immune suppression may play a role in
human skin cancer induction.

phycoerythrin
An extensively used label for immunofluorescence; this
light-gathering plant protein absorbs light efficiently and
emits a brilliant red fluorescence.

phylogenetic-associated residues
Amino acid residues in immunoglobulin variable regions
at a specific position in immunoglobulin (or other protein)
molecules in one or more species.

phylogeny
The evolutionary development of a species.

phytoalexins
Plant substances that are active in phytoimmunity.

phytohemagglutinin (PHA)
A lectin or carbohydrate-binding protein, synthesized by
plants. It cross links human T lymphocyte surface molecules, such as T cell receptors, thereby causing polyclonal
activation and T cell aggregation or agglutination. PHA is
used often in T lymphocyte functional studies to investigate
T cell activation. Clinically, it is employed to determine
whether a patient's T lymphocytes are functional, or it
may be used to induce T lymphocyte mitosis to gather
karyotypic data. PHA is derived from an extract of the red
kidney bean (*Phaseolus vulgaris*) that contains powerful
cell-agglutinating and mitogenic principles. PHA was the
first polyclonal mitogen to be described. It allows lymphocytes to be activated in *in vitro* cultures and the investigation of lymphocyte growth and lymphokine synthesis. PHA
consists of five tetrameric glycoproteins, each of which
contains two different subunits designated ENL and have
molecular weights of 33 and 31.6 kDa, respectively. PHA
stimulates the proliferation of peripheral blood mononuclear cells, notably T cells in the presence of monocytes

acting as accessory cells; these cells do not respond to PHA. PHA binds to glycoproteins on T cell surfaces.

phytoimmunity

Both active and passive immune-like phenomena in plants. Plant substances active in phytoimmunity include phytonicides and phytoalexins. Plant resistance to many diseases is associated with the presence of antibiotic substances in plant tissues. Antibiotic substances are inherent in both susceptible and resistant varieties. They may be constitutional inhibitors present in a plant before contact with a parasite or induced antibiotic substances that arise after contact with a parasite. Defense reactions in plants that are associated with the formation and conversion of antibiotic substances include reactions to wounding and necrotic reactions. Plant resistance to a specific disease is determined by the various antibiotic substances they contain and the synergistic actions of these agents with differing roles in phytoimmunity. Plant varieties differ in the quantities of antibiotic substances present in intact tissues and the intensity of their generation in response to infection. They also differ in the nature of subsequent conversions that may produce a marked increase in antibiotic activity.

phytomitogens

Plant glycoproteins that activate lymphocytes through stimulation of DNA synthesis and induction of blast transformation.

phytonicides

Substances produced in both traumatized and nontraumatized plants that represent factors active in plant immunity. Phytonicides have bactericidal, fungicidal, and protisticidal properties.

PI

Abbreviation for primary immunodeficiency.

picornavirus

Small RNA virus with a naked capsid structure. More than 230 viruses categorized as enteroviruses, rhinoviruses, cardioviruses, and aphthoviruses comprise this family.

picornavirus immunity

Neutralizing antibodies play an important role in protection against picornaviruses as shown by the ability of passively transferred antibodies to block virus replication and disease progression. The early IgM response is less specific than the subsequent IgG and IgA responses. Considerable cross reactivity exists among the different serotypes. Virus neutralization by antibody involves Fc receptor-mediated endocytosis (opsonization) and interactions that prevent virus penetration and uncoating or induce lethal RNA unpackaging. CD4+ T cells have also been shown to be significant in picornavirus infections that induce cell-mediated responses with the production of cytokines. CD4+ and CD8+ T lymphocytes recognize specific epitopes. Picornaviruses evade the immune system through antigenic variation of neutralizing antibody epitopes and may also involve variation at T cell sites and MHC-binding structures that interfere with help for humoral immune responses and cell-mediated killing of infected cells. Vaccines against picornaviruses depend on their ability to induce neutralizing antibodies in the host following administration of a live attenuated virus or a chemically inactivated intact virus.

picryl chloride (1-chloro-2,4,6-trinitrobenzene)

A substance used to add picryl groups to proteins. When applied to the skin of an experimental animal such as a

guinea pig, a solution of picryl chloride may conjugate with skin proteins, where it acts as a hapten and may induce contact (type IV) hypersensitivity.

piecemeal necrosis

Deaths of individual liver cells that are encircled by lymphocytes in chronic active hepatitis.

pigeon breeder's lung

Hypersensitivity pneumonitis. Also called pigeon fancier's lung.

pili

Structures that facilitate adhesion of bacteria to host cells and are therefore direct determinants of virulence.

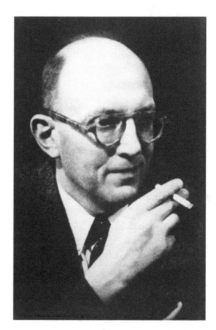

Louis Pillemer.

Pillemer, Louis (1908–1957)

Professor at Western Reserve University (now Case Western Reserve) who described properdin and the alternative pathway of complement activation.

pinocytosis

The uptake by a cell of small liquid droplets, minute particles, and solutes.

Pirquet von Cesenotics, Clemens Peter Freiherr von (1874–1929)

Viennese physician who coined the term *allergy* and described serum sickness and its pathogenesis. He also developed a skin test for tuberculosis. He held academic appointments at Vienna, Johns Hopkins, and Breslau and returned to Vienna in 1911 as director of the University Children's Clinic. (Refer to *Die Serumkrenkheit* [with Schick], 1905; *Klinische Studien über Vakzination und Vakzinale Allergie*, 1907; *Allergy*, 1911.)

pituitary autoantibodies

Autoantibodies most often found in the empty sella syndrome. They are less often found in the sera of patients with pituitary adenomas, prolactinomas, acromegaly, idiopathic diabetes insipidus, Hashimoto's thyroiditis, Graves' disease, and POEMS (polyneuropathy, organomegaly, endocrinopathy, M protein, and skin changes) syndrome. They are also associated with insulin-dependent diabetes mellitus (IDDM)

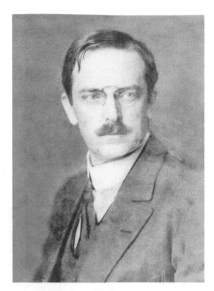

Clemens Peter Freiherr von Pirquet.

and adrenocorticotrophic hormone (ACTH) deficiency. They may portend an unfavorable consequence of pituitary microsurgery for Cushing's disease. Forty-eight percent of children with cryptorchidism may develop autoantibodies against follicle-stimulating hormone (FSH)-secreting and luteinizing hormone (LH)-secreting pituitary cells. Autoantibodies against pituitary hormones have been discovered in 45% of patients with pituitary tumors or empty sella syndrome but not in normal individuals; 100% develop ACTH autoantibodies, and 20% form thyroid-stimulating hormone (TSH) and growth hormone (GH) autoantibodies. Empty sella syndrome may be induced by hypophysitis secondary to pituitary autoantibodies in adults. Autoantibodies against prolactin develop in 16% of patients with idiopathic hyperprolactinemia. Patients with these autoantibodies do not usually have clinical symptoms of hyperprolactinemia.

pituitary hormones
Immunoperoxidase staining of pituitary adenomas with antibodies to adrenocorticotrophic hormone (ACTH), growth hormone (GH), prolactin, follicle-stimulating hormone (FSH), and luteinizing hormone (LH) facilitates definition of their clinical phenotype.

P1 kinase
A serine/threonine kinase activated by interferons α and β. It prevents translation by phosphorylating eIF2, the eukaryotic protein synthesis initiation factor. This facilitates inhibition of viral replication.

PK reaction
Refer to Prausnitz–Küstner reaction.

PK test
Abbreviation for Prausnitz–Küstner reaction.

plague vaccine
Yersinia pestis microorganisms killed by heat or formalin are injected intramuscularly to induce immunity against plague. It is administered in three doses 4 weeks or more apart. The duration of the immunity is approximately 6 months. A live attenuated vaccine, used mainly in Java, has also been found to induce protective immunity. An immunizing preparation is prepared from a crude fraction of killed *Yersinia pestis* plague microorganisms or synthetically from

recombinant proteins. It is rarely used except in a laboratory or for field workers in regions where plague is endemic.

plantibodies
Antibodies derived from plants such as tobacco that may be used in research. They may prove less immunogenic than murine antibodies. Antibody-like substances synthesized by transgenic plants.

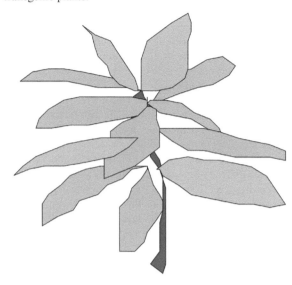

Plant immunity.

plant immunity
Immunity in higher plants consists of an immune state of systemic acquired resistance (SAR) that follows a local infection by pathogenic microorganisms that leads to lesions with death of host cells. SAR encompasses a broad spectrum of bacterial, viral, and fungal agents, as well as the infective pathogen. Various SAR genes encode numerous microbicidal proteins induced by endogenous chemicals that include salicylic acid, which combines with a catalase to increase H_2O_2, which may facilitate defense.

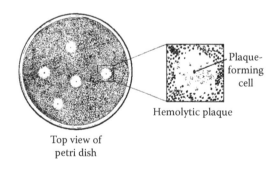

Plaque-forming cell (PFC) assay.

plaque-forming assay
Refer to hemolytic plaque assay.

plaque-forming cell (PFC) assay
Technique for demonstrating and enumerating cells forming antibodies against a specific antigen. Mice are immunized with sheep red blood cells (SRBCs). After a specified period, a suspension of splenic cells from the immunized mouse is mixed with antigen (SRBC) and spread on a suitable semisolid gel medium. After or during incubation at 37°C, complement is added. The erythrocytes that have anti-SRBC

antibody on their surface will be lysed. Circular areas of hemolysis appear in the gel medium. If viewed under a microscope, a single antibody-forming cell can be identified in the center of the lytic area. This assay has several modifications since antibodies other than IgM may fix complement less efficiently. In order to enhance the effects, an antiglobulin antibody called developing antiserum is added to the mixture. The latter technique is called indirect PFC assay.

plaque-forming cells

The antibody-producing cells in the centers of areas of hemolysis observed microscopically during a hemolytic plaque assay. The antibodies they form are specific for red blood cells suspended in the gel medium surrounding them. Once complement is added, the antibody-coated erythrocytes lyse, producing clear areas of hemolysis surrounding the antibody-forming cells. The antibody produced may be specific both for red blood cell surface antigens and also for soluble antigens deliberately coated on their surfaces for assay purposes.

plaque technique

Refer to hemolytic plaque assay and phage neutralization assay.

plasma

A transparent yellow material that constitutes 50 to 55% of blood volume. It is 92% fluid and 7% protein. Inorganic salts, hormones, sugars, lipids, and gases comprise the remaining 1%. Plasma from which fibrinogen and clotting factors have been removed is known as serum.

plasmablast

An immature cell of the plasma cell lineage that reveals distinctive, clumped nuclear chromatin, developing endoplasmic reticulum, and a Golgi apparatus; a B lymphocyte in a lymph node that is beginning to reveal plasma cell features. Manifests increased rough endoplasmic reticulum, Golgi apparatus, and ribosomes.

plasma cell antigen

A murine plasmacyte membrane alloantigen. It may be designated PC-1 or PC-2.

plasma cell dyscrasias

Lymphoproliferative disorders in which monoclonal plasma cell proliferation leads to such conditions as multiple myeloma or to the less ominous extramedullary plasmacytoma. A diverse assemblage of neoplastic diseases characterized by proliferation of a single cell clone producing an M component, a monoclonal immunoglobulin, or immunoglobulin fragment. The cells often have plasma cell morphology but may resemble lymphocytic or lymphoplasmacytic cells.

plasma cell leukemia

A malignancy associated with plasma cells in the circulating blood that constitute greater than 20% of the leukocytes. The absolute plasma cell number is more than 2000 per cubic millimeter of blood. Advanced cases reveal extensive infiltration of the tissue with plasma cells and replacement of the marrow. Reactive plasmacytosis must be considered in the diagnosis.

plasma cells

Terminally differentiated antibody-producing B cells that fail to express MHC class II or mIg and are incapable of receiving further T cell help. Immunoglobulins are present in their cytoplasm, and secretion of immunoglobulin by plasma cells has been directly demonstrated *in vitro*. Increased levels of immunoglobulins in some pathologic conditions are associated with increased numbers of plasma cells and

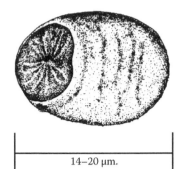

14–20 μm.

Diagram of a plasma cell.

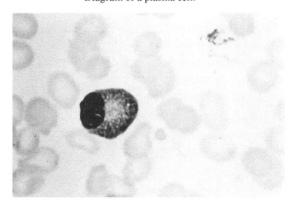

Plasma cell in peripheral blood.

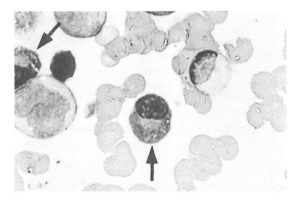

Plasma cell in peripheral blood.

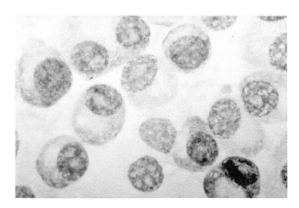

Plasma cells in peripheral blood smear.

conversely their number at antibody-producing sites increases following immunization. Plasma cells develop from B cells and are large, spherical, or ellipsoidal cells, 10 to 20 μm in

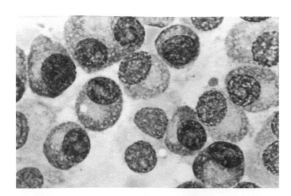

Plasma cells.

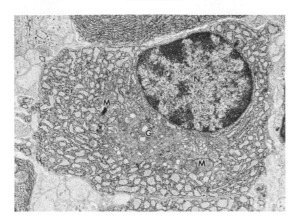

Electron micrograph of plasma cell. N = nucleus. M = mitochondria.
G = Golgi apparatus. ER = endoplasmic reticulum.

size. Mature plasma cells have abundant cytoplasm, which
stains deep blue with Wright's stain, and have an eccentri-
cally located round or oval nucleus, usually surrounded by
a well defined perinuclear clear zone. The nucleus contains
coarse and clumped masses of chromatin, often arranged in a
cartwheel fashion. The nuclei of normal, mature plasma cells
have no nucleoli, but those of neoplastic plasma cells such as
those seen in multiple myeloma have conspicuous nucleoli.
The cytoplasm of normal plasma cells has a conspicuous Golgi
complex and rough endoplasmic reticulum and frequently
contains vacuoles. The nuclear to cytoplasmic ratio is 1:2.
By electron microscopy, plasma cells show very abundant
endoplasmic reticulum, indicating extensive and active protein
synthesis. Plasma cells do not express surface immunoglobulin
or complement receptors which distinguishes them from B
lymphocytes. Plasma cells that are short-lived differentiate
quickly without manifesting isotype switching or somatic
hypermutation leading to the secretion of low affinity IgM
antibodies. Plasma cells that are long-lived differentiate following isotype switching and somatic hypermutation, which leads
to the secretion of high-affinity antibodies that have various
effector functions.

plasmacyte
Plasma cell.

plasmacytoid dendritic cells (PDCs)
Cells with a dendritic-like appearance arising from interfer-
on-synthesizing cells activated in culture by inflammatory
cytokines and products of microbes.

plasmacytoma
A plasma cell neoplasm. Also termed myeloma or multiple myeloma. To induce an experimental plasmacytoma

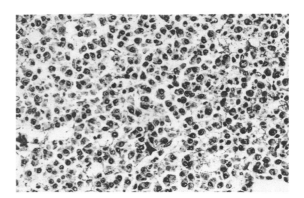

Bone marrow plasmacytoma with pure plasma cell infiltrate.

in laboratory mice or rats, paraffin oil is injected into the
peritoneum. Plasmacytomas may occur spontaneously.
These tumors, composed of neoplastic plasma cells, synthesize and secrete monoclonal immunoglobulins, yielding a
homogeneous product that forms a spike in electrophoretic
analysis of the serum. Plasmacytomas were used extensively to generate monoclonal immunoglobulins prior to
the development of B cell hybridoma technology to induce
monoclonal antibody synthesis at will to multiple antigens.

plasma half-life (T$^{1/2}$)
Determination of the catabolic rate of any component of the
blood plasma. With respect to immunoglobulins, it is the
time required for one half of the plasma immunoglobulins
to be catabolized.

plasma histamine
Even though histamine released from basophils and mast
cells is a critical step in immediate hypersensitivity reactions, plasma histamine levels are rarely determined due to
the short half-life of histamine in plasma. Thus, mast cell
tryptase and thromboxane A$_2$ are the preferred analytes due
to their longer half-lives.

plasmapheresis
A technique in which blood is withdrawn from an individual, the desired constituent is separated by centrifugation,
and the cells are reinjected into the patient; for example,
plasma components may be removed from the circulation of
an individual by this method. The technique is also useful
to obtain large amounts of antibodies from the plasma of
an experimental animal. Plasmapheresis is used therapeutically to rid the body of toxins or autoantibodies in the blood
circulation. Blood taken from the patient is centrifuged, the
cells are saved, and the plasma is removed. Cells are resus-
pended in albumin, fresh normal plasma, or albumin in
saline and returned to the patient. The ill effects of a toxin
or of an autoantibody may be reduced by 65% by removing approximately 2500 mL of plasma. Removal of twice
this amount of plasma may diminish the level of a toxin or
of an autoantibody by an additional 20%. This procedure
has been used to treat patients with myasthenia gravis,
Eaton–Lambert syndrome, Goodpasture's syndrome, hyperviscosity syndrome, post-transfusion purpura, and acute
Guillain–Barré syndrome.

plasma pool
The amount of plasma immunoglobulin per unit of body
weight. This may be designated as milligrams of immunoglobulin per kilogram of body weight.

plasmid

Extrachromosomal genetic structure that consists of a circular, double-stranded DNA molecule that permits the host bacterial cell to resist antibiotics and produce other effects that favor its survival. Plasmid replication is independent of the bacterial chromosome. Plasmids have been used widely in recombinant DNA technology.

plasmin

A serine protease proteolytic enzyme in plasma generated from its inactive precursor plasminogen. It is a 90-kDa enzyme that derives from cleavage of a single arginyl–valyl bond in the C terminal region of plasminogen. It consists of two unequal chains, termed heavy (A) and light (B) chains, linked by a single disulfide bond. The A chain derives from the N terminal region of plasminogen. The B chain carries the serine active site. Plasmin catalyzes the hydrolysis of fibrin; thus, it facilitates the dissolution of intravascular blood clots. In addition to its fibrinolytic activity, plasmin has numerous other functions associated with coagulation, fibrinolysis, and inflammation that include: (1) enhancement of antibody responses to both thymus-dependent and thymus-independent antigens, (2) augmentation of agglutination by lectins, (3) facilitation of the escape of cells from contact inhibition in culture, (4) enhancement of cytotoxicity with or without participation of antibodies, and (5) stimulation of B cell proliferation.

plasminogen

The inactive precursor of the proteolytic enzyme plasmin. Several serine proteases such as urokinase convert it to active plasmin. It is a β globulin widely distributed in tissue, body fluids, and plasma and is a single-chain monomeric molecule. Plasminogen activation occurs in two stages. The GLU plasminogen activation begins with removal of two peptides at the N terminus of the molecule and conversion to Lys-plasminogen. The second step involves the rapid conversion of Lys-plasminogen to Lys-plasmin.

plasminogen activator

An enzyme produced by macrophages that converts plasminogen to plasmin, which degrades fibrin.

platelet

A small (3 μm in diameter) round disk that is derived from bone marrow megakaryocytes and is present in the blood. Platelets function in blood clotting by releasing thromboplastin. They also harbor serotonin and histamine, which may be released during type I anaphylactic hypersensitivity reactions. Complement receptor 1 (CR1) is present on the platelets of mammals other than primates and is significant for immune adherence. Activated platelets cluster to facilitate blood clotting and release cytokines from preformed mRNAs that affect leukocyte migration and function in inflammation.

platelet-activating factor (PAF)

A phospholipid with a molecular weight of about 300 to 500 Da formed by leukocytes, macrophages, mast cells, and endothelial cells that induces aggregation of platelets and promotes amine secretion, aggregation of neutrophils, release of enzymes, and an increase in vascular permeability. Its effect resembles that of IgE-mediated changes in anaphylaxis and cold urticaria. It may also participate in endotoxin shock and is derived from phosphorylcholine. The combination of antigen with the Fab regions of antibody molecules bound through Fc receptors to mast cells, polymorphonuclear leukocytes, and macrophages results in platelet-activating factor (PAF) release. PAF release accompanies anaphylactic shock and apparently mediates inflammation and allergic reactions. PAF induces a transient reduction in blood platelets, causes hypotension, and facilitates vascular permeability, but it has no effects on contracting smooth muscle and have no chemotactic activity. Probably more than a single compound have this activity. PAF is resistant to arylsulfatase B but is sensitive to phospholipases. PAF may induce bronchoconstriction and vascular dilation and leak and may serve as a significant mediator of asthma.

platelet antibodies

Refer to platelet antigens.

platelet antibodies, drug-induced

Amphotericin B, cephalothin, methicillin, pentamidine, trimethoprim-sulfamethoxizole, and vancomycin may all induce the synthesis of antiplatelet antibodies.

platelet antigens

Surface epitopes on thrombocytes that may be immunogenic, leading to platelet antibody formation, which causes such conditions as neonatal alloimmune thrombocytopenia

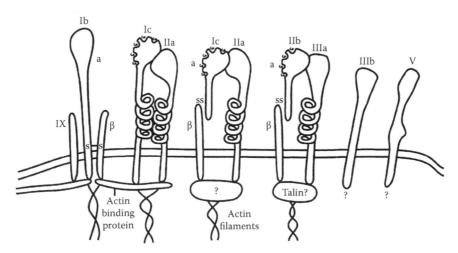

Schematic representation of principal platelet membrane glycoproteins indicating known or suspected complexes, disulfide bonds between chains, calcium-bonding domains, and interactions with cytoskeletal components.

Nomenclature and Phenotype Frequency of Human Platelet Antigens

Antigen System	Glycoprotein (GP) Location	Other Names	Antigens	Other Names	Phenotype Frequency Caucasian	Phenotype Frequency Japanese
HPA-1	GPIIIa	Zw, Pl^A	HPA-1a	Zw^a, Pl^{A1}	97.9	99.9
			HPA-1b	Zw^b, Pl^{A2}	26.5	3.7
HPA-2	GPIb	Ko, Sib	HPA-2a	Ko^b	99.3	NT
			HPA-2b	Ko^a, Sib^a	14.6	25.4
HPA-3	GPIIb	Bak, Lek	HPA-3a	Bak^a, Lek^a	87.7	78.9
			HPA-3b	Bak^b	64.1	NT
HPA-4	GPIIIa	Pen, Yuk	HPA-4a	Pen^a, Yuk^b	99.9	99.9
			HPA-4b	Pen^b, Yuk^a	0.2	1.7
HPA-5	GPIa	Br, Hc, Zav	HPA-5a	Br^b, Zav	99.2	NT
			HPA-5b	Br^{a,} Zav^a, Hc^a	20.6	NT

and post-transfusion purpura. The Pl^{A1} antigen may induce platelet antibody formation in Pl^{A1} antigen-negative individuals. Additional platelet antigens associated with purpura include Pl^{A2}, Bak^a, and HLA-A2.

platelet-associated immunoglobulin G (PAIgG)

PAIgG is present in 10% of normal individuals, in 50% of those with tumors, and in 76% of septic patients and may be induced by graft-vs.-host disease. PAIgG is present in 71% of autologous marrow graft recipients and in 50% of allogeneic marrow graft recipients.

platelet autoantibodies

Platelets possess surface FcRII that combine with IgG or immune complexes. The platelet surfaces can become saturated with immune complexes, as in autoimmune (or idiopathic) thrombocytopenic purpura (ITP) or AITP. Fab-mediated antibody binding to platelet antigens may be difficult to distinguish from Fc-mediated binding of immune complexes to the surface.

platelet-derived growth factor (PDGF)

A low molecular weight protein derived from human platelets that acts as a powerful connective tissue mitogen, causing fibroblast and intimal smooth muscle proliferation. It also induces vasoconstriction and chemotaxis and activates intracellular enzymes. PDGF plays an important role in atherosclerosis and fibroproliferative lesions such as glomerulonephritis, pulmonary fibrosis, myelofibrosis, and other processes. It is comprised of a two-chain (A or B) dimer. It can be an AA or BB homodimer or an AB heterodimer. Human PDGF-AA is a 26.5-kDa A chain homodimeric protein comprised of 250-amino acid residues, whereas PDGF-BB is a 25-kDa B chain homodimeric protein comprised of 218-amino acid residues. In addition to platelets, PDGF is released by activated mononuclear cells, endothelial cells, smooth muscle cells, and fibroblasts. It plays a physiologic role in wound repair and processes requiring accumulation of connective tissue. The three known polypeptide dimers of PDGF include AA, AB, and BB that bind to α or β dimeric tyrosine kinase receptors.

platelet-derived growth factor receptor (PDGF-R)

A glycoprotein in the membrane that has five extracellular domains that resemble those of immunoglobulins. It also has a kinase insert in the cytoplasm. The receptor protein must undergo a conformational change for

signal transduction. A gene on chromosome 4q11 encodes PDGF-R.

platelet endothelial cell adhesion molecule-1 (PECAM-1; CD31)

An antigen that is a single-chain membrane glycoprotein with a molecular weight of 140kD. It is found on granulocytes, monocytes, macrophages, B cells, platelets, and endothelial cells. Although called gpIIa′, it is different from the CD29 antigen. At present the function of CD31 is unknown. It may be an adhesion molecule.

platelet factor 4 (PF-4)

A chemokine that comprises a principal constituent of platelet α granules. Its sequence resembles that of β-thromboglobulin (β-TG) and neutrophil-activating peptide 2 (NAP-2). PF-4 activities include heparin binding, inhibition of angiogenesis, induction of intercellular adhesion molecule 1 (ICAM-1) on endothelial cells, promotion of neutrophil adhesion to endothelium, increased fibrin, fiber formation, inhibition of other chemotactic factor effects, *in vivo* recruitment of neutrophils, fibroblast migration during wound repair, and reversal of con-A-induced suppression of lymphocyte activity.

platelet transfusion

The administration of platelet concentrates prepared by centrifuging a unit of whole blood at low speed to provide 40 to 70 mL of plasma that contains 3 to 4 × 10^{11} platelets. This amount can increase an adult's platelet concentration by 10,000 per cubic millimeter of blood. It is best to store platelets at 20 to 24°C, subjecting them to mild agitation. They must be used within 5 days of collection.

pleiotropic

The production of multiple actions on the same cell type, such as a cytokine that influences the activity of numerous different types of cells.

pluripotency

The versatility to differentiate into one of various different types of cells.

pluripotent stem cell

A continuously dividing, undifferentiated bone marrow cell that has progeny consisting of additional stem cells together with cells of multiple separate lineages. Bone marrow hematopoietic stem cells may develop into cells of the myeloid, lymphoid, and erythroid lineages.

P

PMN
Abbreviation for polymorphonuclear leukocyte.

PM-Scl autoantibodies
Autoantibodies that react with nucleoli and with a complex of 16 (2- to 110-kDa) proteins. They are detected in subjects with homogeneous overlap connective tissue disease marked by Raynaud's phenomenon, scleroderma, myositis, arthritis, and pulmonary restriction. These autoantibodies are closely linked to the major histocompatibility complex (MHC) class II antigen, HLA-DR; PM-Scl autoantibodies represent a good prognostic sign.

pneumococcal 7 valent conjugate vaccine
A pneumococcal vaccine employed to actively immunize infants and small children. The immunizing preparation is composed of antigens derived from seven capsular serotypes of *Streptococcus pneumoniae.*

pneumococcal polysaccharide
A polysaccharide found in the *Streptococcus pneumoniae* capsule that is a type-specific antigen and virulence factor. Serotypes of this microorganism are based upon different specificities in the capsular polysaccharide composed of oligosaccharide repeating units. Glucose and glucuronic acid are the repeating units in type III polysaccharide.

pneumococcal polysaccharide vaccine
A 23-valent vaccine containing capsular polysaccharides of *Streptococcus pneumoniae.* It counters 85 to 90% of the serotypes causing invasive pneumococcal infections. Elderly, immunocompromised, and chronically ill persons are advised to receive the vaccine every 3 years.

pneumococcal vaccine polyvalent (injection)
For vaccination against pneumococcal disease caused by pneumococcal types included in the vaccine. It does not prevent disease caused by capsular types of pneumococcus other than those contained in the vaccine. Purified pneumococcal capsular polysaccharides induce synthesis of an antibody effective in prevention of pneumococcal disease. Clinical trials have proven the immunogenicity of each of the 23 capsular types when tested in polyvalent vaccines. Investigations employing 12-, 14-, and 23-valent pneumococcal vaccines in children 2 years of age and older and adults of all ages revealed immunogenic responses. Protective capsular type-specific antibody usually appears by 3 weeks following vaccination. Antibodies induced by bacterial capsular polysaccharides are mainly by T cell-independent mechanisms. Therefore, responses are generally poor in children below 2 years of age whose immune systems have not yet reached maturity.

pneumococcal 7-valent conjugate vaccine (diphtheria CRM$_{197}$ protein, injection)
A sterile solution of saccharides of the capsular antigens of *Streptococcus pneumoniae* serotypes 4, 6B, 9V, 14, 18C, 19F, and 23F individually conjugated to diphtheria CRM$_{197}$ protein. The polysaccharides are activated chemically to yield saccharides that are directly conjugated to the protein carrier CRM$_{197}$ to form the glycoconjugate by reductive amination. CRM$_{197}$ is a nontoxic variant of diphtheria toxin prepared from *Corynebacterium diphtheriae* strain C7 (β197) cultures grown in a casamino acid and yeast extract-base medium.

Pneumocystis jiroveci (formerly *carinii*)
A fungus that infects immunocompromised subjects such as transplant recipients, patients with AIDS, lymphoma, or leukemia, and other immunosuppressed individuals. It

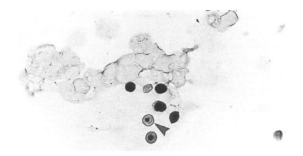

Pneumocystis jiroveci, formerly *Pneumocystis carinii.*

is diagnosed in tissue sections stained with the Gomori–methenamine silver stain. A mannose receptor facilitates uptake of the organism by macrophages. Approximately half of those hospitalized with a first infection by *Pneumocystis jiroveci* pneumonia die. The organism has two major forms (trophozoite and cyst). The trophic form is the smaller (1 to 4 µm), pleomorphic, and present in clusters. The cyst stage is larger (5 to 8 µm) and contains as many as eight intracystic bodies. The two groups of *P. jiroveci* antigens include a large surface complex, designated major surface glycoprotein (MSG), gpA, or gp120, with a molecular weight of 95 to 140 kDa found in organisms derived from human subjects. MSG facilitates the interaction of the microorganisms and host. The other major antigen complex is a glycoprotein of 35 to 45 kDa in human *P. jiroveci.*

PNH
Abbreviation for paroxysmal nocturnal hemoglobinuria.

PNH cells
Red blood cells of patients with paroxysmal nocturnal hemoglobinuria. At weakly acid pH, PNH cells disrupt spontaneously. The ability of complement to lyse these cells is much more pronounced than its action on normal erythrocytes subjected to conditions that promote their lysis by complement.

P nucleotides
Palindromic or P nucleotides are short inverted repeat nucleotide sequences in V–D–J junctions of rearranged immunoglobulin and T cell receptor genes. They are generated from a hairpin intermediate during recombination and contribute to junctional diversity of antigen receptors. Nicking hairpin loop-joining gene segments undergoing V(D)J recombination in the intervening DNA instead of at the precise ends of the coding sequences, a recessed strand end and an overhang are formed. The nucleotides that fill in the spaces on both strands are known as P nucleotides.

POEMS
Abbreviation for polyneuropathy, organomegaly, endocrinopathy, monoclonal gammopathy, and skin alterations; refer to POEMS syndrome.

POEMS syndrome
A condition that manifests polyneuropathy, organomegaly, endocrinopathy, monoclonal gammopathy, and skin alterations. It occurs on a background of sclerosing myeloma, Castleman's disease, and occasionally other lymphoproliferative disorders. The neuropathy is initially distal, symmetrical, mixed, demyelinating, and axonal and involves both motor and sensory fibers. It is progressive and ultimately fatal unless treated. The myeloma is always of the immunoglobulin G (IgG) or IgA type and almost always γ. Elevated cytokine levels may account for many of the symptoms

P

including the organomegaly and the endocrine and pigmentary changes. Tumor necrosis factor (TNF) activates the proopiomelanocortin gene. Both IL1β and TNF-α are osteoclast-activating factors. The levels of vascular endothelial growth factor (VEGF) increase 100-fold. Radiotherapy of isolated solitary plasmacytomas has proven helpful.

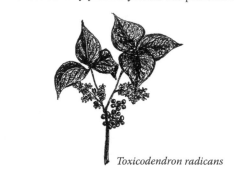

Toxicodendron radicans

Poison ivy.

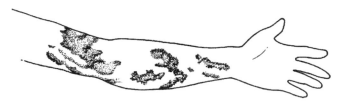

Contact hypersensitivity induced by exposure to poison ivy.

poison ivy

A plant containing urushiol, a chemical that may induce severe contact hypersensitivity of the skin in individuals who come into contact with it. Urushiol is also found in mango trees, Japanese lacquer trees, and cashew plants. It is present in *Toxicodendron radicans* (poison ivy) found in the eastern United States, in *T. diversilobium* (poison oak) found in the western United States, and in *T. vernix* (poison sumac) found in the southern United States. Setting fire to these plants is hazardous because the smoke containing the chemical may induce tracheitis and pulmonary edema in allergic individuals. The chemical may remain impregnated in unwashed clothing and cause reactions in people who come into contact with it over long periods. Pentadecacatechol, a potent contact-sensitizing agent in leaves of the poison ivy plant, is a frequent cause of the contact hypersensitivity.

poison ivy hypersensitivity

Principally type IV contact hypersensitivity induced by urushiols, chemical constituents of poison ivy (*Rhus toxicodendron);* when poison ivy plants containing this chemical come into contact with the skin, the skin becomes hypersensitive. The urushiol acts as a hapten by complexing with skin proteins to induce cellular (type IV) hypersensitivity on contact. Also called delayed-type hypersensitivity.

pokeweed mitogen (PWM)

A lectin extracted from the pokeweed *Phytolacca americana*. It binds carbohydrates and may stimulate human B and T cells. It has been used to promote B cell growth and proliferation in tissue culture, leading to immunoglobulin production. Interleukin-6 (IL6) plays an essential role in PWM-induced immunoglobulin synthesis.

pol

A retrovirus structural gene that codes for reverse transcriptase. The structural genes of human immunodeficiency virus 1 (HIV-1) also include *gag* and *env*.

polar cap

Refer to capping.

poliomyelitis vaccines

The three strains of poliomyelitis virus combined into a live attenuated oral vaccine introduced by Sabin. Replication in the gastrointestinal tract stimulates effective local immunity associated with IgA antibody synthesis. Individuals to be immunized receive three oral doses of the vaccine. The Sabin vaccine largely replaced the Salk vaccine introduced in the early 1950s and composed of the three strains of poliovirus killed with formalin. This vaccine must be administered subcutaneously.

poliovirus

Picornavirus of the genus Enteroviridae. There are three polio serotypes. Polio and other enteroviruses are spread mainly by the fecal–oral route. Poliomyelitis occurs around the world; however, in the western hemisphere the wild-type virus has been eliminated by successful vaccines.

poliovirus vaccine inactivated (IPV, injection)

Used to actively immunize infants, children and adults for prevention of poliomyelitis induced by poliovirus types 1, 2, and 3. The disease produced by these three virus types is spread by the fecal–oral route but may also be disseminated by the pharyngeal route. Poliovirus vaccine, inactivated, leads to the synthesis of neutralizing antibodies against each of the three types of virus, resulting in protective efficacy and antibody responses in most children. It induces secretory antibody (IgA) in the pharynx and gastrointestinal tract and diminishes pharyngeal excretion of poliovirus type 1 from 75% of children with neutralizing antibodies at levels <1:8 to 25% in children with neutralizing antibody levels >1:64. The vaccine may also induce herd immunity in the vaccinated population.

pollen hypersensitivity

Immediate (type I) hypersensitivity that atopic individuals experience following inhalation of pollens such as ragweed in the United States. This is an IgE-mediated reaction that results in respiratory symptoms expressed as hay fever or asthma. Sensitivity to certain pollens can be detected through skin tests with pollen extracts.

polyacrylamide gel

A cross linked medium used in SDS-PAGE (sodium dodecyl sulfate–polyacrylamide gel electrophoresis) and disk gel electrophoresis techniques for protein and nucleic acid separation. Varying the porosity of the polymerized and cross linked acrylamide that forms a gel after solubilization permits molecules of different sizes and charges to be separated.

polyacrylamide gel electrophoresis (PAGE)

Zone electrophoresis that employs a cross linked polyacrylamide gel used in SDS-PAGE and disk gel electrophoretic methods. SDS-PAGE is a method to separate proteins by their molecular weights. Proteins are combined with sodium dodecyl sulfate (SDS) at increased temperature and with a reducing agent to denature the proteins. Electrophoresis is carried out in a transparent synthetic polyacrylamide gel that serves as a molecular sieve. Migration of the protein is inversely proportional to its molecular weight. Coomassie blue is used to stain unlabeled proteins, and autoradiography is used to detect radiolabeled proteins. The molecular weight of an unknown protein can be predicted using standard proteins for comparison.

polyagglutination

The aggregation of erythrocytes by antibodies, autoagglutinins, or alloagglutinins in blood serum. Polyagglutination also refers to aggregation of normal red blood cells treated with neuraminidase and to red blood cells with altered membranes that are improperly aggregated by anti-A or anti-B antibodies. This is linked to altered glycoproteins such as Tn, T, and Cad. Acquired B antigens may also lead to polyagglutination, as can bacterial infections. Serum contaminants including detergents, microbes, metal cations, or silica may also cause polyagglutination. Also called panagglutination.

polyarteritis nodosa

A necrotizing vasculitis of small- and medium-sized muscular arteries that often involves renal and visceral arteries and spares the pulmonary circulation. The disease is often characterized by immune complex deposition in arteries and is often associated with chronic hepatitis B virus infection. Early lesions of the vessels often reveal hepatitis B surface antigen, IgM, and complement components. This uncommon disease has a male-to-female ratio of 2.5 to 1. The mean age at onset is 45 years. Characteristically, the kidneys, heart, abdominal organs, and both peripheral and central nervous systems are involved. Lesions of vessels are segmental and show preference for branching and bifurcation in small- and medium-sized muscular arteries. Usually, the venules and veins are unaffected and only rarely are granulomas formed. Characteristically, aneurysms form following destruction of the media and internal elastic lamina. There is proliferation of the endothelium with degeneration of the vessel wall and fibrinoid necrosis, thrombosis, ischemia, and infarction. Polyarteritis nodosa is also associated with tuberculosis, streptococcal infections, and otitis media. Presenting signs and symptoms include weakness, abdominal pain, leg pain, fever, cough, and neurologic symptoms. There may be kidney involvement, arthritis, arthralgia, or myalgia, and hypertension. Forty percent of patients may have skin involvement manifested as a maculopapular rash. Laboratory findings include elevated erythrocyte sedimentation rate, leukocytosis, anemia, thrombocytosis, and cellular casts in the urinary sediment signifying renal glomerular disease. Angiography is important in revealing the presence of aneurysm and changes in vessel caliber. There is no diagnostic immunologic test, but immune complexes, cryoglobulins, rheumatoid factor, and diminished complement component levels are often found. Biopsies may be taken from skeletal muscle or nerves for diagnostic purposes. Corticosteroids may be used, but cyclophosphamide is the treatment of choice in the severe progressive form.

polyarthritis

Multiple joint inflammation as occurs in rheumatic fever, systemic lupus erythematosus, and related diseases.

polyclonal

Originating from multiple clones.

polyclonal activators

Agents that stimulate numerous lymphocytes without regard to their antigen specificity. The proliferating cells yield products such as immunoglobulins or cytokines. The proliferating cells lack cell-to-cell collaboration that reduces mutations in polyclonal activators. Polyclonal activators use different activation pathways than antigen-stimulated lymphocytes, although pathways overlap and interact. Numerous polyclonal activators have different mechanisms of action on cells of immune systems. Among the polyclonal activators are mitogenic lectins that bind the polysaccharides of surface structures such as phytohemagglutinin (PHA), concanavalin A (con A), and pokeweed mitogen (PWM); bacterial cell wall products that bind lymphocyte receptors such as lipopolysaccharide (LPS); calcium ionophores that alter calcium signals; phosphorylation modifiers that increase stimulatory phosphorylation events such as phorbol myristate acetate; antigen–receptor ligands that bind to nonvariable parts of the receptor mechanism such as staphylococcal protein A; ligands for costimulatory molecules that bind to lymphocytes and favor stimulation such as anti-CD40 and CD40L; and transforming agents that infect cells and cause continued growth or activation such as HIV. Monoclonal activators can be used to access the functional status of a particular lymphocyte population. Some polyclonal activators require more than one type of cell and may even induce inhibition and inactivation of lymphocytes. Numerous interactions occur between antigen-specific and polyclonal forms of lymphocyte activation and inactivation. Costimulation and coinhibition regulate specific immune responses. Defects in signals in these various interactions, especially defects in signaling associated with antagonism and coinhibition, may predispose to autoimmune disease.

polyclonal antibodies

Multiple immunoglobulin responding to different epitopes on an antigen molecule. This multiple stimulation leads to the expansion of several antibody-forming clones whose products represent a mixture of immunoglobulins in contrast to proliferation of a single clone that yields a homogeneous monoclonal antibody product. Polyclonal antibodies represent the natural consequence of an immune response in contrast to monoclonal antibodies that occur *in vivo* in pathologic conditions such as multiple myeloma or are produced artificially by hybridoma technology against one of a variety of antigens.

polyclonal antiserum

Serum that possesses antibodies synthesized by different B cell clones following stimulation by an antigen. Different epitopes on the antigen molecule stimulate this multiplicity of antibodies.

polyclonal hypergammaglobulinemia

An elevation in the blood plasma of γ globulin due to increased quantities of the different immunoglobulin classes rather than an increase of only one immunoglobulin class.

polyclonal lymphocyte activator

Stimulates human lymphocytes. Among the B lymphocytes stimulated are self-reactive ones that are anergic. Lipopolysaccharide (LPS) injection may result in the production of many autoantibodies in mice. Superantigens may cause polyclonal T cell stimulation, which has been suggested to be a mechanism for autoimmunity, but evidence is lacking. Graft-vs.-host reactivity also has many autoimmune-like features. Response of the human body to microbial antigens may lead to an immune response that cross reacts with self antigens. For example, antibodies to streptococci in rheumatic fever may cross react with antigens of the myocardium in humans, leading to myocarditis.

P

If helper T cells are absent, autoreactive B cells may not produce autoantibodies. Antigens consisting of several determinants that include a self epitope that activates helper T cells can result in stimulation of B lymphocytes with autoantibody synthesis.

polyclonal rabbit anti-calretinin

Intended to qualitatively detect normal and malignant mesothelial cells in formalin-fixed, paraffin-embedded tissue sections using light microscopy. Calretinin, a calcium-binding protein with a molecular weight of 29 kDa, is a member of the large family of EF-hand proteins that also include S-100. EF-hand proteins are characterized by a helix–loop–helix fold that acts as a calcium-binding site. Calretinin contains six such EF-hand stretches. It is abundantly expressed in central and peripheral neural tissues, especially in the retina and neurons of the sensory pathways. Calretinin is also consistently expressed in normal and reactive mesothelial cell linings of all serosal membranes, eccrine glands of skin, convoluted tubules of kidney, Leydig and Sertoli cells of the testes, endometrium and ovarian stromal cells, and adrenal cortical cells. Calretinin is also a sensitive and specific indicator of normal and reactive mesothelial cells in effusion cytology. It is useful as part of an immunohistochemical marker panel to distinguish mesothelioma from adeno-carcinoma. The combination of calretinin and E-cadherin was shown to have high sensitivity and specificity in differentiating malignant mesothelioma from metastatic adenocarcinoma to the pleura in one study·

polyclone mitogens

Mitogens that stimulate multiple lymphocyte subpopulations.

polyclone proteins

Protein molecules from multiple cell clones.

polyendocrine autoimmunity

Refer to polyendocrine deficiency syndrome (polygranular autoimmune syndrome).

polyendocrine deficiency syndrome (polyglandular autoimmune syndrome)

Two related endocrinopathies with gonadal failure that may be due to defects in the hypothalamus. Vitiligo and autoimmune adrenal insufficiency are present. Four fifths of the patients have autoantibodies. Type I occurs in late childhood and is characterized by hypoparathyroidism, alopecia, mucocutaneous candidiasis, malabsorption, pernicious

anemia, and chronic active hepatitis. Inheritance is autosomal-recessive. Type II occurs in adults with Addison's disease and autoimmune thyroiditis or insulin-dependent diabetes mellitus.

polyethylene glycol assay for CICs

A method to detect, characterize, and quantitate antigens and antibodies in complexes that sediment in polyethylene glycol. This technique has only borderline clinical utility. In serum sickness conditions, it can detect circulating immune complexes (CICs).

polygenic

Describes several nonallelic genes encoding the same or similar proteins. It may also signify any trait attributable to inheritance of more than one gene.

polygenic inheritance

Phenotypic inheritance based on genetic variation at multiple loci. Numerous genetic loci may contribute to an inherited phenotype. Certain forms of immune responsiveness and susceptibility to selected diseases may be influenced by polygenic inheritance.

poly-Ig receptor

Abbreviation for polymeric immunoglobulin receptor.

polyimmunoglobulin receptor

An attachment site for polymeric immunoglobulins located on the basolateral membranes of epithelial cells and hepatocyte surfaces that facilitate polymeric IgA and IgM transcytosis to the secretions. After binding, the receptor–immunoglobulin complex is endocytosed and enclosed within vesicles for transport. Exocytosis takes place at cell surfaces where the immunoglobulin is discharged into the intestinal lumen. A similar mechanism in the liver facilitates IgA transport into the bile. The receptor–polymeric immunoglobulin complex is released from cells following cleavage near the cell membranes. The receptor segment bound to the polymeric immunoglobulin is known as the secretory component, which can only be used once in the transport process.

polymerase chain reaction (PCR)

A technique to amplify a small DNA segment beginning with as little as 1 µg. The segment of double-stranded DNA is placed between two oligonucleotide primers through many cycles of amplification. Amplification takes place in a thermal cycler, with one step occurring at a high temperature in the presence of DNA polymerase that can withstand the high temperature. Within a few hours,

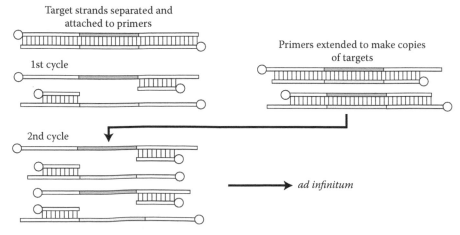

Polymerase chain reaction (PCR).

the original DNA segment is transformed into millions of copies. PCR methodology has been used for multiple purposes including detection of human immunodeficiency virus 1 (HIV-1), prenatal diagnosis of sickle cell anemia, and gene rearrangements in lymphoproliferative disorders among other applications. The technique is used principally to prepare enough DNA for analysis by available methods and is used widely in diagnostic work. PCR has a 99.99% sensitivity.

polymeric Ig

Immunoglobulin molecules comprised of numerous identical H_2L_2 monomers linked by a J chain. Pentameric IgM $[(H_2L_2)5]$, with ten antigen-binding sites and dimeric IgA $[(H_2L_2)2]$ with four, are examples.

polymers

Molecules composed of more than one repeating unit; immunoglobulins composed of more than one basic monomeric four-polypeptide chain unit. IgAs may exist as dimers with two units or as multimers. The IgM molecule is pentameric, containing five monomeric units.

polymorphism

The occurrence of different variants of a gene or trait in a population. The presence of two or more forms such as ABO and Rh blood groups, in individuals of the same species. This is due to two or more variants at a certain genetic locus occurring with considerable frequency in a population. Polymorphisms are also expressed in the human leukocyte antigen (HLA) system, as well as in allotypes of immunoglobulin γ and κ chains. Genetic polymorphism refers to the presence of two or more alleles of a given gene within a population with the variant alleles each appearing at a frequency >1%.

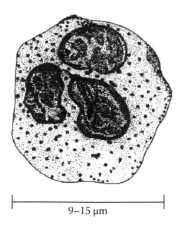

9–15 μm

Schematic representation of a polymorphonuclear leukocyte (PMN).

polymorphonuclear leukocyte (PMN)

White blood cells with lobulated nuclei that are often trilobed. PMNs are of myeloid cell lineage and in mature form may be differentiated into neutrophils, eosinophils, and basophils. This distinction is based on the staining characteristics of their cytoplasmic specific or secondary granules. PMNs measure approximately 13 μm in diameter and are active in acute inflammatory responses.

polymyositis (PM)

An acute or chronic inflammatory disease of muscle, involving fibers of the voluntary muscles; it is twice as common in women as in men. Lymphocytes in polymyositis

Substances Associated with Neutrophils

Azurophil Granules (Primary Granules)	Specific Granules (Secondary Granules)
Bacterial permeability-inducing protein (BPI)	
Cathepsin G	
Cationic antimicrobial protein (CAP) 57	
Cationic antimicrobial protein (CAP) 37	
Defensins:	
HP1	
HP2	
HP3	
Elastase	
Lysozyme	
Myeloperoxidase	Bacterial chemotaxin receptors
Collagenase	
C5a receptors	
Gelatinase	
Lactoferrin	
Lysozyme	
NADPH	
Vitamin B_{12}-binding protein	

Polymorphonuclear leukocyte (PMN).

subjects produce a cytotoxin when incubated with autologous muscle. Biopsies of involved muscle reveal infiltration by lymphocytes and plasma cells. PM characteristically manifests autoantibodies against aminoacyl tRNA synthetases. Antibodies can be demonstrated against the nuclear antigens Jo-1, PM-Scl, and RNP. Patients may develop polyclonal hypergammaglobulinemia. One fifth of patients may develop rheumatoid factors and antinuclear antibodies. Cellular immunity appears important in the pathogenesis, as exemplified by lymphocytes of patients with polymyositis responding to their own muscle antigens as if they were alien. Patients often complain of muscle weakness, especially in the proximal muscles of extremities. To diagnose polymyositis, a minimum of three of the following must be present: (1) shoulder or pelvic girdle weakness, (2) myositis as revealed by biopsy, (3) increased levels of muscle enzymes, and (4) electromyographic findings of myopathy. Corticosteroids have been used to decrease muscle inflammation and increase strength. Methotrexate or other cytotoxic agents may be used when steroids prove ineffective.

polynucleotides

A linear polymer comprised of more than 10 nucleotides joined by 3′,5′-phosphodiester bonds; double-stranded DNA chains that may serve as adjuvants when inoculated with antigens.

polyomavirus immunity

Polyomavirus infections are usually associated with virus reactivation in immunocompromised hosts. Two polyomaviruses, JC virus (JCV) and BK virus (BKV), infect humans. BKV and JCV infect children. In the United States, one half of all children acquire antibodies to BKV during the first 3 years of life and to JCV by the 10th to 12th year of age. Antibody responsiveness is assayed by neutralization, hemagglutination inhibition, and ELISA (enzyme-linked immunosorbent assay). Antibody titers often increase during virus activation. IgM antibodies that are virus-specific have been found in renal allotransplant patients. Cell-mediated immunity develops against BKV. JCV and BKV remain in the body after primary infection. Cell-mediated immunity is believed to prevent or limit virus reactivation in healthy individuals, but the viruses are reactivated in immunosuppressed subjects.

polyreactive antibody

An immunoglobulin molecule that identifies and unites with several different antigens of significantly different configurations with varying affinities.

polyspecific anti-human globulin (AHG)

This is known as the Coombs' reagent consisting of antibodies against human IgG and C3d. It may also contain anti-C3b, anti-C4b, and anti-C4d antibodies. Although it demonstrates only minimal reactivity with IgM and IgA heavy chains, it may interact with these molecules by reacting with their κ or λ light chains. It is used for the direct antiglobulin test.

polyspecificity

The capacity to bind many different antigens. Also termed polyreactivity.

polyvalent

Multivalent.

polyvalent antiserum

An antiserum composed of antibodies specific for multiple antigens.

polyvalent pneumococcal vaccine

An immunizing preparation that contains 23 of the 83 known pneumococcal capsular polysaccharides. It induces immunity for 3 to 5 years and is believed to protect against 90% of the pneumococcal types that induce serious illness in patients over 2 years of age. Children at high risk can be vaccinated at 6 months of age and reinoculated at 2 years of age. The vaccine is especially indicated in high-risk patients such as those with sickle cell disease, chronic debilitating disease, immunological defects, and the elderly. Vaccination against pneumococcal disease is of increasing significance as *Streptococcus pneumoniae* becomes increasingly resistant to antibiotics.

polyvalent vaccine

A vaccine composed of multiple antigens from more than one strain of a pathogenic microorganism or from a mixture of immunogens such as the diphtheria, pertussis, and tetanus toxoid preparation.

popcorn cells

Neoplastic cells in non-Hodgkin lymphoma manifesting a surface phenotype of CD3⁻CD15⁻CD19⁺CD20±. Their immunoglobulin genes manifest somatic hypermutation.

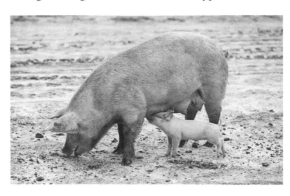

Porcine immunity.

porcine immunity

The pig's immune system differs from those of mice and humans in that pigs have inverted lymph nodes; pig lymphocytes leave lymph nodes in the blood rather than in efferent lymph; pigs have four types of Peyer's patches and small tonsillar papillae in the tongue together with palatine and nasopharyngeal tonsils; and pigs fail to transfer immunoglobulins across the placenta. The pig major histocompatibility complex (MHC) encodes the production of both class I and class II products. Pigs have peripheral blood leukocytes of the same type as found in humans. Unique features of porcine blood leukocytes include a relatively high proportion of γδ T cells, a high CD4⁺/CD8⁺ ratio in adults, and increased frequencies of CD4⁺/CD8⁺ double-positive T cells. Four CD markers have been described, and four classes of immunoglobulins (IgM, IgA, IgG, and IgE) have been identified. Pigs have both αβ T cells and γδ T cells, natural killer (NK) cells, adhesion molecules of the E-selectin type, and cytokines that include interferons, inflammatory cytokines, and chemokines. Other pig cytokines include interleukin-2 (IL2), IL4, IL5, IL10, IL12, granulocyte–macrophage colony-stimulating factor (GM-CSF), and G-CSF, among others.

Porter, Rodney Robert (1917–1985)

British biochemist who with Gerald Edelman received the Nobel Prize in 1972 for their studies of antibodies and their chemical structures. Porter cleaved antibody molecules with the papain enzyme to yield Fab and Fc fragments. He suggested that antibodies have four-chain structures. Fab fragments were shown to have the antigen-binding sites and the Fc fragments conferred the biological properties of the antibody. He also investigated the sequence of complement genes in the major histocompatibility complex (MHC). (Refer to *Defense and Recognition*, 1973.)

Portier, Paul Jules (1866–1962)

French physiologist who, with Richet, was the first to describe anaphylaxis.

positive cross match

The demonstration via serological or flow cytometric techniques of preformed antibodies specific for one or more

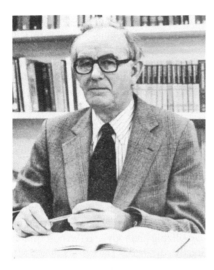

Rodney Robert Porter.

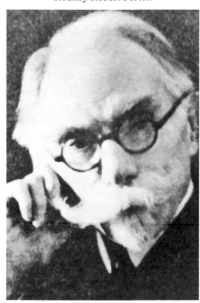

Paul Jules Portier.

HLA molecules on allogeneic donor cells in the blood of a transplant recipient.

positive induction apoptosis

Two central pathways lead to apoptosis: (1) positive induction by ligand binding to plasma membrane receptor; and (2) negative induction by loss of suppressor activity. Each leads to activation of cysteine proteases with homology to IL1β converting enzymes (ICEs or caspases). Positive induction involves ligands related to TNF. Ligands are typically trimeric and bind to cell surface receptors causing aggregation (trimerization) of cell surface receptors. Receptor oligomerization orients their cytosolic death domains into a configuration that recruits adaptor proteins. The adaptor complex recruits caspase-8. Caspase-8 is activated, and the cascade of caspase-mediated disassembly proceeds.

positive selection

Pathway in the thymus that promotes the survival of immature T cells with receptors that recognize self peptide complexed to self MHC with only low affinity/avidity, i.e., those with the greatest capacity to identify nonself peptide complexed to self MHC with high affinity.

Positively selected cells are the only ones permitted to continue their maturation. The resulting cell population is self MHC-restricted and capable of interacting with both self and foreign antigens. NKT cells are also subjected to positive selection in the thymus. It is unclear whether developing B cells with low affinity for self antigen receive survival signals, i.e., are positively selected. Refer to negative selection.

postcapillary venules

Relatively small blood vessels lined with cuboidal epithelium through which blood circulates after it exits capillaries and before it enters veins. They are frequent sites of migration of lymphocytes and inflammatory cells into tissues during inflammation. Recirculating lymphocytes migrate from the blood to lymph through high endothelial venules of lymph nodes.

post-cardiotomy syndrome

A condition that follows heart surgery or traumatic injury. Autoantibodies against heart antigens may be demonstrated by immunofluorescence within weeks of the surgery or trauma. Corticosteroid therapy represents an effective treatment. Patients suffering myocardial infarcts may also develop a similar condition.

post-GC

Designation for a leukemia/lymphoma in which the transformed cells express an activated B cell or memory B cell phenotype. There is a high frequency of somatic hypermutations in the genome.

post-infectious encephalomyelitis

Demyelinating disease following a virus infection that is mediated by autoimmune delayed-type (type IV) hypersensitivity to myelin.

post-infectious iridocyclitis

Inflammation of the iris and ciliary body of the eye. This may occur after a virus or bacterial infection and is postulated to result from an autoimmune reaction.

post-rabies vaccination encephalomyelitis

A demyelinating disease produced in humans actively immunized with rabies vaccine containing nervous system tissue to protect against the development of rabies. Serial injections of rabbit brain tissue containing rabies virus killed by phenol may induce demyelinating encephalomyelitis in a recipient. This method of vaccination was replaced with a vaccine developed in tissue culture that did not contain any nervous tissue.

post-streptococcal glomerulonephritis

An acute proliferative glomerulonephritis that may follow a streptococcal infection of the throat or skin by 1 to 2 weeks. It is usually seen in 6- to 10-year old children, but may occur in adults as well. The onset is heralded by acute nephritis. Ninety percent of patients have been infected with group A β hemolytic streptococci that are nephritogenic— specifically, types 12, 4, and 1, that are revealed by their cell wall M protein. Poststreptococcal glomerulonephritis is mediated by antibodies induced by the streptococcal infection. Most patients show elevated antistreptolysin-O (ASO) titers. Serum complement levels are decreased. Immunofluorescence of renal biopsies demonstrates granular immune deposits that contain immunoglobulin and complement in the glomeruli. This finding is confirmed by electron microscopy. The precise streptococcal antigen has never been identified;

P

however, a cytoplasmic antigen termed endostreptosin together with some cationic streptococcal antigens are found in glomeruli. Subepithelial immune deposits appear as "humps." They are antigen–antibody complexes that may also appear in the mesangium or occasionally in a subendothelial or intramembranous position. These immune deposits stain positively for IgG and complement by immunofluorescence. Affected children develop fever, nausea, oliguria, and hematuria within 2 weeks following a streptococcal sore throat or skin infection. Erythrocyte casts and mild proteinuria may be identified. Periorbital edema and hypertension may be observed upon examination. BUN (blood urea nitrogen) and ASO titer may also be elevated. More than 95% of children with poststreptococcal glomerulonephritis recover, although a few (<1%) develop rapidly progressive glomerulonephritis and a few others develop chronic glomerulonephritis.

post-transfusion graft-vs.-host disease

A condition that resembles post-operative erythroderma and occurs in immunocompetent recipients of blood. Dermatitis, fever, marked diarrhea, pancytopenia, and liver dysfunction are observed.

post-transplant lymphoproliferative disorder (PTLD)

A group of B cell lymphomas occurring in immunosuppressed patients following organ transplantation. It is an uncommon condition occurring in 0.2% of patients within 1 year of transplant, with an annual incidence of 0.04% thereafter. Risk of the disease is higher in children and recipients of heart transplants. It is an uncontrolled proliferation of B lymphocytes following infection with Epstein–Barr virus. Production of IL10, an endogenous anti-T cell cytokine, has also been implicated. In immunocompetent patients, Epstein–Barr virus causes infectious mononucleosis, characterized by proliferation of B lymphocytes, which is controlled by suppressor T cells. However, calcineurin inhibitors such as tacrolimus and cyclosporin used as immunosuppressants in T cell function can prevent the control of B cell proliferation. Depletion of T cells by the use of anti-T cell antibodies in the prevention or treatment of transplant rejection further increases the risk of developing post-transplant lymphoproliferative disorder. Such antibodies include ATG, ALG, and OKT3. Polyclonal PTLD may form tumor masses and present with symptoms due to a mass effect, e.g., symptoms of bowel obstruction. Monoclonal forms of PTLD form a disseminated malignant lymphoma. It may spontaneously regress on reduction or cessation of immunosuppressant medication and can be treated with antiviral therapy. Some cases will progress to non-Hodgkin lymphoma and may be fatal.

post-vaccinal encephalomyelitis

A demyelinating encephalomyelitis occurring approximately 2 weeks following vaccination of infants below 1 year of age and adults with vaccinia virus to protect against smallpox. This rare complication of the smallpox vaccination frequently leads to death.

postzone

Lack of serologic reactivity as a consequence of high dilution of antibody, as in a serial dilution procedure. This is a zone of relative antigen excess.

poxvirus immunity

Multiple antibodies produced in response to poxvirus infection. These antibodies can be detected by numerous assays, including complement fixation, virus neutralization, and ELISA (enzyme-linked immunosorbent assay), among others. Not all these antibodies are protective. Significant are the antibodies that neutralize enveloped or nonenveloped virus infectivity, those that combine with circulating antigens to facilitate immune clearance by phagocytes, and those that with effector cells complement and lyse infected cells. Neutralizing antibody may diminish viremia by acting on extracellular virus. The passive transfer of antibodies has been shown to protect mice and sheep from infection by viruses of this group, but the passive protection is brief and of limited effectiveness compared with active immunization with live virus that induces long-lasting immunity. Cross-reactive neutralizing antibodies may be detected within a week following infection and last for a generation, but the level of neutralizing antibody and the host immune status are not directly correlated. The cell-mediated response is the principal mechanism of protection and recovery from poxvirus diseases. Immune T lymphocytes, monocytes, and macrophages are necessary for regression of ectromelia infection of mice. They develop delayed-type hypersensitivity that is a T cell-mediated response. Vaccinia virus infection of monkeys and hamsters is mediated by natural killer (NK) cells, and by cytotoxic T cells in sheep. Vaccinia virus shows interferon sensitivity. Poxvirus synthesis remains intracellular and is transmitted from one cell to another without exposure to neutralizing antibody, which is effective only against virus budding from infected cells. The virus may also survive in the skin, where epidermal Langerhans' cells process and present antigen to lymphocytes to generate a protective immune response. Poxviruses encode functional homologs of host cell factors that regulate the immune system. Edward Jenner in 1798 showed that a cowpox cross protects against smallpox virus infection. Cowpox vaccinia was invaluable in ridding the world of smallpox; thereafter, it was judged that the effects of the vaccination constituted a liability since smallpox disease had been eliminated. Vaccinia has also been used in the control of pox in various animal species. Vaccinia is currently used as a vector for genes of other viral pathogens in the development of vaccines.

PPD

Purified protein derivative of tuberculin.

PPLOs (pleuropneumonia-like organisms)

Mycoplasma pneumoniae, a microorganism that causes asymptomatic respiratory tract infection or upper respiratory tract inflammation. It spreads in the air. Patients develop headache, muscle pain, chest tenderness, and a low-grade fever. They may manifest cold agglutinin-induced hemolysis.

PRA

Abbreviation for panel reactive antibody.

Prausnitz–Giles, Carl (1876–1963)

German physician who conducted extensive research on allergies. He and Küstner successfully transferred a food allergy with serum. This became the basis for the Prausnitz–Küstner test. He worked at the State Institute for Hygiene in Breslau and spent time at the Royal Institute for Public Health in London early in the 20th century. In 1933, he left Germany and practiced medicine on the Isle of Wight.

Prausnitz–Küstner (PK) reaction (historical)

A skin test for hypersensitivity in which serum containing IgE antibodies specific for a particular allergen is transferred from an allergic individual to a nonallergic recipient by

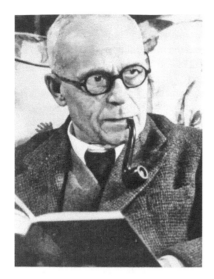

Carl Prausnitz–Giles.

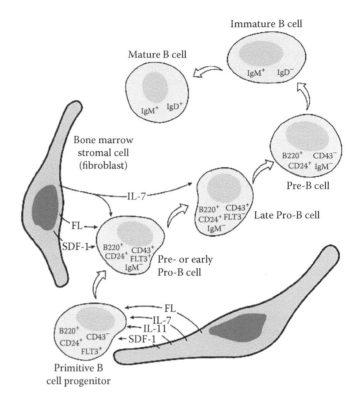

FLT-3 bone marrow B cell lymphopoiesis.

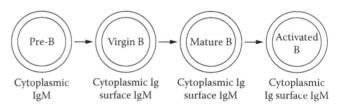

Pre-B cell development.

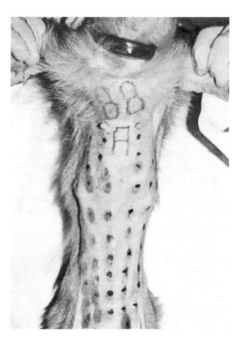

Prausnitz-Küstner reaction to ragweed antigen E in rhesus monkey. Skin sensitized 2 days earlier with human serum from a ragweed-sensitive atopic patient.

intradermal injection. This is followed by injection of the antigen or allergen in question into the same site as the serum injection. Fixation of the IgE antibodies in the "allergic" serum to mast cells in the recipient results in local release of the pharmacological mediators of immediate hypersensitivity that include histamine. It results in a local anaphylactic reaction with a wheal-and-flare response. This test is no longer used because of the risk of transmitting hepatitis or AIDS.

preactivation

A provirus that continues untranscribed in the genome of a host cell because of a lack of host cell stimulation.

pre-B cells

A stage of B cell development characterized by rearrangement of heavy chain genes but not light chain genes. Pre-B cells develop from lymphoid stem cells in the bone marrow. These are large, immature lymphoid cells that express cytoplasmic μ chains but no light chains or surface immunoglobulin and are found in fetal liver and adult bone marrow. They are the earliest cells of the B cell lineage. Antigen is not required for early differentiation of the B cell series. Pre-B cells differentiate into immature B cells, followed by mature B cells that express surface immunoglobulin. Pre-B cell immunoglobulin genes contain heavy chain V, D, and J gene segments that are contiguous. No rearrangement of light chain gene segments has yet occurred. In addition to their cytoplasmic IgM, pre-B cells are positive for CD10, CD19, and HLA-DR markers. Pre-B cells have rearranged heavy but not light chain genes. They express cytoplasmic Ig μ heavy chains and surrogate light chains but not Ig light chains. The pre-B cell receptor consists of μ chains and surrogate light chains. These receptors transmit signals that induce further pre-B cell maturation into immature B cells.

pre-B cell receptor

A maturing B cell lymphocyte receptor comprised of a μ heavy chain, an invariant surrogate light chain, and the Igα/Igβ heterodimer. It is expressed at the pre-B cell stage, and its appearance marks the end of heavy chain gene rearrangement. The two proteins comprising the surrogate light chain include the λ 5 protein, which is homologous to the λ light chain C domain, and the Vpre-B protein, which is homologous to a V domain. Association of the pre-B cell receptor with the Igα and the Igβ signal-transduction proteins forms the pre-B cell receptor complex. Stimulation of proliferation and continued maturation of developing B cells requires pre-B cell receptors.

precipitating antibody

A precipitin.

precipitation

Following the union of soluble macromolecular antigen with a homologous antibody in the presence of electrolytes *in vitro* and *in vivo* that occurs within seconds after contact, complexes of increasing density form in a lattice arrangement and settle out of solution, as in the precipitation or precipitin reaction. The materials needed for a precipitin reaction include antigen, antibody, and electrolyte. The reaction of soluble antigen and antibody in the precipitin test may be observed in liquid or gel media. The reaction in liquid media may be qualitative or quantitative. Following discovery of the precipitin reaction by Kraus, quantitative and semiquantitative measurements of antibody could be made. The term *precipitinogen* is sometimes employed to designate the antigen, and *precipitin* is the antibody in a precipitation reaction.

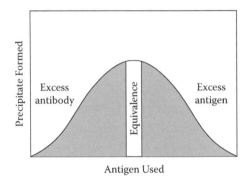

Precipitation curve.

precipitation curve

The milligrams of antibody in a precipitate are plotted on the ordinate and the milligrams of antigen added are plotted on the abscissa of a graph. The precipitin curve contains ascending and descending limbs and zones of antibody excess, equivalence, and antigen excess. By testing with homologous reagents, unreacted antibodies and antigens can be detected in the supernatants. If antigen is homogeneous or if antibodies specific for only one of a mixture of antigens are studied by the precipitin reaction, none of the supernatants contains both unreacted antibodies and unreacted antigens that can be detected. The ascending limb of the precipitin curve represents the zone of antibody excess, where free antibody molecules are present in the supernatants. The descending limb represents the zone of antigen excess, where free antigen is present in the supernatants. Precipitation is maximum in the zone of equivalence (equivalence point)—neither antigen nor antibody can be detected in the supernatants. In contrast to the nonspecific system described above, the presence of more than one antigen–antibody system in a reaction medium may be revealed by a demonstration of unreacted antibody and antigen in certain supernatants. This occurs in cases of overlap between the zone of antigen excess in one antigen–antibody combination with the zone of antibody excess of a separate antigen–antibody system. The lattice theory proposed by Marrack explains how multivalent antigen molecules and bivalent antibodies can combine to yield antigen-to-antibody ratios that differ from one precipitate to another, depending upon the zone of the precipitin reaction in which they are formed. When the ratio of antibody to antigen is above 1.0, a visible precipitate forms; however, when the ratio is less than 1.0, soluble complexes result and remain in the supernatant. The soluble complexes are associated with the descending limb of the precipitin curve. Also termed precipitin curve.

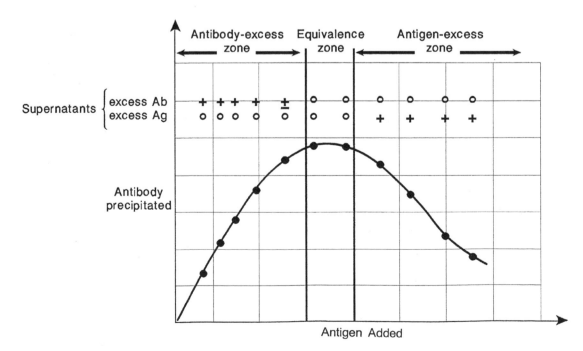

Precipitation curve.

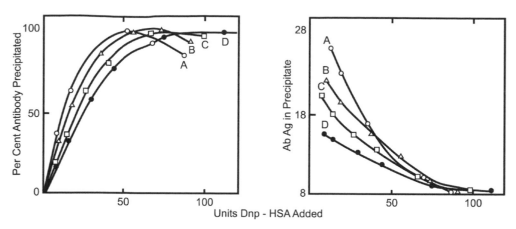

Precipitation curves showing differences in the avidity of four antisera for the same antigen. The order of avidity of the sera is A > B > C > D.

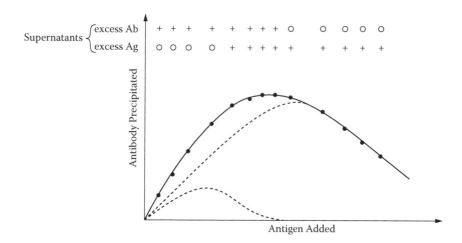

Precipitin curve for multispecific system. The precipitation observed (—•—) is the sum of two or more precipitin reactions (---).

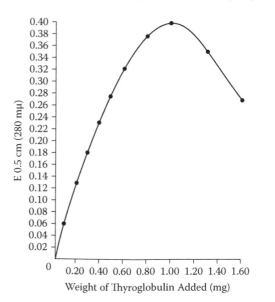

Precipitation curve with human thyroglobulin and homologous antibody.

precipitation in gel media

Oudin in 1946 overlaid antibody incorporated in agar in a test tube with a homologous antigen. A band of precipitation appeared in the gel where the antigen–antibody interaction occurred. Mixtures of antibodies of several specificities were overlaid with a mixture of the homologous antigens, and a distinct band for each resulted. Oudin's technique involves simple or single diffusion in one dimension. In 1953, Oakley and Fulthorpe placed antiserum incorporated into agar in the bottom of a tube, covered this with a layer of plain agar that was permitted to solidify, and then added antigen. This process was double diffusion in one dimension. Double diffusion in two dimensions was developed by Ouchterlony and independently by Elek in 1948. Agar is poured on a flat glass surface such as a microscope slide, glass plate, or Petri dish. Wells or troughs are cut in the agar, and these are filled with antigen and antibody solutions under study. Multiple component systems may be analyzed with this method and cross reactivities may be detected. Double diffusion in agar is a useful method to demonstrate similarity among structurally related antigens. Equidistant holes are punched in agar gel containing electrolyte. Antigen is placed in one well and antiserum in another adjacent to it, and the plates are observed the following day for a precipitation line where antigen and antibody have migrated toward one another and reached equivalent concentrations. A single line implies a single antigen–antibody system. If agar plates containing one central well with others cut equidistant from it at the periphery are employed, a reaction of identity may be demonstrated by placing antibody in the central well and the homologous antigen in adjacent peripheral wells. A confluent line of precipitate is produced in the shape of an arc. This implies that the antigen preparations in adjacent peripheral wells are identical, i.e., they

Tube no.	1	2	3	4	5	6	7
Rabbit antiserum	1 ml.	1 ml.	1 ml.	1 ml.	1 ml.	1 ml.	1 ml.
mg egg albumin (antigen)	0.24	0.18	0.12	0.09	0.06	0.03	0.01

Precipitation reaction in liquid media.

have the same antigenic determinants. If antibodies against two unrelated antigen preparations are combined and placed in the central well and their homologous antigens are placed in separate adjacent peripheral wells, a line of precipitation is produced by each antigen–antibody reaction to give the appearance of crossed sword points. This constitutes a reaction of nonidentity and implies that the antigenic determinants are different in the two samples of antigen. A third pattern known as a reaction of partial identity occurs when two antigen preparations that are related but not the same are placed in separate adjacent wells and an antibody preparation that cross reacts with both is placed in a central well. The precipitation lines between each antigen–antibody system converge, but a spur or extension of one of the precipitation lines occurs. This reaction of partial identity with spur formation implies that the antigen preparations are similar, but that one of them has an antigenic determinant not present in the other. A reaction of identity and nonidentity may be observed simultaneously, implying that two separate antigen preparations have both common and different antigenic determinants.

precipitation reaction
Refer to precipitin test, precipitation, precipitation curve, and precipitation in gel media.

precipitin
An antibody that interacts with a soluble antigen to yield an aggregate of antigen and antibody molecules in a lattice framework called a precipitate. Under appropriate conditions, the majority of antibodies can act as precipitins.

precipitin reaction
Refer to precipitin test, precipitation, precipitation curve, and precipitation in gel media.

precipitin reaction curve
Refer to precipitation curve.

precipitin test
An assay in which antibody interacts with soluble antigen in the presence of electrolyte to produce a precipitate. Both qualitative and quantitative precipitin reactions have been described.

preclinical trials
Assay for toxicity and teratogenicity of an agent or entity in both nonhuman primates and nonprimate animals. May also include efficacy testing.

prednisolone (1,4-pregnadiene-11β,17α, 21-triol-3,20-dione)
A semisynthetic steroid with glucocorticoid action. The molecular configuration into which the immunosuppressive prednisone drug is converted *in vivo*.

prednisone (1,4-pregnadiene-17α,21-diol-3,11,20-trione)
A synthetic steroid with glucocorticoid action. A powerful anti-inflammatory and immunosuppressive agent used in recipients of organ allotransplants.

preemptive immunity
Resistance shown by virus-infected cells to superinfection with a different virus.

pre-GC
Descriptor of a leukemia/lymphoma in which the transformed cells express a naïve B cell phenotype. Somatic mutations in the genome are rare.

preintegration complex
A configuration in the cytoplasm of the host cell that possesses all the components of the HIV core with the exception of the capsid. HIV RT synthesizes the viral DNA rapidly within this configuration. The complex matrix proteins then pilot it into the nucleus.

prekallikrein
A kallikrein precursor. The generation of kallikrein from prekallikrein can activate the intrinsic mechanism of blood coagulation.

premalignant clone
Genetically altered cell clone at a stage before malignant conversion during the progression of carcinogenesis.

premunition
A type of protective immunity characterized by the presence of a few pathogenic microorganisms of a particular species remaining in the body, apparently stimulating a protective immune response. Premunity is associated with certain protozoal diseases such as bovine babesiosis.

preneoplastic clone
A genetically altered cell clone at a stage before development into a tumor during the progression of carcinogenesis.

preprogenitor cells
This pool of cells represents a second step in the maturation of B cells and is induced by nonspecific environmental stimuli. Preprogenitors are immature cells that are unable to mount an immune response but constitute the pool from which specific responsive clones will be selected by a specific antigen. They are present in the bone marrow and peripheral lymphoid organs such as the spleen where they form a minor population. They are characterized by the presence of some surface markers, frequently doublet or triplet surface immunoglobulins, and are capable of stimulation by selected activators. Sometimes termed B1 cells.

present
Refer to antigen presentation.

presentosome
A molecular assemblage on both sides of the endoplasmic reticulum membrane that aids processing of endogenous antigen. Proteasomal degradation yields peptides that are complexed with HSP70, HSP90, or HSP 110 in

the cytosol for conveyance to TAP. Peptides are united to gp96 or PDI in the endoplasmic reticulum on the other side of TAP.

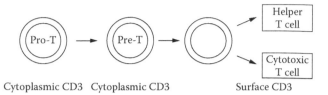

Pre-T cell development.

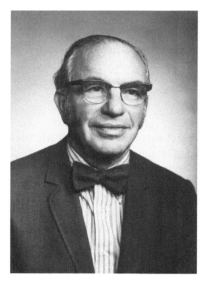

David Pressman.

Pressman, David

Colleague of Linus Pauling and an immunochemist who completed important work at the Roswell Park Memorial Institute in Buffalo, New York.

pre-T α chain (pTα)

Invariant transmembrane T cell receptor α-like chain manifested exclusively by double negative thymocytes. Employed for productivity assays of candidate TCRβ chains. Not requisite for γδ T cell development. Refer to pre-T cell receptor.

pre-T cell

A stage in the maturation of T lymphocytes in the thymus in which cells express the T cell receptor (TCR) β chain, but not the α chain or the CD4 or CD8 markers. The pre-T cell expresses the TCR β polypeptide chain on the cell surface together with the pTa (gp33) molecule to form the pre-T cell receptor.

pre-T cell receptor (pre-TCR)

A receptor on the surfaces of pre-T cells composed of the TCR β chain and the invariant pre-T α chain. This receptor associates with CD3 and ζ molecules to form the pre-T cell receptor complex. It functions similarly to pre-B cell receptors and B cell development in that it delivers signals that stimulate further proliferation, antigen receptor gene rearrangements, and other events related to maturation. It is unknown whether the pre-T cell receptor binds a specific antigen.

pre-TCR activation

Throughout β selection, the swift proliferation of only thymocyte clones that possess functional TCR β chains.

Triggered by pTα signaling induced by an unidentified ligand.

pre-T lymphocyte

Refer to prothymocyte.

prevertebrates

Animals without backbones that evolved from a deuterstome ancestor. Echinoderms (starfish, sea urchins) and protochordates (ascidians and tunicates, including sea squirts) are examples.

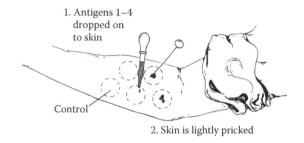

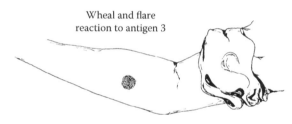

Prick test.

prick test

An assay for immediate (IgE-mediated) hypersensitivity in humans. The epidermal surface of the skin on which drops of diluted antigen (allergen) are placed is pricked by a sterile needle passed through an allergen. The reaction produced is compared with one induced by histamine or another mast cell secretogogue. This test is convenient, simple, and rapid and produces little discomfort in comparison with the intradermal test. It even may be used for infants.

primary agammaglobulinemia

Refer to antibody deficiency syndrome.

primary allergen

The antigenic material that sensitizes a patient who subsequently shows cross sensitivity to a related allergen.

primary biliary cirrhosis (PBC)

A chronic liver disease of unknown cause that affects middle-aged women in 90% of the cases. It involves chronic intrahepatic cholestasis caused by chronic inflammation and necrosis of intrahepatic bile ducts with progression to biliary cirrhosis. It is believed to be autoimmune based on its association with autoimmune conditions and the presence of autoantibodies. Patients develop pruritus, fatigue, steatorrhea, renal tubular acidosis, hepatic osteodystrophy, and increased incidence of hepatocellular carcinoma and breast carcinoma. Four fifths of patients also have a connective tissue or autoimmune diseases such as rheumatoid arthritis, autoimmune thyroiditis, scleroderma, and Sjögren's syndrome. Most patients manifest high titers of antimitochondrial antibodies. IgM in the serum is elevated. Lymphocytic infiltration and intrahepatic bile duct destruction occur. Alkaline phosphatase is greatly increased, in addition to the elevation of IgM and antimitochondrial antibodies. The M2 antimitochondrial antibody is most frequently associated with PBC. In addition to hepatosplenomegaly and skin hyperpigmentation, patients may develop severe jaundice, petechiae, and purpura as the disease progresses. Liver transplantation is the only treatment for end-stage disease.

primary follicle

A densely packed accumulation of resting mature B lymphocytes and macrophages in a network of follicular dendritic cells from secondary lymphoid tissues such as the lymph node cortex or the splenic white pulp, where resting unstimulated B cells develop into germinal centers when stimulated by antigen.

primary granule

Azurophil granule.

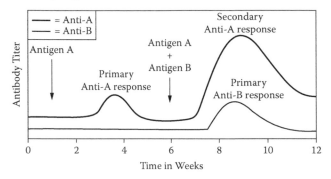

Primary immune response.

primary immune response

The body's adaptive immune response to first contact with antigen. It is characterized by a lag period of a few days following antigen administration before antibodies or specific T lymphocytes are detectable. The antibody produced consists mostly of IgM and is of relatively low titer and low affinity. This is in contrast to the secondary immune response, in which the latent period is relatively brief and IgG is the predominant antibody. The most important component of the primary response is the activation of memory cells that recognize antigen immediately on second encounter with antigen, leading to a secondary response. A similar pattern is followed in cell-mediated responses.

primary immunodeficiency

Diminished immune reactivity attributable to an intrinsic abnormality of T or B lymphocytes. Development failure of a segment of the immune system as a consequence of an inborn genetic mutation.

primary interaction

Antigen and antibody binding that may or may not lead to a secondary visible reaction such as precipitation. Primary antigen–antibody interaction may be measured by equilibrium dialysis, the Farr assay, fluorescence polarization, fluorescence quenching, and selected radioimmunoassays such as radioimmunoelectrophoresis.

primary lymphoid follicles

B cell regions, comprised of resting B lymphocytes, of secondary lymphoid tissues unstimulated by an immune response.

primary lymphoid organ

The site of maturation of B or T lymphocytes. The primary lymphoid organ for B lymphocytes is the bursa of Fabricius in avian species and the bone marrow in adult mammals. By contrast, T cell development occurs in the thymus of all vertebrates. Stem cell maturation in primary lymphoid organs occurs without stimulation by antigen.

primary lymphoid tissues

Bone marrow and thymus, the sites of lymphoid development.

primary lysosome

A lysosome that has not yet fused with a phagosome.

primary nodule

Refer to primary follicle.

primary reaction

The actual binding of antibody, via its Fab or antigen-binding fragment, to its homologous antigen to form an antibody–antigen complex. After initial contact, the union of the two substances takes place almost instantaneously (within milliseconds).

primary response

First response to an immunogen to which the recipient has not been previously exposed. Both B and T lymphocytes are activated by epitopes to proliferate and differentiate into antigen-effector lymphocytes and memory cells. It is principally an IgM response and generates immunologic memory.

primary sclerosing cholangitis (PSC)

A possible autoimmune liver disease characterized by inflammation of the large intra- and extrahepatic bile ducts that eventually leads to strictures and dilatations. The bile ducts eventually become stenotic and small intrahepatic bile ducts disappear. Although its etiology is unknown, chronic portal bacteremia, toxic bile acids, chronic viral infections, ischemic vascular injury, and immunoregulatory disorders have been implicated. Antineutrophil cytoplasmic antibodies (ANCAs) and antinuclear antibodies (ANAs) are principal features of PSC. Of lesser importance are anticolon epithelial autoantibodies. Incidence is predominantly male, in contrast to most autoimmune diseases. Lymphocytes infiltrate and destroy bile ducts. Hypergammaglobulinanemia, circulatory immune complexes, increased metabolism of complement component C3, and classical pathway activation of complement occur.

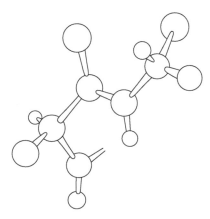

Primary structure.

primary structure

The linear amino acid sequence of a polypeptide or protein molecule.

primary tumor

The original neoplasm arising from the first transformed cell.

primate (nonhuman) immune system

Nonhuman primates represent the best animal models of many human diseases based on the resemblance of their immune system to that of humans. Lymphocyte subsets of human and nonhuman primates have been shown to be similar through the use of leukocyte-specific monoclonal antibodies. Similarities also exist between human and non-human primate major histocompatibility complex (MHC) and T cell receptor (TCR) genes.

prime boost strategy

A vaccination protocol requiring primary vaccination with a recombinant vector or naked DNA vaccine with a subsequent booster injection of a recombinant protein subunit vaccine.

primed

A lymphoid cell or an intact animal exposed once to a specific antigen that mounts a rapid and heightened response upon second exposure to the same antigen. Products of the reaction may be manifested as increased antibody production or heightened cell-mediated immunity against the antigen.

primed lymphocyte

A lymphocyte that has interacted with an antigen *in vivo* or *in vitro*.

primed lymphocyte test (PLT)

Lymphocytes previously exposed or primed to a certain antigen in a primary mixed lymphocyte culture divide rapidly when re-exposed to the same antigen. Using a primed cell, one can determine whether an unknown cell possesses the original stimulating antigen. Cells previously exposed to major histocompatibility complex (MHC) class II human leukocyte antigens (HLAs) can be used in HLA typing for HLA-D region antigens. PLT is an assay for the detection of lymphocyte-associated determinants (LADs). Lymphocytes donated by a normal person can serve as responder cells against the antigens of a known cell type. The test is based on the secondary stimulation of the primed or sensitized lymphocytes. The original stimulator serves as a positive control. The response of the sensitized cell to other cells measured by the incorporation of tritiated thymidine, by comparison with the control, may suggest sharing of HLA-D-associated antigens with the original stimulator cell if high stimulation values result. The HTC typing procedure, on the other hand, implies an antigenic determinant shared between the two cell types when there is little or no response. PLT is a positive typing procedure and has the advantage that homozygous donor cells are not required. Primed or sensitized cells can be prepared and frozen for future use when needed. They can be used to type unknowns within 24 hours which eliminates the 5 to 6 days necessary for a homozygous cell-typing procedure.

primed lymphocyte typing (PLT)

A method to type for HLA-D antigenic determinants. It is a type of mixed lymphocyte reaction in which cells previously exposed to allogeneic lymphocytes of known specificity can be re-exposed to unknown lymphocytes to determine their HLA-DP type, for example.

priming

The activation of antigen-specific naïve lymphocytes following exposure to antigen in an immunogenic form. Primed lymphocytes develop into either armed effector cells or into memory cells capable of responding rapidly to a second exposure to an antigen. The initial interaction of a naïve lymphocyte with a specific epitope that produces a primary immune response.

priming dose

The initial dose of an immunogen administered to an animal for the purpose of inducing an immune response.

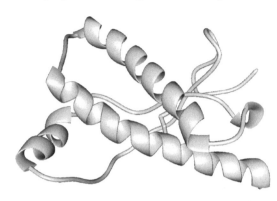

Prion.

prion

An infectious particle comprised of a protein with appended carbohydrate. It is the most diminutive infectious agent known. The three human diseases in which prions have been implicated include kuru, Creutzfeldt–Jakob disease, and Gerstmann–Straussler syndrome. Prions have also been implicated in animal diseases such as sheep and goat scrapie, bovine spongiform encephalopathy, chronic wasting of elk and mule deer, and transmissible mink encephalopathy. Prions do not induce inflammation or stimulate antibody synthesis. They resist formalin, heat, ultraviolet radiation, and other agents that normally inactivate viruses. They possess a 28-kDa, hydrophobic glycoprotein particle that polymerizes, forming an amyloid-like fibrillar structure. Prions produce disease by changing the conformation of their normal protein counterparts in the infected host brain.

PRIST

Abbreviation for paper radioimmunosorbent test, a technique used to assay serum IgE levels. It resembles the radioimmunoabsorbent test except that filter paper discs impregnated with anti-human IgE are used in place of Sephadex® discs.

private antigen

(1) An antigen confined to one major histocompatibility complex (MHC) molecule. (2) An antigenic specificity restricted to a few individuals. (3) A tumor antigen restricted to a specific chemically induced tumor. (4) A low-frequency epitope present on red blood cells of fewer than 0.1% of the population (Pt^a, By, Bp^a, etc.). (5) Human leukocyte antigen (HLA) encoded by one allele such as HLA-B27.

private idiotypic determinant

A determinant produced by a particular amino acid sequence in the immunoglobulin heavy or light chain hypervariable region of an antibody synthesized by only one individual.

private specificity

An epitope found on a protein encoded by a single allele; thus, it is found only on one member of a group of proteins, such as alloantigens of the major histocompatibility complex (MHC), even though it may also apply to other alloantigenic systems.

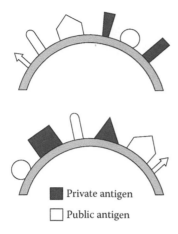

■ Private antigen

□ Public antigen

Public and private antigens.

privileged site

Anatomical location protected from immune effector mechanisms because of the absence of normal lymphatic drainage. Antigenic substances such as tissue allografts may be placed in these sites without evoking immune responses. Privileged sites include the anterior chamber of the eye, the cheek pouch of the Syrian hamster, and the central nervous system. Tissue allografts in these locations enjoy a period of protection from immunologic rejection, as the diffusion of antigen from graft sites to lymphoid tissues is delayed. Immune privilege alters the induction of immunity to antigens first encountered via privileged sites and also inhibits the expression of certain forms of alloimmunity in these same sites.

pro-B cell (progenitor B cell)

Cells that have displayed B cell surface marker proteins but have not yet completed heavy chain gene rearrangement. They are divided into early and late pro-B cells. The earliest stage of B cell development in which a heavy chain D gene segment rearranges to a J gene segment. D_H to J_H joining takes place at the early pro-B cell state and is followed by V_H to DJ_H joining at the late pro-B cell stage. Pro-B cells fail to produce immunoglobulin and express B lineage-restricted surface markers that include CD19 and CD10.

probe hybridization (tissue typing)

A technique used in tissue typing for organ transplantation in which total DNA is isolated from a subject's cells and PCR is conducted with primers that permit generic amplification of all HLA alleles. Hybridization to allele-specific probes permits the identification of sequences of interest.

pro-C3

A polypeptide single chain split into C3 α and β (amino terminal) chains.

pro-C4

A polypeptide single chain split into C4 α, β (amino terminal) and γ (carboxyl terminal) chains.

pro-C5

A polypeptide single chain split into C5 α and β (amino terminal) chains.

procomplementary factors

Serum components of selected species such as swine that resemble complement in their action and confuse evaluation of complement fixation tests.

prodrug

A therapeutic agent that is biologically inactive until metabolized in the body to yield an active drug.

productive infection

An infection in which a pathogenic microorganism proliferates even in the presence of an immune response against it.

productive rearrangement

Immunoglobulin and T cell receptor gene DNA rearrangements that yield a gene capable of governing the production of a functional polypeptide chain.

productivity testing

An assay that involves developing B or T cells of a specific V(D)J combination's functionality by transcribing the newly constructed gene and translating its mRNA. Along with accessory proteins of the pre-B cell receptor or pre-T cell receptor, the chain of interest is expressed on the cell surface and sends a signal to the cell confirming successful recombination.

proenzyme

An inactive enzyme precursor (or zymogen) frequently triggered by enzymatic cleavage in a molecular cascade as in the activation of complement.

professional APC

Refer to professional antigen-presenting cells.

professional antigen-presenting cells

Dendritic cells, macrophages, and B cells capable of initiating responsiveness of naïve T lymphocytes to antigen. These cells display antigenic peptide fragments in association with the proper class of major histocompatibility complex (MHC) molecules and also bear costimulatory surface molecules. Dendritic cells are the most important professional antigen-presenting cells (APCs) for initiating primary T lymphocyte responses.

progenitor cell

A cell no longer containing the capacity for self renewal and which is committed to the generation of a specific cell lineage.

programmed cell death

Apoptosis in which death is activated from within a dying cell. It occurs in lymphocytes deprived of growth factors or costimulators. It is also known as "death by neglect" and "passive cell death," in which mitochondrial cytochrome c is released into the cytoplasm, caspase-9 is activated, and apoptosis is initiated. Refer to apoptosis.

progressive multifocal leukoencephalopathy

A central nervous system disease characterized by demyelination, very little inflammation associated with patches of cortical degeneration, oligodendrogliocytes, intranuclear viral inclusions, aberrant large astrocytes, and reactive fibrillary astrocytes. This condition occurs in immunosuppressed individuals such as those with AIDS or latent virus infections such as measles. Papovavirus (DNA type, often JC) usually causes it.

progressive systemic sclerosis

A connective tissue or collagen-vascular disease in which the skin and submucosal connective tissue become thickened and scarred. Collagen deposition in the skin is increased. The disease is slowly progressive and chronic and may involve internal organs. The female-to-male ratio is 2:1. Although the etiology is unknown, patients demonstrate antinuclear antibodies, rheumatoid factor, and polyclonal hypergammaglobulinemia. No demonstrable immunoglobulin is found at the dermal–epidermal junction. Patients may have altered cellular immunity. The epidermis is thin, dermal appendages atrophy, and rete pegs are lost. Collagen deposition is markedly increased in the reticular dermis, and fibrosis and hyalinization of arterioles are present. The gastrointestinal tract may also reveal increased collagen deposition in the lamina propria, submucosa, and muscularis layers. At the onset, 90% of affected individuals experience Raynaud's phenomenon. Skin changes are usually the initial manifestations, with involvement of the hands, feet, forearms, and face or possibly diffuse involvement of the trunk. A variation of the disease called CREST syndrome consists of calcinosis, Raynaud's disease, esophageal dysmotility, sclerodactyly, and telangiectasia. This form of the disease may become stabilized for a number of years. The skin may exhibit a tight, smooth, waxy appearance in the sclerotic phase with no wrinkles or folds apparent. Ulcers may develop on the fingertips in many patients with a mask-like appearance of the face with thin lips. The skin may become atrophic or return to a normal soft structure. The lungs may be involved, leading to dyspnea on exertion. Pulmonary fibrosis may lead to cor pulmonale. The principal immunologic findings include antinuclear antibodies with a speckled or nucleolar pattern, anticentromere antibodies (in individuals with known CREST syndrome), and the development of antibodies specific for acid-extractable nuclear antigen. Approximately one third of the individuals with diffuse involvement of the trunk reveal antibodies specific for topoisomerase (anti-Scl-70 antibodies).

progressive transformation of germinal centers (PTGC)
Germinal center enlargement in the presence of follicular hyperplasia and loss of the distinct boundary between the mantle zone and the germinal center. Transformed germinal centers contain small lymphocytes with diffuse immunoblasts and histiocytes and often occur in one enlarged lymph node in young men. It is not believed to be neoplastic or portend development of lymphoma although it may be observed in some patients with nodular lymphocyte-predominant Hodgkin disease.

progressive vaccinia
An adverse reaction to smallpox vaccination in children with primary cell-mediated immunodeficiency, such as severe combined immunodeficiency. The vaccination lesion spreads from the site of inoculation and covers extensive areas of the body surface, leading to death.

prokaryote
An organism that contains one linear chromosome rather than a true nucleus.

prokaryotes, immunity in
Numerous antimicrobial agents synthesized and released extracellularly by bacteria exert specific effects on the bacteria. The agents include (1) enzymatically synthesized antibiotics; (2) post-translationally modified peptide antibiotics; (3) protein antibiotics such as bacteriocins, protein exotoxins, and bacteriolytic enzymes; and (4) intemperate or temperate bacterial viruses. After these agents enter bacterial cells, they must remain unchanged to exert their actions. Bacteriocins released by bacteria may inhibit the growth of other sensitive closely related bacteria, yet the strain producing the bacteriocin is usually able to resist its effect through specific immunity peptides or proteins. Antibiotic-synthesizing strains protect themselves from their own products by forming immunity proteins. Immunity to bacteriophage is the failure of an infected bacterial cell to be reinfected by a phage of the same type. Colicins

and bacteriophages and many other substances facilitate bacterial strain competitiveness. Immunity mechanisms are very specific and depend on protein–protein, protein–DNA, or RNA–DNA interactions. Numerous mechanisms confer immunity to prokaryotic organisms against specific bactericidal agents. *Immunity* also refers to replicons carrying transposons. A duplicate of a transposon fails to insert into a replicon already carrying a copy of the same transposon.

promiscuous binding
A docking site that accepts several different ligands with related affinity manifests promiscuous binding.

promoter
(1) The DNA molecular site where RNA polymerase attaches and transcription is initiated. The promoter is frequently situated adjacent to the operator, and upstream from it is an operon. A TATA box and a promoter are both required for immunoglobulin gene transcription.
(2) In tumor biology, a promoter mediates the second or promotion stage in the process of carcinogenesis. It may be a substance that can induce a tumor in an experimental animal that was previously exposed to a tumor initiator, but the promoter alone is not carcinogenic.

properdin (factor P)
A globulin in normal serum that has a central role in activation of the alternative complement pathway. Additional factors such as magnesium ions are required for properdin activity. Properdin is an alternative complement pathway protein that is significant in resistance against infection. It combines with and stabilizes the C3 convertase of the alternate pathway which is designated C3bBb. It is a 441-amino acid residue polypeptide chain with two points where N-linked oligosaccharides may become attached. Electron microscopy reveals it to have a cyclic oligomer conformation. Molecules are composed of six repeating 60-residue motifs that are homologous to 60 amino acids at C7, C8α, and C8β amino carboxyl terminal ends and the C9 amino terminal end.

properdin deficiency
An X-linked recessive disorder involving increased susceptibility to infections by *Neisseria* microorganisms. Males with the deficiency reveal 2% or less of normal serum levels of properdin. In some heterozygous females, the serum properdin level may be only 50%, while in others serum properdin levels are normal.

properdin pathway
An early synonym for alternative pathway of complement activation.

properdin system
An early term for the alternative complement pathway that consists of several proteins that are significant in resistance against infection. The first protein to be discovered was properdin. The properdin system also consists of factor B, a 95-kDa β_2 globulin also known as C3 proactivator, glycine-rich β glycoprotein, or β_2 glycoprotein II. Properdin factor D is a 25-kDa α globulin also called C3 proactivator convertase or glycine-rich β glycoproteinase. The properdin system or alternative pathway does not require the participation of antibody to activate complement. It may be activated by endotoxin or other substances. See alternative complement pathway.

prophylactic immunization
Prevention of disease through active or passive immunization. Active immunization usually induces longer lasting protection.

ProPO system

Prophenoloxidase activating system present exclusively in higher invertebrates. The coagulation sequence is triggered by microbial ligands leading to the activation of serine proteases and hemolymph. The serine proteases split inactive circulating prophenoloxidase (ProPO) and form active phenoloxidase (PO), which is an oxidoreductase that acts on phenols to yield quinines that undergo polymerization nonenzymatically to produce melanin that covers and paralyzes the microorganism in a sequence called the melanization reaction.

Prostacyclin, which is released and helps mediate type I hypersensitivity in tissues.

propylthiouracil

An antithyroid drug that blocks TPO activity.

prostacyclin (PC)

A derivative of arachidonic acid related to prostaglandins. It has a second five-membered ring. It inhibits aggregation

of platelets and is a potent vasodilator. Its actions are the opposite of the actions of thromboxanes.

prostaglandin (PG)

A family of biologically active lipids derived from arachidonic acid through the effects of the cycloxygenase enzyme. Although first described in the prostate gland, prostaglandins are now recognized in most mammal tissues. Their hormonal effects include decreasing blood pressure, stimulating contraction of smooth muscle, regulating inflammation, blood clotting, and the immune response. Prostaglandins are grouped on the bases of their substituted five-membered ring structures. During anaphylactic reactions mediated by IgE on mast cells, PGD_2 is released, producing small blood vessel dilation and constriction of bronchial and pulmonary blood vessels. Mononuclear phagocytes may release PGE_2 after binding of immune complexes to Fc′ receptors. Other effects of PGE_2 include blocking of major histocompatibility complex (MHC) class II molecule expression in T cells and macrophages and inhibition of T cell growth. PGD_2 and PGE_2 both prevent aggregation of platelets. Antiinflammatory agents such as aspirin block prostaglandin synthesis.

prostate-specific antigen (PSA)

A marker in serum or tissue sections for adenocarcinoma of the prostate. PSA is a 33-kDa proteolytic enzyme found exclusively in benign and malignant epithelium of the prostate. Men with PSA levels of 0 to 4.0 ng/mL and

Cycloxygenase pathway of arachidonic acid metabolism which participates in mediation of type I hypersensitivity reactions.

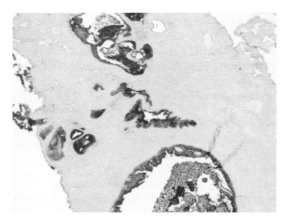

Prostaglandins, which are released and facilitate mediation of type I hypersensitivity reactions.

Prostate-specific antigen (PSA)—prostate.

nonsuspicious digital rectal examinations are generally not biopsied for prostate cancer. Men with PSA levels of 10.0 ng/mL and above typically undergo prostate biopsies. About one half of these men will have prostate cancer. Certain types (bound PSAs) link themselves to other proteins in the blood. Other kinds (free PSAs) float alone. Prostate cancer is more likely to be present in men who have low percentages of free PSA relative to the total amount. This finding is especially valuable in helping differentiate cancer and other benign conditions, thus eliminating unnecessary biopsies among men in the diagnostic gray zone (total PSA levels from 4.0 to 10.0 ng/mL). The PSA molecule is smaller than prostatic acid phosphatase (PAP). In patients with prostate cancer, preoperative PSA serum levels are positively correlated with the disease. PSA is increased in 95% of new cases of prostatic carcinoma, and in 97% of recurrent cases. It is inappropriate to use PSA levels alone to screen asymptomatic males. TUR, urethral instrumentation, prostatic needle biopsy, prostatic infarct, or urinary retention may also result in increased PSA values. PSA is critical for the prediction of recurrent adenocarcinoma in postsurgical patients. In a minority of cases of prostate cancer, especially those confined to the prostate, serum PSA is not elevated. Refinements in PSA testing values increased its diagnostic significance. This includes rate of change of PSA values with time, i.e., PSA velocity, determination of the ratio of serum PSA value and volume of the prostate gland, i.e., PSA density, and the measurement of free versus bound forms of circulating PSA. Free PSA levels >25% suggest a lower risk for cancer; levels below 10% are bothersome.

These parameters may be most useful when PSA levels range between 4.0 and 10.0 ng/ml, the so-called gray zone. PSA is also a useful immunocytochemical marker for primary and metastatic adenocarcinoma of the prostate.

prostatic acid phosphatase (PAP)/prostatic epithelial antigen
Prostate antigens, identifiable by immunoperoxidase staining. They are prostate-specific and -sensitive. Used together, they detect approximately 99% of prostatic adenocarcinomas.

pro-T cell
The earliest identifiable thymocyte recognized by expression of cell surface antigens such as CD2 and CD7 and by CD3 ε protein in the cytoplasm, but absent from cell surfaces. Rearrangement of δ, γ, and β TCR genes accompanies differentiation of pro-T cells into pre-T cells.

protease (HIV)
One of the HIV viral enzymes that splits polyprotein precursors to yield mature viral constituents.

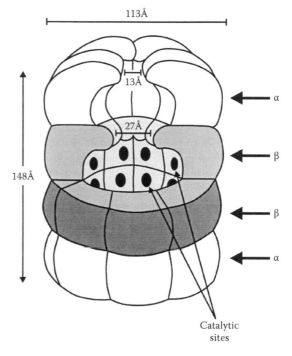

Longitudinal and transverse section through the 20S proteasome composed of two outer and two inner rings. The two outer rings each comprise seven copies of the 25.9-kDa α subunit.

proteasome
A large (650-kDa) organelle in the cytoplasm termed the low molecular mass polypeptide complex. The proteasome is believed to generate peptides by degradation of proteins in the cytosol. It is a cylindrical structure composed of as many as 24 protein subunits that participates in degradation of proteins in the cytosol that are covalently linked to ubiquitin. It is necessary for some protein antigens to be ubiquinated prior to presentation to major histocompatibility complex (MHC) class I-restricted T lymphocytes. Proteasomes that include MHC gene-encoded subunits are especially adept at forming peptides that bind MHC class I molecules. A strategic part of the endogenous antigen processing and presentation pathway. In resting cells, the standard proteasome digests mostly undesired self proteins. In dendritic cells and other cells accompanying inflammation, the immunoproteasome functions to digest foreign proteins.

P

proteasome genes

Two genes in the major histocompatibility complex (MHC) class II region that encode two proteasome sub-units. The proteasome is a protease complex in the cytosol that may participate in the generation of peptides from proteins in the cytosol.

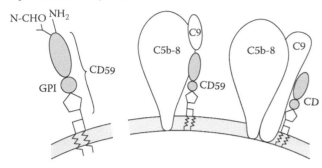

Protectin (CD59).

protectin (CD59)

A protein on cell surfaces that guards host cells from complement-mediated injury. It prevents the formation of the membrane attack complex by inhibiting C8 and C9 binding to the C5b–6–7 complex.

protective antigens

The antigenic determinants of a pathogenic microorganism that stimulate an immune response that can protect a host against an infection by the microorganism. These specific antigenic specificities can be used for prophylactic immunization in vaccines to immunize susceptible hosts against possible future infections.

protective epitopes

Antigenic determinants of a pathogenic microorganism that stimulate a protective immune response against the same microorganism. Refer to protective antigens.

protective immunity

Natural, nonspecific immune mechanisms and actively acquired specific immunity that result in the defense of a host against a particular pathogenic microorganism. Protective immunity may be induced by active immunization with a vaccine prepared from antigens of a pathogenic microorganism or by experiencing a subclinical or clinical infection from the microorganism.

protein A

A *Staphylococcus aureus* bacterial cell wall protein composed of a solitary polypeptide chain whose binding sites manifest affinity for the Fc region of immunoglobulin G (IgG). It combines with IgG_1, IgG_2, and IgG_4 but not IgG_3 subclasses in humans; with the IgG subclasses of mice; and with the IgG of rabbits and certain other species. It has been used extensively for the isolation of IgG during protein purification and for the protection of IgG in immune (antigen–antibody) complexes. Protein A is antiphagocytic, a property that may be linked to its ability to bind the Fc region of an opsonizing antibody. Protein A has been postulated to facilitate escape from the immune response by masking its epitopes with immunoglobulins. It is used for mitogenic stimulation of human B lymphocytes, investigation of lymphocyte Fc receptors, agglutination tests, and the detection and purification of immunoglobulins by the enzyme-linked immunosorbent assay (ELISA) technique.

protein AA

An 8.5-kDa protein isolated by gel filtration and comprised of 76 amino acids. The sequence has no relationship to those of immunoglobulins or other known sequences of human proteins. The sequence of protein AA extracted from various tissues appears identical, but several genetic variants are identified by sequence analysis. The molecule lacks cysteine and accordingly has no cross links. The N terminal residue is arginine (in humans), and in some the second amino acid is phenylalanine. AA also lacks carbohydrate and other attached small molecules. Amyloid protein AA is insoluble in ordinary aqueous solvents. Protein AA is the predominant component in the secondary form of amyloidosis.

protein B

A group B streptococcal protein capable of binding the Fc regions of immunoglobulin A (IgA) molecules. It is used in immunoassays and purification techniques for human serum and secretory IgA. It has the unique capacity to bind specifically to human IgA_1 and IgA_2 subclasses and shows no cross reactivity with other immunoglobulin classes or serum proteins.

protein blotting

Refer to immunoblotting.

protein F

Fusion protein; a 70-kDa glycoprotein believed critical to the generation of an effective immune response against respiratory syncytial virus.

protein G

An antibody-binding protein that combines securely and specifically with certain species of antibody. (1) A group G streptococcus cell wall constituent that combines with IgG Fc regions of four IgG subclasses that may be significant in host resistance to this microorganism. (2) A 90-kDa attachment glycoprotein that is critical in the immune response to respiratory syncytial virus (RSV). G protein antigenic differences are associated with RSV strain differences.

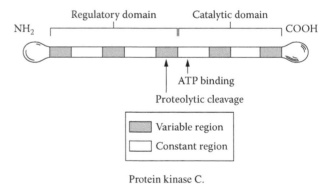

Protein kinase C.

protein kinase C (PKC)

A serine/threonine kinase that Ca^{2+} activates in the cytoplasm of cells. It participates in T and B cell activation and is a receptor for phorbol ester that acts by signal transduction, leading to hormone secretion, enzyme secretion, neurotransmitter release, and mediation of inflammation. It is also involved in lipogenesis and gluconeogenesis and participates in differentiation of cells and tumor promotion.

protein M (M antigen)

Group A streptococcal protein found on fimbriae. It is antiphagocytic and facilitates virulence of streptococci.

protein P

A 23-kDa pentameric protein detectable in amyloid deposits.

protein S

A 69-kDa vitamin K-dependent plasma protein that serves as a cofactor for activated protein C. It occurs as an active single chain protein or as a dimeric protein that is disulfide-linked and inactive. Protein S, in the presence of phospholipid, facilitates protein C inactivation of factor Va and combines with C4b-binding proteins. Protein S deficiency (autosomal-dominant transmission) is characterized clinically by deep vein thrombosis, pulmonary thrombosis, and thrombophlebitis. Laurell rocket electrophoresis is used to assay protein S.

protein SAA

A soluble precursor of AA present in minor quantities in serum. SAA has a molecular weight of 100 kDa and is present in cord blood and during the first three decades of life at an average concentration of 50 ± 40 ng/mL. During the next three decades, SAA shows a slow but steady increase in concentration, with the level doubling in the eighth decade of life. Levels of the serum precursor are elevated in most patients with amyloidosis except in cases of extreme protein dysfunction due to severe nephrosis. Levels reaching 700 ng/mL are detectable in patients with tuberculosis, lymphoma, carcinoma, and leukemia, but SAA levels have no value in the diagnosis of amyloidosis. High levels of SAA are seen in the secondary form of the disease. SAA levels may increase transiently during various infections.

protein separation techniques

Proteins may be purified using both electrophoresis and chromatography. Individual techniques are discussed individually. Refer to affinity chromatography, isoelectric focusing, and SDS–polyacrylamide gel electrophoresis (SDS-PAGE).

protein tyrosine kinases

Enzymes that phosphorylate protein tyrosine residues and participate in signal transduction from several types of cell surface receptors such as B cell and T cell receptors for antigen.

proteinuria

Protein in the urine.

proteolipid protein (PLP) autoantibodies

Proteolipid protein is a principal structural protein of the myelin sheath of the mammalian central nervous system and plays a critical role in myelination. It has been used to induce experimental allergic encephalomyelitis (EAE) in rabbits, producing lesions that resemble those formed in other species following immunization with whole central nervous system (CNS) tissue or myelin basic protein (MBP). The PLP antibody response in rabbits correlates with the clinical and histopathologic severity of experimental and allergic encephalomyelitis. PLP autoantibodies are correlated with a specific subset of multiple sclerosis patients.

proteomics

The study of the total proteins encoded by the genome of an organism. The study of proteins that an organism manifests is called expression proteomics.

***Proteus* immunity**

Proteus mirabilis administered to mice by the transurethral route can induce antibodies that react with purified lipopolysaccharide, flagella, outer membrane protein (OMP), and mannose-resistant *Proteus*-like MR/P fimbriae. Murine vaccination leads to partial immunity. The sera of patients with rheumatoid arthritis also react with *P. mirabilis*. A hexamer peptide within hemolysin is the target of the immunogenic response, probably due to its close similarity to susceptibility sequences of HLA-DR1 and DR4. Several proteins encoded by chromosomal genes serve as *P. mirabilis* virulence factors. These help a host evade immune defenses and lead to cell and tissue injury and include urease and HPM hemolysin. The latter leads to lysis of erythrocytes or epithelial cell membrane injury in culture. The organism also produces four types of fimbriae, surface proteins that have a role in adherence. It also secretes a protease that degrades IgA.

prothrombin antibodies

Antibodies against prothrombin or to the prothrombin–phospholipid complex have been associated with antiphospholipid (APF) syndrome. The test is based on the ability of patient sera to inhibit prothrombin activation to thrombin. Factor Xa or purified snake venom can cleave prothrombin to produce thrombin. Prothrombin antibodies in patient sera inhibit the capacity of these proteins to activate prothrombin. Prothrombin antibodies prevent prothrombin activation but do not interfere with prothrombin activity on fibrin and are therefore associated with thrombosis, not bleeding. Increased concentrations of antibodies against prothrombin increase the risk of deep venous thrombosis and pulmonary embolism in middle-aged men.

prothymocytes

Hematopoietic stem cells from the bone marrow migrate to the thymus via blood circulation and enter through the epithelial cell lining of the cortex. Prothymocytes (pre-T cells) differentiate in the thymus microenvironment. They are educated in the thymus to function as T cells. The four thymic peptide hormones are thymulin, thymosin α, thymosin β, and thymopoietin. These hormones are significant in T lymphocyte proliferation and differentiation. Direct interaction with the thymus epithelium, which expresses human leukocyte antigens (HLAs), is necessary for forming functional T lymphocytes and for learning to recognize major histocompatibility complex (MHC) antigens. Prothymocytes proliferate and migrate from the cortex to the medulla. Some are short-lived and die. The long-lived cells acquire new characteristics and are called thymocytes. They exit the thymus as immature cells and seed specific areas of the peripheral lymphoid organs where they continue to differentiate through a process driven by an antigen. From these areas, they recirculate throughout the body.

protooncogene

A cellular gene that shows homology with a retroviral oncogene. It is found in normal mammalian DNA and governs normal proliferation and probably also differentiation of cells. Mutation or recombination with a viral genome may convert a protooncogene into an oncogene, signifying that it has become activated. Oncogenes may act in the induction and/or maintenance of a neoplasm. Protooncogenes united with control elements may induce transformation of normal fibroblasts into tumor cells. Examples of protooncogenes are c-*fos*, c-*myc*, c-*myb*, c-*ras*, etc. Alteration of the protooncogenes, leading to synthesis of an aberrant gene product, is believed to facilitate their tumorigenesis. An elevation in the quantity of gene product produced is also believed to be associated with tumorigenesis of protooncogenes.

protoplast

A bacterial cell from which the wall has been removed. It includes the cell protoplasm and the cytoplasmic membrane. Lysozyme digestion of Gram-positive bacteria that contain peptidoglycan cell walls yields protoplasts that require hypertonic media for survival. They do not usually multiply. The hypertonic solution protects them from lysis. Protoplasts can also be produced from Gram-positive bacteria by treatment with penicillin or other antibiotics that inhibit cell wall synthesis. Gram-negative bacteria have cell walls composed of a thin peptidoglycan layer enclosed by an exterior membrane of lipopolysaccharide. Protoplasts prepared from Gram-negative bacteria are frequently termed spheroplasts.

protoplast fusion

A technique for DNA transfer from one group of bacteria to others, to myeloma cells, or to other animal cells in culture. The exposure of plasmid-bearing *Escherichia coli* microorganisms to lysozyme and EDTA yields protoplasts that may be fused with myeloma cells by polyethylene glycol treatment.

protostomes

Animals arising from coelomates that developed into higher invertebrates.

protozoa

Microscopic animals that must recognize and eat food. Intricate genetic mechanisms control their surface proteins.

protozoans

Single-celled parasites.

proviral DNA

Refer to provirus.

provirus

The DNA version of a retrovirus integrated into a host cell genome where it may remain inactive transcriptionally for prolonged periods.

provocation poliomyelitis

An uncommon consequence of attempted immunization against poliomyelitis in which paralysis quickly followed injection of vaccines such as those that contained *Bordetella pertussis* or alum.

prozone

In agglutination and precipitation reactions, the lack of agglutination or precipitation in tubes where the antibody concentration is greatest attributable to suboptimal agglutination or precipitation in the region of antibody excess. Agglutination or precipitation becomes readily apparent in the tubes where the same antibody is more dilute. This is known as a prozone or prozone phenomenon. It is attributable to a blocking antibody or antibody combining with individual cells or molecules, as in antibody excess, or to a serum lipid- or protein-induced nonspecific inhibition reaction. Soluble complexes of antigen and antibody may be present in the antibody excess zones of

certain precipitation reactions. Excess antibody coating the surfaces of cells in an agglutination reaction in the antibody excess zone may prevent cross linking, which is requisite for agglutination to become manifest. The prozone represents a false-negative reaction. When a serum sample is believed to contain a certain antibody that is masked or demonstrates a prozone phenomenon, the sample must be diluted serially to demonstrate reactivity in more dilute tubes to avoid reporting a false-negative result.

prozone effect

Refer to prozone.

PRP antigen

Polyribosylribitol capsular polysaccharide; an antiphagocytic cell wall constituent of *Hemophilus influenzae* that provides the microorganism with an effective mechanism to induce disease. Type-specific antibodies that facilitate immunization are requisite for protective immunity against *H. influenzae*. Children under 2 years old are poor producers of anti-PRP antibodies, making them more susceptible to the infection.

PRP-D

Polyribosylribitol–diphtheria toxoid. Refer to Hib.

pruritis

Severe itching.

PSA

Refer to prostate-specific antigen.

pSMAC

Peripheral supramolecular activation complex. The interior pSMAC encircles the cSMAC and accommodates CD2/LFA-3 pairs. The exterior pSMAC encircles the inner pSMAC, accommodates LFA-1/ICAM-1 pairs, and is united to the actin cytoskeleton.

P-selectin

A molecule found in the storage granules of platelets and the Weibel–Palade bodies of endothelial cells. Ligands are sialylated Lewis X and related glycans. P-selectins are involved in the binding of leukocytes to endothelium and platelets to monocytes in areas of inflammation. Also called CD62P.

pseudoalleles

Genes that are closely linked but distinct. They have functional similarity and act as alleles in complementation investigations; crossover studies may separate them.

pseudoallergic reaction

A nonimmunological clinical syndrome characterized by signs and symptoms that mimic or resemble immune-based allergic or immediate hypersensitivity reactions; these reactions are not mediated by specific antibodies or immune lymphoid cells.

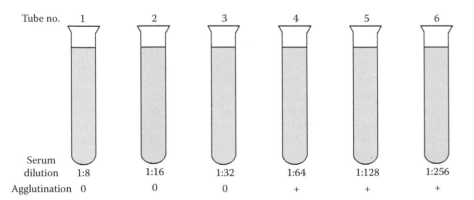

Prozone effect.

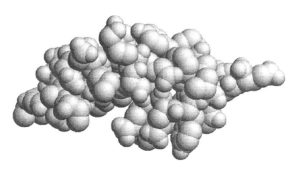

P selection (NMR).

pseudoallergy

An anaphylaxis-like reaction that occurs suddenly, frequently following food ingestion, and represents an anaphylactoid reaction. It may be induced by a psychogenic factor, a metabolic defect, or other nonimmunological cause. This is not an immune reaction and is classified as an anaphylactoid reaction.

pseudogene

A sequence of DNA that is similar to a sequence of a true gene but does not encode a protein due to defects that inhibit gene expression. Pseudogenes represent nonusable or junk DNA. They may result from duplicated genes and have several defects as mutations accumulate.

pseudolymphoma

Hyperplasia of lymphoid tissue involving a uniform accumulation of lymphocytes. Unlike lymphomas, the cells are polyclonal. The architecture of the lymph nodes is well preserved, with distinct cortical germinal centers showing little or minimal capsular infiltration by lymphocytes. Inflammatory cells are detectable between germinal centers, but mitoses occur only within the centers. The reticular framework remains intact. The lymphoid hyperplasia that characterizes pseudolymphoma may be found in various locations such as gastrointestinal tract, lung, breast, salivary gland, mediastinum, skin, soft tissue, and other areas. Pseudolymphomas may occur in individuals who later develop lymphomas.

pseudolymphomatous lymphadenitis

Hyperplasia of lymphoid organs that is similar to lymphoma except that the hyperplasia is reversible.

Pseudomonas aeruginosa immunity

Pseudomonas aeruginosa infection is followed by the development of antibodies that facilitate opsonophagocytosis and protection against subsequent infections. An adequate antibody response is required for protection. Antibody alone may be insufficient because the lungs of patients with cystic fibrosis continue to be chronically colonized even in the presence of potent serum antibody responses to several antigens of this microorganism. Active vaccination is made less desirable by the fact that *P. aeruginosa* infections cannot be reliably predicted; thus, passively administered hyperimmune intravenous immunoglobulin from immunized volunteers has been used to confer protection. Nevertheless, contemporary investigations show that antibodies against lipopolysaccharide (LPS) serotypes and to exotoxin A do not significantly protect recipients.

pseudoparaproteinemia

An elevation of transferrin to levels at least twice normal (200 to 400 mg/dL). Profound iron deficiency anemia leads to this increase. The one molecular form of transferrin in the serum is concentrated into a single band that travels in the β region in serum electrophoresis, giving the appearance of a paraproteinemia. However, a real paraproteinemia is characterized by a spike on serum electrophoresis representing a monoclonal gammopathy.

pseudopodia

Membrane extensions from motile and phagocytic cells.

psoriasis vulgaris

A chronic, recurrent, papulosquamous autoimmune disease attributed to improper functioning of keratinocytes. Marked

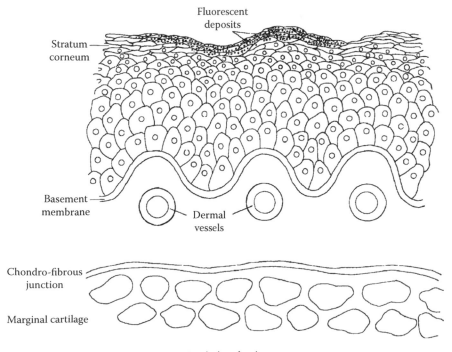

Psoriasis vulgaris.

by erythematous skin lesions that develop a silvery covering. Clinical features include the appearance of discrete, papulosquamous plaques on areas of trauma such as elbows, knees, and scalp, although they may appear elsewhere on the skin. The incidence of HLA-B13 and B17 antigen is relatively high, and T suppressor cell function is decreased. Psoriasis vulgaris may coexist with lupus erythematosus in some individuals. Peripheral blood helper/inducer CD4+ T lymphocytes are significantly decreased in psoriasis patients, who may be treated with psoralens and long-wave ultraviolet radiation. Patients develop Munro microabscesses, hyperkeratosis, parakeratosis, irregular acanthosis, papillary edema, and mild chronic inflammation of the dermis. Focal granular or globular deposits of immunoglobulins and C3 in the stratum corneum are revealed by immunofluorescence. The finely granular deposits principally contain IgG, IgA, and C3 and are deposited in areas where stratum corneum antigens are located. C3 and properdin deposits suggest activation of the alternate complement pathway.

psychoneuroimmunology

The study of central nervous system and immune system interactions in which neuroendocrine factors modulate immune system function. For example, psychological stress arising from bereavement or other causes may lead to depressed immune function through neuroendocrine immune system interaction. Multiple bidirectional interactions exist among the nervous, immune, and endocrine systems. This represents an emerging field of contemporary immunological research.

pTα

Refer to pre-T cell receptor.

PTAP

Purified diphtheria toxoid that has been adsorbed on hydrated aluminum phosphate; it is used to induce active immunity against diphtheria.

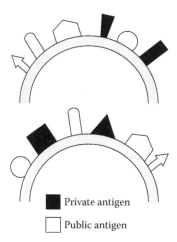

Public and private antigen.

public antigen (supratypic antigen)

An epitope that several distinct or private antigens have in common. A public antigen such as a blood group antigen is present in >99.9% of a population. It is detected by the indirect antiglobulin (Coombs' test). Examples include Ve, Ge, Jr, Gyᵃ, and Okᵃ. Antigens that occur frequently but are not public include MNs, Lewis, Duffy, P, etc. One blood banking problem is finding suitable units of blood for transfusions to recipients who have antibodies against public antigens.

public idiotypic determinant (IdX or CRI)

An idiotypic determinant present on antibody molecules in numerous individuals of one species. It may occur on antibodies with a single antigen specificity but may be present on antibodies with separate specificities as well. The terms IdX or CRI signify that these are cross reacting idiotypic determinants and manifestations of immunoglobulin heavy and light chain amino acid sequence similarities.

public specificity

Specificity of an epitope encoded by two or more alleles of an alloantigenic system. The term most frequently refers to major histocompatibility complex (MHC) determinants such as MHC alleles in which a single epitope is shared by multiple human leukocyte antigen (HLA) molecules. Antigenic products encoded by more than one allele at a single locus may carry public specificities. These specificities may also be encoded by alleles at loci that are separate but related. Thus, epitopes that represent public specificities are shared by two or more proteins in a particular group. For the specificity to be public, it must be found on at least two proteins but may be found on multiple ones.

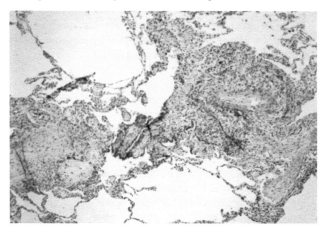

Pulmonary vasculitis. Note the necrosis of endothelial cells and supporting stromal structures with acute and chronic inflammation, as well as the exudation of polymorphonuclear leukocytes (PMNs), eosinophils, and extravasated erythrocytes (35× magnification).

pulmonary vasculitis

Vasculitis characterized by chronic inflammation, necrotizing and non-necrotizing granulomatous inflammation, fibrinoid necrosis, arterial wall medial thickening, and intimal proliferation.

pulsed field gel electrophoresis

A method for separating DNA molecules that vary in size from a few to 4000 kilobase pairs. The direction of the electric field is repeatedly altered, causing the molecules to change direction of migration and enter new pores in a gel. Thus, both small and large DNA molecules migrate through the gel based on size. Migration of the smaller molecules is more rapid than that of the larger molecules.

pulsing

Antigen-presenting cell peptide groove loading with antigen by electroporation.

purified protein derivative (PPD)

A derivative of the growth medium in which *Mycobacterium tuberculosis* has been cultured. It is a soluble protein precipitated from the culture medium by trichloroacetic acid. It is used for tuberculin skin tests.

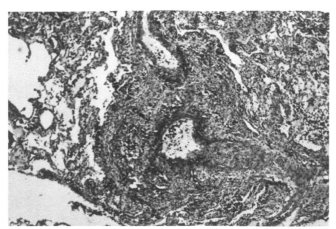

Pulmonary vasculitis. Note necrosis of endothelial cells and supporting stromal structures with acute and chronic inflammation and exudation of polymorphonuclear leukocytes (PMNs), eosinophils, and extravasated erythrocytes (50× magnification).

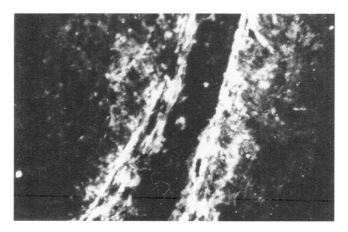

Pulmonary vasculitis. Direct immunofluorescence reveals coalescent and granular deposits of IgM and C3 in the walls of some muscular arteries and occasional large veins consistent with immune complex vasculitis involving large vessels (200× magnification).

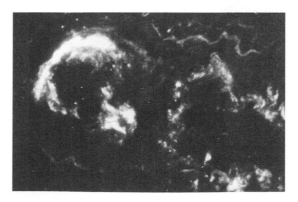

Pulmonary vasculitis. Direct immunofluorescence reveals coalescent and granular deposits of IgM and C3 in the walls of some muscular arteries and occasional large veins consistent with immune complex vasculitis involving large vessels (500× magnification).

purine nucleoside phosphorylase (PNP)

An enzyme involved in purine metabolism. A deficiency of this enzyme leads to the accumulation of purine nucleosides that are toxic for developing T lymphocytes and severe combined immunodeficiency.

purine nucleoside phosphorylase (PNP) deficiency

A type of severe combined immunodeficiency caused by mutant types of PNP that results in the retention of metabolites that have toxic effects on T cells. B lymphocytes appear unaffected and their numbers are normal. All cells of mammals contain PNP, which acts as a catalyst in the phosphorolysis of guanosine, deoxyguanosine, and inosine. Insufficient PNP leads to an elevation in the concentration within cells of deoxyguanosine, guanosine, deoxyguanosine triphosphate (dGTP), and guanosine triphosphate (GTP). dGTP blocks the ribonucleoside-diphosphate reductase enzyme that participates in DNA synthesis. T cell precursors are especially sensitive to death induced by these compounds. PNP is composed of three 32-kDa subunits. Its gene, located on chromosome 14q13.1, codes for a 289-amino acid residue polypeptide chain. Immunologic defects associated with this disorder are characterized by anergy, lymphocytopenia, and diminished T lymphocytes. By contrast, serum immunoglobulin levels and the response following deliberate immunization with various types of immunogens are within normal limits. Inheritance is autosomal-recessive. Treatment is by bone marrow transplantation.

purpura

Purple areas on the skin caused by bleeding into the skin.

purpura hyperglobulinemia

Hemorrhagic areas around the ankles or legs in patients whose serum immunoglobulin levels are strikingly increased. Examples include Waldenström's macroglobulinemia, multiple myeloma, and Sjögren's syndrome.

pyogenic bacteria

Microorganisms, such as Gram-positive staphylococci and streptococci, that induce predominantly polymorphonuclear leukocyte (PMN) inflammatory responses, leading to the formation of pus at sites of infection.

pyogenic infection

An infection associated with the generation of pus. Microorganisms that are well known for their pus-inducing or pyogenic potential include *Streptococcal pyogenes, Staphylococcus aureus, Streptococcus pneumoniae,* and *Hemophilus influenzae.* Antibody-deficient patients and those having defective phagocytic cell capacity show increased susceptibility to pyogenic infections. Patients with complement deficiency such as C3 deficiency, factor I deficiency, etc. are also prone to develop pyogenic infections.

pyogenic microorganisms

Microorganisms that stimulate a large polymorphonuclear leukocyte response to their presence in tissues.

pyrogen

A substance that induces fever. The fever may be either endogenously produced, such as by interleukin-1 (IL1) released from macrophages and monocytes, or an endotoxin associated with Gram-negative bacteria produced exogenously.

pyroglobulins

Monoclonal immunoglobulins that undergo irreversible precipitation upon heating to 56°C. They are usually detected during routine inactivation of complement in serum by heating to 56°C in a water bath. Whereas most immunoglobulins are unharmed at this temperature, pyroglobulins precipitate. This may be attributable to formation of hydrophobic bonds linking immunoglobulin molecules as a consequence of diminished heavy chain polarity. Half of the pyroglobulin-positive subjects have multiple myeloma, and the remaining half have lymphoproliferative disorders such as macroglobulinemia, carcinoma, or systemic lupus erythematosus. The relevance of pyroglobulins to disease is unknown.

pyroninophilic cells

Cells whose cytoplasm stains red with methyl green pyronin stain. This signifies large quantities of RNA in the cytoplasm, indicating active protein synthesis. For example, plasma cells and other protein-producing cells are pyroninophilic.

Q

Q fever

An acute disease caused by *Coxiella burnetii* Rickettsia. Cattle, sheep, goats, and several small marsupials serve as reservoirs. Ticks are the main vectors. The microorganism is highly infectious and multiplies readily to produce clinical infection. The onset is abrupt and accompanied by headaches, high fever, myalgia, malaise, hepatic dysfunction, interstitial pneumonitis, and fibrinous exudate. Q fever may also induce atypical pneumonia, rapidly progressive pneumonia, or be a coincidental finding to a systemic illness. The disease has a relatively low mortality. It is treated successfully with tetracycline and chloramphenicol.

Qa antigens

Class I histocompatibility antigens in mice designated Qa1, Qa2, and Qa10. They are encoded by genes in the QA region of the H-2 complex on the telomeric side. Lymphoid cells express Qa1 and Qa2 antigens, whereas hepatic cells express Q10 antigens. The Qa represents one of two regions of the Tla complex, with Tla representing the second region of this complex.

Qa-2 antigen

An antigen encoded by MHC class I genes that is produced in GPI-linked and soluble secreted forma. It shows little polymorphism and is tissue-specific. Anti-Qa-2 monoclonal antibodies are potent T cell activators in the presence of PMA and cross linking anti-Ig.

Qa locus

A subregion of the murine MHC located on the telomeric side of the H-2 complex in a 1.5 centiMorgan stretch of DNA. The Qa region is a part of the Tla complex which also contains Tla. The Qa region is comprised of 220 kb that encode for class I MHC α chains that associate noncovalently with β2 microglobulin. The Qa region is comprised of eight to ten genes designated Q1, Q2, Q3, etc.

Qa region

Refer to Tla complex.

quantitative gel diffusion test

Estimation of the amount of antibody or antigen by a gel diffusion method such as single radial diffusion or Laurell rocket assay.

quantitative precipitin reaction

An immunochemical assay based on the formation of an antigen–antibody precipitate in serial dilutions of the reactants, permitting combination of antigen and antibody in various proportions. The ratio of antibody to antigen is graded sequentially from one tube to the next. The optimal proportion of antigen and antibody is present in the tube that shows the most rapid flocculation and yields the greatest amount of precipitate. After washing, the precipitate can be analyzed for protein content through procedures such as the micro-Kjeldahl analysis to ascertain nitrogen content, spectrophotometric assay, and other techniques. Heidelberger and Kendall used the technique extensively, employing pneumococcus polysaccharide antigen and precipitating antibody in which nitrogen determinations reflected a quantitative measure of antibody content.

quaternary structure

Four components that are associated. Two or more folded polypeptide chains packed into a configuration such as a tetramer. Quaternary antigenic determinants may be difficult to demonstrate in such structures as hemoglobin molecules.

quaternary syphilis

The stage of syphilis which follows the tertiary stage. It is characterized by a necrotizing encephalitis with tissues rich in spirochetes. End-stage HIV patients who have completely lost cell-mediated immunity against treponemal antigens may show this form of syphilis. Although rare in the past,

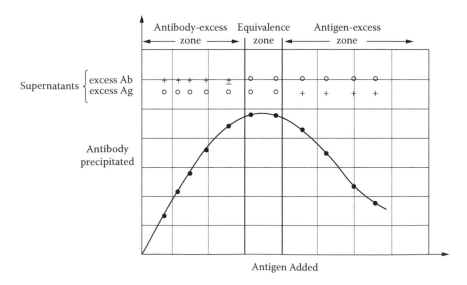

Quantitative precipitin reaction.

Q

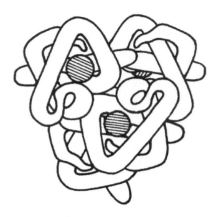

Quarternary structure.

quaternary syphilis is seen more often in AIDS patients also infected with *Treponema pallidum* who show increased susceptibility to neurosyphilis.

Quellung phenomenon

Swelling of the pneumococcus capsule following exposure to antibodies against pneumococci. Refer to Quellung reaction.

Quellung reaction

Swelling of bacterial capsules when the microorganisms are incubated with species-specific antiserum. Examples of bacteria in which this can be observed include *Streptococcus pneumoniae, Hemophilus influenzae, Neisseria,* and *Klebsiella* species. The combination of a drop of antiserum with a drop of material from a patient containing an encapsulated microorganism and the addition of a small loopful of 0.3% methylene blue produces the Quellung reaction. The microorganisms are stained blue and are encircled by a clear halo that resembles swelling, but is in fact antigen–antibody complex produced at the

Quin-2.

surface of the organism. The reaction is due to an alteration of the refractory index.

quenching

When immunofluorescent cell or tissue preparations treated with fluorochrome-labeled antibodies are exposed to ultraviolet light under a microscope, the emission of fluorescent radiation from the fluorochrome label diminishes as a result of quenching. The term may also refer to diminished efficiency of assaying radioactivity in a scintillation counter by such agents as ethanol or hydrogen peroxide (H_2O_2).

Quin-2

A derivative of quinoline that combines with free Ca^{2+} to accentuate fluorescence intensity. It can be introduced into cells as an ester followed by de-esterification. When T or B lymphocytes containing Quin-2 are activated, their fluorescence intensity rises, implying an elevation of free Ca^{2+} in the cytosol.

quinidine (β-quinine; 6′-methoxycinchonan-9-ol)

A stereoisomer of quinine recognized for its cardiac antiarrhythmic effects.

R

R5 viruses

CCR5-binding HIV strains that infect both macrophages and CD4⁺ T cells. Previously known as M-tropic viruses.

RA

Rheumatoid arthritis.

RA-33

A rheumatoid arthritis-specific antigen that is identical to the heterogeneous rhnRNP-A2 ribonucleoprotein.

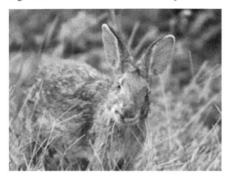

Rabbit immunity.

rabbit immunity

The rabbit immune system is similar to that of the human with only minor variations. Rabbit gut-associated lymphoid tissue (GALT) consists of an appendix, Peyer's patches, and diffuse lymphatic nodules. GALT and other peripheral lymphoid tissues of rabbits contain a permanent lymphatic system with lymph nodes. The rabbit has a prominent spleen and a thymus that undergoes involution in adulthood. Lymphopoiesis originates in the bone marrow, and the maturing cells occupy appropriate tissues and organs. Rabbit leukocytes resemble those of other mammalian mononuclear phagocyte systems. Lymphoid cell populations and circulation routes resemble those of other mammals, making rabbits excellent models for immunological investigations. Rabbit cytokines include migration inhibition factor (MIF), chemotactic factor, migration stimulation factor (MSF), interleukin-1 (IL1), IL2, and tumor necrosis factor (TNF-α). IgM, IgG, IgE, and IgA immunoglobulins and several groups of allotypes have been discovered in rabbits. The rabbit major histocompatibility complex (MHC) has both class I and class II regions. B and T cells, microphages, and polymorphonuclear leukocytes have been described.

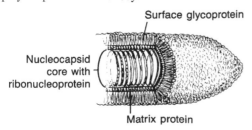

Rabies virus.

rabies

An infection produced by an RNA virus following a bite from an infected animal. The virus passes across the neuromuscular junction and infects a nerve, from which it reaches the central nervous system. It also reaches salivary glands of lower animals. The virus infection leads to cerebral edema, congestion, round cell infiltration of the spinal cord and gray matter in the brain stem, and profound loss of Purkinje cells. Negri bodies are found prominently in the medulla oblongata, hippocampus, and cerebellum. Clinically, the fury associated with the disease is due to irritability of the central nervous system and is accompanied by fever, hyperethesia, and anoxia aggression. The infection may be paralytic. Human rabies is rare in the United States; it is more common in other animals, with most cases in skunks and raccoons. Fewer cases occur in bats, and only 2% each in dogs and cats. The virus is transmitted among humans by inhalation or by corneal transplantation, but not by human bites.

rabies vaccination

Refer to post-rabies vaccination encephalomyelitis.

rabies vaccine

A pre-exposure immunizing preparation that contains killed rabies virus, used primarily for individuals who face rabies as an occupational risk. Following the bite of a rabid animal, both the vaccine and rabies immune globulin containing preformed antibodies are administered. In humans, significant levels of neutralizing antibody can be generated by immunization with a virus grown in tissue culture in diploid human embryo lung cells. A vaccine adapted to chick embryos, especially egg passage material, is used for prophylaxis in animals prior to exposure. The vaccine originally prepared by Pasteur made use of rabbit spinal cord preparations to which the virus became adapted. These preparations were discontinued because of the risk of inducing post-rabies vaccination encephalomyelitis.

Rac

A small guanine nucleotide-binding protein that the guanosine diphosphate (GDP)–guanosine triphosphate (GTP) exchange factor Vav activates during the early stages of T lymphocyte activation. GTP-Rac activates a protein kinase cascade that leads to activation of the stress-activated protein (SAP) kinase, c-Jun N-terminal kinase (JNK), and p38 kinase, which are similar to the mitogen-activated protein (MAP) kinases.

RA cell

Abbreviation for rheumatoid arthritis cell.

radial immunodiffusion

A technique used to ascertain the relative concentration of an antigen. Antigen is placed in a well and permitted to diffuse into agar containing an appropriate dilution of an antibody. The area of the precipitin ring that encircles the well in the equivalence region is proportional to the antigen concentration.

radiation and immunity

Ionizing radiation injures DNA and other cellular constituents. The most radiosensitive cells in the body are the

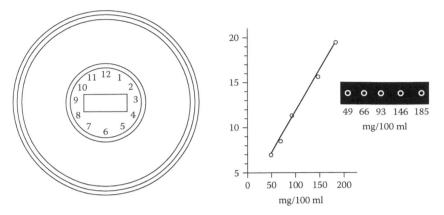

Radioimmunodiffusion.

lymphoid tissues and recirculating lymphocytes. Small doses of radiation can lead to programmed cell death (apoptosis) of lymphocytes and myeloid progenitor cells. Immune system sensitivity to radiation is characterized by (1) the magnitude of the suppression of the primary or secondary immune response, (2) the reduction in size of lymphoid organs, and (3) the diminished number of surviving lymphoid cells. Whereas lymphoid cells are very radiosensitive, selected radioresistant immune functions (and cells) are maintained after significant doses of radiation. The effects of radiation on immunity do not depend on their actions on lymphocytes alone but also on the leukocytes that mediate nonspecific host responses. Microphages and other nondividing cells are relatively radioresistant. They may even be activated following irradiation, revealing enhanced RNA synthesis, enhanced production of cytokines, and increased synthesis and release of lysosomal enzymes. Polymorphonuclear neutrophilic leukocyte phagocytic ability is not decreased by radiation, which may even increase intracellular killing of phagocytized microorganisms. Most mature resting lymphocytes are killed by 80 to 500 rad within hours following radiation. Lymphocytes stimulated by mitogen or antigen become more radioresistant and maintain their functions and viability even following 1000 rad. The thymus is the most radiosensitive lymphoid organ. Radiation is usually more harmful to the antibody response than to delayed-type hypersensitivity (DTH) responses. The irradiation of mice (440 rad) just before antigen exposure leads to immune suppression, whereas the same dose of irradiation 4 days after antigenic challenge leads to increased antibody titers. The *in vivo* secondary immune response is more radioresistant than the primary response. DTH is relatively radioresistant in comparison to antibody production. Most cytotoxic T lymphocytes are radioresistant to doses of several thousand rad. Many immunodeficient conditions have been associated with increased sensitivity to radiation.

radiation bone marrow chimeras

Mice subjected to heavy radiation and then reconstituted with allogeneic bone marrow cells (from a different mouse strain). Thus, their lymphocytes are genetically different from the surroundings in which they develop. These chimeric mice have yielded significant data in the investigation of lymphocyte development.

radiation chimera

Refer to irradiation chimera.

radiation therapy

The destruction of tumor cells by ionizing radiation administered externally as a focused beam or as brachytherapy.

radioallergosorbent test

Refer to RAST.

radioimmunoassay (RIA)

A binder ligand technique used to assay antigen or antibody; it is based on competitive inhibition by a radiolabeled antigen of the binding of an unlabeled antigen to specific antibodies. Minute quantities of enzymes, hormones, and other immunogenic substances can be assayed by RIA. Enzyme immunoassays have largely replaced RIAs because of the problems associated with radioisotope regulation and disposal.

radioimmunodiffusion

A variation of the immunodiffusion technique that uses a radioactively labeled antibody. This enhances the sensitivity

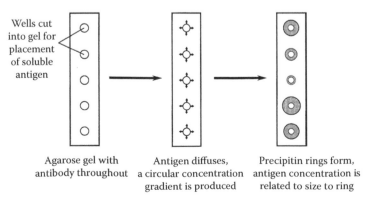

Radioimmunodiffusion.

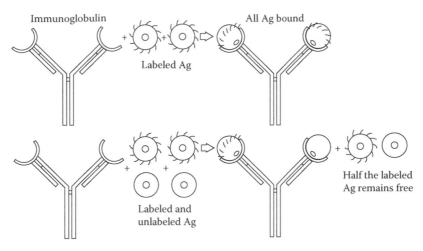

Radioimmunoassay (RIA).

of the results when read by autoradiography. Refer to single radial immunodiffusion.

radioimmunodiffusion test

Refer to single radial immunodiffusion.

radioimmunoelectrophoresis

A type of immunoelectrophoresis that employs radiolabeled antibody or antigen to identify individual precipitin arcs by autoradiography.

radioimmunoprecipitation assay (RIPA)

A method that demonstrates antibodies against viral constituents. Virus grown in culture in the presence of radioactive amino acid is disrupted and incubated with a test sample that may contain antibodies specific for viral antigens. This is followed by polyacrylamide gel electrophoresis of the immunoglobulins in the test sample.

radioimmunoscintigraphy

The use of radiolabeled antibodies to localize tumors or other lesions through radioactivity scanning after injection *in vivo*.

radioimmunosorbent test (RIST)

A solid phase radioimmunoassay to determine serum immunoglobulin E (IgE) concentration. A standard quantity of radiolabeled IgE is added to the serum sample to be assayed. The mixture is then combined with Sephadex® or dextran beads coated with antibody to human IgE. After incubation and washing, the quantity of radiolabeled IgE bound to the beads is measured. The patient's IgE competes with the radiolabeled IgE or antibody attached to the beads. The decrease in labeled IgE attached to the beads compared to a control, in which labeled IgE combines with the beads without competition, represents the IgE concentration. The radioallergosorbent test by comparison assays IgE levels reactive with a specific allergen.

radioimmunotherapy (RIT)

Treatment of cancer with radioimmunoisotopes.

radiolabeling

Radioisotope incorporation into macromolecules has increased the sensitivity of immunoassays 30,000-fold. Radioisotopes permit the detection and quantification of picogram quantities of an antigen or receptor. Radiolabeled antibodies can detect primary binding of antibody to antigen, providing sensitivity and measurements of affinity. They may be used to identify a tumor site or the presence and topography of molecules in a cell membrane. Radiolabeled antigens demonstrated that B cells bind antigen via cell surface immunoglobulin receptors.

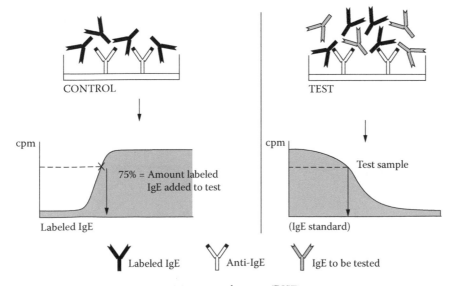

Radioimmunosorbent test (RIST).

radiomimetic drug

An immunosuppressive drug such as an alkylating agent used in the treatment of cancer. Its effect on DNA mimics that of ionizing radiation.

RAG-1 and RAG-2

Refer to recombination-activating genes 1 and 2.

RAG blastocyst complementation

A method employed to test gene function when its null mutation in the body is embryonic lethal. RAG mice are bereft of both T and B cells. The introduction of embryonic stem cells from a particular mutant whose RAG genes are intact into the eight-cell stage blastocyst of a RAG $^{-/-}$ developing embryo results in absorption of new cells by the embryo, which proceeds with normal development following implantation. Different regions of chimeric embryos are the sources of different tissues, leading to viable reconstituted mice that possess lymphoid systems expressing the specific mutation. This technique permits determination of the effect of the mutation on lymphocyte development and function.

RAG recombinases

Recombination activation gene recombinases. RAG-1 and RAG-2 are the main enzymes that facilitate V(D)J gene segment recombination in immunoglobulin and T cell receptor loci. Only developing B and T cells express the RAG genes.

Ragg

Agglutinating activity by rheumatoid factor in the sera of patients with rheumatoid arthritis, as revealed by a positive rheumatoid arthritis (RA) test.

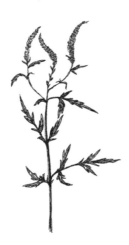

Ambrosia artemisiaefolia, commonly termed ragweed.

ragocyte

Polymorphonuclear leukocytes containing IgG–rheumatoid factor–complement–fibrin conglomerates found in the joints of patients with rheumatoid arthritis. Also called RA cells.

ragweed

Ragweed (genus *Ambrosia*) is distributed throughout the warmer parts of the Western Hemisphere but poses the greatest clinical problem in North America. Airborne ragweed pollen constitutes a troublesome respiratory allergen. It appears in the air in the northern United States and adjacent eastern Canada in late July and reaches levels up to thousands of grains per cubic meter by early September, after which the level declines. Pure ragweed pollinosis has usually subsided by mid-October in the north. Short ragweed (*A. artemisiaefolia*) and giant ragweed (*A. trifida*) range widely from the Atlantic coast to the Midwest, Ozark plateau, and Gulf states. Short ragweed reaches to northern Mexico and is found only sparsely in the Pacific Northwest. Giant ragweed is abundant in the Mississippi Delta and along the flood plains of southeastern rivers. The following ragweed pollen allergens have been characterized:

Allergen Source	Allergen	Molecular Weight (kDa) SDS–PAGE
Ambrosia artemisiaefolia (ragweed)	*AMB* α I (AGE)	38
	AMB α II (AGK)	38
	AMB α III (Ia3)	12
	AMB α IV (Ra4)	23
	AMB α V (Ra5)	5
	AMB α VI (Ra6)	8
	AMB α VII	—
Ambrosia trifida (giant ragweed)	*AMB* T V (Ra6)	4.4

Raji cell assay

An *in vitro* assay for immune complexes in serum. The technique employs Raji cells, a lymphoblastoid B lymphocyte tumor cell line that expresses receptors for complement receptor 1, complement receptor 2, FCγ, and C1q receptors. The cell line does not express surface immunoglobulins.

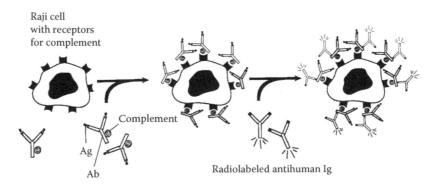

Raji cell assay.

After combination of Raji cells with a serum sample, the immune complex is bound and quantified using radiolabeled F(ab')$_2$ fragments of antibodies against IgG.

Raji cell assay for CIC

One of the least analytically sensitive and least diagnostically specific assays for circulating immune complexes (CICs). Positive results may signify the presence of lymphocyte antibodies, particularly in systemic lupus erythematosus (SLE). Patients with systemic necrotizing vasculitis may appear positive in Raji assays for CICs. This assay has also been used to monitor sarcoidosis patients.

Ramon, Gaston (1886–1963)

French immunologist who perfected the flocculation assay for diphtheria toxin.

Ramon test (historical)

A rough method for assaying the activity of a preparation of diphtheria (or tetanus) toxin. Varying quantities of antitoxin are combined with a constant quantity of toxin *in vitro*. The tubes are placed in a 44 to 46°C water bath and observed often. The test is read by noting the tube in which flocculation occurs first. This is the point of equivalence where antitoxin has neutralized the homologous toxin. This assay is based on the antigenicity of the toxin with which the antitoxin combines, in contrast to toxicity. Thus, it measures combining power and provides an indirect idea of toxicity only insofar as toxicity and antigenicity are positively correlated. Because they are not always closely correlated, this method is less reliable than the *in vivo* technique of Ehrlich that measures the actual toxic effect of the toxin and the ability of the antitoxin to combat it. The Ramon test measures toxin in L$_f$ (flocculating) units. An L$_f$ unit is defined as the amount of toxin that flocculates most rapidly with one unit of antitoxin. The L$_f$ value, in contrast to other L values described, must be calculated. To determine the L$_f$ value for a toxin, the following formula is used.

$$L_f/\text{mL toxin} = ([\text{antitoxin units/mL}] \times [\text{mL antitoxin}]) \div (\text{mL of toxin})$$

Thus, the L$_f$ content of a toxin may be determined if the following values are known: (1) antitoxin units per milliliter of antitoxin, (2) milliliter of antitoxin required for most rapid flocculation with toxin, and (3) milliliter of toxin employed. Although the Ramon flocculation test was classically used to determine the L$_f$ value of toxin, it may be carried out in reverse to assay the antitoxin units in each milliliter of antitoxin not previously standardized. The same formula is applicable:

$$L_f/\text{mL toxin} = ([\text{antitoxin units/mL}] \times [\text{mL antitoxin}]) \div (\text{mL toxin})$$

$$\text{Antitoxin units/mL} = ([L_f/\text{mL toxin}] \times [\text{mL toxin}]) \div (\text{mL antitoxin})$$

Varying quantities of toxin of known L$_f$ value are combined with a constant amount of antiserum. The tube in which flocculation first occurs is the point of equivalence; therefore, the amount of toxin in a milliliter is substituted into the formula together with the known values that include the L$_f$ per milliliter of toxin and the number of milliliters of antitoxin held constant. By simple arithmetic, the antitoxin units per milliliter may then be calculated. In this quantitative precipitin test, antibody dilutions are varied and antigen dilutions remain the same. The first tube where precipitation occurs is considered the end point.

RANA (rheumatoid arthritis-associated nuclear antigen)

An antigen of Epstein–Barr virus (EBV)-immortalized lymphoid cell lines that reacts with sera from patients with rheumatoid arthritis.

RANA (rheumatoid arthritis-associated nuclear antigen) autoantibodies

Patients with rheumatoid arthritis (RA) develop antibodies to Epstein–Barr virus (EBV)-related antigens that include viral capsid antigen, early antigen, EBV nuclear antigen, and rheumatoid arthritis nuclear antigen. RANA antibodies are present in approximately 60% of RA patients, as revealed by incomplete Freund's adjuvant (IFA) or enzyme immunoassay (EIA) techniques using synthetic peptide P62, which is the equivalent of the principal epitope of RANA. The clinical significance of RANA antibodies remains to be determined.

random breeding

The mating of members of a population at random. The genetic diversity arising from random breeding depends on the size of the population. If it is large, genetic diversity will be maintained. If it is small, genetic uniformity will result in spite of random breeding.

RANTES

An 8-kDA protein comprised of 68-amino acid residues. It belongs to the platelet factor-4 (PF-4) superfamily of chemoattractant proteins. RANTES chemoattracts blood monocytes and CD4$^+$/CD45RO$^+$ T cells *in vitro* and is useful in research on inflammation. A chemokine of the β (CC) family, RANTES was first identified by molecular cloning as a transcript expressed in T cells but not B cells. It is the only β chemokine in platelets and demonstrates powerful chemotactic and activating properties for basophils, eosinophils, and natural killer (NK) cells. It has a human immunodeficiency virus (HIV)-suppressive effect and acts synergistically with macrophage inflammatory peptide 1α (MIP-1α) and MIP-1β in the suppression of HIV. Tissue sources include T lymphocytes, monocytes, epithelial cells, mesangial cells, platelets, and eosinophils, among other cell types. Monocytes, T lymphocytes, basophils, eosinophils, natural killer (NK) cells, dendritic cells, and mast cells are targets.

Structure of rapamycin.

rapamycin

Refer to sirolimus. To achieve clinical immunosuppression, rapamycin is effective at one eighth the concentration required for FK506 and at 1% of levels required for cyclosporine.

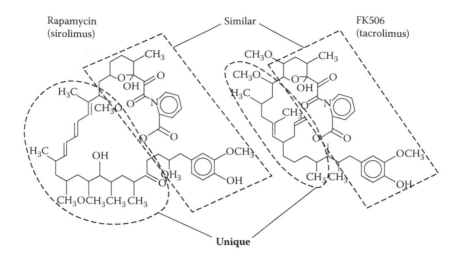

Rapamycin.

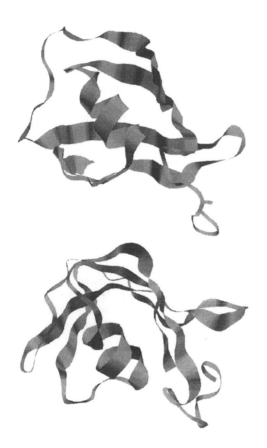

Ras/MAPK signaling pathway

A signal-mediating pathway within cells linked to Ras, a membrane-associated signal transducer that activates ERK1 (extracellular signal regulating kinase 1), a MAPK enzyme. ERK1 activates a constituent of the c-fos AP1 transcription factor. Signaling by Ras/MAPK occurs downstream of TCR engagement.

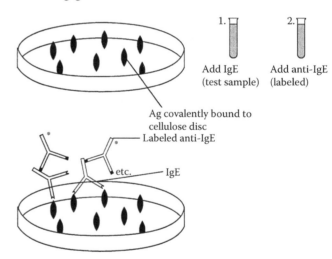

Radioallergosorbent test (RAST).

Rapamycin.

Ras

One of a group of 21-kDA guanine nucleotide-binding proteins with intrinsic GTPase activity that participates in numerous signal transduction pathways in a variety of cells. *Ras* gene mutations may be associated with tumor transformation. Ras is attracted to plasma membranes by tyrosine-phosphorylated adapter proteins during T lymphocyte activation when guanosine diphosphate (GDP)–guanosine triphosphate (GTP) exchange factors are activated. GTP-Ras then activates the mitogen-activated protein (MAP) kinase cascade that results in *fos* gene expression and assembly of AP-1 transcription factor. Refer to small G proteins.

RAST (radioallergosorbent test)

A technique to detect specific IgE antibodies in serum. This solid phase method involves binding of the allergen–antigen complex to an insoluble support such as dextran particles or Sepharose®. The serum is then passed over the allergen support complex that permits specific IgE antibodies in the serum to bind with the allergen. After washing to remove nonreactive protein, radiolabeled anti-human IgE antibody is then placed in contact with the insoluble support, where it reacts with the bound IgE antibody. Both the allergen and anti-IgE antibody must be present in excess for the test to be accurate. The amount of radioactivity on the beads is proportional to the quantity of serum antibody that is allergen-specific.

Raynaud's phenomenon

Episodes of vasospasm in the fingers when the hands are exposed to cold temperatures. The ischemia of the fingers is characterized by severe pallor and often accompanied by pain and paresthesias. It is brought on by cold, emotional stress, or anatomic abnormality. When the condition is idiopathic or primary, it is called Raynaud's disease. Raynaud's phenomenon is seen in several connective tissue diseases including systemic lupus erythematosus and systemic sclerosis. Subjects with cryoglobulinemia may also manifest the phenomenon.

RB200

Refer to lissamine rhodamine.

RCA

Regulator of complement activation.

RCA (regulator of complement activation) locus

A locus on the long arm of chromosome 1 with a 750-kb DNA segment containing genes that encode complement receptor 1, complement receptor 2, C4-binding protein, and decay-accelerating factor. These substances regulate the activation of complement through combination with C4b, C3b, or C3dg. A separate chromosome 1 gene, not in the RCA locus, encodes factor H.

reactation

The resumption of replication of an infectious agent following reactivation of a latent infection that leads to a productive infection that results in disease symptoms.

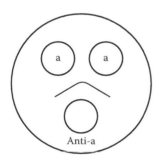

Reaction of identity.

reaction of identity

Double immunodiffusion in two dimensions in gel can reveal that two antigen solutions are identical. If two antigens are deposited into separate but adjacent wells and permitted to diffuse toward a specific antibody diffusing from a third well that forms a triangle with the other two, a continuous arc of precipitation is formed. This reveals the identity of the two antigens.

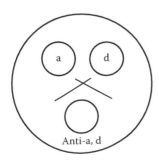

Reaction of nonidentity.

reaction of nonidentity

Double immunodiffusion in two dimensions in gel can reveal that two antigen solutions are nonidentical. If both antigen solutions are deposited into separate but adjacent wells and permitted to diffuse toward a combination of antibodies specific for each antigen diffusing from a third well that forms a triangle with the other two, the lines of precipitation form independently of one another and intersect, resembling crossed swords. This reaction reveals a lack of identity (no epitopes shared) between the antigens detectable by these antibodies.

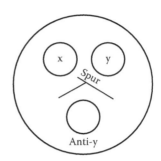

Reaction of partial identity.

reaction of partial identity

Double immunodiffusion in two dimensions in gel can reveal that two antigen solutions share epitopes but are not identical. If each antigen is deposited into separate but adjacent wells and permitted to diffuse toward specific antibodies diffusing from a third well that forms a triangle with the other two, a continuous arc of precipitation manifesting a spur is formed. This demonstrates that the two antigens share some epitopes (shown by the continuous arc) but not others (demonstrated by the spur).

reactive arthritis

Arthritis in the knees, feet, and sacroiliac region attributable to autoimmunity that occurs 1 to 4 weeks following an acute bacterial infection.

reactive lysis

Dissolution of red blood cells not sensitized with antibody. Initiated by C5b and C6 complexes in the presence of C7, C8, and C9. The activation of complement leads to lysis as a "bystander" phenomenon.

reactive nitrogen intermediates

Very cytotoxic antimicrobial substances produced when oxygen and nitrogen combine within phagocytes such as neutrophils and macrophages.

reactive oxygen intermediates (ROIs)

Free radicals derived from nitrogen, including nitric oxide, that destroy microorganisms within phagosomes. Highly reactive compounds that include superoxide anion (O_2), singlet oxygen, hydroxyl radicals (OH), and hydrogen peroxide (H_2O_2) produced in cells and tissues. Phagocytes use ROIs to form oxyhalides that injure ingested microorganisms. Release from cells may induce inflammatory responses leading to tissue injury. Also known as reactive oxygen species (ROS).

reactive oxygen species (ROS)

Oxygen-derived radicals generated in the mitochondria as oxygen is reduced along the electron transport chain. These can be produced by phagocytic cells to kill pathogens, but are also involved in signaling in other cell types. Examples of ROS are nitric oxide (NO); hydroxyl radicals (OH-); and peroxides (H_2O_2). Damage from these toxic species is prevented by antioxidants (ascorbic acid, vitamin E, uric acid, glutathione) and cellular enzymes (superoxide dismutase, catalase, glutathione peroxidase). During oxidative stress, these protective mechanisms are overwhelmed, leading to membrane damage, protein modifications, and apoptosis.

reagin (historical)

(1) Obsolete term for a complement-fixing IgM antibody reacting in the Wassermann test for syphilis. (2) An earlier name for immunoglobulin E (IgE), the anaphylactic antibody in humans that fixes to Fcε receptors on tissue mast cells, leading to the release of histamine and vasoactive amines following interaction with a specific antigen (allergen).

reaginic antibodies

Refer to reagin.

reassortant vaccine

An immunizing preparation prepared by combining antigens from several viruses or from several strains of the same virus.

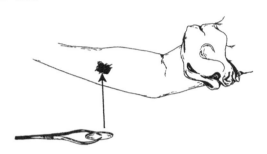

Rebuck skin window.

Rebuck skin window

A clinical method for assessing chemotaxis *in vivo* by making a superficial abrasion of the skin and covering it with a glass slide. The slide is removed several hours later, air dried, and stained for leukocyte content.

receptor

A molecular configuration on a cell surface or macromolecule that combines with molecules that are complementary to it. Examples include enzyme–substrate reactions, T cell receptors, and membrane-bound immunoglobulin receptors of B cells. A receptor is usually a transmembrane molecule that binds to a ligand on a cell surface, leading to biochemical changes within the cell.

receptor-associated tyrosine kinases

Molecules of the Src family with which lymphocyte antigen receptors associate. They bind to the tails of receptors through their SH2 domains.

receptor blockade

The rendering of a B cell anergic as a consequence of interaction of its receptors with large quantities of antigen without cross linking. This diminishes tyrosine kinase activation associated with receptors, which inhibits signaling.

receptor editing

A mechanism whereby rearranged genes in B lineage cells may undergo secondary rearrangement, forming different antigenic specificities. The process involves recombination-activating gene (RAG) reactivation, additional light chain V–J recombinations, and new immunoglobulin (Ig) light-chain synthesis, permitting cells to express a different immunoglobulin receptor that does not react with self. A B cell whose receptors react with self antigen during

development in the bone marrow is provided a narrow window of opportunity to rearrange its light chain gene to prevent apoptosis through alteration of its specificity for antigen as the new light chain replaces the self-reactive one.

receptor-mediated endocytosis

Internalization into endosomes of cell surface receptor-bound molecules, such as B cell receptors, to which antigens are bound and internalized. The interaction of a soluble macromolecule to its corresponding cell surface receptor leads to internalization through clathrin polymerization. When a clathrin-coated pit is invaginated, the receptor and bound macromolecule are enclosed in a clathrin-coated vesicle subjected to the endocytic processing pathway.

recessive lethal gene

A hereditary unit required for humans and other animals to reach adulthood. Death *in utero* or soon after birth results when both copies are defective.

recirculating pool

The continuous recirculation of T and B lymphocytes between the blood and lymph compartments.

recirculation of lymphocytes

The continuous transport of lymphocytes from the blood to secondary lymphoid tissues to lymph and back into the blood. Traffic to the spleen represents an exception, as lymphocytes only enter and exit the spleen via the blood.

recognition phase

The first event in an adaptive immune response when antigen-specific lymphocytes bind to antigens. This phase often occurs in secondary lymphoid tissues such as lymph nodes or spleen where antigens and naïve lymphocytes are present.

recognition unit

Clq facilitates recognition unit binding to cell surface antigen–antibody complexes. To launch the classical complement cascade, Clq must link to two immunoglobulin G (IgG) antibodies through their Fc regions. By contrast, one pentameric IgM molecule attached to a cell surface may interact with Clq to initiate the classical pathway. Binding of Clq activates Clr to become activated Clr*. This, in turn, activates Cls.

recombinant DNA

The physical union of two or more strands of available DNA to form another DNA strand. The term describes the exchange of DNA during meiosis, mitosis, or gene conversion. It may also refer to DNA strands produced *in vitro*.

recombinant DNA technology

The technique of isolating genes from one organism and purifying and reproducing them in another, often accomplished through ligation of genomic or cDNA into a plasmid or viral vector where DNA replication takes place.

recombinant inbred strains

Inbred strains of F_2 generation mice developed by crossing two inbred strains to yield F_1 and then F_2 generations. Progeny of the F_2 generation are inbred until they become homozygous at most loci. The progeny approach complete genetic identity and homozygosity. Recombination occurs during meiosis and consists of crossing over and recombination of parts of two chromosomes. Recombinant inbred strains help to establish genetic linkages. These genetically uniform and homozygous mice offer a means to study the consequences of reassorting various parental genes such as heavy chain genes.

recombinant vaccine

An immunogen preparation for prophylactic immunization composed of products of recombinant DNA methodology prepared by synthesizing proteins employing cloned complementary DNA.

recombinant vector vaccine

An immunizing preparation in which a vector containing the DNA that encodes the vaccine antigen enters host cells and facilitates vaccine antigen translation directly inside them.

recombination-activating genes 1 and 2 (RAG-1 and RAG-2)

Genes that activate immunoglobulin (Ig) gene recombination. Pre-B cells and immature T cells contain them. These genes encode RAG-1 and RAG-2 proteins required for rearrangements of both Ig and T cell receptor (TCR) genes. In the absence of these genes, no Ig or TCR proteins are produced, which blocks production of mature T and B cells.

recombination recognition sequences

DNA sequences situated adjacent to the V, D, and J segments in antigen–receptor loci that are recognized by the RAG-1/RAG-2 component of V(D)J recombinase. The recognition sequences are composed of a highly conserved seven-nucleotide heptamer situated adjacent to the V, D, or J coding sequence followed by a nonconserved 12- or 23-nucleotide spacer and a highly conserved non-nucleotide segment called a nonamer.

recombination signal sequences (RSSs)

Abbreviated stretches of DNA that flank the gene segments that are rearranged to generate a V region exon. They consist of a conserved heptamer and nonamer separated by 12 or 23 base pairs. Gene segments are joined only if one is flanked by an RSS containing a 12-base pair spacer and the other is flanked by an RSS containing a 23-base pair spacer. This is referred to as the 12/23 rule of gene segment joining. Somatic recombination occurs at these sites.

recombinatorial germline theory

Hypothesis proposed by Dreyer and Bennett postulating that variable region and constant region immunoglobulin genes were separated and rejoined in DNA levels. This concept was an important step toward understanding the generation of diversity in the production of antibody molecules, a puzzle finally solved by Tonegawa.

recurring chromosomal translocation

Fusion of part of one chromosome onto part of another. Most frequently associated with hematopoietic malignancies and neoplasms of the same cell type.

red cell-linked antigen antiglobulin test

A passive hemagglutination test in which the red cells serve only as carriers for antigen coated on their surfaces. The test can identify agglutinating or nonagglutinating (incomplete) antibodies by the aggregation or clumping of antigen-bearing red cells. To perform the assay, the test serum is incubated with red cells treated with antigen. The cells are then washed and antibody against human globulin is added.

red marrow

Refer to bone marrow.

red pulp

Areas of the spleen composed of the cords of Billroth and sinusoids. Vascular sinusoids with interspersed large numbers of macrophages, erythrocytes, dendritic cells, a few lymphocytes, and plasma cells comprise red pulp. Macrophages in the red pulp ingest microorganisms, foreign particles, and injured red blood cells.

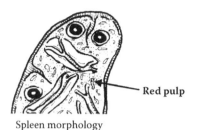

Spleen morphology

Red pulp.

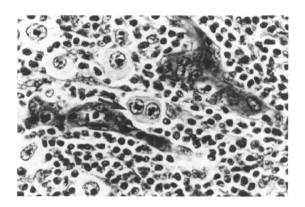

Reed–Sternberg cell.

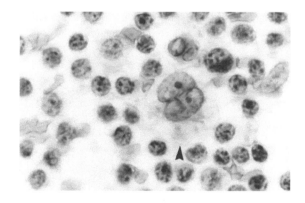

Touch preparation (Reed–Sternberg cell).

Reed–Sternberg cells

Binucleated giant cells that contain prominent nucleoli, classically associated with Hodgkin disease. They constitute a very small percentage of tumor cells in Hodgkin lymphoma. These large CD30+ B lineage cells have a distinctive appearance and manifest variable somatic hypermutation in their immunoglobulin genes.

refractory cancer

A tumor that is not responsive to conventional chemotherapy or radiation treatment.

R

regional enteritis

Inflammatory bowel disease characterized by chronic segmental lymphocytic and granulomatous inflammation of the gastrointestinal tract.

regulator of complement activation (RCA) cluster

A gene cluster on a 950-kb DNA segment of the long arm of chromosome 1 that encodes the CR1, CR2, C4bp, and DAF homologous proteins.

regulators of complement activation (RCAs)

A group of structurally homologous soluble and membrane proteins that interact with C4 and C3 and inhibit activation of complement. They include C4bP, decay-accelerating factor (DAF), membrane cofactor protein (MCP), factors H and I, CR1 gel caps, CR2 gel caps, vitronectin, clusterin, MIRL, and HRF. They are comprised of 60 to 70 amino acid consensus repeat sequences. Also termed complement control proteins (CCPs).

regulatory CD4$^+$ T cells

CD4$^+$ T cells that are antigen-specific and act as T regulatory cells by suppressing immune responses.

regulatory peptides (plants)

Generated as a component of local acquired resistance in plants. They include the ethylene (ET) and jasmonate (JA) plant hormones that mimic inflammatory mediators in mammals, as well as salicylic acid.

regulatory T cells

T lymphocytes that inhibit other immune system cell responses. CD4$^+$ subsets, including T$_{reg}$, Tr1 and Th3 cells, and the CD8$^+$ subset. Ts cells comprise this category. Inhibitory effects demonstrable *in vitro* are attributable to intercellular contacts and secretion of immunosuppressive cytokines. Suppressor T cells are examples of regulatory T cells.

Reiter complement fixation test (historical)

A diagnostic test for syphilis that used an antigen derived from a protein extract of *Treponema pallidum* (Reiter strain) to identify antibodies formed against *Treponema* group antigens.

rejection

An immune response to an organ allograft such as a kidney transplant. *Hyperacute rejection* is due to preformed antibodies and is apparent within minutes following transplantation. Antibodies reacting with endothelial cells cause complement to be fixed, which attracts polymorphonuclear neutrophils and results in denuding of the endothelial linings of vascular walls. This causes platelets and fibrin plugs to block blood flow to the transplanted organ, which becomes cyanotic and must be removed. Only a few drops of bloody urine are usually produced. Segmental thrombosis, necrosis, and fibrin thrombi form in the glomerular tufts, accompanied by hemorrhage in the interstitium and mesangial cell swelling; IgG, IgM, and C3 may be deposited in arteriole walls. *Acute rejection* occurs within days to weeks following transplantation and is characterized by extensive cellular infiltration of the interstitium. These cells are largely mononuclear and include plasma cells, lymphocytes, immunoblasts, macrophages, and neutrophils. Tubules become separated, and the tubular epithelium undergoes necrosis. Endothelial cells are swollen and vacuolated. Vascular edema, bleeding with inflammation, renal tubular necrosis, and sclerosed glomeruli occur. *Chronic rejection* occurs more than 60 days following transplantation and may be characterized by structural changes such as interstitial fibrosis, sclerosed glomeruli, mesangial proliferative glomerulonephritis, crescent formation, and other changes.

relapse

The reoccurrence of clinical manifestations of disease in an individual who was formerly in remission.

relapsing polychondritis

Inflammation of the cartilage, especially that of the external pinnae of the ears, causing them to lose their structural integrity. It appears to have an immunological

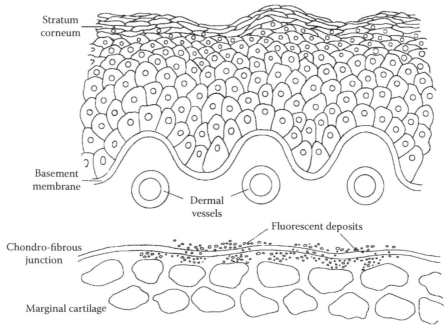

Relapsing polychondritis.

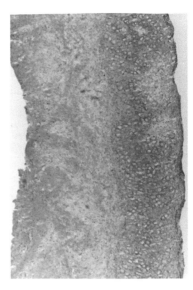

Relapsing polychondritis.

etiology. Anticollagen antibodies may be demonstrated in the sera.

relative risk (RR)

Association of a particular disease with a certain HLA antigen. This represents the chance a person with the disease-associated HLA antigen has of developing the disease compared with that of a person who does not possess the antigen. Relative risk is calculated as follows:

$$RR = \frac{p^+ \times c^-}{p^- \times c^+}$$

where

p^+ = number of patients possessing a particular HLA antigen
c^- = number of controls not possessing the particular HLA antigen
p^- = number of patients not possessing the particular HLA antigen
c^+ = number of controls possessing the particular HLA antigen

The higher the relative risk (above 1), the greater the frequency of the antigen in the patient population.

relative sibling risk

A comparison of the occurrence of a disease among siblings with its occurrence in the general population.

released antigen

Antigen derived from trypanosomes during an infection that may appear in serum. It corresponds to the antigenic type of the trypanosome infecting the individual.

Remicade® (infliximab)

A chimeric IgG$_{1k}$ monoclonal antibody with an approximate molecular weight of 149,100 Da. It is composed of human constant and murine variable regions. Infliximab binds specifically to human tumor necrosis factor α (TNF-α) with an association constant of 10^{10} M^{-1}. Infliximab is produced by a recombinant cell line cultured by continuous perfusion and is purified by a series of steps that includes measures to inactivate and remove viruses.

remission

Clinically undetectable disease following treatment. Remission of a hematopoietic neoplasm is defined as a complete clinical response at least 4 weeks following therapy.

ReoPro® (abciximab)

The Fab fragment of the chimeric human murine monoclonal antibody 7E3. Abciximab binds to the glycoprotein (GP) IIb/IIIa ($\alpha_{IIb\beta3}$) receptors of human platelets and inhibits platelet aggregation. It also binds to the vitronectin ($\alpha_{v\beta3}$) receptors found on platelets and vessel wall endothelial and smooth muscle cells. The chimeric 7E3 antibody is produced by continuous perfusion in mammalian cell culture. The 47,615-Da Fab fragment is purified from cell culture supernatant by a series of steps involving specific viral inactivation and removal procedures, digestion with papain, and column chromatography.

reovirus immunity

Most humans acquire a reovirus-specific antibody response in infancy or early childhood. Reovirus induces strong humoral and cell-mediated immune responses. Reovirus-specific antibodies are directed mainly against the outer capsid protein σ1, yet serum antibodies to other viral proteins are also induced. Reovirus-specific antibodies to the σ1 hemagglutinin protein are mainly serotype-specific. By contrast, reovirus-specific monoclonal antibodies reactive against other external capsid proteins reveal serotype-non-specific neutralizing or hemagglutinin-inhibiting properties. Reovirus-specific monoclonal antibodies can block attachment of the virus to host cells and inhibit internalization and intracellular proteolytic uncoating. Virus-specific cytotoxic T lymphocytes are also elicited in addition to T cell-mediated delayed-type hypersensitivity (DTH) reactions. The DTH response is serotype-specific, whereas CDLs are mainly serotype-nonspecific. These viruses may induce antigen-specific and -nonspecific immunosuppression. Reoviruses can induce specific T cell responses in systemic tissues. A virus-specific B cell response occurs in Peyer's patches, and a cytotoxic T lymphocyte response occurs in Peyer's patches. The ability of reovirus to enter Peyer's patches via M cells indicates that these viruses might be used in a mucosal vaccine.

repeating units

Antigens in which macromolecular configurations are repeated, such as the repeating units of β-1,4-glucose-β-1,3-glucuronic acid in type III pneumococcus polysaccharide. Polysaccharide antigens in the cell walls of Gram-negative bacteria also contain repeating structures. Antigens with such configurations are often thymus-independent.

repertoire

The total antigenic specificity library generated by B or T cells in response to a foreign antigen.

replicative senescence

Cell death at the conclusion of its predestined number of divisions.

reptile immunity

Environmental conditions affect the structures and functional activities of reptile organs including those of the immune system. The reptilian thymus is the first lymphoid organ to develop. It is a bilateral organ lying on both sides of the neck in lizards and anterior to the heart in snakes. It is frequently multilobed in turtles. The thymus is well developed in reptiles collected in nature under the correct

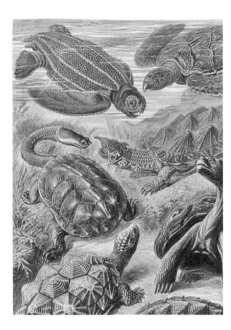

Reptile immunity.

seasonal temperature and other environmental conditions; otherwise, it may reveal degrees of degeneration. The spleen is the most significant peripheral lymphoid organ in reptiles. It becomes lymphopoietic much later than the thymus in lizards, snakes, and tortoises; 50 to 70% of reptile splenic lymphocytes are thymus-derived and located in thymus-dependent areas. Reptiles do not develop germinal centers and nodules found in mammalian secondary lymphoid organs. T and B cell-like cells differ in their sensitivity to environmental conditions. Gut-associated lymphoid tissue (GALT) develops in lizards, snakes, and chelonians. Reptiles do not have tonsils, Peyer's patches, or appendices; they have numerous lymphoid aggregates in the mucosa and submucosa along the gut. In lizards, the esophageal lymphoid aggregates containing T cell-like lymphocytes are greatly affected by seasonal and environmental conditions, whereas the B cell-like cells and GALT in reptiles are resistant to changes in season. The spleen and GALT carry out humoral immune mechanisms. Although reptiles do not have true lymph nodes, their lymphoid systems are homologous to those of mammals except for high sensitivity to ambient conditions. Reptile lymphocytes are strongly responsive to plant mitogens. Lizards and snakes reject skin grafts in a manner similar to mammals. Reptiles also manifest major functional markers of the major histocompatibility complex (MHC). They produce at least two classes of immunoglobulin (Ig) that resemble IgM and a second immunoglobulin of lower molecular weight that is antigenically related to the 7S Ig of birds and amphibians. All reptiles can mount powerful immune responses to various antigens that include bacteria, protozoa, erythrocytes, and proteins. Body temperature is a critical regulator of immune function. Reptiles, in contrast to fish and amphibians, are restricted in the temperature range over which immune responses can occur.

rescue graft

A replacement graft for an original graft that failed.

reservoir

A host or carrier that harbors pathogenic microorganisms without being injured itself; it serves as a source of infection for others. Also termed reservoir host or reservoir of infection.

resident macrophage

A macrophage normally present at a tissue location without being induced to migrate there.

respiratory burst

A process used by neutrophils and monocytes to kill certain pathogenic microorganisms. It involves increased oxygen consumption with the generation of hydrogen peroxide and superoxide anions. This occurs also in macrophages that kill tumor cells. Respiratory burst is characterized by an abrupt elevation in oxygen consumption, followed by metabolic events in neutrophils and mononuclear cells preceding bacteriolysis. Partial reduction of oxygen by this process provides microbicidal oxidants. The initial event is a one-electron reduction of oxygen by membrane-bound oxidase to form a superoxide. The hexose monophosphate shunt reaction that accompanies this reduction liberates an H^+ that unites with the oxygen to produce H_2O_2. Following neutrophil degranulation, NADPH-dependent oxidases fixed to granule membranes activate the formation of inorganic radicals and myeloperoxidase action, leading to the generation of hypochlorous acid, causing the oxidation of nucleic acids, amino acids, and thiols of the microbe. The respiratory burst is reflected in the increased use of oxygen by NADPH oxidases to maintain this antimicrobial activity.

respiratory disease viruses

Influenza, paramyxoviruses, rhinoviruses, pneumoviruses, enteroviruses, coronaviruses, and mastadenoviruses that induce infections of the respiratory tract in humans.

respiratory syncytial virus (RSV)

A frequent cause of severe chest infections in young children who develop wheezing; a paramyxovirus.

respiratory syncytial virus (RSV) immunity

RSV is responsible for 70% of bronchiolitis cases, a common cause of infant hospitalization. Immunoglobulin G (IgG), IgM, and IgA antibodies are formed and can be detected by enzyme immunoassay (EIA). Some heterologous antibody responses occur in primary and recurrent infections with groups A and B RSV. Diagnosis of acute RSV infection is made by antigen detection in nasopharyngeal secretions by fluorescent antibody or EIA methods.

responder animals

Guinea pigs immunized by DNP–PLL or DNP–GL produce significant amounts of anti-DNP antibodies and develop delayed-type hypersensitivity reactions to the conjugate. Conversely, nonresponder animals produce few or no anti-DNP antibodies and do not develop delayed-type hypersensitivity. The capacity to respond to DNP–PLL antigen is a function of a dominant autosomal gene. All guinea pigs of strain 13 are nonresponders, whereas strain 2 guinea pigs and (2×13) F_1 hybrids are responders. The immune response gene present in strain 2 but absent in strain 13 is called the PLL gene.

resting lymphocytes

Under light microscopy, resting lymphocytes appear as a distinct and homogeneous population of round cells, each with a large spherical or slightly kidney-shaped nucleus that occupies most of the cell and is surrounded by a narrow rim of basophilic cytoplasm with occasional vacuoles. The

Resting lymphocyte

Activated lymphocyte

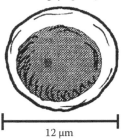
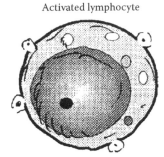

12 μm

Resting lymphocyte.

nucleus usually has a poorly visible single indentation and contains densely packed chromatin. Occasionally, nucleoli can be distinguished. The small lymphocyte variant—the predominant morphologic form—is slightly larger than an erythrocyte. Larger lymphocytes ranging from 10 to 20 μm in diameter are difficult to differentiate from monocytes. They have more cytoplasm and may show azurophilic granules. Intermediate-size forms are also described. Under phase contrast microscopy, living lymphocytes show feeble motility with amoeboid movements that give the cells hand-mirror shapes. The mirror handle is called a uropod. In large lymphocytes, mitochondria and lysosomes are better visualized, and some cells show spherical, birefringent, 0.5-μm diameter inclusions called Gall bodies. Lymphocytes do not spread on surfaces. The different classes of lymphocytes cannot be distinguished by light microscopy. B lymphocytes sometimes show hairy (rough) surfaces under scanning electron microscopy (SEM), but thes are apparently artifacts. Electron microscopy does not provide additional information except for visualization of cellular organelles that are not abundant. This suggests that the small resting lymphocytes are end-stage cells; however, under appropriate stimulation, they are capable of considerable morphologic changes.

restitope

That segment of a T cell receptor that makes contact and interacts with a class II histocompatibility antigen molecule during antigen presentation.

restriction endonucleases

Bacterial products that identify and combine with a short sequence of DNA. The enzyme acts as molecular scissors by cleaving the DNA at the recognition site or at another location. Restriction endonucleases catalyze degradation of foreign DNA. They recognize precise base sequences of DNA and cut it into relatively few fragments, termed restriction fragments. The three major types of restriction endonucleases are (1) type I enzymes that identify specific base sequences but cut the DNA elsewhere (approximately 1000 bp from the recognition site); (2) type II enzymes that identify specific base sequences and cut the DNA within or adjacent to these sequences; and (3) type III endonucleases that identify specific base sequences and cut the DNA approximately 25 bp from the recognition site.

restriction fragment-length polymorphism (RFLP)

Genome diversity in DNA from different subjects revealed by restriction map comparisons. This diversity is based on differences in restriction fragment lengths determined by sites of restriction endonuclease cleavage of the DNA

molecules and revealed by preparing southern blots using appropriate molecular hybridization probes. Polymorphisms may be demonstrated in exons, introns, flanking sequences, or any DNA sequence. Variations in DNA sequence show Mendelian inheritance. Results are useful in linkage studies and can help to identify defective genes associated with inherited disease.

restriction map

A diagram of a linear or circular molecule of DNA that indicates the points where one or more restriction enzymes cleave the DNA. DNA is first digested with restriction endonucleases that split the DNA into fragments that can be separated by gel electrophoresis. Size determination is accomplished by comparison with fragments of known size.

reticular cell

Stroma or framework cells that, with reticular fibers, constitute the lymphoid tissue framework of lymph nodes, spleen, and bone marrow.

reticular dysgenesis

The most severe form of all combined immunodeficiency disorders. Leads to a failure in the development of B cells, T cells, NK cells, and granulocytes. This condition is incompatible with life and leads to early death of affected infants. The only possibility for treatment is hematopoietic stem cell transplantation or bone marrow transplantation. This condition has an autosomal-recessive mode of inheritance.

reticulin antibodies

Antibodies of five separate types of which the R_1 RA is of greatest interest. Immunoglobulin A (IgA) R_1 ARAs show more than 98% specificity for untreated celiac disease; however, sensitivity is only 20 to 25%.

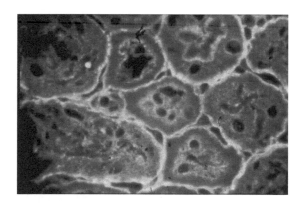

Reticulin autoantibodies.

reticulin autoantibodies

R_1 ARA is the only one of five separate reticulin autoantibodies that has diagnostic and pathogenic significance. IgA R_1 ARAs are highly specific for untreated celiac disease (CD). Approximately 2.6% of healthy children possess reticulin autoantibodies. In IgA-deficient subjects under evaluation for CD, the detection of IgG ARA, IgG gliadin autoantibodies (AGA), and IgG endomysial autoantibodies (EmAs) may be helpful. R_1 ARAs classically disappear 3 to 12 months following the maintenance of a strict gluten-free diet in both adults and children with CD. IgA, ARA, IgA AGA, and IgA EmA may be detected in dermatitis herpetiformis (DH).

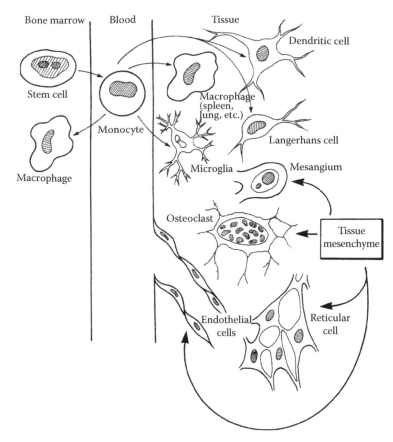

Reticuloendothelial system (RES).

reticuloendothelial blockade

The temporary paralysis of the phagocytic ability of cells of the mononuclear phagocytic system through the injection of excess amounts of inert particles such as colloidal carbon, gold, or iron. After the mononuclear phagocytes have expended their entire phagocytic capabilities by taking up these inert particles, they can no longer phagocytize administered microorganisms or other substances that would normally be phagocytized.

reticuloendothelial system (RES)

A former term for the mononuclear phagocyte system that includes Kupffer's cells lining the sinusoids of the liver and macrophages of the spleen and lymph nodes. Aschoff introduced the term to describe cells that could take up and retain vital dyes and particles injected into the body. In addition to macrophages, less active phagocytic cells such as fibroblasts and endothelial cells were included in the original definition. The principal function of the mononuclear phagocyte system is removal of unwelcome particles from the blood. RES activity may be measured by the elimination rate of radiolabeled molecules or cells such as albumin or erythrocytes coated with antibody.

reticulosis

Refer to lymphoma.

reticulum cell

Refer to reticular cell.

reticulum cell sarcoma

Obsolete term for large cell lymphoma.

retina autoantibodies

Autoantibodies found in ANA-negative patients with cancer-associated retinopathy (CAR) syndrome. These antibodies are specific for five antigens: retinal S, associated with ocular inflammation or uveitis; rhodopsin; interphotoreceptor in retinol-binding protein (IRBP); phosducin; and CAR autoantigen (recoverin), a 23-kDa protein closely associated with CAR syndrome. Retina antibodies are assayed using enzyme immunoassay (EIA), immunoblotting, and dot blotting; there is no known clinical correlation for retina autoantibodies.

Retrovir®

A synthetic nucleoside analog of thymidine in which the 3′ hydroxy group is replaced by an azido group. The FDA approved it for the treatment of human immunodeficiency virus (HIV). The mechanism of action includes the conversion of zidovudine to its active metabolite zidovudine 5′ triphosphate, which inhibits the activity of the HIV reverse transcriptase by competing for utilization with the natural substrate and by its incorporation into viral DNA. Zidovudine is the active component.

retroviral oncogene

The incorporation of a proto-oncogene copy by an integrated retrovirus into its genome may lead to conversion by adjacent regulatory sequences of the proto-oncogene into a

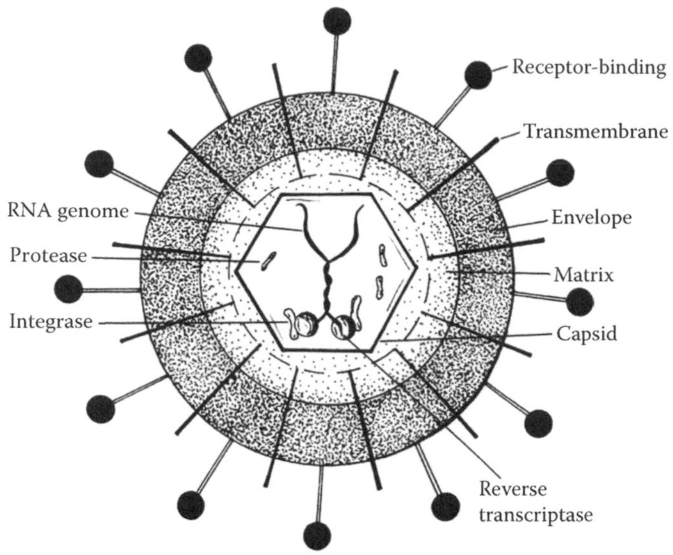

Retrovirus.

retroviral oncogene capable of transforming host cells following infection.

retrovirus

A reverse transcriptase- and integrase-containing virus that permits synthesis of a DNA copy of the viral RNA genome and its incorporation into host cell DNA. Includes human immunodeficiency virus (HIV) and human T cell leukemia virus; an RNA virus that can insert and efficiently express its own genetic information into a host cell through transcription of its RNA into DNA and subsequent integration into the genome of the host cell. Retroviruses are employed in research to deliberately insert foreign DNA into a cell; thus, they have the potential for use in gene therapy when a host cell gene is missing or defective. Retroviruses have been used to tag tumor-infiltrating lymphocytes in experimental cancer treatment.

retrovirus immunity

Refer to human immunodeficiency virus and AIDS.

rev protein

A regulatory protein of the human immunodeficiency virus (HIV) *rev* gene that facilitates passage of viral transcripts from a host cell nucleus to the cytoplasm during HIV replication.

reverse anaphylaxis

Anaphylaxis produced by the passive transfer of serum antibody from a sensitized animal to a normal untreated recipient only after the recipient was first injected with the antigen. Thus, the usual order of administration of antigen and antibody is the reverse of classic anaphylaxis.

reverse genetics approach

The determination of a gene's role in a particular disease by investigating a diseased animal's genome and identifying sustained mutations in its gene.

reverse immunology

Use of computerized algorithms to predict the likelihood of a particular mutation resulting in a strong antigen. Several mutant proteins and peptides have been used to examine the possibility of inducing tumor-specific immunity.

reverse Mancini technique

Refer to reverse radioimmunodiffusion.

reverse passive Arthus reaction

A reaction that differs from a classic Arthus reaction only in that precipitating antibody is injected into an animal intracutaneously and, after an interval of 30 minutes to 2 hours, the antigen is administered intravenously. Antigen rather than antibody diffuses from the blood into the tissues, and antibody rather than antigen diffuses into the tissue where it encounters and interacts with antigen, with the consequent typical changes in the microvasculature and tissues associated with the Arthus reaction.

reverse passive cutaneous anaphylaxis (RPCA)

A passive cutaneous anaphylaxis assay in which the order of antigen and antibody administration is reversed; the antigen is injected first, followed by the antibody. In this case, the antigen must be an immunoglobulin that can fix to tissue cells.

reverse plaque assay

A method to identify antibody-secreting cells regardless of their antibody specificity. The antibody-forming cells are suspended in agarose and incubated at 37°C in Petri plates with sheep red cells coated with protein A. Anti-Ig and complement are also present. Cells synthesizing and secreting immunoglobulin become encircled by Ig–anti-Ig complexes and then link to protein A on erythrocyte surfaces, leading to hemolytic plaques (zones of lysis). Any class of immunoglobulin can be identified by this technique through the choice of the appropriate antibody.

reverse radioimmunodiffusion

A technique to quantify antibody levels that varies from the single radial diffusion test in only one detail: samples are placed in gel containing antigen, and as diffusion takes place, the precipitation rings produced are directly proportional to the antibody concentration.

reverse transcriptase

An enzyme that is a critical component of retroviruses. It translates the RNA genome into DNA before integration

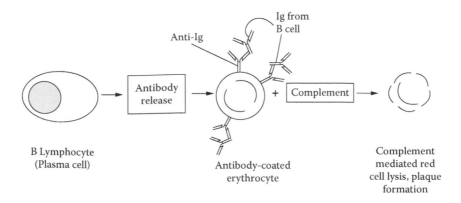

Reverse plaque method.

into host cell DNA. It also permits RNA sequences to be converted into complementary DNA (cDNA) and cloned. Problems in proofreading may lead to introduction of a considerable number of mutations into the DNA. It is encoded by human immunodeficiency virus (HIV), and the purified form is used to clone complementary DNAs encoding a gene of interest from messenger RNA. Inhibitors of the enzyme have been used as therapy for HIV-1 infection.

reverse transcriptase–polymerase chain reaction (RT-PCR)

A technique employed to amplify RNA sequences. Reverse transcriptase is used to convert an RNA sequence into a complementary DNA (cDNA) sequence that is amplified by PCR using gene-specific primers. This technique is a variation of the polymerase chain reaction employed to amplify a complementary cDNA of a gene of interest.

reverse vaccinology

Development of a vaccine antigen based on sequences in a pathogenic organism's genome or proteome that are most likely to represent epitopes that T cells recognize. Also called epitope-driven vaccine design.

RF

Abbreviation for rheumatoid factor.

RFLP (restriction fragment length polymorphism)

Local DNA sequence variations of humans or other animals that may be revealed by the use of restriction endonucleases. These enzymes cut double-stranded DNA at points where they recognize a very specific oligonucleotide sequence, resulting in DNA fragments of different lengths that are unique to each individual. The fragments of different sizes are separated by electrophoresis. The technique is useful for a variety of purposes, such as identifying genes associated with neurologic diseases (e.g., myotonic dystrophy) that are inherited as autosomal-dominant genes or in documenting chimerism. The fragments may also be used as genetic markers to help identify the inheritance patterns of particular genes.

rhabdovirus immunity

Resistance to rabies is in part genetically controlled; in mice, it is controlled by one or two genes. Resistance is a dominant trait. Susceptibility to rabies virus infection varies among species. Immunity may be specific or nonspecific. Interferon plays a critical role. Rhabdoviruses are very susceptible to interferon action. In rabies, no serological evidence of infection is found prior to onset of the disease, which is usually fatal. Vaccination studies have yielded the most data concerning specific immunity. Vaccination during the incubation period, if not repeated, can cause the "early death phenomenon." Passively transferred specific antibodies can protect against rabies. The relative significance of cell-mediated immunity as a protective mechanism remains to be demonstrated, although antibody titers and protection are closely correlated. Protective mechanisms following post-exposure treatment of humans with rabies vaccine involve T lymphocytes. Rabies virus infection progresses silently in the nervous system without inducing any detectable humoral immune response. Use of anti-rabies vaccination must distinguish between preventive vaccination and post-exposure treatment. Several vaccine injections together with specific immunoglobulin inoculation are warranted in post-exposure treatment for humans. Preventive vaccination is usually carried out in veterinary medicine. Contemporary vaccines confer partial or no protection against selected rabies-related virus infections. Only inactivated vaccines are licensed for use in humans. Those previously used that contained nervous tissue were dangerous because their myelin content could have induced hypersensitivity reactions leading to paralysis. Most current vaccines are prepared from virus grown in cell culture. While attenuated virus vaccines have been used in domestic animals in the past, newer potent inactivated vaccines have replaced them. Recombinant vaccines make use of a vaccinia recombinant virus containing the rabies virus glycoprotein gene that induces production of virus glycoprotein in infected cells to induce rabies virus-neutralizing antibodies and protect susceptible hosts. It is active by oral administration.

Rh antigens

Refer to rhesus antigen and to rhesus blood group system.

Rh disease

Refer to erythroblastosis fetalis.

Rh factor

Erythrocyte antigen that determines the Rh blood group system. Refer to rhesus antigen and rhesus blood group system.

Rhazes (Abu Bakr Muhammad ibn Zakariya, 865–932)

Persian philosopher and alchemist who described measles and smallpox as different diseases. He was also a proponent of the theory that immunity is acquired and is often cited as the premier physician of Islam.

rhesus antibody

An antibody reactive with rhesus antigen, especially RhD.

rhesus antigen

Erythrocyte antigen of humans that shares epitopes in common with rhesus monkey red blood cells. Rhesus antigens are encoded by allelic genes. D antigen has the greatest clinical significance as it may stimulate antibodies in subjects

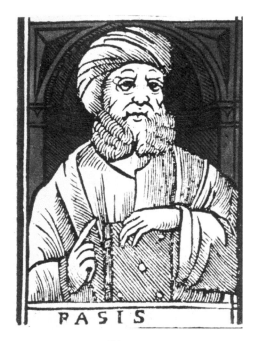

Rhazes.

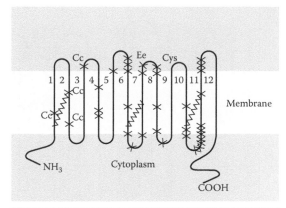

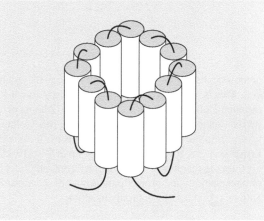

Schematic representation of Cc, Ee, and Dd polypeptide topoloty within the erythrocyte membrane. There are twelve membrane-spanning domains and cytoplasmic N- and C-termini. The linear diagram depicts probable sites of palmitoylation (Cys-Leu-Pro motifs).

not possessing the antigen and induce hemolytic disease of the newborn or cause transfusion incompatibility reactions.

rhesus blood group system

Rhesus monkey erythrocyte antigens such as the D antigen are found on the red cells of most humans who are said to be Rh⁺. This blood group system was discovered by Landsteiner et al. in the 1940s when they injected rhesus monkey erythrocytes into rabbits and guinea pigs. Subsequent studies showed the system to be very complex; the rare Rh alloantigens are still not characterized biochemically. Three closely linked pairs of alleles designated (Dd, Cc, and Ee) are postulated at the Rh locus located on chromosome 1. The Rh system has several alloantigenic determinants. Clinically, the D antigen is the one of greatest concern because RhD⁻ individuals who receive RhD⁺ erythrocytes by transfusion may develop alloantibodies that may lead to severe reactions with further transfusions of RhD⁺ blood. The D antigen also poses a problem

in RhD⁻ mothers who bear children with RhD⁺ red cells inherited from their fathers. The entrance of fetal erythrocytes into the maternal circulation at parturition or trauma during the pregnancy (such as in amniocentesis) can lead to alloimmunization against the RhD antigen that may cause

1. First pregnancy (initial sensitization)   2. Second and third pregnancy (2° and 3° sensitizations)

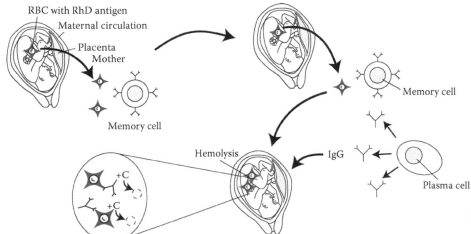

Mechanism of hemolytic disease of the newborn.

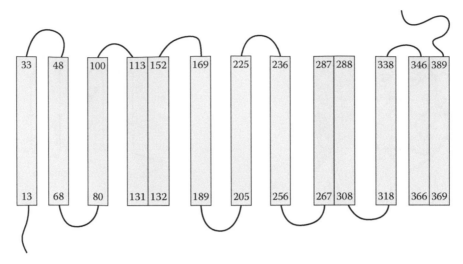

Schematic representation of the suggested molecular structure of Rh polypeptide.

hemolytic disease of the newborn in subsequent pregnancies. This is now prevented by the administration of $Rh_o(D)$ immune globulin to these women within 72 hours of parturition. Further confusion concerning this system has arisen from the use of other designations by the Wiener and Fisher systems. Rh antigens are a group of 7- to 10-kDa, erythrocyte membrane-bound antigens that are independent of phosphatides and proteolipids. Antibodies against Rh antigens do not occur naturally in serum.

Principal *Rh* Genes and Their Frequencies Among Caucasians and African Americans

			Frequency (%)	
Haplotype	Fisher-Race	Wiener	Caucasian	African American
R^1	CDe	Rh_1	42	17
R	Cde	Rh	37	26
R^2	cDE	Rh_2	14	11
R^0	cDe	Rh_o	4	44
r'	Cde	rh'	2	2
rδ	cdE	Rhδ	1	<1
R^z	CDE	Rh^z	Very rare	Very rare
R^y	CdE	rh^y	Very rare	Very rare

rhesus incompatibility
The stimulation of anti-RhD antibodies in an Rh⁻ mother when challenged by RhD⁺ red cells of her baby (especially at parturition) that may lead to hemolytic disease of the newborn. The term also refers to the transfusion of RhD⁺ blood to an Rh⁻ individual who may form antiD antibodies against the donor blood, leading to subsequent incompatibility reactions if given future RhD⁺ blood.

rheumatic
Adjective that describes an inflammatory disease of the joints, muscles, or connective tissues.

rheumatic fever (RF)
An acute, nonsuppurative, inflammatory disease that is autoimmune-mediated and occurs mainly in children a few

weeks after an infection of the pharynx with group A β hemolytic streptococci. M protein, a principal virulence factor associated with specific strains of streptococci, induces antibodies that cross react with epitopes of human cardiac muscle. These antibodies may not produce direct tissue injury, but with other immune mechanisms they evoke acute systemic disease characterized mainly by polyarthritis, skin lesions, and carditis. Although the arthritis and skin lesions resolve, the cardiac involvement may lead to permanent injury to the valves, producing fibrocalcific deformity. Foci of necrosis of collagen with fibrin deposition surrounded by lymphocytes, macrophages, and plump modified histiocytes termed Aschoff bodies are ultimately replaced years later by fibrous scars. Aschoff bodies may be found in any of the three layers of the heart. In the pericardium, they are accompanied by serofibrinous (bread-and-butter) pericarditis. In the myocardium, they are scattered in the interstitial connective tissue, often near blood vessels. Dilatation of the heart and mitral valve ring and inflammation of the endocardium, mainly affecting the left-sided valves, may occur. Small vegetations may form along the lines of closure. Other tissues may be affected, with the production of acute nonspecific arthritis affecting the larger joints. Fewer than half of the patients develop skin lesions such as subcutaneous nodules or erythema marginatum. Subcutaneous nodules that appear at pressure points overlying extensor tendons of extremities at the wrist, elbows, ankles, and knees consist of central fibrinoid necrosis enclosed by a palisade of fibroblasts and mononuclear inflammatory cells. Rheumatic arteritis has been described in coronary, renal, mesenteric, and cerebral arteries and in the aorta and pulmonary vessels. Rheumatic interstitial pneumonitis is a rare complication. Antistreptolysin O (ASO) and antistreptokinase (ASK) antibodies are found in the sera of affected individuals. Myocarditis that develops during an acute attack may induce arrhythmias such as atrial fibrillation or cardiac dilatation with potential mitral valve insufficiency. Long-term antistreptococcal therapy must be given to any patient with a history of rheumatic fever because subsequent streptococcal infections may worsen the carditis.

rheumatoid arthritis
An autoimmune inflammatory disease of the joints defined according to special criteria designated 1 through 7. Criteria 1 through 4 must be present more than 6 weeks. The revised

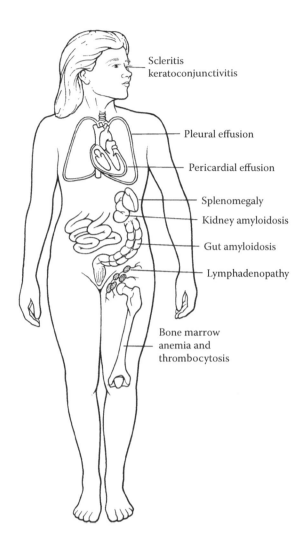

Rheumatoid arthritis.

Labels on figure:
- Scleritis keratoconjunctivitis
- Pleural effusion
- Pericardial effusion
- Splenomegaly
- Kidney amyloidosis
- Gut amyloidosis
- Lymphadenopathy
- Bone marrow anemia and thrombocytosis

criteria for rheumatoid arthritis are as follows: (1) morning stiffness in and around joints lasting at least 1 hour before maximum improvement; (2) soft tissue swelling (arthritis) of three or more joints observed by a physician; (3) swelling (arthritis) of the proximal interphalangeal, metacarpal phalangeal, or wrist joints; (4) symmetric swelling (arthritis); (5) rheumatoid nodules; (6) rheumatoid factors; and (7) roentgenographic erosions. CD4$^+$ T cells, activated B cells, and plasma cells are present in inflamed joint lining (synovium) and multiple proinflammatory cytokines such as IL1 and TNF are found in synovial joint fluid. The disease is accompanied by the production of rheumatoid factor, usually an IgM anti-IgG antibody.

rheumatoid arthritis cell (RA cell)

An irregular neutrophil that contains a variable number of black-staining cytoplasmic inclusions 0.2 to 2.0 µm in diameter. These cells contain IgM rheumatoid factor, complement, IgG, and fibrin and are found in synovial fluids of patients with RA. Although RA cells may constitute 5 to 100% of the neutrophils of RA patients, they may also be present in patients with other connective tissue diseases.

rheumatoid factors (RFs)

An autoantibody present in the sera of patients with rheumatoid arthritis and found with varying frequency in other diseases such as subacute bacterial endocarditis, tuberculosis, syphilis,

sarcoidosis, hepatic diseases, and others. It may also be found in the sera of human allograft recipients and apparently healthy persons. RFs are immunoglobulins, usually of the IgM class and to a lesser degree of the IgG or IgA classes, with reactive specificity for the Fc region of IgG. These anti-immunoglobulin antibodies that may be monoclonal or polyclonal react with the Fc region epitopes of denatured IgG, including the Gm markers. Most RFs are isotype-specific, manifesting reactivity mainly for IgG$_1$, IgG$_2$, and IgG$_4$, and are only weakly reactive with IgG$_3$. Antigenic determinants of IgG that are potentially reactive with RF include (1) subclass-specific or genetically defined determinants of native IgG (IgG$_1$, IgG$_2$, IgG$_4$, and Gm determinants); (2) determinants present on complexed IgG but absent on native IgG; and (3) determinants exposed after enzymatic cleavage of IgG. The Gm determinants are allotypic markers of the human IgG subclasses located in the IgG molecule as follows: in the C$_H$1 domain in IgG$_1$, in the C$_H$2 domain in IgG$_2$, and in C$_H$2 and C$_H$3 domains in IgG$_4$. Although rheumatoid factor titers may not be clearly correlated with disease activity, they may help perpetuate chronic inflammatory synovitis. When IgM rheumatoid factors and IgG target molecules react to form immune complexes, complement is activated, leading to inflammation and immune injury. IgG rheumatoid factors may self associate to form IgG–IgG immune complexes that help perpetuate chronic synovitis and vasculitis. IgG RFs synthesized by plasma cells in the rheumatoid synovia fix complement and perpetuate inflammation. IgG RFs have been shown in microbial infections, B lymphocyte proliferative disorders and malignancies, non-RA patients, and aging individuals. RFs may have a physiologic role in removal of immune complexes from the circulation. They were demonstrated earlier by the Rose–Waaler test and are now detected by the latex agglutination (or RA) test employing latex particles coated with IgG.

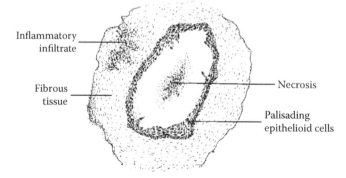

Labels on figure:
- Inflammatory infiltrate
- Fibrous tissue
- Necrosis
- Palisading epithelioid cells

Rheumatoid nodule.

rheumatoid nodule

A granulomatous lesion characterized by central necrosis encircled by a palisade of mononuclear cells and an exterior mantle of lymphocytic infiltrate. The lesions occur as subcutaneous nodules, especially at pressure points such as the elbows in individuals with rheumatoid arthritis or other rheumatoid diseases.

rheumatoid pneumonitis

Diffuse interstitial pulmonary fibrosis that causes varying degrees of pulmonary impairment in 2% of patients with rheumatoid arthritis (RA). It may result from the rare coincidental occurrence of rheumatoid arthritis and interstitial pneumonia. Gold therapy used for RA, smoking, and contact with an environmental toxin may induce interstitial pneumonia.

rhinovirus immunity

Although most rhinovirus infections resolve spontaneously, respiratory tract infections may occur in immunocompromised hosts. There are nearly 100 serotypes of rhinovirus. Studies with human rhinovirus 2 (HRV-2) reveal that HRV-2-specific immunoglobulins in sera and nasal secretions increase 1 to 2 weeks after inoculation. HRV-2 antibodies peak at 35 days after inoculation. Serum neutralizing antibodies remain elevated for many years following infection. Local specific antibodies cannot be detected after 2 years. Preinoculation IgA levels in nasal washings are diminished in those who become infected compared with those who do not. Aspirin and acetaminophen suppress serum antibody responses.

RhLA locus

The major histocompatibility locus in the rhesus monkey.

Rh$_{null}$

Human erythrocytes that fail to express Rh antigens due to the homozygous inheritance of the *Xr* gene that causes a regulator-type defect or the inheritance of an amorphic ($^{-/-}$) gene. The Rh$_{null}$ phenotype is associated with diminished erythrocyte survival.

rhodamine isothiocyanate

A reddish-orange fluorochrome used to label immunoglobulins and other proteins for immunofluorescence studies.

Rh$_o$D immune globulin

Prepared from the serum of individuals hyperimmunized against Rh$_o$D antigen. It is used to prevent the immunization of Rh$^-$ mothers by Rh$_o$D$^+$ erythrocytes of babies, especially at parturition when the babies' red cells enter the maternal circulation in significant quantities, and at other times during pregnancy, such as after a trauma that might introduce fetal blood into the maternal circulation. This prevents hemolytic disease of the newborn in subsequent pregnancies. The dose used is effective in inhibiting immune reactivity against 15 mL of packed Rh$_o$(D)$^+$ red blood cells. It should be administered within 72 hours of parturition. It may also be used following inadvertent or unavoidable transfusion of RhD$^+$ blood to RhD$^-$ recipients, especially women of childbearing age.

Rh$_o$GAM

Refer to Rh$_o$(D) immune globulin.

RIA

Radioimmunoassay.

Ribavirin.

ribavirin (1-β-5-d-ribofuranosyl-1,2,4-triazole-3 carboxamide)

A substance that interferes with mRNA capping of certain viruses, thereby restricting the synthesis of viral proteins. It is used in aerosol form to treat severe respiratory syncytial virus infection in children.

ribosomal autoantibodies

Autoantibodies against ribosomal constituents that are specific to systemic lupus erythematosus (SLE) and occur only rarely in other rheumatic diseases. P (phospho) proteins (P0, P1, and P2) are the most common antigens. These P proteins are also known as A (alanine-rich) proteins. Antibodies to P proteins that are specific for a common carboxyl terminus epitope occur in 12 to 19% of SLE patients. Other ribosomal antigens include L12 protein, L5/5s, S10, Ja, L7, and ribosomal ribonucleoprotein (rRNA). Anti-L7, anti-rRNA, anti-S10, and anti-Ja autoantibodies are more common than those against L12 and L5/5S, which are rare. Immunoblotting techniques reveal autoantibodies to ribosomal proteins in about 42% of SLE and 55% of rheumatoid arthritis (RA) sera. The clinical significance of ribosomal antibodies remains to be determined.

ribosomal P protein (RPP) autoantibodies

Autoantibodies found in 45 to 90% of patients with systemic lupus erythematosus (SLE) with severe depression or psychosis; they are also present in 7 to 20% of SLE patients who are not psychotic. A positive RPP autoantibody test is not diagnostic of lupus psychosis, as approximately 50% of patients with RPP autoantibodies do not have severe behavioral problems. These antibodies are found in Sjögren's syndrome patients with central nervous system (CNS) abnormalities. RPP autoantibodies are rare in systemic sclerosis and when present indicate an overlap with SLE. The clinical significance of these autoantibodies is doubtful. Firm data suggest that RPP autoantibodies may play a role in the pathogenesis of lupus hepatitis.

ribosome

A subcellular organelle in the cytoplasm of a cell that is a site of amino acid incorporation in the process of protein synthesis.

ribozyme

A catalytic RNA segment with the ability to break and form covalent bonds. It combines specifically with and cleaves mRNAs with a complementary sequence, thereby functioning as molecular shears. Employed in treatment to block the expression of selected proteins.

Richet, Charles Robert (1850–1935)

Parisian physician who became a professor of physiology at the University of Paris. He was interested in the physiology of toxins and, with Portier, discovered anaphylaxis, for which he was awarded the Nobel Prize in Physiology or Medicine in 1913. They discovered anaphylaxis in dogs exposed to the toxins of murine invertebrates to which they had been previously sensitized and thus demonstrated an immune-type reaction that was harmful rather than protective. Experimental anaphylaxis was later shown to be similar to certain types of hypersensitivity, lending clinical and theoretical significance to their discovery. (Refer to *L'anaphylaxie*, 1911.)

ricin

A toxic protein found in seeds of *Ricinus communis* (castor bean) plants. It is a heterodimer composed of a 30-kDa α chain that mediates cytotoxicity and a 30-kDa β chain that interacts with cell surface galactose residues that facilitate passage of molecules into cells in endocytic vesicles. Ricin inhibits protein synthesis by linkage of dissociated α chains in cytosols to ribosomes. The ricin heterodimer or its α chain conjugated to a specific antibody serves as an immunotoxin.

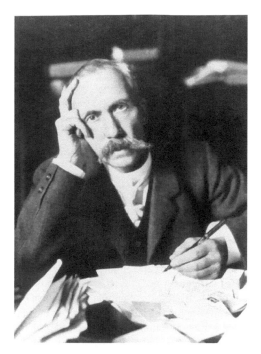

Charles Robert Richet.

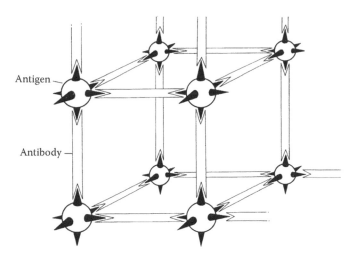

Precipitation test, lattice formation.

Ricinus communis

Refer to ricin.

Rickettsia immunity

The immune response in rickettsial infection involves powerful and persistent humoral and cell-mediated responses. Antibodies act as opsonins that render microorganisms susceptible to destruction by macrophages even though complement and antibody are not bactericidal. Antibody-dependent cellular cytotoxicity has also been demonstrated. Interferon-γ (IFN-γ)-activated macrophages effectively destroy rickettsia. Interferon-γ and to a lesser degree tumor necrosis factor (TNF) can control reproduction of rickettsiae in nonprofessional phagocytes. Protection depends upon cell-mediated immunity rather than antibody alone. Rickettsial infections activate natural killer (NK) cells. Both LAK and cytotoxic T cells can kill rickettsia-infected cells. Numerous attenuated rickettsial and killed subunit vaccines are available.

Rieckenberg reaction

A trypanosome immune adherence test. Anticoagulated blood of an animal that recovered from trypanosomiasis is combined with live trypanosomes. Provided the same antigenic type of trypanosome that produced the infection is used for the test, blood platelets adhere to the trypanosomes.

rinderpest vaccines

Although several types have been used in the past, the most satisfactory contemporary vaccine contains a virus adapted to tissue culture.

ring precipitation test

Refer to ring test.

ring test

A qualitative precipitin test used for more than a century in which soluble antigen (or antibody) is layered onto an antibody (or antigen) solution in a serological tube or capillary tube without agitating or mixing the two layers. If the antigen and antibody are specific for one another, a ring of precipitate will form at the interface. This simple technique was among the first antigen–antibody tests.

RIST

Refer to radioimmunosorbent test.

rituxan

An anti-cancer monoclonal antibody that serves as a type of biotherapy by binding to tumor cells and triggering the immune system to kill target tumor cells rather than using toxic chemicals to accomplish this result. The antibody has been approved by the FDA for use in patients with non-Hodgkin lymphoma.

rituximab

A chimeric murine–human monoclonal IgG_1 (human Fc) that unites with the CD20 molecule on normal and malignant B cells and is used to treat patients with relapsed or refractory low-grade or follicular B cell non-Hodgkin lymphoma. It acts by complement-mediated lysis, antibody-dependent cellular cytotoxicity, and apoptosis of malignant lymphoma cells.

RNA-directed DNA polymerase (reverse transcriptase)

DNA polymerase present in retroviruses such as human immunodeficiency virus (HIV) and Rous sarcoma virus that can use an RNA template to produce DNA. The primer needed must contain a free 3′ hydroxyl group that is base-paired with the template. This produces a DNA–RNA hybrid. Reverse transcriptase is critical in recombinant DNA techniques, as it is employed for first-strand cDNA synthesis.

RNA polymerase (RNAP)

A multiprotein complex comprised of 8 to 14 polypeptides involved in the transcription of different sets of genes into RNA. RNAP I, II, and III direct the synthesis of ribosomal RNA, messenger RNA, and selected small nuclear or cytoplasmic RNAs, including transfer RNA, respectively. Each human RNAP is composed of two large subunits (126 to 192 kDa) and at least six small subunits (14 to 18 kDa), three of which are shared by all three RNAP classes. Autoantibodies against RNAP I and III are very specific for systemic sclerosis and may portend a poor prognosis. Autoantibodies to RNAP II are also associated with systemic sclerosis. Although initially believed to be diagnostic for systemic sclerosis, autoantibodies against RNAP II have also been detected in patients with systemic lupus erythematosus (SLE) and overlap syndromes.

R

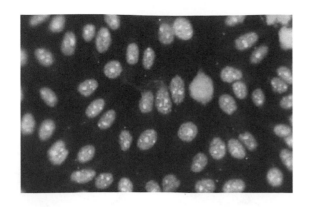

Anti-RNA polymerase autoantibody.

RNA polymerase (RNAP) I, II, and III autoantibodies

RNAP I antibodies found in 4% of systemic sclerosis patients show speckled or punctate nucleolar staining patterns. Autoantibodies are also found in the urine of 46% of patients with systemic lupus erythematosus (SLE) and in 19% of patients with rheumatoid arthritis (RA). Autoantibodies against RNAP I, II, and III are specific for systemic sclerosis (SSc), especially diffuse cutaneous SSc. Clinically, these autoantibodies are associated with increased frequency of heart and kidney involvement and poor 5-year survival. Twenty-three percent of SSc sera contain antibodies against RNAP III, which is a marker for SSc with diffuse or extensive cutaneous involvement. Autoantibodies against RNAP I are present in 4 to 33% of SSc patients and in subjects with SLE or overlap syndromes. Autoantibodies against RNAP II are frequently accompanied by autoantibodies against RNAP I and III.

RNAse protection assay

A technique to detect and quantify messenger RNA (mRNA) copies of specific genes based on nRNA hybridization to radiolabeled RNA probes followed by digestion of the unhybridized RNA with RNAse. Double-stranded RNA duplexes formed as a result of hybridization are resistant to RNAse degradation. Their size depends on the probe length. Gel electrophoresis is used for their separation, and radioautography is employed for their detection and quantification.

RNA splicing

The method whereby nontranslatable RNA sequences (introns) are excised from the primary transcript of a split gene. The translatable sequences (exons) are united to produce a functional gene product.

Ro/SSA and La/SSB

Heterogeneous ribonucleoprotein complexes that consist of antigenic proteins (two principal proteins of 52 kDa [Ro52] and 60 kDa [Ro60] for Ro/SSA and one protein of 48 kDa for La/SSB) associated with small cytoplasmic RNAs (hY-RNAs). Antibodies to Ro/SSA and La/SSB antigens are found frequently in the sera of patients with primary Sjögren's syndrome.

rocket electrophoresis

The electrophoresis of antigen into an agar-containing specific antibody. Through electroimmunodiffusion, lines of precipitation formed in the agar by the antigen–antibody interaction assume the shape of a rocket. The antigen concentration can be quantified because the size of the rocket-like area is proportional to the antigen concentration. This can

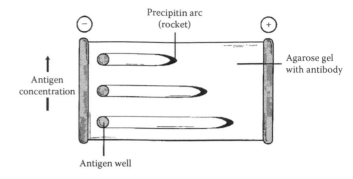

Rocket electrophoresis.

be deduced by comparing with antigen standards. This technique has the advantage of speed. It can be completed within hours instead of longer periods required for single radial immunodiffusion. Also called Laurell rocket electrophoresis.

Rodgers (Rg) antigens

Epitopes of C4d fragments of human complement component C4. They are not intrinsic to erythrocyte membranes. The Chido epitope is found on C4d from C4B, whereas the Rodgers epitope is found on C4A derived from C4d. The Rodgers epitope is Val–Asp–Leu–Leu, and the Chido epitope is Ala–Asp–Leu–Arg. They are situated at residue positions 1188 to 1191 in the C4d region of the C4 α chain. Antibodies against Ch and Rg antigenic determinants agglutinate saline suspensions of red blood cells coated with C4d. Because C4 is found in human serum, anti-Ch and anti-Rg are neutralized by the sera of most individuals that contain the relevant antigens. Ficin and papain destroy these antigens.

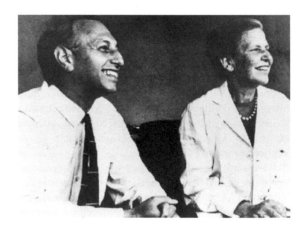

Ivan Roitt (left) with Deborah Doniach (right).

Roitt, Ivan

Roitt, Deborah Doniach, and other colleagues observed a positive precipitation reaction following interaction of sera from Hashimoto's thyroiditis patients and human thyroglobulin *in vitro*. This represented the first proof that humans with thyroid disease had circulating antibodies reactive with thyroglobulin.

Romer reaction (historical)

Romer in 1909 described erythematous swelling following intracutaneous injection of diphtheria toxin in small quantities. The reaction was found to be neutralized by homologous antitoxin. The smallest amount of diphtheria toxin that produced a definite reaction was defined as the minimal reaction dose (MRD). In general, the MRD of a toxin is equivalent to about 1/250 to 1/500 of the MLD (minimal lethal dose). The Lr is the smallest amount of toxin that, after mixing with one unit of antitoxin, will produce a minimal skin lesion when injected intracutaneously into a guinea pig.

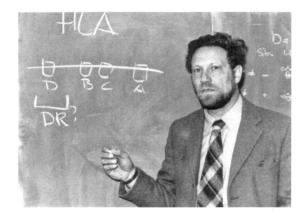

J.J. van Rood.

Rood, J. J. van

Researcher in The Netherlands who wrote his doctoral thesis on leukocyte grouping and techniques. He reported the first two allele systems. He named them 4a and 4b. They were difficult to define because they were "public antigens" shared by many molecules. By testing leukocyte alloantibodies obtained from the sera of a large number of pregnant women against leukocytes from 100 unrelated donors, he developed a systematic approach to decipher the complexity of the HLA system. van Rood and associates described nine HLA antigens and a diallelic system not linked to HLA (the Group Five system). Balner and van Rood showed that leukocyte antigens were transplantation antigens. van Rood made many contributions to HLA research.

roquinimex

An immunomodulating drug capable of augmenting natural killer (NK) cell numbers and reactivity and stimulating various T and B cell functions. It has been used to stimulate immune function in patients after bone marrow transplants. By contrast, it prevents relapses of chronic relapsing allergic encephalomyelitis in animal models of that disease. It also reduces relapses, disease activity, and disease progression in multiple sclerosis patients. If confirmed in further studies, this immunomodulator will have a significant future role in clinical medicine.

Rose, Noel Richard (1927–)

American immunologist and authority on autoimmune disease. Rose and Witebsky discovered experimental autoimmune thyroiditis. Rose's discovery in the mid-1950s that rabbits could be immunized to their own thyroid protein overturned the established dogma of "horror autotoxicus" and showed unequivocally that autoimmunity could cause disease. He and Witebsky also demonstrated that patients with chronic thyroiditis develop similar antibodies to their own thyroid antigens, implicating autoimmunity as the cause of this disease. The initial experiments were followed by others that elucidated the pathogenesis of autoimmune diseases

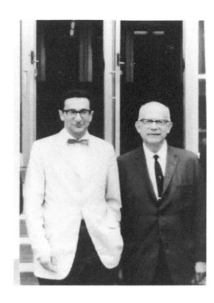

Noel Richard Rose (left) with Ernest Witebsky (right).

in animals and humans. In the 1970s he described the critical role of genetics in conferring susceptibility to autoimmune disease and showed that the major histocompatibility complex includes the major susceptibility gene. In the 1980s, he demonstrated how virus infections can serve as triggers for autoimmune heart disease. His discoveries opened the way to improved treatments and new prevention strategies for this group of diseases. Rose's pioneering investigations initiated the modern era of autoimmune disease research. He served as a professor of microbiology at the State University of New York at Buffalo, professor and chair of immunology and microbiology at Wayne State University, Detroit, and professor and chair of immunology and infectious diseases at The Johns Hopkins University. The author of more than 675 articles and chapters and editor of many books and leading journals, he presently directs The Johns Hopkins Center for Autoimmune Disease Research and the WHO/PAHO Collaborating Center for Autoimmune Disorders.

Rose–Waaler test

Sheep red blood cells are treated with a subagglutinating quantity of rabbit anti-sheep erythrocyte antibody. These particles may be used to identify rheumatoid factor in the sera of rheumatoid arthritis patients. Agglutination of the IgG-coated red cells constitutes a positive test and is based

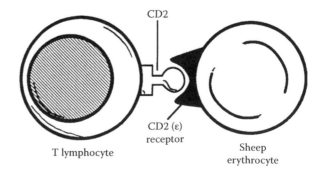

Adhesion of T lymphocyte and sheep red blood cell.

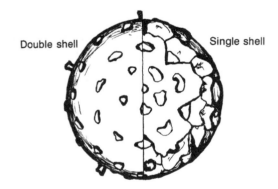

Formation of rosette.

upon immunological cross reactivity of human and rabbit IgG molecules. The test may show positive results in collagen vascular diseases other than rheumatoid arthritis, but it has still proven beneficial for diagnosis.

rosette

Cells of one type surrounding a single cell of another type. The rosette was used as an early method to enumerate T cells (i.e., in the formation of E rosettes, in which CD2 markers on human T lymphocytes adhere to and surround LFA-3 molecules on sheep red cells to give a rosette arrangement). Another example was the use of the EAC rosette consisting of erythrocytes coated with antibody and complement surrounding B cell-bearing Fc receptors or complement receptors on its surface.

Rotavirus.

rotavirus

A double-stranded RNA virus that is encapsulated and belongs to the reovirus family. It is 70 nm in diameter and causes epidemics of gastroenteritis that are usually relatively mild but may be severe in children below 2 years of age.

rouleaux formation

Erythrocytes arranged in the form of stacked coins. This formation is observed when plasma fibrinogen and globulins are increased. It is also seen when sedimentation rate is increased due to monoclonal immunoglobulins, as in multiple myeloma or Waldenström's disease or when dextran is administered. Rouleaux formation may also accompany cryoglobulinemia, sarcoidosis, and cirrhosis. When rouleaux formation interferes with reading weak antigen–antibody reactions, the effect may be diminished by diluting the sample with physiological saline solution.

round cells

Pathologists' term for mononuclear cells, especially lymphocytes, that infiltrate tissues.

Rous sarcoma virus (RSV)

A single-stranded RNA type C oncovirus that produces sarcomas in chickens. It is the typical acute transforming retrovirus. Within its genome are *gag*, *pol*, *env*, and v-*src* genes: *gag* encodes a core protein, *pol* encodes reverse transcriptase, and *env* encodes envelope glycoprotein. V-*scr* is an oncogene associated with the oncogenic capacity of the virus.

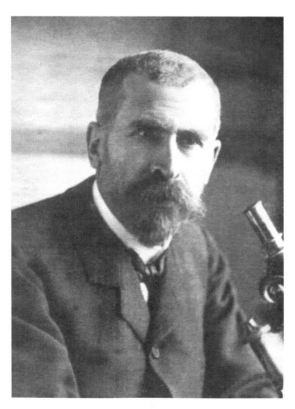

Emile Roux.

Roux, Emile (1853–1933)

A close colleague of Louis Pasteur at the Institut Pasteur in Paris. He showed that the bacterium-free filtrate of the diphtheria bacillus culture contained an exotoxin that produced the disease. He later became director of the Institut Pasteur.

RPR (rapid plasma reagin) test

An agglutination test used to screen for syphilis. Antilipoidal (nontreponemal) antibodies (reagins) develop in a host usually within 4 to 6 weeks after infection with *Treponema pallidum*. Of patients with primary syphilis, 93% develop positive RPR results.

rRNP

Ribosomal P proteins that share a 22-amino-acid sequence at the C terminal that contains an epitope for which anti-rRNP or anti-P antibodies are specific.

Mycophenolate mofetil

RS61443 (mycophenolate mofetil).

RS61443 (mycophenolate mofetil)

An experimental immunosuppressive drug for the treatment of refractory, acute, cellular allograft rejection, and possibly chronic rejection, in renal and other organ allotransplant recipients. Derived from mycophenolic acid, RS61443 interferes with guanosine synthesis, thereby blocking both T cell and B cell proliferation. It acts synergistically with cyclosporin in counteracting chronic rejection and has been reported to prevent FK506- and cyclosporin-A-induced obliterative vasculopathy.

RSV

Abbrevation for respiratory syncytial virus.

rubella vaccine

An attenuated virus vaccine used in the measles–mumps–rubella (MMR) combination or used alone to immunize seronegative women of childbearing age. It is not to be used during pregnancy.

runt disease

The disease process that results when neonatal mice of one strain are injected with lymph nodes or splenic lymphocytes from a different strain. Runt disease is accompanied by weight loss, failure to thrive, diarrhea, splenomegaly, and even death. The immune system of a neonatal animal is immature and reactivity against donor cells is weak or absent. Runt disease is an example of a graft-vs.-host reaction.

runting syndrome

Characterized by wasting, ruffled fur, diarrhea, lethargy, and debilitation. This is a consequence of thymectomy in neonatal mice that develop lymphopenia, lose lymphocytes from their lymphoid tissues, and become immunologically incompetent.

Russell body

A sphere or globule in the endoplasmic reticula of some plasma cells. These immunoglobulin-containing structures are stained pink by eosin.

S

S
Abbreviation for sedimentation coefficient.

S antibody
The sedimentation coefficient of immunoglobulin molecules such as IgG. 6.6S immunoglobulins are usually referred to as 7S immunoglobulins.

7S antibody
The sedimentation coefficient of immunoglobulin molecules such as IgG. 6.6S immunoglobulins are usually referred to as 7S immunoglobulins.

19S antibody
The sedimentation coefficient of the IgM class of immunoglobulins.

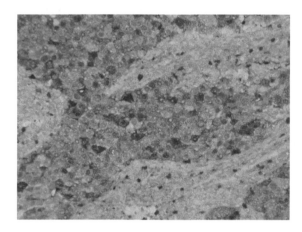

S-100—metastatic melanoma, lymph node.

S-100
A heterodimeric protein composed of α and β chains. It is present in a variety of tissues and is especially prominent in nervous system tissue including brain, neural crest, and Schwann cells. It is also positive in breast ducts, sweat and salivary glands, bronchial glands, serous acini, malignant melanomas, myoepithelium, and neurofibrosarcomas.

S-100 protein
A marker, demonstrable by immunoperoxidase staining, that is extensively distributed in both central and peripheral nervous systems and tumors arising from them, including astrocytomas, melanomas, Schwannomas, etc. Most melanomas express S-100 protein. Such non-neuronal cells as chondrocytes and histiocytes are also S-100-positive.

S-100 protein antibody
A mouse monoclonal antibody specific for S-100 protein that is found in normal melanocytes, Langerhans cells, histiocytes, chondrocytes, lipocytes, skeletal and cardiac muscle, Schwann cells, epithelial and myoepithelial cells of the breast, salivary and sweat glands, and glial cells. Neoplasms derived from these cells also express S-100

protein, albeit nonuniformly. A large number of well differentiated tumors of the salivary gland, adipose and cartilaginous tissue, and Schwann cell-derived tumors express S-100 protein. Most malignant melanomas and cases of histiocytosis X are positive for S-100 protein. Despite the ubiquity of S-100 protein, its demonstration is of great value in the identification of several neoplasms, particularly melanomas.

S protein
A hemolytically active substance encoded by the murine complement locus *C4B*.

S region
The chromosomal segment of the murine MHC containing genes that encode MHC class III molecules including complement component C2, factor B, C4A (Slp), and C4B (Ss). The S locus within this region is the site of genes that encode a 200-kDa protein termed Ss (serum substance) that corresponds to C4 in human serum. Also within the S region is the gene for Slp (sex limited protein, usually found only in male mice), the gene for 21-hydroxylase (an enzyme with no known immune function), and the gene for a serum β globulin. The term also refers to the chromosomal segment between HLA-B and HLA-D where the genes encoding the corresponding human MHC class III molecules are situated.

S value (Sverdberg unit)
The sedimentation coefficient of a protein ascertained by analytical ultracentrifugation.

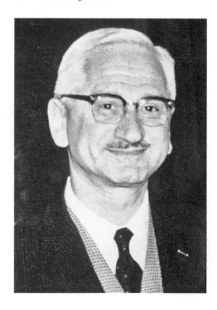

Albert Sabin.

Sabin, Albert (1906–1993)
American physician and immunologist who developed a live attenuated oral vaccine for poliomyelitis that produced

S

local immunity in the intestine. His vaccine largely replaced the earlier Salk vaccine.

Sabin–Feldman dye test

An *in vitro* diagnostic test for toxoplasmosis. Serial dilutions of serum are combined with *Toxoplasma gondii* microorganisms and complement is added. If specific antibodies against *Toxoplasma* organisms are present in the serum, complement interrupts the integrity of the toxoplasma membrane, admitting methylene blue that is added to the system and stains the interior of the organism. The dilution of serum in which one half of the *Toxoplasma* organisms are killed is the titer.

Sabin vaccine

An attenuated live poliomyelitis virus vaccine administered orally to induce local immunity in the gut, which is the natural route of entry of the virus, thereby stimulating local and systemic immunity against the causative agent of the disease.

saccharated iron oxide

Colloidal iron oxide employed to investigate the phagocytic capacity of mononuclear phagocytes.

sacculus rotundus

The lymphoid tissue-rich terminal segments of the ileum of the rabbit; a component of the gut-associated lymphoid tissue (GALT).

sago spleen

The replacement of lymphoid follicles by circular and transparent amyloid deposits in amyloidosis of the spleen.

SAIDS (simian acquired immune deficiency syndrome)

An immunodeficiency of rhesus monkeys induced by retrovirus group D. The animals develop opportunistic infections and tumors. Their CD4 lymphocytes decrease, and they suffer wasting and develop granulomatous encephalitis. The sequence homology between simian immunodeficiency virus (SIV) and human immunodeficiency virus 1 (HIV-1) is minimal, but the sequence homology between SIV and HIV-2 is significant.

saline agglutinin

An antibody that causes the aggregation or agglutination of red blood cells, bacterial cells, or other particles in 0.15 *M* salt solutions without additives.

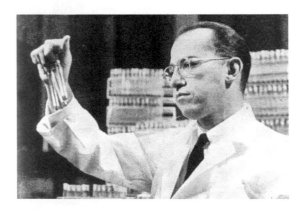

Jonas Salk.

Salk, Jonas (1914–1994)

American physician working at the University of Pittsburgh who prepared the first effective polio vaccine including all three types of viruses inactivated by formaldehyde. It proved safe and effective and was used in 650,000 children in 1954.

Salk vaccine

An injectable, inactivated poliomyelitis vaccine containing virus killed by formalin. It was used for prophylactic immunization against poliomyelitis prior to development of the Sabin oral vaccine.

***Salmonella* immunity**

Natural immunity and adaptive immunity are necessary for survival following primary infection with virulent microorganisms of this genus. *Salmonellae* grow exponentially in the reticuloendothelial system and may reach 10^8 microorganisms—a lethal number, apparently due to endotoxin activity. The balance between strain virulence and host resistance controls the rate at which bacterial cells increase in the reticuloendothelial system. Bone marrow-derived cells, tumor necrosis factor α (TNF-α), interferon-γ (IFN-γ), and interleukin-12 (IL12), but not T lymphocytes, control early growth (plateau phase), after which an immune response phase clears the microorganisms from tissues and provides effective immunity to reinfection. CD4[+] and CD8[+] T lymphocytes along with TNF-α, IFN-γ, and IL12 help clear bacteria from the tissues, but antibody is also required in addition to cell-mediated immunity. The antibody may be directed against lipopolysaccharide (LPS) in animal infections; antibodies to Vi antigen are believed to be significant in humans. The diagnosis of typhoid fever is based on the detection of antibodies to O and H antigens and to Vi antigens in carriers. Immunization with killed *Salmonellae* does not induce cell-mediated immunity and confers less protection than immunization with live organisms that induce both cell-mediated and humoral immunity. Antibody alone is not protective. The protective immunogen is probably LPS O or Vi in *S. typhi,* other protein antigens, or a combination. IgA provides partial immunity. Because killed microorganisms used in vaccines in the past did not induce appropriate cell-mediated immunity and were highly reactogenic, live vaccines of superior efficacy in experimental models are under development.

SALT

Abbreviation for skin-associated lymphoid tissue.

salting out

Salt precipitation of serum proteins such as globulins.

salt precipitation

An earlier method to separate serum proteins based on the principle that globulins precipitate when the concentration of sodium sulfate or ammonium sulfate is less than the concentration at which albumin precipitates. Euglobulins precipitate at concentrations below those at which pseudoglobulins precipitate. Salt precipitation was largely replaced by chromatographic methods using Sephadex® beads and related techniques.

salvage pathway of nucleic acid synthesis

Construction of nucleotides from degraded spent nucleic acids through the actions of adenosine deaminase and purine nucleoside phosphorylase (PIMP).

salvage therapy

An extraordinary effort to rescue a patient with refractory cancer through an innovative or experimental treatment.

Salvarsan (606)

Arsenical compound developed by Paul Ehrlich for the treatment of syphilis.

SAMS

Abbreviation for substrate adhesion molecules.

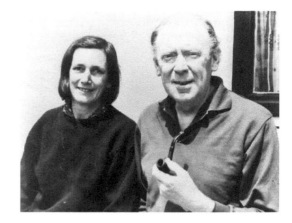

Ruth Sanger (left) and Robert Race (right).

Ehrlich's instructions concerning 606 (salvarsan), the first effective treatment for syphilis.

Sanarelli–Shwartzman reaction

Refer to Shwartzman reaction.

sandoglobulin

Refer to human immune globulin.

sandwich ELISA

A highly specific method in which surface-bound antibody traps a protein by binding to one of its epitopes. An enzyme-linked antibody specific for a different epitope on the protein surface is employed to detect the trapped protein.

sandwich immunoassay

A technique in which the analyte is bound to a solid phase, and a labeled reagent is subsequently bound immunochemically to the analyte.

sandwich methodology

Refer to sandwich technique.

sandwich technique

The identification of antibody or of antibody-synthesizing cells in tissue preparations. Antigen is placed in contact with the tissue section or smear, followed by the application of antibody labeled with a fluorochrome such as fluorescein isothiocyanate (FITC) that is specific for the antigen. This yields a product consisting of antibody layered on both sides of the antigen, in the manner of a sandwich.

Sanger, Ruth (1918–2001)

Ruth Sanger and Robert Race developed the three-allele theory and the CDE nomenclature for the Rh blood group system.

SAPK/JNK signaling pathway

The stress-activated protein kinase/jun N-terminal kinase signaling pathway induced by extracellular stress factors such as osmotic shock, chemical agents, and indirect activation downstream of engagement of the T cell receptor. Leads to stimulation of c-jun, an AP-1 transcription factor constituent.

saponin

A glucoside used for its adjuvant properties to enhance immune reactivity to certain vaccine constituents. It was considered to slow the release of immunogen from an injection site and induce B cells capable of forming antibody at the site of antigen deposition.

Saquinavir mesylate.

Saquinavir mesylate (Invirase)

A protease inhibitor used in the treatment of HIV infections.

SAR

See plant immunity.

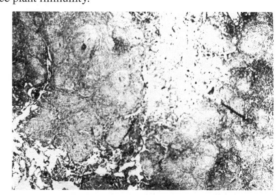

Open lung biopsy showing sarcoidosis.

sarcoma

A tumor that arises from a cell of connective tissue.

sarcoidosis

A systemic granulomatous disease of unknown etiology involving lymph nodes, lungs, eyes, and skin. A granulomatous hypersensitivity reaction resembles that of tuberculosis and fungus infections. Sarcoidosis has a higher incidence in African Americans than in Caucasians and is prominent

S

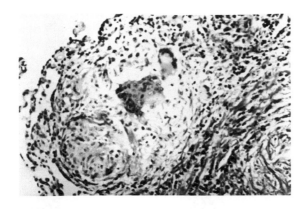

Open lung biopsy showing sarcoidosis.

geographically in the southeastern United States. It exhibits a decrease in circulating T cells. Decreased delayed-type hypersensitivity is manifested as anergy to common skin test antigens. Increased antibody formation leads to polyclonal hypergammaglobulinemia. A marked cellular immune response is observed in local areas of disease activity. Tissue lesions consist of inflammatory cells and granulomas composed of activated mononuclear phagocytes such as epithelioid cells, multinucleated giant cells, and macrophages. Activated T cells are present at the periphery of the granuloma. CD4+ T cells appear to be the immunoregulatory agents governing granuloma formation. Mediators released from T cells nonspecifically stimulate B cells, resulting in the polyclonal hypergammaglobulinemia. The granulomas are typically noncaseating, distinguishing them from those produced in tuberculosis. Patients may develop fever, polyarthritis, erythema nodosum, and iritis. They also may experience loss of weight, anorexia, weakness, fever, sweats, nonproductive cough, and increasing dyspnea on exertion. Pulmonary symptoms occur in more than 90% of patients. Angiotensin-converting enzyme is increased in the sera of sarcoid patients. Disease activity is monitored by measuring the level of this enzyme in serum. The subcutaneous inoculation of sarcoidosis lymph node extracts into patients diagnosed with sarcoidosis leads to a granulomatous reaction in the skin 3 to 4 weeks after inoculation. This served as a diagnostic test of questionable value (known as the Kveim reaction) in the past. Sarcoidosis symptoms can be treated with corticosteroids, but only after disease progression occurs. Sarcoidosis is a relatively mild disease, with 80% of cases resolving spontaneously and only 5% dying of complications. Evidence indicates oligoclonal expansion of αβ T cell subsets and predominant expression of type 1 cytokines—interferon-γ (IFN-γ) and interleukin-2 (IL1-2)—at sites of inflammation, suggesting that sarcoidosis is an antigen-driven, Th1-mediated immune disorder.

sarcoma
A malignant neoplasm arising from connective tissue cells including muscle, bone or cartilage.

Sca-1
Abbreviation for stem cell antigen 1.

SCABs (single-chain antigen-binding proteins)
Polypeptides that join the light chain variable sequence of an antibody to the heavy chain variable sequence of the antibody. All monoclonal antibodies are potential sources of SCABs. They are smaller and less immunogenic than intact heavy chains with immunogenic constant regions. Their potential uses include imaging and treatment of cancer, in cardiovascular disease, as biosensors, and for chemical separations.

scarlet fever
A condition associated with production of erythrogenic toxin by group A hemolytic streptococci associated with pharyngitis. Patients develop strawberry-red tongues and generalized erythematous blanching areas that do not occur on the palms, the soles of the feet, or in the mouth. They may also develop Pastia's lines (petechiae in linear patterns).

Scatchard analysis
A mathematical analytical method to determine the affinity and valence of a receptor–ligand interaction in equilibrium binding.

Scatchard equation
An expression for the union of a univalent ligand with an antibody molecule ($r/c = Kn - Kr$). To obtain the average number of ligand molecules to which an antibody molecule may bind at equilibrium, the bound ligand molar concentration is divided by the antibody molar concentration designated as r. The free ligand molar concentration is represented by c; antibody valence by n; and the association constant by K.

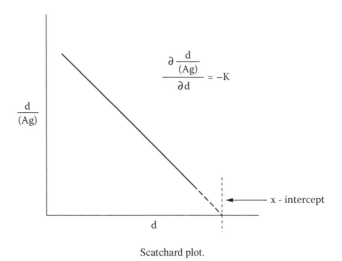

$$\frac{\partial \frac{d}{(Ag)}}{\partial d} = -K$$

$\frac{d}{(Ag)}$

x - intercept

d

Scatchard plot.

Scatchard plot
A graphic representation of binding data obtained by plotting r/c against r (refer to Scatchard equation). The purpose of this plot is to determine intrinsic association constants and ascertain how many noninteracting binding sites each molecule contains. A straight line with a slope of $-K$ indicates that all the binding sites are the same and are independent. The plot should also intercept on the r axis of n. A nonlinear plot signifies that the binding sites are not the same and are not independent. The degree to which the sites are occupied is reflected by the slope ($-K$). An average association constant for ligand binding to heterogeneous antibodies is the reciprocal of the amount of free ligand needed for half saturation of antibody sites.

scavenger receptors
Structures on macrophages and other cell types that bind a variety of ligands and delete them from the blood. Scavenger receptors are especially abundant on Kupffer's cells of the liver.

SCF (stem cell factor)

A substance that promotes growth of hematopoietic precursor cells and is encoded by the murine SI gene. It serves as a ligand for the tyrosine kinase receptor family protooncogene termed c-*kit*. It apparently has a role in embryogenesis in cells linked to migratory patterns of hematopoietic stem cells, melanoblasts, and germ cells.

ScFv

A single chain molecule composed of both heavy and light chain variable regions fastened together by a flexible linker.

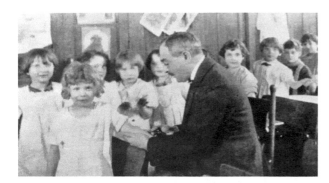

Bela Schick.

Schick, Bela (1877–1967)

Austro-Hungarian pediatrician whose work with von Pirquet resulted in the discovery and description of serum sickness. He developed the test for diphtheria that bears his name. (Refer to *Die Serumkrankheit* [with Pirquet], 1905.)

Schick test

A test for susceptibility to diphtheria. Standardized diphtheria toxin is adjusted to contain 1/50 MLD in 0.1 mL, which is injected intracutaneously into the forearm. Development of redness and induration 24 to 36 hours after administration constitutes a positive test if the condition persists 4 days or longer. The presence of 1/500 to 1/250 or more of a unit of antitoxin per milliliter of patient blood will result in a negative reaction because of neutralization of the injected toxin. Neither redness nor induration appears if a test is negative. An individual with a negative test possesses sufficient antitoxin to protect against infection with *Corynebacterium diphtheria;* a positive test denotes susceptibility. A control is always carried out in the opposite forearm. For this test, diluted toxin is heated to 70°C for 15 minutes and injected intracutaneously. Heating destroys the ability of the toxin to induce local tissue injury, but does not affect the components of the diphtheria bacilli or the medium that may evoke an allergic response. If the size and duration of the reaction at the injection site in the control approximate the reaction in the test arm, the result is negative. If the reaction is at least 50% larger and of longer duration on the test arm compared to the control, the individual is both allergic to the materials in the bacilli or medium and susceptible to the toxin. A positive Schick reaction suggests that diphtheria immunization is needed.

Schistosoma immunity

The immune response to the blood flukes classified as schistosomes is complex. Repeated exposure to schistosome larval antigens may lead to hypersensitivity and cercarial dermatitis (swimmer's itch). Exposure to large numbers of *Schistosoma mansoni* or *S. japonicum* may lead to a serum sickness or immune complex-like disease, whereas immune reactions to later stages of the infection may be associated with resistance against infection. Many of the pathological changes in schistosome infections are linked to deposition of eggs that induce granulomatous reactions in tissues, resulting in fibrosis. The granuloma is a delayed-type hypersensitivity reaction that is T cell-dependent. In addition to the cells expected in a granuloma, eosinophils, lymphocytes, and macrophages are also present. The fibrosis is also egg antigen-induced. Multiple immune parameters are activated by these eggs and their antigens, leading to modulation in chronically infected individuals. Egg antigens may induce protective and immunopathologic responses. Whereas the eggs induce mostly immunopathologic effects, reactions to the schistosomulum are mostly protective of the host. Adult worms from a primary infection can continue to survive in individuals resistant to reinfection with fresh cercariae through "concomitant immunity." Irradiated cercariae can be used to induce immunization of mice and other experimental animals against cercarial challenge. The main target of destructive immunological attack is the migrating schistosomulum. Humans develop concomitant immunity slowly. Resistance is correlated with peripheral blood eosinophilia in *S. haematobium* infections. Infection-protective immunity may be associated in elderly persons with IgE antibodies against adult worm antigens. More than 90% of the surface antigens of the young schistosomulum are carbohydrates. Anti-egg antibodies may cross react with these antigens. Adult worms activate Th1 responses and eggs induce Th2 responses. Protection in mice is mediated mainly by T_h1 cells and can be potentiated with IL12. Tumor necrosis factor α (TNF-α) is associated with granuloma formation. Adult worms are usually not susceptible to immune attack, as they either coat themselves with host-derived macromolecules that mask parasite surface antigens or shed antigenic macromolecules from the outer tegument, rendering their outer surfaces immunologically inert. Although egg identification in human excreta has long been the method of diagnosis, indirect diagnosis using antibody detected by the enzyme-linked immunosorbent assay (ELISA) technique is becoming more common. Schistosome-derived carbohydrate antigens in the blood are also helpful in immunodiagnosis. No vaccine is available to protect against schistosomiasis in humans. Irradiated larvae have been used to immunize cattle.

schistosomiasis

A schistosome infection characteristically followed by a granulomatous tissue reaction.

schistosomiasis vaccines

Schistosomiasis (bilharziasis or snail fever) is the worst human disease induced by a metazoan parasite. Five different species of *Schistosoma* produce the disease. Two isoforms of the schistosome enzyme glutathione-S-transferase have been investigated as candidates for a vaccine. They manifest highly effective immunogens in rat models. Two surface antigens from the migratory larval stage of *S. mansoni* parasites or other molecules appear promising in animal models. Two parasite muscle proteins have also been tested. None of these antigens has reached clinical trials, and no immediate prospect for development of an effective vaccine appears imminent even though the search continues.

schlepper

Landsteiner's term for large macromolecules that serve as carriers for simple chemical molecules serving as haptens. The immunization of rabbits and other animals with a hapten–carrier complex leads to the formation of antibodies specific for the hapten and the carrier. T cells were later shown to be carrier-specific and B cells hapten-specific. Carriers are conjugated to haptens through covalent linkages such as the diazo linkage.

Schultz–Dale test (historical)

Strong contraction of the isolated uterine horn muscle of a virgin guinea pig that has been actively or passively sensitized occurs following the addition of specific antigen to a 37°C tissue bath in which it is suspended. This reaction is the basis for an *in vitro* assay of anaphylaxis termed the Schultz–Dale test. Muscle contraction is caused by the release of histamine and other pharmacological mediators of immediate hypersensitivity following antigen interaction with antibody fixed to tissue cells.

SCID (severe combined immunodeficiency)

Refer to severe combined immunodeficiency syndrome.

SCID (severe combined immunodeficiency, human–mouse)

A murine immunodeficiency in which human immune system elements such as bone marrow and thymic fragments have been introduced. Pluripotent human hematopoietic stem cells differentiate into mature immunocytes in these mice, rendering them useful for investigating lymphocyte development.

SCID (severe combined immunodeficiency, mouse)

An autosomal-recessive mutation expressed as severe combined immune deficiency in the CB-17Icr mouse strain. These mice do not have serum immunoglobulins, yet their adenosine deaminase (ADA) levels are normal. They lack T and B lymphocytes and thus fail to respond to T cell-dependent or -independent antigens when challenged. Likewise, their lymph nodes and spleen cells fail to proliferate following challenge by T or B lymphocyte mitogens. The lymphoid stroma in their lymph nodes and spleen is normal. Even though they exhibit no evidence of T cell-mediated immunity, they have natural killer (NK) cells and mononuclear phagocytes that are normal in number and function. The mutation likewise does not affect myeloid and erythroid lineage cells. B cell development is arrested at the pro-B stage before cytoplasmic or surface immunoglobulins are present. Normal numbers of macrophages are present in the spleen, peritoneum, and liver. The SCID mutation is associated with an intrinsic defect in lymphoid stem cells. The main characteristic of SCID mice is the failure of their lymphocytes to express antigen-specific receptors due to disordered rearrangements of T cell receptors or immunoglobulin genes. The defect in recombination of antigen-specific receptor genes may be associated with the absence of a DNA recombinase specific for lymphocytes in these mice. Attributable to a defect in DNA-PK function requisite for V(D)J recombination. This mouse model may be used to substitute for human experimentation to investigate the effects of anti-HIV drugs and immunostimulants. It is also useful for investigations of neoplasms in hosts lacking effective immune responses.

Scl-70 antibody

An antinuclear antibody found in as many as 70% of patients with diffuse-type scleroderma (progressive systemic sclerosis) who experience extensive and rapid skin involvement and early visceral manifestations.

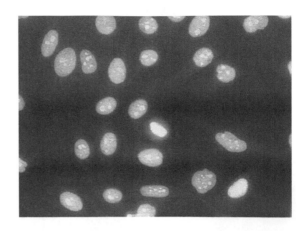

Scl-70 (topoisomerase I) autoantibodies.

Scl-70 (topoisomerase I) autoantibodies

Autoantibodies found in 20 to 40% of diffuse scleroderma patients. Two thirds of patients with these autoantibodies have diffuse scleroderma and 20% of patients with limited scleroderma manifest topoisomerase I autoantibodies. Scl-70 autoantibodies or DR3-DRw52a tissue types represent a 17-fold increase in risk for development of pulmonary fibrosis in scleroderma. These autoantibodies are occasionally found in classical systemic lupus erythematosus (SLE) without manifestations of scleroderma. Topoisomerase I autoantibodies portend a poor prognosis in Raynaud's phenomenon. Silica can induce a scleroderma-like condition. Some patients develop Scl-70 autoantibodies. The preferred technique for detection of IgG autoantibodies against topoisomerase I is enzyme immunoassay (EIA) with immunoblot confirmation. The relevance of an association of topoisomerase I autoantibodies with neoplasms remains to be determined.

scleroderma

Refer to progressive systemic sclerosis.

SCM-1

Single cysteine motif 1 (SCM-1) is a member of the γ (C) family of chemokines. cDNA clones derived from human peripheral blood mononuclear cells stimulated with phytohemagglutinin (PHA) encode SCM-1, which is significantly related to the α and β chemokines. It has only the second and fourth of four cysteines conserved in these proteins. It is 60.5% identical to lymphotactin. SCM-1 and lymphotactin are believed to represent human and mouse prototypes of a γ (C) chemokine family. SCM-1 is expressed by human T cells and spleen.

sCR1 (soluble complement receptor type 1)

A substance prepared by recombinant DNA technology that combines with activated C3b and C4. This facilitates their inactivation by complement factor I. sCR1 significantly diminishes myocardial injury induced by hypoxia in rats.

scratch test

Skin test for the detection of immunoglobulin E (IgE) antibodies against a particular allergen that are anchored to mast cells in the skin. After scratching the skin with a needle, a minute amount of aqueous allergen is applied to the scratch site, and the area is observed for the development of urticaria manifested as a wheal-and-flare reaction. This signifies that the IgE antibodies are specific for the applied allergen and lead to the degranulation of mast cells with release of pharmacologic mediators of hypersensitivity such as histamine.

scurfy mouse

A natural mouse mutant that is a model of human IPEX characterized by rough skin, runting, thrombocytopenia, lymphadenopathy, and elevated susceptibility to infections. A mutation of the FoxP3 gene encoding the scurfin transcription factor leads to failure of T_{reg} cells to function.

SDF-1

Stromal cell-derived factor 1 (SDF-1) is an α (CXC) family chemokine. The stromal cell line PA6 synthesizes SDF-1, which promotes proliferation of stromal cell-dependent pre-B cells of the DW34 stromal cell-dependent pre-B cell clone. Alternative splicing of the *SDF-1* gene yields *SDF-1α* and *SDF-1β*. SDF-1 is believed to be the natural ligand for LESTR (leukocyte-derived seven-transmembrane domain receptor). It is expressed by stromal cells, bone marrow, liver tissue, and muscle.

SDS-PAGE

Polyacrylamide gel electrophoresis in sodium dodecyl sulfate. Refer also to polyacrylamide gel electrophoresis.

SE

Abbreviation for staphylococcal enterotoxins.

second messengers (IP₃ and DAG)

Upon stimulation of the T cell receptor, protein tyrosine kinase (PTK) becomes activated. PTK then phosphorylates phospholipase C (PLC), which in turn hydrolyzes phosphatidylinositol 4,5-bisphosphate (PIP₂). The products of PIP₂ hydrolysis are the intracellular second messengers, inositol 1,4,5-triphosphate (IP₃) and 1,2-diacylglycerol (DAG). IP₃ leads to increased Ca^{2+} release from intracellular stores, and DAG leads to increased levels of protein kinase C. Protein kinase C and Ca^{2+} signals, such as the interaction of CA^{2+}/calmodulin to activate calcineurin, are associated with gene transcription and T cell activation. Second messenger systems are also important in B cell activation as a means of stimulating resting B cells to enter the cell cycle. Through second messenger systems, extracellular signals are received at cell membranes and relayed to nuclei to induce responses at the genetic level.

second set rejection

Second set rejection of an organ or tissue graft by a host who is already immune to the histocompatibility antigens of the graft as a consequence of rejection of a previous transplant of the same antigenic specificity as the second or as a consequence of immunization against antigens of the donor graft. The accelerated second set rejection compared to rejection of a first graft is reminiscent of a classic secondary or booster immune response.

second set response

The accelerated rejection of a second skin graft from a donor that is the same or identical with the first donor. The accelerated rejection is seen when regrafting is performed 12 to 80 days after rejection of the first graft. It is completed in 7 to 8 days and is due to sensitization of the recipient by the first graft.

second signal

The second of two signals required to activate lymphocytes. Lymphocyte activation requires the recognition of antigen by an antigen-specific leukocyte receptor in soluble form by the B cell surface immunoglobulin receptor or complexed to a major histocompatibility complex (MHC) molecule on an antigen-presenting cell by the αβ heterodimer of the T cell receptor (TCR) complex. Following this first signal, lymphocytes do not become fully activated and are turned off, become unresponsive to subsequent receptor stimulation, or undergo apoptosis. A second signal is required to induce a productive immune response. It enhances lymphocyte proliferation and promotes cell survival and/or prevents lymphocyte receptor unresponsiveness. Second signals may potentiate signals transduced by TCR ligation and initiate enhanced proliferation. They may facilitate antigen-driven lymphocyte proliferation and also inhibit the induction of lymphocyte unresponsiveness and/or programmed cell death. These latter costimulatory signals activate intracellular pathways different from those induced by the antigen–receptor complex. Different surface molecules can provide second signals.

secondary allergen

An agent that induces allergic symptoms because of cross reactivity with an allergen to which the individual is hypersensitive.

secondary antibody

An antibody directed against the Fc region of an unlabeled primary antibody that has reacted with an antigen of interest. Application of a labeled secondary antibody after washing away unbound primary antibody permits the detection of primary antibody–antigen complexes.

secondary antibody response

Immunoglobulin M (IgM) appears before IgG in the primary antibody response. The inoculation of an immunogen into an experimental animal primed by previous immunization with the same immunogen produces antibodies following the secondary immunogenic challenge that develop more rapidly, last longer, and reach a higher titer than in the primary response. Antibodies produced in the secondary response are predominantly IgG and reach levels that are 10-fold or greater than those in the primary antibody response.

secondary disease

A condition that occurs in irradiated animals whose cell populations have been reconstituted with histoincompatible, immunologically competent cells derived from allogeneic donor animals. Ionizing radiation induces immunosuppression in the recipients, rendering them incapable of rejecting the foreign cells. Thus, a recipient has two cell populations, its own and the introduced one. Thus, these animals are radiation chimeras. After an initial period of recovery, they develop a secondary runt disease that is usually fatal within 1 month.

secondary follicle

An area in a peripheral lymphoid organ where a germinal center is located. Usually associated with a secondary immune response more often than with a primary one. It forms a ring of concentrically packed B lymphocytes surrounding a germinal center. The infiltration of primary follicles by activated T and B cells results in formation of secondary follicles that lead to germinal centers and facilitation of terminal differentiation of activated B cells into memory B and plasma cells.

secondary granule

A structure in the cytoplasm of polymorphonuclear leukocytes that contains vitamin B_{12}-binding protein, lysozyme, and lactoferrin in neutrophils. Cationic peptides are present in eosinophil secondary granules. Histamine, platelet-activating factor, and heparin are present in the secondary granules of basophils.

S

secondary immune response

A heightened antibody response following second exposure to antigen in animals primed by previous contact with the same antigen. The secondary immune response depends upon immunological memory from the first encounter with antigen. It is characterized by a steep and rapid rise in antibody titer, usually of the immunoglobulin G (IgG) class, accompanied by potent cell-mediated immunity. Protein and glycoprotein immunogens stimulate this type of response. The rapid rise in antibody synthesis is followed by a gradual exponential decline in titer. It begins sooner and develops more rapidly than does the primary immune response. This is also known as the booster response observed following administration of antigens subsequent to the secondary exposure. Refer also to anamnestic response.

secondary immunodeficiency

Immunodeficiency that is not due to a failure or intrinsic defect in the T and B lymphocytes of the immune system. It is a consequence of some other disease process and may be transient or permanent. The transient variety may disappear following adequate treatment, whereas the more permanent type persists. Secondary immunodeficiencies are commonly produced by many effects. For example, those that appear in patients with neoplasms may result from effects of a tumor. Secondary immunodeficiencies may cause an individual to become susceptible to microorganisms that would otherwise cause no problem. They may occur following immunoglobulin or T lymphocyte loss, the administration of drugs, infection, cancer, and effects of ionizing radiation on immune system cells, among other causes.

secondary lymphoid follicle

Areas of secondary lymphoid tissues populated by proliferating B cells responding to antigen.

secondary lymphoid organ

The lymph nodes, spleen, gut-associated lymphoid tissues, and tonsils where T and B lymphocytes interact with antigen-presenting accessory cells such as macrophages, resulting in the generation of an immune response.

secondary lymphoid tissues

Tissues in which immune responses are generated, including lymph nodes, spleen, and mucosa-associated lymphoid tissues. Lymph nodes and spleen are often called secondary lymphoid organs.

secondary lysosome

A lysosome united with a phagosome.

secondary nodule

Refer to secondary follicle.

secondary reactions

The visible effects of antibody–antigen binding such as precipitation, agglutination, flocculation, complement fixation, etc.

secondary response

The anamnestic or memory immune response following second exposure to an antigen in an individual sensitized by a primary immunizing dose of the same antigen. The secondary response occurs more rapidly and is of much greater magnitude than the primary response because of the memory cells that respond to the second challenge. Less costimulation is required by memory lymphocytes than by naïve lymphocytes. Clonal expansion in the primary response increases the frequency of antigen-specific lymphocytes participating in the secondary response, which is more rapid and vigorous than the primary response. Also called booster response.

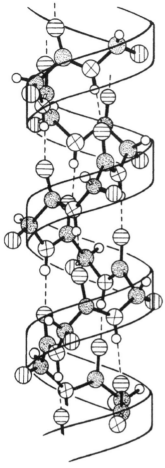

Secondary structure.

secondary structure

Polypeptide chain or polynucleotide strand folding along the axis or backbone of a molecule as a consequence of the formation of intramolecular hydrogen bonds joining carbonyl oxygen and amide nitrogen atoms. Secondary structure is based on the local spatial organization of polypeptide chain segments or polynucleotide strands irrespective of the structures of side chains or the relationship of the segments to one another.

secreted antibody

Refer to secreted immunoglobulin.

secreted immunoglobulin (sIg)

A product of plasma cells that is secreted as free immunoglobulin. It may circulate as a component of blood plasma or become part of the protein contents of other body fluids. This form of immunoglobulin contains a short tail piece and does not possess a transmembrane domain.

Secretor Phenomenon: A, B, and H Substances Detectable in Saliva of Individuals with ABO Blood Groups

Secretors in ABO Blood Group	Antigens in Saliva
O	A, H
A	B, H
B	A, B, H
AB	H

---

secretor

An individual who secretes ABH blood group substances into body fluids such as saliva, gastric juice, tears, ovarian cyst fluid, etc. Secretors constitute at least 80% of the human population. The property is genetically determined and requires that a secretor be homozygous (*Se/Se*) or heterozygous (*Se/se*) for the *Se* gene.

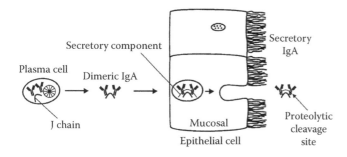

Secretory component.

secretory antibody

A secreted antibody that possesses a tail piece, J chain, and secretory component subjected to post-translational modifications that allow access to body secretions including tears and mucus.

secretory component (SC)

A 75-kDa molecule synthesized by epithelial cells in the lamina propria of the gut that becomes associated with immunoglobulin A (IgA) molecules produced by plasma cells in the lamina propria of the gut as they move across the epithelial cell layer to reach the mucosal surface of intestine to provide local immunity. SCs appear in three molecular forms: as an SIgM and SIgA stabilizing chain, as a transmembrane receptor protein, and as a free secretory component in fluids. SC is a fragment of the poly-Ig receptor that remains bound to Ig following transcytosis across the epithelium and cleavage.

secretory component deficiency

A lack of immunoglobulin A (IgA) in secretions as a consequence of the inability of gastrointestinal tract epithelial cells to produce secretory component to be linked to the IgA molecules synthesized in the lamina propria of the gut. Secretory component normally prevents IgA destruction by proteolytic enzymes in the gut lumen. The disorder is rare and is characterized by protracted diarrhea associated with gut infection.

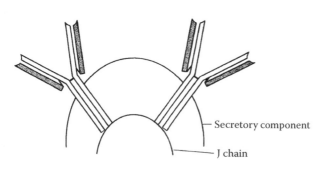

Secretory IgA.

secretory IgA

A dimeric molecule composed of two immunoglobulin A (IgA) monomers joined by a J polypeptide chain and a glycopeptide secretory component that serves as the principal molecule of mucosal immunity. IgA is the only immunoglobulin isotype that can be selectively passed across mucosal walls to reach the lumens of organs lined with mucosal cells. Specific FcαRs that bind IgA molecular dimers are found on intestinal epithelial cells. The FcαR joins the antibody molecule to the basal surface of the epithelial cell exposed to the blood. It is bound to the polyimmunoglobulin receptor on the basolateral surfaces of epithelial cells and facilitates vesicular transport of the anchored IgA across cells to the surface of the mucosa. Once this complex reaches its destination, FcαR (S protein) is split in a manner that permits the dimeric IgA molecule to retain an attached secretory piece that has a strong affinity for mucus, thereby facilitating the maintenance of IgA molecules on mucosal surfaces. The secretory piece also has the important function of protecting the secreted IgA molecules from proteolytic digestion by enzymes of the gut, in addition to its active role in transporting IgA molecules through epithelial cells. Secretory or exocrine IgA appears in the colostrum, intestinal and respiratory secretions, saliva, tears, and other secretions.

secretory immune system

A major component of the immune system that provides protection from invading microorganisms at local sites. Much of the effect is mediated by secretory IgA molecules in the secretions at the mucosal surface. Immunoglobulins may also be in clotted fluids where they protect against microorganisms.

secretory immunoglobulin A (SIgA)

SIgA may interfere with the attachment of bacteria to host cells by coating the microbes. It may also neutralize their exotoxins, inhibit their motility, and agglutinate them. It is not involved in opsonization or lysis of bacteria through complement. Its ability to prevent adherence of such microorganisms as *Vibrio cholerae, Giardia lamblia,* and selected respiratory viruses to mucosal surfaces represents a significant defense mechanism. Although gastric acidity can destroy most microorganisms, it does not destroy *Mycobacterium tuberculosis* and enteroviruses. Gram-negative bacteria may colonize the stomach and small intestine in subjects with achlorhydria. Unconjugated

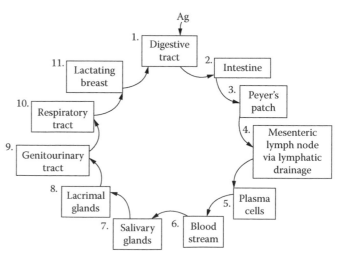

Secretory immune system.

S

bile may prevent bacterial growth in the small gut. Intestinal peristalsis also guards against overgrowth of microorganisms in blind loops.

secretory piece

A 75-kDa polypeptide chain synthesized by epithelial cells of the gut for linkage to immunoglobulin A (IgA) dimers present in body secretions. Secretory component facilitates IgA transport across epithelial cells and protects secretory IgA released into the lumen of the gut from proteolytic digestion by enzymes in the secretions. It is not formed by plasma cells in the lamina propria of the gut that synthesize the IgA molecules with which it combines. Secretory component has a special affinity for mucus, thereby facilitating the attachment of IgA to the mucous membranes. Also called secretory component.

sedimentation coefficient

The rate at which a macromolecule or particle sediments that is equivalent to the velocity per unit centrifugal field: $s = (dx/dt)/w^2x$, where s is the sedimentation coefficient, dx/dt is the velocity, w is the angular velocity, and x is the distance from the axis of the centrifuge rotor. The size, shape, and weight of the macromolecule in question and the concentration and temperature of the solutions (but not the centrifuge speed) determine the sedimentation coefficient. Measurement is in Svedberg units.

sedimentation pattern

The configuration of red blood cells on a test tube or plastic plate bottom at the conclusion of a hemagglutination test. The formation of a covering mat on the curved bottom of a tube or well signifies that agglutination has taken place. The formation of a round button where the red blood cells settled to the midpoint of the bottom of the tube or well and were not retained on the curvature constitutes a negative reaction with no agglutination.

Sedormid™ purpura (historical)

A form of thrombocytopenic purpura occurring in patients who received Sedormid (allyl-isopropyl-acetyl carbamide). The drug served as a hapten complexing with blood platelets. The resulting platelet–drug complex was recognized as foreign by the immune system. Antibodies formed against it lysed blood platelets in the presence of complement, leading to thrombocytopenia followed by bleeding and purpura manifested on the skin. This was a type II hypersensitivity reaction. Sedormid™ is no longer used, but the principle of the hypersensitivity it induced is useful for understanding autoimmunity induced by certain drugs.

segmental exchange

Refer to gene conversion.

selectins

A group of cell adhesion molecules (CAMs) that are glycoproteins and play an important role in the relationship of circulating cells to the endothelium. The members of this surface molecule family have three separate structural motifs: a single N terminal (extracellular) lectin motif preceding a single epidermal growth factor repeat and various short consensus repeat homology units. Selectins are involved in lymphocyte migration. These carbohydrate-binding proteins facilitate adhesion of leukocytes to endothelial cells. A single chain transmembrane glycoprotein located in each selectin molecule has a similar modular structure including the extracellular calcium-dependent lectin domain. The three groups of selectins include

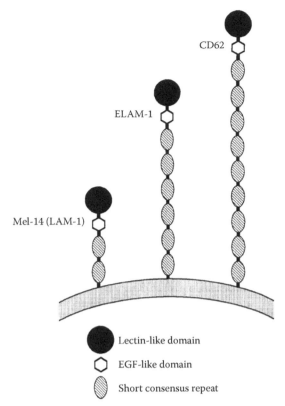

Selectins.

L-selectin (CD62L) expressed on leukocytes; P-selectin (CD62P) expressed on platelets and activated endothelium; and E-selectin (CD62E) expressed on activated endothelium. Under shear forces, the characteristic structural motif is comprised of an N terminal lectin domain, a domain with homology to epidermal growth factor (EGF), and various complement regulatory protein repeat sequences. Refer also to E-selectin, L-selectin, P-selectin, and CD62.

selective IgA and IgG deficiency

This disease that affects both sexes is either X-linked, autosomal-recessive, or acquired later in life. A genetic defect in the switch mechanism may cause immunoglobulin-producing cells to change from immunoglobulin M (IgM) to IgG or IgA synthesis. Respiratory infections with pyogenic microorganisms or autoimmune states that include hemolytic anemia, thrombocytopenia, and neutropenia may occur. Numerous IgM-synthesizing plasma cells are demonstrable in lymph nodes and spleens of affected individuals.

selective IgA and IgM deficiency

A concomitant reduction in both immunoglobulin A (IgA) and IgM concentrations with normal IgG levels. The IgG produced in many individuals may not be protective and recurrent infections may result. The response to many immunogens is inadequate in this disease, which occurs in four males for every female affected.

selective IgA deficiency

The most frequent immunodeficiency disorder affecting approximately 1 in 600 individuals. It is characterized by nearly absent serum and secretory immunoglobulin A (IgA). The IgA level is less than 5 mg/dL, whereas the remaining immunoglobulin class levels are normal or elevated. The disorder is familial or may be acquired in association with measles, other types of virus infection, or toxoplasmosis. Patients may appear normal and asymptomatic or may exhibit some form of an associated disease. IgA is the principal immunoglobulin in secretions and is an important part of the defense of mucosal surfaces; thus, IgA-deficient individuals have increased incidence of respiratory, gastrointestinal, and urogenital infections. They may manifest sinopulmonary infections and diarrhea. Selective IgA deficiency is diagnosed by the demonstration of less than 5 mg/dL of IgA in serum. The etiology is unknown but is believed to be arrested B cell development. B lymphocytes are normal with surface IgA and IgM or surface IgA and IgD. Some patients also have IgG$_2$ and IgG$_4$ subclass deficiencies and are likely to develop infections. IgA-deficient patients show increased incidence of respiratory allergies and autoimmune diseases such as systemic lupus erythematosus (SLE) and rheumatoid arthritis. The principal defect is in IgA B lymphocyte differentiation. A 12-week-old fetus reveals the first IgA B lymphocytes that bear IgM and IgD as well as IgA on their surfaces. At birth, the formation of mature IgA B lymphocytes begins. Most IgA B cells express IgA exclusively on their surfaces, with only 10% expressing surface IgM and IgD in adults. Patients with selective IgA deficiency usually express the immature phenotypes, only a few of which can transform into IgA-synthesizing plasma cells. Patients have increased incidence of HLA-A1, -B8, and -Dw3. Their IgA cells form but do not secrete IgA. The incidence of the disorder is increased in certain atopic individuals. Some patients with selective IgA deficiency form significant titers of antibody against IgA. They may develop anaphylactic reactions upon receiving IgA-containing blood transfusions. They exhibit increased incidence of celiac disease and several autoimmune diseases as noted above. They synthesize normal levels of IgG and IgM antibodies. Autosomal-recessive and autosomal-dominant patterns of inheritance have been described. The deficiency has been associated with several cancers including thymoma, reticulum cell sarcoma, and squamous cell carcinoma of the esophagus and lungs. Certain cases may be linked to drugs such as phenytoin or other anticonvulsants. Some individuals develop antibodies against IgG, IgM, and IgA. γ globulin should not be administered to patients with selective IgA deficiency.

selective IgM deficiency

Immunoglobulin M (IgM) is absent from the serum. Although IgM may be demonstrable on plasma cell surfaces, it is not secreted. This condition may be related to an alteration in secretory peptide or arise from the actions of suppressor T lymphocytes specifically on IgM-synthesizing and -secreting cells. Gram-negative microorganisms may induce septicemia in affected individuals, as the major role of IgM in protection against infection is in the intravascular compartment rather than in extravascular spaces where other immunoglobulin classes may be active.

selective immunoglobulin deficiency

An insufficient quantity of one of the three major immunoglobulins or a subclass of IgG or IgA. The most common is selective IgA deficiency followed by IgG$_3$ and IgG$_2$ deficiencies. Patients suffering from selective immunoglobulin deficiency may appear normal or manifest increased risk for bacterial infections.

selective theory

A hypothesis describing antibody synthesis as a process in which antigen selects cells expressing receptors specific for that antigen. The antigen–cell receptor interaction leads to proliferation and differentiation of a clone of cells that synthesizes significant quantities of antibodies of a single specificity. Selective theories included the 1899 side chain theory of Paul Ehrlich, the natural selection theory proposed by Niels Jerne in 1955, and the cell selection theory Talmage and Burnet proposed in 1957. Burnet named his version the clonal selection theory of acquired immunity; its basic tenets

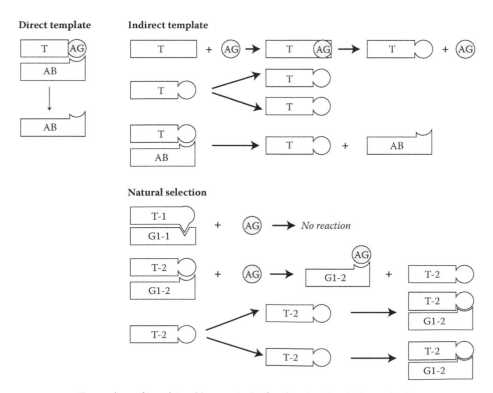

Comparison of template with natural selection theories of antibody synthesis.

have been substantiated by scientific evidence. The selective theories maintained that cells were genetically programmed to react to certain antigenic specificities prior to antigen exposure. These theories are in sharp contrast to the instructive theories postulating that antigen was necessary to serve as a template around which polypeptide chains were folded to yield specific antibodies. The template theory was abandoned when antibody was demonstrated in the absence of antigen.

self antigen

Autoantigen. All normal body constituents to which the immune response would respond were it not for immunologic tolerance to these self epitopes.

self MHC

The major histocompatibility complex (MHC) molecules of a single individual.

self marker hypothesis (historical)

A concept suggested by Burnet and Fenner in 1949 to account for the failure of the body to react against its own antigens. They proposed that cells contained markers that identified them to the host's immunologically competent cells as self. This recognition system was supposed to prevent the immune cells of the host from rejecting its own tissue cells. This hypothesis was later abandoned by the authors and replaced by the clonal selection theory of acquired immunity that Burnet proposed in 1957.

self MHC restriction

The confinement of antigens that an individual's T cells can recognize to complexes of peptides bound to major histocompatibility complex (MHC) molecules in the thymus during T lymphocyte maturation (i.e., self MHC molecules). Positive selection leads to self MHC restriction of the T cell repertoire.

self peptides

Peptides formed from proteins of the body. In the absence of infection, these peptides occupy the peptide binding sites of major histocompatibility complex (MHC) molecules on cell surfaces.

self recognition

The identification of autoantigens by lymphoid cells of the immune system. This is a consequence of the establishment of immunological tolerance of self antigens during fetal development.

self renewal

The capacity of a cell population to restore itself.

self restriction

Refer to MHC restriction.

self tolerance

The body's acceptance of its own epitopes as self antigens. The body is tolerant to these autoantigens that are exposed to lymphoid cells of the host immune system without eliciting an immune response. Tolerance to self antigens is developed during fetal life. Thus, a host is immunologically tolerant to self or autoantigens. Self tolerance is due mainly to inactivation or killing of self-reactive lymphocytes induced by exposure to self antigens. Failure of self tolerance in the normal immune system may lead to autoimmune diseases. Refer also to tolerance and immunologic tolerance.

semisyngeneic graft

A graft that is ordinarily accepted from an individual of one strain into an F_1 hybrid of an individual of that strain mated with an individual of a different strain.

senescent cell antigen

A neoantigen appearing on old red blood cells that binds immunoglobulin G (IgG) autoantibodies. Senescent cell antigen is also found on lymphocytes, platelets, neutrophils, adult human liver cells (in culture), and human embryonic renal cells (in culture). Its appearance on aging somatic cells probably represents a physiologic process to remove senescent and injured cells that fulfilled their functions. Macrophages can identify and phagocytize dying and aging self cells that are no longer functional without disturbing mature healthy cells.

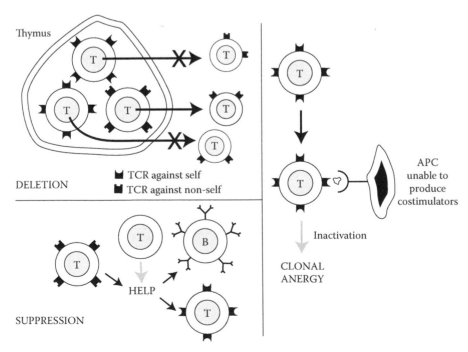

Mechanism of self tolerance.

Takes

1. Autograft

2. Isograft (Syngeneic graft)

A strain   A strain

3. Semisyngeneic Graft

A strain   (A × B)F₁

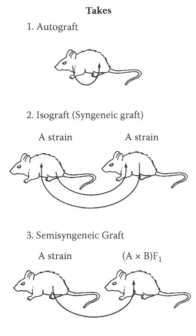

Rejects

1. Allograft

A strain   B strain

2. Semisyngeneic Graft

A strain   (A × B)F₁

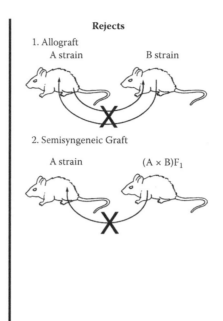

Semisyngeneic graft.

sensitization

(1) Initial exposure of an animal to an antigen so that subsequent or secondary exposure to the same antigen will lead to a greater response. The term is used primarily when the reaction induced is more hypersensitive or allergic than indicative of a protective immune type of response. Thus, an allergic response may be induced in a host sensitized by prior exposure to the same allergen. Linked with immune deviation to Th2 response. (2) Term originally used by investigators who developed the complement fixation test to describe the coating of cells such as red blood cells with specific antibody to "sensitize" them for subsequent lysis by complement. (3) Sensitization associated with organ or tissue transplantation is known as alloimmunization.

sensitized

Immunized. May also refer to red cells *in vitro* that have been treated with specific antibody prior to addition of complement for lysis.

sensitized cell

(1) A cell such as a lymphocyte that has been activated immunologically by interaction with a specific antigen and is known as a primed lymphocyte. (2) Cells such as sheep red blood cells coated with a specific antibody that renders them susceptible to lysis by complement.

sensitized lymphocyte

A primed lymphocyte previously exposed to a specific antigen.

sensitized vaccine

An immunizing preparation containing bacteria treated with their homologous immune serum.

sensitizing agent

An allergen or antigen that elicits a hypersensitivity response.

sensitizing antigen

A substance responsible for inducing hypersusceptibility or exaggerated reactivity to it.

Sephadex™

A trade name for a series of cross linked dextrans used in chromatography.

Sepharose™

A trade name for agarose gels used in electrophoresis.

sepsis

Bloodstream infection that is life threatening and often leads to death. Septic shock may follow infection of the blood with Gram-negative microorganisms through the release of tumor necrosis factor α (TNF-α).

septic shock

Hypotension (systolic blood pressure below 90 mmHg or a decrease in the systolic pressure baseline of more than 40 mmHg) in individuals with sepsis. The shock may be induced by the systemic release of tumor necrosis factor α (TNF-α) following bacterial infection of the blood, frequently with Gram-negative bacteria. Vascular collapse, disseminated intravascular coagulation, and metabolic disorders occur. Septic shock results from the effects of bacterial lipopolysaccharide (LPS) and cytokines, including TNF, interleukin-12 (IL12), and IL1. Also termed endotoxin shock.

septicemia

The presence and persistence of pathogenic microorganisms or their toxins in the blood. Also termed blood poisoning.

sequence motif

A mosaic of nucleotides or amino acids shared by different genes or proteins that frequently have related functions. Sequence motifs in peptides that bind a specific major histocompatibility complex (MHC) glycoprotein are based on the requirements for a particular amino acid to achieve binding to that particular MHC molecule.

sequence-specific priming (SSP)

A method that employs a primer with a single mismatch at the 3′ end that cannot be employed efficiently to extend a DNA strand because the Taq polymerase enzyme during the polymerase chain reaction (PCR) and especially in the first very critical PCR cycles does not manifest 3′–5′ proofreading endonuclease activity to remove the mismatched nucleotide. If primer pairs are designed to have perfectly matched 3′ ends with only a single allele or a single group of alleles

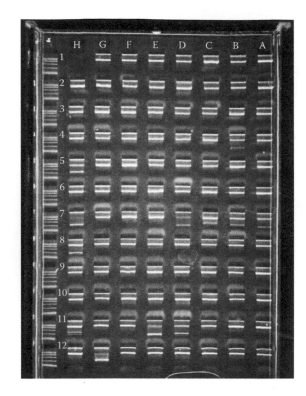

Example of high resolution DRB1 typing using sequence-specific primer methodology. Molecular weight ladder of known base pairs for base pair sizing appears at far left.

and the PCR reaction is initiated under stringent conditions, a perfectly matched primer pair results in an amplification product. A mismatch at the 3′ end primer pair will not provide any amplification product. A positive result (amplification) defines the specificity of the DNA sample. The PCR amplification step provides the basis for identifying polymorphism. The post-amplification processing of the sample consists only of a simple agarose gel electrophoresis to detect the presence or absence of amplified product. DNA-amplified fragments are visualized by ethidium bromide staining and exposure to ultraviolet light. A separate technique detects amplified product by color fluorescence. The primer pairs are selected in such a manner that each allele should have a unique reactivity pattern with the panel of primer pairs employed. Appropriate controls must be maintained.

sequential determinant

An epitope whose specificity is determined by the sequence of several residues within the antigenic determinant rather than by the molecular configuration of the antigen molecule. A peptide segment of approximately six amino acid residues represents the sequential determinant structure.

sequestered antigen

An antigen that is anatomically isolated and not in contact with the immunocompetent T and B lymphoid cells of the immune system. Examples include myelin basic protein, sperm antigens, and lens protein antigens. When a sequestered antigen is released by one or several mechanisms including viral inflammation, it can activate immunocompetent T and B cells. An example of the sequestered antigen release mechanism of autoimmunity is found in experimental and post-infectious encephalomyelitis. Cell-mediated injury represents the principal mechanism in this disease. In vasectomized males,

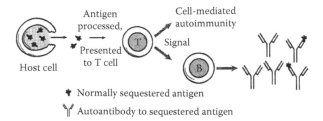

Release of sequestered antigen.

antisperm antibodies are known to develop when sperm antigens become exposed to immunocompetent lymphoid cells. Likewise, lens protein of the eye that enters the circulation as a consequence of crushing injury to the eye or exposure of lens protein to immunocompetent cells inadvertently through surgical manipulation may lead to an antilens protein immune response. Autoimmunity induced by sequestered antigens is relatively infrequent and a rare cause of autoimmune disease.

serial dilution

The successive dilution of antiserum in a row of serological tubes containing physiologic saline solution as diluent to yield the greatest concentration of antibody in the first tube and the lowest in the last tube that contains the highest dilution. For example, a double quantity of antiserum is placed in the first tube, half of which is transferred to the second tube containing an equal volume of diluent. After thorough mixing with a serological pipette, an equivalent amount is transferred to the next tube. The process continues and the volume removed from the last tube in the row is discarded. This represents a doubling dilution.

serial passage

A method to attenuate a pathogenic microorganism but retain its immunogenicity by transfer through several animal hosts, growth media, or tissue culture cells.

serial TC triggering model

A design dependent on the hypothesis that relatively few pMHC complexes can interact successively with enough T cell receptors to yield the sustained signaling requisite for naïve T cell total activation.

seroconversion

The first appearance of specific antibodies against a causative agent in the blood during the course of an infection or following immunization.

serological determinants

Epitopes on cells that react with specific antibody and complement, leading to fatal injuries of cells. Serological determinants are to be distinguished from lymphocyte determinants that are epitopes on cell surfaces to which sensitized lymphocytes are directed, leading to cell destruction. Although the end result is the same, antibodies and lymphocytes are directed to different epitopes on cell surfaces.

serological epitope

An antigenic determinant reactive with a specific antibody or group of antibodies.

serologically defined (SD) antigens

Mammalian cellular membrane epitopes encoded by major histocompatibility complex genes. Antibodies detect these epitopes.

serology

The study of the *in vitro* reactions of antibodies in serum with antigens (usually those of microorganisms inducing infectious disease).

serotherapy

A form of treatment for infectious disease developed almost a century ago in which antiserum raised by immunizing horses or other animals against exotoxin, such as that produced by *Corynebacterium diphtheriae,* was administered to children with diphtheria. This antitoxin neutralized the injurious effects of the toxin; thus, serotherapy was intended for prevention and treatment.

Structural formula of serotonin (5-hydroxytryptamine) released during and participates in the mediation of anaphylactic reactions in some species and not others.

serotonin (5-hydroxytryptamine; 5-HT)

A 176-kDa catecholamine found in mouse and rat mast cells and in human platelets that participates in anaphylaxis in several species such as rabbits, but not in humans. It induces contraction of smooth muscle, enhances vascular permeability of small blood vessels, and induces large blood vessel vasoconstriction. 5-HT is derived from tryptophan by hydroxylation to 5-hydroxytryptophan and decarboxylation to 5-hydroxytryptamine. In humans, gut enterochromaffin cells contain 90% of 5-HT, with the remainder accruing in platelets and the brain. 5-HT is a potent biogenic amine with wide species distribution. It may stimulate phagocytosis by leukocytes and interfere with the clearance of particles by the mononuclear phagocyte system. Immunoperoxidase staining for 5-HT, which is synthesized by various neoplasms, especially carcinoid tumors, is a valuable aid in surgical pathologic diagnosis of tumors producing it.

serotype

The mosaic of epitope of a microorganism defined by specific antibodies.

serotyping

The use of specific antibodies to classify bacterial subtypes based on variations in the surface epitopes of the microorganism. Serotyping has long been used to classify *Salmonella,* streptococci, *Shigella,* and other bacteria. May also describe human alloantigens such as human leukocyte antigen (HLA) and blood group antigens.

serpins

A large family of protease inhibitors.

serum

The yellow-tinged fluid that forms following blood coagulation. Plasma contains fibrinogen, but serum does not; thus, serum is the part of plasma that remains after removal of fibrinogen and clotting factors. Serum contains 35 to 55 mg/mL of serum albumin, approximately 20 mg/mL of immunoglobulins, 3 mg/mL each of transferrin and α-1 antitrypsin, 2.5 mg/mL of α_2 macroglobulin, and 2 mg/mL of haptoglobin. It is more convenient to use serum than plasma in immune reactions since clotting may interfere with certain assays.

serum albumin

The principal protein in serum or plasma. It is soluble in water and in partially concentrated salt solutions such as 50% saturated ammonium sulfate. It is coagulated by heat and accounts for much of the plasma colloidal osmotic pressure. Serum albumin functions as a transport protein for fatty acids, bilirubin, and other large organic anions. It also carries selected hormones including cortisol and thyroxine and many drugs. It is formed in the liver. Levels in the serum decrease under conditions of protein malnutrition or significant liver and kidney disease. In neutral pH, albumin has a negative charge, causing its rapid movement toward the anode during electrophoresis. It is composed of a single 585-amino acid residue chain and has a concentration of 35 to 55 mg/mL. Bovine serum albumin (BSA) and selected other serum albumins have been used as experimental immunogens.

serum amyloid A (SAA) component

A 12-kDa protein in serum that is a precursor of the AA class of amyloid fibril proteins. SAA is formed in the liver and associates with HDL3 lipoproteins in the circulation. It is a 114-amino acid residue polypeptide chain. Its conversion to AA involves splitting of peptides from both amino and carboxyl terminals to yield an 8.5-kDa protein that forms fibrillar amyloid deposits. SAA levels during inflammation may increase 1000-fold.

serum amyloid P (SAP) component

A serum protein that constitutes a minor second component in all amyloid deposits. Under electron microscopy, it appears as a doughnut-shaped pentagon with an external diameter of 9 nm and an internal diameter of 4 nm. Each pentagon has five globular subunits. The amyloid P component in serum consists of two doughnut-shaped structures. Unlike the serum amyloid A component, the P component does not increase during inflammation. It constitutes 10% of amyloid deposits and is indistinguishable from normal α_1 serum glycoprotein. This 180- to 212-kDa substance shows close structural homology with C-reactive protein.

serum antitoxins

Antibodies specific for exotoxins produced by selected microorganisms such as the causative agents of diphtheria and tetanus. Prior to the use of antibiotics, antitoxins were the treatments of choice for diseases produced by the exotoxin products of microorganisms such as *Corynebacterium diphtheriae* and *Clostridium tetani.*

serum hepatitis (hepatitis B)

An infection with a relatively long incubation lasting 2 to 5 months, caused by a double-stranded DNA virus. Transmission may be via administration of serum or blood products. Other high risk groups include drug addicts, dialysis patients, healthcare workers, male homosexuals, and newborns with human immunodeficiency virus (HIV)-infected mothers. Chronic infection may occur in immunosuppressed individuals or those with lymphoid cancer. The infection may be acute or chronic, and hepatocellular carcinoma may be a complication. In acute HBV infection, the hepatocytes may undergo ballooning and eosinophilic degeneration. Focal necrosis of hepatocytes and lymphocytic infiltration of the portal areas and liver parenchyma may occur, in addition to central and mid-zonal necrosis of hepatocytes. Chronic type B hepatitis may progress to cirrhosis and hepatocellular carcinoma. Hepatocellular injury is induced by immunity to the virus. HBsAg, HBeAg, and IgM anti-HBc are present in the serum in acute hepatitis. In the convalescent phase of acute hepatitis, IgG anti-HBs appears in the serum. HBsAg, HBeAg, IgG anti-HBc in

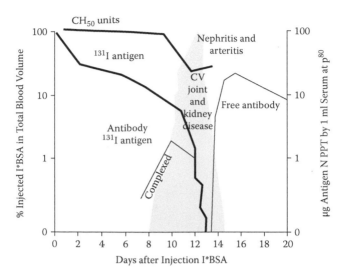

Experimental serum sickness induced by injection of radiolabeled bovine serum albumin (1*BSA) into rabbits by Frank J. Dixon and associates. CH_{50} units, complement activity.

high titer, HBV DNA, and DNA polymerase appear in the serum in the active viral replication phase of chronic hepatitis. In the viral integration phase, HBsAg, anti-HBc, and anti-HBe appear in the serum. Patients with acute hepatitis B often recover completely. Refer to hepatitis B.

serum sickness

A systemic reaction that follows the injection of a relatively large, single dose of serum (e.g., antitoxin). It is characterized by systemic vasculitis (arteritis), glomerulonephritis, and arthritis. The lesions follow deposition in tissues, such as the microvasculature, of immune complexes that form after antibody appears in the circulation between the 5th and 14th days following antigen administration. The antigen–antibody complexes fix complement and initiate a classic type III hypersensitivity reaction resulting in immune-mediated tissue injury. Patients may develop fever, lymphadenopathy, urticaria, and sometimes arthritis. The pathogenesis of serum sickness is a classic type III reaction. Antigen escaping into circulation from the site of injection forms immune complexes that damage small vessels. The antibodies involved in the classic type of serum sickness are of the precipitating variety, usually IgG. They may be detected by passive hemagglutination. Pathologically, serum sickness is a systemic immune complex disease characterized by vasculitis, glomerulonephritis, and arthritis due to the intravascular formation and deposition of immune complexes that subsequently fix complement and attract polymorphonuclear neutrophils to the site through the chemotactic effects of C5a, thereby initiating inflammation. The classic reaction occurring 7 to 15 days after the triggering injection is called the primary form. Similar manifestations appearing only 1 to 3 days following the injection represent the accelerated form of serum sickness and occur in subjects presumably already sensitized. A third (anaphylactic) form develops immediately after injection, apparently due to reaginic IgE antibodies. It usually occurs in atopic subjects sensitized by horse dander or previous exposure to serum treatment. The serum sickness-like syndromes seen in drug allergy have similar clinical pictures and similar pathogenesis. Refer also to type III immune complex-mediated hypersensitivity.

serum spreading factors

In plasma, 65- and 75-kDa glycoproteins that facilitate adherence of cells and the ability of cells to spread and differentiate. Refer to vitronectin.

serum thymic factor (STF)

An obsolete term for thymulin.

serum virus vaccination

An obsolete method of administering an immunizing preparation of an infectious agent such as a live vaccine virus along with an antiserum specific for the virus that was intended to ameliorate the effects of the live infectious agent. The method was abandoned because it was considered dangerous.

severe combined immunodeficient (SCID) mouse

A spontaneous mutation in BALB/c mice characterized by impairment of double-stranded DNA break repair. V(D) J rearrangement is mainly affected, leading to a defective coding joint formation that prevents maturation of B and T lymphocytes. At the molecular level, the SCID mutation is a genetically determined deficiency of the DNA-dependent protein kinase (DNA-PK) that induces DNA break repair by forming an activated complex with the DNA end-binding Ku proteins (p80 and p70) upon association with damaged DNA.

severe combined immunodeficiency (SCID) syndrome

A group of primary immunodeficiencies involving loss of T and B cell functions and sometimes NK cell function as a consequence of genetic defects. The profound immunodeficiency is inherited as an X-linked or autosomal-recessive disease. The thymus has only sparse lymphocytes and Hassall's corpuscles or is bereft of them. Several congenital immunodeficiencies are characterized as SCID. T and B cell lymphopenia and decreased production of IL-2 are observed, as is an absence of delayed-type hypersensitivity, cellular immunity, and normal antibody synthesis following immunogenic challenge. SCID is a disease of infancy and failure to thrive. Affected children frequently die during the first 2 years of life. Clinically, they may develop measles-like rashes, show hyperpigmentation, and develop severe recurrent (especially pulmonary) infections. They face heightened susceptibility to infectious disease agents such as *Pneumocystis carinii*, *Candida albicans*, and others.

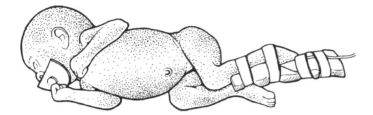

Severe combined immunodeficiency (SCID) syndrome.

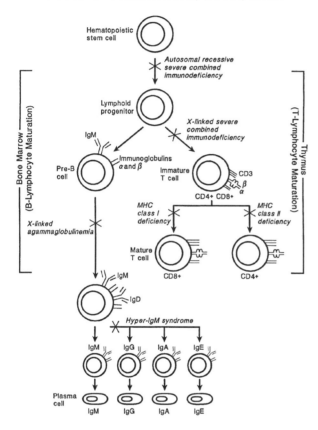

Maturation of T and B lymphocytes.

Even attenuated microorganisms such as those used for immunization (e.g., attenuated poliomyelitis viruses) may induce infection in SCID patients. Graft-vs.-host disease is a problem in patients receiving unirradiated blood transfusions. Maternal–fetal transfusions during gestation or at parturition or blood transfusions at later dates provide sufficient immunologically competent cells entering the SCID patient's circulation to induce graft-vs.-host disease. SCID may be manifested in one of several forms; it is classified as a defect in adenosine deaminase (ADA) and purine nucleoside phosphorylase (PNP) enzymes and in a DNA-binding protein needed for human leukocyte antigen (HLA) gene expression. Treatment is by bone marrow transplantation or gene therapy and enzyme reconstitution in cases caused by a missing gene such as ADA deficiency. X-linked SCID (XSCID), induced by defects in *IL2RG*, the gene encoding the interleukin-2 (IL2) receptor γ chain, is the major genetic form. It occurs in 1 in 50,000 to 100,000 births. Only males, who have single X chromosomes, become ill with XSCID. Females may be carriers, passing along the condition to male offspring. A previously fatal disease, XSCID is now effectively treated by bone marrow transplantation. The cause and pathogenesis of the disease are known and specific gene defects can be identified and traced in patients and at-risk family members.

sex hormones and immunity

Females are more susceptible to certain autoimmune diseases than males, an observation that immediately led to suspicion that sex hormones played a role. The exact mechanisms through which sex steroids interact with the immune system remain to be determined, but sex hormones exert direct effects on immune system cells and indirect effects through cells that control growth and development of the immune system or through organs that are ultimately destroyed by autoimmune reactions. Female mice synthesize more antibodies in response to certain antigens than males, but humans injected with vaccines show essentially identical antibody responses regardless of sex. Murine cell-mediated responses to selected antigens were stronger in females than in males. Sex steroids have profound effects on the thymus. Androgen or estrogen administration to experimental animals led to thymic involution and castration led to thymic enlargement. The thymus is markedly involuted during pregnancy, but achieves its normal size and shape following parturition. Sex steroids have numerous targets including bone marrow and thymus where the precursors of immunity originate and differentiate. Further studies determined how sex hormones control cytokine genes. Sex steroid hormones affect the development and functions of various immune system cells.

sex limited protein

Refer to slp.

Sézary cell

T lymphocytes that form E rosettes with sheep red cells and react with anti-T antibodies. Sézary cells from most individuals show diminished responses to plant mitogens, although those from a few demonstrate normal reactivity. Sézary cells are also poor mediators of T cell cytotoxicity, but they can produce a migration inhibitory factor (MIF)-like lymphokine. Sézary cells do not produce immunoglobulin or act as suppressors. They exert helper effects for immunoglobulin synthesis by B cells.

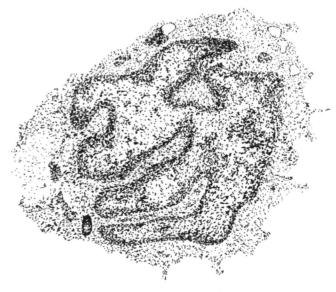

Lymphocyte from a patient with Sézary syndrome.

Sézary syndrome

A disease that occurs in middle age, affecting males more commonly than females. It is a neoplasm (malignant lymphoma of CD4+ T helper lymphocytes with prominent skin involvement). Generalized erythroderma, hyperpigmentation, and exfoliation are observed. Fissuring and scaling of the skin on the palms of the hands and soles of the feet may occur. The peripheral blood and lymph nodes contain the typical cerebriform cells that have nuclei that resemble the brain. Infiltration of the skin by leukocytes is extensive, with prominent clustering in the epidermis forming Pautrier's abscesses. Late in the disease, T immunoblasts may appear. The so-called Sézary cells are T lymphocytes. This syndrome is an advanced type of mycosis fungoides.

SH2 domain

Refer to Src family tyrosine kinases.

shared haplotype

Phenotypic characteristic shared by two siblings based on closely linked genes on one chromosome inherited from each parent. There are four different possibilities of reassortment among offspring, which leads to a particular sibling pair sharing two, one or no haplotypes. Selected haplotypes are in strong linkage disequilibrium between alleles of different loci. According to Mendelian genetics, 25% of siblings will share both haplotypes. Siblings are much more likely to share one or two haplotypes than are unrelated individuals.

sheep red blood cell agglutination test

An assay in which sheep erythrocytes are agglutinated by antibody or are used as carrier particles for an antigen adsorbed to their surfaces, in which case they are passively agglutinated by antibodies specific for the adsorbed antigen.

shift assay

A useful method for identifying protein–DNA interactions that may mediate gene expression, DNA repair, or DNA packaging. The assay can also be used to determine the affinity abundance, binding constants, and binding specificity of DNA-binding proteins. The gel shift assay is performed by annealing two labeled oligonucleotides that contain the test binding sequence, then incubating the duplex with the binding protein. The mixture is then separated on a nondenaturing polyacrylamide gel. Duplexes bound by protein migrate more slowly than unbound duplexes and appear as bands that are shifted relative to the bands from the unbound duplexes. Also called gel mobility shift assay, gel shift assay, gel retardation, or band shift assay.

***Shigella* immunity**

The host protective immune response to *Shigella* infection is poorly understood. Because M cells of the gut take up the microorganisms, secretory immunoglobulin A (IgA) immune responsiveness has been postulated to be protective in shigellosis, but this has been difficult to establish. The immunity induced is type-specific, with reinfection occurring only within different *Shigella* species or serotypes. This immunity is believed to be associated with an immune response to lipopolysaccharide determinants. *Shigella* may destroy antigen-presenting cells in a host following systemic exposure to *Shigella* antigens and toxins before an immune response can be established. Serum IgG has no protective effect. Oral vaccines with attenuated *Shigella* induce type-specific protection. Previous *Shigella* infection leads to specific IgA secretion in breast milk. Antibodies develop early against somatic *Shigella* antigens. Shiga toxin is a multimeric protein comprised of a single enzymatically active A subunit and five B subunits needed for toxin binding. It is synthesized only by *Shigella dysenteriae* type I strains and is an important virulence factor in the pathogenesis of hemolytic–uremic syndrome that may be a complication of infection. Shiga toxin induces IgM antibody responses, but the IgG response is lacking; however, IgG can be raised against Shiga toxin in animal models. Protection against *Shigella* has been associated with the humoral response to lipopolysaccharide (LPS) or plasmid-encoded protein antigens. T cells also become activated *in vivo* during *Shigella* infection. There may be some correlation between T cell activation and disease severity. Local cytokine synthesis is also significant in shigellosis. Increased levels of interleukin-1 (IL1), IL6, tumor necrosis factor (TNF), and interferon-γ (IFN-γ) have been found in stool specimens and plasma of infected patients. Both Th1 and Th2 cytokines are present in shigellosis. Humoral and cytotoxic defense mechanisms may be present during infection. High serum antitoxin titers failed to protect monkeys against intestinal disease following challenge with live *Shigella dysentariae*. Heat-killed whole cell *Shigella* vaccines failed to protect. Post-infection reactive arthritis may occur. Although mucosal secretory IgA is thought to prevent bacterial attachment to the mucosa and neutralize toxins, the significance of these mechanisms in shigellosis has not been proven.

shingles (herpes zoster)

A virus infection that occurs in a band-like pattern according to distribution in the skin of involved nerves. It is usually a reactivation of the virus that causes chickenpox.

SHIV

Simian–human immunodeficiency virus. A SIV$_{mac}$ and HIV-1 chimera capable of infecting macaques, it possesses the HIV genes ENV, Tat, Rev, and Vpu, with its remaining genes derived from SIV$_{mac}$.

shocking dose

The amount of antigen required to elicit a particular clinical response or syndrome.

shock organ

An organ involved in a specific reaction such as an anaphylactic reaction.

short-lived lymphocytes

Lymphocytes with lifespans of 4 to 5 days, in contrast to long-lived lymphocytes that may exist in blood circulation from months to years.

Shulman, Sidney

Professor of microbiology and immunology at the University of Buffalo who performed important work on immune aspects of human infertility.

Shwartzman, Gregory (1896–1965)

Russian–American microbiologist who described systemic and local reactions that follow injection of bacterial endotoxins. The systemic Shwartzman reaction, a nonimmunologic phenomenon, is related to disseminated intravascular coagulation. The local Shwartzman reaction in skin resembles the immunologically based Arthus reaction in appearance. (Refer to *Phenomenon of Local Tissue Reactivity and Its Immunological and Clinical Significance*, 1937.)

Shwartzman (or Shwartzman–Sanarelli) reaction

A nonimmunologic phenomenon in which endotoxin (lipopolysaccharide) induces local and systemic reactions.

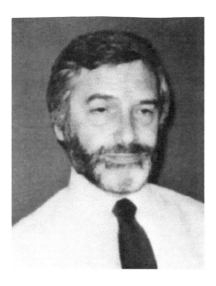

Sidney Shulman.

Following the initial or preparatory injection of endotoxin into the skin, polymorphonuclear leukocytes accumulate and are then thought to release lysosomal acid hydrolases that injure the walls of small vessels, preparing them for the second provocative injection of endotoxin. The intradermal injection of endotoxin into the skin of a rabbit followed within 24 hours by the intravenous injection of the same or a different endotoxin leads to hemorrhage at the local site of the initial injection. Although the local Shwartzman reaction may resemble an Arthus reaction in appearance, the Arthus reaction is immunological and the Shwartzman reaction is not. In the Shwartzman reaction, the time between the first and second injections is insufficient to induce an immune reaction in a previously unsensitized host. There is also a lack of specificity: different endotoxins may be used for first and second injections. The generalized or systemic Shwartzman reaction again involves two injections of endotoxin; however, both are administered

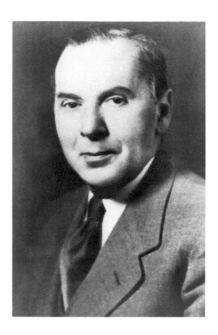

Gregory Shwartzman.

intravenously, one 24 hours following the first. The generalized Shwartzman reaction is the experimental equivalent of disseminated intravascular coagulation found in a number of human diseases. Following the first injection, sparse fibrin thrombi are formed in the vasculature of the lungs, kidney, liver, and capillaries of the spleen. The reticuloendothelial system is blocked, as its mononuclear phagocytes proceed to clear thromboplastin and fibrin. Administration of the second dose of endotoxin while the reticuloendothelial system is blocked leads to profound intravascular coagulation because the mononuclear phagocytes are unable to remove the thromboplastin and fibrin. Bilateral cortical necrosis of the kidneys and splenic hemorrhage and necrosis are observed. Neither platelets nor leukocytes are present in the fibrin thrombi that are formed. The

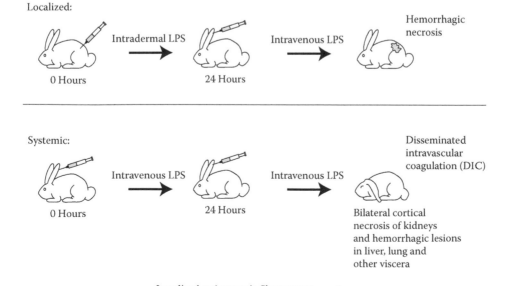

Localized and systemic Shwartzman reaction.

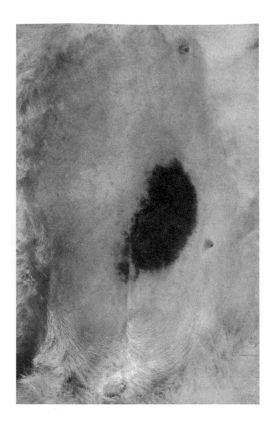

Ventral view of a rabbit in which the localized Shwartzman reaction was induced with endotoxin. Note hemorrhage and necrosis.

Shwartzman reaction may be induced by two sequential exposures to LPS or IL-1.

sia test (historical)

A former qualitative test for macroglobulinemia in which patient serum was placed in water in one tube and in saline in another tube. Precipitation of the serum in water attributable to the low water solubility of immunoglobulin M (IgM) but not in saline constituted a positive test.

sialophorin (CD43)

A principal glycoprotein present on the surfaces of thymocytes, T cells, selected B lymphocytes, neutrophils, platelets, and monocytes. Monocyte and lymphocyte sialophorin is a 115-kDa polypeptide chain. The platelet and neutrophil sialophorin is a 135-kDa polypeptide chain that differs from the first form only in carbohydrate content. Galactose β1–3 galactosamine in O-linked saccharides bound to threonine or serine amino acid residues represents a site of attachment for sialic acid in thymocytes in the medulla and in mature T cells. Incomplete sialylation of thymocytes in the thymic cortex accounts for their binding to peanut lectin. The more thoroughly sialylated structures on T cells and thymocytes in the medulla fail to bind lectin. In humans, the sialophorin molecule is composed of 400 amino acid residues: a 235-residue extracellular domain, a 23-residue transmembrane portion, and a 123-residue domain in the cytoplasm. Antibodies specific for CD43 can activate T cells. The T cells of patients with Wiskott–Aldrich syndrome have defective sialophorin.

sicca complex

A condition characterized by dryness of mucous membranes, especially of the eyes, producing keratoconjunctivitis attributable to decreased tearing that results from lymphocytic infiltration of the lachrymal glands, and by dry mouth (xerostomia), associated with decreased formation of saliva as a result of lymphocytic infiltration of the salivary glands producing obstruction of the duct. Sicca complex is most frequently seen in patients with Sjögren's syndrome, but it also may be seen in sarcoidosis, amyloidosis, hemochromatosis, vitamin A and C deficiencies, scleroderma, and hyperlipoproteinemia types IV and V.

sicca symptoms

Symptoms marked by dry eyes leading to blurry vision, dry mouth (xerostomia) and dry throat, leading to swallowing difficulties, and dry nose and skin.

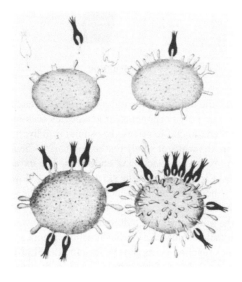

DIAGRAMMATIC REPRESENTATION OF THE SIDE-CHAIN THEORY
(PLATES I AND II)

Fig. 1 "The groups [the haptophore group of the side-chain of the cell and that of the food-stuff or the toxin] must be adapted to one another, *e.g.*, as male and female screw (PASTEUR), or as lock and key (E. FISCHER)."

Fig. 2 ". . . the first stage in the toxic action must be regarded as being the union of the toxin by means of its haptophore group to a special side-chain of the cell protoplasm."

Fig. 3 "The side-chain involved, so long as the union lasts, cannot exercise its normal, physiological, nutritive function . . ."

Fig. 4 "We are therefore now concerned with a defect which, according to the principles so ably worked out by . . . Weigert, is . . . [overcorrected] by regeneration."

Side-Chain Theory

Paul Ehrlich's side-chain theory, developed in 1900, was the first selective theory of antibody synthesis. Although elaborate in detail, the essential feature of the theory was that cells of the immune system possess the genetic capability to react to all known antigens and that each cell on the surface bears receptors with surface haptophore side chains. On combination with antigen, the side chains would be cast off into the circulation and new receptors would replace old ones. These cast-off receptors represented antibody molecules in the circulation. Although far more complex than this explanation, the importance of the theory was in the amount of research stimulated trying to disprove it. Nevertheless, it was the first effort to account for the importance of genetics in immune responsiveness at a time when Mendel's basic studies had not yet been rediscovered by De Vries.

side chain theory

In 1899, Paul Ehrlich postulated that a cell possessed highly complex chemical aggregates with attached groupings or side chains whose normal function was to anchor nutrient

S

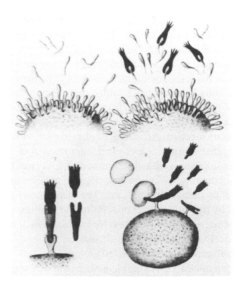

DIAGRAMMATIC REPRESENTATION OF THE SIDE-CHAIN THEORY
(cont.)

Fig. 5   ". . . the antitoxins represent nothing more than the side-chains reproduced in excess during regeneration and therefore pushed off from the protoplasm—thus coming to exist in a free state."

Fig. 6   [The free side-chains (circulating antitoxins) unite with the toxins and thus protect the cell.]

Fig. 7   ". . . two haptophore groups must be ascribed to the 'immune-body [haemolytic amboceptor], one having a strong affinity for a corresponding haptophore group of the red blood corpuscles, . . . and another . . which . . . becomes united with the 'complement' . . ."

Fig. 8   "If a cell . . . has, with the assistance of an appropriate side-chain, fixed to itself a giant [protein] molecule . . . there is provided [only] one of the conditions essential for the cell nourishment. Such . . . molecules . . are not available until . . . they have been split into smaller fragments This will be . . . attained if . . . the 'tentacle' . . . possesses . . . second haptophore group adapted to take to itself ferment-like materia . . ."

Side-Chain Theory

Side-Chain Theory, continued.

substances to the cell prior to internalization. These side chains or receptors were considered to permit cellular interaction with substances in the extracellular environment. Antigens were postulated to stimulate cells by attachment to the receptors. Because antigens played no part in the normal cell economy, the receptors were diverted from their normal function. Stimulated by this derangement of their normal mechanism, cells produced excessive new receptors of the same type as those thrown out of action. The superfluous receptors were shed into the extracellular fluids and constituted specific antibodies with the capacity to bind homologous antigens. Ehrlich proposed a haptophore group that reacted with a corresponding group of an antigen, as in neutralization of toxin by antitoxin. For reactions such as agglutination or precipitation, he postulated that another (ergophobe) group determined the change in antigen after the antibody was anchored by its haptophore group. Ehrlich proposed receptors with two haptophore groups: one that attached to antigen and the other to complement. The group that combined with the cell or other antigen was called the cytophilic group, and the group that combined with complement was the complementophilic group. Ehrlich called these types of receptors amboceptors because both groups were supposed to be of the haptophore type. He considered a toxin to have a haptophore group and a toxophore group. Detoxification without loss of antitoxin-binding capacity led Ehrlich to believe that a toxophore group was altered while the haptophore group

remained intact. His theory assumed that each antibody-forming cell had the ability to react to every antigen in nature. The demonstration by Landsteiner that antibodies could be formed against substances manufactured in a laboratory and never present in nature led to abandonment of the side chain theory although its basic premise as a selective hypothesis rather than an instructive theory was ultimately proven correct.

side effect

An unwanted reaction to a drug administered to achieve a desirable curative or other effect.

signal hypothesis

A proposed mechanism for selection of secretory proteins by and for transport through the rough endoplasmic reticulum. The free heavy and light chain leader peptide is postulated to facilitate the joining of polyribosomes forming these molecules to the endoplasmic reticulum. The hypothesis also cites the release of heavy and light polypeptide chains through the endoplasmic reticulum membrane into the cisternal space followed by immunoglobulin secretion after the immunoglobulin molecule has been assembled and to the pathways whereby proteins reach their proper cellular destinations. Important to protein targeting is the signal sequence—a short amino acid sequence at the amino terminus of a polypeptide chain. This signal sequence directs the protein to the proper destination in a cell and is removed during passage or when the protein arrives at its final location.

signal joint

A structure produced by the precise joining of recognition signal sequences during somatic recombination that produces T cell receptor (TCR) and immunoglobulin (Ig) genes. The DNA sequence produced by uniting of blunt RSS ends after V(D)J recombination of gene segments.

signal pathway DNA-binding proteins

Because DNA-binding proteins are made in genes distant to their sites of activity, they are designated trans-acting. These proteins are transcription factors that interact with enhancers and promoters by binding to unique nucleotide sequences. Due to these interactions, DNA-binding proteins regulate the transcription of the genes under the influence of each promoter or enhancer. They are important means of signal transduction through which external stimuli induce responses at the nuclear level.

signal peptide

The small leader sequence of amino acids that shepherds the heavy or light chain through the endoplasmic reticulum and is cleaved from the nascent chains prior to assembly of a completed immunoglobulin molecule.

signal recognition particle
autoantibodies (SRP autoantibodies)

Autoantibodies against SRP such as mitochondrial, ribosomal, and certain cytoplasmic autoantibodies that stain Hep-2 cell cytoplasm and can be assayed by radioimmunoprecipitation assay (RIPA), enzyme immunoassay (EIA), and cytoplasmic (non-Jo-1) fluorescence in approximately 4% of polymyositis/dermatomyositis (PM/DM) patient sera. SRP autoantibodies characterize a homogeneous group of patients with similar clinical features (typically black females with acute onsets of severe polymyositis together with cardiac involvement and resistance to therapy, including corticosteroids); mortality is 75% at 5 years. SRP autoantibodies are not usually detected in patients with arthritis, dermatomyositis, pulmonary fibrosis, or Raynaud's phenomenon.

S

signal sequence

Refer to signal hypothesis.

signal transducer and activator of transcription (STAT)

A protein signaling molecule and transcription factor in response to cytokines binding to type I and type II cytokine receptors. STATs exist as inactive monomers in cell cytoplasm and are transported to cytoplasmic tails of cross linked cytokine receptors where they are tyrosine-phosphorylated by Janus kinases (Jaks). Phosphorylated STAT proteins dimerize and migrate to nuclei where they bind to specific sequences in the promoter regions of various genes and activate their transcription. Different cytokines activate different STATs.

signal transduction

Process whereby signals received on cell surfaces, such as by the binding of antigen to its receptor, are transmitted into cell nuclei, resulting in altered gene expression.

silencer sequence

Blocks transcription of the T cell receptor α chain. This sequence is found 5′ to the α chain enhancer in non-T cells and in those with $\gamma\delta$ receptors.

silencers

Nucleotide sequences that downregulate transcription, functioning in both directions over a distance.

silica adjuvants

Silica crystals and hydrated aluminum silicate (bentonite) were occasionally used in the past to enhance immune responses to certain antigens. They were considered to exert a central action on the immune system rather than serving as depot adjuvants, although bentonite can delay the distribution of antigen from its site of inoculation by surface adsorption.

silicate autoantibodies

Autoantibodies stimulated by silicone plastic polymers used for breast implants in cosmetic and reconstructive surgery, vascular prostheses, and joint repair and replacement. Silicone-induced human adjuvant diseases characterized by autoimmune-disease-like symptoms, granulomas, and serological abnormalities have been reported since 1964. Some individuals with breast and joint implants reportedly developed delayed-type hypersensitivity to silicone plastic as interpreted by refractile particles in phagocytes and passage between lymphocytes and macrophages. Women who develop implant ruptures or leakage of silicone gel implants may develop high titers of silicone autoantibodies as measured using silicate-coated plates in enzyme immunoassay (EIA). Only 4% of 249 patients with silicone breast implants developed immunoglobulin G (IgG) binding to fibronectin–laminin adsorbed to silicone and only 2% showed IgG binding to silicone film alone. Thus, patients occasionally develop antibodies against fibronectin and laminin denatured by silicone. Whereas 30% of 40 of symptomatic women with silicone breast implants formed IgG antibodies that reacted with bovine serum albumin (BSA)-bound silicate, 9% (8 of 91) of asymptomatic patients with silicone breast implants also formed these antibodies in low concentrations.

silicosis

The inhalation of silica particles over a prolonged period produces a chronic, nodular, densely fibrosing pneumoconiosis that has an insidious onset and progresses even in the absence of continued exposure to silica dust. Lymphocytes and alveolar macrophages are quickly attracted to the particles that are phagocytized by the macrophages. Some macrophages remain in the interstitial tissue or pulmonary lymphatic channels. Interaction of macrophages and silica particles leads over time to collagenous fibrosis and fibrosing nodules. The silica dust–macrophage interaction may cause the secretion of interleukin-1 (IL1) that recruits T helper cells producing IL2, which induces proliferation of T lymphocytes that in turn produce a variety of lymphokines. Thus, immunocompetent cells mediate the collagenous reaction. Activated T cells interact with B lymphocytes that synthesize increased amounts of IgG, IgM, rheumatoid factor, antinuclear antibodies, and circulating immune complexes. Collagenous silicotic nodules may coalesce, producing fibrous scars. The disease may be complicated by rheumatoid arthritis, pulmonary tuberculosis, emphysema, and other diseases. No increased incidence of lung cancer is associated with silicosis.

simian immunodeficiency virus (SIV)

This virus causes a disease resembling human acquired immune deficiency syndrome (AIDS) in rhesus monkeys. The SIV sequence reveals significant homology with human immunodeficiency virus 2 (HIV-2), a cause of AIDS in western Africa.

Simonsen phenomenon

A graft-vs.-host reaction in chick embryos that develop splenomegaly following inoculation of immunologically competent lymphoid cells from adult chickens. Splenic lymphocytes are increased and represent a mixture of both donor and host lymphocytes.

simple allotype

An allotype that differs from another allotype in the sequence of amino acids at one or several positions. Alleles at one genetic locus often encode simple allotypes.

Simulect™ (basiliximab)

A chimeric (murine–human) monoclonal antibody (IgG$_{1k}$), produced by recombinant DNA technology that functions as an immunosuppressive agent, specifically binding to and blocking the interleukin-2 receptor α (IL2Rα; also known as CD25 antigen) chain on the surfaces of activated T lymphocytes. Based on the amino acid sequence, the calculated molecular weight of the protein is 144 kDa. It is a glycoprotein obtained from fermentation of an established mouse myeloma cell line genetically engineered to express plasmids containing the human heavy and light chain constant region genes and mouse heavy and light chain variable region genes encoding the RFT5 antibody that binds selectively to IL2Rα. Basiliximab (the active ingredient) is water-soluble. The Simulect product is a sterile lyophilisate available in 6-mL colorless glass vials. Each vial contains 20 mg basiliximab, 7.21 mg monobasic potassium phosphate, 0.99 mg disodium hydrogen phosphate (anhydrous), 1.61 mg sodium chloride, 20 mg sucrose, 80 mg mannitol, and 40 mg glycine to be reconstituted in 5 mL of sterile water for injection, USP. No preservatives are added.

single chain Fv fragment

A genetically engineered structure consisting of a heavy chain V region linked by a stretch of synthetic peptide to a light chain V region.

single cysteine motif-1 (SCM-1)

A member of the γ (C) family of chemokines. cDNA clones derived from human peripheral blood mononuclear cells stimulated with PHA encode SCM-1, which is significantly related to the α and β chemokines. It has only the second and fourth of four cysteines conserved in these proteins. It is 60.5% identical to lymphotactin. SCM-1 and lymphotactin are believed to represent human and mouse prototypes of a γ (C) chemokine family. SCM-1 is expressed by human T cells and spleen.

single diffusion test

A type of gel diffusion test in which antigen and antibody are placed in proximity and one diffuses into the other, leading to the formation of a precipitate in the gel. This is in contrast to double diffusion in which antigen and antibody diffuse toward each other.

single domain antibodies

Antibodies capable of binding epitopes with high affinity even though they do not possess light chains. They are cloned from heavy chain variable regions and can be produced in days to weeks in contrast to monoclonal antibodies that require weeks to months to develop. Their relatively small size is a further advantage. Single domain antibodies with antigen-specific VH domains are expected to find wide application in the future.

single hit theory

The hypothesis that hemolysis of red blood cells sensitized with specific antibody is induced by perforation of the membrane by complement at only one site rather than at multiple sites on the membrane.

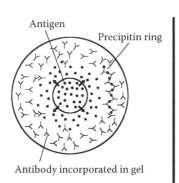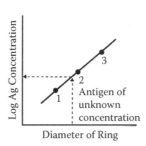

Single immunodiffusion (Mancini technique).

single immunodiffusion

(1) A technique in which antibody is incorporated into agar gel and antigen is placed in a well cut into the surface of the antibody-containing agar. Following diffusion of the antigen into the agar, a ring of precipitation forms at the point where antigen and antibody reach equivalence. The diameter of the ring is used to quantify the antigen concentration by comparison with antigen standards. (2) The addition of antigen to a tube containing gel into which specific antibody has been incorporated. Lines of precipitation form at the site of interaction between equivalent quantities of antigen and antibody.

single locus probe (SLP)

A probe that hybridizes at only one locus. SLPs identify a single locus of variable number of tandem repeats (VNTRs) and permit detection of a region of DNA repeats found in the genome only once and located at a unique site on a certain chromosome. An individual may have only two alleles that SLPs will identify, as each cell of the body will have two copies of each chromosome, one from each parent. When the lengths of related alleles on homologous

chromosomes are the same, the DNA typing pattern will have only a single band; therefore, the use of an SLP may yield a single- or double-band result from each individual. Single locus markers such as the pYNH24 probe developed by White may detect loci that are highly polymorphic, exceeding 30 alleles and 95% heterozygosity. SLPs are used in resolving cases of disputed parentage.

single nucleotide polymorphism (SNP)

A single nucleotide variation in a gene that leads to an allelic amino acid difference in the corresponding protein.

single-positive thymocyte

A late stage of T cell development in the thymus in which maturing T cell precursors express CD4 or CD8 molecules but not both. The thymocites have matured from the double-positive stage and are present principally in the medulla.

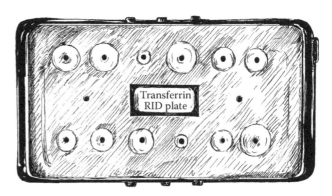

Single radial immunodiffusion.

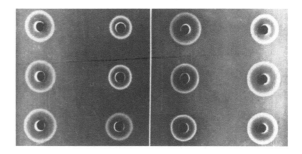

Single radial immunodiffusion.

single radial immunodiffusion

A technique to quantify antigens. Antibody is incorporated into agar in plates, wells are cut, and precise quantities of antigen are placed in the wells. The antigen is permitted to diffuse into the agar containing antibody and produce a ring of precipitation upon interaction with the antibody. As diffusion proceeds, an excess of antigen develops in the area of the precipitate which causes it to dissolve, only to form again at a greater distance from the site of origin. At the point where antigen and antibody reach equivalence in the agar, a precipitation ring is produced. The ring encloses an area proportional to the concentration of antigen measured 48 to 72 hours following diffusion. Standard curves are employed using known antigen standards. The antigen concentration is determined from the diameter of the precipitation ring. This method can detect as little as 1 to 3 µg/mL of antigen. Known also as the Mancini technique.

S

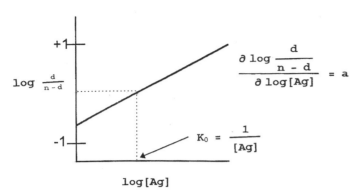

Plot of Sips distribution function.

Sips distribution

Frequency distribution of antibody association constants in a heterogeneous mixture. The Sips distribution is very similar to Gaussian (normal) distribution. It is employed to analyze data from antigen–antibody reactions measured by equilibrium dialysis.

Sips plot

Data representation produced in assaying ligand binding to antibodies by plotting $\log r/(n - r)$ against $\log c$. A straight line signifies that the data are in agreement with the Sips equation. The slope signifies heterogeneity of antibody affinity.

sirolimus

A powerful immunosuppressive drug derived from a soil fungus, *Streptomyces hygroscopicus*, on *Rapa Nui* (Easter Island), also known as rapamycin. It binds immunophilins and inhibits calcineurin and resembles FK506 in structure, but has a different mechanism of action. It does not inhibit interleukin synthesis by activated T cells; it blocks responses of T cells to cytokines. It suppresses B and T lymphocyte proliferation, lymphokine synthesis, and T cell responsiveness to interleukin-2 (IL2). It is a powerful inhibitor of B cell proliferation and immunoglobulin synthesis. It blocks the mononuclear cell proliferative response to colony-stimulating factors. It is effective as an immunosuppressant when used alone or in combination with other agents such as corticosteroids, cyclosporine, tacrolimus, and mycophenolate mofetil in preventing rejection of solid organ allografts. It may be useful in treating steroid-refractory acute and chronic graft-vs.-host disease in hematopoietic stem cell transplant recipients. Sirolimus-eluding coronary stents have been used effectively to reduce restenosis in patients with advanced coronary artery disease, due to its antiproliferative effects. Myelosuppression, hepatotoxicity, diarrhea, and hypertriglyceridemia are toxic effects. To achieve clinical immunosuppression, rapamycin is effective at concentrations one eighth those required for FK506 and 1% of the levels required for cyclosporin. An immunosuppressive agent that inhibits T lymphocyte activation and proliferation that occurs following antigenic and cytokine (IL2, IL4, and IL15) stimulation by a mechanism distinct from other immunosuppressive agents. It also inhibits antibody production. Sirolimus binds to immunophilin in cells, FK binding protein-12 (FKBP-12), to form an immunosuppressive complex. The sirolimus:FKBP-12 complex affects calcineurin activity. It binds to and inhibits

activation of mTOR, the mammalian target of rapamycin, an important regulatory kinase. This blockage suppresses cytokine-driven T cell proliferation, resulting in inhibition of G_1 to the S phase of the cell cycle. It prolongs survival of allografts of kidney, heart, skin, islet, small bowel, pancreatic–duodenal, and bone marrow transplants, reverses acute rejection of heart and kidney allografts in rats, and prolongs graft survival in presensitized rats. In selected studies, the immunosuppressive effect lasted up to 6 months after therapy was discontinued, representing an alloantigen-specific tolerization effect. It has also been used in animal models of autoimmune disease.

SIRS

Abbreviation for soluble immune response suppressor.

site-directed mutagenesis

A laboratory procedure that involves the substitution of amino acids in a protein whose function is defined for the purpose of localizing a certain activity.

SIV (simian immunodeficiency virus)

A lentivirus of primates that resembles human immunodeficiency virus 1 (HIV-1) and HIV-2 in morphology and attraction to cells that bear CD4 molecules such as lymphocytes and macrophages. SIV also shares with these human viruses the additional genes lacking in other retroviruses, including *vip*, *rev*, *upr*, *tat*, and *nef*. SIV induces the classic cytopathologic alterations of the type produced by HIV, and can also induce chronic disease following a lengthy latency. SIVmac239 is an SIV clone that induces a disease resembling acquired immune deficiency syndrome (AIDS) in monkeys.

SIV$_{mac}$

Simian immunodeficiency virus capable of infecting macaque monkeys.

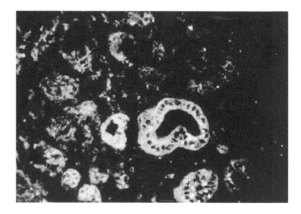

Sjögren's syndrome. Salivary gland. Antibody to ductal epithelium.

Sjögren's syndrome

A condition in which immunologic injury to the lacrimal and salivary glands leads to dry eyes (keratoconjunctivitis sicca) and dry mouth (xerostomia). The condition may occur alone as sicca syndrome (primary form) or with an autoimmune disease such as rheumatoid arthritis (secondary form). The lacrimal and salivary glands show extensive lymphocytic infiltration and fibrosis. Most of the infiltrating cells are CD4+ T cells, but some B cells (plasma cells) that form antibody are present. Approximately 75% of the patients form rheumatoid factor. The lupus erythematosus

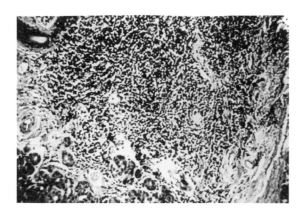

Sjögren's syndrome.

(LE) cell test is positive in 25% of patients. Numerous antibodies are produced, including autoantibodies against salivary duct cells, gastric parietal cells, thyroid antigens, and smooth muscle mitochondria. Antibodies against ribonucleoprotein antigens are termed Ro/SSA and La/SSB. Approximately 90% of the patients have these antibodies. Anti-SSB shows greater specificity for Sjögren's syndrome than do anti-SSA antibodies that also occur in SLE. Patients who have Sjögren's syndrome with rheumatoid arthritis may have antibodies to rheumatoid-associated nuclear antigen (RANA). A positive correlation exists between HLA-DR3 and primary Sjögren's syndrome and between HLA-DR4 and secondary Sjögren's syndrome associated with rheumatoid arthritis. Genetic predisposition, viruses, and disordered immunoregulation may play a role in pathogenesis. About 90% of the patients are 40- to 60-year old females. In addition to dry eyes and mouth and associated visual or swallowing difficulties, 50% of the patients show parotid gland enlargement. Drying of the nasal mucosa is accompanied by bleeding, pneumonitis, and bronchitis. A lip biopsy to examine minor salivary glands is needed to diagnose Sjögren's syndrome. Inflammation of the salivary and lacrimal glands was previously called Mikulicz's disease. Mikulicz's syndrome is enlargement of the salivary and lacrimal glands due to any cause. Enlarged lymph nodes that reveal a pleomorphic cellular infiltrate with many mitoses are typical of Sjögren's syndrome and have been referred to as pseudolymphoma. Patients have a 40-fold greater risk than others for lymphoid neoplasms.

skin autoantibodies
Autoantibodies detectable by immunofluorescence associated with selected bullous skin diseases and useful for categorizing them. The three principal categories of bullous skin diseases are intraepidermal bullae with an immunological etiology, subepidermal bullae with immunological pathogenesis, and nonimmune bullous disorders.

skin-associated lymphoid tissue (SALT)
Diffuse epidermal T cells, including αβ and γδ T cells and dendritic (Langerhans) cells together with dermal αβ T cells, fibroblasts, macrophages, and lymphatic vessels.

skin-fixing antibody
An antibody such as immunoglobulin E (IgE) retained in the skin following local injection as in passive cutaneous anaphylaxis. Antibody with this property was referred to previously as reagin before IgE was described.

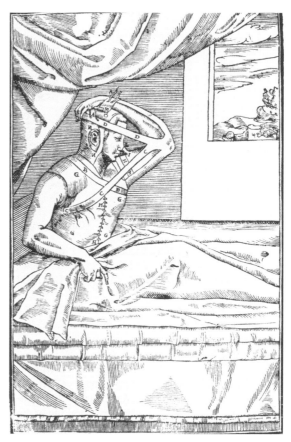

Early depiction of skin grafts from forehead, neck, and cheek used to restore mutilation of the nose, ear, and lip.

skin graft
Skin from an individual (autologous graft) or donor skin applied to areas of the body surface that have undergone third-degree burns. A patient's keratinocytes may be cultured into confluent sheets that can be applied to the affected areas, although these may not "take" because of the absence of type IV collagen 7S basement membrane sites for binding and fibrils to anchor the graft.

skin immunity
The skin, the largest organ of the body, shields the interior environment from a hostile exterior. The skin defends the host through stimulation of inflammatory and local immune responses. Antigen applied to or injected into the skin drains to the regional lymph nodes through the skin's extensive lymphatic network. Cells of the epidermis and papillary and reticular dermis play critical roles in the skin's immune function. Keratinocytes (epidermal epithelial cells) secrete various cytokines such as granulocyte–macrophage colony-stimulating factor (GM-CSF), interleukin-1 (IL1), IL3, IL6, and tumor necrosis factor (TNF). T lymphocytes in the skin may secrete interferon-γ (IFN-γ) and other cytokines that cause these epithelial cells to synthesize chemokines that lead to leukocyte chemotaxis and activation. Stimulation by IFN-γ may also lead to expression of major histocompatibility complex (MHC) class II molecules. Other epidermal cells include Langerhans' cells that form an extensive network in the epidermis that permits their interaction with any antigen entering the skin. The few lymphocytes in the epidermis are principally CD8+ T

Cutaneous immune system and its cellular components.

cells, often with restricted antigen receptors. In mice, they are mostly γδ T cells. Skin lymphocytes and macrophages are mostly in the dermis. The T cells are of CD4$^+$ and CD8$^+$ phenotypes and often perivascular.

skin-reactive factor (SRF)

A lymphokine that induces vasodilation and increased vascular permeability when injected into the skin.

skin-sensitizing antibody

An antibody, usually of the immunoglobulin E (IgE) class, that binds to the Fc receptors of mast cells in the skin, thereby conditioning the area for a type I immediate hypersensitivity reaction following cross linking of the IgE Fab regions by a specific allergen (antigen). In guinea pig skin, human IgG$_1$ antibodies may be used to induce passive cutaneous anaphylaxis.

skin-specific histocompatibility antigen

A murine skin minor histocompatibility antigen termed Sk that can elicit rejection of skin but not other tissues following transplantation from one parent into the other parent that has been irradiated and rendered a chimera by previous injection of F$_1$ spleen cells. The two parents are from different inbred strains of mice. The rate of rejection is relatively slow. Immunologic tolerance of F$_1$ murine spleen cells to the skin epitope of the parent in which they are not in residence is abrogated following residence in the opposite parent.

skin test

Any of several assays in which a test substance is injected into the skin or applied to it to determine host response. Skin tests have long been used to determine hypersensitivity or immunity to a particular antigen or product of a microorganism. Examples include the tuberculin test, the Schick test, the Dick test, the patch test, the scratch test, etc.

skin window

A method for observing sequential changes in cells during the development of acute inflammation. Following superficial abrasion of an area of skin, sterile cover slips are applied, removed at specified intervals thereafter, stained, and observed microscopically for the types of cells present. The first cells to appear are polymorphonuclear neutrophils that comprise most of the cell population within 3 to 4 hours of the induced injury. By contrast, a cover slip removed after 12 hours reveals mononuclear cells such as lymphocytes, plasma cells, and monocytes. Removal after 24 hours reveals mostly monocytes and macrophages. Also termed a Rebuck window, named for the researcher who perfected the method.

skin window of Rebuck

Refer to skin window.

SLE

Abbreviation for systemic lupus erythematosus.

slide agglutination test

The aggregation of particulate antigen using red blood cells, microorganisms, or latex particles coated with antigen within 30 seconds following contact with specific antibody. The reactants are usually mixed by rocking the slide back and forth, and agglutination is observed macroscopically and microscopically. The test has been widely used for screening but is unable to distinguish reactions produced by cross reacting antibodies that can be ruled out in a tube test that allows dilution of the antiserum.

slide flocculation test

Refer to slide agglutination test.

slot blot analysis

A quick technique to detect gene amplification by determining the DNA content of a solution by electrophoresis. The technique is similar to dot blot, except that a slot instead of a punched-out hole is cut in the agar.

slow reacting substance of anaphylaxis (SRS-A)

A 400-kDa acidic lipoprotein derived from arachidonic acid that induces the slow contraction of bronchial smooth muscles and is produced following exposure to certain antigens. It is composed of leukotrienes LTC$_4$, LTD$_4$, and LTE$_{4\text{ that}}$ produce the effects observed in anaphylactic reactions. SRS-A is released *in vitro* in effluents from synthesized lung tissues of guinea pigs, rabbits, and rats perfused with antigen. It has also been demonstrated in human lung tissue and nasal polyps. It contracts smooth muscles of guinea pig ileum. *In vitro,* it also increases vascular permeability upon intracutaneous injection and decreases pulmonary compliance by a mechanism independent of vagal reflexes. It enhances some smooth muscle effects of histamine. The sources of SRS-A are mast cells and certain other cells; it is found in immediate (type I) hypersensitivity reactions. SRS-A is not stored in a preformed state and is sequentially synthesized and released. The effects have a latent period before becoming manifest. Antihistamines do not neutralize the effects of SRS-A.

slow viruses

Agents that induce infectious encephalitis following a lengthy latency. Slow viruses consist of conventional viruses and prions that are composed of subverted cell proteins. Among the conventional viruses group is measles, which induces subacute sclerosing panencephalitis; papovavirus, which induces progressive multifocal leukoencephalopathy; and rubella, which induces rare progressive rubella panencephalitis. The agents that cause kuru and Creutzfeldt–Jakob disease are among the nonconventional group of slow viruses.

slp

Abbreviation for sex limited protein encoded by genes at the C4A complement locus in mice. It is restricted to males but may be induced in females by androgen administration.

Sm (anti-Smith) antibodies

Antibodies that occur in approximately 29% of patients with systemic lupus erythematosus (SLE) and are specific for this disease. They are specific for polypeptides of U1, U2, and U4–U6 small nuclear ribonucleoproteins (snRNPs) that are significant in pre-mRNA splicing. Anti-Sm antibodies do not show the increase in titer observed with anti-double-stranded DNA antibodies during exacerbations of the disease.

Sm (anti-Smith) autoantibodies

Anti-Sm autoantibodies recognize a subset of the protein components of U1 snRNP. Anti-Sm antibodies recognize a group of proteins (B′/B, D, E, F, and G) that form a stable subparticle (the Sm core particle) associated with U1 snRNP and a series of other snRNPs, the most abundant of which are the U2, U5, and U4/U5. The assembly of these proteins and RNAs into macromolecular complexes is responsible for the patterns found on protein and RNA immunoprecipitation.

SMAA

Solid matrix antibody–antigen complex. A vaccine comprised of monoclonal antibodies against a vaccine epitope. The antibodies are bound chemically to microbeads after which the vaccine antigenic determinant interacts with the monoclonal antibodies. A microbead coated with monoclonal antibodies against different epitopes can exhibit epitopes of both B and T cells.

SMAC

Supramolecular activation complex. The point of contact between a T cell and an antigen-presenting cell where accumulation of stabilized lipid rafts and activated T cell receptors occurs; also known as the immunological synapse. The SMAC possesses a concentric triple ring construct comprised of the cSMAC, inner pSMAC, and outer pSMAC ("c" indicates central; "p" indicates peripheral).

small blues

Blue aggregates of acellular debris observed in clinical histocompatibility testing using microlymphotoxicity. Small blues appear in the wells of tissue-typing trays and arise from an excess of Trypan blue mixed with protein. They are technical artifacts.

small G proteins

Monomeric G proteins, including Ras, that function as intracellular signaling molecules downstream of many transmembrane signaling events. In active form they bind GTP (guanosine triphosphate) and hydrolyze it to GDP (guanosine diphosphate) to become inactive.

small lymphocyte

One of the five types of leukocytes in the peripheral blood; they measure 6 to 8 μm in diameter. In Wright's and Giemsa-stained blood smears, the nucleus stains dark blue and is encircled by a narrow rim of robin's egg blue cytoplasm. Although most lymphocytes look alike, they differ greatly in origin and function and in other features as well. Under light microscopy, T and B lymphocytes and the E rosette subpopulations look the same but they have different phenotypic surface markers and differ greatly in function. A common designation for resting T and B lymphocytes that are recirculating.

small pre-B cells

Pre-B cells undergoing light chain gene rearrangements.

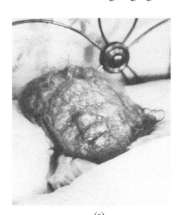 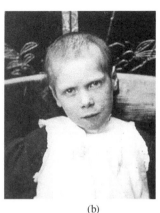

(a)   (b)

(a) Small eruptions on the face of a smallpox patient. (b) Same patient following recovery.

smallpox

Refer to variola.

smallpox vaccination

The induction of active immunity against smallpox (variola) by immunization with a related agent, vaccinia virus, obtained from vaccinia vesicles on calf skin. Shared, and therefore cross reactive, epitopes in the vaccinia virus provide protective immunity against smallpox. This ancient disease has now been almost entirely eliminated worldwide; laboratory stocks are maintained in Atlanta, Georgia, and Moscow although they were supposed to have been destroyed after the virus was sequenced. Smallpox vaccination was developed by Edward Jenner, an English physician, whose method diminished mortality from 20% to <1%. Following application of vaccinia virus by a multiple-pressure method, vesicles occur at the site of application in 6 to 9 days. Maximum reactivity is observed by day 12. In the past, initial vaccinations were given to 1- to 2-year old children, with revaccination after 3 years. Children with cell-mediated immunodeficiency syndromes sometimes developed complications such as generalized vaccinia spreading from the site of inoculation. Postvaccination encephalomyelitis also occurred occasionally in adults and in babies prior to their first birthdays. The procedure was contraindicated in subjects experiencing immunosuppression due to any cause.

smallpox vaccine

An immunizing preparation prepared from the lymph of cowpox vesicles obtained from healthy vaccinated bovines. This vaccine is no longer used because smallpox has been practically eradicated.

Smith, Theobald (1859–1934)

Smith was an American investigator who with David E. Salmon found that pigeons inoculated with heat-killed cultures of hog cholera bacilli developed immunity. Smith and Salmon reasoned from this discovery that immunity could

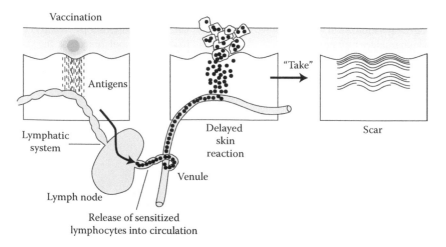

Smallpox vaccination.

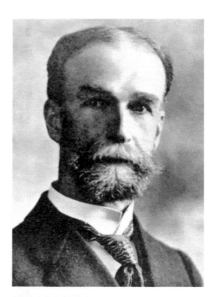

Theobald Smith.

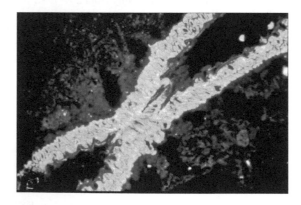

Smooth muscle antibodies (SMAs).

be induced by exposure of the body to chemical substances or toxins produced by bacteria causing the disease.

smooth muscle antibodies (SMAs)

Autoantibodies belonging to the immunoglobulin M (IgM) or IgG class found in the sera of 60% of patients with chronic active hepatitis. Among patients with biliary cirrhosis, 30% may also be positive for these antibodies. Low

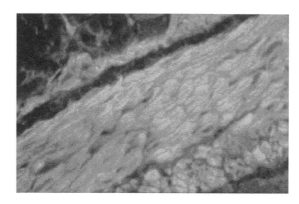

Smooth muscle antibodies (SMAs).

titers of smooth muscle antibodies may be found in certain viral infections of the liver. The anti-actin variety of smooth muscle antibodies is especially associated with autoimmune liver disease, while SMAs directed to intermediate filaments may appear in virus-induced liver disease. The presence of SMAs is not predictive of the development of liver disease and is not helpful for prognosis in autoimmune patients with chronic active hepatitis.

SNagg

Agglutinating activity by rheumatoid factor in certain normal sera, as revealed by a positive RA (rheumatoid arthritis) test.

sneaking through

The successful growth of a sparse number of transplantable tumor cells inoculated into a host in contrast to the induction of tumor immunity and lack of tumor growth in the same host if larger doses of the same cells are administered.

Snell–Bagg mice

A mutant strain (dw/dw) of inbred mice with pituitary dwarfism. Characteristics are a diminutive thymus, deficient lymphoid tissue, and decreased cell-mediated immune responsiveness.

Snell, George Davis (1903–1996)

American geneticist who shared the 1980 Nobel Prize in Medicine or Physiology with Jean Dausset and Baruj Benacerraf for their work on genetically determined structures of cell surfaces that regulate immunologic reactions. Snell's major contributions were in the field of mouse genetics, including discovery of the H-2 locus (with Gorer) and

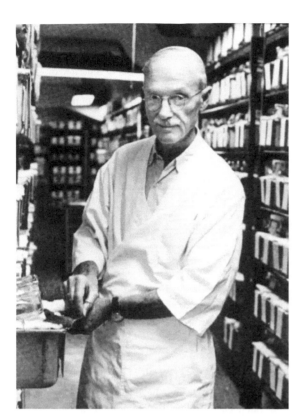

George Davis Snell.

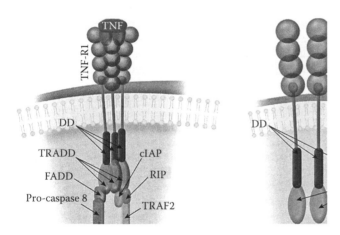

(a) TNF-RI-initiated apoptosis and activation of NF-κB. (b) SODD silencing of TNF-RI signaling.

the development of congenic mice. He made many seminal contributions to transplantation genetics and received the Gairdner Award in 1976. (Refer to *Histocompatibility* [with Dausset and Nathenson], 1976.)

SOD

Abbreviation for superoxide dismutase.

SODD (silencer of death domains)

The tumor necrosis factor (TNF) receptor superfamily contains several members with homologous cytoplasmic domains known as death domains (DDs). The intercellular DDs are important in initiating apoptosis and other signaling pathways following ligand binding by the receptors. In the absence of ligand, DD-containing receptors are maintained in an inactive state. TNF-RI contains a cytoplasmic DD required for signaling pathways

associated with apoptosis and NF-κB activation. Jiang et al. identified a widely expressed 60-kDa protein they named SODD (silencer of death domains) associated with the DDs of TNF-RI and -DR3. Overexpression of SODD suppresses TNF-induced cell death and NF-κB activation, demonstrating SODD's role as a negative regulatory protein for these signaling pathways. TNF-induced receptor trimerization aggregates the DDs of TNF-RI and recruits the adapter protein TRADD. This in turn promotes the recruitment of the DD-containing cytoplasmic proteins FADD, TRAF2, and RIP to form an active TNF-RI signaling complex. In contrast, SODD acts as a silencer of TNF-RI signaling and does not interact with TRADD, FADD, or RIP. It is associated with the DD of TNF-RI and maintains TNF-RI in an inactive, monomeric state. TNF-induced aggregation of TNF-RI promotes the disruption of the SODD–TNF-RI complex. SODD does not interact with the DDs of other TNF receptor superfamily members such as Fas, DR4, DR5, and TNF-RII. SODD association with TNF-RI may represent a general model for the prevention of spontaneous TNF signaling by other DD-containing receptors.

solid organ transplant

The surgical transfer of a kidney, heart, lung, liver or skin from a donor to a recipient.

solid phase radioimmunoassay

The attachment of antigen (or antibody) to an insoluble support that can be used to capture antibodies (or antigens) in a specimen to be assayed. Antibodies in a serum sample are exposed to excess antigen on an insoluble support and sufficient time is allowed for antigen–antibody interaction. This is followed by washing and the application of radiolabeled anti-Fc antibodies specific for the Fc regions of the captured antibodies. Quantification of the bound antibody is determined from the amount of radioactivity adhering to the insoluble support. Various materials may be used as supports. These include Sepharose™ beads or tissue-culture-plate wells. An unrelated protein must be used to coat the insoluble support prior to application of the specific antibody to saturate areas of the insoluble support where antigen is not located.

solitary plasmacytoma of bone

A plasma cell dyscrasia characterized by a single plasma cell neoplasm in the bone marrow.

solubilized water-in-oil adjuvant

A water-in-oil emulsion adjuvant composed of a small-volume aqueous phase compared to the volume of oil. A mixture of aqueous and oil phases results in an emulsion that is stabilized by the addition of emulsifying agents.

soluble antigen

An antigen solubilized in an aqueous medium.

soluble complex

An immune (antigen–antibody) complex formed in excess antigen and rendered soluble. Antigen excess prevents lattice formation *in vitro* and *in vivo.* Soluble complexes may produce tissue injury *in vivo,* which is more severe if complement has been fixed. C5a attracts neutrophils, and capillary permeability is increased. PMNs, platelets, and fibrin are deposited on the endothelium, followed by thrombosis and necrosis. Immune complexes induce type III hypersensitivity reactions.

S

soluble cytokine receptors

IL1 type I-R, IL1 type II-R, IL2Rα, IL2Rβ, IL4R, IL5Rα, IL6Rα, gp130 IL6Rβ ciliary neurotrophic factor (CNF)-Rα, and growth hormone R. Most of these function by blocking ligand binding.

soluble liver antigen (cytokeratin autoantibodies)

Autoantibodies that react with liver but not kidney as revealed by immunofluorescence. They are found in a subgroup of patients with chronic autoimmune hepatitis (AIH) with negative antinuclear antibodies (ANAs) and negative liver–kidney microsome 1 (LKM-1) autoantibodies and a low prevalence of autoantibodies against smooth muscle mitochondria and liver membrane antigens. These autoantibodies are believed to be identical to LP2 autoantibodies present in 45% of patients with cryptogenic chronic active hepatitis.

somatic

Pertaining to the body wall; of the body.

somatic antigen

An antigen, such as the O antigen, that is part of the structure of a bacterial cell.

somatic cell hybrid

The union of two or more sets of chromosomes into a single large nucleus as a consequence of fusion of multiple heterokaryon nuclei.

somatic gene conversion

Nonreciprocal exchange of sequences between genes. A portion of the donor gene or genes is copied into an acceptor gene, leading to alteration only in the acceptor gene. It serves as a mechanism to generate diverse immunoglobulins in nonhuman species.

somatic gene therapy

A potential therapy to treat or cure inherited immunodeficiency diseases. Stem cells derived from a patient are transfected with a normal copy of the defective gene of the patient. The stem cells now equipped with a good copy of the defective gene are reinfused into the patient's circulation.

somatic hybrid selection

Selection of somatic cell hybrids with required characteristics by complementation.

somatic hypermutation

The induced increase in frequency of mutation in rearranged variable region DNA of immunoglobulin genes in activated B cells. The high frequency introduction of single or double nucleotide substitutions into the V exons of Ig genes, leading to elevated numbers of random point mutations in the V regions of Ig proteins. This increase leads to the synthesis of variant antibodies, some of which have higher affinities for antigen. Somatic mutation may occur in germinal centers. Only somatic cells are affected. Somatic hypermutation is not inherited through germline transmission. T cell receptor genes do not undergo somatic hypermutation.

somatic mutation

A genetic variation in a somatic cell that is heritable by its progeny. Increased somatic mutation enhances diversity of the light and heavy chain variable regions of an antibody. Immunoglobulin G (IgG) and IgA antibodies reveal somatic mutations more often than IgM antibodies. Such a mutation is a mechanism whereby point mutations can be introduced into the rearranged immunoglobulin variable region genes during B lymphocyte activation and proliferation.

somatic recombination

DNA recombination whereby functional genes encoding variable regions of antigen receptors are produced during lymphocyte development. A limited number of inherited or germline DNA sequences that are first separated from each other are assembled together by enzymatic deletion of intervening sequences and relegation. This process takes place only in developing B or T cells. Also called somatic rearrangement.

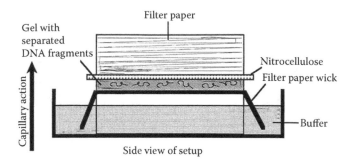

Southern blotting.

southern blotting

A procedure to identify DNA sequences. Following extraction of DNA from cells, it is digested with restriction endonucleases to cut the DNA at precise sites into fragments. This is followed by separation of the DNA segments according to size by electrophoresis in agarose gel, denaturation with sodium hydroxide, and transfer of the single-stranded DNA to a nitrocellulose membrane by blotting. This procedure is followed by hybridization with an ^{35}S- or ^{32}P-radiolabeled probe of complementary DNA. Alternatively, a biotinylated probe may be used. Autoradiography or substrate digestion identifies the location of the DNA fragments that have hybridized with the complementary DNA probe. Specific sequences in cloned and in genomic DNA can be identified by southern blotting. DNA analysis is referred to as a southern blot; RNA analysis is referred to as a northern blot; and protein analysis is referred to as a western blot. A northwestern blot is one in which RNA–protein hybridizations are formed.

southwestern blot

A method that combines southern blotting to identify DNA segments with western immunoblotting that characterizes proteins. A protein may be hybridized to a molecule of single-stranded DNA bound to a membrane. Southwestern blotting is helpful in delineating nuclear-transcription-related proteins.

SP-40,40

A heterodimeric serum protein derived from soluble C5–C9 complexes that may modulate the cell lysing action of the membrane attack complex (MAC).

spacer

Refer to the 12/23 rule.

species specificity

Cellular or tissue antigens present in one species only and not found in other species.

specific granule

A secondary granule in the cytoplasms of polymorphonuclear leukocytes that contains lysozyme, vitamin B$_{12}$-binding protein, neutral proteases, and lactoferrin. It is

Opsonic–promote ingestion and killing by phagocytic cells (IgG)
Block attachment (IgA)
Neutralize toxins
Agglutinate bacteria–may aid in clearing
Render motile organisms nonmotile
Abs only rarely affect metabolism or growth of bacteria (Mycoplasma)
Abs, combining with antigens of the bacterial surface, activate the complement cascade, thus inducing an inflammatory response and bringing fresh phagocytes and serum Abs into the site
Abs, combining with antigens of the bacterial surface, activate the complement cascade, and through the final sequences the membrane attack complex (MAC) is formed involving C5b–C9

Antimicrobial actions of antibodies.

Specific immune response to extracellular bacteria.

smaller and fuses with phagosomes more quickly than does the azurophil granule.

specific immune response to extracellular bacteria

Antibodies are the primary agents that protect the body against extracellular bacteria. Microbial cell wall polysaccharides serve as thymus-independent antigens that stimulate specific immunoglobulin M (IgM) antibody responses. Cytokine production may even permit switching from IgM to IgG production. Protein antigens of extracellular bacteria primarily stimulate active CD4+ T cells. Toxins of extracellular bacteria may activate multiple CD4+ T lymphocytes. A bacterial toxin that stimulates an entire family of T lymphocytes that express products of a certain family of v_{beta} T lymphocyte receptor genes is referred to as a superantigen. Immune stimulation of this type may lead to the production of abundant quantities of cytokines that lead to pathologic sequelae. The resistance mechanism against extracellular

bacteria regrettably may include two reactions that produce tissue injury: acute inflammation and endotoxin shock. In addition, late in the course of a bacterial infection, pathogenic antibodies may appear. The multiple lymphocyte clones stimulated by bacterial endotoxins or superantigens may lead to the production of autoimmunity through overriding specific T cell bypass mechanisms. Autoreactive lymphocytes may also be activated during this process.

specific immunity

An immune state in which antibodies or specifically sensitized or primed lymphocytes recognize an antigen and react with it. By contrast, immunologically competent cells may interact with antigens to produce specific immunosuppression referred to as immunologic tolerance.

specificity

Recognition by an antibody or lymphocyte receptor of a specific epitope in the presence of other epitopes for which the antigen-binding site of the antibody or lymphoid cell receptor is specific.

speckled pattern

A type of immunofluorescence produced when serum from a patient with one of several connective tissue diseases is placed in contact with the human epithelial cell line HEp-2 and "stained" with fluorochrome-labeled goat or rabbit antisera against human immunoglobulin. The speckled pattern of fluorescence occurs in mixed connective tissue disease, lupus erythematosus, polymyositis, sicca syndrome, Sjögren's syndrome, drug-induced immune reactions, and rheumatoid arthritis. It is the most frequent pattern and shows the greatest variations of immunofluorescent nuclear staining. The speckles are classified as (1) fine speckles associated with anticentromere antibody; (2) coarse speckles associated with antibodies against the nonhistone nuclear proteins Scl-70, nRNP, La/SSB, and Sm; and (3) large speckles that may be limited to 3 to 10 per nucleus, are seen in undifferentiated connective tissue disease, and represent IgM antibody against class H3 histones.

spectratyping

Selected types of DNA gene segments that give a repetitive spacing of three nucleotides or one codon.

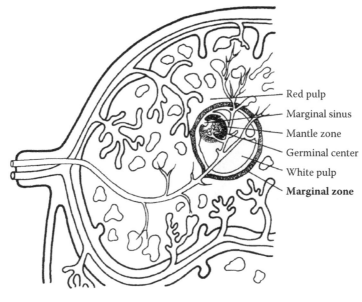

Spleen.

S

spectrotype

In isoelectric focusing analysis, the arrangement of bands in a gel that is characteristic for a single protein or category of proteins. An antibody spectrotype on an isoelectric focusing gel may signify that it is the product of a particular antibody-synthesizing clone.

sperm antibodies

Antibodies specific for the heads or tails of sperm. These antibodies are synthesized by 3% of infertile males and 2 to 9% of infertile females. The titer of antibody against sperm and infertility are positively correlated. Treatment includes corticosteroid therapy or the use of a condom to permit waning of immunologic memory in the female or washing of sperm prior to insemination.

sperm autoantibodies

Antibodies against human sperm can be formed in both sexes and play a role in infertility. Not all antibodies against spermatozoa interfere with sperm function and fertilization. Antibodies in cervical mucus or on sperm are associated with a reduction in cervical mucus penetration. Vasectomy causes the production of sperm autoantibodies. In vasectomized men, immunoglobulin A (IgA) sperm antibodies on all sperm and a heightened immune response (antibody titer >1:256) are associated with conception failure. Assays for circulating sperm antibodies vary in sensitivity and specificity. The variables to be considered include class of immunoglobulin and different sperm antigens, among others. Of the various methods to measure sperm antibodies, the direct immunobead test (dIBT) is the method of choice. It is based on rosette formation by viable sperm and plastic beads coated with antiserum to human immunoglobulins and allows measurement of class-specific antibodies (IgG, IgM, or IgA) and antibody attachment sites (heads or tails). Antibodies can be measured in cervical mucus, seminal plasma, serum, and in an antibody complex on the surfaces of donor sperm. The measurement of sperm antibodies on sperm is the preferred technique. Three major sperm surface glycoproteins have been identified. Sperm antibodies include those reactive with galactosyl transferase.

spheroplast

A Gram-negative bacterial protoplast that contains outer membrane remains.

spherulin

An antigen derived from spherules of *Coccidioides immitis* used for the delayed-type hypersensitivity skin test for coccidioidomycosis.

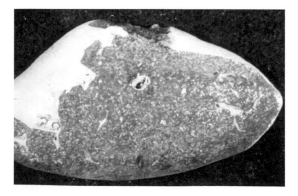

Spleen, gross specimen.

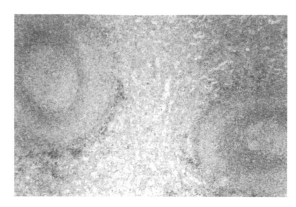

Spleen follicle with central follicular artery.

spleen

An encapsulated organ in the abdominal cavity that has important immunologic and nonimmunologic functions. Vessels and nerves enter the spleen at the hilum, as in lymph nodes, and travel part of their course within the fibrous trabeculae that emerge from the capsule. The splenic parenchyma has two regions that are functionally and histologically distinct. The white pulp consists of a thick layer of lymphocytes surrounding the arteries that have left the trabeculae. They form periarterial sheaths that contain mainly T cells. The sheaths then expand along their course to form well developed lymphoid nodules called malpighian corpuscles. The red pulp consists of a mesh of reticular fibers, continuous with the collagen fibers of the trabeculae. These fibers enclose an open system of sinusoids that drain into small veins and are lined by endothelial cells with reticular properties. The endothelium is discontinuous, leaving small slits through which cells must pass during transit. Within the sinusoidal mesh are red blood cells, macrophages, lymphocytes, and plasma cells. The red pulp between adjacent sinusoids forms pulp cords, sometimes called the cords of Billroth. The marginal zone consists of a poorly defined area between the white and red pulp where the periarterial sheath and lymphoid nodules merge. The blood vessels branch, and at the periphery of the marginal zone the blood empties into the pulp. Lymphocytes of the marginal zone are mainly T cells. They surround the periphery of the lymphoid nodules that comprise B cells. In this marginal region, the T and B cells contact each other. Some B cells may convert into immunoblasts. Further maturation to plasma cells occurs in the red pulp. Active follicles contain germinal centers in which lymphoblasts may be generated. They are discharged into sinusoids, and plasma cells may form. The spleen also contains dendritic cells that have long cytoplasmic extensions and serve as antigen-presenting cells, interacting with lymphocytes. The spleen filters blood as the lymph nodes filter the lymph. The spleen is active in the formation of antibodies against intravenously administered particulate antigens. It has numerous additional functions, including the sequestration and destruction of senescent red blood cells, platelets, and lymphocytes.

splenic cords

A network of collagen that encircles accumulations of erythrocytes, reticular cells, fibroblasts, macrophages, and lymphocytes in the spleen.

spliceosomal snRNP autoantibodies

Sm autoantibodies are reactive with Sm core proteins (B, V, E) common to U1 snRNP, U2 snRNP, and other uridine-rich snRNPs (U4/U6, U5, U7, and U11/U12). Use of the *U1 snRNP autoantibodies* term should be restricted to autoantibodies reactive with non-Sm protein epitopes characteristic of individual snRNPs (70K, A, and C for U1; AN and BO for U2; 120-kDa/150-kDa for U4/U6). Sm autoantibodies occur in 20 to 30% of Caucasian adults and children with systemic lupus erythematosus (SLE) and in 30 to 40% of Asians and blacks with SLE. Mixed connective tissue disease (MCTD) is characterized by U1 snRNP (100%) and occasionally accompanied by U2 snRNP (approximately 15%) autoantibodies.

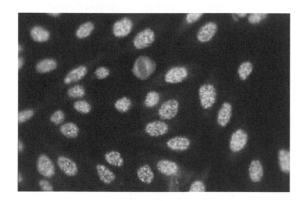

SS-A/Ro antibodies.

splits

Human leukocyte antigen (HLA) subtypes. For example, the base antigen HLA-B12 can be subdivided into splits HLA-B44 and HLA-B45. The *split* term designates an HLA initially believed to be a private antigen but later shown to be a public antigen. The former designation can be placed in parentheses following its new designation, e.g., HLA-B44(12).

split thickness graft

A skin graft that is only 0.25 to 0.35 mm thick and consists of epidermis and a small layer of dermis. These grafts vascularize rapidly and last longer than regular grafts. They are especially useful for burns, contaminated skin areas, and sites that are poorly vascularized. Thick split thickness grafts are further resistant to trauma, produce minimal contraction, and permit some sensation, but graft survival is poor.

split tolerance

(1) Specific immunological unresponsiveness (tolerance) affecting the B cell (antibody) limb or the T lymphocyte (cell-mediated) limb of the immune response. The unaffected limb is left intact to produce antibody or respond with cell-mediated immunity, depending on which limb has been rendered specifically unresponsive to the antigen in question. (2) The induction of immunologic tolerance to some epitopes of allogeneic cells, leaving the remaining epitopes capable of inducing an immune response characterized by antibody production and/or cell-mediated immunity. (3) T cell tolerance to a specific tolerogen may be induced, whereas B cell reactivity remains intact.

sponges

Even the most primitive invertebrates (marine sponges) can discriminate self from nonself, leading to rejection

Splits

Original Broad Specificities	Splits and Associated Antigens
A2	A203#, A210#
A9	A23, A24, A2403#
A10	A25, A26, A34, A66
A19	A29, A30, A31, A32, A33, A74
A28	A68, A69
B5	B51, B52
B7	B703#
B12	B44, B45
B14	B64, B65
B15	B62, B63, B75, B76, B77
B16	B38, B39, B3901#, B3902#
B17	B57, B58
B21	B49, B50, B4005#
B22	B54, B55, B56
B40	B60, B61
B70	B71, B72
Cw3	Cw9, Cw10
DR1	DR103#
DR2	DR15, DR16
DR3	DR17, DR18
DR5	DR11, DR12
DR6	Dr13, DR14, DR1403#, DR1404#
DQ1	DQ5, DQ6
DQ3	DQ7, DQ8, DQ9
Dw6	Dw18, Dw19
Dw7	Dw11, Dw17

of parabiosed fingers of different colonies in 7 to 9 days. Species-specific glycoproteins of sponge cells are used for identification of self and inhibition of hybrid colony formation. Placed in apposition to one another, nonidentical sponge colonies become necrotic at interfaces. Second grafts undergo accelerated rejection.

spongiform encephalopathies

Fatal prion diseases. The brain becomes sponge-like. This category includes variant Creutzfeldt-Jakob disease (vCJD) in humans, scrapie in sheep, and bovine spongiform encephalopathy (BSE, also known as mad cow disease) in cattle.

spontaneous autoimmune thyroiditis (SAT)

Spontaneous autoimmune thyroiditis (SAT) in the obese strain (OS) of chicken constitutes an animal model of Hashimoto's thyroiditis in humans. Many mononuclear cells infiltrate the thyroid gland, leading to disruption of the follicular architecture. Immunodysregulation is critical in the etiopathogenesis of SAT. Endocrine abnormalities play a role in pathogenesis. Disturbances in communication between the immune and endocrine systems occur. Dysregulation leads to hyperreactivity of the immune system which, combined with a primary genetic defect-induced alteration of the thyroid gland, leads to autoimmune thyroiditis. Both T and B lymphocytes are significant in the pathogenesis of SAT. T cell effector mechanisms have greater influence than humoral factors in initiating the disease, and most lymphocytes infiltrating the autoimmune thyroid are mature cells. Autoantibodies play a minor role

S

in the pathogenesis and T cells rather than B cells of OS chickens are defective.

spontaneous cancer

A malignant neoplasm that arises in a laboratory animal without experimental intervention.

spontaneous remission

The reversal of progressive growth of a neoplasm with inadequate or no treatment. Spontaneous remission occurs only rarely.

sporadic cancer

A malignant neoplasm of humans induced by somatic cell rather than germ cell transformation.

spot ELISA

An assay that is a variation on standard enzyme-linked immunosorbent assay (ELISA). It is used primarily for the detection of immunoglobulin-secreting cells (ISCs) or cytokine-secreting cells (CSCs), although future applications may include detection of specific hormone-secreting cells. As in standard ELISA, the starting point is a plastic or nitrocellulose vessel coated with antigen or capture antibody. The ISC or CSC of interest is added and then removed following sufficient incubation time for the cell to secrete its immunoglobulin or cytokine. The secreted product binds locally to the capture protein and is subsequently detected by enzyme-linked antibody. Finally a substrate that yields an insoluble product is added, and the resulting colored precipitate is quantified.

S protein

An 83-kDa serum protein in humans that prevents generation of the membrane attack complex (MAC) of complement. The S protein molecule is comprised of one 478-amino acid residue polypeptide chain. Its mechanism of action is to inhibit insertion of the C5b67 complex into the membrane of a cell by first linking three of its molecules to each free C5b67 complex. It also inhibits C9 from polymerizing on C5b678 complexes. Refer also to vitronectin.

SP thymocyte

Single positive thymocyte that expresses either CD4$^+$ with a surface phenotype of CD4$^+$CD8$^-$ or CD8$^+$ with a surface phenotype of CD4$^-$CD8$^+$.

sprue

Refer to gluten-sensitive enteropathy.

spur

An extension of a precipitation line observed in a two-dimensional double immunodiffusion assay such as the Ouchterlony test. It represents a reaction of partial identity between two antigens that cross react with an antibody.

squalene

A substance synthesized when cholesterol is converted to fat. It is present in selected cosmetics and foods. Squalene has immunologic adjuvant properties and has been used in experimental vaccines as an adjuvant to facilitate response to an immunogen; adjuvants are incorporated into certain vaccines to improve the response to the vaccine constituents. Not all vaccines, however, contain adjuvants; some do not require adjuvants to induce protective immunity in recipients. Aluminum compounds are common adjuvants in licensed vaccines. Some vaccines administered to military personnel during the Gulf War, including anthrax, botulinum toxoid, hepatitis B, and tetanus–diphtheria vaccines, contained aluminum compounds as adjuvants. The presence of antibodies to artificial squalene in the sera of Gulf War veterans has been interpreted by some investigators to imply that squalene or its antibodies may have contributed to these illnesses. The investigators believe that squalene was used as an adjuvant, a claim that has been denied by the U.S. Department of Defense. Squalene is not approved by the FDA for use as an adjuvant in anthrax or any other vaccine.

SRBCs

Abbreviation for sheep red blood cells.

Src homology 2 (SH-2) domain

A 100-amino acid residue, three-dimensional domain structure found in numerous signaling proteins that allows specific noncovalent interactions with other proteins by linking to phosphotyrosines. A unique binding specificity for each SH-2 domain is determined by amino acid residues adjacent to the phosphotyrosine on the target protein. SH-2 domains serve as important sites of protein interaction during early signaling events in T and B lymphocytes.

Src homology 3 (SH-3) domain

A 60-amino acid residue, three-dimensional domain structure found in numerous signaling proteins that facilitates the binding of proteins to one another. SH-3 domains bind to proline residues and function in concert with SH-2 domains on the same protein molecules.

S region

The chromosomal segment of the murine major histocompatibility complex (MHC) containing genes that encode MHC class III molecules, including complement component C2, factor B, C4A (Slp), and C4B (Ss). The S locus within this region contains genes that encode a 200-kDa protein termed Ss (serum substance) that corresponds to C4 in the sera of humans. Also within the S region can be found the gene for Slp (sex limited protein), a protein usually found only in male mice; the gene for 21-hydroxylase, an enzyme with no known immune function; and the gene for a serum β globulin. This term likewise refers to the chromosomal segment that lies between HLA-B and HLA-D, where the genes encoding the corresponding human MHC class III molecules are situated.

SRS-A

Abbreviation for slow-reacting substance of anaphylaxis.

SRV-1

A simian acquired immune deficiency syndrome (AIDS) virus type D that shows little similarity with human immunodeficiency 1 (HIV-1); however, both contain genes that resemble one another. This strain was responsible for an infection among a colony of macaques in California.

SRY

The protein coded for by the sex-determining region of the Y chromosome, known as the *sry* gene in humans. It is equivalent to the testis-determining gene of the Y chromosome. The corresponding protein in mice is called Sry. The murine *sry* gene can cause transgenic female mice to become phenotypic males when the gene is inserted into them.

SS-A

Anti-RNA antibody that occurs in patients with Sjögren's syndrome. The antibody may pass across the placenta in a pregnant female and be associated with heart block in her infant.

SS-A/Ro

An antigen in the cytoplasm to which 25% of patients with lupus erythematosus and 40% of patients with Sjögren's syndrome synthesize antibodies.

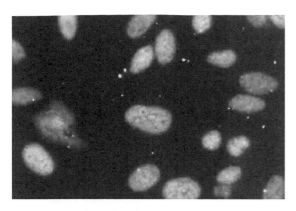

SS-B autoantibodies.

SS-A/Ro antibodies

Antibodies against SS-A/Ro antigen, which consists of 60-kDa and 52-kDa polypeptides associated with Ro RNAs. They may be demonstrated by immunodiffusion in the sera of 35% of patients with systemic lupus erythematosus and 60% of patients with Sjögren's syndrome.

SS-B

An anti-RNA antibody detectable in patients with Sjögren's syndrome and other connective tissue (rheumatic) diseases.

SS-B/La

An antigen in the cytoplasm to which patients with Sjögren's syndrome and lupus erythematosus form antibodies. Anti-SS-B antibodies may portend a better prognosis in patients with lupus erythematosus.

SS-B/La antibodies

Antibodies to SS-B/La antigen, a 48-kDa nucleoplasmic phosphoprotein associated with selected Ro small RNA (Ro hY1–hY5). These antibodies may be demonstrated by enzyme immunoassay (EIA) in Sjögren's syndrome that is primary or secondary to rheumatoid arthritis or in systemic lupus erythematosus.

SSPE

Abbreviation for subacute sclerosing panencephalitis.

Ss protein

A hemolytically active substance encoded by the murine complement locus C4B.

SSS III

One of more than 70 types of specific soluble substances comprising the polysaccharide in capsules of *Streptococcus pneumoniae,* commonly known as pneumococcus. It was used extensively by Michael Heidelberger and associates to perfect the quantitative precipitation reaction.

staphylococcal enterotoxins (SEs)

Bacterial cell constituents that cause food poisoning and activate numerous T lymphocytes by binding to major histocompatibility complex (MHC) class II molecules and the Vβ domains of selected T cell receptors, thus qualifying staphylococcal enterotoxins to be classified as superantigens.

staphylococcal protein A

A substance derived from the cell walls of *Staphylococcus aureus* that interacts with IgG_1, IgG_2, and IgG_4 subclasses. It stimulates human B cell activation.

***Staphylococcus* immunity**

Most individuals synthesize antibodies reactive with staphylococcal antigens that include cell wall-associated teichoic acid and the α-hemolysin extracellular protein. These antibodies are not protective against staphylococcal infections. They may be of some use in diagnosis, but a significant increase in antibody titer is required. High titers of antibodies against toxic shock syndrome toxin (TSST), enterotoxins, and exfoliatins are protective. These toxins are immunomodulatory and mitogenic and induce cytokine synthesis. No effective staphylococcal vaccine has been developed.

STAT transcription factors

Signal transducers and activators of transcription. Proteins activated to become transcription factors through the Janus kinases previously activated by cytokine receptor interaction.

status asthmaticus

A clinical syndrome characterized by diminished responsiveness of asthmatic patients to drugs to which they were formerly sensitive. Patients may not respond to adrenergic bronchodilators and are hypoxemic. Treatment is with oxygen, aminophylline, and methylprednisone.

status thymolymphaticus (historical)

A clinical condition described a half century ago as pathological enlargement of the thymus. Regrettably, it was treated with radiotherapy. Physicians then did not realize that the thymus enlarges under such physiologic conditions, at times attaining a weight of 15 to 25 g at puberty. This enlargement was followed by subsequent involution of the gland. Individuals subjected to radiation therapy were at increased risk of developing thyroid and breast cancer.

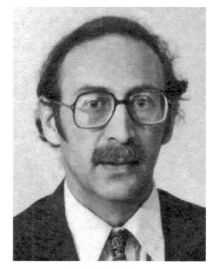

Alfred D. Steinberg.

Steinberg, Alfred

Authority on autoimmunity who worked formerly at the National Institutes of Health, Bethesda, Maryland.

stem cell factor (SCF)

A bone marrow stromal cell transmembrane protein that binds to c-Kit, a signaling receptor found on developing B cells and other developing leukocytes.

stem cells

Relatively large cells with cytoplasmic rims that stain with methyl green pyronin, nuclei that have thin chromatin strands and contain nucleoli that are pyroninophilic. They are found in hematopoietic tissues such as bone marrow. These stem cells constitute part of the colony-forming unit (CFU) pool;

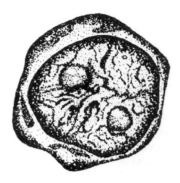

Stem cell.

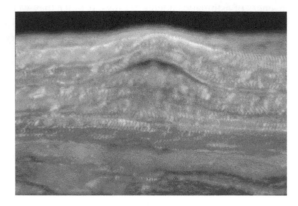

Striational autoantibodies.

individual cells can differentiate and proliferate under favorable conditions. Pluripotent stem cells (CFU-S) are capable of differentiating into committed precursor cells of the granulocyte and monocyte lineage (CFU-C), of erythropoietic lineage (CFU-E and BFUE), and of megakaryocyte lineage (CFU-Mg). Lymphocytes, like other hematopoietic cells, are generated in bone marrow. The stem cell compartment is composed of a continuum of cells that includes the most primitive, with the greatest capacity for self renewal and the least evidence of cell cycle activity, to the most committed with a lesser capacity for self renewal and the most evidence of cell cycle activity. Stem cells are multipotential precursors with the capacity to yield differentiated cell types with different functions and phenotypes; however, their proliferative capacity is limited.

steric hindrance

Interference between the interaction of the paratope of an antibody molecule with the homologous epitopes on antigen molecules of varying sizes based on the shapes of the two reactants. Whereas IgM molecules potentially have an antigen-binding capacity of ten, only some of these may be able to interact with relatively large antigen molecules bearing epitopes because of their shapes. By contrast, relatively small antigen molecules may permit their epitopes to bind with more paratopes on IgM molecules. Steric hindrance also refers to the blocking of ligand binding when a receptor site is already occupied by another ligand.

steric repulsion

Refer to van der Waals forces and London forces.

steroid cell antibodies

Immunoglobulin G (IgG) antibodies that interact with antigens in the cytoplasm of cells, producing steroids in the ovary, testes, placenta, and adrenal cortex. Patients with Addison's disease along with ovarian failure or hypoparathyroidism develop these antibodies that are rarely associated with primary ovarian failure in which organ-specific and nonorgan-specific autoantibodies are prominent.

stiff man syndrome (SMS)

Progressive involuntary axial and lower limb rigidity that disappears during sleep. It results from an imbalance between descending inhibitory γ amino butyric acid (GABA)-ergic and excitatory aminergic pathways. Sixty percent of SMS patients have circulating antibody against glutamic acid decarboxylase (GAD), an enzyme that has 65- and 67-kDa isoforms. GAD is a major antigenic target in insulin-dependent diabetes mellitus (IDDM). Antibody levels to GAD are 100- to 500-fold higher in SMS than in IDDM. SMS anti-GADs bind to both linear epitopes and epitopes that depend on protein conformation. SMS is associated with other autoimmune diseases including myasthenia gravis, pernicious anemia, vitiligo, autoimmune adrenal failure, ovarian failure, thyroid disease, and IDDM.

stimulated macrophage

A macrophage activated *in vivo* or *in vitro*. *Activated macrophage* is the preferred term.

stochastic models

Designs characterized by chance events without external direction or regulation.

Stormont test

A double intradermal tuberculin test.

strain

Genetically identical animals such as mice or rats used in medical research.

street virus

A natural or genetically unmodified virus such as rabies that can be isolated from animals.

streptavidin

A protein isolated from streptomyces that binds biotin. This property makes streptavidin useful in the immunoperoxidase reaction used extensively in antigen identification in histopathologic specimens, especially in surgical pathologic diagnosis.

Streptobacillus immunity

Although immune responses are induced in subjects infected with *Streptobacillus moniliformis*, the exact mechanisms and relative contribution of antibody remain to be determined. In mouse experiments, antibody confers only partial immunity to challenge with the microorganism. Inactivated *S. moniliformis* vaccines induce only partial protection against challenge.

streptococcal M protein

A cell wall protein of virulent *Streptococcus pyogenes* microorganisms that interferes with phagocytosis and also serves as a nephritogenic factor.

Streptococcus immunity

The most effective host resistance against pneumococcal (*Streptococcus pneumoniae*) infection is the synthesis of immunoglobulin G (IgG) or IgM that interacts with capsular polysaccharide, opsonizing the bacteria for ingestion and killing by professional phagocytes. Anticapsular antibody develops following colonization or infection. Most individuals have low resistance as reflected by their lack of antibodies to most of the commonly infecting pneumococcal serotypes even though normal adults may have sufficient antibodies against phosphocholine-containing epitopes of the pneumo-coccal cell wall. This antibody does not appear protective in human subjects; reaction between the antibody and the bacterial cell wall occurs beneath the capsule. The comple-ment fragments and bound Fc are inaccessible to phago-cytic cells. Vaccines to prevent streptococcal infections are hindered by the systemic local and systemic reactions that follow administration of large does of M protein given in an effort to induce type-specific antibody responses. This may be attributable to M proteins serving as superantigens. Heart-reactive epitopes have been removed from M proteins, which has made possible immunization with purified M protein preparations to induce type-specific opsonic antibodies that do not cross react with heart antibodies. Immunization pro-tocols also included attempts to stimulate antibodies against lipoteichoic acid, the adherence constituent of streptococci, but these efforts have been limited by the poor immunogenic-ity of this component. Vaccination with capsular polysaccha-rides is effective in preventing pneumococcal infection.

streptolysin O test

Refer to ASO.

stress and immunity

Stressors can alter many facets of the immune response. Numerous bidirectional pathways of communication con-nect the immune system and the brain, and stress may function through this neuroimmune network to influence immune responses. However, the different types of stress and different means of stress perception lead to the produc-tion of different combinations of autonomic activations and hormones. Immune system-derived information may act on the nervous system, such as during an infection, and may also trigger changes in behavior patterns that resemble stress-associated behavior. The immune system may serve as a sensory organ, transmitting to the brain information about antigens through lymphocyte-derived hormones while being modulated by neural factors (stress related or otherwise). Immune, neural, and psychosocial realms may be coordinated as coherent processes allow identification of the context, interpretation, and meaning of stress for an individual to determine the effects on immunity.

stress proteins

Stress proteins are characterized into major families, gener-ally by molecular weights. Heat shock proteins show a high degree of sequence homology throughout the phylogenetic spectrum and are among the most highly conserved proteins in nature. Heat shock protein 70 from mycobacteria and humans reveals 50% sequence homology. In spite of this homology, subtle differences exist in the functions, inducibil-ity, and cellular locations of related heat shock proteins for a given species. Although major stress proteins accumulate to very high levels in stressed cells, they are present at low to moderate levels in unstressed cells, indicating that they play a role in normal cells. In addition to increased synthesis, many heat shock proteins change their intracellular distri-bution in response to stress. An important characteristic is their capacity to function as molecular chaperones, reflecting their capacity to bind to denatured proteins, preventing their aggregation; this helps explain the functions of heat shock proteins under normal conditions and in stress situations.

striational antibodies

Antibodies demonstrable in 80 to 100% of myasthenia gravis (MG) patients with thymoma; they are not present in 82 to

100% of patients with MG who do not have thymoma. If stria-tional antibodies are not demonstrable in a patient with MG, the individual probably does not have thymoma. One quarter of patients with rheumatoid arthritis receiving penicillamine therapy develop immunoglobulin M (IgM) striational antibod-ies. Patients receiving immunosuppressive therapy may also be monitored for striational antibodies to detect the development of autoimmune reactions following bone marrow transplantation.

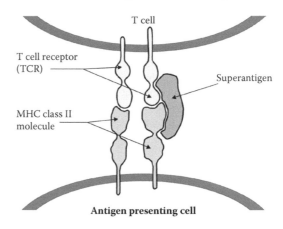

Superantigen.

striational autoantibodies (StrAbs)

Autoantibodies associated with thymoma in patients with myasthenia gravis (MG). Thymoma occurs in 10% of MG patients and MG occurs in 15 to 80% of patients with thymoma. Striational antibodies react with proteins in the contractile constituents of skeletal muscle. The relevant epitopes remain to be demonstrated. Autoantigens reactive with striational autoantibodies include actin, α-actinin, myosin, and titin (connectin). The ryanodine receptor (sarcoplasmic reticulum calcium release channel protein). Striational autoantibodies can be detected by immunofluo-rescence using cryostat sections of skeletal muscle—the method of choice for striational autoantibody screening. These autoantibodies are most often found in MG patients over 60 years of age. The autoantibodies are present in 80 to 90% of patients with both MG and thymoma, in approxi-mately 30% of patients with acquired (adult onset) MG, and in 24% of patients with thymoma without clinical signs of MG. Striational autoantibodies are absent in more than 70% of patients with MG without thymoma; thus, they are very sensitive and specific for thymoma in MG patients, and their absence rules out a diagnosis of thymoma in MG.

stromal cells

Sessile cells that form an interconnected network that gives an organ structural integrity but also provides a specific inductive microenvironment that facilitates differentiation and maturation of incoming precursor cells. Stromal cells and their organization are fully as complex as the cells whose development they regulate. For example, stromal cells of the thymus are the best characterized with respect to their role in T lymphocyte maturation.

***Strongyloides* hyperinfection**

Strongyloides stercoralis larvae may invade the tissues of immunosuppressed patients with enteric strongyloides infection to produce this condition.

Strongyloides immunity

Immunoglobulin G (IgG), IgA, and IgE classes form in response to antigens of *Strongyloides stercoralis* filariform larvae. The principal humoral responses of the IgG$_4$ subclass may be directed to more than 50 different 15- to 100-kDa antigens. The remaining IgG subclasses recognize fewer than 20 antigens. Zinc endopeptidase together with 31- and 28-kDa proteins are antigens that induce specific immune responses, but they are not protective against dissemination in the host. Patients without detectable humoral responses remain asymptomatic. Immunocompromised patients with disseminated infection may manifest high titers of parasite-specific antibodies. Impaired cell-mediated immunity has been claimed by some to facilitate parasite dissemination, but this has not been proven, especially as patients with acquired immune deficiency syndrome (AIDS) have not developed this as an opportunistic infection.

STS

Abbreviation for serological test for syphilis.

St. Vitus dance (chorea)

Involuntary muscular twitching movements that may occur in acute rheumatic fever.

subacute sclerosing panencephalitis

A slow virus disease that occurs infrequently as a complication of measles and produces progressively destructive injury to the brain through slow replication of defective viruses.

subexon

A small exon possessing splice donor and acceptor sites that is spliced at the RNA level with other small subexons to produce a complete constant exon in the Igh locus.

subset

A subpopulation of cells such as T lymphocytes in samples of peripheral blood. Subsets are identified by immunophenotyping with monoclonal antibodies and by flow cytometry. The cells are separated based on their surface CD (cluster of differentiation) determinants, such as CD4, which identifies helper/inducer T lymphocytes, and CD8, which identifies suppressor/cytotoxic T lymphocytes.

substance P (SP)

A tachykinin that may induce joint inflammation when released at local sites. It facilitates synthesis by monocytes of interleukin-1 (IL1), IL6, and tumor necrosis factor α (TNF-α) and stimulates synovial cells to produce prostaglandins. Its receptor is designated NK1. Substance P is a principal component of the neuroimmune axis and axon reflex. It is a mediator of neurogenic inflammation, causing vasodilatation and plasma extravasation. It induces histamine release from mast cells; lymphocyte proliferation; immunoglobulin and cytokine secretion from B lymphocytes and monocytes, respectively; macrophage stimulation; immune complex formation; eosinophil peroxidase secretion; and chemotaxis in response to platelet-activating factor (PAF). SP induces polymorphonuclear leukocyte (PMNL) chemotaxis, phagocytosis, respiratory burst activity, exocytosis, and antibody-mediated cell cytotoxicity. It elevates superoxide production in PMNLs and facilitates TNF-dependent IL8 secretion. SP derived from primary afferent nerves has a proinflammatory effect on neutrophils, leading to increased adhesion to bronchial epithelial cells in acute and chronic bronchitis. SP levels are increased in the sputum of asthmatic and chronic bronchitis patients and those with nasal allergies. It increases PMNL infiltration into the skin in allergic contact dermatitis and enhances PGD$_2$ and leukotriene C4 release from human nasal mucosa and skin mast cells. In vessels, SP induces intercellular adhesion molecule 1 (ICAM-1) expression on vascular endothelial cells. It induces degranulation of mast cells and facilitates transendothelial migration.

substrate adhesion molecules (SAMs)

Extracellular molecules that share a variety of sequence motifs with other adhesion molecules. Most prominent are segments similar to the type III repeats of fibronectin and immunoglobulin-like domains. In contrast to other morphological regulatory molecules, SAMs do not have to be made by the cells that bind them. SAMs can link and influence the behavior of one another. Examples include glycoproteins, collagens, and proteoglycans.

subunit vaccine

An immunizing preparation comprised of a specific component of a pathogen, such as a viral protein or bacterial polysaccharide. The vaccine employs whole micromolecules or large macromolecular fragments that contain the protective epitopes.

sugar cane worker's lung

Refer to bagassosis and farmer's lung.

suicide, immunological

The use of an antigen deliberately labeled with high-dose radioisotope to kill a subpopulation of lymphocytes with receptors specific for that antigen following antigen binding.

sulfite sensitivity

Sulfites or sulfiting agents (such as sulfur dioxide, bisulfite salt, and metabisulfite salt) broadly used as food additives that can induce reactions marked by angioedema, laryngeal edema, asthma, and anaphylaxis. Sulfite reactions occur in atopic and selected nonatopic patients but are more commonly observed in chronic asthma. The hyperreactivity to sulfur dioxide generated from sulfites is believed to involve afferent cholinergic receptors in the tracheobronchial tree, IgE-mediated reactions in a few patients, and sulfite oxidase deficiency. Kinins are believed to play a role in mediation of bronchial constriction. Treatment includes cromolyn to stabilize mast cells; atropine to block cholinergic sensitivity; and cyanocobalamin to assist sulfite oxidation in sulfite oxidase-deficient patients. Diagnosing sulfite sensitivity is based on metabisulfite challenge.

Sulzberger–Chase phenomenon

The induction of immunological unresponsiveness to skin-sensitizing chemicals such as picryl chloride by feeding an animal (e.g., guinea pig) the chemical in question prior to application to the skin. Intravenous administration of the chemical may also block the development of delayed-type hypersensitivity when the same chemical is later applied to the skin. Simple chemicals such as picryl chloride may induce contact hypersensitivity when applied to the skin of guinea pigs. The unresponsiveness may be abrogated by adoptive immunization of a tolerant guinea pig with lymphocytes from one that has been sensitized by application of the chemical to the skin without prior oral feeding.

superantigen

An antigen such as a bacterial toxin that is capable of stimulating multiple T lymphocytes, especially CD4$^+$ T cells, leading to the release of relatively large quantities of cytokines. A protein that unites simultaneously with an invariant site

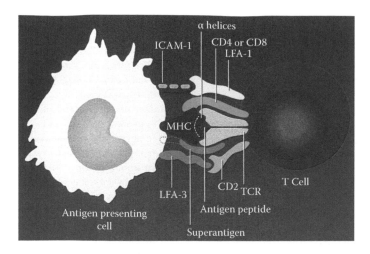

Cellular and molecular interactions in antigen presentation.

on the MHC protein outside the peptide-binding groove and with the CDR2 of selected TCRβ chains. Selected bacterial toxins may stimulate all T lymphocytes that contain a certain family of Vβ T cell receptor (TCR) genes. Superantigens may induce proliferation of 10% of CD4+ T cells by combining with the TCR Vβ and the MHC HLA-DR α-1 domain. Superantigens are thymus-dependent (TD) antigens that do not require phagocytic processing. Instead of fitting into the TCR internal groove where a typical processed peptide antigen fits, superantigens bind to the external regions of αβ TCRs and simultaneously link to DP, DQ, or DR molecules on antigen-presenting cells. Superantigens react with multiple TCR molecules with similar peripheral structures. Thus, they stimulate multiple T cells that augment protective T and B cell antibody responses. This enhanced responsiveness to antigens such as toxins produced by staphylococci and streptococci is an important protective mechanism in an infected individual. Several staphylococcal enterotoxins are superantigens and may activate many T cells, resulting in the release of large quantities of cytokines to produce a clinical syndrome resembling septic shock.

superinfection immunity

The inability of two related organisms (for example, plasmids) to invade a host cell at the same time.

superoxide anion

A free radical formed by the addition of an electron to an oxygen molecule, causing it to become highly reactive. This process takes place in inflammation or is induced by ionizing radiation. The anion is formed by reduction of molecular oxygen in polymorphonuclear neutrophils (PMNs) and mononuclear phagocytes. The hexose monophosphate shunt activation pathway enhances superoxide anion generation. Superoxide anion interacts with protons, additional superoxide anions, and hydrogen peroxide. Oxidation of one superoxide anion and reduction of another may lead to the formation of oxygen and hydrogen peroxide. Superoxide dismutase found in phagocytes catalyzes this reaction. Injury induced by superoxide anion is associated with age-related degeneration. It may also serve as a mutagen with implications for carcinogenesis. It plays a pivotal role in the ability of mononuclear phagocytes and neutrophils to kill microorganisms through their oxidative microbicidal functions.

superoxide dismutase

An enzyme that defends an organism against oxygen-free radicals by catalyzing the interactions of superoxide anions with hydrogen ions to yield hydrogen peroxide and oxygen.

suppressin

A 63-kDa, single polypeptide chain molecule with multiple disulfide linkages and a phagocytic index (PI) of 8.1. It is produced by the pituitary and lymphocytes and is a negative regulator of cell growth. It inhibits lymphocyte proliferation and is more effective on T cells than on B cells. Suppressin has properties similar to transforming growth factor β (TGF-β), although it is structurally different. Antisuppressin antibody leads to T or B cell proliferation.

suppression

Immunologic unresponsiveness that may be specific or general and attributable to products produced by selected lymphocytes or by the administration of immunosuppressive drugs such as for organ transplantation.

suppressor CD4+ T cells

Refer to regulatory CD4+ T cells.

suppressor cell

A lymphoid cell subpopulation that can diminish or suppress the immune reactivity of other cells. An example is the CD8+ suppressor T lymphocyte subpopulation detectable by monoclonal antibodies and flow cytometry in peripheral blood lymphocytes.

suppressor/inducer T lymphocyte

A subpopulation of T lymphocytes that fail to induce immunosuppression but are claimed to activate suppressor T lymphocytes.

suppressor macrophage

Macrophage activated by its response to an infection or neoplasm in the host from which it was derived. It can block immunologic reactivity *in vitro* through production of prostaglandins, oxygen radicals, and other inhibitors produced via arachidonic acid metabolism.

suppressor T cell factor (TSF)

A soluble substance synthesized by suppressor T lymphocytes that diminishes or suppresses the functions of other lymphoid cells. The suppressor factor downregulates immune reactivity. TSF is also an abbreviation for suppressor T cell factor.

suppressor T cells (Ts cells)

A T lymphocyte subpopulation that diminishes or suppresses antibody formation by B cells or downregulates the ability of T lymphocytes to mount cellular immune responses. Ts cells may induce suppression specific for antigen or idiotype or nonspecific suppression. Some CD8$^+$ T lymphocytes diminish T helper CD4$^+$ lymphocyte responsiveness to endogenous and exogenous antigens, leading to suppression of the immune response. An overall immune response may be a consequence of a balance between helper T lymphocyte and suppressor T lymphocyte stimulation. Suppressor T cells are also significant in the establishment of immunologic tolerance and are particularly active in response to unprocessed antigen. The inability to confirm the presence of receptor molecules on suppressor cells has cast a cloud over the suppressor cell; however, functional suppressor cell effects are indisputable. Some suppressor T lymphocytes are antigen-specific and important in the regulation of T helper cell function. Like cytotoxic T cells, T suppressor cells are major histocompatibility complex (MHC) class I-restricted. T cells may act as suppressors of various immune responses by forming inhibitory cytokines.

supratypic antigen

Refer to public antigen.

suramin

Antrypol, 8,8′-(carbonyl-*bis*-(imino-3,1-phenylenecarbonylimino))-*bis*-1,3,5-naphthalene trisulfonic acid; a therapeutic agent for African sleeping sickness produced by trypanosomes. Of immunologic interest is its ability to combine with C3b, thereby blocking binding of factors H and I. The drug also blocks complement-mediated lysis by preventing attachment of the membrane attack complex of complement to the membranes of cells.

surface antigen

Epitopes on a cell surface such as the bacterial antigens Vi and O.

surface immunoglobulin

All immunoglobulin isotypes may be expressed on the surfaces of individual B cells but only one isotype is expressed at any one time, with the exception of unstimulated mature B lymphocytes that coexpress surface IgM (sIgM) and surface IgD (sIgD). Refer to B lymphocyte receptor.

surface marker

A protein on a cell surface that reveals a cell type or stage of differentiation.

surface phagocytosis

Facilitation of phagocytosis when microorganisms become attached to the surfaces of tissues, blood clots, or leukocytes.

surface plasmon resonance (SRP)

A phenomenon that is the basis for instruments designed to measure macromolecular interactions in real time. It measures alterations in the refractive index of a medium surrounding a receptor immobilized on a solid support that occur when a ligand binds. SRP is useful in the analysis of antigen–antibody interactions and can be employed to determine kinetic parameters (association–dissociation rate constants) and equilibrium binding constants and also measure concentrations, perform epitope mapping, and determine antibody isotypes.

surface secretions

Lysozyme induces lysis of bacterial cells by breaking the linkage connecting *N*-acetyl muraminic acid and *N*-acetylglucosamine in the walls of Gram-positive bacterial cells. Lactoferrin interrupts metabolism of bacterial iron.

surrogate light chains (SLC)

Invariant light chains that are structurally homologous to κ and λ light chains and associate with pre-B cell μ heavy chains. They are the same in all B cells. V regions are absent in surrogate light chains. Low levels of cell surface μ chain and surrogate light chain complexes are believed to participate in stimulation of κ or λ light chain synthesis and maturation of B cells. This complex of two non-rearranging polypeptide chains (V pre-B and λ5) synthesized by pro-B cells associate with the Igμ heavy chain to form the pre-B cell receptor.

Sustiva™

A human immunodeficiency virus 1 (HIV-1)-specific, non-nucleoside, reverse transcriptase inhibitor. It is FDA approved for the treatment of HIV. The mechanism of action includes noncompetitive inhibition of HIV-1 reverse transcriptase by efavirenz, the active component of the drug that exerts no inhibitory effect on HIV-2 reverse transcriptase.

SV40 (simian virus 40)

An oncogenic polyoma virus. It multiplies in cultures of rhesus monkey kidney and produces cytopathic alterations

	SV40$_{(1)}$	SV40$_{(1)}$	SV40$_{(1)}$
Immunize (Inactive Tumor)			
Challenge (Live Tumor)	SV40$_{(1)}$	SV40$_{(2)}$	Murine leukemia virus (MuLV)
Result	No growth	No growth	Murine leukemia virus (MuLV) Growth

SV40.

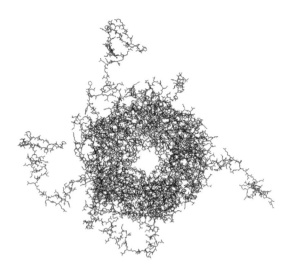

SV40. Resolution = 3.1 Å.

in African green monkey cell cultures. Inoculation into newborn hamsters leads to the development of sarcomas. SV40 has 5243 base pairs in its genome. It may follow either of two patterns of life cycle according to the host cell. In permissive cells such as those from African green monkeys, the virus-infected cells are lysed, causing the escape of multiple viral particles. Lysis does not occur in nonpermissive cells infected with the virus. By contrast, they may undergo oncogenic transformation in which SV40 DNA sequences become integrated into the genome of the host cell. Cells that are transformed have characteristic morphological features and growth properties. SV40 may serve as a cloning vector. It is a diminutive icosahedral papovavirus that contains double-stranded DNA. It may induce progressive multifocal leukoencephalopathy and is useful for the *in vitro* transformation of cells as a type of "permissive" infection ultimately resulting in lysis of infected host cells.

S value (Svedberg unit)
The sedimentation coefficient of a protein ascertained by analytical ultracentrifugation.

Svedberg unit (S)
A sedimentation coefficient unit equal to 10^{-13} seconds. Whereas most immunoglobulin molecules such as IgG sediment at 7S, the pentameric IgM molecule sediments at 19S.

Sweet's syndrome (acute febrile neutrophilic dermatosis)
A syndrome with neutrophilia, fever, and erythematous and painful skin plaques with pronounced dermal neutrophilic inflammation. About 10 to 15% of the cases may have an underlying malignant disease such as a myeloid proliferative disorder, acute myelogenous leukemia, or other tumor. The cutaneous lesions may become vesicular, and pustular skin lesions resemble those in bowel bypass syndrome. Patients may develop arthritis, myalgia, conjunctivitis, and proteinuria. Immunofluorescence reveals IgG, IgM, and C3 in some lesions. Systemic steroid treatment has proven effective in improving skin lesions.

Swiss agammaglobulinemia
A type of severe combined immunodeficiency (SCID) that has an autosomal-recessive mode of inheritance. Patients usually die during infancy as consequences of severe diarrhea, villous atrophy, and malabsorption with disaccharidase deficiency. Because of severely impaired humoral

and cellular immune defense mechanisms, patients face increased susceptibility to various opportunistic infections such as those induced by *Pneumocystis carinii, Candida albicans,* measles, varicella, and cytomegalovirus. Patients are also at increased risk of developing graft-vs.-host disease following blood transfusion. A stem cell defect leads to diminished numbers of T and B lymphocytes. Patients have elevated liver enzymes, lymphopenia, anemia, and diarrhea, causing an electrolyte imbalance. They are usually treated with antibiotics, γ globulin, and HLA-6 antigen match bone marrow transplants.

Swiss-type immunodeficiency
Refer to Swiss agammaglobulinemia.

Swiss type of severe combined immunodeficiency
A condition resulting from a defect at lymphocytic stem cell level that produces cellular abnormalities that affect both T and B cell limbs of the immune response, culminating in impaired cell-mediated immunity and humoral antibody responsiveness following challenge by appropriate immunogens. The mode of inheritance is autosomal-recessive. Refer also to severe combined immunodeficiency syndrome.

switch
The change within an immunologically competent B lymphocyte from synthesizing one isotype of heavy polypeptide chain such as μ to another isotype such as γ during differentiation. The switch signal comes from T cells. Isotype switching does not alter the antigen-binding variable region of the chain at the N terminus.

switch cells
A subset of T lymphocytes that governs isotype differentiation of B lymphocytes exiting the Peyer's patches to ensure that they become immunoglobulin A (IgA)-producing plasma cells when they home back to the lamina propria of the intestine from the systemic circulation.

switch defect disease
Refer to hyperimmunoglobulin M syndrome.

switch region
The amino acid sequence between the constant and variable portions of light and heavy polypeptide immunoglobulin chains. This segment is encoded by D and J genes and controls recombination associated with immunoglobulin class switching. Specific switch region sequences are critical for switching from one immunoglobulin isotype (class) to another. During isotype switching, the active heavy chain V region exon undergoes somatic recombination with a 3′ constant region gene at a switch region of DNA.

switch recombination
Immunoglobulin isotype switching mechanism. Based on pairing of switch regions located 5′ of each C_H exon (other than Cs). The C_H switch region, an original component of the $V(D)J$-C gene, couples with the downstream C_H exon's switch region, leading to excision of the intervening C_H exons. This is followed by union of the $V(D)J$ exon with the new C_H exon. Selected cytokines including TGFβ, INFγ, and IL4 and germline transcripts govern C_H exon selection.

switch site
Breakage points on a chromosome where gene segments unite during gene rearrangement. In immunology, a switch site is an abbreviated DNA sequence 5′ to each gene encoding a heavy chain C region. It serves as an identification site

for V region gene translocation in the process of switching gene expression from one immunoglobulin heavy chain class to another. Numerous switch sites exist for each gene encoding the C region.

SXY-CIITA regulatory system

Regulates MHC class I and II molecule expression. SXY controls promoters of genes governing expression of MHC class I and II molecules. SXY permits construction of the RFS/X2BP/NF-Y endosome on the promoter. CIITA (class II transactivator) serves as a transcription factor uniting with the RFX/X2BP/NF-Y complex.

Syk PTK

A 72-kDa phosphotyrosine kinase (PTK) found on B cells and myeloid cells that is homologous to the ZAP-70 PTK found on T cells and NK cells. Syk and ZAP-70 play roles in the functions of distinct antigen receptors.

sympathetic nervous system autoantibodies

Complement-fixing sympathetic ganglia (CF-SG) autoantibodies and complement-fixing adrenal medullary (CF-ADM) autoantibodies present in some prediabetic and insulin-dependent diabetic patients are associated with decreased catecholamine response. Patients with insulin-dependent diabetes mellitus (IDDM) may manifest CF autoantibodies against vagus nerve that correlate with the presence of CF-SG and CF-ADM autoantibodies. CF-V autoantibodies (parasympathetic nervous system autoantibodies) may also be found in patients with IDDM, but their clinical significance remains to be determined.

sympathetic ophthalmia

Uveal inflammation of a healthy uninjured eye in an individual who sustains a perforating injury to the other eye. The uveal tract reveals an infiltrate of lymphocytes and epithelioid cells and granuloma formation occurs. The mechanism suggested is autoimmunity expressed as T lymphocyte-mediated immune reactivity against previously sequestered antigens released from the patient's other (injured) eye.

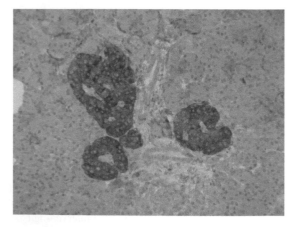

Synaptophysin—pancreas.

synaptophysin

A neuroendocrine differentiation marker detectable by the immunoperoxidase technique used in surgical pathologic diagnosis. Tumors in which it is produced include ganglioneuroblastoma, neuroblastoma, ganglioneuroma, paraganglioma, pheochromocytoma, medullary carcinoma of the thyroid, carcinoid, and tumors of the endocrine pancreas.

syncytia formation

The generation of large multinucleated structures created by the fusion of a large number of uninfected cells by a virus infected cell.

synergism

Mutual assistance, e.g, the finding that the combined effect of two cytokines is greater than the action of either one alone.

syngeneic

Implication of genetic identity between identical human twins or among members of inbred strains of mice and other species. The term is used principally to refer to transplants between genetically identical members of a species. Syngeneic individuals possess the same alleles at all genetic loci.

syngeneic preference

The better growth of neoplasms when they are transplanted to histocompatible recipients than when they are transplanted in histoincompatible recipients. Refer also to allogeneic inhibition.

syngraft

A transplant from one individual to another within the same strain; also called isograft.

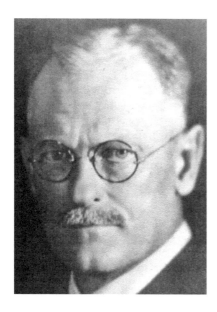

Martin J. Synnott.

Synnott, Martin J.

In 1912, Synott developed the idea for the formation of a Society of Vaccine Therapists that later became the American Association of Immunologists.

synthetic antigen

An antigen derived exclusively by laboratory synthesis and not obtained from living cells. Synthetic polypeptide antigens have backbones consisting of amino acids that usually include lysine. Side chains of different amino acids are attached directly to the backbone and are then elongated with a homopolymer or conversely attached via the homopolymer. They have contributed much to our knowledge of epitope structure and function. They have well defined specificities determined by arrangement, number, and nature of amino acid components of the molecule, and they may be made more complex by further coupling to haptens or derivatized with various compounds. Molecule

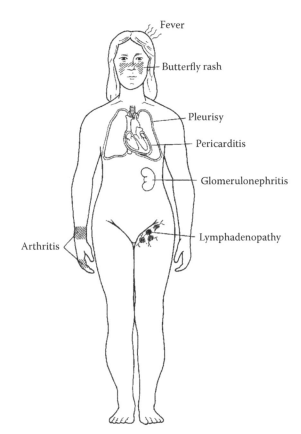

Systemic lupus erythematosus (SLE).

size is less critical with synthetic antigens than with natural antigens. Thus, molecules as small as those of *p*-azobenzenearsonate coupled to three L-lysine residues (750 kDa molecular weight) or even of *p*-azobenzenearsonate-*N*-acetyl-L-tyrosine (451 kDa) may be immunogenic. Specific antibodies are markedly stereospecific, and no cross reaction occurs (e.g., between poly-D-alanyl and poly-L-alanyl determinants). Studies employing synthetic antigens demonstrated the significance of aromatic charged amino acid residues in proving the ability of synthetic polypeptides to induce immune responses.

synthetic polypeptide antigens

Antigens having a backbone consisting of amino acids that usually include lysine. Side chains of different amino acids are attached directly to the backbone and then elongated with a homopolymer or attached via the homopolymer. They have contributed much to our knowledge of epitope structure and function. They have well defined specificities determined by the arrangement, number, and nature of the amino acid components. They may be made more complex by further coupling to haptens or derivatized with various compounds. The size of the molecule is less critical with synthetic antigens than with natural antigens. Molecules as small as p-azobenzenearsonate coupled to three L-lysine residues (750 molecular weight) or p-azobenzenearsonate-N-acetyl-L-tyrosine (451 M.W.) may be immunogenic. Specific antibodies are markedly stereospecific, and no cross reaction occurs, for example, between poly-D-alanyl and poly-L-alanyl determinants. Studies employing synthetic antigens demonstrated the significance of aromatic charged amino acid residues in proving the ability of synthetic polypeptides to induce immune responses.

synthetic vaccines

Substances used for prophylactic immunization against infectious disease prepared by artificial techniques such as DNA cloning or peptide synthesis.

systemic acquired resistance (SAR)

An immune state of a plant that enables it to resist attack by a broad range of pathogens. Elevated concentrations of nitric oxide (NO), salicylic acid, and pathogenesis-related (PR) proteins mediate SAR.

systemic anaphylaxis

Type I immediate anaphylactic hypersensitivity mediated by immunoglobulin E (IgE) antibodies anchored to mast cells that become cross linked by homologous antigen (allergen), causing release of the pharmacological mediators of immediate hypersensitivity and producing lesions in multiple organs and tissue sites. This is in contrast to local anaphylaxis in which effects are produced in isolated anatomical locations. The intravenous administration of a serum product, antibiotic, or other substance against which the patient has anaphylactic IgE-type hypersensitivity may lead to the symptoms of systemic anaphylaxis within seconds and prove lethal.

systemic autoimmune disease

Refer to systemic autoimmunity.

systemic autoimmunity

The formation of antibodies specific for self constituents leading to type III hypersensitivity in which immune complexes are deposited in tissues, leading to pathological sequelae. The prototype for systemic autoimmune disease is systemic lupus erythematosus (SLE) in which autoantibodies specific for DNA, RNA, and proteins associated with nucleic acids form immune complexes deposited in small blood vessels, fix complement, and incite inflammation, leading to vascular injury.

systemic immunoblastic proliferation

A condition characterized by gene translocation and immature lymphocyte proliferation. Patients manifest rash, dyspnea, hepatosplenomegaly, and lymphadenopathy and show increased incidence of immunoblastic lymphoma.

systemic inflammatory response syndrome (SIRS)

The systemic effects of disseminated bacterial infection. Mild and severe forms have been described. The mild form is characterized by fever, neutrophilia, and an increase in acute phase reactants. Lipopolysaccharide (LPS) and other bacterial products may stimulate these changes that are mediated by innate immune system cytokines. Severe SIRS is characterized by disseminated intravascular coagulation, adult respiratory distress syndrome, and septic shock.

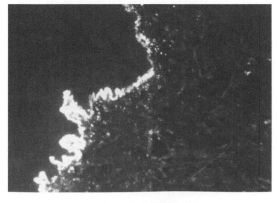

Lupus band test.

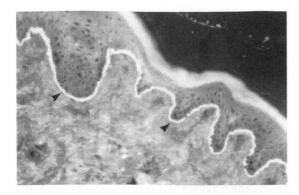

Lupus erythematosus. Immune deposits at dermal–epidermal junction.

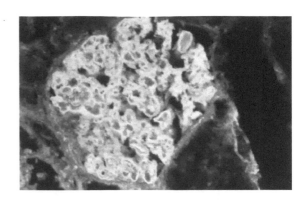

Systemic lupus erythematosus (SLE). Diffuse immune deposits on peripheral capillary loops.

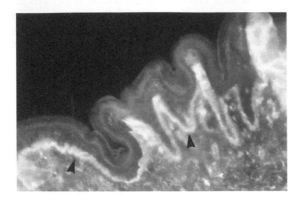

Systemic lupus erythematosus (SLE). Immune deposits at dermal–epidermal junction.

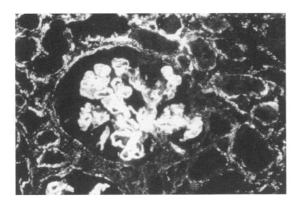

Diffuse proliferative lupus nephritis.

systemic lupus erythematosus (SLE)

The prototype of connective tissue diseases that involves multiple systems and an autoimmune etiology. It has an acute or insidious onset. Patients may experience fever, malaise, loss of weight, and lethargy. All organ systems may be involved. Patients form a plethora of autoantibodies, especially antinuclear autoantibodies. SLE is characterized by exacerbations and remissions. Patients often have injuries of the skin, kidneys, joints, and serosal membranes. SLE occurs in 1 in 2500 people in certain populations and has a female-to-male predominance of 9:1. Its cause remains unknown. Antinuclear antibodies produced in SLE fall into four categories: (1) antibodies against DNA, (2) antibodies against histones, (3) antibodies to nonhistone proteins bound to RNA, and (4) antibodies against nucleolar antigens. Indirect immunofluorescence is used to detect nuclear fluorescence patterns that are characteristic for certain antibodies, such as homogeneous or diffuse staining that reveals antibodies to histones and deoxyribonucleoprotein; rim or peripheral staining that signifies antibodies against double-stranded DNA; speckled patterns that indicate antibodies to non-DNA nuclear components including histones and ribonucleoproteins; and the nucleolar pattern, in which fluorescent spots are observed in the nucleus and reveal antibodies to nucleolar RNA. Antinuclear antibodies most closely associated with SLE are anti-double-stranded DNA and anti-Sm (Smith). The disease appears to have a genetic predisposition associated with DR2 and DR3 genes of the major histocompatibility complex (MHC) in Caucasians of North America. Genes other than human leukocyte antigen (HLA) genes are also important. In addition to the anti-double-stranded DNA and anti-Sm antibodies, other immunologic features of the disease include depressed serum complement levels, immune deposits in glomerular basement membranes and at the dermal–epidermal junction, and the presence of other autoantibodies. Of all the immunologic abnormalities, the hyperactivity of B cells is critical to pathogenesis. B cell activation is polyclonal, leading to the formation of antibodies against self and nonself antigens. SLE also involves a loss of tolerance to self constituents, leading to the formation of antinuclear antibodies. The polyclonal activation leads to antibodies of essentially all classes in immune deposits found in renal biopsy specimens by immunofluorescence. In addition to genetic factors, hormonal and environmental factors are important in producing B cell activation. Nuclei of injured cells react with antinuclear antibodies, forming a homogeneous structure called an LE or hematoxylin body usually found in neutrophils that have phagocytized the denatured nuclei of injured cells. Tissue injury is mediated mostly by an immune complex (type III hypersensitivity). Autoantibodies specific for erythrocytes, leukocytes, and platelets also induce injury through a type II hypersensitivity mechanism. Acute necrotizing vasculitis involves small arteries and arterioles present in tissues. Fibrinoid necrosis is classically produced. Most SLE patients exhibit renal involvement that may take several forms; diffuse proliferative glomerulonephritis is the most serious. Subendothelial immune deposits in the kidneys are typical and may exhibit a "wire-loop" appearance to a thickened basement membrane. In the skin, immunofluorescence can demonstrate deposition of immune complexes and complement at the dermal–epidermal junction. Immune deposits in the skin are especially prominent in sun-exposed areas. Joints may be involved, but the synovitis is nonerosive. Typical female patients have butterfly rashes over the bridges of their noses along with fever and pain in peripheral joints. However, the presenting complaints vary widely. Patients may have central nervous system involvement, pericarditis, or other serosal cavity inflammation. Pericarditis may be present along with involvement of the myocardium or cardiac valves to produce Libman–Sacks endocarditis. Splenic enlargement, pleuritis, and pleural effusion or interstitial pneumonitis, and other organ or system involvement may be observed. Patients may also develop antiphospholipid antibodies called lupus anticoagulants. They may be associated with a false-positive VDRL (Venereal Disease Research Laboratory) test for syphilis. A drug such as hydrazaline may induce a lupus-like syndrome; however, the antinuclear antibodies produced in drug-induced lupus are often specific for histones, a finding not commonly found in classic SLE. Lupus erythematosus induced by drugs remits when the drug is removed. Discoid lupus is a form limited to the skin. Corticosteroids have proven very effective in suppressing immune reactivity in SLE. In more severe cases, cytotoxic agents such as cyclophosphamide, chlorambucil, and azathioprine have been used. Refer to LE cell.

systemic lupus erythematosus, animal models

The main lupus models include inbred murine strains. They are best suited for investigation because their serologic, cellular, and histopathologic characteristics closely resemble those of the corresponding human disease. The three principal types of lupus-prone mice include New Zealand (NZB, NZW, and their F1 hybrid), BXSB, and MRL mice. In addition, single autosomal-recessive mutations termed *gld* (generalized lymphoproliferative disease) and *lprcg* (*lpr*-complementing gene) have been described.

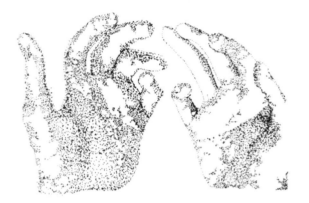

Systemic sclerosis.

systemic sclerosis

Refer to progressive systemic sclerosis.

systemic type III hypersensitivity

Refer to type III hypersensitivity.

T

T1DM

Abbreviation for type 1 diabetes mellitus.

T2DM

Abbreviation for type 2 diabetes mellitus.

T4 count

An abbreviated clinical term designating the number of CD4⁺ T cells in the blood. Normal value is 800 to 1100 CD4⁺ T cells/mm³ blood.

T-200

An obsolete term for leukocyte common antigen (CD45).

TAA

Abbreviation for tumor-associated antigen.

TAB vaccine

An immunizing preparation used to protect against enteric fever. It is composed of *Salmonella typhi* and *S. paratyphi* A and B microorganisms killed by heat and preserved with phenol. The bacteria used in the vaccine are in the smooth specific phase and contain both O and Vi antigens. The vaccine is administered subcutaneously. Lipopolysaccharide from the Gram-negative bacteria may induce fever in vaccine recipients. If *S. paratyphi* C is added, the vaccine is known as TABC. If tetanus toxoid is added, it is referred to as TABT.

Tac

A cell surface protein on T lymphocytes that binds interleukin-2 (IL2). It is a 55-kDa polypeptide (p55) expressed on activated T lymphocytes. Tac is an abbreviation for T activation. The p55 Tac polypeptide combines with IL2 with a K_d of about $10^{-8}M$. Interaction of IL2 with p55 alone does not lead to activation. IL2 binds to a second protein termed p70 or p75 that has a higher binding affinity to p55. T cells expressing p70 or p75 alone are stimulated by IL2. Cells that express both receptor molecules bind IL2 more securely and can be stimulated with a relatively lower IL2 concentration compared to stimulation when p70 or p75 alone interacts with IL-2. Anti-Tac monoclonal antibody can inhibit T cell proliferation.

Tac antigen

Refer to CD25.

TACI (transmembrane activator and CAML-interactor)

A tumor necrosis factor (TNF) receptor family member that serves as one of the two major receptors for BLyS. Dendritic cells, B cells, and T cells all express the TACI receptor, which is believed to be important for receiving signals from BLyS.

tacrolimus

An immunosuppressive polypeptide agent administered to allotransplant recipients to suppress their T cells through inhibition of signal transduction from T cell receptors. Refer to FK506.

T activation

The use of bacterial neuraminidase to cleave *N*-acetyl (sialic acid) residue to uncover masked or hidden antigenic determinants (epitopes). This permits agglutination of the treated cells by natural antibodies in the blood of most individuals. Aged blood can be used to detect T activation.

Taenia solium immunity

Pre-encystment (early) immunity is defined as the immune response at the oncosphere penetration site. Late post-oncospheral or post-encystment immunity is the immune response at the final establishment site. Secretory immunoglobulin A (IgA) in gut secretions likely attacks invading oncospheres, as it is resistant to intestinal enzymes. Mast cells surround invading oncospheres and developing larvae, suggesting that IgE may react with antigen, leading to degranulation of cells whose products cause increased vascular permeability. This would permit IgG antibodies to reach the invading site. Eosinophils also surround invading oncospheres, but no evidence indicates that they induce injury. When newly hatched oncospheres reach their establishment site, they transform from a stage in which they are highly vulnerable to attack to one in which they are completely resistant. Both humoral and cellular responses to *T. solium* are heterogeneous in pigs and humans. Ninety percent of the serum antibody is IgG. The *T. solium* cysticerci induce a chronic granulomatous reaction in pig muscle with extensive eosinophil infiltration and degranulation. T cell immunity to larval cestodes remains to be demonstrated. Larval cestodes may contain blocking antibodies on the surface. Molecular mimicry is also believed to represent an evasive strategy whereby this parasite avoids the host immune response. Some larvae produce inhibitors of proteolytic enzymes such as trypsin and chymotrypsin and some may induce immunosuppression of the host. Vaccination with living eggs can induce complete protection against challenge infection, but egg supplies are limited. This has been remedied by the development of recombinant taeniid vaccine antigens that have been able to induce protection in animals.

TAFs

Abbreviation for toxoid antitoxin floccules.

T agglutinin

An antibody that occurs naturally in the sera of humans. It agglutinates red blood cells expressing T antigen as a result of their exposure to bacteria or treatment with neuraminidase. This antibody is of interest in transfusion medicine as it may confuse blood grouping or cross matching by giving a false-positive reaction when red blood cell suspensions contaminated with microorganisms are used.

tag

A molecular label employed to render unitary antigen–antibody combinations detectable. Substances frequently used as tags include radioisotopes, enzymes, fluorochromes, and electron-dense materials that may be united covalently to the antigen or antibody portion of a complex.

Tagliacozzi, Gaspare (1545–1599)

Physician of Bologna who wrote a famous book on skin grafting titled *De curtorum chirurgia per insitionem*. His

T

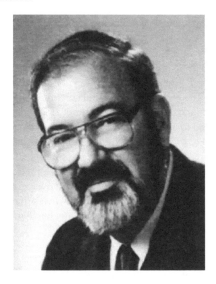

Gaspare Tagliacozzi.

book showed in detail his methods and included illustrations of his instruments and methods of bandaging. He drew analogies from the agricultural practices of grafting in explaining his technique. He understood that xenografts were impossible and allografts were highly unlikely to unite, if only because of the awkwardness of keeping the two parts in close contact so that a graft could take.

tail peptide

An immunoglobulin heavy polypeptide chain carboxyl terminus separate from the carboxyl terminal domain. Tail peptides are present in membrane-anchored immunoglobulins. Tail peptides of 20 amino acids are present in secreted IgM and IgA molecules. IgG and IgE molecules do not contain tail peptides.

Takatsy method

A technique that employs tiny spiral loops on the end of a handle similar to wire loops used by bacteriologists. The loops are carefully engineered to retain precise volume when immersed in liquid and are used to prepare doubling dilutions of test liquids in microtiter wells of test plates. As the loops are passed from one well to the next, the spiral motion helps discharge the contents into the well diluent and mix it. A single operator can manipulate several loops at one time using a single plastic plate with multiple wells. This method has been applied to hemagglutination assays.

Takayasu's arteritis

Inflammation and stenosis involving large- and intermediate-sized arteries including the aortic arch. The disease occurs in the 15- to 20-year old age group and exhibits a 9:1 female predominance. Mononuclear and giant cells infiltrate all layers of the walls of involved arteries,

reflecting true panarteritis. Intimal proliferation, fibrosis, elastic lamina disruption, and media vascularization may be present. The disease begins with an inflammatory phase, followed within several weeks up to 8 years by a chronic occlusive phase. In the initial inflammatory phase, patients develop fever, malaise, weakness, night sweats, arthralgias, and myalgias. Symptoms in the chronic phase are related to ischemia of involved organs. Vascular insufficiency is indicated by decreased or absent radial, ulnar, and carotid pulses. Approximately one third of the patients may have cardiac symptoms such as palpitations and congestive heart failure secondary to hypertension. IgG, IgA, and IgM may be elevated, and the erythrocyte sedimentation rate is usually increased. Corticosteroids may be helpful in controlling inflammation. Cyclophosphamide has been successfully used in cases not responsive to corticosteroid therapy.

take

The successful grafting of skin that adheres to a recipient graft site 3 to 5 days following application. This is accompanied by neovascularization, as indicated by a pink appearance. Thin grafts are more likely to take than thicker grafts, but a thin graft must contain some dermis to be successful. The term *take* also refers to an organ allotransplant that has survived hyperacute and chronic rejection.

Norman Talal

Authority on autoimmune diseases, University of Texas, San Antonio.

Norman Talal.

Talmage, David Wilson (1919–)

American physician and investigator who developed the cell selection theory of antibody formation in 1956. His work was a foundation for Burnet's subsequent clonal selection theory. After training in immunology with Taliaferro in Chicago, where he became a professor in 1952, Talmage became the chairman of microbiology in 1963 and dean of medicine in 1968 at the University of Colorado. He was appointed director of the Webb–Waring Institute in Denver in 1973. In addition to his investigations of antibody formation, he studied heart transplantation tolerance. (Refer to *The Chemistry of Immunity in Health and Disease* [with Cann], 1961.)

Tamiflu®

Refer to oseltamivir.

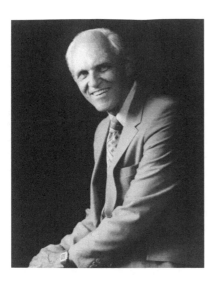

David Wilson Talmage.

Tamm–Horsfall glycoprotein (uromodulin)

A 616-amino acid glycoprotein that produces immunosuppressive effects *in vitro*. It is formed by the kidneys and contains 30% carbohydrate. It may appear in normal human urine. In plasma cell dyscrasia patients, it may combine with Bence–Jones proteins to form multimeric aggregates that may lead to hypercalcemia and hypercalciuria.

tandem immunoelectrophoresis

A variation of crossed immunoelectrophoresis in which the material to be analyzed is placed in one well cut in a gel and a reference antigen is placed in a second well. After electrophoresis in one direction, it is repeated at a right angle, driving antigens that have been separated into another gel containing specific antibodies. Planes of precipitation form and are observed to determine whether they share identity with the reference antigen.

tanned red cell test

A passive hemagglutination assay in which red blood cells are used only as carrier particles for soluble antigens. Agglutination of the cells by specific antibody signifies a positive reaction. To render erythrocytes capable of adsorbing soluble protein antigens to their surfaces, the cells are treated with a weak tannic acid solution. This promotes cell surface attachment of the soluble protein antigen.

tanned red cells

The treatment of a suspension of erythrocytes with a 1:20,000 to 1:40,000 dilution of tannic acid that renders their surfaces capable of adsorbing soluble antigen. They are widely used as passive carriers of soluble antigens in passive hemagglutination reactions. By adding toluene diisocyanate, the protein can become covalently bound to the red cell surface; however, this is not necessary for routine hemagglutination reactions.

T antigen

(1) An erythrocyte surface antigen shielded from interaction with the immune system by an *N*-acetyl-neuraminic acid residue. An antibody is formed against this antigen after bacterial infection has diluted the neuraminic acid residue. Antibodies produced can cause polyagglutination of red cells bearing the newly revealed T antigen. (2) Several 90-kDa nuclear proteins that combine with DNA and are critical in transcription and replication of viral DNA in the lytic cycle. T antigen participates in the change from early to late stages of transcription. (3) An epitope that shares homology at the N terminal sequence with the SV40 virus T antigen.

T1 antigen

Refer to CD5.

T3 antigen

Refer to CD3.

T4 antigen

Refer to CD4.

T8 antigen

Refer to CD8.

TAP

Abbreviation for transporter of antigen processing. A heterodimeric protein situated in the rough endoplasmic reticulum membrane that conveys HSP-chaperoned peptides from the cytosol into the rough endoplasmic reticulum lumen where they are loaded onto MHC class I molecules. It is a critical constituent of endogenous antigen processing and presentation.

TAP 1 and 2 genes

Refer to transporter in antigen processing (TAP) 1 and 2 genes.

TAPA-1

A serpentine membrane protein that crosses a cell membrane four times. It is one of three proteins comprising the B cell coreceptor. It is also call CD81.

tapasin (TAP-associated protein)

A chaperone molecule critical to major histocompatibility complex (MHC) class I molecule assembly. Tapasin participates in the assembly of peptide–MHC class I molecule complexes in the endoplasmic reticulum. It is a rough endoplasmic reticulum protein that unites TAP and the MHC class I α chain at two separate binding sites. Believed to stabilize empty MHC class I heterodimers in a configuration appropriate for peptide loading. Cells deficient in this protein have unstable MHC class I cell surface molecules.

tapioca adjuvant (historical)

An immunologic adjuvant consisting of starch granules to which molecular antigen was absorbed. This permitted the adjuvant–antigen complex to form a depot in the tissues from which the antigen was slowly released to stimulate a sustained antibody response.

Taq polymerase

Thermus aquaticus polymerase. A heat-resistant DNA polymerase that greatly facilitates use of the polymerase chain reaction (PCR) to amplify minute quantities of DNA from various sources into a sufficiently large quantity that can be analyzed.

target cell

A cell that serves as the object of an immune attack mediated by antibodies and complement or by specific immune effector T cells, effector NK cells, and other effector cells and molecules. A target cell must bear an antigen for which the antigen-binding regions of the antibody molecules or T cell receptors are specific. Examples include virus-infected cells that are targets of cytotoxic T cells, leading to target cell death and the facilitation of antibody synthesis by B cells that are targets of effector CD4 T helper lymphocytes.

Tat

The transactivator protein product of the *tat* gene of human immunodeficiency virus (HIV). It increases the rate of transcription of viral RNA. Activation of latently infected cells leads to synthesis. Tat protein binds to a transcriptional enhancer in the long terminal repeat of the provirus, increasing proviral genome transcription. It activates proviral DNA transcription by interfering with premature transcription termination. It also facilitates apoptosis of infected host cells and hinders survival signaling.

TATA
Abbreviation for tumor-associated transplantation antigen.

TATA box
An oligonucleotide sequence comprised of thymidine–adenine–thymidine–adenine found in numerous genes that are transcribed often or rapidly.

tat gene
A retrovirus gene found in HIV-1. The Tat transactivating protein encoded by this gene gains access to the nucleus and activates viral proliferation. Additional retroviral genes become activated. Mesenchymal tumors may be induced by *tat* genes in experimental animals.

TB
Abbreviation for tuberculosis.

T–B cell cooperation
Cooperation of B cells and helper T cells that leads to B cell proliferation and differentiation into plasma cells that synthesize and secrete specific antibody. B cell immunoglobulin receptors react with protein antigen, followed by endocytosis, antigen processing, and presentation to helper T lymphocytes. Their antigen-specific T cell receptors recognize processed antigen only in the context of major histocompatibility complex (MHC) class II molecules on B cell surfaces during antigen presentation. CD4+ helper T cells secrete lymphokines, including interleukin-2 (IL2),

that promote B cell growth and differentiation into plasma cells that secrete specific antibody. T cells are required for B cells to be able to switch from forming immunoglobulin M (IgM) to synthesizing IgG or IgA. B and T lymphocytes recognize different antigens. B cells may recognize peptides, native proteins, or denatured proteins. T cell recognition systems are more complex in that a peptide antigen may be presented to them only in the context of MHC class II or class I histocompatibility molecules. Hapten–carrier complexes have been successfully used in delineating the different responses of B and T cells to each part of this complex. Immunization of a rabbit or other animal with a particular hapten–carrier complex will induce a primary immune response; a second injection of the same conjugate will induce a secondary immune response. However, linkage of the same hapten to a different carrier elicits a much weaker secondary response in an animal primed with the original hapten–carrier complex. This is termed the carrier effect. B lymphocytes recognize the hapten, and T lymphocytes the carrier.

TBI
Abbreviation for total body irradiation.

T cell activation
Response of mature naïve T cells to antigen presented to them by professional antigen-presenting cells, resulting in T lymphocyte proliferation and differentiation into effector T cells.

T cell antigen receptors
The two types of T cell antigen receptors are TCR1, which appears first in ontogeny, and TCR2. TCR2 is a heterodimer of α and β polypeptides. TCR1 consists of γ and δ

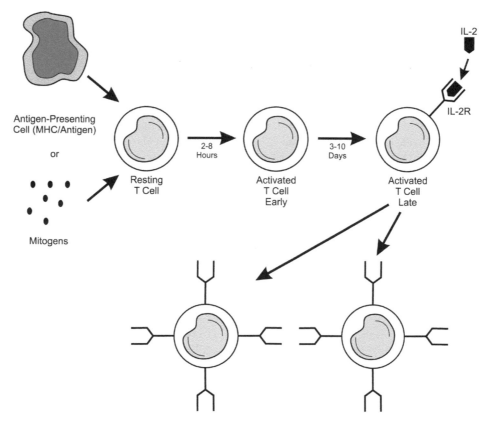

T cell activation.

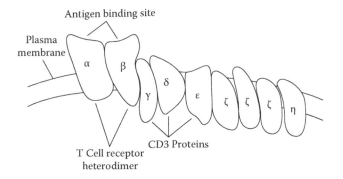

Antigen binding site

Plasma membrane

α   β

δ

γ   ε   ζ   ζ   ζ   η

CD3 Proteins

T Cell receptor heterodimer

T cell antigen receptor.

polypeptides. Each of the two polypeptides comprising each receptor has a constant and a variable region (similar to immunoglobulin). Reminiscent of the diversity of antibody molecules, T cell antigen receptors can likewise identify a tremendous number of antigenic specificities (estimated to be able to recognize 10^{15} epitopes). The TCR is comprised of a minimum of seven receptor subunits whose production is encoded by six separate genes. Following transcription, these subunits are assembled precisely. Assimilation of the complete receptor complex is requisite for surface expression of TCR subunits. Numerous biochemical events are associated with activation of a cell through a TCR. These events ultimately lead to receptor subunit phosphorylation. T cells may be activated by the interaction of antigen, in the context of MHC, with the T cell receptor. This involves transmission of a signal to the interior through the CD3 protein to activate the cell.

T cell antigen-specific suppressor factor

A soluble substance produced by a suppressor T cell after it has been activated. This suppressor factor has been claimed

to bind antigen and cause the immune response to be suppressed in an antigen-specific manner.

T cell areas

Regions of secondary tissues occupied predominantly by T lymphocytes.

T cell chemotactic factor

Former term for interleukin-8 (IL8).

T cell clonal expansion

Clonal expansion of T lymphocytes after initial encounter with antigen is a critical mechanism of the effector limb of the immune response. This permits the immune system to respond to a broad spectrum of pathogens. Clonal expansion is closely regulated to prevent inappropriate responses. Increased clonal expansion is desirable during the early course of an infection and in the prevention of growth and survival of T cells mediating autoimmune disease.

T-cell-dependent (TD) antigen

An immunogen that is much more complex than the T-cell-independent (TI) antigens. TD antigens are usually proteins, protein–nuclear protein conjugates, glycoproteins, or lipoproteins. They stimulate all five classes of immunoglobulin, elicit anamnestic or memory responses, and are present in most pathogenic microorganisms. These properties ensure that an effective immune response can be generated in a host infected with these pathogens.

T cell development

Stem cells in the bone marrow that are destined to develop into T cells migrate to the thymus, where they undergo maturation and development. These precursors of T cells possess unrearranged T cell receptor (TCR) genes and do not express CD4 or CD8 markers. Thymocytes (developing T cells) are found first in the outer cortex, where their numbers increase; the TCR genes are rearranged; and CD3, CD4, CD8, and TCR molecules are expressed on the surface. During maturation, these cells pass from the

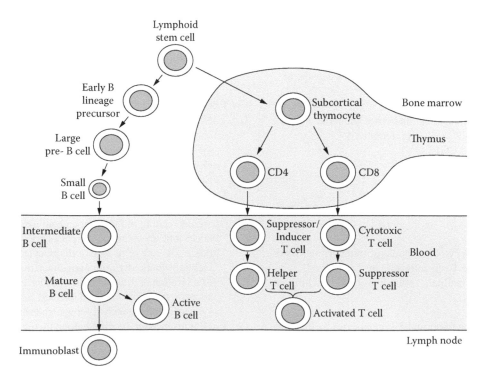

Thymus cell differentiation—T cell maturation.

T

cortex to the medulla. As maturation proceeds, CD4⁻/ CD8⁻ (double-negative) T cells develop into CD4⁺/CD8⁺ and become CD4⁻/CD8⁻ or CD4⁻/CD8⁺ single-positive T cells. Somatic rearrangement of variable, diversity (β), and joining gene segments in the area of C gene segments leads to the production of functional genes that encode TCR γ and δ polypeptides. Many T cell specificities result from the numerous combinations possible for joining separate gene segments in addition to various mechanisms for junctional diversity. Somatic rearrangement of germline genes is also responsible for the functional genes that encode TCR α and β polypeptides. While fewer V genes are in the γ and δ loci and junction diversity is greater, the mechanisms to produce γδ diversity resemble those for the αβ receptor. A few cortical thymocytes express γδ receptors. Thereafter, a line of developing T lymphocytes expresses numerous αβ TCR receptors. The β chains appear first, followed by α chains of TCRs. The β chain associates with an invariant pre-T α surrogate α chain. Signals transduced by the pTαβ receptor facilitate expression of CD4 and CD8 and facilitate expansion of immature thymocytes. CD4⁺/CD8⁺ cortical thymocytes first express αβ receptors. Self major histocompatibility complex (MHC) restriction and self tolerance develop as consequences of the interactions of cortical epithelial cells and nonlymphoid cells derived from the bone marrow that both express MHC. This leads to selection of T cells to be saved. During positive selection, CD4⁺/CD8⁺ TCR αβ thymocytes recognize peptide–MHC complexes on thymic epithelial cells with low avidity. This saves them from programmed cell death (apoptosis). Recognition of self peptide–MHC complexes on thymic antigen-presenting cells with avidity by CD4⁺/CD8⁺ TCR αβ thymocytes leads to apoptosis. Most cortical thymocytes are killed during selection. The αβ thymocytes that remain undergo maturation and proceed to the medulla, where they become CD4⁺/CD8⁻ or CD4⁻/CD8⁺ single-positive cells. During residence in the medulla, they become helper or cytolytic cells prior to their journey to the peripheral lymphoid tissues, where they function as self MHC-restricted helper T cells or precytotoxic T lymphocytes capable of responding to foreign antigen.

T cell domains
Specific areas in lymph nodes and other lymphoid organs where T lymphocytes localize preferentially.

T cell growth factor (TCGF)
Refer to interleukin-2 (IL2).

T cell growth factor 1
Interleukin-2 (IL2).

T cell growth factor 2
Interleukin-4 (IL4).

T cell help
Facilitation through cytokines and costimulatory signals or B cell and cytotoxic T cell activation by T helper cells. Th1 and Th2 cytokines facilitate antibody isotype switching in B cells.

T cell hybridomas
The immortalization of normal T lymphocytes by fusion with continuously replicating tumor cells. Fusion randomly immortalizes T lymphocytes regardless of their antigen specificity and genetic restrictions to form a T cell hybridoma. This represents one of two methods to isolate

and propagate T cell lines in clones of defined specificity. The other technique is to span clones of normal immune T lymphocytes stimulated with appropriate antigens and antigen-presenting cells. The hybridoma technique has an advantage over T cell cloning in the relative ease in securing relatively large numbers of T cells of interest and their biologically active products. Lymphokines and other regulatory molecules along with their nRNA and DNA represent T cell hybridoma products. This technology has facilitated evaluation of T cell receptors and their antigen recognition mechanisms. The adoptive (passive) transfer of autoantigen-specific T cell hybridomas in mice can induce autoimmune diseases.

T cell immunodeficiency syndrome (TCIS)
Decreased immune function as a consequence of complete or partial defects in T lymphocyte functioning. Patients develop recurrent opportunistic infections and may manifest cutaneous anergy, wasting, diminished life expectancy, growth retardation, and increased likelihood of developing graft-vs.-host disease. They may have serious or even fatal reactions following immunization with BCG or live virus vaccines and face increased likelihood of malignancy. T cell immunodeficiencies are usually more profound than B cell immunodeficiencies and have no effective treatment. This group of disorders includes thymic hypoplasia (DiGeorge syndrome), cellular immunodeficiency with immunoglobulins, and defects of T lymphocytes caused by deficiency of purine nucleoside phosphorylase and lack of inosine phosphorylase.

T cell-independent (TI) antigen
An immunogen that is simple in structure, often a polysaccharide such as the polysaccharide of the pneumococcus, a dextran polyvinyl hooter, or a bacterial lipopolysaccharide. This antigen elicits an IgM response only and fails to stimulate an anamnestic response. It is not found in most pathogenic microbes.

T cell leukemia
Adult T cell leukemia/lymphoma.

T cell leukemia viruses
Retroviruses such as HTLV-I (human T lymphocyte virus I) that induce human T cell leukemia, and HTLV-II, which has been associated with hairy cell leukemia.

T cell lymphoma (TCL)
Neoplastic proliferation of T lymphocytes diagnosed by determining whether rearrangement of the genes encoding the T lymphocyte receptor β chain has occurred.

T cell maturation
Refer to thymus cell differentiation figure.

T cell migration
Cells leaving the thymus migrate to all peripheral lymphoid organs seeding in the T-dependent regions of the lymph nodes and spleen and at the peripheries of lymphoid follicles. The rate of release of thymocytes from the thymus increases markedly after antigenic stimulation. The patterns of migration of T cells and B cells have been studied by adoptive transfer of labeled purified cells into irradiated syngeneic mice matched for age and sex.

T cell non-antigen-specific helper factor
A substance that provides nonspecific help to T lymphocytes.

T cell priming
Mature naïve T cell stimulation by antigen presented to them by professional antigen-presenting cells.

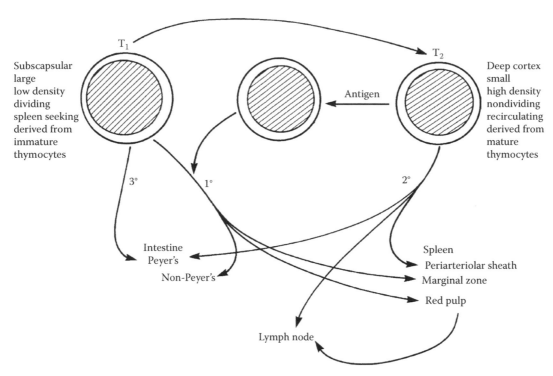

Migration patterns of thymus cells.

T cell receptor (TCR)

A T cell surface structure composed of a disulfide-linked heterodimer of highly variable α and β chains expressed at cell membranes as a complex with invariant CD3 chains. Most T cells that bear this type of receptor are termed αβ T cells. A second receptor known as γδ TCR is comprised of variable γ and δ chains expressed with CD3 on a smaller subset of T lymphocytes that recognize different types of antigens. Both types of receptors are expressed with a disulfide-linked homodimer of ζ chains. Both αβ and γδ receptors on cell surfaces are associated with complexes of invariant CD3 and ζ chains that have a signaling function. The TCR is a receptor for antigen on CD4⁺ and CD8⁺ T lymphocytes that recognizes foreign peptide–self MHC molecular complexes on the surfaces of antigen-presenting cells. In the predominant αβ TCR, each of the two disulfide-linked transmembrane α and β polypeptide chains bears one N terminal Ig-like variable (V) domain, one Ig-like constant (C) domain, a hydrophobic transmembrane region, and a short cytoplasmic region. Refer also to T lymphocyte antigen receptor, T cell receptor genes, and T cell receptor, γδ.

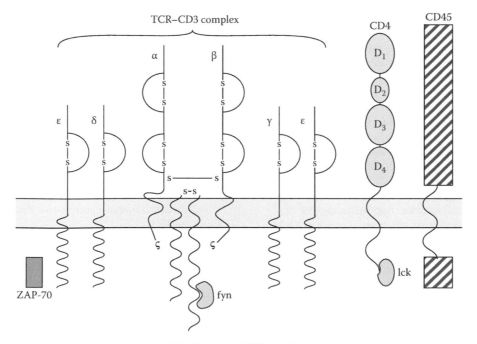

T cell receptor–CD3 complex.

T

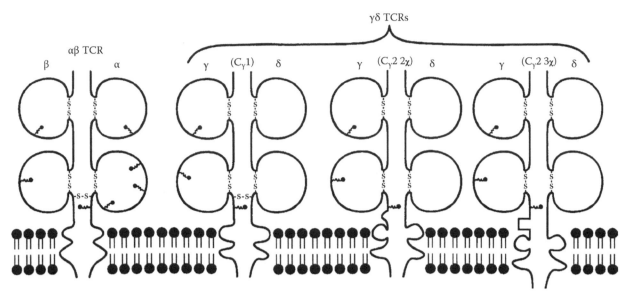

T cell receptor showing αβ and γδ receptors.

T cell receptor α chain (TCRα)
One of the two polypeptide chains comprising the predominant type of T cell receptor.

T cell receptor β chain (TCRβ)
One of the two polypeptide chains comprising the predominant type of T cell receptor.

T cell receptor (TCR) complex
The combination of T cell receptor α and β chains and the invariant signaling proteins CD3 γ, δ, and ε and the ζ chain.

T cell receptor γδ (TCR γδ)
A far less common receptor than the αβ TCR. It is composed of γ and δ chains and occurs on the surfaces of early thymocytes and less than 1% of peripheral blood lymphocytes. The γδ TCR appears on double-negative CD4⁻/CD8⁻ cells. Thus, the γδ heterodimer resembles its αβ counterpart in possessing V and C regions but has less diversity. TCR specificity and diversity are attributable to the multiplicity of germline V gene segments subjected to somatic recombination in T cell ontogeny, leading to a complete TCR gene. Cells bearing the γδ receptor often manifest target cell killing that is not major histocompatibility complex (MHC) restricted. Monoclonal antibodies to specific TCR V regions are undergoing investigation for possible use in treating autoimmune diseases. γδ T cells are sometimes found associated with selected epithelial surfaces, especially in the gut. The TCR complex is composed of the antigen-binding chains associated at cell level with the signal transduction molecules CD3, ζ, and η.

T cell receptor (TCR) genes
Four separate sets of genes encode the antigen–MHC binding region of the T cell receptor. Approximately 95% of peripheral T lymphocytes express α and β gene sets. Only about 5% of circulating peripheral blood T cells and a subset of T lymphocytes in the thymus express γ and δ genes. The αβ chains or γδ chains encoded by their respective genes form intact T cell receptors and are associated with γ, δ, ε, ζ, and ἡ chains that comprise the CD3 molecular complex. The arrangement of TCR genes resembles that of genes that encode immunoglobulin heavy chains. The TCR δ genes are located in the centers of the α genes. V, D,

and J segment recombination permits TCR gene diversity. Rearrangement of a V α segment to a J α segment yields an intact variable region. Two sets of D, J, and C genes exist at the β locus. During joining, marked diversity is achieved by V–J, V–D–D–J, and V–D–J rearrangements. Humans have eight V γ, three J γ, and an initial C γ gene. Before reaching Cγ2, there are two more J γ genes. The δ locus contains five V δ, two D δ, and six J δ genes. TCR gene recombination occurs via mechanisms that resemble those of B cell genes. B and T lymphocytes have essentially the same rearrangement enzymes. TCR genes do not undergo somatic mutation, which is essential to immunoglobulin diversity.

T cell replacing factor (TRF)
An earlier term for B cell differentiation factor derived from CD4⁺ helper T lymphocytes that permits B lymphocytes to synthesize antibody without the presence of T lymphocytes.

T cell rosette
E rosette.

T cells
T lymphocytes that mature in the thymus and are responsible for cell-mediated immunity. Their cell surface receptor for antigen is designated T cell receptor (TCR). Cells derived from hematopoietic precursors that migrate to the thymus, where they undergo differentiation that continues to completion in the various lymphoid tissues or during their circulation to and from these sites. T cells are primarily involved in the control of the immune responses by providing specific cells capable of helping or suppressing such responses. They also fulfill other functions related to cell-mediated immune phenomena. Refer to T lymphocyte.

T cell specificity
Refer to MHC restriction.

T cell system
Mediates self–nonself recognition. Appeared earlier in evolution than did antibodies that are essentially confined to vertebrates. Vertebrate T and B lymphocyte responses are clearly defined. Separate developmental sites have been identified. The appearance of a true thymus in bony fishes (teleosts), amphibians, reptiles, birds, and mammals was accompanied

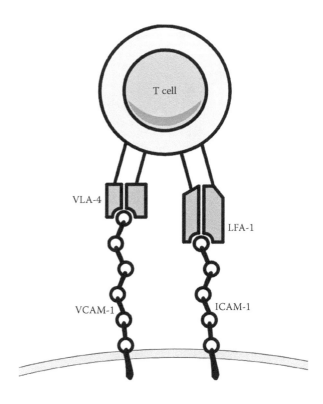

Activated endothelial cell.

by MHC molecules, cytotoxic T cells, cell-mediated immunity, and allograft rejection. T cell-dependent, rapid anamnestic antibody responses of high affinity and heterogeneity are confined to warm blooded vertebrates such as mammals and birds.

T cell tolerance

The processing and presentation of self proteins complexed with major histocompatibility complex (MHC) molecules on antigen-presenting cells of the thymus. The immature T lymphocytes exiting the thymus are tolerant to self antigens. Tolerance of T cells to tissue antigens not represented in the thymus is maintained by peripheral tolerance and is attributable to clonal anergy in which antigen-presenting cells recognize antigen in the absence of costimulation. Thus, cytokines are not activated to stimulate T cell responses. The activation of T lymphocytes by high antigen concentration may lead to their deaths through Fas-mediated apoptosis. Regulatory T lymphocytes may also suppress the reactivity of T lymphocytes specific for self antigens. Interleukin-10 (IL10), transforming growth factor β (TGF-β), or another immunosuppressive cytokine produced by T lymphocytes reactive with self may facilitate tolerance. Clonal ignorance may also be important in preventing autoimmune reactivity.

T cell vaccination (TCV)

A technique to modulate immune response in which T lymphocytes are administered as immunogens. The vaccine is composed of T cells specific for the target autoantigen in an autoimmune response to be modulated. For example, antimyelin basic protein CD4$^+$/CD8$^-$ T cells serving as a vaccine were irradiated (1500 R) and injected into Lewis rats. Vaccination with the attenuated anti-MBP T cells induced resistance against subsequent efforts to induce experimental allergic encephalomyelitis (EAE) by active immunization with myelin basic protein in adjuvant. This technique may even induce resistance against EAE adoptively transferred

by active anti-MBP T cells. This method was successfully applied to other disease models of adjuvant arthritis, collagen-induced arthritis, experimental autoimmune neuritis, experimental autoimmune thyroiditis, and insulin-dependent diabetes mellitus (IDDM). TCV was demonstrated to successfully abort established autoimmune disease and spontaneous autoimmune disease in the case of IDDM.

TCGF (T cell growth factor)

Interleukin-2 (IL2).

TCRαβ transgenic mouse (TCR tg)

A murine transgenic model produced by incorporating into its germline DNA the rearranged genes that encode specific TCRα and β chains that constitute a TCR recognizing a specific pMHC. Most T cells in each TCR Tg mouse express the same TCR protein and same specificity for antigen.

TCR complex

Antigen receptor of T lineage cells. In αβ T cells, the complex is comprised of αβ TCR in addition to CD3γε, CD3δε, CD3ζζ, CD3ζη, or CD3ζ–Fc ε RIγ. In γδ T cells, the complex is comprised of a γδ TCR, two CD3γε heterodimers, and CD3ζζ, CD3ζη, or CD3ζ–FcεRIγ.

TCR tickling

Protracted but slight activation of the T cell receptors of resting naïve T cells by self-pMHC complexes presented in lymph nodes. Inhibits apoptotic death usually induced in naïve mature T cells without specific antigen. May have a role in maintaining memory T cells.

Tc cells

Cytotoxic T lymphocytes that identify nonself peptide presented by an MHC class I molecule on a target cell surface. Once activated, Tc cells become cytotoxic T lymphocyte effector cells that fatally injure target cells via perforin/granzyme-mediated cytotoxicity or secreted cytotoxic cytokines. Tc cells are usually CD8 coreceptor-positive.

Tc lymphocyte

Refer to cytotoxic T lymphocyte.

TD antigen

Abbreviation for thymus-dependent antigen.

T-dependent antigen

Refer to thymus-dependent antigen.

TdT

Abbreviation for terminal deoxynucleotidyl transferase.

TDTH lymphocyte

A delayed-type hypersensitivity T lymphocyte.

Tec kinase

A family of src-like tyrosine kinases that play a role in activation of lymphocyte antigen receptors through activation of PLC-γ. Btk in B lymphocytes, which is mutated in X-linked agammaglobulinemia (XLA) and human immunodeficiency disease, and ltk in T lymphocytes are examples of other Tec kinases.

telencephalin

An immunoglobulin superfamily member with nine immunoglobulin-like domains that is expressed in the central nervous system. It is a human α$_{1β2}$ ligand that has a high homology with intercellular adhesion molecule 1 (ICAM-1) (50%) and ICAM-3 (55%) in the first five amino terminal domains. The clustered location for ICAM-1, ICAM-3, and telencephalin is on human chromosome 19. Their corresponding α chain receptors are located on chromosome 16.

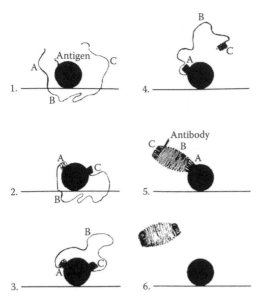

Template theory.

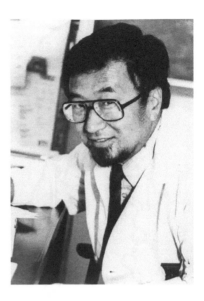

Paul Terasaki, a pioneer in human histocompatibility.

template theory (historical)

An instructive theory of antibody formation that requires that antigen be present during antibody synthesis. According to the refolding template theory, uncommitted and specific globulins may become refolded on the antigen, serving as a template for it. The cell thereupon releases complementary antibodies that rigidly retain their shapes through disulfide bonding. This theory was abandoned when it became clear that the specificity of antibodies in all cases is due to the particular arrangement of their primary amino acid sequences. The template theory could not explain immunological tolerance or the anamnestic (memory) immune response.

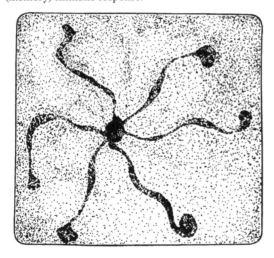

Tenascin.

tenascin

A matrix protein produced by embryonic mesenchymal cells. It facilitates epithelial tissue differentiation and consists of six identical 210-kDa proteins.

Terasaki, Paul (1929–)

American immunologist who began his career in transplantation immunology as a postdoctoral research fellow under Peter Medawar in London in 1957. On returning to UCLA in 1959, he perfected the microcytotoxicity test, which was important in identification of the HLA system. He established the usefulness of HLA in cross matching and detection of presensitization in organ grafting. The principal theme of his research has concerned evaluation of the role of HLA matching in transplantation. His more recent work has been in establishing the role of HLA antibodies in chronic rejection. Terasaki has played a significant international role in tissue typing as director of Tissue Typing at UCLA and directro of the Regional Organ Procurement Agency in southern California. He is one of the world's leading researchers in HLA and transplantation. The company he founded, One Lambda, Inc., has made key contributions to HLA technology.

terminal complement complex

A sequence remains the same whether activation is initiated via the classical, alternative, or lectin pathway. Following cleavage of C5 by the classical or alternative C5 convertase, the terminal complement components C6, C7, C8, and C9 are sequentially but nonenzymatically activated, resulting in the formation of a terminal complement complex (TCC). TCC can be generated on a biologic target membrane as potentially membranolytic membrane attack complex (MAC) or in extracellular fluids as nonlytic SC5b–9 in the presence of S protein (also called vitronectin). Both forms consist of C5b and the complement proteins C6, C7, C8, and C9. Although some lytic activity is expressed by the C5b–8 complex, efficient lysis is dependent on an interaction with C9, facilitated by the α moiety of C8.

terminal complement complex (TCC) deficiency

The hereditary deficiency of a terminal complement component leads to inability to form a functional terminal complement complex with absence of hemolysis and bactericidal activity. Patients with meningococcal infections frequently exhibit terminal complement deficiencies, suggesting that the cytolytic activity of the complement system is critical in resistance to *Neisseria meningitidis*.

terminal complement components

The C5 through C9 constituents of the complement system that assemble to produce the membrane attack complex (MAC).

terminal deoxynucleotidyl transferase

Terminal deoxynucleotidyl transferase (TdT) is an enzyme catalyzing the attachment of mononucleotides to the 3′ terminus of DNA. It thus acts as a DNA polymerase. It is present in immature B and T lymphocytes but not demonstrable in mature lymphocytes. TdT is present both in the nuclear and soluble fractions of thymus and bone marrow. It can also incorporate ribonucleotides into DNA. In mice, two forms of TdT can be separated from a preparation of thymocytes and are designated peak I and peak II. They have similar enzymatic activities and appear to be serologically related but display significant differences in biologic properties. Peak I appears constant in various strains of mice and at various ages, while peak II varies greatly. In some strains, peak II remains constant up to 6 to 8 months of age; in others, it declines immediately after birth. Eighty percent of bone marrow TdT is associated with a particular fraction of bone marrow cells separated on a discontinuous bovine serum albumin (BSA) gradient. This fraction represents 1 to 5% of the total marrow cells but is O antigen-negative. These cells become O-positive after treatment with the thymopoietin thymic hormone, suggesting that they are precursors of thymocytes. Thymectomy is associated with rapid loss of peak II and a slower loss of peak I in this bone marrow cell fraction. TdT is detectable in T cell leukemia, 90% of common acute lymphoblastic leukemia cases, and half of acute undifferentiated leukemia cells. Approximately one third of chronic myeloid leukemia cells in blast crisis and a few cases of pre-B cell acute lymphoblastic leukemia show cells that are positive for TdT. This marker is rarely seen in cases of chronic lymphocytic leukemia. In blast crisis, some cells may simultaneously express lymphoid and myeloid markers. Indirect immunofluorescence procedures can demonstrate TdT in immature B and T lymphocytes. It inserts nontemplated nucleotides (N nucleotides) into the junctions between gene segments during T cell receptor and immunoglobulin heavy-chain gene rearrangement.

terminal transferase

Refer to DNA nucleotidyl exotransferase.

termination of tolerance

The unresponsive states of several forms of tolerance may be terminated by appropriate experimental manipulation. (1) Tolerance to heterologous γ globulin can be terminated by normal thymus cells; however, this is only possible in adoptive transfer experiments with cells of tolerant animals 81 days after the induction of tolerance and after supplementation with normal thymus cells. By this time, B cell tolerance vanishes, and only the T cells remain tolerant. Similar experiments at an earlier date do not terminate tolerance. (2) Allogeneic cells injected when B cell tolerance has vanished or has not yet been induced can also terminate or prevent tolerance. The mechanism is not specific and involves the allogeneic effect factor with activation of the unresponsive T cell population. (3) *Lipopolysaccharide (LPS),* a polyclonal B cell activator, can terminate tolerance if the B cells are competent. LPS can bypass the requirements for T cells in response to the immunogen by providing the second (mitogenic) signal required for response. The termination of tolerance by LPS does not involve T cells. LPS may also circumvent tolerance to self by a similar mechanism. (4) *Cross-reacting immunogens* (a heterologous protein in aggregated form or a different heterologous

protein) also are capable of terminating tolerance to a soluble form of a protein. Termination occurs by a mechanism that bypasses the unresponsive T cells and is obtainable at time intervals after tolerization when the responsiveness of B cells is restored. The antibody produced to the cross-reacting antigen also reacts with the tolerogenic protein and is indistinguishable from the specificity produced by this protein in the absence of tolerance.

tertiary granule

A structure in the cytoplasm of polymorphonuclear neutrophils (PMNs) in which complement receptor 3 precursor, acid hydrolase, and gelatinase are located.

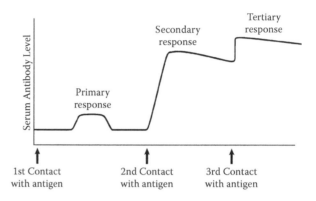

Tertiary immune response.

tertiary immune response

An immune response induced by a third (second booster) administration of antigen. It closely resembles the secondary (or booster) response.

tertiary immunization

The immune response following the third injection of the same immunogen.

tertiary lymphoid tissue

Inflamed peripheral tissues in which postcapillary venules have been modified to allow ingress of leukocytes including effector and memory lymphocytes.

tertiary reaction

May result from either primary or secondary interactions of antibody with antigen including *in vivo* biological manifestations of antibody reactivity. Some *in vitro* secondary interactions such as cytophilic reactions (adherence of antibody via its Fc to a cell surface) may, when occurring *in vivo,* give rise to tertiary manifestations. Because reactions occur *in vivo,* they tend to be very complex and subject to many variables. In an immune response, antibodies are directed against specific confirmational areas on antigen molecules known as antigenic determinants. Antigens are macromolecules that stimulate antibody production. Antibody populations directed against these macromolecules are notoriously heterogenous with respect to their antibody specificity and affinity because antibodies to different antigenic determinants may be present simultaneously in the sera. Bivalent and multivalent antibodies directed against multideterminant antigens result in the formation of large antibody–antigen aggregates of type $(Ab)_x(Ag)_y$ varying in size, complexity, and solubility. Landsteiner devised a method whereby an immune response could be directed against small molecules of known structure and called them haptens. They were too small to initiate an immune response alone, but were capable of reacting with the products of an immune response. He chemically coupled haptens to large biological macromolecules (he called carriers) such as ovalbumin, producing conjugated antigens capable of stimulating an immune response. The nonvalent hapten in pure form along with serum antibodies could then be used to study antibody–hapten interactions without the complications of multideterminant macromolecular antigens. These antibody populations were still heterogenous with respect to structure to class, subclass, and so on. Isolation of monoclonal antibodies derived from the sera of multiple myeloma patients led to sequencing and x-ray diffraction studies of homogenous antibody populations. Hybridoma technology now provides a mechanism to produce monoclonal homogenous antibodies *in vitro*.

tertiary response

The consequence of a third injection of an immunogen into an animal.

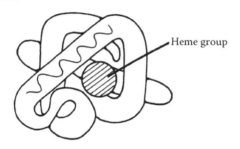

Tertiary structure.

tertiary structure

The folding of a polypeptide chain as a result of the interactions of its amino acid side chains that may be situated near or far along the chain. This three-dimensional folding occurs in globular proteins. Tertiary structure also refers to the spatial arrangement of protein atoms regardless of their relationship to atoms in adjacent molecules.

test dosing

A method to determine whether an individual has type I anaphylactic hypersensitivity to various drugs (e.g., penicillin) or antisera prior to administration. The procedure is not without danger, as even scratch tests with highly diluted penicillin preparations in highly sensitized subjects have been known to produce fatal anaphylactic shock.

testicular autoimmunity

Natural animal models of infertility include beagles and mink. A colony of developed mink contains approximately 20 to 30% infertile males that develop circulating antibodies to acrosomal antigens of spermatozoa that may be detected in their sera. Heavy granular deposits of immunoglobulin G (IgG) and/or C3 have been found in the basal lamina of the seminiferous tubules in 71% of mink with late infertility. Immunoglobulins eluted from these deposits contained antibodies to the acrosome of mink spermatozoa. Spermatozoal antigens were not detected in the immune deposits.

tetanus

A disease in which the exotoxin of *Clostridium tetani* produces tonic muscle spasm and hyperreflexia, leading to tris (lock jaw), generalized muscle spasms, spasm of the glottis, arching of the back, seizures, respiratory spasms, and paralysis. Tetanus toxin is a neurotoxin. The disease occurs 1 to 2 weeks after tetanus spores are introduced into deep wounds that provide anaerobic growth conditions.

tetanus antitoxin

Antibody raised by immunizing horses against *Clostridium tetani* exotoxin. It is used to treat or prevent tetanus in individuals with contaminated lesions. Anaphylaxis or serum sickness (type III hypersensitivity) may occur in individuals receiving second injections because of sensitization to horse serum proteins following initial exposure to horse antitoxin. One solution has been the use of human antitetanus toxin of high titer. Treatment of the IgG fraction yields F(ab$_2$) fragments that retain all of the toxin neutralizing capacity with diminished antigenicity of the antitoxin preparation.

tetanus toxin

The exotoxin synthesized by *Clostridium tetani*. It acts on the nervous system, interrupting neuromuscular transmission and preventing synaptic inhibition in the spinal cord. It binds to disialosyl ganglioside, a nerve cell membrane glycolipid. The effects of tetanus toxin are countered by specific antitoxin.

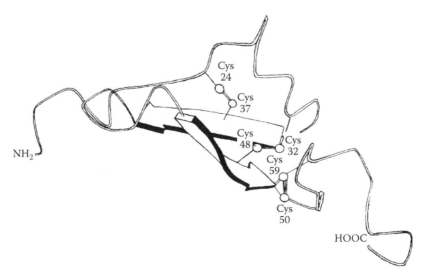

Transforming growth factor α (TGF-α). The structure was determined by a combination of two-dimensional NMR distance geometry and restrained molecular dynamics using the GROMOS program. United atoms were used for all nonpolar hydrogen atoms and are not included in this coordinate entry.

tetanus toxoid

Formaldehyde-detoxified toxins of *Clostridium tetani.* Tetanus toxoid is an immunizing preparation. Individuals with increased likelihood of developing tetanus as a result of deep, penetrating wounds caused by rusty nails or other contaminated objects are immunized by subcutaneous inoculation. The preparation is available in fluid and adsorbed forms. It is included with diphtheria toxoid and pertussis vaccine in a mixture known as DTP, DPT, or triple vaccine. It is employed to routinely immunize children under 6 years old.

tetanus vaccine

An immunizing preparation to protect against *Clostridium tetani.* Refer to DTaP vaccine.

tetramethylrhodamine isothiocyanate

A red fluorochrome used in immunofluorescence.

tetraparental chimera

The deliberate fusion of two-, four-, or eight-cell-stage murine blastocysts ultimately yields a chimera mouse with contributions from four parents. These animals are of great value in studies of immunological tolerance.

tetraparental mouse

An allophenic mouse.

Texas red

A fluorochrome derived from sulforhodamine 101. It is often used as a second label in fluorescence antibody techniques where fluorescein, an apple green label, is also used. This provides two-color fluorescence.

TFA antigens

Antigens in rabbits and rats that result from changes in liver cell components arising from exposure to the halothane anesthetic. Rats administered halothane intraperitoneally expressed maximum amounts of the 100-, 76-, 59-, and 57-kDa antigens after 12 hours. The antigens were still detectable after 7 days. TFA antigen expression varies in humans as a consequence of variability of hepatic cytochrome P-450 isoenzyme profiles.

(TG)AL

Tyrosine and glutamic acid polymers fasten as side chains to a poly-L-lysine backbone through alanine residues. This substance is a synthetic antigen.

TGF-α (transforming growth factor α)

A polypeptide produced by transformed cells. It shares approximately one third of its 50-amino acid sequence with epidermal growth factor (EGF). TGF-α has a powerful stimulatory effect on cell growth and promotes capillary formation.

TGF-β (transforming growth factor β)

Five TGF-βs in the C terminal regions of proteins are structurally similar. They are designated TGF-β_1 through TGF-β_5 and have similar functions with respect to their regulation of cellular growth and differentiation. After formation as secretory precursor polypeptides, TGF-β_1, TGF-β_2, and TGF-β_3 molecules are altered to form a 25-kDa homodimeric peptide. The ability of TGF-β to regulate growth depends on the type of cell and whether other growth factors are also present. TGF-β also regulates deposition of extracellular matrix and cell attachment to it. It induces fibronectin, chondroitin/dermatin sulfate proteoglycans, collagen, and glycosaminoglycans. TGF-β also promotes the formation and secretion of protease inhibitors. It has been shown to increase the rate of wound healing and induce granulation tissue. It also stimulates proliferation of

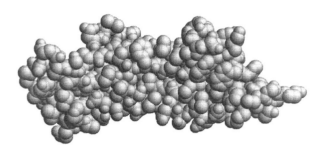

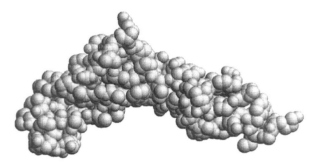

Human transforming growth factor β_2. Resolution = 1.8 Å.

osteoblasts and chondrocytes. TGF-β inhibits bone marrow cell proliferation and also blocks interferon-α-induced activation of natural killer (NK) cells. It diminishes interleukin-2 (IL2) activation of lymphokine-activated killer (LAK) cells. TGF-β decreases cytokine-induced proliferation of thymocytes and also decreases IL2-induced proliferation and activation of mature T lymphocytes. It inhibits T cell precursor differentiation into cytotoxic T lymphocytes. It may reverse the activation of macrophages by preventing the development of cytotoxic activity and superoxide anion formation necessary for antimicrobial effects. It may also diminish major histocompatibility complex (MHC) class II molecule expression and it decreases Fcε receptor expression in allergic reactions. TGF-β has potential value as an immunosuppressant in tissue and organ transplantation, and it may protect bone marrow stem cells from the injurious effects of chemotherapy. It may have use as an anti-inflammatory agent based on its ability to inhibit the growth of T and B cells. It also has potential as a treatment for selected autoimmune diseases. It diminishes myocardial damage associated with coronary occlusion, promotes wound healing, and may be of value in restoring collagen and promoting formation of bone in patients with osteoporosis. TGF-β is produced by activated Th2 cells, mononuclear phagocytes, and other cells. Its main effect is to inhibit proliferation and differentiation of T cells, inhibit macrophage activation, and counteract pro-inflammatory cytokines.

TGFs (transforming growth factors)

Polypeptides produced by virus-transformed 3T3 cells that induce various cells to alter their phenotypes.

T globulin

A serum protein found after hyperimmunization of horses. It is a γ_1 7S globulin that appears as a prominent band of immunoglobulin (Ig) when the serum is electrophoresed. It may be a subtype of IgG.

Th cells

Helper T lymphocytes that identify nonself peptide presented in the context of MHC class II molecules displayed

T

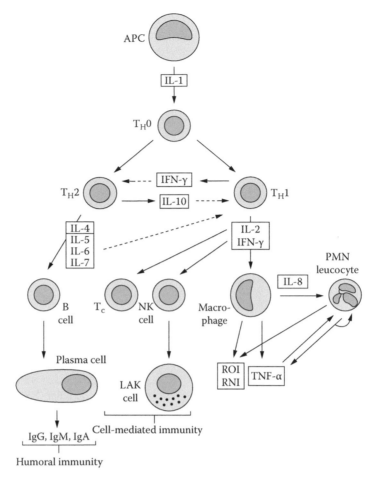

Th0 cells.

by antigen-presenting cells. Effector Th cells are designated as Th1 or Th2 with respect to phenotype. Th1 cells synthesize IFNγ and IL2 and are active against intracellular bacteria and viruses. They also mediate isotype switching to IgG1 and IgG3 in humans. Th2 cells synthesize IL4, IL5, IL10, and IL13; combat extracellular bacteria and parasites; and facilitate isotype switching to IgA, IgE and IgG4. Th cells usually manifest CD4 coreceptors.

Th1/Th2 differentiation

The pathway whereby Th cells proliferate to synthesize IFN-γ- and IL4-secreting Th0 cells that become Th1 or Th2 effector cells based on other transcription factors and cytokines. T-bet and IL12 can induce differentiation of Th0 cells into Th1 effector lymphocytes. GATA-3 and IL4 can induce differentiation of Th0 cells into Th2 effector lymphocytes.

Th3 cells

CD4$^+$ regulatory T cells that synthesize large quantities of TGF-β.

Th17 cells

A recently discovered unique subset of CD4 T cells that synthesize IL17 and are distinct from Th1 and Th2. Th17 cells are of central importance to the pathogenesis of inflammatory diseases and autoimmune diseases. They develop via cytokine signals distinct from and antagonized by products of the Th1 and T2 lineages. IL23, TGF-β, IL6, IL7, and their receptors are important for the development of the Th17 lineage. Expression of RORγt transcription factor directs Th17 differentiation. Th17 development

depends on the pleiotropic cytokine TGF-β that is also linked to regulatory T cell function. In pathogen-driven inflammation, naïve T cells that recognize foreign antigen may receive signals from regulatory T cells (TGF-β) to induce Th17 development, whereas the pathogen-induced signal that acts with TGF-β to switch the response to Th17 (IL6) also subverts T$_{reg}$ dominance and facilitates T$_{reg}$ expansion that could block further T effector differentiation as the inflammatory inducing pathogen is cleared. TGF-β synthesis may initiate development of T$_{reg}$ that may maintain dominant suppressive function in the absence of pathogenic challenges but facilitate Th17 effector development when needed. Key transcription factors include T-bet that specifies Th1, GATA-3 that specifies Th2, and FOXp3 that specifies T$_{reg}$ development. IL17 cytokines are products of two of the three arms of effector CD4$^+$ T cell lineages: IL17A and IL17F in Th17 and IL25 in Th2. Innate immune cell products that control Th17 responses include new members of the IL12 family cytokines, IL23 and IL27; and IL6, prototype for IL12 cytokines. IL27 and SOC3 are negative regulators for the development of Th17 cells. The Th17 lineage is implicated in multiple auto-inflammatory disorders and a possible role in allograft rejection.

T$_h$0 cells

A murine and human CD4$^+$ T cell subset based on cytokine production and effector functions. Th0 cells synthesize multiple cytokines. They are responsible for effects intermediate of those of Th1 and Th2 cells, based on the cytokines synthesized and the cells responding. Th0 cells may be precursors of Th1 and Th2 cells.

T$_h$1 cells

A murine and human CD4$^+$ T cell subset based on cytokine production and effector functions. Th1 cells synthesize interferon-γ (IFN-γ), IL2, and tumor necrosis factor β (TNF-β). They are mainly responsible for cellular immunity against intracellular microorganisms and for delayed-type hypersensitivity reactions. They affect IgG$_{2a}$ antibody synthesis and antibody-dependent, cell-mediated cytoxicity. Th1 cells activate host defense mediated by phagocytes. Intracellular microbial infections induce Th1 cell development, which facilitates elimination of the microorganisms by phagocytosis. Th1 cells induce synthesis of antibody, which activates complement and serves as an opsonin that facilitates phagocytosis. The IFN-γ they produce enhances macrophage activation. The cytokines released by Th1 cells activate natural killer (NK) cells, macrophages, and CD8$^+$ T cells. Their main function is to induce phagocyte-mediated defense against infections, particularly by intracellular microorganisms. Also termed inflammatory T cells.

T$_h$2 cells

A murine and human CD4$^+$ T cell subset based on cytokine production and effector functions. Th2 cells synthesize interleukin-4 (IL4), IL5, IL6, IL9, IL10, and IL13. Their main function is to induce antibody synthesis by B cells. They greatly facilitate IgE and IgG$_1$ antibody responses and mucosal immunity by synthesis of mast cell and eosinophil growth and differentiation factors and facilitation of IgA synthesis. IL4 facilitates IgE antibody synthesis. IL5 is an eosinophil-activating substance. IL10, IL13, and IL4 suppress cell-mediated immunity. Th2 cells are principally responsible for host defense exclusive of phagocytes. They are crucial for IgE and eosinophil responses to helminths and for allergy attributable to activation of basophils and mast cells through IgE.

T$_h$17 (hypothesis)

A concept to explain T cell-mediated tissue injury including organ-specific autoimmunity triggered by microbial infection. The identification of novel cytokines of the IL17 and IL12 families has permitted identification of factors that specify differentiation of a new effector T cell lineage known as T$_h$17 that provides a new mechanism of adaptive immunity and a unifying model to explain many aspects of immune regulation, immune pathogenesis, and host defense. The T$_h$17 pathway involves the actions of pleiotropic cytokines including transforming growth factor-β (TGF-β) and IL6. IL17 is a T cell-expressed pleiotropic cytokine that exhibits a high degree of homology to a protein encoded by the ORF13 gene of herpes virus Saimiri. Both recombinant and natural IL17 occur as disulfide linked homodimers. IL17 exhibits multiple biological activities on a variety of cells, including the induction of IL6 and IL8 production in fibroblasts, activation of NF-κB, and costimulation of T cell proliferation. IL17 is an essential inflammatory mediator in the development of autoimmune diseases. Neutralization of IL17 with monoclonal antibody can ameliorate the disease course. Also called CTLA-8.

thalidomide

An immunomodulatory agent whose effects vary under different conditions, but may be related to suppression of excessive TNF-α synthesis and downmodulation of selected cell surface adhesion molecules involved in leukocyte migration. A drug originally used as a sedative, it was withdrawn in the 1960s as a consequence of disastrous teratogenic effects when used during pregnancy. However, it is again in use because of its significant immunomodulatory effects. It inhibits angiogenesis and exerts anti-inflammatory and immunomodulatory actions. It inhibits tumor necrosis factor α (TNF-α), diminishes phagocytosis by neutrophils, increases IL10 synthesis, alters expression of adhesion molecules, and facilitates cell-mediated immunity through interaction with T cells. Presently used to treat multiple myeloma, it has potential for treatment of myelodysplastic syndrome, acute myelogenous leukemia and graft-vs.-host disease. Toxicities include teratogenesis, peripheral neuropathy, constipation, fatigue, rash, hypothyroidism, and increased risk of deep vein thrombosis.

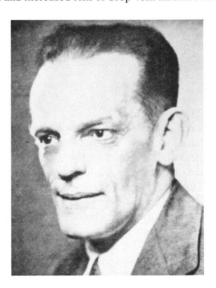

Max Theiler.

Theiler, Max (1899–1972)

South African virologist who received a Nobel Prize in 1951 for his development of vaccines against yellow fever.

Theileria immunity

Immunity against these tick-transmitted intracellular protozoan parasites of domestic animals depends upon the protection of cell-mediated immune responses. Humoral immune responses directed against schizonts and piroplasms are insignificant in the development of natural protective immunity. Animals that recover may be resistant to homologous challenge and develop immunity that persists 3 to 5 years. Infection with sporozoites and the development of schizonts are critical for the development of natural immunity. Live attenuated, subunit, and recombinant vaccines have been used. *Theileria annulata* live vaccine is prepared from attenuated cell lines that produce infection in cattle without causing disease and induce protective immunity. *T. parva* subunit vaccine contains p67 antigen, the recombinant form of which protects 70% of immunized cattle against experimental challenge.

Theiler's virus myelitis

Murine spinal cord demyelination considered an immune-based consequence of a viral infection.

theliolymphocyte

A small intraepithelial lymphocyte associated with intestinal epithelial cells.

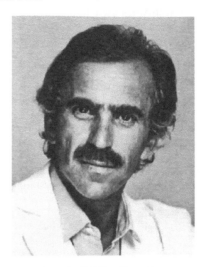

Argyrios N. Theofilopoulos.

Argyrios N. Theofilopoulos

Authority on autoimmunity at Scripps Research Institute, LaJolla, California.

theophylline (1,3,dimethylxanthine)

A compound used to treat acute bronchial asthma because of its powerful smooth muscle relaxing activity. Aminophylline, a salt of theophylline, is another smooth muscle relaxant used to induce bronchodilation in the treatment of asthma.

therapeutic antisera

Serum antibody preparations employed to protect against or treat disease. They are distinct from antibody or antisera preparations used for the serological identification of microorganisms. Therapeutic antisera such as horse antitoxins against diphtheria were widely used early in the 20th century. A few specific antisera such as tetanus antitoxin are still used.

therapeutic vaccination

A vaccine administered to alleviate a pre-existing allergic or autoimmune condition, cancer, or other disease.

***Thermoactinomyces* species**

Gram-positive, endospore-forming microorganisms that *Aspergillus fumigatus,* are the most common causes of the hypersensitivity pneumonitis (HP) known as farmer's lung (FL). Other thermophilic actinomycetes also play a role in the pathogenesis of this disease. Antibodies reactive with a 55-kDa band are frequent in the sera of patients with FL, but the significance is not known.

Thomas, Edward Donnall (1920–)

American hematologist whose fundamental investigations of bone marrow transplantation led to his winning a Nobel Prize for Medicine or Physiology with J. E. Murray in 1990.

thoracic duct

A canal that leads from the cisterna chyli, a dilated segment of the thoracic duct at its site of origin in the lumbar region, to the left subclavian vein.

thoracic duct drainage

The deliberate removal of lymphocytes through drainage of lymph from the thoracic duct with a catheter.

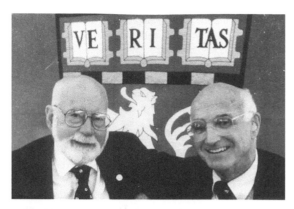

E. Donnall Thomas and Joseph E. Murray, recipients of the 1990 Nobel Prize for Physiology or Medicine for their work during the 1950s and 1960s on reducing the risk of organ rejection by the human immune system. In 1954, at the Peter Bent Brigham Hospital, Murray performed the first successful organ transplant of a kidney from one identical twin to another. Two years later, Thomas performed the first successful transplant of bone marrow by administering a drug that prevented rejection. Thomas and Murray made significant discoveries that "enabled the development of organ and cell transplantation into a method for the treatment of human disease" (from Nobel Assembly citation).

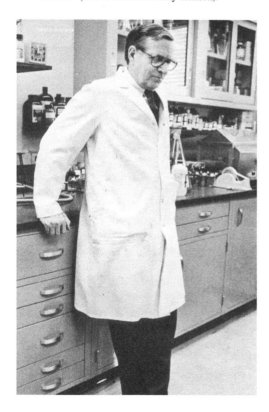

Lewis Thomas.

Thomas, Lewis

Distinguished American physician who served as Chair of Pathology at Yale, as administrator at New York University Medical Center, and as director of Sloan-Kettering-Memorial Medical Center in New York City. He wrote popular books on medicine and had a special interest in tumor immunology.

thorotrast (thorium dioxide 32THOT)

A radiocontrast medium that yields α particles. It is no longer in use because neoplasia have been attributed to its use.

It induced hepatic angiosarcoma, cholangiocarcinoma, and hepatocellular carcinoma in some patients who received it and it is known to produce other neoplasms. It has been used in experimental animal studies involving the blockade of the reticuloendothelial system. It is removed by the reticuloendothelial (mononuclear phagocyte) system.

three-signal model of lymphocyte activation
A prototype accounting for the requirement by most lymphocytes of three coordinated signals for total activation. The signals are antigen recognition, costimulation, and cytokine signaling. Usually, T cells require engagement by pMHC for the first signal; costimulation by interaction of CD28 with B7-1/B7-2 for the second signal; and cytokine signaling, often by IL2, as the third. B cells require interaction of their receptors with antigen as the first signal; costimulation by interaction of CD40 or CD40L expressed by an activated antigen-specific Th cell as the second signal; and cytokine signaling via cytokines released from Th cells as the third.

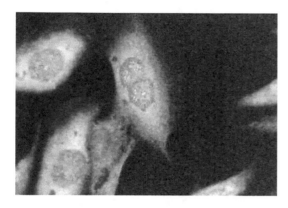

Threonyl transfer RNA synthetase antibodies.

threonyl transfer RNA synthetase antibodies
Antibodies against threonyl tRNA synthetase (threonyl RS) protein that show high specificity for myositis. They were demonstrated in 4% of polymyositis/dermatomyositis patients. Antithreonyl RS antibodies have also been linked to the antisynthetase syndrome characterized by fever, Raynaud's phenomenon, symmetrical arthritis, interstitial lung disease, myositis, and mechanic's hands.

threonyl transfer RNA synthetase autoantibodies
Autoantibodies (PL-7) to the 80-kDa threonyl tRNA synthetase protein that are highly specific for myositis. PL-7 autoantibodies have been found with autoantibodies against aminoacyl tRNA synthetases including histidyl, alanyl, isoleucyl, and glycyl tRNA synthetases, and are associated with the antisynthetase syndrome characterized by acute onset steroid-responsive myositis with interstitial lung disease, fever, symmetrical arthritis, Raynaud's phenomenon, and mechanic's hands.

thrombocyte
Blood platelet.

thrombocytopenia
Diminished blood platelet numbers with values below 100,000/cm³ of blood compared to a normal value of 150,000 to 300,000/cm³. This decrease in blood platelets can lead to bleeding.

thrombocytopenic purpura, idiopathic
An autoimmune disease in which antiplatelet autoantibodies destroy platelets. Splenic macrophages remove circulating platelets coated with immunoglobulin G (IgG) autoantibodies at an accelerated rate. Thrombocytopenia occurs although the bone marrow increases platelet production, which can lead to purpura and bleeding. The platelet count may fall below 20,000 to 30,000/μL. Antiplatelet antibodies are detectable in sera and on platelets. Platelet survival is decreased. Splenectomy is recommended in adults. Corticosteroids facilitate a temporary elevation in platelet count. This disease is characterized by decreased blood platelets, hemorrhage, and extensive thrombotic lesions.

thrombocytosis
Elevated blood platelet numbers with values exceeding 600,000/cm³ of blood compared to a normal value of 150,000 to 300,000.

thromboxanes
A group of biologically active compounds that play a physiological role in homeostasis and a pathophysiological role in thromboembolic disease and anaphylactic reactions. They are cyclopentane derivatives of polyunsaturated fatty acids derived by isomerization from prostaglandin endoperoxide PGH_2, the immediate precursor. The isomerizing enzyme is called thromboxane synthetase. The active compound, thromboxane A_2, is unstable, degraded to thromboxane B_2, which is stable but inactive on blood vessels, but has polymorphonuclear cell chemotactic activity. The short notations are TXA_2 and TXB_2. Both compounds represent the major pathway of conversion of prostaglandin endoperoxide precursors. The level of TXA_2, derived from prostaglandin G_2 generated from arachidonic acid by cyclooxygenase, increases following injury to vessels. TXA_2 stimulates a primary hemostatic response and is a potent inducer of platelet aggregation, smooth-muscle contraction, and vasoconstriction. TXA_2 was previously called rabbit aorta contacting substance (RACS). It is isolated from lung perfusates during anaphylaxis. It appears to be a peptide containing fewer than ten amino acid residues. Thromboxane formation in platelets is associated with the dense tubular system. Polymorphonuclear neutrophils (PMNs) and spleen, brain, and inflammatory granulomas have been demonstrated to produce thromboxanes.

thy (θ)
Epitope found on murine thymocytes and most murine T lymphocytes.

θ antigen
Refer to Thy-1 antigen.

Thy-1
A murine and rat thymocyte surface glycoprotein found also in neuron membranes of several species. Thy-1 was originally called θ alloantigen. Thy.1 and Thy.2 are the allelic forms. A substitution of one amino acid, arginine or glutamine, at position 89 represents the difference between Thy1.1 and Thy1.2. Mature T cells and thymocytes in mice express Thy-1. The genes encoding Thy-1 are present on chromosome 9 in mice. Although few human lymphocytes express Thy-1, it is present on the surfaces of neurons and fibroblasts.

Thy-1 antigen
A murine isoantigen present on the surfaces of thymic lymphocytes and on thymus-derived lymphocytes found in peripheral lymphoid tissues. Central nervous system tissues may also express Thy-1 antigen.

Thy-1+ dendritic cells
Cells derived from the T lymphocyte lineage and found within the epithelium of murine epidermis.

T

thymectomy

Surgical removal of the thymus, leading to failure to develop cell-mediated and humoral immunity to thymus-dependent antigens in mice thymectomized as neonates. T cells fail to develop, lymphoid tissues atrophy, and the failure to gain weight are characteristic of runt or wasting disease.

thymic alymphoplasia

Severe combined immune deficiency (SCID) transmitted as an X-linked recessive trait.

thymic anlage

The tissue that gives rise to thymic stroma during embryogenesis.

thymic cortex

Refer to thymus.

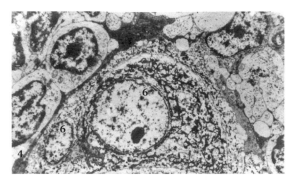

Two type 6 large medullary epithelial cells (6) adjacent to the Hassall's corpuscle and two type 4 epithelial cells (4) in the medulla (magnification, 7000×).

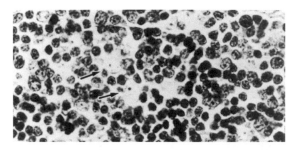

Thymic epithelial cells: cortex. Cortical type epithelial cells have large, round to oval, clear nuclei and conspicuous nucleoli.

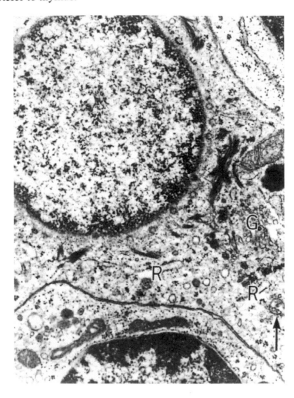

Type 2 "pale" epithelial cell in outer cortex (9000× magnification). R = profiles of RER. G = Golgi complex. Arrow = multivesicular body.

thymic epithelial cells (TECs)

Cells present in the cortex and to a lesser degree in the medulla of the thymus. They are derived from the third and fourth pharyngeal pouches. They affect maturation and differentiation of thymocytes through the secretion of thymopoietin, thymosins, and serum thymic factors. TECs express both major histocompatibility complex (MHC) class I and class II molecules. They secrete interleukin-7 (IL7) required for early T lymphocyte development during positive selection. Maturing T lymphocytes must recognize self peptides bound to TEC surface MHC molecules to avoid programmed cell death. TECs mediate positive and negative selection through presentation of self ligands in the thymus.

thymic hormones

Soluble substances synthesized by thymic epithelial cells that promote thymocyte differentiation. They include thymopoietin and thymosins—peptides that help regulate differentiation of T lymphocytes.

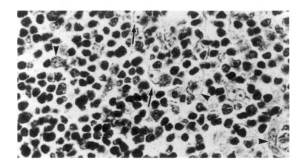

Thymic epithelial cells: cortico-medullary junction. Cortical type epithelial (arrows) and medullary type (arrowheads) are intermingled.

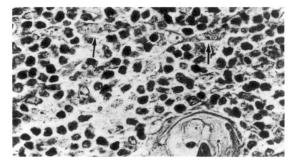

Thymic epithelial cells: medulla. Fusiform epithelial cells have spindle-shaped nuclei, coarse chromatin structure, and interconnecting cell processes. A Hassall's corpuscle can be seen in the lower section of the photomicrograph.

thymic hormones and peptides

Polypeptides extracted from thymus glands include thymulin, thymopoietin, thymic humoral factor (THF), and thymosins. Only thymulin has been characterized as

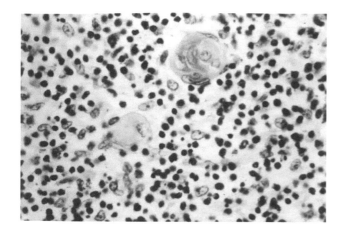

Hassall's corpuscle.

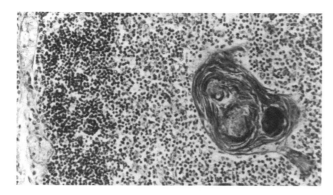

Normal thymus. This child's thymus shows the dense cortex composed predominantly of lymphocytes and the less dense medulla with few lymphocytes. Note the Hassall's corpuscle.

a hormone that fits the accepted classical endocrine and physiological criteria: it is thymus-restricted and -regulated in its secretions.

thymic humoral factors (THFs)

Soluble substances such as thymosins, thymopoietin, and serum thymic factor that are synthesized by the thymus and govern differentiation and function of lymphocytes.

thymic hypoplasia

An immunodeficiency that selectively affects the T cell limb of the immune response. Early symptoms soon after birth may stem from associated parathyroid abnormalities leading to hypocalcemia and heart defects that may lead to congestive heart failure. Lymphopenia is present, with diminished T cell numbers. T lymphocyte function cannot be detected in peripheral blood T cells. Antibody levels and functions vary. The condition has been successfully treated by thymic transplantation. Some patients with DiGeorge syndrome may have normal B cell immunity. The others may have diminished immunoglobulin levels and may not form specific antibody following immunization. Patients may exhibit fish-shaped mouths and abnormal faces with low-set ears, hypertelorism, and antimongoloid eyes, in addition to the factors mentioned above.

thymic involution

Following puberty, inhibition of double-negative (CD4-/CD8-) thymocyte proliferation leads to the progressive loss of thymic tissue mass and function. Tissue replacement is mainly by fat deposits.

thymic leukemia (TL) antigen

Epitope on thymocyte membrane of TL+ mice. As the T lymphocytes mature, antigen disappears, but resurfaces if leukemia develops. TL antigens are specific and are normally present on the surfaces of thymocytes of certain mouse strains. They are encoded by a group of structural genes located at the Tla locus, in the linkage group IX, very near the D pole of the H-2 locus on chromosome 17. There are three structural TL genes, one of which has two alleles. The TL antigens are numbered from 1 to 4, specifying four antigens: TL.1, TL.2, TL.3, and TL.4. TL.3 and TL.4 are mutually exclusive; their expression is under the control of regulatory genes apparently located at the same Tla locus. Normal mouse thymocytes belong to three phenotypic groups: Tl-, Tl.2, and Tl.1, 2, 3. Development of leukemia in mice induces a restructuring of the TL surface antigens of thymocytes with expression of TL.1 and TL.2 in TL- cells, expression of TL.1 in TL.2 cells, and expression of TL.4 in TL- and TL.2 cells. When normal thymic cells leave the thymus, the expression of TL antigen ceases. Thus, thymocytes are TL+ (except TL-) and the peripheral T cells undergo antigenic modulation. In transplantation experiments, TL+ tumor cells underwent antigenic modulation. Tumor cells exposed to homologous antibody stop expressing the antigen and thus escape lysis when subsequently exposed to the same antibody plus complement.

thymic medullary hyperplasia

Germinal centers present in the thymic medullae in patients with myasthenia gravis; however, normal thymus glands occasionally contain germinal centers, although most do not.

thymic nurse cells

Relatively large epithelial cells near thymic lymphocytes that are believed to play a significant role in T lymphocyte maturation and differentiation.

thymic stroma

Thymic reticular epithelial cells and connective tissue that constitute the principal microenvironment for development of T cells.

thymic stromal-derived lymphopoietin (TSLP)

A cytokine isolated from a murine thymic stromal cell line that possesses a primary sequence distinct from other known cytokines. The cDNA encodes a 140-amino acid protein that includes a 19-amino acid signal sequence. TSLP stimulates B220+ bone marrow cells to proliferate and express surface μ. It synergizes with other signals to induce thymocyte and peripheral T cell proliferation but is not mitogenic for T cells alone.

thymin

A hormone extracted from the thymus whose activity resembles that of thymopoietin.

thymocyte

T cell precursors that develop in the thymus beginning with a double-negative (CD4-/CD8-) stage followed by a double-positive (CD4+/CD8+) phase and finally become single-positive as CD4+/CD8- or CD4-/CD8+ prior to release into the periphery as mature CD4+ or CD8+ T lymphocytes.

thymoma

A rare benign neoplasm of epithelial cells often with associated thymic lymphoproliferation. Half of these tumors occur in patients with myasthenia gravis. They may also be associated with immunodeficiency.

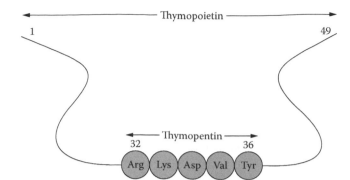

Structure of thymopoietin and thymopentin.

thymopentin (TP-5)

A synthetic pentapeptide, Arg–Lys–Asp–Val–Tyr, that corresponds to amino acid residues 32 through 36 of the thymopoietin thymic hormone. Thymopentin is the minimal fragment that can produce the biological activities of thymopoietin, i.e., thymopentin is the active site of thymopoietin. The cell-mediated immune response is a host defense mediated by antigen-specific T lymphocytes with nonspecific cells of the immune system. It offers protection against intracellular bacteria, viruses, and neoplasms and mediates graft rejection. It may be transferred passively with primed T lymphocytes.

thymopoietin

A 49-amino acid polypeptide thymic hormone secreted by epithelial cells in the thymus. It affects neuromuscular transmission and immune regulation and also induces early T lymphocyte differentiation. Thymopentin functions biologically to normalize immune imbalances related to hypo- or hyper-responsiveness that may be related to thymic involution arising from age, thymectomy, or other factors. It is a 7-kDa protein that facilitates the expression of Thy-1 antigen on T lymphocytes that may interfere with neuromuscular transmission, an effect noted in patients with myasthenia gravis who often develop thymoma.

thymosin

A 12-kDa protein hormone produced by the thymus gland that may provide T lymphocyte immune function in thymectomized animals.

thymosin α-1 (thymopoietin)

A hormone produced by the thymus that stimulates T lymphocyte helper activity. It induces production of lymphokines such as interferon and macrophage-inhibiting factor and enhances Thy-1.2 and Lyt-1, -2, -3 antigens of T lymphocytes. It may also alter thymocyte terminal deoxynucleotidyl-transferase (TdT) concentrations.

thymotaxin

Refer to β₂ microglobulin.

thymulin

A nonapeptide (Glu–Ala–Lys–Ser–Gln–Gly–Ser–Asn) extracted from sera of humans and pigs and from calf thymus. Thymulin shows a strong binding affinity for T cell receptors on lymphocyte membranes. Its zinc-binding property is associated with biological activity. Its enhancing action is reserved exclusively for T lymphocytes. It facilitates the functions of several T lymphocyte subpopulations but mainly enhances T suppressor lymphocyte activity. Formerly called FTS.

thymus

A triangular bilobed structure enclosed in a thin fibrous capsule and located retrosternally. Each lobe is subdivided by prominent trabeculae into interconnecting lobules and comprises two histologically and functionally distinct areas, cortex and medulla. The cortex consists of a mesh of epithelial–reticular cells enclosing densely packed large lymphocytes. It has no germinal centers. The epithelial cell component is of endodermal origin; the lymphoid cells are of mesenchymal origin. Prothymocytes that migrate from the bone marrow to the subcapsular regions of the cortex are influenced by this microenvironment that directs their further development. The education process is exerted by hormonal substances produced by thymic epithelial cells. The cortical cells proliferate extensively. Some are short-lived and die. The surviving cells acquire characteristics of thymocytes. The cortical cells migrate to the medulla, then to the peripheral lymphoid organs, sites of their main residence. The medullary areas of the thymus are even richer in epithelial cells, and the lymphocytes in the medulla are loosely packed. The lymphocytes are small cells ready to exit the thymus. Some remnants of epithelial islands, called Hassall's corpuscles, are histologically identifiable and are

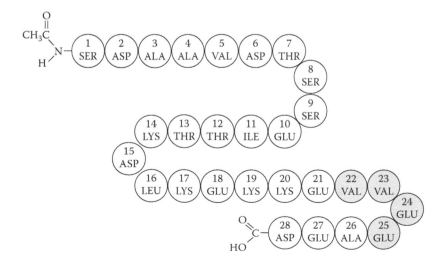

Structure of thymosin α-1.

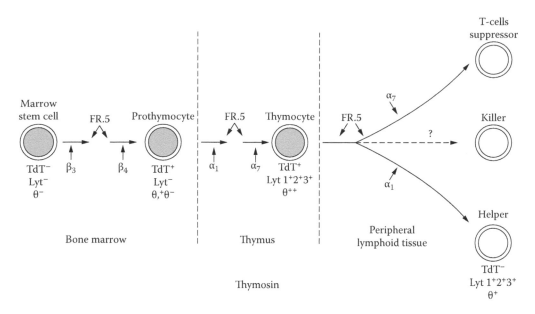

Proposed site of action of thymosin polypeptides on maturation of T cell subpopulations.

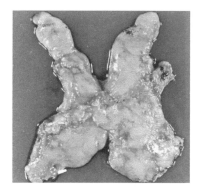

Normal adult thymus. The thymus often shows an X- or H-shaped configuration.

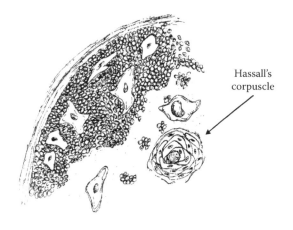

Hassall's corpuscle.

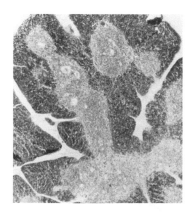

The normal thymus of infant showing lobulation and sharp separation of cortex from the stalk-like medulla (40× magnification).

markers for thymic tissue. The blood supply to the cortex comes from capillaries that form anastomosing arcades. Drainage is mainly through veins; the thymus has no lymphatic vessels. The thymus develops from the branchial pouches of the pharynx at about 6 weeks of embryonal age.

In most species, it is fully developed at birth. In humans, the weight of the thymus at birth is 10 to 15 g. It continues to increase in size, reaching a maximum (30 to 40 g) at puberty. It then begins to involute with increasing age, but remains functional. The medulla involutes first with pyknosis and beading of the nuclei of small lymphocytes, giving a false impression of an increased number of Hassall's corpuscles. The cortex atrophies progressively. The blood–thymus barrier protects thymocytes from contact with antigen. Lymphocytes reaching the thymus are prevented from contact with antigen by a physical barrier. The first level is represented by capillary walls with endothelial cells inside the pericytes outside the lumen. Potential antigenic molecules that escape the first level of control are taken over by macrophages present in the pericapillary space. Further protection is provided by a third level, represented by a mesh of interconnecting epithelial cells that enclose the thymocyte population. The effects of thymus and thymic hormones on the differentiation of T cells are demonstrable in animals congenitally lacking a thymus (nu/nu animals), in neonatally or adult thymectomized animals, and in

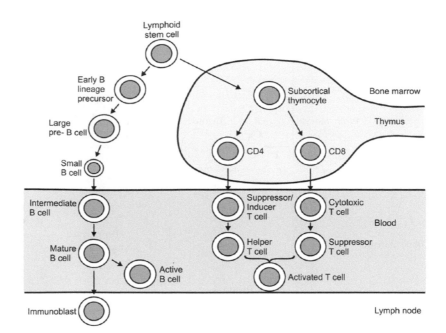

T cell maturation.

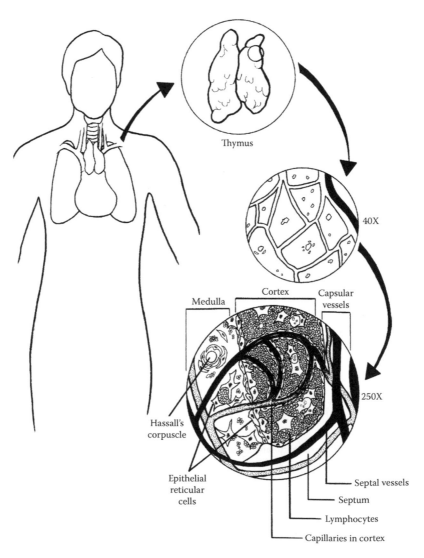

Human thymus: location and histology, with an enlarged view of its histology.

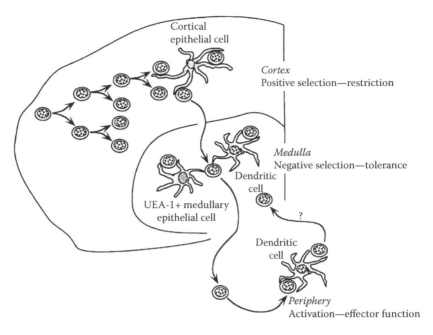

A model for thymic compartment specialization.

subjects with immunodeficiencies involving T cell function. Differentiation is associated with surface markers, the presence or disappearance of which characterizes the different stages of cell differentiation. Proliferation of the subcapsular thymocytes is extensive. Most of these cells die, but the remaining cells continue to differentiate, become smaller, and move through interstices in the thymic medulla. Fully developed thymocytes pass through the walls of the postcapillary venules to reach the systemic circulation and seed in the peripheral lymphoid organs. Some recirculate, but do not return to the thymus.

thymus cell differentiation

Stem cell maturation and differentiation into mature T lymphocytes in the thymus are accompanied by the appearance and disappearance of specific surface CD antigens. In humans, the differentiation of CD38+ stem cells into early thymocytes is signaled by the appearance of CD2 and CD7, followed by the transferrin receptor marker; expression of

CD1 identifying thymocytes in the mid-stage of differentiation when T cell receptor genes γ and δ and later α and β rearrange; and expression of CD3, CD4, and CD8 surface antigens by thymocytes. CD1 usually disappears at this time. Ultimately, the CD4+/CD8+ and CD4−/CD8+ subpopulations that both express the CD3 pan-T cell marker appear. An analogous maturation of T cells takes place in mice.

thymus cell education

Thymus cell differentiation.

thymus-dependent (TD) antigen

An immunogen that requires antigen-specific T lymphocyte cooperation for B cells to synthesize specific antibodies. The immunogen binds to the receptors of B cells to induce activation but is unable to induce B cell differentiation or immunoglobulin production without direct intercellular contact with a primed helper T cell. T cell cooperation is required for B cells to synthesize specific antibodies. Presentation of thymus-dependent antigen to

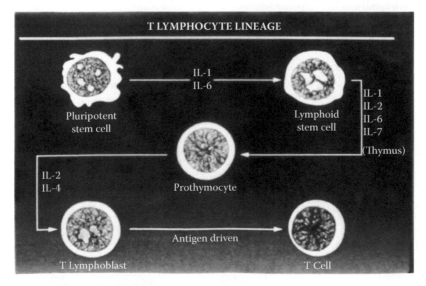

Differentiation of a stem cell into a mature T cell.

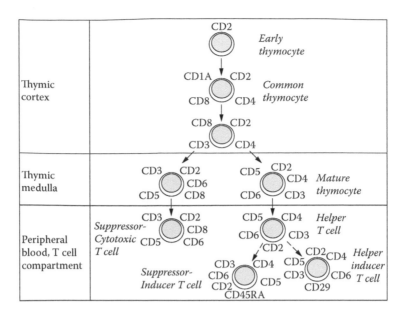

T cell maturation showing the addition of CD (cluster of differentiation) markers and position of T cell (in thymus or periphery) when marker is added.

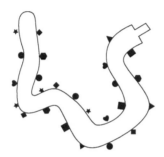

Thymus-dependent (TD) antigen.

	T Cell-dependent antigen	T Cell-independent antigen
Structural properties	Complex	Simple
Chemistry	Proteins; protein-nucleoprotein conjugates; glycoproteins; lipoproteins	Polysaccharide of pneumococcus; dextran polyvinyl pyrolidone; bacterial lipo-polysaccharide
Antibody class-induced	IgG, IgM, IgA (+IgD and IgE)	IgM
Immunological memory response	Yes	No
Present in most pathogenic microbes	Yes	No

Thymus-dependent (TD) antigen.

T cells must be in the context of major histocompatibility complex (MHC) class II molecules. Thymus-dependent antigens include proteins, polypeptides, hapten–carrier complexes, erythrocytes, and many other antigens that have diverse epitopes. T-dependent antigens contain some epitopes that T cells recognize and others that B cells identify. T cells produce cytokines and cell surface molecules that induce B cell growth and differentiation into antibody-secreting cells. Humoral immune responses to T-dependent antigens are associated with isotype switching, affinity maturation, and memory. The response to thymus-dependent antigens shows only minor heavy-chain isotype switching or affinity maturation, both of which require helper T cell signals.

thymus-dependent (TD) areas

Regions of peripheral lymphoid tissues occupied by T lymphocytes: the paracortical areas of lymph nodes, the zones between nodules and Peyer's patches, and the centers of splenic malpighian corpuscles. These regions contain small lymphocytes derived from circulating cells that reach these areas by passage through high endothelial venules. Proof that these anatomical sites are thymus-dependent is the lack of lymphocytes in these areas exhibited by animals thymectomized as neonates. Likewise, humans and animals with thymic hypoplasia or congenital aplasia of the thymus reveal no T cells in these areas.

thymus-dependent (TD) cells

Lymphoid cells that mature only under the influence of the thymus.

thymus-dependent lymphocyte

Refer to thymus-dependent (TD) cells.

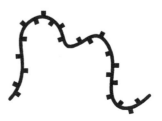

Thymus-independent (TI) antigen.

thymus-independent (TI) antigen

An immunogen that can stimulate B cells to synthesize antibodies without participation by T cells. These antigens are less complex than thymus-dependent antigens. They are often polysaccharides that contain repeating epitopes or lipopolysaccharides (LPSs) derived from Gram-negative microorganisms. Thymus-independent antigens induce IgM synthesis by B lymphocytes without cooperation by T cells. They do not stimulate immunological memory. Humoral immune responses to T-independent antigens show only minor heavy chain isotype switching or affinity maturation, both of which require helper T cell signals. TI antigens are classified as TI-1, which have intrinsic B cell activating activity, or TI-2, which have multiple identical epitopes that cross link B cell receptors. Murine TI antigens are classified as TI-1 or TI-2. LPS, which activates murine B cells without participation by T or other cells, is a typical TI-1 antigen. Low LPS concentrations stimulate synthesis of specific antigen; high concentrations activate growth and differentiation of essentially all B cells. TI-2 antigens include polysaccharides, glycolipids, and nucleic acids. When T lymphocytes and macrophages are depleted, no antibody response develops against them. Somatic hypermutation and memory B cell development are lacking. The antigens induce a low affinity primary IgM response. TI-1 antigens are usually large polymeric proteins that interact with B cell receptors, leading to B cell activation without T cell help. TI-2 antigens, usually polysaccharides composed of repetitive elements, interact with B cell receptors but are incapable of completely activating B cells without cytokines provided by bystander cells.

thymus-replacing factor (TRF)

Interleukin-5 (IL5).

thyroglobulin

A thyroid protein demonstrable by immunoperoxidase staining that serves as a marker for papillary and/or follicular thyroid carcinomas.

thyroglobulin autoantibodies

Autoantibodies found in the sera of patients with such thyroid disorders as chronic lymphocytic (Hashimoto's) thyroiditis (76 to 100%), primary myxedema (72%), hyperthyroidism (33%), colloid goiter (7%), adenoma (28%), thyroid cancer based on type (13 to 65%), pernicious anemia (27%), autoimmune diseases, e.g., Addison's disease (28%), and diabetes mellitus (20%). Thyroglobulin autoantibodies can be detected in normal subjects, diminishing their clinical usefulness; 18% of women have these antibodies that increase in frequency up to 30% as they age. They are much less prevalent in men (approximately 3 to 6%), in whom they also increase with age. Enzyme immunoassay (EIA), immunoradiometric assay (IRMA), and chemiluminescence (CL) are the assays of choice for these autoantibodies.

thyroid antibodies

Autoantibodies present in patients with Hashimoto's thyroiditis or thyrotoxicosis (Graves' disease) that are organ-specific for the thyroid. Antibodies against thyroglobulin and autoantibodies against the microsomal antigen of thyroid acinar cells may appear in patients with autoimmune thyroiditis. Antibodies against thyroid-stimulating hormone (TSH) receptors appear in patients with Graves' disease and cause stimulatory hypersensitivity.

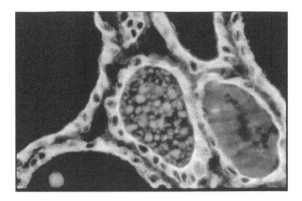

Thyroid autoantibodies.

They mimic the action of TSH. They are IgG molecules known as long-acting thyroid stimulator (LATS). LATS levels are increased in many patients with thyrotoxicosis or Graves' disease.

thyroid autoantibodies

Autoantibodies found in patients with Hashimoto's thyroiditis or thyrotoxicosis (Graves' disease) that are organ-specific for the thyroid. Antibodies against thyroglobulin and autoantibodies against the microsomal antigen of thyroid acinar cells may appear in patients with autoimmune thyroiditis. Antibodies against TSH receptors appear in Graves' disease patients and cause stimulatory hypersensitivity. They mimic the action of TSH. They are IgG molecules known as long-acting thyroid stimulator (LATS). LATS levels are increased in many patients with thyrotoxicosis or Graves' disease.

thyroid gland

Endocrine tissue encircling the trachea that synthesizes and releases thyroxine, a hormone that regulates the rate of metabolism.

thyroid autoimmunity animal models

Spontaneous and experimentally induced thyroiditis are the two models used in research. Spontaneous models of thyroiditis include OS chickens, BUF and BB rat strains, NOD mice, and a special colony of beagle dogs. Genetic and environmental factors contribute to autoimmune thyroid disease. Genetic susceptibility to thyroid autoimmunity is multifaceted and diverse. Major histocompatibility complex (MHC) class II genes are the principal genetic determinants of susceptibility in most species. Autoimmunity commences as a response to a restricted region of the thyroglobulin molecule, but a number of epitopes are present in that region. Autoimmunity differs among species. Experimental thyroiditis in mice is produced mainly by cytotoxic T cells; antibodies play a significant pathogenetic role in spontaneous thyroiditis of OS chickens.

thyroiditis, autoimmune

Hashimoto's disease (chronic thyroiditis) is an inflammatory disease found most frequently in middle-aged to older women. Extensive lymphocyte infiltration of the thyroid completely replaces the normal glandular structure of the organ. The numerous plasma cells, macrophages, and germinal centers give the appearance of node structure within the thyroid. B cells and CD4+ T lymphocytes comprise the principal infiltrating lymphocytes. Thyroid function is first increased as the inflammatory reaction injures thyroid

T

follicles, causing them to release thyroid hormones. This stage is soon replaced by hypothyroidism in the later stages of Hashimoto's thyroiditis. Patients with this disease have enlarged thyroid glands. Circulating autoantibodies against thyroglobulin and thyroid microsomal antigen (thyroid peroxidase) are present. Cellular sensitization to thyroid antigens may also be detected. Thyroid hormone replacement therapy is given for the hypothyroidism that develops.

thyrotoxicosis

Disease of the thyroid characterized by hyperthyroidism with elevated levels of thyroid hormones in the blood and thyroid gland hyperplasia or hypertrophy. Thyrotoxicosis may be autoimmune, as in Graves' disease, in which diffuse goiter may be observed. Autoantibodies specific for thyroid antigens mimic thyroid-stimulating hormones (TSHs) by stimulating thyroid cell function. In addition, patients with Graves' disease develop ophthalmopathy and proliferative dermopathy. The disease occurs predominantly in females (70 females to 1 male) and usually appears in the 30- to 40-year old age group. In Caucasians, it is a disease associated with DR3. Patients may develop nervousness, tachycardia, and other symptoms of hyperthyroidism. They also have increased levels of total and free T3 and T4 along with a diffuse and homogeneous uptake of radioactive iodine. Three types of antithyroid antibodies occur: (1) thyroid-stimulating immunoglobulin, (2) thyroid growth-stimulating immunoglobulin, and (3) thyroid binding-inhibitory immunoglobulin. Their presence confirms a diagnosis of Graves' disease. The thyroid gland may be infiltrated with lymphocytes. Long-acting thyroid stimulator (LATS) is classically associated with thyrotoxicosis. It is an IgG antibody specific for thyroid hormone receptors. It induces hyperactivity by combining with TSH receptors.

thyrotropin

Thyroid-stimulating hormone (TSH).

thyrotropin receptor autoantibodies

Autoantibodies specific for thyrotopin receptor (TSHR) are very heterogeneous. Some TSHR antibodies stimulate the receptor and are associated with Graves' disease (hyperthyroidism). Others are inhibitory. Thyrotopin-binding inhibitory immunoglobulin (TBII) antibodies bind to TSHR and inhibit binding of TSH to receptors. Thyroid-stimulating antibodies (TSAbs) mimic TSH and induce thyroid cells to increase cAMP production in a bioassay. Long-acting thyroid stimulator (LATS), a growth-promoting immunoglobulin (IgG) found in Graves' disease, interacts with TSHR. TSHR antibodies are measured by receptor assays. TS antibodies are 95% in Graves' disease and correlate closely with disease activity. TSB antibodies are associated closely with atrophic gastritis and severe hypothyroidism, yet atrophic thyroiditis may occur in their absence. TBII and TS Bantibodies occur in nongoiterous autoimmune thyroiditis. Placental passage of TSHR antibodies may induce transient hypo- or hyperthyroidism.

thyroxine

A hormone synthesized and released by the thyroid gland that regulates cell metabolism, body temperature, use of energy, and normal functioning of the central nervous and cardiovascular systems.

TI antigen

Abbreviation for T-independent (Td) antigen.

TI-1 antigen, TI-2 antigen

Refer to thymus-independent antigen.

tight junction

Juncture between the apical poles of epithelial cells that blocks the passive diffusion of pathogenic microorganisms, macromolecules, and peptides but can be unblocked by cytokine signaling.

tight skin 1 (Tsk1) mouse

A mouse strain developed from a spontaneous dominant mutation in the inbred B10.D2(58N)/Sn strain that represents a genetically transmitted model of systemic sclerosis. The effects of the Tsk1 mutation include excessive accumulation of collagen in the dermis and various internal organs, thereby mimicking major aspects of human systemic sclerosis. The principal visceral changes in Tsk1/+ occur in the lungs and heart. Lungs are greatly distended and histologically resemble human emphysema with little fibrosis. Alveolar spaces are markedly dilated with thin disrupted walls and subpleural cysts and bullae. Myocardial hypertrophy with increased collagen deposition is present.

tight skin 2 (Tsk2) mouse

A mouse strain with features resembling those of both human systemic sclerosis and the original tight skin mutation of the mouse, Tsk1.

TIL

Abbreviation for tumor-infiltrating lymphocyte.

tine test

A human tuberculin test involving intradermal inoculation of dried, old tuberculin using a four-pointed applicator that introduces the test substance 2 mm below the surface.

tingible body

Nuclear debris present in macrophages of lymph node, spleen, tonsil germinal centers, and the dome of the appendix.

tingible body macrophages

Phagocytic cells that engulf apoptotic B cells. They form in large numbers at the height of a germinal center response.

TIR domain

Toll/IL-1R domain present in Toll-like receptor cytoplasmic tails, IL1R, and selected plant pattern recognition molecules. Possesses no intrinsic tyrosine kinase activity but acquires the MyD88 adaptor protein.

Tiselius, Arne W. K. (1902–1971)

Swedish chemist educated at the University of Uppsala, where he also conducted research. In 1934, he was at the Institute for Advanced Study in Princeton, and in 1946 he worked for the Swedish National Research Council. He was awarded the Nobel Prize in Chemistry in 1948 and became president of the Nobel Foundation in 1960. With Elvin A. Kabat, he perfected the electrophoresis technique and classified antibodies as γ globulins. He also developed synthetic blood plasmas.

tissue-fixed macrophage

Histiocyte.

tissue-specific antigen

An antigen restricted to cells of one type of tissue. Tissue-specific or organ-specific autoantibodies occur in certain types of autoimmune diseases. Organ-specific or tissue-specific antibodies are often not species-specific. For example, autoantibodies against human thyroglobulin may cross react with the corresponding molecules of other species. The antigen may be a protein or carbohydrate epitope present only in a particular tissue or subcellular site. When

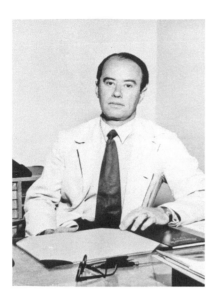

Arne W.K. Tiselius.

expressed inappropriately in a neoplastic cell, it may be called a tumor-associated antigen.

tissue transglutaminase autoantibodies

Immunoglobulin A (IgA) autoantibodies against tissue transglutaminase (tTG) that have a close correlation with active celiac disease. tTG is an intracellular enzyme found in the endomysium and is released after cellular injury or wounding. The enzyme facilitates deamidation of extracellular proteins including gluten peptides, leading to enhanced T cell stimulatory activity. tTG antibodies are transient, disappearing when gluten is eliminated from the diet and mucosal healing occurs. Available data suggest that tTG autoantibodies are very specific for celiac disease.

tissue typing

The identification of major histocompatibility complex (MHC) class I and class II antigens on lymphocytes by serological and cellular techniques. The principal serological assay is microlymphocytotoxicity using microtiter plates containing predispensed antibodies against human leukocyte antigen (HLA) specificities to which lymphocytes of unknown specificity plus rabbit complement and vital dye are added. Following incubation, the wells are scored according to the relative proportion of cells killed. This method is employed for organ transplants such as renal allotransplants. For bone marrow transplants, the earlier mixed lymphocyte culture (MLC, also called mixed lymphocyte reaction) procedure was performed to determine the relative degree of histocompatibility or histoincompatibility between donor and recipient. The older cellular and serological techniques have been replaced largely by molecular (DNA) typing procedures employing polymerase chain reaction (PCR) methodology and DNA or oligonucleotide probes, especially for MHC class II typing. Sequence-specific primer (SSP) technology is the current choice for molecular typing. In addition to PCR-based probe hybridization techniques, restriction fragment length polymorphisms and direct amplicon analysis methods are also employed. Panel-reactive antibody analysis by Luminexx® or an equivalent instrument is useful also for antibody identification in post-transplant monitoring.

titer

An approximation of the antibody activity in each unit volume of a serum sample. The term is used in serology. Titer is determined by preparing serial dilutions of antibody to which a constant amount of antigen is added. The end point is the highest dilution of antiserum in which a visible reaction with antigen (e.g., agglutination) can be detected. Titer is expressed as the reciprocal of the serum dilution that defines the end point. If agglutination occurs in a tube containing a 1:240 dilution, the antibody titer is said to be 240, that is, the serum contains approximately 240 units of antibody per milliliter of antiserum. Titer provides only an estimate of antibody activity. For absolute amounts of antibody, quantitative precipitation or other methods must be employed.

TL (thymic leukemia) antigen

An epitope on the thymocyte membranes of TL+ mice. As the T lymphocytes mature, this antigen disappears, but it resurfaces if leukemia develops. TL antigens are specific and normally present on surfaces of thymocytes of certain mouse strains. They are encoded by a group of structural genes located at the Tla locus, in the linkage group IX, very near the D pole of the H-2 locus on chromosome 17. One of the three structural TL genes has two alleles. The TL antigens are numbered from 1 to 4, specifying four antigens: TL.1, TL.2, TL.3, and TL.4. TL.3 and TL.4 are mutually exclusive. Their expression is under the control of regulatory genes, apparently located at the same Tla locus. Normal mouse thymocytes belong to three phenotypic groups: TL, TL.2, and TL.1, 2, 3. Development of leukemia in mice induces a restructuring of the TL surface antigens of thymocytes with expression of TL.1 and TL.2 in TL cells, expression of TL.1 in TL.2 cells, and expression of TL.4 in both TL and TL.2 cells. When normal thymic cells leave the thymus, the expression of TL antigen ceases. Thus, thymocytes are TL (except the TL strains) and the peripheral T cells are TL. In transplantation experiments, TL tumor cells undergo antigenic modulation. Tumor cells exposed to the homologous antibody stop expressing the antigen and thus escape lysis when subsequently exposed to the same antibody plus complement.

Tla antigen

Murine major histocompatibility complex (MHC) class I histocompatibility antigen encoded by genes situated near the Qa region on chromosome 17. Thymocytes may express products of up to six alleles. Leukemia cells may aberrantly express Tla antigens.

Tla complex

Genes that map to the major histocompatibility complex (MHC) region telomeric to H2 loci on chromosome 17 in mice. These genes encode MHC class I proteins such as Qa and Tla that have no known immune function. Qa and Tla proteins that closely resemble H2 MHC class I proteins in sequence associate noncovalently with β_2 microglobulin. Expression of Qa and Tla proteins, unlike expression of MHC H-2 class I proteins, is limited to only selected mouse cells. For example, only hepatocytes express Q10 protein, only selected lymphocyte subpopulations such as activated T lymphocytes express Qa-2 proteins, and T lymphocytes express Tla proteins. Thus, Qa and Tla class I molecules differ in structure and expression from the remaining MHC class I genes and proteins in mice. This may account

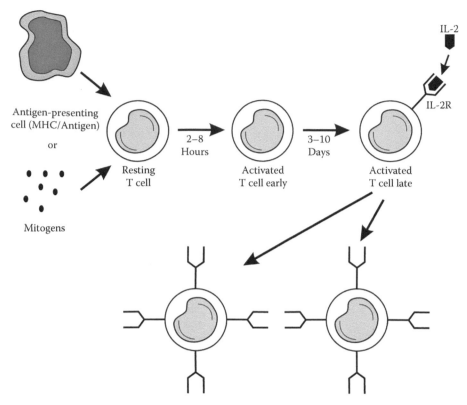

Antigen-presenting
cell (MHC/Antigen)

or

Mitogens

Resting
T cell

2–8
Hours

Activated
T cell early

3–10
Days

Activated
T cell late

IL-2

IL-2R

T lymphocyte (T cell) activation.

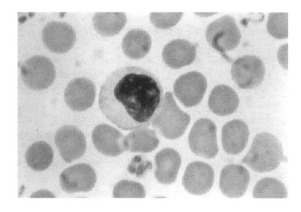

T lymphocyte (T cell) in peripheral blood.

for their failure to function in antigen presentation to T
lymphocytes.

TLR1–10
Refer to Toll-like receptors.

T lymphocyte (T cell)
A thymus-derived lymphocyte that confers cell-mediated
immunity and cooperates with B lymphocytes, enabling
them to synthesize antibody specific for thymus-dependent
antigens, including switching from IgM to IgG and/or IgA
production. T lymphocytes exiting the thymus recirculate
in the blood and lymph and in peripheral lymphoid organs.
They migrate to the deep cortices of lymph nodes. Those
in the blood may attach to postcapillary venule endothelial
cells of lymph nodes and to the marginal sinus in the spleen.
After passing across the venules into the splenic white pulp
or lymph node cortex, they reside there for 12 to 24 hours,

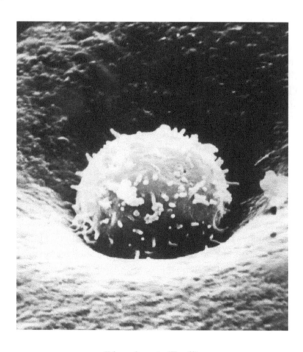

T lymphocyte (T cell).

exit by the efferent lymphatics, proceed to the thoracic duct,
and then proceed to the left subclavian vein where they
enter the blood circulation. Mature T cells are classified on
the basis of their surface markers, such as CD4 and CD8.
CD4+ T lymphocytes recognize antigens in the context of
MHC class II histocompatibility molecules. CD8+ T lymphocytes recognize antigen in the context of MHC class I
histocompatibility molecules. CD4+ T cells participate in the

afferent limb of the immune response to exogenous antigen delivered to them by antigen-presenting cells. This stimulates the synthesis of interleukin-2 (IL2), which activates CD8+ T cells, natural killer (NK) cells, and B cells, thereby orchestrating an immune response to the antigen. Thus, they are termed helper T lymphocytes. They also mediate delayed-type hypersensitivity reactions. CD8+ T lymphocytes include cytotoxic and suppressor cell populations. They react to endogenous antigen and often express their effector function via a cytotoxic mechanism (e.g., against a virus-infected cell). Other molecules on mature T cells in humans include the E rosette receptor CD2 molecule, T cell receptor, pan-T cell marker termed CD3, and transferrin receptors.

T lymphocyte antigen receptor (TCR)

The two types of T cell antigen receptors are TCR1 (appears first in ontogeny) and TCR2. TCR2 is a heterodimer of α and β polypeptides. TCR1 consists of γ and δ polypeptides. Each of the two polypeptides comprising each receptor has a constant and a variable region (similar to immunoglobulin). Reminiscent of the diversity of antibody molecules, T cell antigen receptors can likewise identify a tremendous number of antigenic specificities (estimated at 10^{15} epitopes). The TCR is composed of a minimum of seven receptor subunits whose production is encoded by six separate genes. Following transcription, these subunits are assembled precisely. Assimilation of the complete receptor complex is requisite for surface expression of TCR subunits. Numerous biochemical events are associated with activation of a cell through the TCR. These events ultimately lead to receptor subunit phosphorylation. T cells may be activated by the interaction of antigen in the context of the major histocompatibility complex (MHC) with T cell receptors, involving transmission of a signal to the interior through the CD3 protein to activate cells.

T lymphocyte–B lymphocyte cooperation

The association of T and B cells through a number of receptor–ligand interactions at the surfaces of both cell types, culminating in the synthesis by B cells of antibody specific for thymus-dependent antigens.

T lymphocyte clone

Daughter cells of one T lymphocyte derived from the blood or spleen that are added to culture medium and activated by antigen. T cells stimulated by the antigen form blasts that can be separated from the remaining T cells by density gradient centrifugation. T cells that have responded to antigen are diluted, and aliquots are dispensed into tissue culture plates to which antigen and interleukin-2 (IL2) are added. Each well contains a single lymphocyte. This method provides individual T cell clones.

T lymphocyte-conditioned medium

A cell culture medium containing multiple lymphokines released from T cells stimulated by antigens or lectins.

T lymphocyte hybridoma

Produced by fusing a murine splenic T cell and an AKR strain BW5147 thymoma cell using polyethylene glycol (PEG). The hybrid cell clone is immortal and releases interleukin-2 (IL2) when activated by antigen provided by an antigen-presenting cell.

T lymphocyte receptor

Refer to T lymphocyte antigen receptor.

T lymphocyte subpopulation

A subset of T cells that have a specific function and express a specific cluster of differentiation (CD) markers or other antigens on their surfaces. Examples include the CD4+ helper T lymphocyte subset and the CD8+ suppressor/cytotoxic T lymphocyte subset.

T lymphocytes

Synonym for T cells. T lymphocyte precursors are detectable in a human fetus at 7 weeks of gestation. Between weeks 7 and 14 of gestation, thymic changes begin to imprint thymic lymphocytes as T cells. The maturation (mediated by hormones such as thymosin, thymulin, and thymopoietin II) may be followed by identification of surface (cluster of differentiation [CD]) markers detectable by immunophenotyping. CD3, a widespread T cell marker, serves as a signal transducer from the antigen receptor to the cell interior. Thus, CD3 is intermittently associated with the T cell receptor for antigen. T lymphocytes in the medulla initially express both CD4 and CD8 class markers but these cells later differentiate into CD4+ helper cells or CD8+ suppressor cells. The CD4+ cells characterized by 55-kDa surface markers communicate with macrophages and B cells bearing major histocompatibility complex (MHC) class II molecules during antigen presentation. The CD8+ suppressor/cytotoxic cells interact with antigen-presenting cells bearing MHC class I molecules.

T lymphocyte–T lymphocyte cooperation

Signals from one T lymphocyte subpopulation to another, e.g., isotype class switching in the regulation of immunologic responsiveness.

Tm

Membrane immunoglobulin heavy chain tail (C terminal) polypeptide.

T6 marker

A chromosome of CBA/H-T6 inbred mice discovered in an irradiated male. It has been used as a cell marker to trace cells transferred to other mice. Its length is abbreviated and it has a secondary constriction adjacent to the centromere.

TNF

Abbreviation for tumor necrosis factor.

TNF-α

Abbreviation for tumor necrosis factor α.

TNF-β

Abbreviation for tumor necrosis factor β.

TNF receptor-associated factors (TRAFs)

Adaptor molecules that interact with cytoplasmic domains in TNF receptor molecules. This family includes tumor necrosis factor (TNF)-RII, lymphotoxin (LT) β receptor, and CD40. Cytoplasmic motifs in these receptors bind separate TRAFs that interact with other signaling molecules, resulting in transcription factor AP-1 and NF-κB transcription factors.

TNF receptor-associated periodic syndrome (TRAPS)

A primary autoinflammatory immunodeficiency defined by repeated episodes of severe localized inflammation and extended bouts of fever. Attributable to TNGR1 mutations that lead to uncontrolled activation of the TNRF1 pathway.

TNF receptors

Tumor necrosis factor (TNF) receptors interact with three structurally related ligands: TNF-α, lymphotoxin α (LTα) or TNF-β, and LTβ. Two of the three have the designations CD120a (type I, p55 or p60 receptor) and CD120b (type II, p75 or p80 receptor). The third is designated LTβ receptor (LTβ-R), type III TNF receptor, or TNFR-RP. TNF receptors may be cell-bound or soluble. CD120a and CD120b

T

may bind cell-bound and soluble forms of homotrimers of TNF-α and LTα. CD120b binds more effectively to cell-bound TNF-α. LTβ-R binds only to heterotrimers of LTα and LTβ. CD120a, CD120b, and LTβ-R represent single transmembrane type I proteins. Activation of CD120a in tissue cultured cells by antibody induces numerous TNF effects. CD120b may be important in immunoregulatory activities of TNFs.

TNF-related activation-induced cytokine
See TRANCE (RANK ligand).

TNFR1 pathway
Abbreviation for tumor necrosis factor receptor pathway. An intracellular signaling circuit in which a ligand unites with TNFR1 and leads to cell death or survival based on the signals involved. TRADD, FADD, caspase-8, and caspase-3 cascades mediate death signaling. TRADD, TRAF2/RIP, and the cIAPs causing NF-KB activation and SAPKIJNK signaling pathways mediate survival signaling.

TNP
Abbreviation for trinitrophenol group.

togavirus immunity
Lifelong immunity is induced by infection with a number of togaviruses. Attenuated vaccines have been used to successfully control Venezuelan equine encephalitis virus in horses. Induction of vaccinal immunity in livestock can protect humans through vaccination of the intermediate host. Antibodies against E1 and E2 proteins can neutralize and passively protect against α virus infection in mice and monkeys. Nonstructural protein antibodies can recognize surface components of infected cells. Anti-NS-1 antibodies are highly efficient in activating complement on cell surfaces, leading to lysis of infected cells. Maturation of these viruses from infected cells is by budding through the cytoplasmic membrane. The recognition of nonstructural proteins on infected cell surfaces by T lymphocytes is a significant immunity mechanism. Vaccinia virus live vaccines expressing nonstructural proteins have been used experimentally. E1 proteins of α viruses participate in cell surface adsorption and fusion. E2 proteins contain significant virulence determinants.

tolerance
Active state of unresponsiveness by lymphoid cells to a particular antigen (tolerogen) as a result of their interaction with the antigen. Immune responses to all other immunogens are unaffected. Tolerance is acquired nonresponsiveness to a specific antigen. When inoculated into a fetus or a newborn, an antigenic substance will be tolerated by the recipient in a manner that prevents manifestations of immunity when the individual is challenged with the antigen as an adult. This treatment has no suppressive effect on responses to other unrelated antigens. Immunologic tolerance is much more difficult to induce in adults whose immune systems are fully developed. However, it can be accomplished by administering repetitive minute doses of protein antigens or administering them in large quantities. Mechanisms of tolerance induction have been the subjects of numerous investigations. Clonal deletion is one of these mechanisms. Helper T or B lymphocytes may be inactivated or suppressor T lymphocytes may be activated in the process of

tolerance induction. Clonal anergy and clonal balance are other complex mechanisms proposed to account for self tolerance in which an animal body accepts its own tissue antigens as self and does not reject them. Nevertheless, certain autoantibodies form under physiologic conditions and are not pathogenic; autoimmune phenomena may form under disease conditions and play a significant role in the pathogenesis of autoimmune disease. An immunological adaptation to a specific antigen is distinct from unresponsiveness, the genetic or pathologic inability to mount a measurable immune response. Tolerance involves lymphocytes as individual cells; unresponsiveness is an attribute of the whole organism. The humoral or cell-mediated response may be affected individually or in concert with tolerance. The genetic form of unresponsiveness has been demonstrated with the immune response to synthetic antigens and led to characterization of the immune response (Ir) locus of the major histocompatibility complex (MHC). The immune response of experimental animals (classified as high, intermediate, or nonresponder) is not defective but is not reactive to the particular antigen. In some cases, suppressor cells prevent the development of an appropriate response. Unresponsiveness may also be the result of immunodeficiency states, some with clinical expression, or may be induced by immunosuppressive therapy such as that following x-irradiation, chemotherapeutic agents, or antilymphocyte sera. Tolerance currently has a broader connotation and is intended to represent all instances in which an immune response to a given antigen is not demonstrable. Immunologic tolerance refers to a lack of response as a result of prior exposure to antigen. It may be peripheral which, when abrogated, may lead to autoimmune disease, or central. Refer to immunological tolerance, self tolerance, central tolerance, and peripheral tolerance.

tolerization
The process of rendering an animal tolerant to a specific antigen.

tolerogen
A foreign antigen recognized by a T or B lymphocyte that can induce immunologic tolerance, i.e., this antigen renders lymphocytes refractory to activation. The production of tolerance rather than immunity in response to antigen depends on such variables as physical state of the antigen (soluble or particulate), route of administration, level of maturation of the recipient's immune system, and immunologic competence. Soluble antigens administered intravenously will favor tolerance in many situations as opposed to particulate antigens injected into the skin that may favor immunity. Tolerogens may be orally administered antigens or large doses of protein administered without adjuvants. Immunologic tolerance with cells is easier to induce in a fetus or neonate than in an adult animal that would be more likely to develop immunity rather than tolerance.

tolerogenic
The capacity of a substance such as an antigen to induce immunological tolerance.

tolerogenic dendritic cells
They cause naïve T cells to become anergic rather than activated and/or activate T_{reg} cells induced *in vitro* by

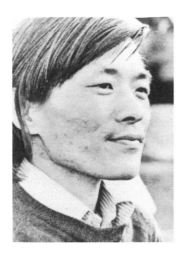

Susumu Tonegawa.

tolerosome

A modified membrane complex of T cell receptors stimulated by antigen, CD3 chains, costimulatory and adhesion molecules, coreceptors, and additional signaling molecules linked with lipid rafts in an anergic T cell. These constituent signaling molecules are distinct from those present in the immunosomes of activated T cells.

Toll-like receptors

Receptors on the surfaces of phagocytes and other cells that signal the activation of macrophages responding to microbial products such as endotoxins in a natural or innate immune response. They are structurally homologous and share signal transduction pathways with the type I interleukin-1 (IL1) receptor. This family of membrane-bound pattern recognition receptors has been conserved in evolution. Lipopolysaccharide (LPS), host stress ligands, peptidoglycan, bacterial flagellin, viral dsRNA, viral ssRNA, and bacterial CpG nucleotides serve as ligands for selected

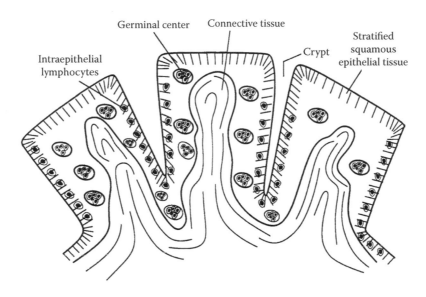

Histology of the tonsil.

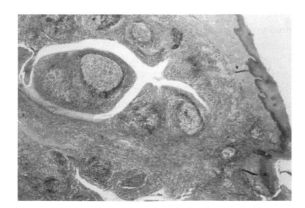

Tonsil.

interaction of dendritic cells with Ts cells or culture with low levels of GM-CSF, elevated IL10, or TGFβ, or with pharmacologic agents such as cyclosporine A, aspirin, or corticosteroids that block NF-κB signaling. Also called modulated dendritic cells.

TLRs. While selected TLRs such as TLR2 and TLR4 are expressed on the cell surface, others such as TLR7 and TLR9 are found in endosomal vesicle membranes. TLR interaction activates dendritic cell maturation and the synthesis of defensins by epithelial cells.

tolmetin

(1-methyl-5-*p*-toluoylpyrrole-2-acetic acid). An anti-inflammatory agent effective in treating juvenile rheumatoid arthritis, rheumatoid arthritis, and ankylosing spondylitis.

Tonegawa, Susumu (1939–)

Japanese-born immunologist working in the United States. He received the Nobel Prize in 1987 for his research on immunoglobulin genes and antibody diversity. He and his colleagues were responsible for the discovery of immunoglobulin gene C, V, J, and D regions and their rearrangement.

tonsil

Lymphoid tissue masses at the intersection of the oral cavity and the pharynx (in the oropharynx). Tonsils contain mostly B lymphocytes and are classified as secondary lymphoid organs. There are several types, designated as palatine, flanked by the palatoglossal and palatopharyngeal arches; pharyngeal, adenoids in the posterior pharynx; and lingual, at the base of the tongue. Waldeyer's ring in the nasopharynx is composed of the five tonsils: nasopharyngeal, two lingual and two palatine.

topoisomerase I

A 100-kDa nuclear enzyme that induces autoantibodies. It is concerned with the relaxation of supercoiled DNA, by nicking and releasing one strand of the DNA duplex.

TORCH panel

A general serologic screen to identify antenatal infection. Elevated levels of immunoglobulin M (IgM) in a neonate reflect *in utero* infection. The panel may be refined by determining IgM antibodies specific for certain microorganisms. TORCH is an acronym for toxoplasma, other, rubella, cytomegalic inclusion virus, herpes (and syphilis). False-positive and false-negative reactions occur in quantitative screening. A positive TORCH panel is indicative of *in utero* infection that may bring major consequences. Toxoplasmosis may result in microglial nodules, thrombosis, necrosis, and blocking of the foramina, leading to hydrocephalus. Rubella may cause hepatosplenomegaly, congenital heart disease, petechiae and purpura, decreased birth weight, microcephaly, cataracts, and central nervous system manifestations including seizures and bulging fontanelles. Cytomegalovirus is characterized by hepatosplenomegaly, hyperbilirubinemia, microcephaly, thrombocytopenia at birth followed later by deafness, mental retardation, learning disabilities, and other manifestations. Herpes simplex can lead to premature birth. Central nervous system manifestations include seizures, chorioretinitis, flaccid or spastic paralysis, and coma. Syphilis is an addendum to the TORCH designation. Congenital syphilis has increased in recent years and is not associated with specific clinical findings.

tositumomab

An anti-CD20 monoclonal antibody labeled with iodine 131 (^{131}I), used to treat patients with CD20-positive follicular non-Hodgkin lymphoma refractory to standard therapy. Toxicities include severe cytopenias including thrombocytopenia and neutropenia.

total body irradiation (TBI)

The administration to hematopoietic cell transplant recipients of sufficient ionizing radiation over the whole body to destroy hematopoietic cells in the bone marrow.

total lymphoid irradiation (TLI)

A technique to induce immunosuppression in which lymphoid organs are irradiated and other organs are protected from irradiation. This method has been used to treat lymphomas.

totipotent

Having the potential for developing in various specialized ways in response to external and internal stimuli; of a cell or part.

toxic complexes

Increased levels of circulating immune complexes may be harmful and trigger type III hypersensitivity reactions. The soluble complexes are pathogenic. The classic description regards such complexes as toxic, and the *toxic complexes* term appeared frequently in the literature. Such complexes are characterized by (1) formation in a zone of moderate antigen excess, (2) lack of cytotropic affinity for tissues of the antibody in the complex, and (3) ability of the complex

to activate the complement system. Complex formation is associated with conformational changes in the antibody molecule. The activity of the complex depends on the antibody, not on the antigen. Antibodies produced in some species such as rabbits, humans, and guinea pigs have these properties. Antibodies of other species such as bovines, chickens, and horses are inactive in this respect. Fixation of the complexes occurs via the Fc portion of the antibody in the complex. The complexes stick to cells and basement membranes, causing injury to the endothelia of small vessels. The injury may occur at the local site of antigen injection or may be systemic when antigen is injected intravenously. The chain of events characteristic for inflammation is set in motion with liberation of vasoactive amines and involvement of polymorphonuclear leukocytes.

toxic epidermal necrolysis

A hypersensitivity reaction to certain drugs such as allopurinol, nonsteroidal anti-inflammatory drugs, barbiturates, sulfonamides such as sulfmethoxazole–trimethoprim, carbamazepine, and other agents. It may closely resemble erythema multiforme. Patients develop erythema, subepidermal bullae, and open epidermal lesions. They become dehydrated, show electrolyte imbalances, and often develop abscesses with sepsis and shock. Toxic epidermal necrolysis may also be observed in a hyperacute type of graft-vs.-host reaction, especially in babies receiving bone marrow transplants.

toxic shock syndrome

A potentially lethal acute systemic toxic reaction in which the patient manifests shock, skin exfoliation, conjunctivitis, and diarrhea resulting from the excessive production of cytokines by CD4$^+$ T cells activated by the bacterial superantigen toxic shock syndrome toxin 1 (TSST-1), secreted by *Staphylococcus aureus*. Linked to the improper use of feminine hygiene products.

toxin

A usually immunogenic poison that stimulates production of antibodies called antitoxins that have the ability to neutralize the harmful effects of the toxin eliciting their synthesis. A toxin molecule synthesized by a pathogenic microorganism may kill a host cell, inhibit its metabolism, or modify host immune responses against the pathogen. The general groups of toxins include (1) bacterial toxins produced by microorganisms such as those causing tetanus, diphtheria, botulism, and gas gangrene, including toxins of staphylococci; (2) phytotoxins including plant toxins such as ricin of the castor bean, crotein, and abrin derived from the Indian licorice seed Gerukia; and (3) zootoxins such as snake, spider, scorpion, bee, and wasp venoms.

toxin neutralization (by antitoxin)

Toxicity is titrated by injection of laboratory animals, and the activity of antitoxins is evaluated by comparison with standard antitoxins of known protective ability. Antitoxin combines with toxin in varying proportions, depending on the ratio in which they are combined, to form complexes that prove nontoxic when injected into experimental animals. Mixing of antitoxin and toxin in optimal proportions may result in flocculation. If toxin is added to antitoxin in several fractions at intervals instead of all at once, more antitoxin is required for neutralization than would be necessary if a single addition of toxin were made. This means that toxins are polyvalent. This phenomenon is explained by the ability of toxin to combine with antitoxin in multiple proportions.

Neutralization does not destroy the reacting toxin. In many instances, toxin may be recovered by dilution of the toxin–antitoxin mixture. The effect of heat on a zootoxin is illustrated by the destruction of cobra venom antitoxin if cobra venom (toxin)–antivenom (antitoxin) mixtures are subjected to boiling. The venom or toxin remains intact. Because toxins have specific affinities for certain tissues, e.g., the high affinity of tetanus toxin for nervous tissue, antitoxins are believed to act by binding toxins before they have the opportunity to combine with specific tissue cell receptors.

toxin-1 (TSST-1)

A toxic bacterial product secreted by *Staphylococcus aureus* and implicated in toxic shock syndrome.

***Toxocara canis* immunity**

The human immune response to the domestic dog roundworm or *Toxocara canis* includes the development of antibodies useful for immunodiagnosis to detect infection. The seroprevalence rate in the United States general population is 2.8% for adults and 23.1% for children. The immune response is also characterized by development of eosinophilic granulomata which may appear throughout the body except for the brain. Larvae within liver granulomata may be killed. *T. canis* infection induces powerful Th2 responses in experimental animals. No vaccine is available.

toxoid

Treatment of a microbial toxin with formaldehyde to inactivate toxicity while leaving the immunogenicity (antigenicity) of the preparation intact. Toxoids are prepared from exotoxins produced in diphtheria and tetanus. They are used to induce protective immunization against adverse effects of the exotoxins in question.

toxoid–antitoxin floccules

An immunizing preparation used to induce active immunity against diphtheria in subjects who are hypersensitive to alum-precipitated toxoid alone. The preparation consists of diphtheria toxoid combined with diphtheria antitoxin in the presence of minimal excess antigen. Horse serum in the preparation may induce hypersensitivity to horse protein in some subjects.

***Toxoplasma gondii* immunity**

Both humoral and cell-mediated responses follow infection with *T. gondii*. The cellular immune response is the principal mediator of resistance to infection, although both types of responses confer resistance. Antibodies activate complement by the classical pathway to lyse extracellular parasites. Tachyzoites coated with immunoglobulin within macrophages are killed. Monocytes and neutrophils also mediate effective killing. While antibodies mediate only a partial protective effect, cell-mediated immunity is critical for survival of the host during acute infection. Activation of macrophages by interferon-γ (IFN-γ) is a principal effector mechanism in toxoplasma infection. Macrophages kill by both oxidative and nonoxidative pathways. Natural killer (NK) and T cells are essential components of the efferent limb of the protective cell-mediated immune response. CD8+ T cells produce IFN-γ to activate macrophages, and CD4+ T cells synthesize interleukin-2 (IL2), which facilitates IFN-γ synthesis by CD8+ T cells. NK cells also produce IFN-γ that helps induce a Th1-type response (IL2 and IFN-γ synthesis) of CD4+ T cells. Transforming growth factor β (TGF-β) and IL10 downregulate IFN-γ production by NK cells during infection. AIDS patients may develop toxoplasmic encephalitis,

indicating the significance of their lost cell-mediated immunity. Tachyzoites in the acute stage of infection are the principal targets for the protective immune response. They induce both antigen-specific and nonspecific suppressor cells to inhibit induction of the immune response to the parasite. No vaccine for *T. gondii* is available.

toxoplasmosis

A disease induced by the *Toxoplasma gondii* protozoan parasite.

Tp44 (CD28)

A T lymphocyte receptor that regulates cytokine synthesis, thereby controlling responsiveness to antigen. Its significance in regulating T lymphocyte activation is demonstrated by the ability of monoclonal antibody against CD28 receptor to block T cell stimulation by specific antigen. During antigen-specific activation of T lymphocytes, stimulation of the CD28 receptor occurs when it combines with the B7/BB1 coreceptor during the interaction of T and B lymphocytes. CD28 is a T lymphocyte differentiation antigen that four fifths of CD3/Ti+ lymphocytes express. It is a member of the immunoglobulin superfamily. CD28 is found only on T lymphocytes and plasma cells. The 134 extracellular amino acids have transmembrane domains and brief cytoplasmic tails in the CD28 monomers.

TPA

Abbreviation for tissue plasminogen activator.

TPHA

Refer to *Treponema pallidum* hemagglutination assay.

TPI

Refer to *Treponema pallidum* immobilization test.

T piece

Refer to secretory piece.

TR1

Refer to regulatory T cell.

Tr1 cells

CD4+ regulatory T cells that secrete IL10 and diminutive quantities of TGF-β.

trace labeling

Refer to isotopic labeling.

traffic area

Thymus-dependent area.

TRAFs (TNF receptor-associated factors)

Signal transducing molecules composed of at least six members that bind to various tumor necrosis factor (TNF) family receptors (TNFRs). They all share a TRAF domain in common and play a critical role as signal transducers between upstream members of the TNFR family and downstream transcription factors.

TRAIL (TNF-related apoptosis-inducing ligand)

A member of the tumor necrosis factor (TNF) family of cytokines. Several TRAIL receptors have been identified, including decoy receptors that function to antagonize TRAIL-induced apoptosis.

TRALI (transfusion-related acute lung injury)

A form of acute respiratory distress syndrome (ARDS), with a reasonably good prognosis, that often occurs within hours following a blood transfusion. It is attributable to leukocyte antibodies and is an acute pulmonary reaction leading to noncardiac pulmonary edema. Mortality is 10% as opposed to 50 to 60% for other forms of ARDS. Eighty percent of TRALI patients experience rapid resolution of pulmonary infiltrates and restoration of arterial

T

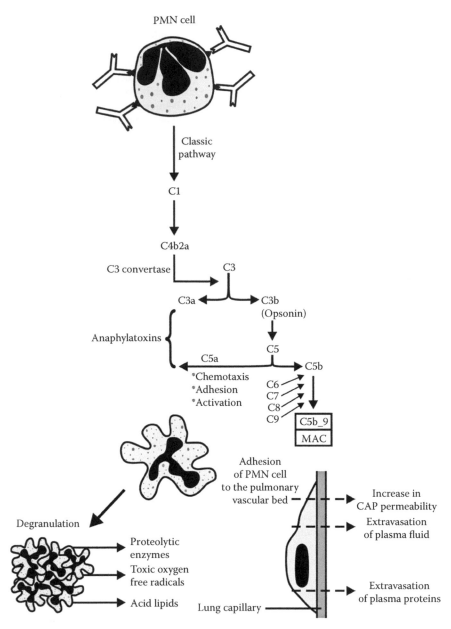

Molecular and cellular events that lead to production of transfusion-related acute lung injury (TRALI) believed to be a form of adult respiratory distress syndrome (ARDS).

blood gas values to normal within 96 hours; 17% retain pulmonary infiltrates for a week following the transfusion reactions. TRALI reactions occur in 1 in 5000 units of blood transfused. Leukoagglutinating antibodies and some lymphocytotoxins have been implicated. The offending antibody is passively transfused in donor plasma rather than donor leukocyte reaction with recipient antibody. Both donor granulocyte antibodies and donor lymphocytes antibodies have been implicated in TRALI reactions. Sixty-five percent of cases studied revealed the presence of human leukocyte antigen (HLA)-specific antibodies, but HLA antibodies may be present in donor plasma and not cause TRALI reactions. Donor plasma implicated in TRALI reactions is often from multiparous females and individuals who received multiple blood transfusions. It is difficult to explain the pathophysiology of a mechanism whereby such a small amount of antibody can induce a

severe clinical reaction unless it initiates an amplification mechanism such as activation of complement. Such a mechanism could cause the formation of C5a, which attaches to granulocytes and alters their membranes so that they adhere nonspecifically to various surfaces. Once these cells are sequestered in the pulmonary vascular bed, they may become activated and release proteolytic enzymes in toxic oxygen metabolites, leading to acute lung injury. Pulmonary sequestration of granulocytes may lead to further endothelial injury and microvascular occlusion. The activation of complement, generation of C5a, and pulmonary sequestration of granulocytes when blood comes into contact with hemodialysis membranes further support a role for complement activation. In summary, TRALI depends on the simultaneous presence of antibody, complement, and antigen-positive cells and leads to extensive capillary leakage.

TRANCE (RANK ligand)

TNF-related activation-induced cytokine (TRANCE) is a member of the tumor necrosis factor (TNF) family and is involved in regulating the functions of dendritic cells and osteoclasts. RANK is the cell surface signaling receptor for TRANCE. Osteoprotegerin also binds TRANCE and serves as a decay receptor that counterbalances the effects of TRANCE.

transcobalamin II deficiency

Infants deficient in transcobalamin II, the main transport protein for vitamin B_{12}, develop megaloblastic anemia and agammaglobulinemia. B lymphocytes require vitamin B_{12} for terminal differentiation. B_{12} therapy corrects the deficiency that has an autosomal-recessive mode of inheritance.

transcobalamin II deficiency with hypogammaglobulinemia

An association of transcobalamin II deficiency with hypogammaglobulinemia, gastrointestinal, and hematologic disorders. This condition is inherited as an autosomal-recessive trait. Patients may manifest macrocytic anemia, thrombocytopenia, leukopenia, and malabsorption resulting from small intestinal mucosal atrophy. Transcobalamin II is a protein needed for vitamin B_{12} transport in the blood. Circulating B lymphocytes are normal, but plasma cells are absent from the bone marrow. Affected subjects often fail to produce antibodies following immunogenic challenge. T cell responsiveness to phytohemagglutinin (PHA) and skin tests are within normal limits. Intramuscular replacement therapy with vitamin B_{12} has improved immunoglobulin levels in the blood and rendered immunization against common antigens successful. The defect in the ability of B cells to undergo clonal expansion and mature into antibody-producing B cells is related to a deficiency in the transcobalamin II necessary for the passage of vitamin B_{12} to the internal environments of cells.

transcription

RNA synthesis using a DNA template.

transcription factors

Proteins that unite with motifs in promoters and initiate, support, or block gene transcription. Examples are: NF-κB, NF-AT, CIITA, IRF, AP-1 (c-fos/c-jun), c-myc, CREB, CBF, Ikaros, PU-1, Tcf-1, Lef-1, GATA-3 and T-bet.

transcriptomics

Science concerned with the total RNA an organism produces.

transcytosis

The conveyance of a molecule from one cell surface area to the opposite cell surface via intracellular transport vesicles, e.g., the active transport of molecules across epithelial cells. Immunoglobulin A (IgA) molecules are transported by transcytosis across intestinal epithelial cells in vesicles formed on basolateral surfaces and fuse with apical surfaces in contact with the intestinal lumen.

transduction

The use of a virus to transfer genes, such as the use of a bacteriophage to convey genes from one bacterial cell to another. Other viruses such as retroviruses may also transfer genes from one cell type to another.

transfection

The transfer of double-stranded DNA extracted from neoplastic cells for the purpose of producing phenotypic alterations of malignancy in the recipient cells.

transfectoma

Antibody-synthesizing cells generated by introducing genetically engineered antibody genes into myeloma cells using genomic DNA.

transfer factor (TF)

A substance in extracts of leukocytes that is as effective as viable lymphoid cells in transferring delayed-type hypersensitivity. The active principle is not destroyed by treatment with DNase or RNase. Originally described by H.S. Lawrence, TF has been the subject of numerous investigations. It is dialyzable and its weight is <10 kDa. It has been separated on Sephadex®. Following demonstration of its role in humans, TF was shown to transfer delayed-type hypersensitivity in laboratory animals. It is capable of transferring cell-mediated immunity and delayed-type hypersensitivity between members of numerous animal species. It thus became possible to transfer delayed-type hypersensitivity across species barriers using TF. The identification of purified TF remains a major challenge, but the combination of TF with specific antigen has been demonstrated. Urea treatment of a solid phase immunosorbent permits its recovery. Thus, specific TF is generated in an animal immunized with a specific antigen. T helper lymphocytes produce TF, which combines with T suppressor cells and Ia antigen on B lymphocytes and macrophages. It also interacts with antibody specific for V region antigenic determinants. It may be a fragment of the T cell receptor for antigen. TF has been used as an immunotherapeutic agent for many years to treat patients with various types of immunodeficiencies. It produces clinical improvement in numerous infectious diseases caused by viruses and fungi. It also improves cell-mediated immunity and delayed-type hypersensitivity response (i.e., it restores decreased cellular immunity to some degree).

transferrin

A protein that combines with and competes for iron with bacteria.

transferrin receptor (T9)

The receptor on cell membranes for the 76-kDa transferrin protein in serum that serves as a conveyor of ferric (Fe^{3+}) iron. Monoclonal antibody can detect transferrin receptors on activated T lymphocytes, even though resting T cells are essentially bereft of this receptor. Primitive thymocytes also express it. Transferrin receptor is comprised of two identical 100-kDa polypeptide chains fastened together by disulfide bonds. The transferrin receptor gene is located on chromosome 3p12-ter in humans.

transformation

A heritable alteration in a cell as a consequence of investigative manipulation. (1) Lymphocyte transformation is the stimulation of a resting lymphocyte with a lectin, antigen, or lymphokine to undergo blast transformation associated with cell division, proliferation, and differentiation. This process can be assayed quantitatively by adding ^{3}H (thymidine) to the cell culture which becomes incorporated into the DNA. (2) Genetic transformation by DNA occurs when nonvirulent living pneumococci become virulent after taking up DNA from dead pneumococci by transformation. (3) Cells can undergo neoplastic transformation in culture and acquire the capacity for unrestricted proliferation, thereby resembling neoplastic cells.

transforming growth factor α (TGF-α)

Refer to TGF-α.

transforming growth factor β (TGF-β)

Refer to TGF-β.

T

transfusion

The transplantation of blood cells, platelets, and/or plasma from the circulation of one individual to another. Acute blood loss due to hemorrhage or the replacement of deficient cell types due to excess destruction or inadequate formation are indications for transfusion. With the description of human blood groups by Landsteiner in 1900, the transfusion of blood from one human to another became possible. This ability ushered in the field of transfusion medicine concerned with substitution therapies with human blood, protein deficiencies, and blood loss. Peripheral blood cell and plasma collection, processing, storage, compatibility matching, and transfusion are routine procedures in medical centers throughout the world. The descriptions of other blood group systems followed the initial description of the ABO types. Modern blood group serology and immunohematology laboratories consider all aspects of allo- and autoantibodies against red cells in clinical transfusion. Blood-borne viruses are recognized as critical risk factors in transfusion. In recent years, the rate of viral transmission through transfusions has greatly diminished with the development of adequate screening for human immunodeficiency virus (HIV), hepatitis viruses, and other infectious agents.

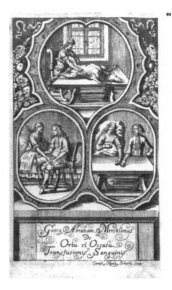

Engraved title page from G.A. Merklin's *Tractatio Med: Curiousa de Ortu et Sanguinis,* 1679. This is one of the best early depictions of blood transfusion. (From the Cruse Collection, Middleton Library, University of Wisconsin.)

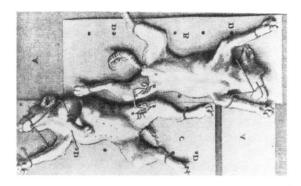

Early dog blood transfusion.

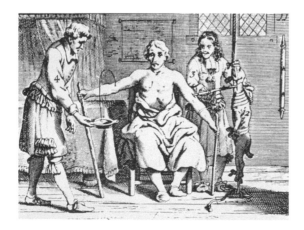

Transfusion of patient with animal blood. (From Scultatus, courtesy of National Library of Medicine.)

transfusion-associated graft-vs.-host disease (TAGVHD)

Infused immunocompetent T lymphocytes react against histoincompatible immune system cells of a recipient. This is likely to occur in patients who have been immunocompromised or are receiving chemotherapy for tumors. Patients

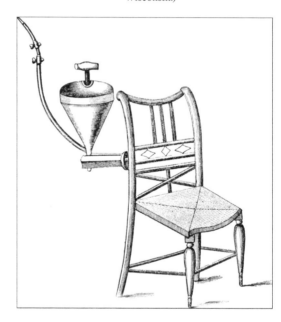

Transfusion chair developed by James Blundell, the father of modern blood transfusion therapy.

may develop skin rashes and have profound pancytopenia and altered liver function tests. Three weeks following transfusion, 84% may die. To avoid graft-vs.-host reactivity induced by a transfusion, any blood product containing lymphocytes should be subjected to 1500 rad prior to administration.

transfusion effect

Facilitation of organ transplant acceptance by a recipient who received prior blood transfusions from individuals sharing an HLA-DR allotype with the organ donor.

transfusion reactions

Immune and nonimmune reactions that follow the administration of blood. Transfusion reactions with immune causes are considered serious and occur in 1 in 3000 transfusions. Patients may develop urticaria, itching, fever, chills, chest pains, cyanosis, and hemorrhage; some may even collapse. The appearance of these symptoms and a temperature increase of 1°C signal the need to halt the transfusion. Immune noninfectious transfusion reactions include allergic urticaria (immediate hypersensitivity); anaphylaxis, as in the administration of blood to immuno-globulin A (IgA)-deficient subjects, some of whom develop anti-IgA antibodies of the IgE class; and serum sickness, in which the serum proteins such as immunoglobulins induce the formation of precipitating antibodies that lead to immune complex formation. Transfusion reactions may cause intravascular lysis of red blood cells and when severe may lead to renal injury, fever, shock, and disseminated intravascular coagulation.

transgenes

Foreign genes that are artificially and deliberately intro-duced into a germline. Refer to transgenic mice.

transgenic

An organism in which DNA from another organism has been inserted into its genome via recombinant DNA techniques. Transgenic animals are usually produced by microinjection of DNA into the pronuclei of fertilized eggs, with the DNA integrating at random.

transgenic animal

An animal into whose genome a foreign gene has been intro-duced. Introduction of the exogenous gene into a mouse can be achieved by microinjection into a pronucleus of a recently fertilized egg or through retroviruses. The egg that received the foreign gene is transferred to the oviduct of a pseudopreg-nant female. If the gene becomes integrated into a chromo-some, it is passed on to the progeny through the germline and will be expressed in all cells. Natural transcriptional promoters and enhancers or exogenous regulatory elements engineered into it may control expression of a transgene.

transgenic line

A transgenic mouse strain in which the transgene is stably integrated into the germline and therefore inherited in Mendelian fashion by succeeding generations.

transgenic mice

Mice that carry a foreign gene that was artificially and deliberately introduced into their germline. The added genes are termed transgenes. Fertilized egg pronuclei receive microinjections of linearized DNA. These are placed in pseudopregnant female oviducts and develop-ment proceeds. About one fourth of the mice that develop following injection of several hundred gene copies into pronuclei are transgenic. These mice are used to study genes not usually expressed *in vivo* and alterations in genes that are developmentally regulated to express normal genes and cells where they are not usually expressed. Transgenic mice are also used to delete certain populations of cells with transgenes that encode toxic proteins. They are highly significant in immunologic research.

transgenic mouse

A mouse developed from an embryo into which foreign genes were transferred. Transgenic mice have provided much valuable data related to immunological tolerance, autoimmune phenomena, oncogenesis, developmental biol-ogy, and related topics. The transgene has been introduced and stably incorporated into germline cells, ensuring that it can be passed on to progeny. A specific DNA sequence is injected into the pronuclei of fertilized mouse eggs. Transgenes insert randomly at chromosomal breakpoints and are inherited as simple Mendelian traits. Studies with transgenic mice have yielded much data about cytok-ines, cell surface molecules, and intracellular signaling molecules.

transgenic organism

An animal or plant into which foreign genes that encode specific proteins have been inserted. Controlling the site of gene insertion has not yet been accomplished. Insertion into some positions may even lead to activation of the host's own structural genes.

transgenics

The transfer of needed genes into an organism for the pur-pose of providing a missing protein that these genes encode.

transient hypogammaglobulinemia of infancy

A delay in the onset of antibody synthesis by a 2-1/2- to 3-year old child in whom maternal antibodies passed across the placenta have already disappeared. Helper T cell func-tion is impaired, yet B cell numbers are at physiologic levels.

translation

The synthesis of a peptide chain using amino acids to produce proteins.

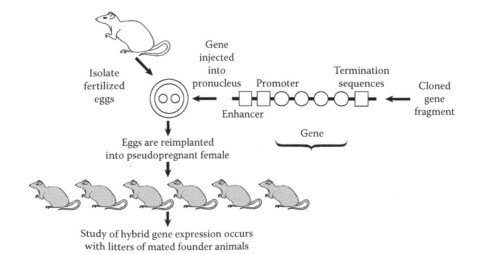

Transgenic mice.

translocation

A chromosomal aberration in which one segment of a chromosome has become joined to another chromosome. B and T cell rearranging genes are frequently sites of translocation in B cell and T cell tumors.

transmissible spongiform encephalopathy (TSE) immunity

Paradoxically, a functional immune system is requisite for efficient experimental transmission of scrapie and for TDE agents to pass from one species to another. Immunologically immature mice are less susceptible to scrapie than older mice; SCID mice are refractory to infection. PHA and BCG increase susceptibility to infection. Interferon, antilymphocyte serum, neonatal thymectomy, and whole body radiation fail to alter the incubation period.

transplant rejection

Refer to transplantation rejection.

transplantation

The replacement of an organ or other tissue such as bone marrow with organs or tissues derived ordinarily from a nonself source such as an allogeneic donor. Organs include kidney, liver, heart, lung, pancreas (including pancreatic islets), intestine, and skin. Bone matrix and cardiac valves have also been transplanted. Bone marrow transplants are used for nonmalignant conditions such as aplastic anemia and to treat certain leukemias and other malignant diseases.

transplantation antigens

Histocompatibility antigens that stimulate an immune response in the recipient that may lead to rejection.

transplantation immunology

The study of immunologic reactivity of a recipient to transplanted organs or tissues from a histoincompatible recipient. Effector mechanisms of transplantation rejection and transplantation immunity consist of cell-mediated immunity and/or humoral antibody immunity, depending on the category of rejection. For example, hyperacute rejection of an organ such as a renal allograft is mediated by preformed antibodies and occurs soon after the vascular anastomosis is completed. By contrast, acute allograft rejection is mediated principally by T lymphocytes and occurs during the first week after transplantation. There are instances of humoral vascular rejection mediated by antibodies as a part of the acute rejection in response. Chronic rejection is mediated by a cellular response.

transplantation rejection

The consequences of cellular and humoral immune responses to a transplanted organ or tissue that may lead to loss of function and necessitate removal of the transplanted organ or tissue. Transplantation rejection episodes occur in many transplant recipients but are controlled by such immunosuppressive drugs as cyclosporine, rapamycin, and FK506 or by monoclonal antibodies against T lymphocytes.

transport piece

Refer to secretory piece.

transporter associated with antigen processing (TAP)

A TAP-binding heterodimeric protein in the rough endoplasmic reticulum membrane that transports peptides from the cytosol to the endoplasmic reticulum lumen. It is comprised of TAP 1 and TAP 2 subunits that bind peptides to major histocompatibility complex (MHC) class I molecules. Genes in the MHC class II region must be expressed for MHC class I molecules to be assembled efficiently. TAP 1 and 2 are postulated to encode components of a heterodimeric protein pump that conveys cytosolic peptides to the endoplasmic reticulum. They associate with MHC class I heavy chains.

transudation

The movement of electrolytes, fluid, and proteins of low molecular weight from intravascular spaces to extravascular spaces as in inflammation.

trastuzumab

A recombinant DNA-derived humanized monoclonal antibody that selectively binds with high affinity in a cell-based assay to the extracellular domain of the human epidermal growth factor receptor 2 protein (HER-2/*neu*). The antibody is an IgG$_{1\kappa}$ that contains human framework regions with the

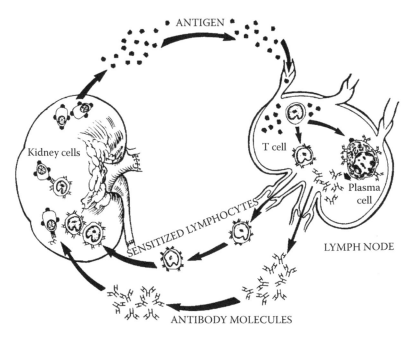

Rejection.

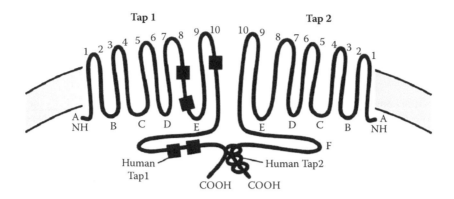

Topology of TAP1 and TAP2 proteins.

complementarity-determining regions of a murine antibody (4D5) that binds to HER-2. Commercially distributed as HERCEPTIN®. It prevents binding by the natural ligand and downregulates the receptor. It is used to treat metastatic breast cancer in which the tumors overexpress HER-2/*neu*.

T_{reg} cells

CD4+/CD25+ regulatory T cells that are positive for CTLA-4 but fail to secrete significant quantities of cytokines. Through intercellular interactions, they can anergize T cells nonspecifically. They may render antigen-presenting cells tolerogenic through downregulation of their costimulatory molecules.

***Treponema* immunity**

Infection with *Treponema pallidum* induces both cellular and humoral immune responses. The humoral response is characterized by the synthesis of phospholipid and treponemal antibodies detected in the serological diagnosis of syphilis. Flocculation tests have long been used to detect phospholipid and cardiolipin antibodies. They make use of a cardiolipin–lecithin–cholesterol antigen in the VDRL (Venereal Disease Research Laboratory) test. Cardiolipin F antibody specific for host cell mitochondrial cardiolipin (autoantibody) is also associated with syphilis but not used in diagnosis. Treponemal antibodies that appear with cardiolipin antibodies after infection are detectable by immunofluorescence and remain detectable in a host for many years. Autoantibodies against tissue phospholipids and other tissue components also occur in *T. pallidum*-infected hosts. The cell-mediated immune response consists of macrophage activation and induction of CD8+ and CD4+ T cells. The cell-mediated immunity appears to be more important than the humoral response.

***Treponema pallidum* hemagglutination assay (TPHA)**

A test for antibodies specific for *Treponema pallidum* used formerly to diagnose syphilis. *T. pallidum* antigens are coated onto sheep red blood cells treated with tannic acid and formalin. Aggregation of antigen-coated red cells signified the presence of antibody.

***Treponema pallidum* immobilization test (TPI)**

A diagnostic test for syphilis in which living, motile *Treponema pallidum* microorganisms are combined with a sample of serum presumed to contain specific antibody. Complement is also present. If the serum sample contains anti-*Treponema* antibody, the motile microorganisms become immobilized. This test is much more specific for the diagnosis of syphilis than complement fixation tests such as the early Wassermann reaction. It is rarely used because living *T. pallidum* microorganisms are not readily available and handling them is hazardous.

TRF

Abbreviation for T cell replacing factor.

***Trichuris trichiura* immunity**

Human immune responses against these worm infections include specific immunoglobulin G (IgG), IgA, and IgE antibody responses. The IgG level increases with the level of infection, but elevated IgA levels may be associated with diminished worm burdens. The cellular response remains to be defined. Macrophages release tumor necrosis factor α (TNF-α), and an IgE-mediated release of mast cell mediators contributes to inflammation and enteropathy associated with infection. In mice, the immune response to *T. muris* consists of a powerful T cell response that leads to premature expulsion of worms from the intestine. Primary infections are followed by the development of resistance to reinfection. Immunity can be passively transferred with CD4+ T cells or immune sera. Inflammatory responses are not believed to contribute to immunity. Murine strains that effectively eliminate the infection develop responses mediated by Th2 cells. No vaccine is available for *Trichuris*.

Trinitrophenyl group.

trinitrophenyl (picryl) group

A chemical grouping that may serve as a hapten when linked to a protein through –NH₂ groups by reaction with picryl chloride or trinitrobenzene sulfonic acid.

triple response of Lewis

Skin change of immediate hypersensitivity determined by striking the skin with a sharp object such as the side of a ruler. The first (stroke) response is caused by the production of histamine and related mediators at the point of contact. The second response is a flare resembling a red halo produced by vasodilation. The third response is a wheal characterized by swelling and blanching induced by histamine from mast cell degranulation. The swelling is attributable to edema between the junctions of cells that become rich in protein and fluid.

triple vaccine

An immunizing preparation composed of three components and used to protect infants against diphtheria, pertussis (whooping cough), and tetanus. It consists of diphtheria toxoid, pertussis vaccine, and tetanus toxoid. The first of four doses is administered between 3 and 6 months of age. The second dose is administered 1 month later, and the third dose is given 6 months after the second. A booster injection is given when a child begins school.

Triton X-100

A surface-active quaternary ammonium salt (isooctyl phenoxy polyethoxy ethanol) used as a detergent, emulsifier, wetting agent, and surfactant.

trophoblast

A layer of cells in the placenta that synthesizes immunosuppressive agents. The cells are in contact with the uterine lining.

tropical eosinophilia

A hypersensitivity to filarial worms manifested in the lungs and reported in the Near and Far East. Patients develop wheezing, productive cough, and a cellular infiltrate consisting of eosinophils, lymphocytes, and fibroblasts. Fibrosis may result.

Trypan blue

A vital dye used to stain lymphoid cells, especially in the microlymphocytotoxicity test used for human leukocyte antigen (HLA) tissue typing. Cell membranes whose integrity has been interrupted by antibody and complement permit the dye to enter and stain the cells dark blue. By contrast, viable cells with intact membranes exclude the dye and remain as bright circles of light under a microscope. Dead cells stain blue.

Trypan blue dye exclusion test

A test for viability of cells in culture. Living cells exclude Trypan blue by active transport. When membranes have been interrupted, dye enters the cells, staining them blue, indicating the cells are dead. The method can be used to calculate the percent of cell lysis induced.

trypanosome adhesion test

Selected mammalian red blood cells or bacteria may stick to the surfaces of trypanosomes when specific antibody and complement are present. This characteristic was used in the past as a test for antibodies to trypanosomes.

trypanosome immunity

Vaccination against African sleeping sickness known as trypanosomiasis has thus far been unattainable. Although the antigen that induces a protective humoral response is well known as a surface glycoprotein that covers the entire trypanosome, the organism repeatedly changes the antigenic structure of this glycoprotein (variant surface glycoprotein, VSG), thereby evading destruction by the host immune response. Only a single VSG is expressed by a trypanosome at one time. Trypanosomes that express the same VSG are classified as belonging to the same variable antigenic type (VAT). Only short-term immunity can be induced by allowing cattle to become infected by fly bites and then treating the infection as soon as the parasitemia

becomes patent. The powerful humoral response in trypanosomal infections is characterized by the appearance of immunoglobulin M (IgM) and IgG antibodies associated with the elimination of each VAT. These antibodies kill parasites and clear them from the blood by complement activation by way of the classic pathway and opsonization, which results in uptake by the Kupffer's cells of the liver. The immune response in experimental mice consists of both T-dependent and T-independent components. Lymphocyte responsiveness is profoundly depressed in trypanosome infections.

tryptic peptides

Peptides formed by tryptic digestion of protein.

Ts

(1) Suppressor T lymphocyte. (2) Secreted immunoglobulin heavy chain tail (C terminal) polypeptide.

Ts1, Ts3 lymphocytes

Suppressor T lymphocyte subpopulations.

TsF

Abbreviation for suppressor T cell factor.

Ts cells

CD8$^+$/D57$^+$/CD28$^-$ regulatory T cells considered to downregulate immune responses. Interaction of a Ts cell with an antigen presenting cell pMHC leads to tolerization of the antigen presenting cell through suppression of B7 expression and upregulation of ILT3 and ILT4. CD4$^+$ Th0 cells are rendered anergic and/or develop into T_{reg} cells after interaction with the antigen presenting cells. When Ts cells become activated, they synthesize a Th0-like profile of cytokines.

TSA

Abbreviation for tumor-specific antigen.

TSF

T cell suppressor factor.

TTF-1 (8G7G3/a), mouse

Thyroid transcription factor-1 is useful in differentiating primary adenocarcinoma of the lung from metastatic carcinomas from the breast and malignant mesothelioma. It can also be used to differentiate small cell lung carcinoma from lymphoid infiltrates.

tube agglutination test

An agglutination assay that consists of serial dilutions of antiserum in serological tubes to which a particulate antigen such as a microorganism is added.

tuberculid

A hypersensitivity skin reaction to mycobacteria. The lesion may be a papulonecrotic tuberculid with sterile papules ulcerated in the center and obliterative vasculitis, or crops of small red papules with sarcoid-like appearances that represent lichen scrofulosorum.

tuberculin

A sterile solution containing a group of proteins derived from culture medium in which *Mycobacterium tuberculosis* microorganisms have been grown. It has been used for almost a century as a skin test preparation to detect delayed-type (type IV) hypersensitivity to infection with *M. tuberculosis*. Many tuberculin preparations have been used in the past, but only old tuberculin (OT) and purified protein derivative (PPD) are still used. While OT is a heat-concentrated filtrate of the culture medium in which *M. tuberculosis* was grown, PPD of tuberculin is a trichloroacetic acid precipitate of the growth medium. Tuberculin is a mitogen for murine B lymphocytes and also a T lymphocyte mitogen.

tuberculin hypersensitivity

A form of bacterial allergy specific for a product in culture filtrates of *Mycobacterium tuberculosis* which, when injected into the skin, elicits a cell-mediated delayed-type (type IV) hypersensitivity response. Tuberculin-type hypersensitivity is mediated by CD4+ T lymphocytes. After intracutaneous inoculation of tuberculin extract or purified protein derivative (PPD), an area of redness and induration develops at the site in 24 to 48 hours in individuals subjected to present or past interaction with *M. tuberculosis.*

tuberculin reaction

A test of *in vivo* cell-mediated immunity. Robert Koch observed localized skin lesions of tuberculous guinea pigs inoculated intradermally with broth from a culture of tubercle bacilli. The body's immune response to infection with the tubercle bacillus is signaled by the appearance of agglutinins, precipitins, opsonins, and complement-fixing antibodies in the serum. This humoral response is, however, not marked, and such antibodies are present in low titer. The most striking response is the development of delayed-type hypersensitivity (DTH) that plays a protective role in preventing reinfection with the same organism. Subcutaneous inoculation of tubercle bacilli in a normal animal produces no immediate response, but in 10 to 14 days a nodule develops at the site of inoculation. The nodule then becomes a typical tuberculous ulcer. The regional lymph nodes become swollen and caseous. In contrast, a similar inoculation in a tuberculous animal induces an indurated area at the site of injection within 1 to 2 days. This becomes a shallow ulcer that heals promptly. No swelling of the adjacent lymphatics is noted. The tubercle bacillus antigen responsible for DTH is wax D, a lipopolysaccharide–protein complex of bacterial cell walls. The active peptide consists of diaminopimelic acid, glutamic acid, and alanine. Testing for DTH to the tubercle bacillus is done with tuberculin, a heat-inactivated culture extract containing a mixture of bacterial proteins, or with PPD, a purified protein derivative of culture in nonproteinaceous media. Each compound alone is capable of sensitizing the recipient. The protective role of DTH is supported by the observation that in positive reactors living cells are usually free of tubercle bacilli and the bacteria are present in necrotic areas, separated by an avascular barrier. By contrast, in infected individuals producing negative reactions, the tubercle bacilli are found in great numbers in living tissues. The reaction is permanently or transiently negative in individuals whose cell-mediated immune responses are transiently or permanently impaired.

tuberculin test

The 24- to 48-hour response to intradermal injection of tuberculin. If positive, it signifies delayed-type (type IV) hypersensitivity to tuberculin and implies cell-mediated immunity to *Mycobacterium tuberculosis*. The intradermal inoculation of tuberculin or purified protein derivative (PPD) produces an area of erythema and induration within 24 to 48 hours in positive individuals. A positive reaction signifies the presence of cell-mediated immunity to *M. tuberculosis* as a consequence of past or current exposure to the microorganism; however, tuberculin is not a test for the diagnosis of active tuberculosis.

tuberculin-type reaction

A cell-mediated delayed-type hypersensitivity skin response to an extract such as candidin, brucellin, or histoplasmin.

Individuals who experience positive reactions have delayed-type hypersensitivity or cell-mediated immunity mediated by T lymphocytes following contact with the microorganism in question.

tuberculosis immunization

The induction of protective immunity through injection of an attenuated vaccine containing bacille Calmette-Guérin (BCG). This vaccine was more widely used in Europe than in the United States in attempts to provide protection against tuberculosis. A local papule develops several weeks after injection in individuals who were previously tuberculin-negative. The vaccine is not administered to positive individuals. The vaccine is claimed to protect against development of tuberculosis, although not all authorities agree on its efficacy for this purpose. In recent years, oncologists have used BCG vaccine to reactivate the cellular immune systems of patients bearing neoplasms in the hope of facilitating antitumor immunity.

tubular basement membrane autoantibodies

Autoantibodies specific for tubular basement membranes (TBMs). They are detectable by immunofluorescence in some renal allotransplant patients following certain types of drug therapy and occasionally without a known cause. In human tubulointerstitial nephritis (TIN), TBM autoantibodies generated react with a major 58-kDa antigen (TIN antigen) and minor 160-, 175-, and 300-kDa antigens related to laminin and entactin/nidogen. Twenty-two percent of patients with various types of interstitial nephritis manifest autoantibodies against TIN antigen. Normal urine may reveal human TBM antigens that are capable of inducing TIN in rats. TBM autoantibodies are only rarely detected in human cases of TIN, but they are often prominent as glomerular basement membrane (GBM) autoantibodies in patients with Goodpasture's syndrome. TBM autoantibodies are of unknown clinical significance.

tuftsin

A leukokinin globulin-derived substance that enhances phagocytosis. It is a tetrapeptide comprised of Thr–Lys–Pro–Arg. The leukokinin globulin from which it is derived represents immunoglobulin Fc receptor residues 289 through 292. Tuftsin is formed in the spleen. Its actions include neutrophil and macrophage chemotaxis, enhancing phagocyte motility, and promoting oxidative metabolism. It also facilitates antigen processing.

tuftsin deficiency

A tetrapeptide that stimulates phagocytes. Tuftsin is split from an immunoglobulin by the action of one proteolytic enzyme in the spleen that cleaves the carboxyl terminus between residues 292 and 293 and another enzyme (leukokinase) confined to neutrophil membranes that splits the molecule between positions 288 and 289. Thus, tuftsin deficiency, which is transmitted as an autosomal-recessive trait, results from a lack of this splenic enzyme. Although γ globulin has been used, there is no known treatment.

tumor

A neoplasm developing as a consequence of uncontrolled cell proliferation. Benign tumors are self-limiting, whereas malignant tumors may be invasive.

tumor antigens

Cell surface proteins on tumor cells that can induce a cell-mediated and/or humoral immune response. Refer also to tumor-associated antigens and tumor-specific antigens.

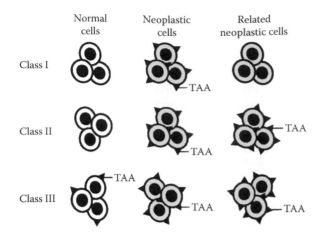

Tumor-associated antigens (TAAs) among normal and neoplastic cells.

tumor-associated antigens

Epitopes of selected tumor cells that are also found on certain types of normal cells. They may be protein or carbohydrate molecules expressed in abnormal concentration, location, or time in a tumor cell compared with expression in a healthy differentiated cell in the tissue of origin. Normal cellular genes that have become dysregulated encode tumor-associated antigens. Examples include normal cellular proteins, differentiation antigens, tissue type-specific antigens, embryonic antigens, and idiotypic antigens. Certain antigens designated CA-125, CA-19-9, and CA195, among others may be linked to certain tumors such as lymphomas, carcinomas, sarcomas, and melanomas, but the immune response to these tumor-associated antigens is not sufficient to mount a successful cellular or humoral immune response against the neoplasm. Three classes of tumor-associated antigens have been described. Class 1 antigens are very specific for a certain neoplasm and absent from normal cells. Class 2 antigens are found on related neoplasms from separate individuals. Class 3 antigens are

found on malignant and normal cells but show increased expression in neoplastic cells. Assays of clinical value will probably be developed for class 2 antigens, as they are associated with multiple neoplasms and are rarely found in normal individuals.

tumor enhancement

The successful establishment and prolonged survival (conversely, the delayed rejection) of a tumor allograft, especially in mice, as a consequence of contact with specific antibody.

tumor hypoxia

Diminished oxygen pressure that develops in parts of a tumor that has outgrown its blood supply. Sensitivity to radiation and chemotherapy become less effective as tumor cells undergo hypoxia.

tumor imaging

An experimental and clinical technique employed to localize neoplastic lesions using a labeled antibody or its fragment. Tumor imaging is based on the presence of an antigen expressed only on a tumor cell or exhibits a significant difference in amount and/or distribution between tumor and normal tissues.

tumor immunity

A number of experimentally induced tumors in mice express numerous specific transplantation antigens that can induce an immune response leading to the destruction of neoplastic cells *in vivo*. Lymphocytes play a critical role in the immunological destruction of many antigenic tumors. Both cell-mediated and antibody-mediated immune responses to human neoplasms have been identified and their targets characterized in an effort to develop clinically useful immunotherapy.

tumor immunotherapy

Immunological surveillance, first proposed by Paul Ehrlich 100 years ago, is believed to be a protective mechanism against the development of neoplasias in intact healthy subjects. Significant suppression of the immune system from any cause may favor tumor development. Contemporary attempts at therapeutic modification of the immune response include the use of immune response

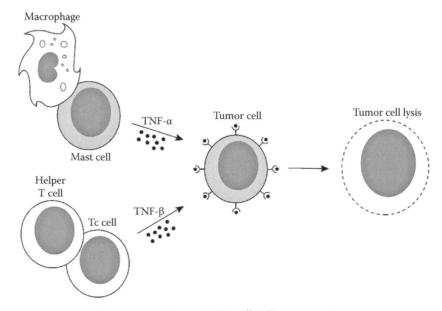

Tumor necrosis factor (TNF)-mediated immune reaction.

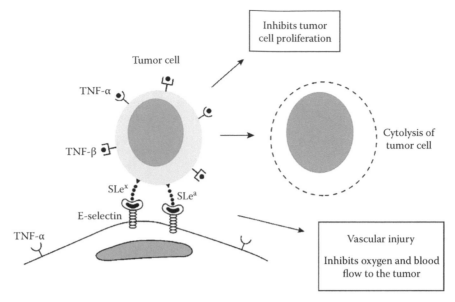

Tumor necrosis immunotherapy.

modifiers, monoclonal antibodies, cancer vaccines, and gene therapy. Genetically engineered cytokines such as interleukin-2 (IL2) and interferon-α (IFN-α) have been used to activate the immune system. Early hopes for success have now abated. Interferons have some proven efficacy in the management of melanoma, renal cell carcinoma, and hairy cell leukemia and as adjuvant therapy in certain hematological malignancies such as low-grade lymphoma and myeloma. Although IL2 has been used in the past to treat renal cell carcinoma and melanoma with the generation of tumor-infiltrating lymphocytes (TILs) and lymphokine-activated killer (LAK) cells, it has toxic physiologic effects. Monoclonal antibodies as anticancer agents are promising but have problems with delivery to targets and reactions to murine antibodies along with difficulties in linking therapeutic war heads to these "smart bombs." Bispecific antibodies have been used to cross link targets to immune effector cells to activate a cell-mediated antitumor response. Current cancer vaccines include autologous cell lines, allogeneic cell lines, genetically modified tumor cells, glycoproteins, stripped glycoproteins, peptides, antitumor idiotypes, and polynucleotides encoding tumor antigens. Gene therapy may be used to modify tumor cells to express costimulatory molecules such as B7-1 to help initiate a cell-mediated response against a neoplasm.

tumor-infiltrating lymphocytes (TILs)

Cytotoxic T lymphocytes within a tumor mass. T lymphocytes isolated from the tumor they are infiltrating. They are cultured with high concentrations of interleukin-2 (IL2), leading to expansion of these activated T lymphocytes *in vitro*. TILs are very effective in destroying tumor cells and have proven much more effective than lymphokine-activating killer (LAK) cells in experimental models; they have 50 to 100 times the antitumor activity produced by LAK cells. TILs have been isolated and grown from multiple resected human tumors, including those from kidney, breast, colon, and melanoma. In contrast to the non-B/non-T LAK cells,

TILs nevertheless are generated from T lymphocytes and phenotypically resemble cytotoxic T lymphocytes. TILs from malignant melanoma exhibit specific cytolytic activity against cells of the tumor from which they were extracted, whereas LAK cells have a broad range of specificity. TILs appear unable to lyse cells of melanomas from patients other than those in whom the tumor originated. TILs may be tagged so that they may be identified later.

tumor necrosis factor α (TNF-α)

A cytotoxic monokine produced by macrophages stimulated with bacterial endotoxin. TNF-α participates in inflammation, wound healing, and remodeling of tissue. TNF-α, which is also called cachectin, can induce septic shock and cachexia. It is a cytokine comprised of 157-amino acid residues. It is produced by numerous types of cells including monocytes, macrophages, T lymphocytes, B lymphocytes, natural killer (NK) cells, and other types stimulated by endotoxins or other microbial products. The genes encoding TNF-α and TNF-β (lymphotoxin) are located on the short arm of chromosome 6 in humans in the major histocompatibility complex (MHC) region. High levels of TNF-α are detectable in the blood circulation very soon following administration of endotoxin or microorganisms. The administration of recombinant TNF-α induces shock, organ failure, and hemorrhagic necrosis of tissues in experimental animals, including rodents, dogs, sheep, and rabbits, closely resembling the effects of lethal endotoxemia. TNF-α is produced during the first 3 days of wound healing. It facilitates leukocyte recruitment, induces angiogenesis, and promotes fibroblast proliferation. It can combine with receptors on selected tumor cells and induce their lysis. TNF mediates the antitumor action of murine natural cytotoxic (NC) cells which distinguishes their functions from those of natural killer (NK) and cytotoxic T cells. TNF-α was termed cachectin because of its ability to induce wasting and anemia when administered on a chronic basis to experimental animals. Thus, it mimics the action in patients with cancer and chronic infection with human immunodeficiency virus

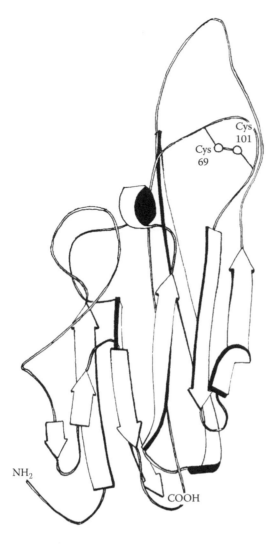

Molecular model of a TNF-α (cachectin) human recombinant form. Resolution = 2.6 Å. The molecule exists as a trimer in which the three subunits are related by approximately threefold symmetry.

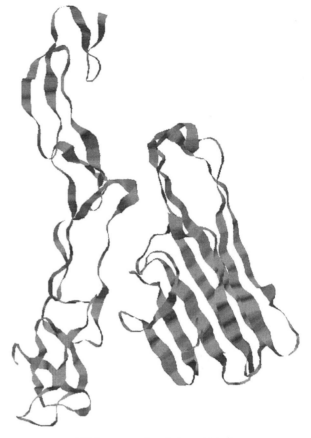

TNF receptors. Resolution = 2.85 Å.

(HIV) or other pathogenic microorganisms. It can induce anorexia that may lead to death from malnutrition. Both TNF-α and TNF-β are cytotoxic for tumor cells but not normal cells. TNF induces vascular endothelial cells to express new adhesion molecules, induces macrophages and endothelial cells to secrete chemokines, and facilitates apoptosis of target cells. Large amounts of TNF produced during severe infections may lead to systemic effects that include fever, synthesis of acute phase proteins by the liver, and cachexia. Very large quantities of TNF may induce intravascular thrombosis and shock. Of all its biological effects, the cytotoxic effects of TNF-α and its induction of apoptosis are the most important. Its specific receptor is tumor necrosis factor receptor (TNFR). TNF has powerful immunoregulatory, cytotoxic, antiviral and procoagulatory properties. It may facilitate cell survival and affects hematopoiesis.

tumor necrosis factor β (TNF-β)
A 25-kDa protein synthesized by activated lymphocytes. It can kill tumor cells in culture, induce expression of genes, stimulate proliferation of fibroblasts, and mimic most of the actions of TNF-α (cachectin). It participates in inflammation and graft rejection and was previously termed lymphotoxin. TNF-β and TNF-α have approximately equivalent affinities for TNF receptors. Both 55- and 80-kDa TNF receptors bind TNF-β. TNF-β has diverse effects that include killing some cells and causing proliferation of others. It is the mediator whereby cytolytic T cells, natural killer cells, lymphokine-activated killer cells, and helper–killer T cells induce fatal injuries to their targets. TNF-β and TNF-α have been suggested to play a role in acquired immune deficiency syndrome (AIDS), possibly contributing to its pathogenesis.

tumor necrosis factor (TNF) family
Tumor necrosis factor (TNF) is responsible for lipopolysaccharide (LPS)-induced hemorrhagic necrosis of tumors in animals. It was subsequently identified as cachectin, a factor responsible for wasting during parasitic infections or neoplasia. TNF cDNA cloning and purification of TNF protein showed that TNF is related structurally to lymphotoxin, a product of activated T lymphocytes called LTα (formerly TNF-β). The TNF designation now refers to what was formerly TNF-α. Both TNF and LTα are synthesized by different cells. They occupy the same receptors and can produce similar biological activities. LTα forms a heterocomplex with LTβ. This complex requires a different receptor (LTβ receptor) and performs biologic functions different from those of LTα alone. TNF and LTα are the first described members of the large TNF family of ligands and receptors that also includes LTβ, the Fas/Apo1 receptor and its ligand, TRAIL/Apo2L and its receptor, CD40, and many others.

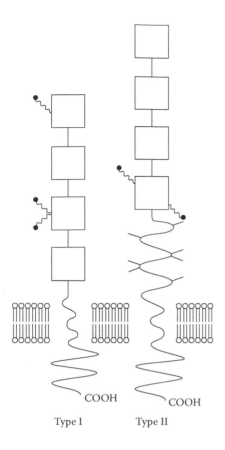

TNF receptors designated type I (CD120a) and type II (CD120b). Both the 55-kDa type I and the 75-kDa type II receptors bind TNF-α and TNF-β (lymphotoxin). These receptors belong to the NGRF/TNFR superfamily. Their extracellular domains contain four cysteine-rich repeats.

tumor necrosis factor (TNF) receptors

A receptor for tumor necrosis factor composed of 461-amino acid residues and an extracellular domain that is rich in cysteine. Cell surface receptors for TNF-α and TNF-β (LTα) are expressed by most cell types. Of the two TNF receptors, TNF-RI mediates most biologic effects of TNF-N (TNF-RII). TNF receptors possess cysteine-rich extracellular motifs that include Fas and CD40. These receptors have essentially no homology in their intracellular domains.

Soluble types I and II have been described in urine and serum. With the exception of erythrocytes and resting T cells, TNF receptors are found on most types of cells. Whereas the type I p55 receptor is widely distributed on various cell types, the type II p75 receptor appears confined to hematopoietic cells. The human p55 receptor contains three potential N-linked glycosylation sites; the type II p75 form contains only two.

tumor promoter

Refer to phorbol esters.

tumor regression

A decrease in size or remission of a malignant tumor as a consequence of anticancer therapy; regression may occur spontaneously without treatment.

tumor rejection antigen

An antigen that is detectable when transplanted tumor cells are rejected; also called tumor transplant antigen.

tumor-specific antigen (TSA)

An antigen present on tumor cells but not found on normal cells. Murine tumor-specific antigens can induce transplantation rejection in mice. Encoded by mutated cellular genes or viral oncogenes.

tumor-specific determinants

Epitopes present on tumor cells and also identifiable in varying quantities and forms on normal cells.

tumor-specific transplantation antigen (TSTA)

Epitopes that induce rejection of tumors transplanted among syngeneic (histocompatible) animals.

tumor suppressor genes

Genes such as *p53* and *PTEN* that encode cellular proteins that prevent cells from becoming neoplastic; their absence promotes carcinogenesis.

TUNEL assay (TdT-dependent dUTP–biotin nick end labeling)

A technique that identifies apoptotic cells *in situ* by fragmentation of their DNA. Immunohistochemical staining with enzyme-linked streptavidin identifies biotin-tagged dUTP added to the free 3′ ends of the DNA fragments by the terminal deoxynucleotidyl transferase (TdT) enzyme.

TUNEL-based assays

DNA fragments can be stained *in situ* by using terminal deoxynucleotidyl transferase (TdT) to polymerize labeled nucleotides onto the ends of nicked DNA (TdT-dependent

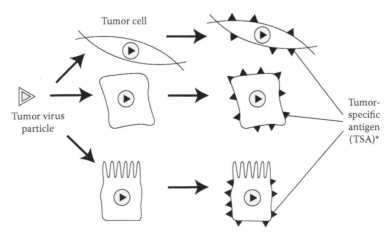

Tumor-specific antigens (TSAS).* Each tumor induced by a single virus will express the same TSA on the cell surface despite the morphology of the cell.

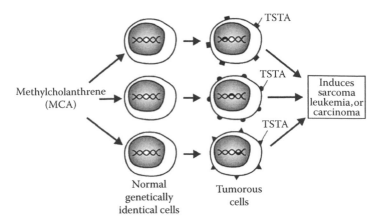

Each genetically identical cell develops unique antigenic specificity to MCA.

Tumor-specific transplantation antigens (TSTAs).

dUTP–biotin nick end labeling, TUNEL). For example, following TdT labeling, biotinylated nucleotides may be detected with a chromogenic or fluorometric-conjugated streptavidin, or brominated nucleotides may be detected with a highly sensitive, biotinylated anti-BrdU antibody and chromogenic-conjugated streptavidin.

tunicates

Tunicates, including the sea-squirt *Amphioxus*, manifest hemopoietic cells that are self-renewing, lymphoid-type cells and a single MHC that governs rejection of foreign grafts.

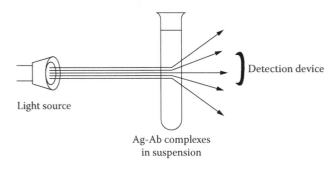

Turbidimetry.

turbidimetry

Quantification of a substance in suspension based on the ability of the suspension to reduce forward light transmission.

Tween®

A nonionic detergent.

Tween 80®

Polyoxyethylene sorbitan monooleate; an emulsifying agent used in cultures of mycobacteria and in water-in-oil-in-water emulsion adjuvants as a stabilizing agent.

twelve/twenty-three rule (12/23 rule)

Immunoglobulin or T cell-receptor gene segments can be joined only if one has a recognition signal sequence with a 12-base-pair spacer and the other has a 23-base-pair spacer. V(D)J recombination takes place only between gene segments whose apposition unites a 12-recognition signal sequence with a 23-recognition signal sequence. RAG recombinases only recognize gene segments with pairing of opposing types of these sequences.

two-dimensional gel electrophoresis

A technique to separate proteins by isoelectric focusing in one dimension, followed by sodium dodecyl sulfate– polyacrylamide gel electrophoresis (SDS-PAGE) on a slab gel at right angles to the first dimension. Large numbers of distinct proteins can be separated and identified by this technique.

two-signal hypothesis

The concept that lymphocyte activation requires two separate signals, the first mediated by antigen and the second by microbial products or constituents of the natural or innate immune response to microorganisms. The first signal mediated by antigen guarantees that the immune response will be specific. The second known as costimulation and induced by microorganisms or innate immune responses ensures that immune responses are induced when required, for example, defending against microorganisms or other offending agents but not against self antigens or harmless components. The second costimulatory signal is frequently mediated by professional antigen-presenting cell membrane molecules including B7 proteins.

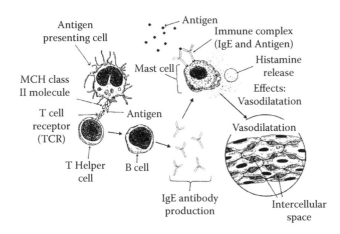

Events that follow degranulation of mast cells in tissues. Vasodilatation of capillaries is followed by changes associated with type I hypersensitivity reactions.

type I anaphylactic hypersensitivity

A hypersensitivity reaction mediated by immunoglobulin E (IgE) antibodies reactive with specific allergens (antigens

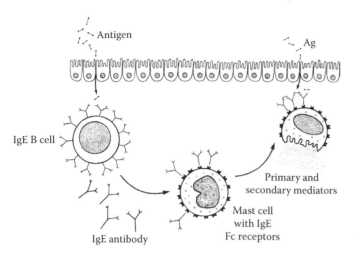

Type I hypersensitivity reaction in which antigen molecules cross link IgE molecules on surfaces of mast cells, resulting in their degranulation and release of primary and secondary mediators of anaphylaxis.

that induce allergy) attached to basophil or mast cell Fcε receptors. Cross linking of the cell-bound IgE antibodies by antigen is followed by mast cell or basophil degranulation and the release of pharmacological mediators including vaso-active amines such as histamine that causes increased vascular permeability, vasodilation, bronchial spasm, and mucous secretion. Secondary mediators of type I hypersensitivity include leukotrienes, prostaglandin D_2, platelet-activating factor, and various cytokines. Systemic anaphylaxis is a serious clinical problem and can follow the injection of protein antigens such as antitoxins or of drugs such as penicillin.

type I cytokine receptors

Cytokine receptors that possess conserved structural motifs in their extracellular domains and bind cytokines that fold into four α-helical strands. They include growth hormone, interleukin-2 (IL2), IL3, IL4, IL5, IL6, IL7, IL9, IL11, IL13, IL15, granulocyte–macrophage colony-stimulating factor (GM-CSF), and G-CSF. Some of these receptors have ligand-binding chains and one or more signal-transducing chains. The same structural motifs are found in all these chains. When bound to their cytokine ligands, type I

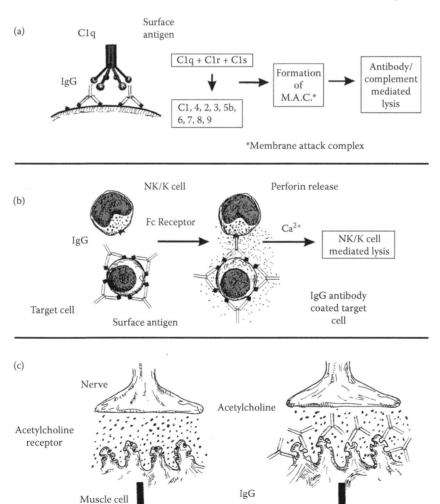

Three forms of type II hypersensitivity.(a) Antibody and complement-mediated lysis of a nucleated cell as a consequence of formation of the membrane attack complex (MAC). (b) Antibody-dependent, cell-mediated cytotoxicity through the action of a natural killer (NK) or killer (K) cell with surface antibody specific for a target cell. (c) Inhibition of transmission of nerve impulses by antibodies against acetylcholine receptors as occurs in myasthenia gravis.

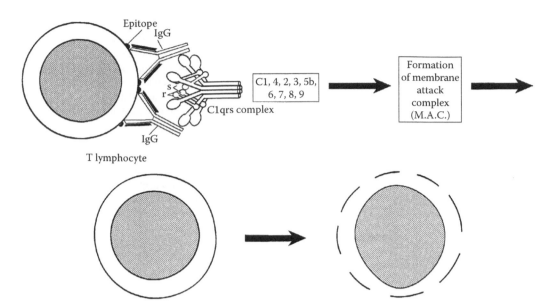

Action of specific IgG antibody on surface epitopes of a T lymphocyte, leading to antibody–complement-mediated lysis of the cell.

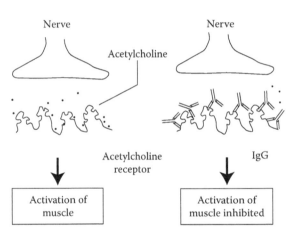

Interference by acetylcholine receptor (AChR) antibodies with chemical transmission of a nerve impulse. AChR antibodies are IgG autoantibodies that cause loss of function of AChRs that are critical to chemical transmission of nerve impulses at neuromuscular junctions. This event represents a type II mechanism of hypersensitivity according to the Coombs and Gell classification. AChRs are heterogeneous; some show specificity for antigenic determinants other than those that serve as acetylcholine or α-bungarotoxin binding sites. As many as 85 to 95% of myasthenia gravis patients may manifest AChR antibodies.

cytokine receptors become dimerized. They signal through JAK–STAT (Janus kinase–signal transducer and activator of transcription) pathways.

type 1 diabetes mellitus (T1DM)

Insulin-dependent diabetes mellitus in which injury to pancreatic β islet cells leads to loss of insulin synthesis associated with autoimmunity. Associated with insulitis and antibodies against pancreatic β islet cell antigens.

type 2 diabetes mellitus (T2DM)

Noninsulin-dependent diabetes mellitus characterized by normal insulin production but failure of host cells to respond to it. Not attributable to autoimmunity.

type I interferons (IFN-α, IFN-β)

Cytokines synthesized by virus-infected cells that inhibit replication of virus by infected cells and alert bystander uninfected cells to arm themselves against infection. A cytokine family of proteins comprised of several of the IFN-α variety that are structurally similar together with a single IFN-β protein. All the type I interferons manifest potent antiviral activity. Mononuclear phagocytes represent the principal source of IFN-α, whereas IFN-β is synthesized by numerous cell types that include fibroblasts. The same cell surface receptor binds both IFN-α and IFN-β, both of which have similar biologic effects. Type I interferons block viral replication, potentiate the lytic activity of natural killer (NK) cells, enhance major histocompatibility complex (MHC) class I expression on virus-infected cells, and induce the development of human Th1 cells.

type II antibody-mediated hypersensitivity

A type of hypersensitivity induced by antibodies and which appears in three forms. The classic type of hypersensitivity involves the interaction of antibody with cell membrane antigens followed by complement lysis. These antibodies are directed against antigens intrinsic to specific target tissues. Antibody-coated cells also have increased susceptibility to phagocytosis. Examples of type II hypersensitivity include the antiglomerular basement membrane antibody that develops in Goodpasture's syndrome and antibodies that develop against erythrocytes in Rh incompatibility, leading to erythroblastosis fetalis or autoimmune hemolytic anemia. A second variety of type II hypersensitivity is antibody-dependent cell-mediated cytotoxicity (ADCC). Natural killer (NK) cells that have Fc receptors on their surfaces may bind to the Fc regions of immunoglobulin G (IgG) molecules. They may react with surface antigens on target cells to produce lysis of the antibody-coated cells. Complement fixation is not required and does not participate in this reaction. In addition to NK cells, neutrophils, eosinophils, and macrophages may participate in ADCC. A third form of type II hypersensitivity involves antibodies against cell surface receptors that interfere with function, as in the case of antibodies against acetylcholine receptors in motor endplates of skeletal muscle in myasthenia gravis. This interference

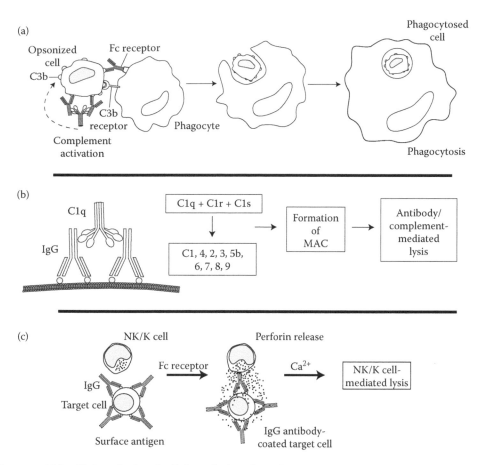

Forms of type II hypersensitivity. (a) Opsonization of cells by antibody and complement components and ingestion by phagocytes. (b) Antibody–complement-mediated lysis of a nucleated cell as a consequence of formation of a membrane attack complex (MAC). (c) Antibody-dependent, cell-mediated cytotoxicity through the action of a natural killer (NK) or killer (K) cell with surface antibody specific for a target cell.

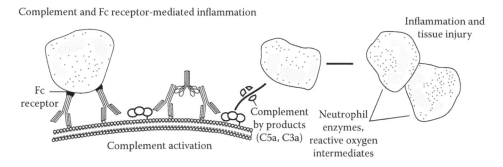

Inflammation induced by antibody binding to Fc receptors of leukocytes and by complement breakdown products.

with neuromuscular transmission results in muscular weakness, ultimately affecting the muscles of respiration and producing death. By contrast, stimulatory antibodies develop in hyperthyroidism (Graves' disease); they react with thyroid-stimulating hormone receptors on thyroid epithelial cells to produce hyperthyroidism.

type II interferon
Synonym for interferon-γ (IFN-γ).

type III immune complex-mediated hypersensitivity
A type of hypersensitivity mediated by antigen–antibody–complement complexes. Antigen–antibody complexes can stimulate an acute inflammatory response that leads to complement activation and polymorphonuclear neutrophil (PMN) leukocyte infiltration. The immune complexes are formed by exogenous antigens such as those from microbes or by endogenous antigens such as DNA, a target for antibodies produced in systemic lupus erythematosus (SLE). Immune complex-mediated injury may be systemic or localized. In the systemic variety, antigen–antibody complexes are produced in the circulation, deposited in the tissues, and initiate inflammation. Acute serum sickness occurred in children treated with diphtheria antitoxin early in the 20th century as a consequence of antibodies produced against horse

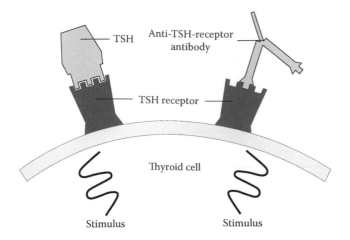

Third form of type II hypersensitivity. Long-acting thyroid stimulator (LATS), an IgG antibody specific for the thyroid-stimulating hormone (TSH) receptor, leads to continuous stimulation of thyroid parenchymal cells, causing hyperthyroidism. The IgG antibody mimics the action of TSH.

Schematic representation of the formation and deposition of immune complexes in vessel walls in type III hypersensitivity

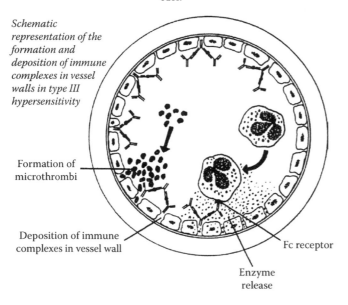

Type III immune complex-mediated hypersensitivity.

serum protein. When immune complexes are deposited in tissues, complement is fixed and PMNs are attracted to the site. Their lysosomal enzymes are released, resulting in tissue injury. Localized immune complex disease, sometimes called the Arthus reaction, is characterized by acute immune complex vasculitis with fibrinoid necrosis in the walls of small vessels.

type IV cell-mediated hypersensitivity

A form of hypersensitivity mediated by specifically sensitized cells. Antibodies participate in type I, II, and III reactions; T lymphocytes mediate type IV hypersensitivity. Two types of reactions mediated by separate T cell subsets are observed. Delayed-type hypersensitivity (DTH) is mediated by CD4$^+$ T cells, and cellular cytotoxicity is mediated principally by CD8$^+$ T cells. A classic delayed hypersensitivity reaction is the tuberculin or Mantoux reaction. Following exposure to *Mycobacterium tuberculosis,* CD4$^+$ lymphocytes recognize the antigens of the microbe complexed with major histocompatibility complex (MHC) class II molecules on the surfaces of antigen-presenting cells that process the mycobacterial antigens. Memory T cells develop and remain in the circulation for prolonged periods. When tuberculin antigen is injected intradermally, sensitized T cells react with the antigen on the surface of the antigen-presenting cell, undergo transformation, and secrete lymphokines that lead to manifestations of hypersensitivity. Unlike antibody-mediated hypersensitivity, lymphokines are not antigen-specific. In T-cell-mediated cytotoxicity, CD8$^+$ T lymphocytes kill antigen-bearing target cells. Cytotoxic T lymphocytes play a significant role in resistance to viral infections. MHC class I molecules present viral antigens to CD8$^+$ T lymphocytes as a viral peptide–class I molecular complex that is transported to the surfaces of infected cells. Cytotoxic CD8$^+$ cells recognize this action and lyse the target before the virus can replicate, thereby stopping the infection.

typhoid vaccination

Refer to TAB vaccine.

typhoid vaccine

Following ingestion, virulent strains of *Salmonella typhi* can penetrate the stomach acid barrier, colonize the intestinal tract, pass through the lumen, and gain access to the lymphatic system and bloodstream to produce disease. *S. typhi*'s ability to induce disease and a protective immune response depends on the presence of a complete lipopolysaccharide in the microorganisms. Two forms of immunizing preparation are currently in use. One is a live attenuated *S. typhi* strain (Ty2la) used as an oral vaccine administered in four doses to adults and children over 6 years of age. It affords protection for 5 years. It is contraindicated in patients taking antimicrobial drugs and patients with acquired immune deficiency syndrome (AIDS). A second type of the vaccine for parenteral use is prepared from the capsular polysaccharide of *S. typhi*. It is administered to

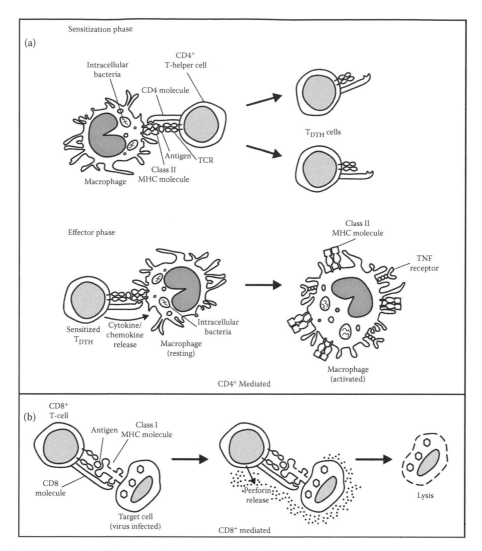

Type IV (cell-mediated) hypersensitivity. (a) Skin tuberculin reactivity mediated by CD4+ helper/inducer T cells represents a form of bacterial allergy. (b) Cytotoxic action of CD8+ T cells against a virus-infected target that presents antigen via class I major histocompatibility complex (MHC) molecules to its T cell receptor (TCR), resulting in the release of perforin and granzyme molecules that lead to target cell lysis. TNF = tumor necrosis factor.

6-month old children and is divided into two doses spaced 4 weeks apart. It is effective 55 to 75% of the time and lasts 3 years.

typhus vaccination

Protective immunization against typhus transmitted by lice or fleas and Rocky Mountain spotted fever by the administration of inactivated vaccines. Rickettsiae prepared in chick embryo yolk sacs or tissues are treated with formaldehyde to render them inactive. Rather than provide protective immunity to prevent the disease, these vaccines condition the host to experience a milder form than occurs in a nonvaccinated host.

typhus vaccine

An immunizing preparation that contains killed rickettsiae microorganisms of a strain or strains of epidemic typhus rickettsiae.

tyrosine kinase

An enzyme that phosphorylates proteins on tyrosine residues. Enzymes of this family play a critical role in T and B cell activation. Lck, Fyn, and ZAP-70 are the principal tyrosine kinases critical for T cell activation. Blk, Fyn, Lyn, and Syk are the main tyrosine kinases critical for B cell activation.

U

U antigen

A rare MNs erythrocyte antigen present in fewer than 1% of African Americans and absent from Caucasian red blood cells. When U antigen is not present, s antigen is not expressed. Membrane sialoglycoprotein and glycophorins A and B are requisite for U antigen expression.

U1 snRNP antibodies

Antibodies against 70-kDa A and C protein constituents of the U1 small nucleoribonuclear proteins (U1 snRNPs). They are commonly found in mixed connective tissue disease (MCTD) or other syndromes related to systemic lupus erythematosus (SLE) but rarely found in SLE. These antibodies were formerly designated as RNP (ribonucleoprotein) or nRNP (nuclear RNP) antibodies.

U1 snRNP autoantibodies

Autoantibodies against protein constituents (70-kDa A and C) of the U1 small nuclear ribonucleoproteins (U1 snRNPs) often found in systemic lupus erythematosus (SLE)–overlap syndromes including mixed connective tissue disease (MCTD) and less often SLE. U1 snRNP autoantibodies were formerly termed RNP (ribonucleoprotein) or nRNP (nuclear RNP) antibodies. Thirty-eight percent of sera that react with protein constituents of U1 snRNPs also interact with the RNA portions of snRNP particles. These U1 RNP antibodies are present only in SLE and SLE–overlap syndromes. Unlike dsDNA antibodies, titers of antibodies against 70-kDa or A constituents of U1 snRNP are not helpful in monitoring disease activity or predicting SLE flares. High-titer RNP antibodies are not linked to an increased risk of fetal loss in SLE. Sm antibody sera do not contain U1 RNA antibodies; 60% of sera with U1 smRNP antibodies have small quantities of Sm antibodies and may be designated anti-RNP/Sm sera. Besides U1 smRNP and Sm antibodies, a less common U1/U2 snRNP antibody reactive with U1-A and U2-B proteins is present in SLE and SLE–overlap syndromes. Specific T lymphocyte and antibody epitopes are present in the 70-kDa protein of U1 snRNP. These epitopes are recognized in MCTD and to a lesser degree in other systemic rheumatic diseases.

U2 snRNP antibodies

Antibodies against small nuclear ribonucleoparticles, composed of U2 snRNA and eight other polypeptides. Anti U2 sera that react with β polypeptides are often present in overlap syndromes with myositis and may be associated with antibodies against U1 snRNP polypeptides (70-kDa A and C). U1 snRNP antibodies that interact with 70-kDa polypeptide were previously designated RNP or nRNP and are principal features of mixed connective tissue disease.

U2 snRNP autoantibodies

Antibodies against U2 snRNP (small nuclear ribonucleoproteins) composed of U2 snRNA and eight associated polypeptides. A′ and B′ are unique to U2 snRNP and six (B′, B, D, E, F, and G) are shared with U1 and other snRNP.

Patients who have overlap syndromes with features of myositis often manifest U2-specific antibodies that react with B′ with or without A′. These patients may also have antibodies against U1 snRNP polypeptide (70-kDa A and C).

ubiquitin

A 7-kDa protein found free in the blood or bound to cytoplasmic, nuclear, or membrane proteins united through isopeptide bonds to numerous lysine residues. Ubiquitin combines with a target protein and marks it for degradation. It is a 76-amino-acid residue polypeptide found in all eukaryotes but not in prokaryotes. Ubiquitin is found in chromosomes covalently linked to histones, although the function is unknown. Ubiquitin is present on the lymphocyte homing receptor gp90Mel-14.

ubiquitin antibodies

Antibodies present in 79% of patients with systemic lupus erythematosus (SLE) that may facilitate the diagnosis of SLE when double-stranded DNA (dsDNA) antibodies are also present. Ubiquitin antibodies may be inversely related to dsDNA antibodies and disease activity. Immunohistochemical staining revealed the presence of intracellular ubiquitinated filamentous inclusions in human chronic neurodegenerative diseases (e.g., in the motor cortex and spine in motor neuron disease and in brain cortical regions in one of the major newly recognized forms of dementia, diffuse Lewy body disease). Ubiquitinated filamentous inclusions have also been observed in some liver and viral diseases (e.g., I hepatocytes in alcoholic liver disease and in Epstein–Barr virus [EBV]-transformed human lymphocytes). Ubiquitin-protein conjugates have been found in the primary (azurophilic) lysosome-related granules in mature polymorphonuclear neutrophils.

ubiquitination

The covalent linkage of several molecules of ubiquitin, a small polypeptide, to a protein. Ubiquitinated protein is marked for proteolytic degradation by proteasomes involved in major histocompatibility complex (MHC) class I antigen processing and presentation.

ubiquitin autoantibodies

Autoantibodies against ubiquitin, a highly conserved protein of 76 amino acids found universally in eukaryotic cells present among antibodies of 29 to 79% of patients with systemic lupus erythematosus (SLE) patients. An inverse correlation is believed to exist between ubiquitin antibodies assicuated with disease activity and dsDNA antibodies. Enzyme immunoassay (EIA) and immunoblotting are the methods of choice to detect ubiquitin autoantibodies. Renal biopsies in 29% of lupus nephritis patients reveal ubiquitin autoantibodies which points to a possible role in lupus nephritis.

UCHL1 anti-human T cell (CD45RO)

A mouse monoclonal antibody that recognizes specifically the 180-kDa isoform of CD45 (leukocyte common antigen). The 180-kDa glycoprotein occurs on most thymocytes and

U

activated T cells but only a proportion of resting T cells. This antibody and antibodies to the high molecular-weight form of CD45 (CD45R) seem to define complementary, largely nonoverlapping populations in resting peripheral T cells demonstrating heterogeneity within the CD4 and CD8 subsets. The antibody labels most thymocytes, a subpopulation of resting T cells within both the CD4 and CD8 subsets, and mature activated T cells. Cells of the myelomonocytic series (e.g., granulocytes and monocytes) are also labeled, whereas most normal B and natural killer (NK) cells are consistently negative. Weak cytoplasmic staining is, however, seen in cases of centroblastic and immunoblastic lymphoma.

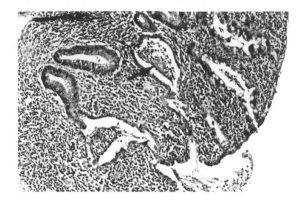

Ulcerative colitis; crypt abscess.

ulcerative colitis (immunologic colitis)

An ulcerative condition that may involve the entire colon but does not significantly affect the small intestine. Neutrophils, plasma cells, and eosinophils infiltrate the colonic mucosa, followed by ulceration of the surface epithelium, loss of goblet cells, and formation of crypt abscess. The etiology is unknown. An immune effector mechanism is believed to maintain chronic disease. Serum immunoglobulins and peripheral blood lymphocyte counts are usually normal. Complexes present in the blood are relatively small and contain IgG, although no antigen has been identified. The complexes may be merely aggregates of immunoglobulin G (IgG). Patients have diarrhea with blood and mucus in stools. The signs and symptoms are intermittent, and the severity of colon lesions varies. Lymphocytes are cytotoxic for colon epithelial cells. Antibodies against *Escherichia coli* may cross react with colonic epithelium; whether such antibodies play a role in etiology and pathogenesis remains to be proven.

ultracentrifugation

The separation of cell components, including organelles and molecules, through high-speed centrifugation reaching 6000 rpm with a gravitational force of up to 500,000 *g*. In differential velocity centrifugation, a stepwise increase in gravitational force removes selected components. Following centrifugation of a cellular homogenate at 600 *g* for 10 minutes to isolate the nuclei, further spinning at 15,000 *g* for 5 minutes permits isolation of mitochondria, lysosomes, and peroxisomes. Respinning at 100,000 *g* for 1 hour permits isolation through sedimentation of the plasma membrane, microsomal fraction, endoplasmic reticulum, and large polyribosomes. Respinning at 300,000 *g* for 2

hours permits sedimentation of ribosomal subunits and small polyribosomes. This leaves the cytosol—the soluble portion of the cytoplasm. Separation can also be achieved by sucrose density gradient ultracentrifugation. Combining cesium chloride with the molecules to be analyzed permits the molecules to migrate to a particular density equivalent. Ultracentrifugation may function as an analytical method for identifying proteins that differ in sedimentation coefficient or as a preparative method to separate proteins based on their densities and shapes.

ultrafiltration

The passage of solutions or suspensions through membranes with minute pores of graded sizes.

umbrella effect

The masking, by relatively large amounts of immunoglobulin G (IgG), of low immunoglobulin light chain concentrations in early IgM macroglobulinemia and IgA myeloma, observed in immunoelectrophoresis. Immunofixation electrophoresis, employing fluorochrome-labeled antibodies, can resolve this masking effect.

undifferentiated connective tissue disease

A prodromal phase of a collagen vascular or connective tissue disease during which the principal clinical manifestations have not yet become apparent.

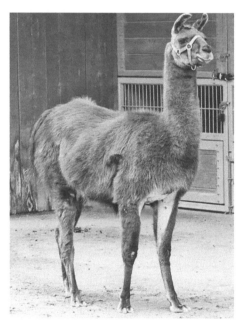

Ungulate immunity.

ungulate immunity

Ungulates develop immune systems similar to those of most other mammalian species. The thymus and bone marrow serve as the sources for generation of T and B cells, respectively. A feature unique to ruminant ungulates is the major role played in primary B cell development by the ileal Peyer's patch, which is a single structure in the terminal ileum. Ruminants have a higher proportion of γδ T cells than other species. Ungulate immunoglobulins consist of IgG$_1$, IgG$_2$, IgM, IgA (serum), IgA (secretory), and IgE isotypes. IgA antibodies predominate on mucosal surfaces; mammary glands produce milk that is different in immunoglobulin content compared to other species. No immunoglobulin transport takes place across the placenta. The colostrum contains very high levels of IgG₁ and very little IgA. The IgA in milk is derived from the plasma. A biliary pump removes IgA from serum for delivery by way of the bowel to the gut lumen. Whereas immunologic tissues are well developed before birth, differentiation of peripheral organs does not occur until antigenic stimulation occurs in extrauterine life. This antigenic stimulation is followed by the development of follicles and germinal centers. Because ungulates do not receive immunoglobulin prenatally from their mothers, they are born agammaglobulinemic. However, large amounts of maternal IgG are concentrated in mammary glands just prior to parturition and are ingested and absorbed intact into the circulation by suckling neonates. In addition to antibodies in the colostrum that are transferred to neonates, cells and other soluble factors in milk are also important in passive protection.

unidentified reading frame (URF)

An open reading frame (ORF) that does not correlate with a defined protein.

unitarian hypothesis

The view that one type of antibody produced in response to an injection of antigen may induce agglutination, complement fixation, precipitation, and lysis based on the type of ligand with which it interacted. This contrasts with the earlier belief that separate antibodies accounted for every type of serological reactivity described above. Usually, more than one class of immunoglobulin may manifest a particular serological reactivity such as precipitation.

univalent

A single binding site.

univalent antibody

An antibody molecule with one antigen-binding site. Although incapable of leading to precipitation or agglutination, univalent antibodies or Fab fragments resulting from papain digestion of an immunoglobulin G (IgG) molecule may block precipitation of antigen by a typical bivalent antibody.

universal donor

A blood group O RhD⁻ individual whose erythrocytes express neither A nor B surface antigens. These red blood cell fail to elicit hemolytic transfusion reactions in recipients with A, B, AB, or O blood groups. However, group O individuals serving as universal donors may express other blood group antigens on their erythrocytes that will induce hemolysis. It is preferable to use type-specific blood for transfusions, except during disasters or emergencies.

universal recipient

An ABO blood group individual whose cells express antigens A and B and serum does not contain anti-A and anti-B antibodies. Thus, red blood cells containing any of the ABO antigens may be transfused to these individuals without inducing a hemolytic transfusion reaction (i.e., from an individual with type A, B, AB, or O). It is best if a universal recipient is Rh⁺ (has the RhD antigen on erythrocytes) to avoid a hemolytic transfusion reaction; however, blood group systems other than ABO may induce hemolytic reactions in universal recipients. Thus, it is best to use type-specific blood for transfusions.

unprimed

Animals or cells that have had no previous contact with a particular antigen.

unproductive rearrangements

DNA rearrangements of T cell receptor and immunoglobulin genes that produce a gene incapable of encoding a functional polypeptide chain.

unresponsiveness

The failure to respond to an immunogenic (antigenic) stimulus. Unresponsiveness may be antigen-specific as in immunological tolerance or nonspecific as a consequence of general suppression of the immune system by whole-body irradiation or immunosuppressive drugs such as cyclosporine.

uromodulin Tamm–Horsfall protein

An 85-kDa α₁ acid glycoprotein produced in Henle's ascending loop and distal convoluted tubules by epithelial cells. It is a powerful immunosuppressive protein based upon N-linked carbohydrate residues. It inhibits proliferation of T cells induced by antigen and monocyte cytotoxicity. Uromodulin is a ligand for interleukin-1α (IL1α), IL1β, and tumor necrosis factor (TNF).

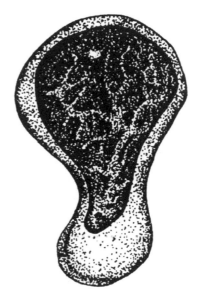

Uropod.

uropod

Lymphocyte cytoplasm extending as an elongated tail or pseudopod in locomotion. A uropod may resemble the handle of a hand mirror. The plasma membrane covers its cytoplasm.

urticaria

Pruritic skin rash identified by localized elevated, edematous, erythematous, and itching wheals with pale centers encircled by red flares. It is due to the release of histamine and other vasoactive substances from mast cell cytoplasmic granules arising from immunologic sensitization or physical or chemical factors. It is a form of type I immediate hypersensitivity mediated by immunoglobulin E (IgE) antibodies in humans. The action of allergen or antigen with IgE antibodies anchored to mast cells may lead to this form of cutaneous anaphylaxis or hives. The wheal is due to leakage of plasma from venules; the flare is caused by neurotransmitters. Also called hives.

urushiols

Catechols of poison (*Rhus toxicodendron*) plants that act as allergens to produce contact hypersensitivity (i.e., contact dermatitis at skin sites touched by urushiol-bearing plants).

U

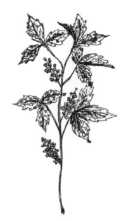

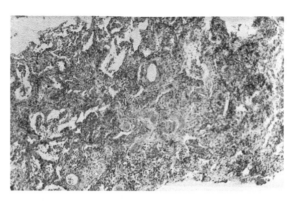

Usual interstitial pneumonitis (UIP). Histopathology reveals fibrosis and inflammation, numerous plasma cells, fibroblasts, histiocytes, and vascular destruction.

Rhus toxicodendron, now commonly called *Toxicodendron radicans*.

The cutaneous lesion is T cell-mediated and classified as type IV hypersensitivity. The four *Rhus* catechols differ according to pentadecyl side-chain saturation and induce type IV delayed hypersensitivity. They are present in such plants as poison oak, poison sumac, and poison ivy.

US28

A member of the G protein-coupled receptor family, the chemokine receptor branch of the rhodopsin family. It is expressed in late phases of lytic infections of leukocytes. Tissue sources include human cytomegalovirus (CMV) DNA and CMV-infected human fibroblasts. Ligands include COS-7 cells transfected with US28-bound ^{125}I-MCP-1 and ^{125}I-RANTES. Also called human CMV G-protein-coupled receptor.

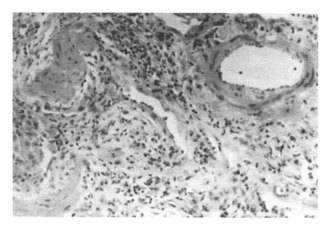

Usual interstitial pneumonitis (UIP).

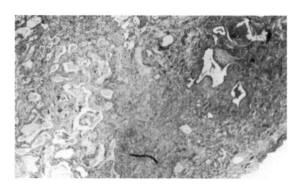

Usual interstitial pneumonitis (UIP). Biopsy reveals idiopathic pulmonary fibrosis. Histopathology reveals a bronchus with chronic lymphocytic infiltrate, interstitial inflammation, fibrosis, and edema. Only a few air spaces are irregularly located.

usual interstitial pneumonia (UIP)

Lung disease associated with interstitial inflammation and fibrosis that lead to progressive insufficiency. It is the most frequent type of idiopathic interstitial pneumonitis and is known by various names including Hamman–Rich syndrome. It is believed to have an immunologic basis, with 20% of the cases associated with collagen vascular diseases such as rheumatoid arthritis, progressive systemic sclerosis, and systemic lupus erythematosus. Autoantibodies include

antinuclear antibodies and rheumatoid factor. Immune complexes may be found in the blood, alveolar walls, and bronchoalveolar lavage fluid, yet the antigen remains unknown. Alveolar macrophages are believed to become activated after phagocytizing immune complexes, possibly followed by the release of cytokines that attract neutrophils that cause injuries of alveolar walls, leading to interstitial fibrosis. Pathological symptoms include chronic inflammation of interstitial spaces and extensive alveolar damage of normal lung parenchyma. Areas of diffuse alveolar damage contain infiltrates of lymphocytes and plasma cells in alveolar walls and hypoplasia of type II pneumocytes. Fibrosis varies from mild to severe, leading even to honeycomb lung in severe cases. The distal acinus shrinks and proximal bronchioles dilate as fibrosis may be accompanied by pulmonary hypertension. UIP may occur over a 5- to 10-year period with development of dyspnea on exertion and dry cough. The disease may follow acute viral infection of the respiratory tract in one third of patients or in rare cases involve acute fulminating interstitial inflammation and fibrosis leading to Hamman–Rich syndrome that may lead to death. Treatment modalities include corticosteroids or cytophosphamide in lung transplantation.

uveitis

Uveal tract inflammation involving the uvea, iris, ciliary body, and choroid of the eye. It may be associated with Behçet's disease, sarcoidosis, and juvenile rheumatoid arthritis.

V

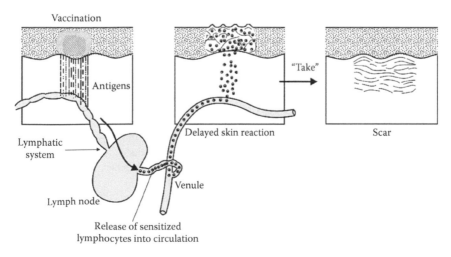 (top right corner: V)

V28

An orphan chemokine receptor expressed in neural and lymphoid tissue and on the THP-1 cell line. The tissue sources are peripheral blood mononuclear cells.

vaccinable

Capable of being vaccinated successfully.

vaccinate

To inoculate with a vaccine to induce immunity against a disease.

vaccination

Immunization against infectious disease through the administration of vaccines that produce active (protective) immunity in humans and other animals. It may be induced with killed, attenuated, or nonpathogenic forms of a pathogenic agent or its antigens to generate protective adaptive immune responses characterized by antigen-specific memory T cells and memory B cells specific for the pathogen. Subsequent exposure to the pathogen will then induce a secondary or anamnestic response.

vaccine

Live attenuated or killed microorganisms, or their parts or products containing antigens, that stimulate a specific immune response consisting of protective antibodies and T cell immunity. A vaccine should stimulate a sufficient number of memory T and B lymphocytes to yield effector T cells and antibody-producing B cells. It should also be able to stimulate high titers of neutralizing antibodies. Injection of a vaccine into a nonimmune subject induces active immunity against the modified pathogen. Other than macromolecular components, a vaccine may consist of a plasmid that contains a cDNA encoding an antigen of a microorganism. Other vaccines include anti-insect vector vaccines, fertility control vaccines, peptide-based preparations, anti-idiotype preparations, and DNA vaccines. No antiparasite vaccine manufactured by conventional technology is in use at present. Vaccines may be prepared from weakened or killed microorganisms, inactivated toxins, toxoids derived from microorganisms, or immunologically active surface markers of microorganisms. They can be administered intramuscularly, subcutaneously, intradermally, orally, or intranasally, as single agents or in combination. An ideal vaccine should be effective, well tolerated, easy and inexpensive to produce, easy to administer, and convenient to store. Vaccine side effects include fever, muscle aches, and injection site pain and are usually mild. Reportable adverse reactions to vaccines include anaphylaxis, shock, seizures, active infection, and death.

vaccine extraimmunization

The administration of excessive or repeated doses of a vaccine to children or adults—usually a consequence of poor recordkeeping.

vaccinia

A cowpox-derived virus known as *Poxvirus officinale* used to induce active immunity against smallpox through vaccination. It differs from cowpox and smallpox viruses in minor antigens.

vaccinia gangrenosa

Chronic progressive vaccinia.

vaccinia immune globulin

Hyperimmune γ globulin used to treat dermal complications of smallpox vaccination such as eczema vaccinatum and progressive vaccinia. It is no longer used because smallpox has been eradicated.

vaccinia virus

Refer to vaccinia.

vaginal mucus agglutination test

An assay for antibodies in bovine vaginal mucus from animals infected with *Campylobacter fetus, Trichomonas fetus,* and *Brucella abortus.* The mucus can be used in the same manner as serum for slide or tube agglutination employing the etiologic microorganisms as antigens.

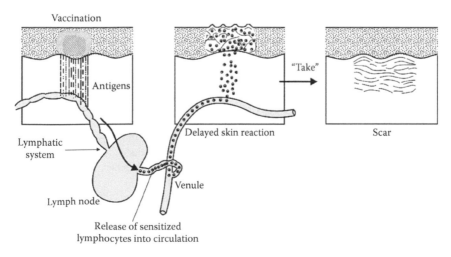

Vaccination against smallpox.

V

valence

The number of antigen-binding sites on an antibody molecule or the number of antibody-binding sites on an antigen molecule. The valence equals the maximum number of antigen molecules that can combine with a single antibody molecule. Antigens are usually multivalent; most antibodies are bivalent. Immunoglobulin M (IgM) has a valence as high as 10. The valence of IgA differs depending on its level of polymerization. Antibodies of the IgG, IgD, and IgE classes have valences of 2. Due to steric hindrance, antibodies usually bind less antigen than would be expected based on valence. Antibody molecules are bivalent or multivalent; T lymphocyte receptors are univalent.

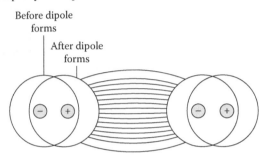

van der Waals forces.

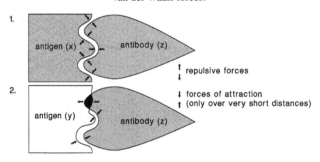

Antibody affinity.

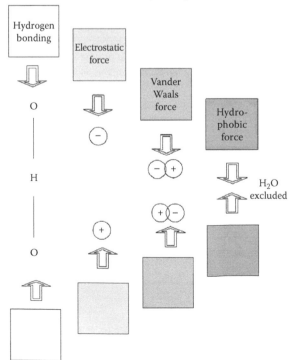

Attractive forces binding antigen to antibody.

van der Waals forces

Weak forces of attraction among atoms, ions, and molecules. It is active only at short distances and varies inversely to the seventh power of the distance between ions or molecules. Thus, van der Waals forces may be important in antigen–antibody binding. A consequence of oscillation of polarities in the outer electron clouds of two nearby atoms, leading to the formation of attractive/repulsive forces between them.

variability plot

Refer to Wu–Kabat plot.

variable (V) domain

An Ig or TCR chain N terminal domain encoded by the corresponding variable (V) exon. The variable domains of Ig heavy and light chains and TCR-α and -β chains characterize the variable regions and antigen-binding sites of Ig and TCR molecules. Paired amino terminal variable domains of Ig and T cell receptor polypeptide chains constitute the antigen-binding site.

variable (V) exon

Gene coding sequence for the variable domain of an Ig or TCR protein. The Igk, Igl, TCR-α and TCR-δ loci V exons are assembled randomly from V and J gene segments, whereas the Igh, TCR-β and TCR-γ are comprised of V, D and J gene segments.

variable (V) gene segment

The immunoglobulin or T cell receptor gene DNA sequence that encodes the V domain's approximately first 95 amino acids. The germline genome contains numerous different V gene segments. To construct a complete exon that encodes a V domain, it is necessary to rearrange one V gene segment to link with a J or a rearranged DJ gene segment.

variable lymphocyte receptors (VLRs)

GPI-anchored cell surface receptors expressed by primitive Agnatha lymphocytes. They undergo somatic variation.

variable (V) region

The part of an immunoglobulin molecule or T cell receptor in the N terminal portion of its constituent polypeptide chains that reveal a high level of amino acid variability and defines antigen recognition. Isoforms with different antigen specificities vary in amino acid sequence. The segment of an immunoglobulin molecule or antibody formed by the variable domain of a light polypeptide (κ or λ) or heavy polypeptide (α, γ, μ, δ, or ε) chain, sometimes called the Fv region, and encoded by the V gene. This region of the molecule is responsible for the specificity of the antigen bound. The antigen-binding variable sequences are present in the extended loop structures or hypervariable segments. Refer also to the variable region (V) of T cell receptor α, β, γ, and δ chains that contain variable amino acid sequences.

variable surface glycoproteins (VSGs)

Surface coat constituents of African trypanosomes. By a process similar to gene conversion, a trypanosome may alter its surface glycoprotein coat by expressing different glycoprotein genes.

varicella

A human herpesvirus type 3 (HHV-3) induced in acute infection, usually occurring in children below 10 years of age. Anorexia, malaise, low fever, and a prodromal rash follow a 2-week incubation. Erythematous and pruritic papules appear in crops and intensify for 3 to 4 days. Complications include viral pneumonia, secondary bacterial infection, myocarditis, thrombocytopenia, glomerulonephritis, and other conditions. HHV-3 may become latent when chicken-pox resolves. Its DNA may become integrated into dorsal route ganglion cells. Varicella may be associated with the onset of herpes zoster or shingles later in life.

varicella (chickenpox) vaccine

An immunizing preparation comprised of attenuated vari-cella virus.

varicella–zoster virus immunity

Varicella–zoster virus (VZV) causes two illnesses: chicken-pox or varicella and shingles or herpes zoster. Chicken-pox is the primary infection, and reactivation of the virus in adulthood causes shingles, a dermatomal exanthem. The immune response to chickenpox includes an IgM response at the end of the incubation period when a vesicular rash appears. Immunofluorescence can be used to detect VZV-specific antibodies reacting with the outer membranes of live VCV-infected cells. The initial antibodies are specific for VCV gB and are followed quickly by antibodies to gH and gE. Chickenpox patients also develop a cellular immune response that reacts with the same viral glycopro-teins recognized by the antibody and a regulatory protein called IE62. Chickenpox patients develop lymphocyte proliferative responses to VZV gE, gI, gB, gH, and IE62 antigens. CD8$^+$ class I-restricted T cells and CD4$^+$ class-II-restricted T cells mediate VZV-specific cytotoxicity. The VZV cellular immune responses control the severity of the chickenpox exanthem in normal individuals. A latent VZV infection develops in most children, in whom the virus remains dormant in the dorsal root ganglia for many years. In senior adult years, the virus may become reacti-vated and induce herpes zoster (shingles) associated with the decreased immunity that accompanies increasing age. In the period prior to the development of zoster, anti-VZV glycoprotein antibody is greatly diminished in serum and cellular immunity is likewise decreased. Cells synthesiz-ing IFN-γ (Th1 cells) diminish more than those producing interleukin-4 (IL4) (Th2 cells). Several weeks after the appearance of herpes zoster, high titers of VZV-specific antibody appear along with increased lymphoproliferative response to VZV antigens. Varicella–zoster immune globu-lin (VZIG) of high titer can prevent chickenpox if injected intermuscularly. It is important to give the globulin within 3 to 4 days after exposure to chickenpox. A live attenuated varicella vaccine is available in the United States, Europe, and Japan. Vaccination is followed by the development of both humoral and cellular immune responses.

variola (smallpox)

Variola major is a *Poxvirus variolae*-induced disease that has been almost eliminated worldwide. This virus-induced disease causes vesicular and pustular skin lesions, leading to disfigurement, and produces viremia and toxemia. In the past, approximately one third of unvaccinated people succumbed to the disease. Variola minor (alastrim) is a mild form of smallpox produced by a different strain that is so weak it cannot induce the formation of pox on the chick chorioallantoic membrane. The term *variola* describes both the smallpox virus and the disease it causes.

variolation (historical)

The intracutaneous inoculation of pus from lesions of smallpox victims into healthy nonimmune subjects to produce smallpox immunity. In China, lesional crusts were ground to a powder and inserted into the nostrils. The procedure protected some individuals, but often caused life-threatening smallpox infections. Jenner's introduction of cowpox vaccination to protect against smallpox rendered variolation obsolete.

vascular addressins

Mucin-like molecules on endothelial cells that bind selected leukocytes to certain anatomical sites. They govern the selective homing of leukocytes to specific locations. The cellular adhesion molecules on high endothelial venules (HEVs) facilitate extravasation of lymphocytes at particular anatomical sites. HEVs of the various lymphoid organs and tissues express different addressins on their surfaces and signal only lymphocytes with appropriate complementary homing receptors.

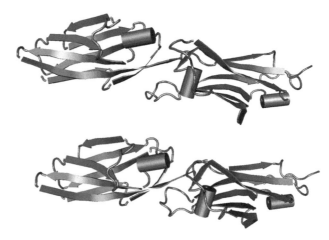

Integrin-binding fragment of VCAM-1.

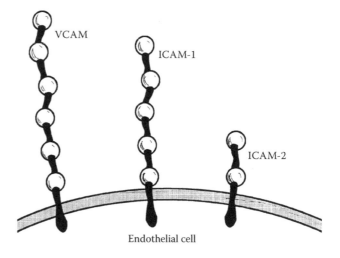

Vascular cell adhesion molecule 1 (VCAM-1).

vascular cell adhesion molecule 1 (VCAM-1)

A molecule that binds lymphocytes and monocytes. It is found on activated endothelial cells, dendritic cells, tissue macrophages, bone marrow fibroblasts, and myoblasts. VCAM-1 belongs to the immunoglobulin gene superfam-ily and is a ligand for VLA-4 (integrin α_4/β_1) and integrin α_4/β_7. It plays an important role in leukocyte recruitment to inflammatory sites; facilitates lymphocyte, eosinophil, and monocyte adhesion to activated endothelium; and participates in lymphocyte–dendritic cell interaction in the immune response.

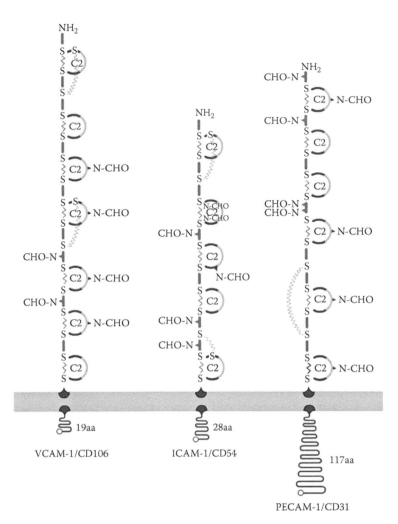

Vascular cell adhesion molecule 1 (VCAM-1).

vascular permeability factors

Substances such as serotonins, histamines, kinins, and leukotrienes that increase spaces between cells of capillaries and small vessels, facilitating losses of protein and cells into the extravascular fluid.

vasculitis

Inflammation of the wall of a blood vessel that may be accompanied by necrosis. Vasculitis with an immunologic basis is often associated with immune complex disease, in which deposition of complement-fixing microprecipitates in the vessel wall may attract polymorphonuclear neutrophils and lead to tissue injury associated with acute inflammation.

vasectomy

Vasectomy causes autoimmunity to spermatozoa antigens in various species including monkeys, guinea pigs, rabbits, and mice. Autoimmune responses to spermatozoa in vasectomized men led to concerns about the safety of the procedure. Cohort investigations of vasectomized men established vasectomy as a safe contraceptive procedure even though the mechanisms of vasectomy-induced autoimmunity remain elusive. Animal studies have revealed that autosensitization to spermatozoal autoantigens can occur without the use of adjuvants or other agents or processes designated as "dangerous" agents.

vasoactive amines

Amino group-containing substances that include histamine and serotonin (5-hydroxytryptamine) induce vasodilation of the peripheral vasculature and increase the permeability of capillaries and small vessels. This promotes the influx of inflammatory leukocytes into tissues.

vasoactive intestinal peptide (VIP)

A 28-residue neuropeptide member of the secretin–glycogen group of molecules found in nerve fibers of blood vessels, smooth muscles, and upper respiratory tract glands. It activates adenylate cyclase and produces vasodilatation and increases cardiac output, glycogenolysis, and bronchodilation while preventing release of macromolecules from mucus-secreting glands. VIP may be increased in pancreatic islet G cell tumors. A deficiency of VIP aggravates bronchial asthma; asthmatic patients usually do not have VIP.

vasoconstriction

Diminished blood flow as a consequence of contraction of precapillary arterioles.

vasodilatation

Increased blood flow through capillaries as a consequence of precapillary arteriolar dilatation.

Vaughn, Victor Clarence

A professor at the University of Michigan who championed the cause of laboratory researchers as vital to the interdisciplinary goals of the American Association of Immunologists.

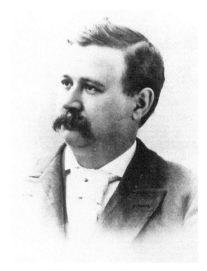

Victor Clarence Vaughn.

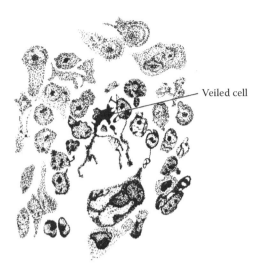

Veiled cell.

V(D)J recombinase

Enzymes required to recombine VDJ segments. An enzyme that can identify and splice the V (variable), J (joining), and in some cases D (diversity) gene segments that confer antibody diversity. This collection of enzymes makes possible the somatic recombination events that produce functional antigen receptor genes in developing T and B lymphocytes. Some, including recombination-activating genes (RAG)-1 and RAG-2, are present only in developing lymphocytes; others are ubiquitous DNA repair enzymes.

V(D)J recombination

The formation of unique variable (V) exons by site-specific recombination at the DNA level of pre-existing Ig and TCR loci of V,D, and J gene segments. Accomplished by the recognition, cutting and rejoining of heptamer–nonamer recombination signal sequences (RSSs) that flank these gene segments. When three segments are involved, the D and J gene segments are linked first, followed by the joining of V to the DJ unit.

V(D)J recombination class switching

A mechanism to generate multiple-binding specificities by developing lymphocytes through exon recombination from a conservative number of gene segments known as variable (V), joining (J), and diversity (D) at seven different loci that include μ, κ, and λ for B cell immunoglobulin genes and α, β, γ, and δ genes for T cell receptors.

VDRL (Venereal Disease Research Laboratory) test

Reaginic screening for syphilis. VDRL antigen is combined with a patient's heat-inactivated serum and the combination is observed for flocculation by light microscopy after 4 minutes. Reaginic assays are helpful to screen for early syphilis and are usually positive in secondary syphilis, although the results are more variable in tertiary syphilis. VDRL is negative in approximately half of the neurosyphilis cases. Reaginic tests for syphilis may be biologically false positive in cases of malaria, lupus erythematosus, and acute infections. Biologic false-positive VDRL tests may also be seen in some cases of hepatitis, infectious mononucleosis, rheumatoid arthritis, and even pregnancy.

V domain

Refer to variable region.

V gene segment

Refer to variable (V) gene segment.

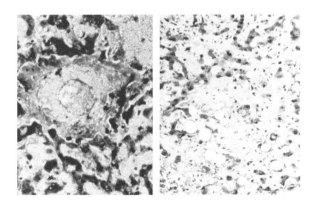

Venoocclusive disease (VOD) accompanying graft-vs.-host disease of the liver. Left: Early VOD showing concentric subendothelial widening and sublobular central venules with degeneration of surrounding pericentral hepatocytes. No depositions of fibrin and factor VIII are apparent. Right: Late lesion of VOD showing fibrous obliteration of central venules and sinusoids by combination of types 3, 1, and even type 4 collagens.

vector

A DNA segment employed for cloning a foreign DNA fragment. A vector should be able to reproduce autonomously in a host cell, possess one or more selectable markers, and have sites for restriction endonucleases in nonessential regions that permit DNA insertion into the vector or replacement of a segment of the vector. Plasmids and bacteriophages may serve as cloning vectors.

veiled cell

A mononuclear phagocytic cell that serves as an antigen-presenting cell. It is found in the afferent lymphatics and marginal sinuses. It may manifest interleukin-2 (IL2) receptors in the presence of granulocyte–macrophage colony-stimulating factor (GM-CSF).

veno-occlusive disease (VOD)

Serious liver complication after marrow transplantation. Histopathology of early VOD reveals concentric subendothelial widening and sublobular central venules with degeneration of surrounding pericentral hepacytes along with depositions of fibrin and factor VIII. Late lesions show fibrous obliteration of central venules and sinusoids by combinations of type 3, 1, and even type 4 collagen. The clinical diagnosis is reasonably accurate based on the combination of jaundice, ascites, hepatomegaly, and encephalopathy in

V

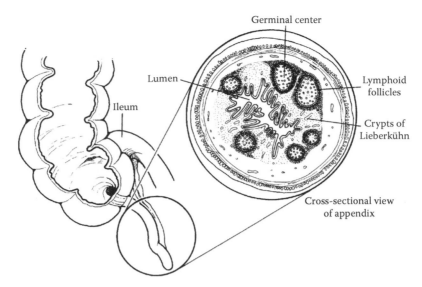

Vermiform appendix.

the first 2 weeks after the transplant. The incidence may be higher among older patients with diagnoses of acute myelogenous leukemia (AML) or chronic myelogenous leukemia (CML) and hepatitis. The mortality rate of VOD is relatively high at 32%.

venom

A poisonous substance produced by selected species such as snakes, arthropods, and bees. The poison is transmitted by bite or sting. At least 100 species of fish inject venoms that are hazardous to humans including sharks, rays, catfish, weever fish, scorpion fish, and stargazers.

vermiform appendix

A lymphoid organ situated at the ileocecal junction of the gastrointestinal tract.

very late activation antigens (VLA molecules)

β_1 integrins that have the CD19 β chain in common. They were originally described on T lymphocytes grown in long-term culture and subsequently found on additional types of leukocytes and on cells other than blood cells. VLA proteins facilitate leukocyte adherence to vascular endothelium and extracellular matrix. Resting T lymphocytes express VLA-4, VLA-5, and VLA-6. VLA-4 is expressed on multiple cells that include thymocytes, lymphocytes in blood, B and T cell lines, monocytes, natural killer (NK) cells, and eosinophils. The extracellular matrix ligand for VLA-4 and VLA-5 is fibronectin, and for VLA-6 it is laminin. The binding of these molecules to their ligands gives T lymphocytes costimulator signals. VLA-5 is present on monocytes, memory T lymphocytes, platelets, and fibroblasts. It facilitates B and T cell binding to fibronectin. VLA-6, found on platelets, T cells, thymocytes, and monocytes, mediates platelet adhesion to laminin. VLA-3 is a laminin receptor, binds collagen, and identifies fibronectin. It is present on B cells, the thyroid, and the renal glomeruli. Platelet VLA-2 binds to collagen only. Endothelial cell VLA-2 combines with collagen and laminin. Lymphocytes bind through VLA-4 to high endothelial venules and endothelial cell surface proteins (VCAM-1) in areas of inflammation. VLA-1 present on activated T cells, monocytes, melanoma cells, and smooth muscle cells binds collagen and laminin.

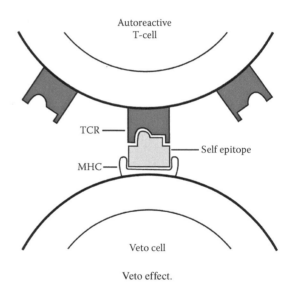

Veto effect.

vesiculation

Development of minute intraepidermal fluid-filled spaces, i.e., vesicles seen in contact dermatitis.

veto cells

A proposed population of cells suggested to facilitate maintenance of self tolerance through veto of autoimmune responses by T cells. A veto cell would neutralize the function of an autoreactive T lymphocyte. A T cell identifies itself as an autoreactive lymphocyte by recognizing the surface antigen on the veto cell. No special receptors with specificity for the autoreactive T lymphocyte are required for the veto cell to render the T lymphocyte nonfunctional. Contemporary research suggests the existence of a veto cell that can eliminate cytotoxic T lymphocyte (CTL) precursors reactive against allogeneic major histocompatibility complex (MHC) class I molecules or antigens presented in association with self MHC class I molecules.

V gene

Gene encoding the variable region of immunoglobulin light or heavy chains. Although it is not in proximity to the

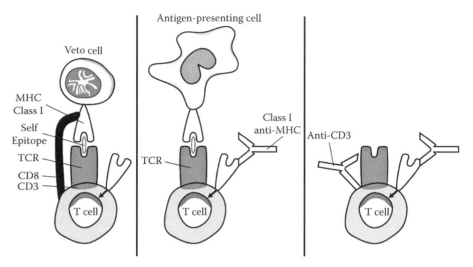

The three mechanisms of the veto effect.

C gene in germline DNA, in lymphocyte and plasma cell DNA the V gene lies near the 5′ end of the C gene from which it is separated by a single intron.

V gene segment

DNA segment encoding the first 95 to 100 amino acid residues of immunoglobulin and T cell polypeptide chain variable regions. The two coding regions in the segment are separated by a 100- to 400-bp intron. The first 5′ coding region is an exon that codes for a brief untranslated mRNA region and the first 15 to 18 signal peptide residues. The second 3′ coding region is part of an exon that codes for terminal 4 signal peptide residues and 95 to 100 variable region residues. A J gene segment encodes the rest of the variable region. A D gene segment is involved in encoding immunoglobulin heavy chain and T cell receptor β and δ chains.

V$_H$ region

The variable region of immunoglobulin heavy chain; that part of a variable region encoded for by the *VH* gene segment.

viability techniques

Methods employed to determine the viability of cells maintained *in vitro*. Of the many dyes used for viability assays, anionic Trypan blue is the most frequently employed. For example, the viability of leukocytes suspended in balanced salt solution is evaluated based on their ability to exclude Trypan blue from cell interiors. Leukocytes are counted in a hemacytometer and the percentage of viability is calculated by dividing the number of unstained viable cells by the number of all cells counted (stained and unstained).

Vi antigen

A virulence antigen linked to *Salmonella* microorganisms. It is found in the capsule and interferes with serological typing of the O antigen, a heat-stable lipopolysaccharide of enterobacteriaceae.

Vibrio cholerae immunity

Vibrio cholerae induces disease by production of virulence factors and toxins. Protective antigens have been identified

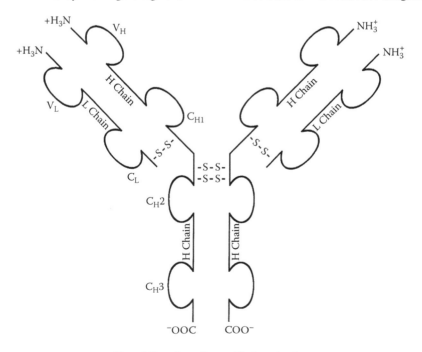

V$_H$ and V$_I$ regions of an antibody molecule.

and vaccine development is progressing. Mucosal immunity is mediated by secretory IgA antibodies necessary for protection. *V. cholerae* is noninvasive, thus antibodies block adherence and inhibit colonization. They neutralize the toxin or inhibit binding to specific receptors. The intestinal immune response begins in lymphoid follicles where mononuclear cells are responsible for phagocytic uptake of antigen from the intestine. Live microorganisms are more effective immunogens than killed ones. An initial infection with cholera yields long-lasting immunity. The most important protective agent is the O antigen of lipopolysaccharide (LPS). Antibodies to TCP are protective but are biotype-restricted as a consequence of biotype-specific antigenic variation in the major structural subunit. The other protective antigen is the B subunit of CT. The major epidemic strain now appears to be 0139, which increases the significance of anti-LPS immunity; this new strain has the virulence of the original 01 El Tor strains. Immunity against non-LPS antigens is far less important than to a specific LPS type. Non-LPS antigens are less immunogenic than the LPS antigen.

Videx®

A synthetic purine nucleoside analogue approved by the FDA to treat human immunodeficiency virus (HIV). The mechanism of action includes the activation of didanosine to dideoxyadenosine 5′-triphosphate, which inhibits the activity of HIV-1 reverse transcriptase by competing with the natural substrate and by incorporation into viral DNA. Didanosine is the active component.

Vif (HIV)

A protein of human immunodeficiency virus that stabilizes recently synthesized HIV DNA and aids its passage to the nucleus. It inhibits CEM-15 packaging into virions.

vimentin

A 55-kDa intermediate filament protein synthesized by mesenchyma cells such as vascular endothelial cells, smooth muscle cells, histiocytes, lymphocytes, fibroblasts, melanocytes, osteocytes, chondrocytes, astrocytes, and occasional ependymal and glomerular cells. Malignant cells may express more than one intermediate filament. For example, immunoperoxidase staining may reveal vimentin and cytokeratin in breast, lung, kidney, or endometrial adenocarcinomas.

vinblastine

A chemotherapeutic alkaloid that leads to lysis of rapidly dividing cells by disruption of mitotic spindle microtubules. It is used to treat leukemia, Hodgkin disease, lymphoproliferative disorders, and malignancies.

vincristine

A chemotherapeutic alkaloid that lyses proliferating cells via disruption of mitotic spindles. It is used to treat leukemia and other malignancies.

vinyl chloride (VC)

A synthetic resin that represents a toxin of immunologic significance in occupational exposure. It is associated with mixed connective tissue disease. Autoantibodies are formed against ribonucleoproteins (RPs). Human leukocyte antigen (HLA) disease association studies have implicated HLA-DR5 of haplotype A1B8 and HLA-DR3 with these syndromes. Oxidized metabolites of VC are highly reactive and bind to sulfhydryl groups, amino radicals, and nucleotides. VC can induce oxidative cell injury and may

enhance the immunogenicity of self molecules. Oxidizing agents may inactivate T suppressor cells. Cell surface thiols influence the activities of lymphocytes. The reduction of disulfide bridges to thiols is linked to increased cellular activity. By contrast, thiol oxidation to disulfides decreases cell responsiveness. CD8+ T cells are more sensitive to thiol blockers and oxidants than CD4+ T cells. Exposure to VC, mercury, iodides, and toxic oils may pose interactions with cellular thiols, leading to preferential inactivation of CD8+ T suppressor cells.

Viracept®

An inhibitor of the human immunodeficiency virus 1 (HIV-1) protease that prevents cleavage of the *gag–pol* polyprotein, resulting in the production of noninfectious virus. The FDA has approved it for the treatment of HIV. Nelfinavir mesylate is the active component.

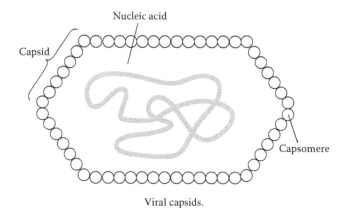

Viral capsids.

viral capsids

Envelope antigens that inhibit adherence and invasion of host cells. Antibodies may also act as opsonins that increase the attractiveness of viral particles to phagocytic cells. Secretory IgA antibody is important in neutralizing viruses on mucosal surfaces. Complement also facilitates phagocytosis and may be significant in viral lysis.

viral hemagglutination

Selected viruses may combine with specific receptors on surfaces of red cells from various species to produce hemagglutination. The ability of antiviral antibodies to inhibit this reaction constitutes hemagglutination inhibition, which serves as an assay to quantify the antibodies. One must be certain that inhibition is due to the antibody and not to nonspecific agents such as mucoproteins with myxoviruses or lipoproteins with arborviruses. Blood sera to be assayed by this technique must have the inhibitor activity removed by treatment with neuraminidase or acetone extraction, depending on the chemical nature of the inhibitor. The attachment of virus particles to cells is termed hemadsorption. Among viruses causing hemagglutination are those that induce influenza and parainfluenza, mumps, Newcastle disease, smallpox and vaccinia, measles, St. Louis encephalitis, western equine encephalitis, Japanese B encephalitis, Venezuelan equine encephalitis, West Nile fever, dengue viruses, respiratory syncytial virus, and some enteroviruses. Herpes simplex virus can be absorbed to tanned sheep red cells and hemagglutinated in the presence of specific antiserum against the virus. This method is termed indirect virus hemagglutination.

viral immunity

Congenital immunodeficiency patients have demonstrated the relative significance of various constituents of the immune system. Subjects with isolated defects of cell-mediated immunity contract severe and often fatal viral infections that include measles and chickenpox. By contrast, individuals with isolated immunoglobulin deficiencies usually recover normally from most viral infections except enteroviruses that may lead to chronic infection of the central nervous system. Certain generalizations may be reached concerning viral immunity: antibodies act mainly by neutralizing virions, rendering them noninfectious. By contrast, cell-mediated immunity is against virus antigens present in infected cells. Antibody prevents primary infection and reinfection through neutralization of viruses on mucosal surfaces and limiting their spread in body fluids; cell-mediated immunity eliminates intracellular infection and limits reactivation of persistent viruses. The immune system may be considered in three phases: immediate (<4 hours), early (4 to 96 hours), and late (>96 hours). It may also be divided into humoral and cell-mediated components that include both specific and nonspecific mechanisms.

viral interference

Resistance of cells infected with one virus to infection by a second virus.

Viramune®

A non-nucleoside reverse transcriptase inhibitor approved by the FDA to treat human immunodeficiency virus (HIV). Nevirapine, the active component, binds directly to reverse transcriptase and blocks the RNA- and DNA-dependent polymerase activities by causing disruption of the catalytic site of the enzyme. Nevirapine has no inhibitory effect on HIV-2 reverse transcriptase.

virgin B cells

Virgin B cells have never interacted with antigen and must have two separate types of signals to proliferate and differentiate. The antigen provides the first signal through interaction with surface membrane immunoglobulin (Ig) molecules on specific B lymphocytes. Helper T cells and their lymphokines provide the required second type of signal. Polysaccharides and lipids, as nonprotein antigens, induce IgM antibody responses without antigen-specific T-cell help, while protein antigens that are helper T cell-dependent lead to the production of immunoglobulin of more than one isotype and of high affinity in addition to immunologic memory.

virion

Complete virus particle.

viroid

A 100-kDa, 300-bp subviral infectious RNA particle composed of a circular single-stranded RNA segment that induces disease in certain plants. Viroids may be escaped introns.

viropathic

Host tissue injury resulting from infection by a pathogenic virus.

virosome

A vaccine comprised of a spherical artificial virus employed to direct vaccine antigens directly into a host cell. It consists of a liposome containing the vaccine antigen and hemagglutinin and neuraminidase proteins of influenza. It has membrane fusion properties, conformational stability, and ability to invade host cells of the native virus. The antigen is present in the virosome lumen or chemically cross linked to its surface.

virulence

The pathogenicity of a microorganism to invade host tissues as indicated by the severity of the disease it causes.

virulence genes

Genes that govern the expression of multiple other genes with changing environmental conditions such as temperature, pH, osmolarity, etc. An example is the *toxR* gene of *Vibrio cholerae* that coordinates 14 other genes of this microorganism.

virus

An infectious agent that ranges from 10^6 D for the smallest viruses to 200×10^6 for larger ones such as the pox viruses. Viruses contain single- or double-stranded DNA or RNA that may be circular or open and linear. The nucleic acid is enclosed by a protein coat (capsid) composed of a few characteristic proteins. Most viruses are helical or icosahedral and may include a lipid envelope containing viral proteins. Viruses may be incubated with cells in culture, where they produce characteristic cytopathic effects. Inclusion bodies may be produced in cells infected by viruses, which infect host cells through specific receptors. Examples of this specificity include cytomegalovirus linking to β_2 microglobulin, Epstein–Barr virus (EBV) linking to C3d receptor (CR2), and HIV-1 binding to CD4. These submicroscopic acellular pathogens are composed of either a DNA or RNA nucleic acid genome enclosed in a protein coat. To replicate, the virus must invade a host cell and use its protein synthesis machinery that a virus lacks but is required for independent life. Also called a virion.

virus-associated hemophagocytic syndrome

An aggressive hemophagocytic state occurring in both immunocompromised and nonimmunocompromised individuals, usually those with herpetic infections such as cytomegalovirus (CMV), Epstein–Barr virus (EBV), and herpesvirus. It may also occur in adenovirus and rubella infections, brucellosis, candidiasis, leishmaniasis, tuberculosis, and salmonellosis. Lymphadenopathy, hepatosplenomegaly, pulmonary infiltration, skin rash, and pancytopenia are present. The disease is sometimes confused with malignant histiocytosis, lymphoma, sinus histiocytosis, and lymphomatoid granulomatosis.

virus neutralization test

A test based on the ability of a specific antibody to neutralize virus infectivity. It may be employed to measure the titer of antiviral antibody. It may be performed *in vivo* using susceptible animals or chick embryos or *in vitro* in tissue culture.

virus neutralizing capacity

The ability of serum to prevent virus infectivity. Neutralizing antibody is usually of the IgM, IgG, or IgA class.

viscosity

The physical consistency of a fluid such as serum based on the size, shape, and conformation of its molecules. Molecular charge, sensitivity to temperature, and hydrostatic state affect viscosity.

vitamin A

Vitamin A may serve as an adjuvant to elevate antibody responses to soluble protein antigens in mice. The adjuvant effect is produced whether administered orally or parenterally.

vitamin A and immunity

A deficiency of vitamin A compromises acquired, adaptive, antigen-specific immunity. The deficiency has been linked

V

to atrophy of thymus, spleen, lymph nodes, and Peyer's patches, pointing to major alterations of immune effector cell mechanisms. Vitamin A deficiency is also associated with impaired ability to form antibody responses to T cell-dependent antigens such as tetanus toxoid, proteins, and viral infections. It is also linked to decreased antibody responsiveness to T cell-independent antigens such as pneumococcal and meningococcal polysaccharides. Vitamin A deficiency also compromises natural innate immunity because it is necessary for maintenance of mucosal surfaces, the first line of defense against infection. Immune effector cells that mediate nonspecific immunity include polymorphonuclear cells, macrophages, and natural killer (NK) cells. Neutrophil phagocytosis is diminished by vitamin A deficiency, and viral infections are more severe because of diminished cytolytic activity by NK cells.

vitamin B and immunity

B complex vitamins differ greatly in chemical structures and biological actions. Vitamin B_6 deficiency induces marked changes in immune function, especially in the thymus. Thymic hormone activity is diminished and lymphopenia occurs. Vitamin B_6 deficiency suppresses delayed cutaneous hypersensitivity responses, primary and secondary T cell mediator cytotoxicity, and skin graft rejection. It also impairs humoral immunity and the number of circulating lymphocytes is decreased. Folate and vitamin B_{12} deficiencies are linked to diminished host resistance and impaired lymphocyte function. Pantothenic acid deficiency suppresses humoral antibody responses to antigens. Thiamin, biotin, and riboflavin deficiencies induce moderate interference with immune function. Riboflavin deficiency diminishes humoral antibody formation in response to antigen. Intake of micronutrients, including B complex vitamins at doses two to three times higher than the U.S. recommended daily allowance (RDA) help maintain optimal immune function in healthy elderly adults.

vitamin C and immunity

Ascorbic acid (vitamin C) is necessary for proper functioning of cells, tissues, and organs. It is an antioxidant and a cofactor in many hydroxylating reactions. The immune system is sensitive to levels of vitamin C intake. Leukocytes have high concentrations of ascorbate that are used rapidly during infection and phagocytosis, indicating the role of vitamin C in immunity. Vitamin C facilitates neutrophil chemotaxis and migration, induces interferon synthesis, maintains mucus membrane integrity, and plays a role in the expression of delayed-type hypersensitivity. High-dose vitamin C supplementation is believed to increase T and B lymphocyte proliferation. It diminishes nonspecific extracellular free radical injury and autotoxicity after the oxidative burst activity of stimulated neutrophils. It further enhances immune function indirectly by maintaining optimal levels of vitamin E.

vitamin D and immunity

Calcitriol, the hormonal form of vitamin D, plays a significant regulatory role in cell differentiation and proliferation of the immune system. It mediates its action through specific intracellular vitamin D_3 receptors (VDRs). Among the numerous effects of calcitriol on the immune system are the inhibition of cytokine release from monocytes, prolongation of skin allograft survival in mice, inhibition of autoimmune encephalomyelitis and thyroiditis in mice, potentiation of murine primary immune responses, restoration of defective macrophage and lymphocyte functions in vitamin D-deficient patients with rickets, restoration of lymphocyte proliferation, and interleukin-2 (IL2) synthesis in human dialysis patients, among many others.

vitamin E and immunity

Vitamin E is required by the immune system. It is a major antioxidant that protects cell membranes from free radical attack and is effective in preventing biological injury by immunoenhancement. Vitamin E in high doses diminishes $CD8^+$ T cells and increases the $CD4^+$ to $CD8^+$ T cell ratio; increases total lymphocyte count; and stimulates cytotoxic natural killer (NK) cells, phagocytosis by macrophages, and mitogen responsiveness. Its immunostimulatory action renders it useful for therapeutic enhancement of immune responses. The effect of vitamin E on the immune system depends on its interaction with other antioxidant and preoxidant nutrients, polyunsaturated fatty acids, and other factors that affect immune response, including age and stress. Vitamin E stimulation of immunity is particularly important in the elderly because infectious disease and tumor incidence increase with age. Vitamin E facilitates host defense by inhibiting increases in tissue prostaglandin synthesis from arachidonic acid during infection. *In vitro*, vitamin E has been shown to stimulate interleukin-2 (IL2) and interferon γ (IFN-γ) by mitogen-stimulated lymphocytes. Vitamin E prevents lipid peroxidation of cell membranes which may be a mechanism to enhance immune responses and phagocytosis.

vitiligo

Loss of skin or hair pigmentation as a consequence of autoantibodies against melanocytes. The Smyth chicken is a partially inbred line that exhibits a post-hatching depigmentation of feathers as a consequence of an autoimmune process; 95% of the depigmented chicks have detectable autoantibodies several weeks prior to the appearance of depigmentation. The autoantigen is a tyrosinase-related protein. Smyth chicken amelanosis and human vitiligo are similar in that their onset is in early adulthood and is often associated with other autoimmune diseases, especially those of the thyroid gland. Vitiligo may also result from a polygenic disorder or sporadically. It is a syndrome marked by acquired loss of pigmentation in a usually symmetrical but spotty distribution, usually involving the central face and lips, genitalia, hands, and extremities. Skin pigmentation is produced by melanin, which is present in melanosomes that are transferred to keratinocytes to protect the skin against light. The two stages in the production of vitiligo may be sequential. Type I vitiligo is marked by decreased melanocyte tyrosinase activity, and type II vitiligo is characterized by destruction of melanocytes. Melanocytes and keratinocytes in the borders of vitiligo lesions exhibit increased intercellular adhesion molecule 1 (ICAM-1) expression.

vitronectin

A 65-kDA cell adhesion glycoprotein found in serum at a concentration of 20 mg/L. It combines with coagulation and fibrinolytic proteins and with C5b67 complex to block its insertion into lipid membranes. Vitronectin appears in basement membranes along with fibronectin in proliferative vitreoretinopathy. It decreases nonselective lysis of autologous

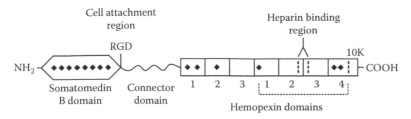

Vitronectin.

◆ = Cysteine residues

cells by insertion of soluble C5b67 complexes from other cell surfaces. Also called epibolin and protein S.

V(J) recombination

Class switching.

Vκ

The variable region of an immunoglobulin κ light chain. This symbol may be used to signify the part of a variable region encoded by the *Vκ* gene segment.

Vλ

The variable region of an immunoglobulin λ light chain. The symbol may designate the part of a variable region encoded by the *Vλ* gene segment.

VLA-4

An integrin molecule found on T lymphocyte surfaces that binds to mucosal cell adhesion molecules.

VLA receptors

A family of integrin receptors found on cell surfaces. They consist of α and β transmembrane chain heterodimers. VLA-binding sites are located at the Arg–Gly–Asp sequences of vitronectin and fibronectin. VLA receptors occur principally on T lymphocytes. They also bind laminin and collagen and participate in cell–extracellular matrix interactions.

VLIA (virus-like infectious agent)

A mycoplasma, possibly synergistic with HIV-1, leading to profound immunodeficiency, named *Mycoplasma incognitos*.

V$_L$ region

The variable region of an immunoglobulin light chain. The symbol may be used to designate the segment encoded by the *VL* gene.

v-*myb* oncogene

A genetic component of an acute transforming retrovirus that leads to avian myeloblastosis. It represents a truncated genetic form of c-*myb*.

Vogt–Koyanagi–Harada (VKH) syndrome

Uveal inflammation with acute iridocyclitis, choroiditis, and retinal detachment. Initial manifestations include headache, dysacusis, and sometimes vertigo. Scalp hair may show patchy loss or whitening. Vitiligo and poliosis occur often. The development of delayed-type hypersensitivity to melanin-containing tissue has been postulated. Apparently, pigmented constituents of the eye, hair, and skin are altered by some type of insult in a manner that leads to a delayed-type hypersensitivity response. Possible autoantigens are soluble substances from the retinal photoreceptor layer. Uveal tissue extracts have been used in delayed-hypersensitivity skin tests. Antibodies to uveal antigens may be present, but they are not specific for VKH. Hereditary factors play a predisposing role. Asians have a predisposition to VKH, a common cause of uveitis in Japan. VKH syndrome is closely

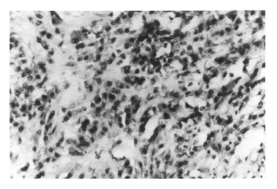

Hematoxylin and eosin (H&E) stained eye section showing extensive mononuclear cellular infiltrate of lymphocytes and plasma cells.

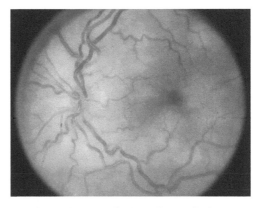

Vogt–Koyanagi–Harada (VKH) funduscopic examination reveals venous engorgement and serous retinal detachment.

associated with HLA-DR4. Corticosteroids, chlorambucil, cyclophosphamide, and cyclosporin A have been used for treatment.

Vollmer test (historical)

A tuberculin patch test employing gauze treated with tuberculin.

voltage-gated calcium channel autoantibodies

Autoantibodies specific for voltage-gated calcium channels (VGCCs) located on presynaptic nerve terminals are generated during an autoimmune disease associated with small cell lung cancer (SCLC) known as Lambert–Eaton myasthenic syndrome (LEMS). Although the exact role of N-type VGCC autoantibodies remains to be determined, they may contribute to disturbance of autonomic neurotransmitter release associated with LEMS.

von Krough equation

A mathematical equation to ascertain serum hemolytic complement titer. It correlates complement with the extent of lysis of red blood cells coated with anti-erythrocyte antibodies under standard conditions.

Vpr (HIV)

A protein of the human immunodeficiency virus that facilitates passage of HIV DNA to the nucleus. It promotes G2 arrest and activation of the intrinsic apoptotic pathway.

VpreB

Refer to pre-B cell receptor.

VpreB and λ5

Proteins produced at the early pro-B cell stage of B cell development required for regulation of μ chain expression on cell surfaces. VpreB and λ5 replace immunoglobulin light chains in pre-B cells and play an important role in B cell differentiation.

Vpu (HIV)

A protein of the human immunodeficiency virus that combines with recently synthesized CD4 in the cytoplasm of host cells and targets it for ubiquitin-mediated degradation by proteasomes. It leads to formation of ion channels in the membranes of host cells to permit virus release. It interferes with the synthesis of MHC class I and increases susceptibility to the Fas-mediated apoptotic pathway.

V region

Refer to variable region.

V region subgroups

Individual chain V region subdivisions based on significant homology in amino acid sequence.

V$_T$ region

T lymphocyte antigen receptor variable region.

W

w

Symbol for *workshop* used for histocompatibility (HLA) antigen and cluster of differentiation (CD) designations when new antigenic specificities have not been conclusively decided. After authorities agree upon the specificities, the *w* is removed from the designation.

Waaler–Rose test

Refer to Rose–Waaler test.

Waldenström, Jan Gosta (1906–)

Swedish physician who described the macroglobulinemia that now bears his name. He received the Gairdner Award in 1966.

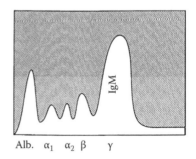

Waldenström's macroglobulinemia.

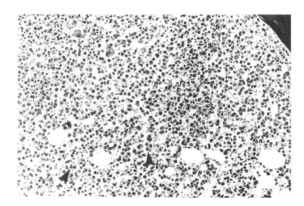

Waldenström's macroglobulinemia with IgM spike.

Waldenström's macroglobulinemia

This paraproteinemia is second in frequency only to multiple myeloma and usually occurs in people over 50 years of age. It manifests in various clinical forms. Most features of the disease relate to the oversynthesis of monoclonal IgM. Relatively mild cases may be characterized by anemia and weakness or pain in the abdomen resulting from enlargement of the spleen and liver. A major difference from multiple myeloma is a lack of osteolytic lesions of the skeleton, although patients may have peripheral lymphadenopathy. On bone marrow examination, many kinds of cells are found with characteristics of plasma cells and lymphocytes constituting so-called lymphocytoid plasma cells. Many are transitional or intermediate between one type or another. Patients may develop bleeding disorders due to paraproteins in their circulation. The more severe forms are characterized by features that resemble chronic lymphocytic leukemia or even lymphosarcoma with a rapidly fatal course. Many individuals may develop anemia. The large molecules of IgM (molecular weight approaching one million) lead to increased blood viscosity. Central nervous system and visual difficulties may also be manifested.

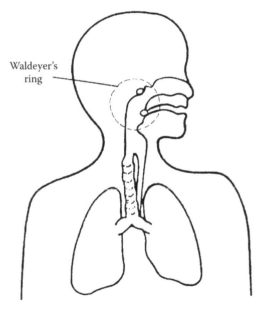

Waldeyer's ring.

Waldeyer's ring

A circular arrangement of lymphoid tissue composed of tonsils and adenoids encircling the pharynx–oral cavity junction.

warm agglutinin disease

Immunoglobulin G (IgG)-induced autoimmune hemolysis. Two fifths of cases are secondary to other diseases such as neoplasia, including chronic lymphocytic leukemia and ovarian tumors. It may also be secondary to connective tissue diseases such as lupus erythematosus, rheumatoid arthritis, and progressive systemic sclerosis. Patients experience hemolysis leading to anemia with fatigue, dizziness, palpitations, exertion dyspnea, mild jaundice, and splenomegaly and manifest positive Coombs' antiglobulin tests. Their erythrocytes appear as spherocytes and schistocytes, and they show evidence of erythrophagocytosis. Erythroid hyperplasia of the bone marrow is observed, and lympho-proliferative disease may be present. Glucocorticoids and blood transfusions are used for treatment. Approximately 66% of patients improve after splenomectomy, but they often relapse. Three quarters survive for a decade.

warm antibody

An antibody that reacts best at 37°C. It is usually an immu-noglobulin G (IgG) agglutinin and shows specificity for selected erythrocyte antigens including Kell, Duffy, Kidd, and Rh. It may be associated with immune hemolysis.

Wassermann, August von (1866–1925)

German physician who, with Neisser and Bruck, described the first serological test (Wassermann reaction) for syphilis. (Refer to *Handbook der Pathogenen Mikroorganismen* [with Kolle], 1903.)

Wassermann reaction

A complement fixation assay used extensively in the past to diagnose syphilis. Cardiolipin extracted from ox heart serves as the antigen that reacts with antibodies in patients with syphilis. Biologic false-positive reactions using this test require the use of such confirmatory tests as the FTA–ABS (fluorescence *Treponema* antibody absorption), Reiter's complement fixation, or *Treponema pallidum* immobiliza-tion. Both FTA and TPI tests use *T. pallidum* as the antigen.

waste disposal hypothesis

The concept that selected cases of autoimmunity may be attributable to a failure to clear apoptotic cells. The release of autoantigens from these accumulated cells in the tissues may activate autoimmune reactions.

wasting disease

Neonatal thymectomy in mice can lead to a chronic and eventually fatal disease characterized by lymphoid atrophy and weight loss. Animals may develop ruffled fur, diarrhea, and hunched appearance. Gnotobiotic (germ-free) animals fail to develop wasting disease following neonatal thymec-tomy. Thymectomy of animals that are not germ-free may lead to fatal infection resulting from greatly decreased cell-mediated immunity. Wasting disease is also called runt disease. Wasting may appear in immunodeficiency states such as AIDS as well as in graft-vs.-host (GVH) reactions.

wax D

A high molecular weight (70-kDa) glycolipid and peptido-glycolipid extracted from wax fractions of *Mycobacterium tuberculosis* isolated from humans. It is soluble in chloro-form and insoluble in boiling acetone and has the adjuvant properties that *Mycobacterium tuberculosis* organisms add to Freund's adjuvant preparations. Thus, wax D can be used to replace mycobacteria in adjuvant preparations to enhance cellular and humoral immune responsiveness to antigen.

Webb, Gerald Bertram

Colorado Springs scientist who named the American Association of Immunologists and served two terms as its first president.

Wegener's granulomatosis

Necrotizing sinusitis with necrosis of both the upper and lower respiratory tract. The disease is characterized by granulomas, vasculitis, granulomatous arteritis, and glomerulonephritis and is believed to have an immunologi-cal etiology, although this remains to be proven. Patients develop antineutrophil cytoplasmic antibodies (cANCAs). The disease may be treated successfully in many subjects by cyclophosphamide therapy.

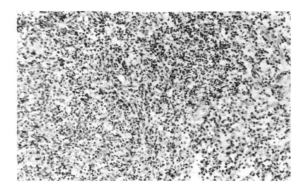

Inflammation of ethmoid and maxillary sinuses.

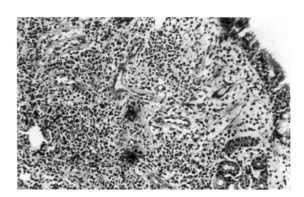

Necrosis in respiratory epithelium.

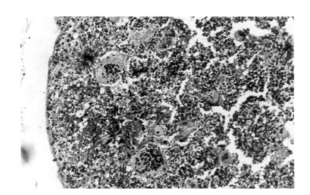

Giant cells in respiratory epithelium.

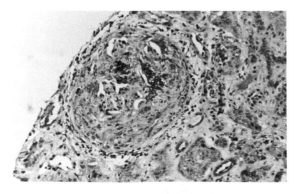

Obsolescent renal glomerulus in Wegener's granulomatosis.

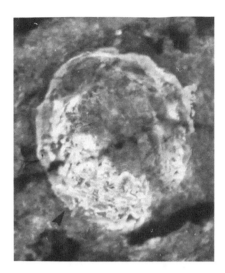

Immunofluorescence of renal glomerulus in Wegener's granulomatosis.

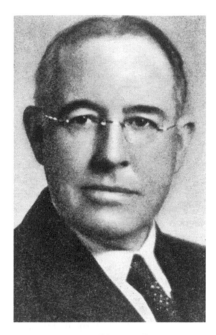

Harry Gideon Wells.

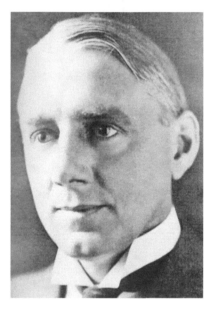

Gerald Bertram Webb.

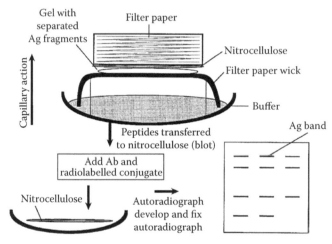

Western blot.

Weibel–Palade bodies

P-selectin granules found in endothelial cells. P-selectin is translocated rapidly to the cell surface following activation of an endothelial cell by such mediators as histamine and C5a.

Weil–Felix reaction

A diagnostic agglutination test in which *Proteus* bacteria are agglutinated by the sera of patients with typhus. The reaction is based upon the cross reactivity of the carbohydrate antigen shared by *Rickettsiae* and selected *Proteus* strains. Various rickettsial diseases may be diagnosed based on the reaction patterns of antibodies in the sera of patients with rickettsial disease with O-agglutinable strains of *Proteus* OX19, OX2, and OX12.

Wells, Harry Gideon

A professor of pathology at the University of Chicago who wrote an important early book in the 1920s titled *Chemical Aspects of Immunity*.

western blot (immunoblot)

A method to identify antibodies against proteins of precise molecular weight. It is widely used as a confirmatory test for HIV-1 antibody following screening via the ELISA assay. Following separation of proteins by one- or two-dimensional electrophoresis, they are blotted or transferred to a nitrocellulose or nylon membrane followed by exposure to biotinylated or radioisotope-labeled antibody; the antigen under investigation is revealed by either a color reaction or autoradiography, respectively.

wheal-and-flare reaction

An immediate hypersensitivity, IgE-mediated human reaction to an antigen. Application of antigen by a scratch test in a hypersensitive individual may be followed by erythema (red flare) and edema (wheal). Atopic subjects whose allergies have hereditary components experience the effects of histamine and other vasoactive amines released from mast cell granules following cross linking of surface immunoglobulin E (IgE) molecules by antigen or allergen. Refer to urticaria.

Whipple's disease

A disorder characterized immunologically by massive infiltration of the lamina propria with periodic acid Schiff stain (PAS)-positive macrophages. Secondary T cell abnormalities are observed. This is a rare infectious disease produced by one or more microorganisms that remain unidentified. Diagnosis is established by intestinal biopsy, showing microorganisms and numerous macrophages containing microbial cell wall debris in their cytoplasm. The cellular infiltration is associated with "clubbed" villi, lymphatic obstruction, malabsorption, and protein-losing enteropathy. Loss of lymphocytes into the gastrointestinal tract as a result of lymphatic obstruction may be associated with the development of lymphopenia and secondary T cell immune deficiency.

white graft rejection

Accelerated rejection of a second skin graft performed 7 to 12 days after rejection of the first. It is characterized by lack of vascularization of the graft and its conversion to a white eschar. The characteristic changes are seen by day 5 after the second procedure. The transplanted tissue is rendered white because of hyperacute rejection, such as in the case of a skin or kidney allograft. Preformed antibodies occlude arteries following surgical anastomosis, producing infarction of the tissue graft.

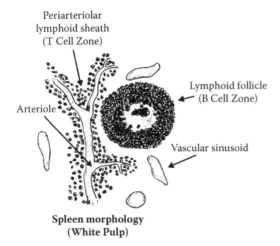

**Spleen morphology
(White Pulp)**

White pulp.

white pulp

The periarteriolar lymphatic sheaths encircled by small lymphocytes that are mainly T cells surrounding germinal centers composed of B lymphocytes and B lymphoblasts in normal splenic tissue. Following interaction of B cells in the germinal centers with antigen in the blood, a primary immune response is generated within 24 hours, revealing immunoblastic proliferation and enlargement of germinal centers.

white pulp diseases

Lymphoproliferative diseases that express major anatomical changes in the splenic white pulp. They include histiocytic lymphoma, lymphocytic leukemia, and Hodgkin disease.

whooping cough vaccine

Refer to pertussis vaccine.

Widal reaction

Bacterial agglutination test used to diagnose enteric infections caused by *Salmonella*. Doubling dilutions of patient serum are combined with a suspension of microorganisms known to cause enteric fever such as *S. typhi*, *S. paratyphi* B, and *S. paratyphi* A and C. The test microorganisms should be motile and smooth and in the specific phase. Formalin-treated suspensions are used to assay H agglutinins, and alcohol-treated suspensions assay O agglutinin. The Widal test is positive after the 10th day of the disease. Results may be false-positive if an individual previously received a TAB vaccine. Thus, it is important to repeat the test and observe a rising titer rather than merely observe a single positive test. Widal originally described the test to diagnose *S. paratyphi* B infection.

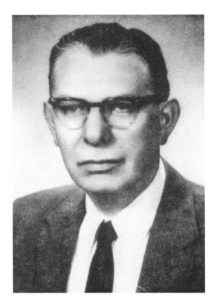

Alexander Wiener.

Wiener, Alexander

Co-discoverer with Landsteiner of the Rh blood group system.

wild mouse

A mouse that is free in the environment and has not been raised under laboratory conditions.

window

(1) The period between exposure to a microorganism and the appearance of serologically detectable antibody. It is observed in hepatitis B and in human immunodeficiency virus 1 (HIV-1) infections. In hepatitis B, a "core window" occurs in active but unidentified infection. The hepatitis B surface antigen (HBsAg) can no longer be detected, and the antibody against hepatitis B surface antigen (anti-HB$_s$) has not reached sufficiently high levels to be detected. (2) The period between the first infection with HIV-1 and synthesis of anti-p24 and anti-p41 antibodies in amounts measurable by the enzyme-linked immunosorbent assay (ELISA). Use of the polymerase chain reaction (PCR) to demonstrate the p24 antigen can be useful to indicate infection during the window. The window period in HIV-1 infection may be 3 to 9 months and may reach 36 months. Blood donated for transfusion in the United States is assayed for anti-HIV-1 p24 antibody; thus, these units of blood may be in the HIV-1 infection window.

Winn assay

A method to determine the ability of lymphoid cells to inhibit the growth of transplantable tumors *in vivo*. Following incubation of lymphoid cells and tumor cells *in vitro*, the mixture is injected into the skin of X-irradiated

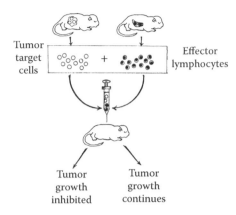

Winn assay.

mice. Growth of the transplanted cells follows. T lymphocytes that are specifically immune to the tumor cells will inhibit tumor growth and provide information related to tumor immunity.

wire loop lesion

Thickening of capillary walls as a result of subendothelial immune complex deposits situated between the capillary endothelium and the glomerular basement membrane. Wire loop lesions are seen in diffuse proliferative lupus nephritis and are characteristic of class IV lupus erythematosus. They may also be seen in progressive systemic sclerosis and appear with crescent formation, necrosis, and scarring.

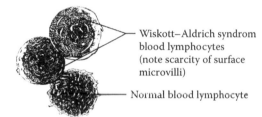

Wiskott–Aldrich syndrom blood lymphocytes (note scarcity of surface microvilli)

Normal blood lymphocyte

Wiskott–Aldrich syndrome.

Wiskott–Aldrich syndrome

X-linked recessive immunodeficiency disease of infants characterized by thrombocytopenia, eczema, and increased immunoglobulin A (IgA) and IgE levels. It is a consequence of mutations in the WAS protein (WASP) that may have a role in the survival and/or function of hematopoietic stem cells, platelets, and lymphocytes. This protein connects several membrane receptors to the cytoskeleton. A defect in this protein could cause abnormal cellular morphology or defective lymphocyte activation signals. Cell-mediated immunity and delayed hypersensitivity are decreased, and the antibody response to polysaccharide antigens is defective, with only minute quantities of IgM appearing in the serum. The condition may involve inability to recognize processed antigen. It is a genetic disease characterized by defective interactions of T cells and B cells. Male patients may have small platelets with no surface glycoprotein Ib. There is increased susceptibility to infection by pyogenic bacteria. IgA and IgE are increased and IgM is diminished, although IgG serum concentrations are usually normal. Under electron microscopy, T lymphocytes appear bereft of markedly fimbriated surfaces of normal T cells.

T lymphocytes have abnormal sialophorin. Patients may have increased incidence of malignant lymphomas. Bone marrow transplantation corrects the deficiency.

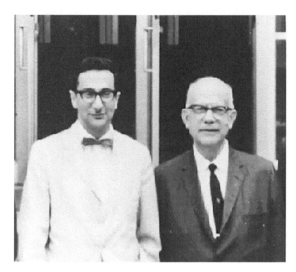

Noel Rose (left) and Ernest Witebsky (right), members of the Buffalo Immunology Group.

Witebsky, Ernest (1901–1969)

German-American immunologist and bacteriologist who made significant contributions to transfusion medicine and concepts of autoimmune diseases. He was a direct descendant of the Ehrlich school of immunology, having worked at Heidelberg with Hans Sachs, Ehrlich's principal assistant, in 1929. He went to Mt. Sinai Hospital in New York in 1934 and became a professor at the University of Buffalo in 1936, where he remained until his death. A major portion of his work on autoimmunity was the demonstration with Noel R. Rose of experimental autoimmune thyroiditis.

Witebsky's criteria

According to criteria suggested by Ernest Witebsky, an autoimmune response should be considered as a cause of a human disease if (1) it is regularly associated with that disease, (2) immunization of an experimental animal with the antigen from the appropriate tissue causes an immune response (formation of antibodies or development of allergy), (3) the animal develops pathological changes associated with this response that are basically similar to those of humans, and (4) the experimental disease can be transferred to a nonimmunized animal by serum or lymphoid cells.

worms

Four types of cells are present in the earthworm coelom, all of which are phagocytic. Some cells participate in allograft rejection, whereas others synthesize antibacterial substances.

Wright, Almroth Edward (1861–1947)

British pathologist and immunologist who graduated as a doctor of medicine from Trinity College, Dublin in 1889. He became a professor of pathology at the Army Medical School in Netley in 1892 and became associated with the Institute of Pathology at St. Mary's Hospital Medical School, London, in 1902. He and Douglas formulated a theory of opsonins and perfected an antitoxoid inoculation

W

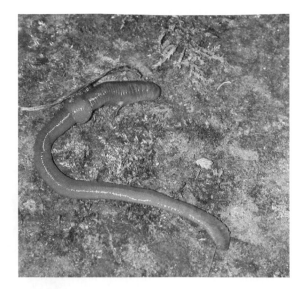

Worms.

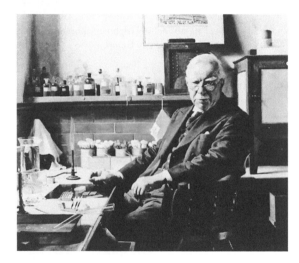

Almroth Edward Wright.

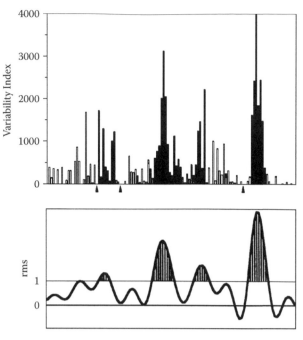

Variability of TCR β chains. Variability indices calculated according to the modified formula are plotted for the 159 TCR β chains from database 1.

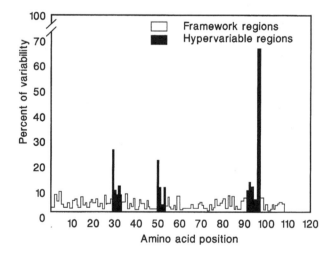

Wu-Kabat plot.

system. He studied immunology in Frankfurt-am-Main under Paul Ehrlich and made important contributions to the immunology of infectious diseases and immunization. He played a significant role in the founding of the American Association of Immunologists. His published works include *Pathology and Treatment of War Wounds*, 1942; *Researches in Clinical Physiology*, 1943; and *Studies in Immunology* (2 volumes), 1944.

Wu–Kabat plot

A graph that demonstrates the extent of variability at individual amino acid residue positions in immunoglobulin and T cell receptor (TCR) variable regions. Division of the different amino acid numbers at a given position by the frequency of the amino acid that occurs most commonly at that position gives the index of variability (from 1 to 400). To show the variability graphically, a biograph is prepared in which the index is plotted at each residue position. This plot indicates the extent of variability at each position and is useful in localizing immunoglobulin and TCR hypervariable regions. This analytic method revealed that the most variable residues of immunoglobulin heavy or light chains are clustered in three hypervariable regions.

W, X, Y boxes (MHC class II promoter)

Three conserved sequences found in the promoter region of the HLA-DRα chain gene. The X box contains tandem regulatory sequences designated X1 and X2. Any cell that expresses major histocompatibility complex (MHC) class II molecules will have all three boxes interacting with binding proteins. Decreased or defective production of some of these binding proteins can lead to bare lymphocyte syndrome.

X

X cell

See XYZ cell theory.

X4 viruses

HIV strains that have become incapable of infecting macrophages and preferentially attack CD4⁺ T lymphocytes. Previously called T-tropic viruses.

xenoantibodies

Antibodies formed in one species that are specific for antigens of a separate species.

xenoantibody

An antibody specific for xenoantigen.

xenoantigen

Tissue antigens of one species that induce an immune response in members of a different species. Antigen of a xenograft. Also called heteroantigen.

xenobiotics

Exposure of humans to xenobiotics including chemicals and drugs may lead to autoimmune responses resembling responses to infections with microorganisms, but true autoimmune disease is observed less frequently. Various animal models of autoimmunity such as drug-induced lupus have been induced by chemicals. The models do not correspond exactly to the human disease although renal autoimmune disease caused by metals shows close similarity in animals and humans. Isoniazid, hydralazine, and procainamide have been implicated in drug-induced lupus. Iodine administration to experimental animals prone to spontaneous autoimmune thyroiditis favors the development of this disease. Toxic oil syndrome has been induced in B10.S mice by the intraperitoneal administration of oleic acid anilide. HgCl₂ administration to rats, mice, and rabbits led to the production of autoimmune kidney disease. Streptozotocin administration induced an experimental model of insulin-dependent diabetes mellitus in animal models. The halothane anesthetic induced liver changes in rabbits and rats that led to the formation of halothane antigens. Complete Freund's adjuvant can induce adjuvant arthritis in rats. Xenobiotics are nonliving substances derived from drugs, metals, or industrial or natural chemicals that may interact with self proteins to yield neo-antigens.

xenogeneic

Tissues or organs transplanted from one species to a genetically different species (e.g., a baboon liver transplanted to a human). It refers to the genetic relationship of an individual of one species to a member of a different species.

xenograft

A tissue or organ graft from a member of one species (donor) to a member of a different species (recipient); also called a heterograft. Antibodies and cytotoxic T cells reject xenografts several days following transplantation.

Xenopus

Anuran amphibian that serves as an excellent model for investigating the ontogeny of immunity. Comparative immunologic research employs isogeneic and inbred families of this amphibian. *Xenopus* is especially useful for studying the role of the thymus in immune ontogeny because early thymectomy of free-living larvae does not lead to runting.

xenoreactive

A T cell or antibody response to an antigen of a graft derived from another species. T lymphocytes may recognize an intact xenogenic major histocompatibility complex (MHC) molecule or a peptide from a xenogeneic protein bound to a self MHC molecule.

xenotransplantation

Organ or tissue transplantation between members of different species. Xenogeneic transplantation may involve concordant or discordant donors, according to the phylogenetic distance between the species involved. Natural preformed antibodies in a recipient specific for donor endothelial antigens that lead to hyperacute rejection of most vascularized organ transplants now occur in discordant species combinations. The immune response to a xenotransplant resembles the response to an allotransplant; however, greater antigenic differences exist between donor and host in xenotransplantation than in allotransplantation. Previously termed heterotransplantation. The procedure is under investigation

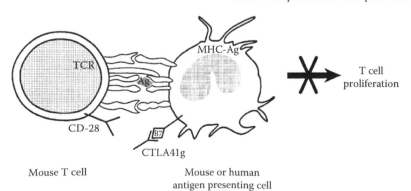

Induction of tolerance to xenogenic tissue graft.

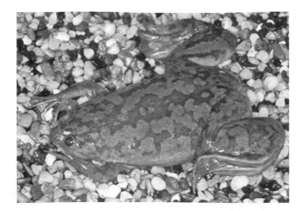

Xenopus.

to potentially increase the supply of organs for human transplantation.

xenotype

Molecular variations based on differences in structure and antigenic specificity. Examples include membrane antigens of cells or immunoglobulins from separate species.

xenozoonosis

Transmission of an infection that may be a consequence of xenotransplantation. Such infections may involve infection of recipient cells with endogenous retroviral sequences from donor cells, giving rise alone or after recombination with human endogenous retroviral sequences to previously unknown pathogenic viruses. Such new viruses may be pathogenic for humans other than the xenograft recipient.

xeroderma pigmentosum (XP)

A rare disorder attributable to *XPA-XPG* gene mutations that participate in the nucleotide excision pathway of DNA repair. It is associated with profound sensitivity to sunlight and variable CID.

Xg^a

The sex-linked blood antigen is an antibody more common in women than in men. It is specific for the Xg^a antigen, in recognition of its X-borne pattern of inheritance. The table below shows phenotype frequencies in Caucasian males and females. The antibody is relatively rare and has not been implicated in hemolytic disease of the newborn or hemolytic transfusion reaction although it can bind complement and may occasionally serve as an autoantibody. Anti-Xg^a antibodies may be of value in identifying genetic traits transmitted in association with the X chromosome.

Xg^a: Sex-Linked Blood Antigen

Phenotype	Reaction with Anti-Xg^a	Phenotype Frequency Male	Female
Xg (a+)	+	65.6	88.7
Xg (a–)	0	34.4	11.3

***xid* gene**

An X-chromosome mutation. When homozygous, it leads to diminished responsiveness to some thymus-independent antigens, a limited decrease in responsiveness to thymic-dependent antigens, and defective terminal differentiation of B cells. Many autoimmune features are diminished when

the *xid* gene is bred into autoimmune mouse strains. These include reduced anti-DNA antibody levels, diminished renal disease, and increased survival.

X-linked agammaglobulinemia (XLA)

A disease of Btk tyrosine kinase characterized by increased susceptibility to infections beginning most often during the first year of life when transferred maternal immunoglobulin is catabolized. Arrested B cell development at the pre-B cell stage blocks formation of mature B cells and antibody synthesis. Serum analysis reveals a pronounced decrease in immunoglobulin levels of all isotypes. IgA is usually undetectable and a humoral response to recall antigens is virtually absent. B lymphocyte and plasma cell numbers are markedly decreased, whereas T lymphocyte subsets show a relative increase. The defect is caused by a differentiation arrest confined to the B cell lineage, distinguishing XLA from most other immunoglobulin deficiencies. B lineage cells in all organs are affected, resulting in reduced sizes of lymph nodes and tonsils. The defective gene encodes a cytoplasmic tyrosine kinase, designated Btk. Mutation analysis confirms the diagnosis and can be used to identify healthy carriers. Treatment consists of antibiotics to combat ongoing infections and γ globulin substitution as a prophylaxis.

X-linked hyper-IgM syndrome

Refer to hyperimmunoglobulin M syndrome.

X-linked lymphoproliferative disease (XLP)

A combined immunodeficiency involving T and B lymphocytes. It is exacerbated following exposure to Epstein–Barr virus (EBV), one of the eight known human herpesviruses. In older children and adults, EBV is the causative agent of infectious mononucleosis, frequently a self-limiting polyclonal lymphoproliferative disease with an excellent prognosis. In immunosuppressed individuals, EBV infection may lead to life-threatening lymphoproliferative disorders and lymphoma. EBV has been primarily associated with certain malignancies such as endemic Burkitt's lymphoma (BL), nasopharyngeal carcinoma (NPC), certain B and T cell lymphomas, and approximately 50% of Hodgkin disease. The XLP (*LYP*) gene locus has been mapped to Xq25. In general, XLP has an unfavorable prognosis, but transplantation of hematopoietic stem cells from a suitable donor may cure this immunodeficiency. The SAP/SH2D1A gene is altered. The two sets of target molecules for this small SH2 domain-containing protein include (1) a family of hematopoietic cell surface receptors (SLAM family), and (2) a second phosphorylated adapter molecule. EAT-2, a SAP-like protein, also interacts with these surface receptors. SAP/SH2D1A is a natural inhibitor of SH2-domain-dependent interactions with SLAM family members. Dysgammaglobulinemia and B cell lymphoma can occur without prior EBV infection. The SAP/SH2D1A gene controls signaling via SLAM surface receptors, thereby playing a critical role in T cell and antigen-presenting cell (APC) interactions during viral infections. XLP leads to an inability to control EBV infections. It is characterized by cytotoxic T lymphocyte-mediated immunopathologic injury in response to EBV infections.

X-linked lymphoproliferative syndrome

A type of infectious mononucleosis in X-linked immunodeficiency patients who manifest Epstein–Barr virus nuclear antigen (EBNA)-positive lymphoid cells, polyclonal B lymphocyte proliferation, and plasma blasts. The disease may be caused by an inability to combat Epstein–Barr virus, leading to a fatal outcome.

X-linked severe combined immunodeficiency (XSCID)

A condition characterized by T cell development failure during an early intrathymic stage, resulting in a lack of production of mature T cells or T cell-dependent antibody. It is a consequence of a defect in a gene that encodes portions of receptors for different cytokines such as inherited mutations in the common γ chains of the receptors for interleukin-2 (IL2), IL4, IL7, IL9, and IL15, resulting in impaired ability to transmit signals from the receptor to intracellular proteins.

x-ray crystallography

A method to analyze protein structure at the atomic level. Monochromatic X-rays from a rotating anode x-ray generator or a synchrotron are directed to bombard a crystallized protein. Although most x-rays pass through the crystal, some are deflected after striking atoms of the protein to produce a detectable and reproducible pattern. Analysis of the diffraction reveals information about the positions and orientations of the atoms in the crystal.

XYZ cell theory (historical)

An earlier concept of antibody synthesis proposing (1) an immunocompetent X cell that had not participated previously in a specific immune response, (2) a Y cell activated immunologically by X cell interaction with antigen, and (3) a Z cell that synthesized antibodies following second contact with antigen.

Y

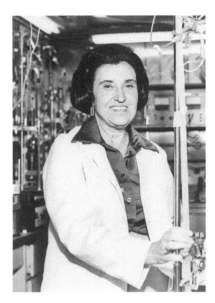

Rosalyn Sussman Yalow.

Yalow, Rosalyn Sussman (1921–):

American investigator who shared the 1977 Nobel Prize with Guillemin and Schally for endocrinology research and perfection of the radioimmunoassay (RIA) technique. With Berson, Yalow made an important discovery of the role of antibodies in insulin-resistant diabetes. Her technique provided a test to estimate nanogram or picogram quantities of various types of hormones and biologically active molecules, thereby advancing basic and clinical research.

Y cell

See XYZ cell theory.

yellow fever vaccine

An immunizing preparation that contains a live attenuated strain of yellow fever virus that protects against this mosquito-borne tropical, viral, hemorrhagic fever; a lyophilized attenuated vaccine prepared from the 17D strain of live attenuated yellow fever virus grown in chick embryos. A single injection may confer immunity that persists for a decade.

yellowjacket venom

A hymenopteran insect (bee, wasp, ant) toxin that may induce anaphylactic shock (type I hypersensitivity), possibly leading to death, in victims of insect bites. The release of vasoactive amines may lead to urticaria, tightness in the chest, chills, fever, and even cardiovascular collapse.

***Yersinia* immunity**

Both humoral and cell-mediated immune responses develop in yersiniosis. The antibody is directed mainly to lipopolysaccharide. Antibodies in patients with *Yersinia* infection are specific for numerous epitopes. The antibodies persist for months and in some cases even years. Reactive arthritis, a frequent postinfection complication, is strongly associated with HLA-B27 antigen. The immune response against the infectious agents is believed to have a significant role in the pathogenesis of *Yersinia*-triggered reactive arthritis. No effective vaccine is available for *Yersinia* infection.

Z

ZAP-70

A T cell cytoplasmic tyrosine kinase that constitutes part of the T cell receptor signal transduction pathway.

ZAP-70 (ζ-associated protein of 70 kDa) deficiency

A rare autosomal-recessive type of severe combined immunodeficiency syndrome (SCID) that features a selective absence of CD8⁺ T cells and abundant CD4⁺ T lymphocytes in the peripheral blood that do not respond to T cell receptor (TCR)-mediated stimuli *in vitro*. Peripheral T cells from patients manifest defective T cell signaling attributable to inherited mutations within the kinase domain of the TCR-associated protein tyrosine kinase (PTK) ZAP-70. ZAP-70 deficiency shows that PTKs, and especially ZAP-70, are necessary for the physiologic development and function of T cells in humans. The condition is marked by CD8 lymphocytopenia but presents during infancy with severe, recurrent, frequently fatal infections resembling those in SCID patients. Patients have normal or elevated numbers of circulating CD3⁺/CD4⁺ T lymphocytes but essentially no CD8⁺ T cells. The T cells fail to respond to mitogens or to allogeneic cells *in vitro* or to form cytotoxic T lymphocytes. By contrast, natural killer (NK) activity is normal, and they have normal or elevated numbers of B cells and low to elevated serum immunoglobulin concentrations. The thymus may have normal architecture with normal numbers of double-positive (CD4⁺/CD8⁺) thymocytes but no CD8 single-positive thymocytes. The condition results from mutations in the gene encoding ZAP-70, a non-*src* PTK important in T cell signaling.

Z cell

See XYZ cell theory.

ζ (zeta) associated protein of 70 kDa (ZAP-70)

A 70-kDa tyrosine kinase present in the cytosol and believed to participate in maintaining T lymphocyte receptor signaling. It belongs to the *src* family of cytoplasmic protein tyrosine kinases and is requisite for early signaling in antigen-induced T lymphocyte activation. It binds to cytoplasmic tail phosphorylated tyrosines of the ζ chain of the T cell receptor complex. This is followed by phosphorylation of adapter proteins that recruit other signaling cascade components. It is similar to *syk* in B lymphocytes. Refer also to *lck*, *fyn*, and ZAP (phosphotyrosine kinases in T cells).

ζ (zeta) chain

A T cell receptor complex expressed as a transmembrane protein in T lymphocytes that contains immunoreceptor tyrosine-based activation motifs (ITAMs) in its cytoplasmic tail and binds ZAP-70 protein tyrosine kinase during T lymphocyte activation.

ζ (zeta) potential

The collective negative charge on erythrocyte surfaces that causes them to repulse one another in cationic medium. Some cations are red cell surface-bound; others are free

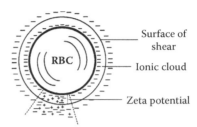

The ζ (zeta) potential surrounding red blood cells.

in the medium. The boundary of shear is between the two cation planes, where the ζ potential may be determined as negative millivolts (–mV). IgM antibodies have optimal ζ potentials of –22 to –17 mV, and IgG antibodies have optimum levels of –11 to –4.5 mV. The fewer the absolute millivolts, the less the space between cells in suspension. The addition of certain proteins such as albumin to the medium diminishes the ζ potential.

Ziagen®

A carbocyclic synthetic nucleoside analog approved by the FDA for the treatment of human immunodeficiency virus (HIV). The mechanism of action includes activation of abacavir to carbovir triphosphate, which inhibits the activity of HIV-1 reverse transcriptase by competing with the natural substrate deoxyguanosine triphosphate (dGTP) and its incorporation into viral DNA. Abacavir is the active component.

zidovudine (3′-azido-3′-deoxythymidine, AZT)

A reverse transcriptase inhibitor that is a thymidine analog approved by the FDA to treat acquired immune deficiency syndrome (AIDS). The mechanism of action includes phosphorylation of the drug *in vivo* to 3′-azido-3′-deoxythymidine triphosphate. This combines with human immunodeficiency virus (HIV) reverse transcriptase, which leads to cessation of DNA elongation.

zinc

An element of great significance to the immune system and to other nonantigen-specific host defenses. The interleukins of the immune system play a role in zinc distribution and metabolism. As a constituent of the active sites in multiple metalloenzymes, zinc is critical in chemical processes within lymphocytes and leukocytes. Its role in the reproduction of cells is critical for immunological reactions because nucleic acid synthesis depends, in part, on zinc metalloenzymes. Zinc facilitates cell membrane modification and stabilization. Zinc deficiency is associated with reversible dysfunction of T lymphocytes in humans. Thymic hormonal function requires zinc; a deficiency causes atrophy of the thymus and other lymphoid organs and is associated with decreased lymphocytes in the T cell areas of lymphoid tissues. Lymphopenia is also present. Anergy develops in zinc-deficient patients and signifies disordered cell-mediated immunity as a consequence of the deficiency.

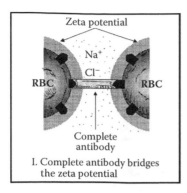

I. Complete antibody bridges the zeta potential

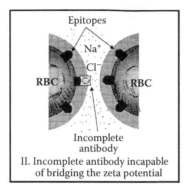

II. Incomplete antibody incapable of bridging the zeta potential

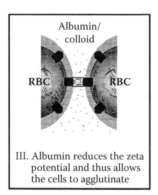

III. Albumin reduces the zeta potential and thus allows the cells to agglutinate

Comparison of ability of complete antibody to bridge the ζ potential with the inability of complete antibody to do so.

Zidovudine.

The synthesis of antibodies to T-cell-dependent antigens is decreased. In zinc deficiency, a selective decline in the number of CD4+ helper T cells is observed, as are strikingly decreased proliferative responses to phytomitogens, including phytohemagglutinin (PHA). Zinc deficiency is

also associated with decreased formation of monocytes and macrophages and altered chemotaxis of granulocytes. Wound healing is impaired in deficient individuals, who also show greatly increased susceptibility to infectious diseases that are especially severe.

zinc and immunity

Zinc is found in all tissues and fluids of the body. It is mainly an intracellular ion, over 95% is found within cells; 60 to 80% of the cellular zinc is located in the cytosol. About 85% of the total body zinc is present in skeletal muscles and bones. Zinc is absorbed all along the small intestine but is taken up primarily in the jejunum. It has catalytic, structural, and regulatory functions. Catalytic roles are present in all six classes of enzymes. More than 50 enzymes require zinc for normal activity; its role in zinc metalloenzymes is usually structural. Regulation of gene expression is also a significant biochemical function. Classic symptoms of zinc deficiency in experimental animals include retarded growth, depressed immune function, skin lesions, depressed appetite, skeletal abnormalities, and impaired reproduction. In humans, zinc deficiency causes severe growth retardation and sexual immaturity. Acute zinc toxicity may occur with intake in the range of 1 to 2 g, which leads to gastric distress, dizziness, and nausea. High chronic intake from supplements (150 to 300 mg/day) may impair immune function and reduce concentrations of high density lipoprotein cholesterol. High intakes of zinc have been used to treat Wilson's disease, a copper accumulation disorder. Zinc is believed to induce synthesis of metallothionein in intestinal mucosal cells. Zinc is relatively nontoxic, but the chronic use of zinc supplements may induce nutrient imbalances and physiological effects. Diagnosis of zinc deficiency is difficult because of the lack of a sensitive, specific indicator. Stress, infection, food intake, short-term fasting, and hormonal status all influence plasma zinc levels. Zinc deficiency is best assessed by using a combination of dietary, static, and functional signs of depletion. Red meat and shellfish constitute the best food sources.

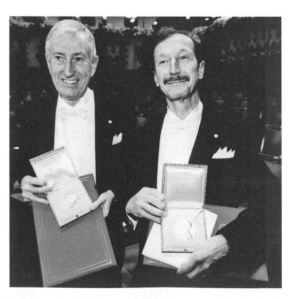

Peter Doherty and Rolf Zinkernagel, Nobel Laureates in Medicine, for their work on major histocompatibility complex (MHC) restriction.

Zinkernagel, Rolf (1944–) and Doherty, Peter (1944–)

Recipients of the 1996 Nobel Prize for Physiology or Medicine for demonstration of MHC restriction. In an investigation of how T lymphocytes protect mice against lymphocytic choriomeningitis virus (LCMV) infection, they found that T cells from mice infected by the virus killed only infected target cells expressing the same major histocompatibility complex (MHC) class I antigens but not those expressing a different MHC allele. They found that murine cytotoxic T cells (CTL) would lyse only virus-infected target cells if the effector and target cells were H-2 compatible. This significant finding had broad implications, demonstrating that T cells recognize a virus only in conjunction with MHC molecules and not directly.

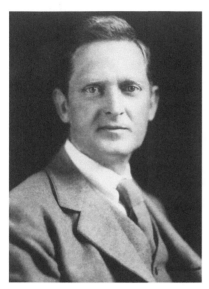

Hans Zinsser.

Zinsser, Hans (1878–1940)

A leading American bacteriologist and immunologist and educator at Columbia, Stanford, and Harvard. His work in immunology involved hypsersensitivity, plague immunology, formulation of the unitarian theory of antibodies, and demonstration of differences between tuberculin and anaphylactic hypersensitivity. His famous text, *Microbiology* (with Hiss, 1911), has been through two dozen editions since its first appearance.

zippering

A mechanism in phagocytosis in which the phagocyte membrane covers a particle by a progressive adhesive interaction. Evidence in support of this process comes from experiments in which capped B cells are only partially internalized, whereas those coated uniformly with anti-IgG opsonizing antibody are engulfed fully.

zirconium granuloma

A tissue reaction in axillary regions of subjects who use solid antiperspirants containing zirconium. The granuloma develops as a consequence of sensitization to zirconium.

zonal centrifugation

The separation of molecules according to size based on molecular mass and centrifugation time.

zone electrophoresis

The separation of proteins on cellulose acetate (or on paper) based upon charge when an electric current is passed through the gel.

zone of antibody excess

The part of the precipitin reaction curve that depicts the sparse immune complexes that may form when the number of antibody-combining sites is greater than the number of antigenic epitopes.

zone of antigen excess

That part of the precipitin reaction curve that depicts the sparse immune complexes that form little or no precipitate when the number of antigenic epitopes is greater than the number of antibody-combining sites.

zone of equivalence

That point in a precipitin antigen–antibody reaction *in vitro* at which the ratio of antigen to antibody is equivalent, i.e., the numbers of antigenic epitopes and antibody-combining sites are approximately equal. The supernatant contains neither free antigen nor antibody. All molecules of both compounds have reacted to produce antigen–antibody precipitate. When a similar reaction occurs *in vivo*, immune complexes are deposited in the microvasculature and serum sickness develops.

zoonosis

Cross-species infection; an animal disease transmissible to humans.

zygosity

Characterization of heredity traits in terms of gene pairing in a zygote from which an individual develops.

zymogen

The inactive state in which an enzyme may be synthesized. Proteolytic cleavage of the zymogen may lead to active enzyme formation.

zymosan

A complex polysaccharide derived from dried cell walls of the *Saccharomyces cerevisiae* yeast that activates the alternative complement pathway. It binds to C3b and is useful in investigations of opsonic phagocytosis.

Appendix I

Mouse CD Chart

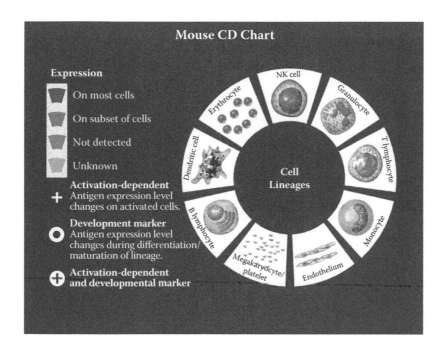

A I

Antigen Clones offered by BD Biosciences **Alternate names of antigen**	*Gene*	Component of Molecular Weight Family/Superfamily	Ligands/ Substrates	Antigen Distribution	Functions of Antigens
CD1d 1B1, 3C11 **CD1.1, CD1.2, Ly-38**	*Cd1d1*	 43-49 kDa CD1/MHC	Lipid/glycolipid Ag		Antigen presentation
CD2 RM2-5 **LFA-2, Ly-37**	*Cd2*	 45-58 kDa CD2 Ig	CD48		Activation/costimulation; adhesion
CD3 17A2 **T3**		T-cell receptor 			Signal transduction
CD3δ **CD3d, CD3 δ chain**	*Cd3d*	T-cell receptor 20 kDa Ig			Signal transduction
CD3ε 145-2C11, 500A2 **CD3e, CD3 ε chain**	*Cd3e*	T-cell receptor 20 kDa Ig			Signal transduction
CD3γ **CD3g, CD3 γ chain**	*Cd3g*	T-cell receptor 25 kDa Ig			Signal transduction *For CD3ζ see CD247
CD4 GK1.5, H129.19, RM4-5, RM4-4 **L3T4**	*Cd4*	T-cell receptor complex 55 kDa Ig	MHC class II		Signal transduction; receptor/coreceptor
CD5 53-7.3 **Ly-1, Lyt-1, Ly-12**	*Cd5*	 67 kDa SRCR	CD72		Adhesion; immunoregulation
CD5.1 H11-86.1 **Ly-1.1**	*Cd5[a]*	 67 kDa SRCR	CD72		Immunoregulation
CD6 	*Cd6*	 100- and 128-130 kDa SRCR	CD166		Activation/costimulation; adhesion; differentiation/development
CD7 	*Cd7*	 40 kDa Ig			Immunoregulation
CD8a 53-6.7, 5H10-1 **Ly-2, Lyt-2**	*Cd8a*	T-cell receptor complex 38 kDa Ig	MHC class I		Signal transduction; receptor/coreceptor
CD8b H35-17.2 **Ly-3, Lyt-3**	*Cd8b*	T-cell receptor complex 30 kDa Ig	MHC class I		Signal transduction; receptor/coreceptor
CD8b.2 53-5.8 **Ly-3.2**	*Cd8b[b]*	T-cell receptor complex 30 kDa Ig	MHC class I		Signal transduction; receptor/coreceptor
CD9 KMC8 **p24**	*Cd9*	 21, 24 kDa TM4			Activation/costimulation

Antigen Clones offered by BD Biosciences **Alternate names of antigen**	*Gene*	Component of Molecular Weight Family/Superfamily	Ligands/ Substrates	Antigen Distribution	Functions of Antigens
CD10 R103 **CALLA, MME, NEP**	*Mme*	100 kDa Metalloproteinase	Peptides		Enzymatic activity; differentiation/ development
CD11a 2D7, M17/4 **Ly-15, Ly-21, Integrin α_L chain**	*Itgal*	LFA-1 180 kDa Integrin	CD54; CD 102		Adhesion; differentiation/ development
CD11b M1/70 **Integrin α_M chain, Ly-40**	*Itgam*	Mac-1 (aka CR3) 170 kDa Integrin	CD54; iC3b; fibronectin		Adhesion
CD11c HL3 **Integrin α_x chain**	*Itgax*	p150, 95 (aka CR4) 150 kDa Integrin	iC3b; fibronectin		Adhesion
CD13 R3-242 **Aminopeptidase N, gp 150**	*Anpep*	140-150 kDa Metalloproteinase	L-leucyl-β-naphthylamine		Enzymatic activity
CD14 rmC5-3 **Mo2, LPS receptor**	*Cd14*	53-55 kDa Leucine-rich repeat	LPS/LPB complex		Receptor/coreceptor
CD15 SSEA-1, FAL, Lewis X	*Fut4*		CD62E?		Adhesion
CD16 2.4G2 **FcγRIII, FcγRIIIα, Ly-17**	*Fcgr3*	40-60 kDa Ig	mouse IgG		Ig Fc receptor
CD18 GAME-46, C71/16, M18/2 **Integrin β_2 chain**	*Itgb2*	LFA-1, Mac-1, & p150, 95 95 kDa Integrin	varies, see CD11a, b, c		Signal transduction; adhesion
CD19 1D3, MB19-1 **B4**	*Cd19*	CD19/CD21/CD81 complex 95 kDa Ig			Signal transduction; receptor/coreceptor
CD20 **Ly-44, B1**	*Ms4a2*	33-37 kDa Cd20/FcεRIβ			Activation/costimulation; differentiation/ development
CD21 7G6 **CR2**	*Cr2*	CD19/CD21/CD81 complex 150 kDa RCA	C3d		C' regulation
CD22.2 Cy34.1 **Lyb-8.2, Siglec-2**	*Cd22b*	140-160 kDa Siglec	N-glycolyl neuraminic acid		Adhesion; immunoregulation; receptor/coreceptor
CD23 B3B4 **FcεRII, Ly-42**	*Fcer2a*	45-49 kDa C-type lectin	IgE		Ig Fc receptor
CD24 30-F1, J11d, M1/69 **Heat stable antigen, Ly-52, Nectadrin**	*Cd24a*	35-52 kDa	CD62P		Activation/costimulation; adhesion

A I

Antigen Clones offered by BD Biosciences **Alternate names of antigen**	*Gene*	Component of Molecular Weight Family/Superfamily	Ligands/ Substrates	Antigen Distribution	Functions of Antigens
CD25 PC61, 7D4, 3C7 **Ly-43, IL-2 receptor α chain, p55**	*Il2ra*	IL-2 receptor 50-60 kDa CCP-like	IL-2		Activation/costimulation; receptor/coreceptor
CD26 H194-112 **Dipeptidyl peptidase, DPP IV, THAM**	*Dpp4*	220 kDa Dipeptidyl-peptidase	Polypeptides		Activation/costimulation; adhesion; enzymatic activity
CD27 LG.3A10	*Tnfrsf7*	Homodimer 45 kDa TNFR	CD70		Activation/costimulation; receptor/coreceptor
CD28 37.51	*Cd28*	Homodimer 65-80 kDa Ig	CD80; CD86		Signal transduction; activation/costimulation; receptor/coreceptor
CD29 9EG7, KMI6, Ha2/5, HMβ1-1 **Integrin β₁ chain, VLAβ, gpIIa**	*Itgb1*	VLA-1, VLA-6; $\alpha_v\beta_1$, $\alpha_7\beta_1$, $\alpha_8\beta_1$, $\alpha_9\beta_1$ integrins 130 kDa Integrin	Varies, see CD49a-f and CD51		Signal transduction; adhesion; differentiation/ development
CD30 mCD30.1 (*aka* 2SH12-5F-2D) **Ki-1**	*Tnfrsf8*	105-120 kDa TNFR	CD153		Immunoregulation; receptor/coreceptor; cytotoxicity?
CD31 MEC 13.3, 390 **PECAM-1, gpIIa, endoCAM**	*Pecam*	130-140 kDa Ig	CD38; vitronectin receptor		Adhesion; angiogenesis
CD32 2.4G2 **FcγRII, Ly-17, Ly-m20**	*Fcgr2b*	40-60 kDa Ig	mouse IgG		Ig Fc receptor; phagocytosis
CD33 Siglec-3	*Cd33*	67 kDa Siglec	Sialylated glyco- proteins?		Adhesion
CD34 RAM34 (*aka* 49E8) **Mucosialin**	*Cd34*	90, 105-120 kDa Sialomucin	CD62L		Adhesion
CD35 8C12, 7G6 **CR1, C3b receptor**	*Cr2*	190 kDa RCA	C3b		C' regulation; phagocytosis
CD36 Scavenger receptor	*Cd36*	88 kDa Class B scavenger receptor	Oxidized LDL		Adhesion; receptor/coreceptor; phagocytosis
CD37	*Cd37*	TM4			
CD38 90 **T10**	*Cd38*	42 kDa	CD31		Activation/costimulation; enzymatic activity
CD39 **NTPDase-1**	*Entpd1*		ATP; ADP		Enzymatic activity

Antigen Clones offered by BD Biosciences **Alternate names of antigen**	*Gene*	Component of Molecular Weight Family/Superfamily	Ligands/ Substrates	Antigen Distribution	Functions of Antigens
CD40 HM40-3, 3/23 **gp39 receptor**	*Tnfrsf5*	 45-50 kDa TNFR	CD154		Activation/costimulation; immunoregulation
CD41 MWReg30 **Integrin α$_{IIb}$ chain**	*Itga2b*	α$_{IIb}$β$_3$ integrin (GPIIb-IIIa) 105 kDa Integrin	Fibronectin; fibrinogen; von Willebrand factor; thrombospondin		Adhesion; hemostasis
CD42a GPIX	*Gp9*	GPIb/IX/V Complex 20 kDa Leucine-rich repeat			Adhesion; hemostasis
CD42b GPIbα	*Gp1ba*	GPIb/IX/V Complex 145 kDa Leucine-rich repeat	Von Willebrand factor		Adhesion; hemostasis
CD42c GPIbβ	*Gp1bb*	GPIb/IX/V Complex 24 kDa Leucine-rich repeat			Adhesion; hemostasis
CD42d GPV	*Gp5*	GPIb/IX/V Complex 88 kDa Leucine-rich repeat			Adhesion; hemostasis
CD43 S7, 1B11 **Leukosialin, Ly-48, sialophorin**	*Spn*	 115 and 130 kDa Sialomucin	CD54		Signal transduction, adhesion
CD44 IM7, KM114, TM-1 **Pgp-1, Ly-24**	*Cd44*	 85-95 kDa Core/link proteoglycan	Hyaluronate; collagen; fibro- nectin; laminin; osteopontin		Activation/costimulation; adhesion
CD45 30-F11, 69 **Ly-5, T200, LCA**	*Ptprc*	 180-240 kDa RPTP			Signal transduction
CD45.1 A20 **Ly-5.1**	*Ptprc^a*	 180-240 kDa RPTP			Signal transduction
CD45.2 104 **Ly-5.2**	*Ptprc^b*	 180-240 kDa RPTP			Signal transduction
CD45R RA3-6B2 **B220**	*Ptprc*	 220 kDa RPTP			Signal transduction
CD45RA 14.8	*Ptprc*	 220, 235 kDa RPTP			Signal transduction
CD45RB 16A (*aka* C363, 16A)	*Ptprc*	 200-240 kDa RPTP			Signal transduction
CD45RC DNL-1.9	*Ptprc*	 200-240 kDa RPTP			Signal transduction

A I

Antigen Clones offered by BD Biosciences **Alternate names of antigen**	Gene	Component of Molecular Weight Family/Superfamily	Ligands/ Substrates	Antigen Distribution	Functions of Antigens
CD45RO	*Ptprc*	180 kDa RPTP			Signal transduction
CD46	*Mcp*	41 kDa RCA	C3b		C' regulation
CD47 miap301 **Integrin-associated protein (IAP)**	*Itgp*	β₃ integrins 50 kDa Ig	CD172a		Signal transduction?; activation/costimulation; adhesion
CD48 HM48-1 **BCM1, sgp-60**	*Cd48*	45 kDa CD2 Ig	CD2; CD244; Enteric bacteria		Activation/costimulation; adhesion
CD49a Ha31/8 **Integrin α₁ chain**	*Itga1*	VLA-1 200 kDa Integrin	Laminin; collagen		Adhesion; differentiation/ development
CD49b HMα2, Ha1/29, DX5 **Integrin α₂ chain**	*Itga2*	VLA-2 165 kDa Integrin	Laminin; collagen; fibronectin		Adhesion; differentiation/ development
CD49c 42 **Integrin α₂ chain**	*Itga3*	VLA-3 Integrin	Fibronectin; laminin; collagen		Adhesion; differentiation/ development
CD49d R1-2, 9C10(MFR4.B), DATK32, SG31 **Integrin α₄ chain**	*Itga4*	VLA-4 (LPAM-2), LPAM-1 150-155 kDa Integrin	VCAM-1; fibronectin; MAdCAM-1; invasin		Adhesion; differentiation/ development
CD49e 5H10-27(MFR5), HMα5-1 **Integrin α₅ chain**	*Itga5*	VLA-5 135 kDa Integrin	Fibronectin		Adhesion; differentiation/ development
CD49f GoH3 **Integrin α₆ chain**	*Itga6*	VLA-6, α₆β₄ integrin(TSP-180) 120 kDa Integrin	Laminin		Adhesion; differentiation/ development
CD50 **ICAM-3**	*Icam3*	Ig	Unknown in mouse		
CD51 H9.2B8, RMV-7, 21 **Integrin α_v chain**	*Itgav*	Vitronectin receptor; α_vβ₁, α_vβ₅, α_vβ₆, and α_vβ₈ integrins 125 kDa Integrin	Vitronectin; fibronectin; fibrinogen; thrombospondin; von Willebrand factor; CD31		Activation/costimulation; adhesion; differentiation/ development
CD52 **CAMPATH-1, B7**	*Cd52*	12 kDa			
CD53 OX-79	*Cd53*	35-45 kDa TM4			Signal transduction?; differentiation/ development?

Antigen Clones offered by BD Biosciences **Alternate names of antigen**	Gene	Component of Molecular Weight Family/Superfamily	Ligands/ Substrates	Antigen Distribution	Functions of Antigens
CD70 FR70 **CD27 Ligand**	Tnfsf7	30-33 kDa TNF	CD27		Activation/costimulation
CD71 C2 (C2F2) **Transferrin receptor**	Trfr	180-190 kDa	Transferrin		Activation/costimulation; metabolism
CD72 10-1.D.2, K10.6, JY/93 **Lyb-2, Ly-m19**	Cd72	90 kDa C-type lectin	CD5; CD100		Activation/costimulation; differentiation/ development
CD73 TY/23 **NT, ecto-5'-nucleotidase**	Nt5	69 kDa	NMP		Enzymatic activity
CD74 In-1 **Ia-associated invariant chain (ii)**	Ii	Ia-associated chondroitin sulfate proteoglycan 31, 41 kDa	CD44; MHC class II		Antigen presentation; differentiation/ development
CD79a HM47 **Igα, mb-1, Ly-54**	Iga	B-cell receptor complex 30-35 kDa Ig			Signal transduction
CD79b HM79b **Igβ, B29**	Igb	B-cell receptor complex 30-40 kDa Ig			Signal transduction; differentiation/ development
CD80 16-10A1, 1G10 **B7/BB1, B7-1, Ly-53**	Cd80	55 kDa Ig	CD28; CD152		Activation/costimulation; immunoregulation
CD81 2F7, Eat1, Eat2 **TAPA-1**	Cd81	CD19/CD21/CD81 complex 26 kDa TM4			Activation/costimulation; adhesion; differentiation/ development
CD82 **C33 Ag, KAI1**	Kai	TM4			Activation/costimulation
CD83	Cd83	Ig			Activation/costimulation
CD84	Cd84	Cd2 Ig			
CD86 GL1, PO3 **B7-2, B70, Ly-58**	Cd86	80 kDa Ig	CD28; CD152		Activation/costimulation; immunoregulation
CD87 **uPA Receptor**	Plaur		uPA		Adhesion; receptor/coreceptor

A I

Antigen Clones offered by BD Biosciences Alternate names of antigen	Gene	Component of Molecular Weight Family/Superfamily	Ligands/ Substrates	Antigen Distribution	Functions of Antigens
CD88 **C5a Ligand, C5aR**	C5r1	 G-protein coupled	C5a		Activation/costimulation; C' regulation
CD90 G7 **Thy-1, θ, T25**	Thy1	 25-30 kDa Ig			Signal transduction; activation/costimulation; adhesion; differentiation/ development
CD90.1 HIS51, OX-7 **Thy-1.1, θ-AKR**	Thy1a	 25-30 kDa Ig			Signal transduction; activation/costimulation; adhesion; differentiation/ development
CD90.2 53-2.1, 30-H12 **Thy-1.2, θ-C3H**	Thy1b	 25-30 kDa Ig			Signal transduction; activation/costimulation; adhesion; differentiation/ development
CD91 **LRP, A2MR**	Lrp1	 600 kDa LDLR	LDL; LRPA1; α_2M; apo E; Gp96		Antigen presentation; hemostasis; metabolism
CD94 18d3	Klrd1	CD94/NKG2 heterodimers C-type lectin	Qa-1/Qdm		Antigen recognition; immunoregulation
CD95 Jo2, 13 **Fas, APO-1**	Tnfrsf6	 45 kDa TNFR	Cd178		Apoptosis
CD97 	Cd97	 EGF-TM7	CD55		
CD98 H202-141 **4F2, Ly-10, RL-388**	Cd98	 120 kDa 			Activation/costimulation; immunoregulation?
CD100 30 **Semaphorin H, coll-4**	Sema4d	 150 kDa Semaphorin	Cd72; Plexin-B1		Immunoregulation
CD102 3C4(mIC2/4) **ICAM-2, Ly-60**	Icam2	 55-68 kDa Ig	LFA-1		Activation/costimulation; adhesion
CD103 2E7, M290 **Integrin α_{IEL} chain**	Itgae	$\alpha_{IEL}\beta_7$ integrin 150 kDa (and 20 kDa?) integrin	E-cadherin		Activation/costimulation; adhesion; differentiation/ development
CD104 346-11A **Integrin β_4 chain**	Itgb4	$\alpha_6\beta_4$ integrin (TSP-180) 205 kDa 	Laminin		Adhesion
CD105 MJ7/18 **Endoglin**	Eng	 180 kDa TGFR	TGF-β		Adhesion; receptor/coreceptor

Antigen Clones offered by BD Biosciences **Alternate names of antigen**	*Gene*	Component of Molecular Weight Family/Superfamily	Ligands/ Substrates	Antigen Distribution	Functions of Antigens
CD106 429 (MVCAM.A) **VCAM-1**	*Vcam*1	 100-110 kDa; 47 kDa GPI-linked Ig	VLA-4		Adhesion; differentiation/ development
CD107a 1D4B **LAMP-1**	*Lamp*1	 100-140 kDa Lamp	Collagen?; laminin?; fibronectin?		Adhesion?
CD107b ABL-93 **LAMP-2**	*Lamp*2	 100-110 kDa Lamp			Adhesion?
CD110 Thrombopoietin receptor, c-mpl	*Mpl*	 CKR			Differentiation/development
CD111 **PRR1, nectin-1**	*Pvrl*1	 Ig	α-herpesviruses		Adhesion
CD112 **PRR2, nectin-2**	*Pvs*	 Ig			Adhesion
CD114 **G-CSF Receptor**	*Csf3r*	 95-125 kDa CKR	G-CSF		Signal transduction; differentiation/ development; receptor/coreceptor
CD115 **M-CSF Receptor, CSF-1R, c-fms, Fim-2**	*Csf1r*	 165 kDa RTK	M-CSF		Signal transduction; differentiation/ development; receptor/coreceptor
CD116 **G-CSF Receptor α chain**	*Csf2ra*	GM-CSF Receptor CKR	GM-CSF		Signal transduction; differentiation/ development; receptor/coreceptor
CD117 2B8, ACK45 **c-kit, Steel factor receptor, dominant white spotting**	*Kit*	 145-150 kDa Ig, RTK	c-Kit Ligand (*aka* Steel, stem cell, or mast cell growth factor)		Signal transduction; adhesion; differentiation/ development; receptor/coreceptor
CD118 **IFN-α/β Receptor, type 1 IFN-R, IFN-a Receptor**	*Ifnar*	 CKR	IFN-α; IFN-β		Immunoregulation?; receptor/coreceptor
CD119 GR20, 2E2 **IFN-γ Receptor α chain**	*Ifnar*	IFN-γ Receptor 85-95 kDa CKR	IFN-γ		Immunoregulation; receptor/coreceptor
CD120a 55R-170, 55R-593, 55R-286 **TNFR1, TNF-R55**	*Tnfrsf1a*	 55-60 kDa TNFR	TNF; LT-α3 (*aka* TNF-β)		Signal transduction; apoptosis; receptor/coreceptor
CD120b TR75-32, TR75-54, TR75-89 **TNFR2, TNF-R75**	*Tnfrsf1b*	 75-80 kDa TNFR	TNF; LT-α3 (*aka* TNF-β)		Signal transduction; apoptosis; necrosis; receptor/coreceptor

A I

Antigen — Clones offered by BD Biosciences — Alternate names of antigen	Gene	Component of — Molecular Weight — Family/Superfamily	Ligands/Substrates	Antigen Distribution	Functions of Antigens
CD121a — 35F5, 12A6, JAMA-147 — **IL-1 Receptor, Type I**	*Il1r1*	— / 80 kDa / Ig	IL-1α; IL-1β		Signal transduction; activation/costimulation; receptor/coreceptor
CD121b — 1F6, 4E2 — **IL-1 Receptor, Type II**	*Il1r2*	— / 60 kDa / Ig	IL-1α; IL-1β		Immunoregulation; receptor/coreceptor
CD122 — TM-β1, 5H4 — **IL-2 and IL-15 Receptor β chain**	*Il2rb*	IL-2 and IL-15 receptors / 85-100 kDa / CKR	IL-2; IL-15		Signal transduction; immunoregulation; receptor/coreceptor
CD123 — 5B11 — **IL-3 Receptor α chain**	*Il3ra*	IL-3 receptor / 60-70 kDa / CKR	IL-3		Differentiation/development?; receptor/coreceptor
CD124 — mIL4R-M1 — **IL-4 Receptor α chain**	*Il4ra*	IL-4 and IL-3 receptors / 138-145 kDa / CKR	IL-4; IL-13		Signal transduction; receptor/coreceptor
CD125 — **IL-5 Receptor α chain**	*Il5ra*	IL-5 receptor / 60 kDa / CKR	IL-5		Activation/costimulation; immunoregulation?; receptor/coreceptor
CD126 — D7715A7 — **IL-6 Receptor α chain**	*Il6ra*	IL-6 receptor / 80 kDa / CKR, Ig	IL-6		Differentiation/development; immunoregulation; receptor/coreceptor
CD127 — B12-1, SB/14 — **IL-7 Receptor α chain**	*Il7r*	IL-7 receptor / 65-75 kDa / CKR	IL-7		Signal transduction; differentiation/development; receptor/coreceptor
CD128 — **IL-8 Receptor α chain, CXCR2**	*Cmkar2*	— / — / α-chemokine receptor	MIP2; KC; (human IL-8)		Activation/costimulation; receptor/coreceptor
CD130 — **gp 130, Common β chain**	*Il6st*	IL-11, OSM, CNTF & LIF receptors / 130 kDa / CKR			Signal transduction
CD131 — JORO50 — **AIC2A & AIC2B, β$_{IL-2}$ and β$_C$**	*Csf2rb1* and *Csf2rb2*	IL-3, IL-5, & GM-CSF receptors / 110-120 kDa(AIC2A); 120-140 kDa(AIC2B) / CKR	IL-3 (for AIC2A)		Signal transduction; receptor/coreceptor
CD132 — 4G3, 3E12, TUGm2 — **Common γ chain**	*Il2rg*	IL-2, IL-4, IL-7, IL-9 and IL-15 receptors / — / CKR			Signal transduction
CD133 — **AC133, Prominin**	*Prom*	— / — / 5-TM			
CD134 — OX-86 — Ly-70, OX-40 antigen, **ACT35 antigen**	*Tnfrsf4*	— / 50 kDa / TNFR	OX-40 Ligand		Activation/costimulation

Antigen Clones offered by BD Biosciences **Alternate names of antigen**	*Gene*	Component of Molecular Weight Family/Superfamily	Ligands/ Substrates	Antigen Distribution	Functions of Antigens
CD135 A2F10.1 **Flk-2, Flt3, Ly-72**	*Flt3*	135-150 kDa Ig, RTK	flt3 Ligand		Differentiation/ development; receptor/coreceptor
CD137 1AH2 (*aka* 53A2) **4-1BB, Ly-63**	*Tnfrsf9*	30 kDa (monomer); 55 kDa (dimer); or 110 kDa (tetramer) TNFR	4-1BBL; fibronectin; laminin; vitronectin; collagen IV		Antigen presentation; signal transduction; activation/costimulation; adhesion
CD138 281-2 **Syndecan-1**	*Sdc1*	31 kDa core protein Glycosaminoglycan	Interstitial matrix proteins		Adhesion
CD140a APA5 **PDGF Receptor α chain, PDGFR-a**	*Pdgfra*	PDGF receptor homodimer and heterodimer 180 kDa CKR, RTK	PDGF A Chain; PDGF B Chain		Signal transduction; differentiation/ development; receptor/coreceptor
CD140b 28 **PDGF Receptor β chain, PDGFR-b**	*Pdgfrb*	PDGF receptor homodimer and heterodimer 180 kDa CKR, RTK	PDGF B Chain		Signal transduction; differentiation/ development; receptor/coreceptor; chemotaxis
CD141 **Thrombomodulin**	*Thbd*	C-type lectin	Thrombin		Hemostasis
CD142 **Tissue Factor, Coagulation Factor III**	*F3*	Serine protease cofactor	Plasma factor VII/VIIa		Differentiation/ development?; hemostasis; angiogenesis
CD143 **Angiotensin coverting enzyme, dipeptidyl peptidase**	*Ace*	Peptidylpeptidase	Angiotensin I		Enzymatic activity
CD144 11D4.1 **VE-Cadherin**	*Cdh5*	125 kDa Cadherin	Cd 144		Adhesion; angiogenesis
CD146	*Mcam*	Ig			Adhesion
CD147 **Basigin, HT7, neurothelin, gp42**	*Bsg*	Ig			Adhesion
CD148 **PTPβ2, ByP**	*Ptprj*	FNIII, PTP			Signal transduction
CD150 **IPO-3**	*Slam*	Ig			Signal transduction
CD151 **SFA-1, PETA-3**	*Cd151*	TM4			Hemostasis?

A I

Antigen Clones offered by BD Biosciences Alternate names of antigen	Gene	Component of Molecular Weight Family/Superfamily			Ligands/ Substrates	Antigen Distribution	Functions of Antigens
CD152 9H10, UC10-4F10-11 **CTLA-4, Ly-56**	Cd152		33-37 kDa	Ig	CD80; CD86		Immunoregulation
CD153 RM153 **CD30 Ligand**	Tnfsf8		40 kDa	TNF	CD30		Activation/costimulation; immunoregulation
CD154 MR1 **gp39, CD40 Ligand, Ly-62**	Tnfsf5		39 kDa	TNF	CD40		Activation/costimulation
CD156a MS2, ADAM 8	Adam8		89 kDa	Metalloproteinase			Adhesion; enzymatic activity
CD156q TACE, ADAM17	Adam17		130 kDa	Metalloproteinase	TNF-α; APP; CD62L		Adhesion; enzymatic activity; receptor/coreceptor
CD157 Ly-65, Bp-3, BST-1	Bst1		38-48 kDa	ADP-ribosylcyclase			Adhesion?
CD159a 20d5 **NKG2A, NKG2B**	Klrc1	Cd94/NKG2 heterodimers	38 kDa	C-type lectin	Qa-1/Qdm		Antigen recognition; signal transduction
CD160 BY55	Cd160			Ig			
CD161a NKR-P1A	Ly55a						
CD161b PK136 NKR-P1B	Ly55b		81 kDa	C-type lectin			
CD161c PK136 **NKR-P1C, NK-1.1, Ly-55**	Ly55c		76-80 kDa	C-type lectin			Activation/costimulation
CD162 2PH1 P-selectin-IgG fusion protein **P-selectin glycoprotein Ligand (PSGL-1)**	Selpl		160 kDa	Sialomucin	CD62P		Adhesion
CD163	Cd163			SRCR			
CD164 MGC-24, A115, A24	Cd164						Adhesion
CD166 ALCAM, DM-GRASP	Alcam		120 kDa	Ig	CD6		Activation/costimulation; adhesion; differentiation/development?

Antigen Clones offered by BD Biosciences **Alternate names of antigen**	*Gene*	Component of Molecular Weight Family/Superfamily	Ligands/ Substrates	Antigen Distribution	Functions of Antigens
CD167a **Cak, Nep**	*Ddr1*	 RTK			Adhesion
CD168 **RHAMM**	*Hmmr*	 			Adhesion
CD169 **Sialoadhesin, Siglec-1**	*sn*	 Siglec	CD43; CD162		Adhesion
CD170 **Siglec-5**	*Siglec5*	 Siglec			Adhesion
CD171 17 **L1**	*L1cam*	 			Adhesion
CD172a P84 **SIRPα, SHPS-1, BIT, P84** **Antigen**	*Ptpns1*	 77, 86 kDa Ig	CD47		Signal transduction; adhesion
CD178 MFL3, MFL4, 33 **CD95L, Fas Ligand**	*Tnfsf6*	 TNF	CD95		Signal transduction; activation/costimulation; differentiation/development; apoptosis; cytotoxicity?
CD178.1 Kay-10 **mFasL. 1**	*Tnfsf6*	 TNF	CD95		Signal transduction; activation/costimulation; differentiation/development; apoptosis; cytotoxicity?
CD179a **VpreB**	*Vpreb1*	Pre-B cell receptor 16 kDa Ig			Differentiation/ development
CD179b LM34 **λ5**	*Vpreb2*	Pre-B cell receptor 22 kDa Ig			Differentiation/ development
CD180 RP/14 **RP105**	*Ly78*	RP105/MD-1 complex 105 kDa Leucine-rich repeat			Signal transduction
CD183 **CXCR3**	*Cmkar3*	 Chemokine receptor	IP-10; 6Ckine; Mig; I-TAC		Receptor/coreceptor; chemotaxis
CD184 2B11/CXCR4 **CXCR4**	*Cmkar4*	 Chemokine receptor	SDF-1		Receptor/coreceptor; chemotaxis
CD195 C34-3448 **CCR5**	*Cmkbr5*	 Chemokine receptor	MIP-1α; MIP-1β; RANTES; MCP-1		Receptor/coreceptor; chemotaxis
CD197 **CCR7**	*Cmkbr7*	 Chemokine receptor	SLC		Receptor/coreceptor; chemotaxis

A I

Antigen (Clones offered by BD Biosciences / Alternate names of antigen)	Gene	Component of	Molecular Weight	Family/Superfamily	Ligands/Substrates	Antigen Distribution	Functions of Antigens
CD200 — OX-90, OX-2 Ag	Mox2			Ig	CD200 receptor		Immunoregulation
CD201 — CCD41, EPCR, Protein C Receptor	Procr			CD1/MHC	Protein C		Receptor/coreceptor; hemostasis
CD202 — 33, Endothelial-specific receptor tyrosine kinase, Tie2	Tek			RTK			Differentiation/development
CD203c — Ly-41, PC-1	Enpp1		220 kDa	E-NPP	Extracellular nucleotides		Enzymatic activity
CD204 — Macrophage scavenger receptor	Scvr			Class A scavenger receptor	LPS; collagen; LDL?		Adhesion
CD205 — DEC-205, Ly-75	Ly75		205 kDa	C-type lectin			Antigen presentation
CD206 — Macrophage mannose receptor	Mrc1		175 kDa	C-type lectin	High-mannose carbohydrates		Antigen presentation
CD210 — 1B1.3a, IL-10 receptor, CRF2-4	Il10ra, Il10rb			CKR	IL-10		Immunoregulation; receptor/coreceptor
CD212 — 114, IL-12R β chain	Il12rb1	IL-12 receptor		CKR	IL-12		Immunoregulation; receptor/coreceptor
CD213a1 — NR4, IL-13R α1 chain	Il13ra1	IL-13 and IL-4 receptors		CKR	IL-13		Immunoregulation; receptor/coreceptor
CD213a2 — IL-13R α2 chain	Il13ra2	IL-13 receptor		CKR	IL-13		Immunoregulation; receptor/coreceptor
CD217 — IL-17R	Il17r				IL-17; vIL-17		Immunoregulation; receptor/coreceptor
CD220 — 46, Polyclonal, Insulin receptor	Insr		130 kDa, 95 kDa	RTK	Insulin		Receptor/coreceptor; metabolism
CD221 — IGF-IR	Igf1r			RTK	IGF-I; Insulin		Receptor/coreceptor; metabolism
CD222 — IGF-IIR, CI-MP R	Igf2r		220-250 kDa	RTK	IGF-II; mannose-6-phosphate residues; retinopic acid; TGF-β LAP		Receptor/coreceptor; metabolism

A I

Antigen Clones offered by BD Biosciences Alternate names of antigen	Gene	Component of Molecular Weight Family/Superfamily		Ligands/ Substrates	Antigen Distribution	Functions of Antigens
CD223 C9B7W **Ly-66, LAG3**	*Lag3*		Ig	MHC class II		Immunoregulation
CD224 **γ-glutamyl transpeptidase**	*Ggtp*			Glutathione		Enzymatic activity
CD227 EMA	*Muc1*					
CD228 **MTf, p97**	*Mfi2*					
CD229 **Lgp 100, T100, Ly-9**	*Ly9*	100 kDa, 150 kDa	Cd2 Ig			
CD229.1 30C7 **Lgp100, Ly-9.1**	*Ly9ᵃ*	100 kDa	Cd2 Ig			
CD230 **Prion protein**	*prnp*					Differentiation/ development
CD231 **TALLA, A15**	*Tm4sf2*		TM4			
CD232 **Plexin C1, Vespr**	*plxnc1*		Plexin			
CD233 **AE1, band 3**	*slc4a1*		SLC			Metabolism
CD234 **Duffy blood group, DARC**	*Dfy*			Chemokines		Receptor/coreceptor; chemotaxis
CD235a **Glycophorin A**	*Gypa*					
CD236R **Glycophorin C**	*Gypc*					
CD238 **Kell blood group, endo-thelin-3-converting enzyme**	*Kel*	Kell/Kx antigen complex 110 kDa Neutral endopeptidase		big ET3		Enzymatic activity
CD239 **Lutheran blood group**	*Lu*		Ig	Laminin 10/11		Adhesion

A I

Antigen Clones offered by BD Biosciences Alternate names of antigen	Gene	Component of Molecular Weight Family/Superfamily	Ligands/ Substrates	Antigen Distribution	Functions of Antigens
CD240 **Rh30, Rh antigen**	*Rhced*	Rh blood group Rh			Metabolism
CD241 **Rh50, Rh-associated glycoprotein**	*Rhag*	Rh blood group 50 kDa Rh			Metabolism
CD243 **P-glycoprotein 1, Mdr1**	*Abcb*1	 ABC transporter, MDR/TAP	Drugs, dyes		Enzymatic activity; metabolism
CD244.2 2B4 **2B4 Antigen**	*Nmrk*[b]	 66 kDa CD2 Ig	CD48		Signal transduction
CD246 **Anaplastic lymphoma kinase**	*alk*	 RTK	Unknown		Enzymatic activity
CD247 1ζ3A1, 1η4F2, 8d3 **CD3z, CD3 ζ chain**	*Cd3z*	T-cell receptor 16, 21, 32, 42 kDa			Signal transduction

Appendix II

Complement Pathways

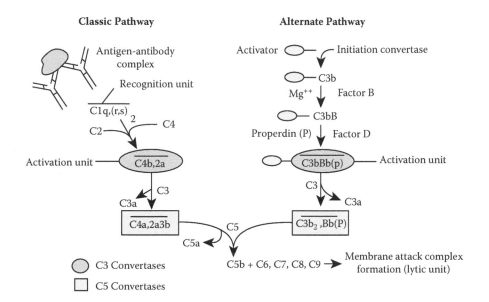

Classic Pathway

Antigen-antibody complex

Recognition unit

$\overline{C1q,(r,s)}_2$

C2 — C4

Activation unit — $\overline{C4b,2a}$

C3a C3

$\overline{C4a,2a3b}$

C5a

○ C3 Convertases

☐ C5 Convertases

Alternate Pathway

Activator ○— ↗ Initiation convertase

○— C3b

Mg^{++} ↓ Factor B

○— C3bB

Properdin (P) ↓ Factor D

○ $\overline{C3bBb(p)}$ — Activation unit

C3 C3a

$\overline{C3b_2,Bb(P)}$

C5

C5b + C6, C7, C8, C9 → Membrane attack complex formation (lytic unit)

Appendix III

Cytokines and Their Receptors

Appendix III. Cytokines and their receptors.						
Family	Cytokine (alternative names)	Size (no. of amino acids and form)	Receptors (c denotes common subunit)	Producer cells	Actions	Effect of cytokine or receptor knock-out (where known)
Colony-stimulating factors	G-CSF	174, monomer*	G-CSFR	Fibroblasts and monocytes	Stimulates neutrophil development and differentiation	G-CSF, G-CSFR: defective neutrophil production and mobilization
	GM-CSF (granulocyte macrophage colony stimulating factor)	127, monomer*	CD116, βc	Macrophages, T cells	Stimulates growth and differentiation of myelomonocytic lineage cells, particularly dendritic cells	GM-CSF, GM-CSFR: pulmonary alveolar proteinosis
	M-CSF (CSF-1)	α: 224 active β: 492 forms are γ: 406 homo- or heterodimeric	CSF-1R (c-fms)	T cells, bone marrow stromal cells, osteoblasts	Stimulates growth of cells of monocytic lineage	Osteopetrosis
Interferons	IFN-α (at least 12 distinct proteins)	166, monomer	CD118, IFNAR2	Leukocytes, dendritic cells	Antiviral, increased MHC class I expression	CD118: impaired antiviral activity
	IFN-β	166, monomer	CD118, IFNAR2	Fibroblasts	Antiviral, increased MHC class I expression	IFN-β: increased susceptibility to certain viruses
	IFN-γ	143, homodimer	CD119, IFNGR2	T cells, natural killer cells	Macrophage activation, increased expression of MHC molecules and antigen processing components, Ig class switching, supresses T_H2	IFN-γ, CD119: decreased resistance to bacterial infection and tumors
Interleukins	IL-1-α	159, monomer	CD121a (IL-1RI) and CD121b (IL-1RII)	Macrophages, epithelial cells	Fever, T-cell activation, macrophage activation	IL-1RI: decreased IL-6 production
	IL-1β	153, monomer	CD121a (IL-1RI) and CD121b (IL-1RII)	Macrophages, epithelial cells	Fever, T-cell activation, macrophage activation	IL-1β: impaired acute-phase response
	IL-1 RA	152, monomer	CD121a	Monocytes, macrophages, neutrophils, hepatocytes	Binds to but doesn't trigger IL-1 receptor, acts as a natural antagonist of IL-1 function	IL-1RA: reduced body mass, increased sensitivity to endotoxins (septic shock)
	IL-2 (T-cell growth factor)	133, monomer	CD25α, CD122β, CD132 (γc)	T cells	T-cell proliferation	IL-2: deregulated T-cell proliferation, colitis IL-2Rα: incomplete T-cell development autoimmunity IL-2Rβ: increased T-cell autoimmunity IL-2Rγc: severe combined immunodeficiency
	IL-3 (multicolony CSF)	133, monomer	CD123, βc	T cells, thymic epithelial cells	Synergistic action in early hematopoiesis	IL-3: impaired eosinophil development. Bone marrow unresponsive to IL-5, GM-CSF
	IL-4 (BCGF-1, BSF-1)	129, monomer	CD124, CD132 (γc)	T cells, mast cells	B-cell activation, IgE switch, induces differentiation into T_H2 cells	IL-4: decreased IgE synthesis
	IL-5 (BCGF-2)	115, homodimer	CD125, βc	T cells, mast cells	Eosinophil growth, differentiation	IL-5: decreased IgE, IgG1 synthesis (in mice); decreased levels of IL-9, IL-10, and eosinophils
	IL-6 (IFN-β2, BSF-2, BCDF)	184, monomer	CD126, CD130	T cells, macrophages, endothelial cells	T- and B-cell growth and differentiation, acute phase protein production, fever	IL-6: decreased acute phase reaction, reduced IgA production
	IL-7	152, monomer*	CD127, CD132 (γc)	Non-T cells	Growth of pre-B cells and pre-T cells	IL-7: early thymic and lymphocyte expansion severely impaired

*May function as dimers

Family	Cytokine (alternative names)	Size (no. of amino acids) and form	Receptors (c denotes common subunit)	Producer cells	Actions	Effect of cytokine or receptor knock-out (where known)
	IL-9	125, monomer	IL-9R, CD132 (γc)	T cells	Mast-cell enhancing activity, stimulates T$_H$2	Defects in mast-cell expansion
	IL-10 (cytokine synthesis inhibitory factor)	160, homodimer	IL-10Rα, IL-10Rβc (CRF2-4, IL-10R2)	Monocytes	Potent suppressant of macrophage functions	IL-10 and IL20Rβc-: reduced growth, anemia, chronic enterocolitis
	IL-11	178, monomer	IL-11R, CD130	Stromal fibroblasts	Synergistic action with IL-3 and IL-4 in hematopoiesis	IL-11R: defective decidualization
	IL-12 (NK-cell stimulatory factor)	197 (p35) and 306 (p40c), heterodimer	IL-12Rβ1c +IL-12Rβ2	Macrophages, dendritic cells	Activates NK cells, induces CD4 T-cell differentiation into T$_H$1-like cells	IL-12: impaired IFN-γ production and T$_H$1 responses
	IL-13 (p600)	132, monomer	IL-13R, CD132 (γc) (may also include CD24)	T cells	B-cell growth and differentiation, inhibits macrophage inflammatory cytokine production and T$_H$1 cells, induces allergy/asthma	IL-13: defective regulation of isotype specific responses
	IL-15 (T-cell growth factor)	114, monomer	IL-15Rα, CD122 (IL-2Rβ) CD132 (γc)	Many non-T cells	IL-2-like, stimulates growth of intestinal epithelium, T cells, and NK cells, enhances CD8 memory T cell survival	IL-15: reduced numbers of NK cells and memory phenotype CD8+ T cells IL-15Ra: lymphopenia
	IL-16	130, homotetramer	CD4	T cells, mast cells, eosinophils	Chemoattractant for CD4 T cells, monocytes, and eosinophils, anti-apoptotic for IL-2-stimulated T cells	
	IL-17A (mCTLA-8)	150, homodimer	IL-17AR (CD217)	Th17, CD8 T cells, NK cells, γδ T cells, neutrophils	Induces cytokine production by epithelia, endothelia, and fibroblasts, proinflammatory	IL-17R: reduced neutrophil migration into infected sites
	IL-17F (ML-1)	134, homodimer	IL-17AR (CD217)	Th17, CD8 T cells, NK cells, γδ T cells, neutrophils	Induces cytokine production by epithelia, endothelia, and fibroblasts, proinflammatory	
	IL-18 (IGIF, interferon-α inducing factor)	157, monomer	IL-1Rrp (IL-1R related protein)	Activated macrophages and Kupffer cells	Induces IFN-γ production by T cells and NK cells, promotes T$_H$1 induction	Defective NK activity and TH1 responses
	IL-19	153, monomer	IL-20Rα +IL-10Rβc	Monocytes	Induces IL-6 and TNF-α expression by monocytes	
	IL-20	152	IL-20Rα +ILa10Rβc; IL-22Rαc +IL-10Rβc	TH1 cells	Stimulates keratinocyte proliferation and TNF-α production	
	IL-21	133	IL-21R, +CD132(γc)	TH2 cells	Induces proliferation of B, T and NK cells	Increased IgE production
	IL-22 (IL-TIF)	146	IL-22Rαc+ IL-10Rβc	NK cells	Induces liver acute-phase proteins, pro-inflammatory agents	
	IL-23	170 (p19) and 306 (p40c), heterodimer	IL-12Rβ1 +IL-23R	Dendritic cells	Induces proliferation of memory T cells, increased IFN-γ production	Defective inflammation
	IL-24 (MDA-7)	157	IL-22Rαc +IL-10Rβc; IL-20Rα+ IL-10Rβc	Monocytes, T cells	Inhibits tumor growth	
	IL-25 (IL-17E)	145	IL-17BR (IL-17Rh1)	TH2 cells, mast cells	Promotes T$_H$2 cytokine production	Defective T$_H$2 response
	IL-26(AK155)	150	IL-20Rα +IL-10Rβc	T cells (type 1), NK cells		
	IL-27	142 (p28) and 209 (EBI3), heterodimer	WSX-1 +CD130c	Monocytes, macrophages, dendritic cells	Induces IL-12R on T cells via T-bet induction	EBI3: reduced NKT cells. WSX-1: overreaction to *Toxoplasma gondii* infection and death from inflammation

Family	Cytokine (alternative names)	Size (no. of amino acids) and form	Receptors (c denotes common subunit)	Producer cells	Actions	Effect of cytokine or receptor knock-out (where known)
	IL-28A,B (IFN-λ2,3)	175	IL-28Rαc +IL-10Rβc		Antiviral	
	IL-29 (IFN-λ1)	181	IL-28Rαc +IL-10Rβc		Antiviral	
	LIF (leukemia inhibitory factor)	179, monomer	LIFR, CD130	Bone marrow stroma, fibroblasts	Maintains embryonic stem cells, like IL-6, IL-11, OSM	LIFR: die at or soon after birth; decreased hematopoietic stem cells
	OSM (OM, oncostatin M)	196, monomer	OSMR or LIFR, CD130	T cells, macrophages	Stimulates Kaposi's sarcoma cells, inhibits melanoma growth	OSMR: defective liver regeneration
TNF family	TNFα· (cachectin)	157, trimers	p55 (CD120a), p75 (CD120b)	Macrophages, NK cells, T cells	Promotes inflammation, endothelial activation	p55: resistance to septic shock, susceptibility to *Listeria*, STNFαR: periodic febrile attacks
	LT-α (lymphotoxin-α)	171, trimers	p55 (CD120a), p75 (CD120b)	T cells, B cells	Killing, endothelial activation	TNF-β: absent lymph nodes, decreased antibody, increased IgM
	LT-β	Transmembrane, trimerizes with LT-α	LTβR or HVEM	T cells, B cells	Lymph node development	Defective development of peripheral lymph nodes, Peyer's patches, and spleen
	CD40 ligand (CD40L)	Trimers	CD40	T cells, mast cells	B-cell activation, class switching	CD40L: poor antibody response, no class switching, diminished T+cell priming (hyper IgM syndrome)
	Fas ligand (FasL)	Trimers	CD95 (Fas)	T cells, stroma(?)	Apoptosis, Ca^{2+}-independent cytotoxicity	Fas, FasL: mutant forms lead to lymphoproliferation, and autoimmunity
	CD27 ligand (CD27L)	Trimers (?)	CD27	T cells	Stimulates T-cell proliferation	
	CD30 ligand (CD30L)	Trimers (?)	CD30	T cells	Stimulates T- and B-cell proliferation	CD30: increased thymic size, alloreactivity
	4-1BBL	Trimers (?)	4-1BB	T cells	Co-stimulates T and B cells	
	Trail (AP0-2L)	281, trimers	DR4, DR5 DCR1, DCR2 and OPG	T cells, monocytes	Apoptosis of activated T cells and tumor cells	tumor-prone phenotype
	OPG-L (RANK-L)	316, trimers	RANK/OPG	Osteoblasts, T cells	Stimulates osteoclasts and bone resorption	OPG-L: osteopetrotic, runted, toothless OPG: osteoporosis
	APRIL	86	TAC1 or BCMA	Activated T cells	B-cell proliferation	Impaired IgA-class switching
	LIGHT	240	HVEM, LT,R	T cells	Dendritic cell activation	Defective CD8+ T-cell expansion
	TWEAK	102	TWEAKR (Fn14)	macrophages, EBV transformed cells	Angiogenesis	
	BAFF (CD257, BlyS)	153	TAC1 or BCMA or BR3	B cells	B-cell proliferation	BAFF: B-cell dysfunction
Unassigned	TGFβ1	112, homo- and heterotrimers	TGFβR	Chondrocytes, monocytes, T cells	Inhibits cell growth, anti-inflammatory, induces switch to IgA production	TGF-β: lethal inflammation
	MIF	115, monomer	MIF-R	T cells, pituitary cells	Inhibits macrophage migration, stimulates macrophage activation, induces steroid resistance	MIF: resistance to septic shock, hyporesponsive to Gram-negative bacteria

Appendix IV

Chemokines and Their Receptors

Appendix IV. Chemokines and their receptors.				
Chemokine systematic name	**Common names**	**Chromosome**	**Target cell**	**Specific receptor**
CXCL (†ELR⁺)				
1	GROα	4	Neutrophil, fibroblast, melanoma cell	CXCR2
2	GROβ	4	Neutrophil, fibroblast, melanoma cell	CXCR2
3	GROγ	4	Neutrophil, fibroblast, melanoma cell	CXCR2
5	ENA-78	4	Neutrophil, endothelial cell	CXCR2>>1
6	GCP-2	4	Neutrophil, endothelial cell	CXCR2>1
7	NAP-2 (PBP/CTAP-IIIβ-B44TG)	4	Fibroblast, neutrophil, endothelial cell	CXCR2
8	IL-8	4	Neutrophil, basophil, CD8, T cell subset, endothelial cell	CXCR1, 2
14	BRAK/bolekine	5	T cell, monocyte, B cell	Unknown
15	Lungkine/WECHE	5	Neutrophil, epithelial cell, endothelial cell	Unknown
(†ELR⁻)				
4	PF4	4	Fibroblast, endothelial cell	CXCR3B (alternative splice)
9	Mig	4	Activated T cell ($T_H1 > T_H2$), natural killer cell, B cell, endothelial cell, plasmacytoid dendritic cell	CXCR3A and B
10	IP-10	4	Activated T cell ($T_H1 > T_H2$), natural killer cell, B cell, endothelial cell	CXCR3A and B
11	I-TAC	4	Activated T cell ($T_H1 > T_H2$), natural killer cell, B cell, endothelial cell	CXCR3A and B, CXCR7
12	SDF-1α/β	10	CD34+ bone marrow cell, thymocytes, monocytes/macrophages, naive activated T cell, B cell, plasma cell, neutrophil immature dendritic cells, mature dendritic cells, plasmacytoid dendritic cells	CXCR4, CXCR7
13	BLC/BCA-1	4	Naive B cells, activated CD4 T cells, immature dendritic cells, mature dendritic cells	CXCR5>>CXCR3
16	(None)	17	Activated T cell, natural killer T cell, endothelial cells	CXCR6
CCL				
1	I-309	17	Neutrophil (TCA-3 only), T cell, monocyte	CCR8
2	MCP-1	17	T cell, monocyte, basophil, immature dendritic cells, natural killer cells	CCR2
3	MIP-1α	17	Monocyte/macrophage, T cell ($T_H1 > T_H2$), natural killer cell, basophil, immature dendritic cell, eosinophil, neutrophil, astrocyte, fibroblast, osteoclast	CCR1, 5
4	MIP-1β	17	Monocyte/macrophage, T cell ($T_H1 > T_H2$), natural killer cell, basophil, immature dendritic cell, eosinophil, B cell	CCR5>>1
5	RANTES	17	Monocyte/macrophage, T cell (memory T cell > T cell; $T_H1 > T_H2$), natural killer cell, basophil, eosinophil, immature dendritic cell	CCR1, 3, 5
6	C10/MRP-1	11 (mouse only)	Monocyte, B cell, CD4⁺ T cell, natural killer cell	CCR 1
7	MCP-3	17	T cell, monocyte, eosinophil, basophil, immature dendritic cell, natural killer cell	CCR1, 2, 3, 5, 10
8	MCP-2	17	T cell, monocyte, eosinophil, basophil, immature dendritic cell, natural killer cell	CCR2, 3, 5>1
9	MRP-2/MIP-1γ	11 (mouse only)	T cell, monocyte, adipocyte	CCR1
11	Eotaxin	17	Eosinophil, basophil, T_H2 cell	CCR3>>CCR5
12	MCP-5	11 (mouse only)	Eosinophil, monocyte, T cell, B cell	CCR2
13	MCP-4	17	T cell, monocyte, eosinophil, basophil, dendritic cell	CCR1, 2, 3>5
14a	HCC-1	17	Monocyte	CCR1, 5
14b	HCC-3	17	Monocyte	Unknown

Chemokine systematic name	Common names	Chromosome	Target cell	Specific receptor
15	MIP-5/HCC-2	17	T cell, monocyte, eosinophil, dendritic cell	CCR1, 3
16	HCC-4/LEC	17	Monocyte, T cell, natural killer cell, immature dendritic cell	CCR1, 2, 5
17	TARC	16	T cell ($T_H2 > T_H1$), immature dendritic cells, thymocyte, regulatory T cell	CCR4>>8
18	DC-CK1/PARC	17	Naive T cell > activated T cell, immature dendritic cells, mantle zone B cells	Unknown
19	MIP-3β/ELC	9	Naive T cell, mature dendritic cell, B cell	CCR7
20	MIP-3α/LARC	2	T cell (memory T cell > T cell), peripheral blood mononuclear cell, immature dendritic cell, activated B cells, natural killer T cells	CCR6
21	6Ckine/SLC	9	Naive T cell, B cell, thymocytes, natural killer cell, mature dendritic cells	CCR7
22	MDC	16	Immature dendritic cell, natural killer cell, T cell ($T_H2 > T_H1$), thymocyte, endothelial cells, monocyte, regulatory T cell	CCR4
23	MPIF-1/CK-β\8	17	Monocyte, T cell, resting neutrophil	CCR1, 5
24	Eotaxin-2/MPIF-2	7	Eosinophil, basophil, T cell	CCR3
25	TECK	19	Macrophage, thymocytes, dendritic cell, intraepithelial lymphocyte, IgA+ plasma cell D118	CCR9
26	Eotaxin-3	7	Eosinophil, basophil, fibroblast	CCR3
27	CTACK	9	Skin homing memory T cell, B cell	CCR10
28	MEC	5	T cell, eosinophil, IgA+B cell	CCR10>3
C and CX3C				
XCL 1	Lymphotactin	1 (1)	T cell, natural killer cell	XCR1
XCL 2	SCM-1β	1	T cell, natural killer cell	XCR1
CX3CL 1	Fractalkine	16	Activated T cell, monocyte, neutrophil, natural killer cell, immature dendtritic cells, mast cells, astrocytes, neurons	CX3CR1

Chromosome locations are for humans. Chemokines for which there is no human homolog are listed with the mouse chromosome.

† ELR refers to the three amino acids that precede the first cysteine residue of the CXC motif. If these amino acids are Glu-Leu-Arg (ie ELR+), then the chemokine is chemotactic for neutrophils; if they are not (ELR–) then the chemokine is chemotactic for lymphocytes.

Appendix V

Human Leukocyte Differentiation Antigens

CD	Gene Locus	Epithelial Cell	Endothelial Cell	Erythrocyte	Platelet	Granulocyte	Macrophage/Monocyte	Stem Cell/Precursor	NK Cell	Dendritic Cell	B Cell	T Cell	MW (kDa)	Description and Function	Ligand/receptor/substrate/associated molecule	HLDA Section	Alternative Name	CD
CD1a	1q22-q23			–	–	–	⊕		–		⊕	⊕	49/–	Non-peptide antigen presenting molecules; involved in lymphocyte activation; related to thymic T-cell development.		T	R4	CD1a
CD1b	1q22-q23			–	–	–	⊕		–		⊕	⊕	45/–	Non-peptide antigen presenting molecules; involved in lymphocyte activation; related to thymic T-cell development.		T	R1	CD1b
CD1c	1q22-q23			–	–	–	⊕		–		+	⊕	43/–	Non-peptide antigen presenting molecules; involved in lymphocyte activation; related to thymic T-cell development. Expressed by a subset of peripheral blood B cells.		T	M241, R7	CD1c
CD1d	1q22-q23	+c		–	–	–			–		+	⊕		Non-peptide antigen presenting molecules; involved in lymphocyte activation; related to thymic T-cell development.		T	R3	CD1d
CD1e	1q22-q23			–	–	–			–					Non-peptide antigen presenting molecules; involved in lymphocyte activation; related to thymic T-cell development.		T	R4	CD1e
CD2	1p13		–	–	–	–	–	–	+			+	50/–	Receptor for CD58, CD48, CD59 and CD15; adhesion and signal-transducing molecule.		T	E-rosette R T11, LFA-2	CD2
CD3	11q23	–	–	–	–	–	–	–	+		–	+	20–26	Associated with T-cell receptor α/β or γ/δ dimer; signal transduction; assembly and expression of the T-cell receptor complex.		T	T3	CD3
CD4	12pter-p12	–	–	–	–	–	+	–	–		–	+	55	Co-receptor in antigen-induced T-cell activation; thymic differentiation; regulation of T-B lymphocyte adhesion; primary receptor for HIV; binds to MHC class II. Also expressed in peripheral blood monocytes, tissue macrophages, granulocytes.	MHC Class II, gp120,IL-16	T	L3T4, W3/25	CD4
CD5	11q13			–	–	–	–		–		+	+	58/67	Co-stimulatory molecule; receptor for constitutive (CD72) and inducible (gp35-37) B-cell specific molecules.	CD72,BCR, gp35-37	T	T1, Tp67, Leu-1	CD5
CD6	11q13			–	–	–	–		–		+	+	–/105-130	Adhesion molecule. In thymocyte resistance to apoptosis and in positive selection; important in T mature cell response to both alloantigen and self-antigen.	CD166	T	T12	CD6
CD7	17q25.2-q25.3	–	–	–	–	–	–	+	+		–	+	40	Possible co-activation/adhesion modulating molecule.		T	gp40	CD7
CD8α	2p12	–	–	–	–	–	–	+	+		–	+	68/30–34	Co-receptor molecule; binds to MHC class I.	MHC I, Lck	T	Leu2, T8	CD8α
CD8β	2p12	–	–	–	–	–	–	–	–		–	+		Co-receptor molecule; binds to MHC class I.		T	CD8, Leu2, Lyt3	CD8β
CD9	2p13	+	+	–	+	+	+	+	–	+	+	⊕	/24,26	Modulates cell adhesion and migration; triggers platelet activation; expressed on eosinophils and basophils.	CD63, CD81,CD82	Platelet	p24, DRAP-1, MRP-1	CD9
CD10	3q25.1-q25.2	+	–	–	–	–	+	+	+	+	+	+	100/–	Zinc Metalloprotease; neutral endopeptidase; regulator of B-cell growth and proliferation by hydrolysis of peptides with proliferative/anti-proliferative effects.		B	CALLA, NEP, gp100	CD10
CD11a	16p11.2		–	–	–	+	+		+		+	+	170/180	Intracellular adhesion and co-stimulation; binds to ICAM-1, ICAM-2, ICAM-3; expressed on eosinophils and basophils.	ICAM-1,2,3	Adhesion structure	LFA-1a Integrin αL	CD11a
CD11b	16p11.2			–	–	+	+		+		+	+	165/170	Adherence of polymorphonuclear neutrophils and monocytes to fibrinogen, iCAM-1 endothelium; extravasation; chemotaxis; apoptosis.	iC3b, Fibrinogen	Adhesion structure	Integrin αM Mac-1a	CD11b
CD11c	16p11.2		–	–	–	+	+		+		+	+	145/150	Adherence of polymorphonuclear neutrophils and monocytes to fibrinogen, iCAM-1 endothelium; binds iC3b-coated particles.	iC3b	Adhesion structure	Integrin αX, p150:95a	CD11c
CDw12				–	–	+	+	–	+			–	150-160/120	Function unknown.		Myeloid	p90-120	CDw12

CD	Chromosome					Expression						MW (kDa)	Function	Ligand / CD	Family	Other names
CD13	15q25-q26	+	+	–	–	+	+	+	–	–	–	–	150/–	Acts as receptor for coronavirus which causes upper respiratory tract infections; involved in interactions between human CMV and target cells; CD13 auto-Ab associated with GVHD.	APN, Gp150	Myeloid	APN, Gp150
CD14	5q31.1	+	+	–	–	+	+	–	–	–	–	–	53/55	Receptor for lipopolysaccharide (endotoxin).	LPS	Myeloid	LPS-R
CD15		–	–	–	–	+	+	–	–	–	–	–		May be important for direct carbohydrate-carbohydrate interactions.		Carbohydrate	X-hapten, Lewis X
CD15s		–	+	–	+	+	+	+	+	+	⊕	+		Expressed on myelomonocytic leukemia, some lyphocytic leukemia cells and on adenocarcinomas.	CD62 selectin	Carbohydrate and Lectin	Sialyl Lewis X
CD15u		+	+	–	+	+	+	+	–	+	⊕	+		CD15 subgroups involved with different carbohydrate to carbohydrate cell adhesion.	E-selectins	Carbohydrate and Lectin	3' sulpho Lewis X
CD15su		+	+	–	+	+	+	+	+	+	⊕	+		CD15 subgroups involved with different carbohydrate to carbohydrate cell adhesion.	P-selectins	Carbohydrate and Lectin	6 sulpho-sialyl Lewis X
CD16	50-65/–	–	+	–	+	+	+	+	+	–	–	–	50-65/–	Low affinity receptor for IgG. Major histocompatibility complex.	L-selectins	NK	FcγRIIIa
CD16b	N/A	+	+	–	+	+	+	–	–	+	+	+	N/A	Function unknown.	Fc	NK	FcγRIIIb
CDw17	150-160/120				+				+	+	+	+	150-160/120	Possible role in phagocytosis. Expressed in basophils.	Fc	Myeloid	None
CD18	21q22.3	+	–	–	+	+	+	–	+	+	+	+	90/95	Leukocyte adhesion.	CD11a,b,c	Adhesion structure	Integrin β2
CD19	16p11.2	–	–	–	–	–	–	+	+	+	+	–	90	A critical signal transduction molecule that regulates B lymphocyte development, activation and differentiation.	CD2,CD81, CD225	B	B4
CD20	11q12-q13.1	–	–	–	–	–	–	–	+	+	+	+	37/35	Regulation of B lymphocyte activation and proliferation by regulating transmembrane Ca2+ conductance and cell cycle progression.		B	B1, Bp35
CD21	1q32	+	+	–	–	–	–	+	+	–	+	–	130-145	Receptor for EBV and C3d, C3dg and iC3b; subset of immature thymocytes; CD21 is part of a large signal transduction complex that also involves CD19, CD81 and Leu1.	C3d,CD23, CD19,CD81	B	CR2, EBV-R, C3dR
CD22	19q13.1	–	–	–	+	–	–	+	–	–	+	–	135	Adhesion molecule; signaling molecule; antibody treatment of leukemia and lymphoma.	p72syk,p53/56lyn,SHP1	B	Bl-CAM, Lyb8
CD23	19p13.3	–	–	–	–	–	–	+	–	–	+	–	50-45	Low affinity IgE receptor; regulates IgE synthesis; triggers monokine release; serum soluble CD23 level is a significant prognostic marker in CLL.	IgE, CD21, CD11b,CD11c	B	FcRII, B6, BLAST-2
CD24	6q21	+	+	–	+	–	–	+	–	–	+	–	41/38	Function unknown; homologous to mouse heat stable antigen; P-selectin on human carcinomas is involved in carcinoma binding to platelets.	P-selectin	B	BBA-1, HSA
CD25	10p15-p14	–	–	–	–	+	+	–	+	⊕	+	+	55	IL-2 receptor α chain; associated with CD122 and CD132.	IL-2	CK/CKR	Tac antigen, IL-2Rα
CD26	2q24.3	+	–	–	–	–	–	–	+	+	+	+	120	Co-stimulatory molecule in T cell activation; associated marker of auto-immune diseases, adenosine deaminase-deficiency and HIV pathogenesis.	Adenosine deaminase	T	DPP IV ectoenzyme
CD27	12p13	+	–	–	+	–	–	–	+	+	+	+	110-120	Mediates a co-stimulatory signal for T cell activation. Involved in murine T cell development.	CD70,TRAF5,TRAF2	T	T14, S152
CD28	2q33	–	–	–	–	–	–	–	–	–	+	+	90	Co-stimulates T cell proliferation and cytokine production with CD3; co-stimulates T cell effector function and T cell dependent antibody production.	CD80,CD86	T	Tp44, T44
CD29	10p11.2	+	–	–	+	+	+	+	+	+	+	+	110-130	Critical molecule for embryogenesis and development; essential to the differentiation of hematopoietic stem cells; associated with tumor progression and metastasis/invasion.	VCAM-1 and MAdCAM-1	Adhesion structure	Platelet GPIIa, β-1 integrin
CD30	1p36	–	–	–	+	+	–	–	+	⊕	⊕	⊕	120	Member of TNFR family, involved in negative selection of T cells in thymus and TCR mediated cell death; expressed on R-S cells in Hodgkin's lymphomas.	CD153 TRAF1,2,3,5	Non-lineage	Ber-H2, Ki-1
CD31	17q23	+	+	–	+	+	+	+	+	+	+	+	130-140	Adhesion receptor with signaling function that participates in an adhesion cascade; transendothelial migration cell-cell adhesion.	CD38	Adhesion structure	PECAM-1, endocam

CD	Alternative Name	HLDA Section	Ligand/receptor/substrate/associated molecule	Description and Function	MW (kDa)	T Cell	B Cell	Dendritic Cell	NK Cell	Stem Cell/Precursor	Macrophage/Monocyte	Granulocyte	Platelet	Erythrocyte	Endothelial Cell	Epithelial Cell	Gene Locus
CD32	FcγRII	Non-lineage	phosphatases	Regulates B cell function; major player in immune complex-induced tissue damage.	40	–	+		–		+	+	+	–	–	–	1q23
CD33	P67	Myeloid	Sugar chains	Diagnosis of acute myelogenous leukemia; negative selection for human self-regenerating hematopoietic stem cells.	67	–	–	–	–	+	+	+	–	–	–	–	19q13.3
CD34	gp 105-120	Adhesion structure	L-selectin	Cell adhesion; CD34 also expressed on embryonic fibroblasts and nervous tissue.	105-120	–	–	+	–	+	–	–	–	–	+	–	1q32
CD35	CR1, C3b/C4b receptor	Myeloid	C3b, C4b, iC3, iC4	C3b/C4b receptor; promotes phagocytosis (immune adherence); plays a major role in removal of immune complexes; regulates complement activation.	160-250	+	+	+	–	+	+	+	–	+	–	–	1q32
CD36	GpIIb, GPV	Platelet	Thrombo-spondin	Recognition and phagocytosis of apoptotic cells; involved in platelet adhesion and aggregation; cytoadherence of plasmodium falciparum-infected erythrocytes.	90	–	+	+	+	+	+	+	+	+	+	+	7q11.2
CD37	gp52-40	B	CD53,CD81, CD82,MHC II	Involved in signal transduction.	40-52/40-52	+	+				+	+		–			19p13-q13.4
CD38	ADP-ribosyl cyclase, T10	B	ADP/ATP	Regulates cell activation and proliferation; involved in lymphocyte and endothelial cell adhesion.	45/45	+	+	+	+	+	+	–				+	4p15
CD39	None	B	ADP/ATP	May protect cells from lytic effects of extracellular ATP.	80/80	⊕	+	+	+	+	+					+	10q24
CD40	Bp50	B	CD40L	Involved in B-cell growth, differentiation and isotype switching; potent rescue signal from apoptosis; promotes cytokine production.	85/48	–	+	+	+	+	+	–	–	–	+	+	20q12-q13.2
CD41	GPIIb, αIIb integrin	Platelet	Fg, Fn, vWF	CD41/CD61 complex plays a central role in platelet activation and aggregation.	135/120,23	–	–	–	–	+	–	–	+	–	–	–	17q21.32
CD42a	GPIX	Platelet	vWF, Thrombin	Forms complex with GPIbα, GPIbβ and GPV, which binds to vWF and thrombin.	22/17-22	–	–	–	–	+	–	–	+	–	–	–	3q21
CD42b	GPIbα	Platelet	vWF, Thrombin	Forms complex with GPIX, GPIbβ and GPV, which binds to vWF and thrombin.	160/145	–	–	–	–	+	–	–	+	–	–	–	17pter-p12
CD42c	GPIbβ	Platelet	vWF, Thrombin	Forms complex with GPIX, GPIbα and GPV, which binds to vWF and thrombin.	160/24	–	–	–	–	+	–	–	+	–	–	–	22q11.21
CD42d	GPV	Platelet	vWF, Thrombin	Forms complex with GPIX, GPIbα and GPIbβ, which binds to vWF and thrombin.	82/82	–	–	–	–	+	–	–	+	–	–	–	3
CD43	Sialophorin, leukosialin	Non-lineage	Hyaluronan	Anti-adhesion molecules mediates repulsion between leukocytes and other cells; under some circumstances it may act as an adhesion molecule.	95-135/95-135	+	–	+	+	+	+	+	+	–	–	–	16p11.2
CD44	ECMRII, H-CAM,Pgp-1	Adhesion structure	Hyaluronan	An adhesion molecule in lymphocyte-endothelial cell interaction; a differentiation antigen during lymphopoiesis; a potential marker of malignancy and metastasis.	85/–	+	+	+	+	+	+	+	–	+	–	+	11p13
CD44R	CD44v, CD44v9	Adhesion structure	Hyaluronan	Involved in adhesion of leukocytes and endothelial cells; leukocyte homing.	85-200/–	–	–	–	–	+	⊕	+	–	+	+	+	11p13
CD45	LCA, T200	Non-lineage	p56ˡᶜᵏ, p59ᶠʸⁿ, Src kinases	Critical requirement for TCR and BCR mediated activation; possible requirement for receptor-mediated activation in other leukocytes.	180-220/–	+	+	+	+	+	+	+	–	–	–	–	1q31-q32
CD45RA		Non-lineage	p56ˡᶜᵏ, p59ᶠʸⁿ, Src kinases	Critical requirement for TCR and BCR mediated activation; expressed on resting/naive T cells; possible requirement for receptor-mediated activation in other leukocytes.	220	+	+	+	+	+	+	–	–	–	–	–	1q31-q32
CD45RB		Non-lineage	p56ˡᶜᵏ, p59ᶠʸⁿ, Src kinases	Critical requirement for TCR and BCR mediated activation; possible requirement for receptor-mediated activation in other leukocytes.	220	+	+	+	+	+	+	+	–	+	–	–	1q31-q32

CD	Location	MW (kDa)	Function	Ligand / Association	Lineage	Other names
CD45RC	1q31-q32	220	Critical requirement for TCR and BCR mediated activation; possible requirement for receptor-mediated activation in other leukocytes.	$p56^{lck}$, $p59^{fyn}$, Src kinases	Non-lineage	
CD45RO	1q31-q32	180	Critical requirement for TCR and BCR mediated activation; expressed on activated/memory T cells; possible requirement for receptor-mediated activation in other leukocytes.	$p56^{lck}$, $p59^{fyn}$ Src kinases	Non-lineage	UCHL-1
CD46	1q32	52-58/64-68	Co-factor for factor I proteolytic cleavage of C3b and C4b.	SCR	Non-lineage	MCP
CD47	3q13.1-q13.2	45-60/50-55	Adhesion molecule; thrombospondin receptor.	SIRP	Adhesion structure	gp42, IAP, OA3
CD47R	3q13.1-q13.2	120/-	CDw149 mAbs actually recognized with low affinity the CD47 glycoprotein.	SCR	Non-lineage	MEM-133
CD48	1q21.3-q22	45/45	Adhesion molecule; acts as an accessory molecule for γ/δ T-cell recognition; as predicted for α/β T-cell antigen recognition.	CD2, lck, fyn	Non-lineage	Blast-1, Hu lym3
CD49a	5	200/200	Adhesion receptor.	Collagen, Laminin-1	Adhesion structure	VLA-1α, α1 integrin
CD49b	5q23-31	150/160	Adhesion molecule.	Collagen, Laminin	Adhesion structure	VLA-2α, GPIa
CD49c	17q21.31	145-150/125,30	Component of adhesion receptor; associates with TM4 family of protein; may be involved in signal transduction.	laminin-5, Fn, Collagen	Adhesion structure	VLA-3α, α3 integrin
CD49d	2q31-q32	145/150	Cell adhesion; lymphocyte migration; tethering or rolling and homing of T cells.	CD106, MAdCAM	Adhesion structure	VLA-4α, α4 integrin
CD49e	12q11-q13	160/135,25	Adhesion molecule.	Fibronectin, Invasin	Adhesion structure	VLA-5α, α5 integrin
CD49f	2p14-q14.3	150/125	Component of adhesion receptor; CD49f/CD29-mediated T cell binding to laminin receptor provides a co-stimulatory signal to T cells for activation and proliferation.	Laminins, invasin	Adhesion structure	VLA-6α, α6 integrin, gplc
CD50	19p13.3-p13.2	110-140/-	Co-stimulatory molecule; regulates LFA-1/ICAM-1 and integrin-β1-dependent pathways adhesion; soluble form can be detected in the blood.	LFA-1, Integrin αd/β2	Adhesion structure	ICAM-3
CD51	2q31-q32	150/124,24	Involved in cell adhesion and signal transduction; role in bone metabolism and apoptosis; possible role in infection.	Arg-Gly-Asp	Platelet	Integrin αv, VNR-α
CD52	1p36	25-29/25-29	CD52 antibodies are remarkably lytic for target cells, both with human complement and by antibody-dependent cellular cytotoxicity.		Non-lineage	CAMPATH-1, HE5
CD53	1p31-p12	32-42/-	Signal transduction; CD53 cross-linking promotes activation of B cells.	VLA-4, HLA-DR	Non-lineage	
CD54	19p13.3-p13.2	90/95	Involved in immune reaction and/or inflammation; receptor for Rhinovirus or RBCs infected with malarial parasite; soluble form can be detected in the blood.	LFA-1, Mac-1, Rhinovirus	Adhesion structure	ICAM-1
CD55	1q32	55-70/80	Complement regulation by decay acceleration; ligand or protective molecule in fertilization; involved in signal transduction; soluble form can be detected in plasma and body fluid.	SCR, CD97	Non-lineage	DAF
CD56	11q23-q24	140	Homophilic and heterophilic adhesion.	NCAM, Heparin sulfate	NK	Leu-19, NKH-1, NCAM
CD57		110-115	Cell-cell adhesion.	L-selectin, P-selectin, Laminin	NK	HNK1, Leu-7
CD58	1p13	55-70	Mediates adhesion between killer and target cells, antigen presenting cells and T cells; activation of killer cells; co-stimulatory molecule.	CD2	Adhesion structure	LFA-3
CD59	11p13	18-25	Associates with C9, inhibiting incorporation into C5b-8 preventing the completion of MAC formation.	C8-α, C9, lck, fyn	Non-lineage	1F5Ag, H19

CD	Gene Locus	Epithelial Cell	Endothelial Cell	Erythrocyte	Platelet	Granulocyte	Macrophage/Monocyte	Stem Cell/Precursor	NK Cell	Dendritic Cell	B Cell	T Cell	MW (kda)	Description and Function	Ligand/receptor/substrate/associated molecule	HLDA Section	Alternative Name	CD
CD60a		−		−	+	+	+				+	+		Induces mitochondrial permeability transition during apoptosis; marker for malignant melanomas.		Carbohydrate and Lectin	GD3	CD60a
CD60b		+				+	+	+			+	+	90-94/120	mAbs immunoreactive to CD60b have co-mitogenic activity of synovial T lymphocytes; also observed on some breast carcinomas and melanomas.	9-0-acetyl-GD3	Carbohydrate and Lectin	9-0-acetyl GD3	CD60b
CD60c						+	+				+	+		T cell activation receptor; T cell activation by CD60c does not require co-stimulatory signals.	7-0-acetyl GD3	Carbohydrate and Lectin	7-0-acetyl GD3	CD60c
CD61	17q21.32		+		+		+						90-110	CD41/61 mediates attachment of cells to diverse matrix proteins.	fibrinogen	Platelet	GP IIIa, β3 integrin	CD61
CD62E	1q22-q25		+										115	Mediates leukocyte rolling on activated endothelium at inflammatory sites; may support cell adhesion during hematogenous metastasis and play a role in angiogenesis.	(CD15s)	Adhesion structure	E-selectin	CD62E
CD62L	1q23-q25					+			+		+	+	74	Mediates lymphocyte homing to high endothelial venules or peripheral lymphoid tissue and leukocyte rolling on activated endothelium at inflammatory sites.	CD34, GlyCAM-1,M	Adhesion structure	L-selectin	CD62L
CD62P	1q22-q25		+		+	+	+	−		+			120	Interaction of CD62P and CD162 mediates tethering and rolling of leukocytes on the surface of activated endothelial cells; mediates rolling of platelets on endothelial cells.	CD162, CD24	Platelet	P-selectin, GMP-140	CD62P
CD63	12-q12-q13	−	−	−	−	+	+		−	+	−	−	40-60	CD63 gene may play a role in tumor suppression; expression of CD63 in melanoma cells reduces metastasis.	VLA-3, VLA-6, CD81	Platelet	LIMP, MLA1, gp55	CD63
CD64	1q21.2-q21.3	−	−	−	−	+	+	+	−	+	−	−	72	Receptor-mediated endocytosis of IgG-antigen complexes; antigen capture for presentation to T cells. ADCC.	IgG	Myeloid	FCRI	CD64
CD65														Function unknown.	E-selectin	Myeloid	Ceramide, VIM-2	CD65
CD65s				−		+	+		−		−	−		VIM2 antibody has been described to inhibit phagocytosis and to induce phagocyte calcium flux and oxidative burst.	Possibly E- or P-selectin	Myeloid	Sialylated-CD65, VIM2	CD65s
CD66a	19q13.2	+		−		+	+		−		−	−	140-180	Homophilic and heterophilic adhesion; E-selectin binding; capable of activating granulocytes; functions as a receptor for Neisseria gonorrhea.		Myeloid	NCA-160, BGP	CD66a
CD66b	19q13.2					+							95-100	Capable of heterophilic adhesion and transmembrane signaling; capable of activating neutrophils.		Myeloid	CD67, CGM6, NCA-95	CD66b
CD66c	19q13.2	+		−		+	+						90	Homophilic and heterophilic adhesion, E-selectin binding; capable of activating granulocytes; functions as a receptor for Neisseria gonorrhea.		Myeloid	NCA, NCA-50/90	CD66c
CD66d	19q13.2					+							35	Capable of activating granulocytes. Functions as a receptor for Neisseria gonorrhea.		Myeloid	CGM1	CD66d
CD66e	19q13.2-q13.2	+											180-200	Homophilic and heterophilic adhesion.		Myeloid	CEA	CD66e
CD66f	19q13.2	+		−	−								54-72	Unclear, may be involved in immune regulation and regulation and protection of fetus from maternal immune system; necessary for successful pregnancy.		Myeloid	SP-1, PSG	CD66f
CD68	17p13			−		+c	+c	+c		+c	+c	+c	110	Lysosomal membrane glycoprotein (LAMP 1 group); possible receptor.	LDL	Myeloid	gp110, macrosialin	CD68
CD69	12p13-p12				+	⊕	⊕		⊕	⊕	⊕	⊕	60	Involved in lymphocyte, monocyte and platelet activation.		NK	AIM, EA 1, MLR3, gp34/28	CD69
CD70	19p13	−	−	−	−	−			−	−	⊕	⊕	55-170	Co-stimulation of T and/or B cells; enhances the proliferation of cytotoxic T cells and cytokine production. Co-stimulates B cell proliferation and Ig production.	CD27	Non-lineage	Ki-24	CD70

CD	Other names	Non-lineage	Ligand	Function	MW (kDa)	Chromosome
CD71	T9, Transferrin receptor	—	Transferrin	Controls the supply of iron uptake during proliferation.	190	3q26.2-qter
CD72	Ly-19.2, Ly-32.2, Lyb-2	B	CD5	Plays a role in downregulation of signaling through the BCR on B cells as a regulator of signaling thresholds.	43/39	9p
CD73	Ecto-5-nucleotidase	B	AMP	Hydrolyzes adenosine monophosphate into adenosine; can mediate co-stimulatory signals in T cell activation.	69-72	6q14-q21
CD74	invariant chain	B	HLA-DR, CD44	Intracellular sorting of MHC class II molecules; also known as Class II specific chaperone Ii.	41	5q32
CD75	sialo-masked lactosamine	Carbohydrate and Lectin		CD75 is newly clustered including CDw75 and CDw76. CDw76 has been deleted.		
CD75s	a2,6 sialylated lactosamine	Carbohydrate and Lectin	CD22 (proposed)	May be involved in regulation of CD95-mediated apoptosis and may be important for infection by a lymphotropic virus.		
CD77	Pk antigen/ BLA/CTH/Gb3	B	Receptor for Shiga toxin	Cross-linking of CD77 induces apoptosis in Burkitt's lymphoma cells.	1	
CD79a	Ig α/MB1	B	Ig/CD5/CD19/ CD22/CD79b	Transmits signals into cytoplasm upon antigen-binding to surface Igs.	-/40-45	19q13.2
CD79b	Ig β/B29, BCR	B	Ig/CD5/CD19/ CD22/CD79a	B cell antigen receptor (BCR) mediates the response of B cells to foreign antigens and determines the fate of B cell during development and differentiation.	-/37	17q23
CD80	B7-1/BB1	B	CD28/CD152 (CTLA-4)	Co-regulation of T-cell activation with CD86.	60/-	3q13.3-q21
CD81	TAPA-1	B	Leu-13/ CD19/CD21	Member of CD19/CD21/Leu-13 signal transduction complex. #Only on eosinophils, not neutrophils.	26/-	11p15
CD82	4F9/C33/IA4/ KAI1/R2	B		Signal transduction. #Also associates with MHC class I & II, β1 integrins, CD4 and CD8.	45-90/-	11p11.2
CD83	HB15	B	Unknown	Function unknown.	-/43	6p23
CD84	None	B	Unknown	Function unknown, some indication that it may be a signaling molecule.	68-80	1q24
CD85a*	ILT5/LIR3/HL9	Dendritic cell	HLA class I	Contains ITIM sequences in cytoplasmic tail; involved in the suppression of NK-mediated cytotoxicity.		19q13.4
CD85b*	ILT8	NK	FcRγ	Involved with activation of NK-mediated cytotoxicity.		19q13.4
CD85c*	LIR8	NK	FcRγ	Involved with activation of NK-mediated cytotoxicity.		19q13.4
CD85d*	ILT4/LIR2/ MIR10	Dendritic cell	HLA class I	Contains ITIM sequences in cytoplasmic tail; involved in the suppression of NK-mediated cytotoxicity.	110	19q13.4
CD85e*	ILT6/LIR4	NK	FcRγ	Involved with activation of NK-mediated cytotoxicity.		19q13.4
CD85f*	ILT11	NK	FcRγ	Involved with activation of NK-mediated cytotoxicity. Mainly expressed on PBL.		19q13.4
CD85g*	ILT7	NK	FcRγ	Involved with activation of NK-mediated cytotoxicity.		19q13.4
CD85h*	ILT1/LIR7	NK	FcRγ	Involved with activation of NK-mediated cytotoxicity. Expressed on myeloid cells and some NK cells.		19q13.4
CD85i*	LIR6a	NK	FcRγ	Involved with activation of NK-mediated cytotoxicity.		19q13.4

CD	Alternative Name	HLDA 7 Section	Ligand/receptor/substrate/associated molecule	Description and Function	MW (kDa)	T Cell	B Cell	Dendritic Cell	NK Cell	Stem Cell/Precursor	Macrophage/Monocyte	Granulocyte	Platelet	Erythrocyte	Endothelial Cell	Epithelial Cell	Gene Locus	CD
CD85j*	ILT2/LIR1/MIR7	Dendritic cell	HLA class I	Contains ITIM sequences in cytoplasmic tail; involved in the suppression of NK-mediated cytotoxicity.	110	+	+	+	+	–	+	+	–	–	–	–	19q13.4	CD85j*
CD85k*	ILT3/LIR5/HM18	Dendritic cell	HLA class I	Ligation of CD85K induces an inhibitory signal via recruitment of SHP-1 phosphatase.	60	–	–	+	–	+	+	+	–	–	–	–	19q13.4	CD85k*
CD85l*	ILT9	NK	FcRγ	Binds FcRγ.													19q13.4	CD85l*
CD85m*	ILT10	NK	FcRγ	Binds FcRγ.													19q13.4	CD85m*
CD86	B7-2/B70	B	CD28/CD152 (CTLA-4)	Co-regulator of T cell activation with CD80.	-/80	⊕	⊕	+	–	–	+	–	–	–	+	–	3q21	CD86
CD87	uPAR	Myeloid	uPA/Pro-uPA/Vitronectin	CD87 serves as the cellular receptor for pro-uPA and uPA.	35-68/32-66	+	–	+	+	–	+	+	–	–	+	+	19q13	CD87
CD88	C5aR	Myeloid	C5a/C5a(desArg)	C5a-mediated inflammation; activation of granulocytes.	43/-	–	–	+	–	–	+	+	–	–	+	+	19q13.3-q13.4	CD88
CD89	IgA FC receptor	Myeloid	IgA1/IgA2	Induces phagocytosis, degranulation, respiratory burst and the killing of microorganisms.	45-100/45-100	–	–	–	–	–	+	+	–	–	–	–	19q13.2-q13.4	CD89
CD90	Thy-1	Endothelial cell	CD45/lck/fyn/P100	May contribute to lymphocyte co-stimulation, inhibition of stem cell proliferation/differentiation and neuron memory formation.	25-35/25-35	–	–	–	–	+	–	–	–	–	+	–	11q22.3-q23	CD90
CD91	ALPHA2M-R/LRP	Myeloid	ALPHA2M/LDLs	Endocytosis-mediating receptor expressed in coated pits. #Expressed on erythroblast/reticulocytes.	600/-	–	–	–	–	+#	+	–	–	–	–	+	12q13-q14	CD91
CD92	None	Myeloid	Unknown	Function unknown.	70/70	+	+	–	–	–	+	+	–	–	+	+		CD92
CDw93	None	Myeloid	Unknown	Function unknown.	110/120	–	–	–	–	–	+	+	–	–	+	–		CDw93
CD94	Kp43	NK	HLA class I	Assembled with other C-type lectins (NKG2) forms inhibitory or activating receptors for HLA class I.	70,30	+	–	–	+	–	+	–	–	–	–	–	12q13	CD94
CD95	APO-1, FAS, TNFRSF6	Cytokine Receptor	Fas ligand	Receptor molecule for Fas ligand, which mediates apoptosis-inducing signals.	45,90,200/45	+	+	–	+	–	+	+	–	–	–	+	10q24.1	CD95
CD96	TACTILE	NK		Adhesion of activated T and NK cells during the late phase of immune response; Weakly expressed by peripheral resting NK or T cells, upregulated after activation.	160/-	⊕	–		⊕		–							CD96
CD97	None	Non-lineage	CD55	Member of the EGF-TM7 family; Weakly expressed on resting lymphocytes, upregulated by activation.	/28, 75-85	⊕	⊕	+	⊕	–	+	+	–	–	+	–	19p13.2-p13.12	CD97
CD98	4F2, FRP-1, RL-388	Non-lineage	actin	Possible amino acid transporter; broad reactivity on activated and transformed cells, not hematopoietic specific, and found at lower levels on quiescent cells.	125/80,45	+	+	–	+	–	+	+	–	–	+	+	11q13	CD98
CD99	MIC2, E2	T		Modulates T-cell adhesion; induces apoptosis of double-positive thymocytes; expressed on all hemological cells and present on many other cell types.	32/32	+	+	–	+	–	+	–	+	+	+	+	Xp22.32, Yp11.3	CD99
CD99R	CD99 Mab restricted	T		Modulates T-cell adhesion; induces apoptosis of double-positive thymocytes.	32/32	+	–	–	+	–	+	+	–	–	+	+	9q22-q31	CD99R
CD100	SEMA4D	Non-lineage	CD45, serine kinase	Co-stimulatory molecule for T-cells; increases PMA, CD3 and CD2 induced T cell proliferation; Soluble form is 120kd.	300/150	+	+	–	+	–	+	+	–	–	–	–	9q22-q31	CD100

AV

CD	Other names	Category	Ligand / Associated	Function	MW	Location
CD101	IGSF2, P126, V7	Myeloid		Co-stimulatory molecule; antibodies against CD101 inhibit allogenic T-cell responses and co-stimulate T-cell proliferation with suboptimal anti-CD3 activation.	240/120	1p13
CD102	ICAM-2	Adhesion structure	LFA-1, CD11b/CD18	Provides co-stimulatory signal in immune response; lymphocyte recirculation; expressed on some resting lymphocytes.	55-65/	17q23-q25
CD103	HML-1, Integrin αE	Adhesion structure	E-cadherin; Integrin β7	Expressed on intestinal intraepithelial lymphocytes, lamina propria T cells in intestine; stimulation of PBL with PHA induce CD103 expression.	175/150,25	17p13
CD104	β4 Integrin chain, TSP-180	Adhesion structure	laminins(I,II, IV,V), CD49f	Hemidesmosomal CD49f/CD104 ($\alpha6\beta4$ integrin) plays an important role in the adhesion of epithelia to basement membranes. #CD4-CD8- pre-T cells.	205/220	17q11-qter
CD105	Endoglin	Endothelial cell	TGF-β 1, TGF-β 3	Regulatory component of the TGF β receptor complex; modulator of cellular responses to TGF-1 β.	180/90	9q33-q34.1
CD106	VCAM-1, INCAM-110	Endothelial cell	integrin α4β 1	Leukocyte adhesion, transmigration and co-stimulation of T-cell proliferation; expressed on activated endothelial cells, follicular dendritic cells, and certain tissue macrophages. #	110/110	1p32-p31
CD107a	LAMP-1	Platelet		Possible role in cell adhesion; highly metastatic tumor cells express more LAMP molecules on the cell surface than poorly metastatic cells; expressed on lysosomal membrane.	100/120	13q34
CD107b	LAMP-2	Platelet		Possible role in cell adhesion; highly metastatic tumor cells express more LAMP molecules on the cell surface than poorly metastatic cells; expressed on lysosomal membrane.	100/120	Xq24
CD108	SEMA7A, JMH	Non-lineage	CD232	Function unknown; carries JMH blood group antigen; expressed at low levels on circulating lymphocytes, at moderately high levels by lymphoblasts and lymphoblastic cell lines.	76/80	15q22.3-q23
CD109	8A3, 7D1, E123	Endothelial cell		Function unknown.	170/170	
CD110	TPO-R, MPL, C-MPL	Platelet	TPO	Receptor for TPO. Receptor binding results in the prevention of apoptosis, stimulation of cell growth and differentiation of megakaryocyte and platelet formation.	82-92/	1p34
CD111	HveCPRR1, PVRL1, Nectin1	Myeloid	gD, nectin3, Afadin	Intercellular adhesion molecule; involved in epithelial cell physiology; pan-alphaherpes virus entry receptor.	~75	11q23-q24
CD112	HveB,PRR2, PVRL2,Nectin2	Myeloid	PRR3, Afadin	Homophilic adhesion receptor that could play a role in the regulation of hematopoietic/endothelial cell functions; involved in cell to cell spreading of viruses.	72,64/72,64	19q13.2-13.4
CD114	CSF3R,G-CSFR, HG-CSF	Myeloid	G-CSF, Jak1, Jak2	Regulates myeloid proliferation and differentiation.	130	1p35-p34.3
CD115	c-fms, CSF-1R, M-CSFR	Myeloid	CSF-1	Receptor for CSF-1 (macrophage colony stimulating factor); mediates all of the biological effects of this cytokine.	150	5q33.2-33.3
CD116	GM-CSFRα	CK/CKR	GM-CSF	Primary binding subunit of GM-CSF with low affinity and binds it with high affinity when it is coexpressed with the common beta subunit CDw131.	80	Xp22.32 or Yp11.3
CD117	c-KIT SCRF	CK/CKR	SCF, MGF, KL	Growth factor receptor, tyrosine kinase.	145	4q11-q12
CDw119	IFNγR, IFNγRa	CK/CKR	IFNγ	Interferon γ binding.	80-95	6q23-q24
CD120a	TNFRI, p55	CK/CKR	TNF,TRADD, TRAF,RIP,LTa	Programmed cell death anti-viral activity; receptor for TNF.	55	12p13.2
CD120b	TNFRII, p75, TNFR p80	CK/CKR	TNF,TRADD, TRAF,RIP,LTa	Programmed cell death anti-viral activity; receptor for TNF.	75	1p36.3-p36.2
CD121a	IL-1R type 1	CK/CKR	Il-1α and Il-1β	IL-1 signaling.	75-85/75-85	2q12
CD121b	IL-1R type 2	CK/CKR	IL-1β,IL-1Rα, IL-1α	Negative regulator of IL-1.	60-68/60-68	2q12-q22
CD122	IL2Rβ	CK/CKR	IL-2, IL-15, (CD25,CD132)	Critical component of IL-2 and IL-15-mediated signaling.	70-75/	22q13.1

CD	Alternative Name	HLDA Section	Ligand/receptor/substrate/associated molecule	Description and Function	MW (kDa)	T Cell	B Cell	Dendritic Cell	NK Cell	Stem Cell/Precursor	Macrophage/Monocyte	Granulocyte	Platelet	Erythrocyte	Endothelial Cell	Epithelial Cell	Gene Locus	CD
CD123	IL-3Rα subunit	CK/CKR	IL-3	Primary low affinity binding subunit of IL-3 receptor.	70	−	−	+	−	+	+	+	−	−	+		Xp22.3 or Yp11.3	CD123
CD124	IL-4R	CK/CKR	IL-4, IL-13	Receptor subunit for IL-4 and IL-13; #expression on B cells is up-regulated by LPS, anti-IgM or IL-4; #on T cells is increased by stimulation with ConA or IL-4.	140/-	⊕#	⊕#	−	−		+	+	−	−	−		16p11.2-12.1	CD124
CD125	IL-5Rα	CK/CKR	IL-5	Low affinity receptor for IL-5; alpha chain of IL-5 receptor; expressed on eosinophils and basophils.	60/-	−	⊕		−		−	+	−	−	−		3p26-p24	CD125
CD126	IL-6R	CK/CKR	IL-6	Required, in association with gp130(CD130), for mediating biological activities of interleukin-6; expressed on hepatocytes and some non-hematopoietic cells.	80/80	+	⊕		−		+	−	−	−	−		1q21	CD126
CD127	IL-7Rα	CK/CKR	IL-7, CD132, fyn,lyn,Jak1	Specific receptor for IL-7; expression down-regulated following T cell activation.	65-90/-	+	+			+							5p13	CD127
CD128a	IL-8RA, CXCR1	CK/CKR	IL-8	Critical regulators of IL-8 mediated neutrophil chemotaxis and activation; potential role in angiogenesis.	44-59/67-70	+	−		+	−	+	+	+		+		2q35	CD128a
CD128b	IL-8RB, CXCR2	CK/CKR	IL-8	Critical regulators of IL-8 mediated neutrophil chemotaxis and activation; potential role in angiogenesis.	44-59/67-70	+	−		+	−	−	+	+		+		2q35	CD128b
CD130	gp130	CK/CKR	Oncostatin M	Required for transducing biological activities of IL-6, IL-11, LIF, ciliary neutrophilic factor, oncostatin M, and cardiotrophin-1.	130-140/130-140	+	+	−	+	+	+	+	+	−	+		5q11	CD130
CD131	Common beta subunit	CK/CKR	CD123, CD125,CD116	Key signal transducing molecule of the IL-3, GM-CSF and IL-5 receptors; expressed on early B cells and early progenitors.	120-140/-	−	−		−	+	+	+					22q13.1	CD131
CD132	IL-2Rγ	CK/CKR	IL-12	Common subunit of IL-2, IL-4, IL-7, IL-9, IL-15 receptors; mutation causes X-linked severe combined immunodeficiency (XSCID).	65-70/-	+	+		+	+	+	+	+	−	+		Xq13.1	CD132
CD133	AC133	Stem Cell	N/A	Used for positive selection of hematopoietic stem and progenitor cells for transplantation studies.	120	−	−	−	−	+	−	−	−	−	+	+	4p16.2	CD133
CD134	OX40	CK/CKR	OX40 ligand	Receptor for OX40 ligand; co-stimulatory signal transducer of T-cell receptor-mediated activation, cell adhesion.	48-50/-	⊕	−	−			−	+					1p36	CD134
CD135	Flt3, FLK2, STK1	CK/CKR	FL	Receptor tyrosine kinase; co-stimulatory molecule; survival receptor; growth factor receptor for early hematopoietic progenitors.	130/155-160	−	−			+				−			13q12	CD135
CDw136	MSP-R, RON	CK/CKR	MSP, HGFl	Chemotactic migration, morphological change, cell growth, cytokine induction, phagocytosis, and cell differentiation.	180/150,40	⊕					+					+	13p21.3	CDw136
CDw137	4-1BB, ILA	CK/CKR	4-1BB ligand	Receptor for 4-1BB ligand; co-stimulatory molecule.	85/39	⊕	+		−		+	+				+	1p36	CDw137
CD138	Syndecan1	B		Extracellular matrix receptor; co-receptor for fibroblast growth factor signaling receptors; #expressed on plasma cells.	-/165-150	−	+#		−		+	+	−	−	+	+	2p24.1	CD138
CD139	None	B		Function unknown.	209/228	−	+	+	−	+	+	+	+	+				CD139
CD140a	PDGF a receptor	Endothelial Cell	PDGF	Involved in signal transduction associated with PDGF receptors; expressed on mesenchymal cells.	160,180/-	−			−		−	−	+	+	+		4q11-q13	CD140a
CD140b	PDGF B receptor	Endothelial Cell	PDGF	Involved in signal transduction associated with PDGF receptors; expressed on mesenchymal cells.	160,180/-	−	−		−	+	+	+	+	−	+		5q31-q32	CD140b
CD141	Thrombomodulin	Endothelial Cell	Thrombin, protein C	Critical for activation of protein C and initiation of the protein C anticoagulant pathway; co-factor in the thrombin-mediated activation of protein C.	75/105	−	−		−	+	+	+	+	−	+	+	20p12-cen	CD141

CD	Other names	Lineage	Ligand	Function	MW												Chromosome	CD
CD142	Tissue factor	Endothelial Cell	Factor VIIIa, Factor Xa/TFPI	Initiator of the blood clotting cascade; cell surface receptor/cofactor for factor VII; can be induced by inflammory mediators.	45-47/ 45-47	−	−		−		−	−	−		+	+	1p22-p21	**CD142**
CD143	ACE	Endothelial Cell	ANG-1, Bradykinin	Angiotensin-converting enzyme, peptidyl dipeptidase, is necessary for spermatozoa to bind to eggs.	90,170/ 90,170	+	−		−		−	−	−	−	+	+	17q2	**CD143**
CD144	VE-cadherin, Cadherin-5	Endothelial Cell	β-catenin, p120 CAS	Controls endothelial permeability, growth, migration and contact inhibition of cell growth; expressed only on endothelial cells.	135/ 130	−	−	−	−		−	−	−	−	+	−		**CD144**
CDw145	None	Endothelial Cell		Highly expressed on endothelial cells; antibodies were originally raised against human urinary bladder carcinoma cells.	25,90, 110				−		−	−	−	−	+			**CDw145**
CD146	Muc 18 S-endo	Endothelial Cell		Potential adhesion molecule; expressed by melanoma, smooth muscle and intermediate trophoblasts.	118/ 130	⊕	−		−		−	−	−	−	+		11q23.3	**CD146**
CD147	Neurothelin, OX-47	Endothelial Cell		Potential adhesion molecule; involved in regulation of T cell function	50-60/ 55-95	+	+		+		+	+	+	+	+		19p13.3	**CD147**
CD148	HPTPn, p260 DEP-1	Non-lineage		HPTP-etc/Dep-1 involved in contact inhibition of cell growth; chromosomal location region frequently detailed in carcinomas	200-260/ 200-260	+		+			+	+	+		+		11p11.2	**CD148**
CD150	SLAM-1, IPO-3	Non-lineage	Tyrosine phosphatase CD45	An important molecule associated with intracellular adaptor protein SAP. Absence of SAP causes X-linked lymphoproliferative disease.	65-85/ 75-95	+	+	+	−		−	−	−	−	+		1q22-q23	**CD150**
CD151	PETA-3	Platelet	β1 integrins	Integrin-associated protein; transmembrane signaling.	32/-	−	−	−		+	−	−	+		+	+	11p15.5	**CD151**
CD152	CTLA-4	T		Receptor for CD80/CD86. Negative regulator of T-cell activation.	50/33	⊕	⊕	−	−		−	−	−				2q33	**CD152**
CD153	CD30L	T	CD30	Co-stimulatory signal for peripheral blood T cells.	40	+		−			⊕	+					9q33	**CD153**
CD154	CD40L, gp39, TRAP-1, T-BAH	T	ligand for CD40	Essential for germinal center formation and antibody class switching; co-stimulatory molecule; regulator of TH1 generation and function.	33	⊕	−	−	−		−			−	−		Xq26	**CD154**
CD155	PVR	Myeloid	Polio virus receptor	Possible interaction with CD44.	60-90			−			+		−				19q13.2	**CD155**
CD156a	CD156, ADAM8, MS2	Myeloid	Myeloid	Possible involvement in extravasation of leukocytes.	-/69						+	+					10q26.3	**CD156a**
CD156b	TACE, ADAM17	Adhesion structure	pro-TNF, pro-TGFα, MAD2	Cleaves the transmembrane form of TNF-α to yield the soluble active form.	100-120	+	−	+	−	−	+	+	−	−	+	−	2p25	**CD156b**
CD157	Mo5, BST-1	Myeloid		A sister molecule of CD38, a type II membrane protein with identical ectoenzyme activity; a distribution complementary to that of CD38.	42-45			+		+	+	+			+			**CD157**
CD158a[†]	KIR2DL1, p58.1	NK	HLA-Cw4,2,5,6	Contains ITIM sequences in cytoplasmic tail. Involved in the suppression of NK-mediated cytotoxicity.	58/58	+			+								19q13.4	**CD158a[†]**
CD158b1[†]	KIR2DL2, p58.2	NK	HLA-3,1,7,8	Contains ITIM sequences in cytoplasmic tail. Involved in the suppression of NK-mediated cytotoxicity.	58/58	+			+								19q13.4	**CD158b1[†]**
CD158b2[†]	KIR2DL3, p58.3	NK	HLA-Cw3, 1, 7, 8	Contains ITIM sequences in cytoplasmic tail; involved in the suppression of NK-mediated cytotoxicity.	58/58	+			+								19q13.4	**CD158b2[†]**
CD158c[†]	KIR2DS6, KIRX	NK		Contains ITIM sequences in cytoplasmic tail; involved in the suppression of NK-mediated cytotoxicity.		+			+								19q13.4	**CD158c[†]**
CD158d[†]	KIR2DL4	NK		Function unknown.					+								19q13.4	**CD158d[†]**
CD158 e1/e2[†]	KIR3DL1/S1, p70	NK	HLA-Bw4	Involved in the suppression of NK-mediated cytotoxicity (KIR3DL1); expressed on subsets of NK and cytotoxic cells	70/70	+			+								19q13.4	**CD158 e1/e2[†]**
CD158f[†]	KIR2DL5	NK		Contains ITIM sequences in cytoplasmic tail; involved in the suppression of NK-mediated cytotoxicity.		+			+								19q13.4	**CD158f[†]**

AV

CD	Alternative Name	HLDA Section	Ligand/receptor/substrate/associated molecule	Description and Function	MW (kDa)	T Cell	B Cell	Dendritic Cell	NK Cell	Stem Cell/Precursor	Macrophage/Monocyte	Granulocyte	Platelet	Erythrocyte	Endothelial Cell	Epithelial Cell	Gene Locus
CD158g†	KIR2DS5	NK		Associated with KARAP/DAP12; involved in the activation of NK-mediated cytotoxicity.		+			+								19q13.4
CD158h†	KIR2DS1, p50.1	NK	HLA-C	Associated with KARAP/DAP12; involved in the activation of NK-mediated cytotoxicity.		+			+								19q13.4
CD158i†	KIR2DS4, p50.3	NK	HLA-C	Associated with KARAP/DAP12; involved in the activation of NK-mediated cytotoxicity.	50/50	+			+								19q13.4
CD158j†	KIR2DS2, p50.2	NK	HLA-C	Associated with KARAP/DAP12; involved in the activation of NK-mediated cytotoxicity.		+			+								19q13.4
CD158k†	KIR3DL2, p140	NK	HLA-A	Contains ITIM sequences in cytoplasmic tail; involved in the suppression of NK-mediated cytotoxicity.	140/70	+			+								19q13.4
CD158z†	KIR3DL7, KIRC1	NK	HLA-C	Contains ITIM sequences in cytoplasmic tail; involved in the suppression of NK-mediated cytotoxicity.		+			+								19q13.4
CD159a	NKG2A	NK	HLA-E	CD94/CD159a heterodimer constitutes a potent negative regulator of NK- and T-lymphocyte activation programs; expressed on subsets of NK and CD8+ (γδ) cells.	70/43	+			+								12p12.3-p13.1
CD160	BY55, NK1, NK28	T	MHC class I	Cross-linking CD160 with certain mAbs triggers co-stimulatory signals in CD8 T lymphocytes. CD160 is also expressed on all intestinal intraepithelial lymphocytes.	80/27	+	−		+								1q42.3
CD161	NKR-P1A	NK		NK cell cytolytic activity; Regulation of thymocyte precursor proliferation.	80/40	+	−	−	+			−	−	−	−	−	
CD162	PSGL-1	Adhesion structure	P-selectin	Binds P- and L-selectins; can mediate leukocyte rolling.	160-250/110-120	+	+			+	+	+	−	−	−		
CD162R	PEN5	NK	L-selectin	Post-translational modification of the P-selectin glycoprotein ligand-1 (CD162); Developmentally regulated marker of both immune and neural cells.	240/140				+								
CD163	M130,GHI/61, RM3/1	Myeloid		Expressed on tissue macrophages and LPS activated monocytes.	110	−	+	−			⊕	−	−	−	−	−	
CD164	MGC-24, MUC-24	Adhesion structure		Facilitating the adhesion of human CD34+ cells to stroma and by negatively regulating CD34+CD38- progenitor cell proliferation.	160/80	+	+			+	+	−		−	−	+	
CD165	Ad2, gp37	Adhesion structure		Adhesion of thymocytes to thymic epithelial cells; expressed on many T cell acute lymphoblastic leukemia (ALL).	37/42					−	+	−	+	−		+	
CD166	ALCAM, KG-CAM	Adhesion structure	binds CD6	Adhesion receptor.	100-105/100-105	⊕	+				⊕	−			+	+	
CD167a	DDR1	Adhesion structure	Collagen	Adhesion molecule, DDR1 overexpression in several human cancers suggests a function in tumor progression.	52-62	+	+	+			+					+	6p21.3
CD168	RHAMM	Adhesion structure	CD44	Involved in adhesion of early thymocyte progenitors to matrix and its interaction with HA can mediate signals to other cell adhesion molecules.	52-125	−	−	+		+	+						5q33.2
CD169	Sialoadhesin/Siglec-1	Adhesion structure	MUC1, CD206	Mediates cell-cell, cell matrix interaction; may facilitate phagocytosis.	180/200			+			+						20p13
CD170	Siglec-5	Adhesion structure	Terminal sialic acid residues	Adhesion molecule; as a pattern or self/non-self recognition receptor and mediates negative signals into the cell.	140			+				+					19q13.3
CD171	N-CAM, L1	Adhesion structure	CD56,CD24	Neuronal cell recognition molecule L1 involved in cell adhesion, cell spreading and motility. Also acts as a co-stimulatory molecule on lymphocytes.	200-230	+	+	+			+				+		Xq28

CD172	SIRP-1a	Adhesion structure	CD47	Adhesion molecule; binds to CD47 and may mediate inhibitory signals via the ITIM/SHP-2.	65			+		+	+	+					20p13	**CD172**
CD173	Blood group H type 2	Carbohydrate and Lectin		Biosynthetic precursor of A and B antigen; carcinoma-associated antigen; may be involved in the homing process of hematopoietic stem cells to the bone marrow.					−	+				+	+			**CD173**
CD174	Lewis Y	Carbohydrate and Lectin		New hematopoietic progenitor cell marker; may be involved in the homing process of hematopoietic stem cells to the bone marrow.					−	+						+		**CD174**
CD175	Tn	Carbohydrate and Lectin	TFRA	Tumor-specific antigen expressed on various carcinomas; histo-blood group-related carbohydrate antigen; precursor of the blood groups ABO and TF antigen.		−	−		−	+						+		**CD175**
CD175s	Sialyl-Tn (s-Tn)	Carbohydrate and Lectin	TFRA	Tumor-specific antigen expressed on various carcinomas; histo-blood group-related carbohydrate antigen; precursor of the blood groups ABO and TF antigen.		−	+		−	+					+	+		**CD175s**
CD176	TF Antigen	Carbohydrate and Lectin	TFRA	Pan-carcinoma antigen tumor antigen marker; may be involved in metastasis of tumor cells.	120-198		−			+				+	+	+		**CD176**
CD177	NB1, HNA-2a	Myeloid		NB antigens play a critical role in autoimmune neonatal neutropaenia and auto-immune neutropaenia; polymorphic; expressed in 89-97% of healthy individuals.	49-55/56-64							+						**CD177**
CD178	Fas Ligand	CKR	CD95(Fas)	Involved in Fas/Fas ligand interaction, apoptosis, regulates immune responses. #Expressed on immature dendritic cells.	27-40/27-40	⊕	−	+#	+		−	+	−	−	+	+	1q23	**CD178**
CD179a	VpreB	B	CD179b, μ heavy chain	Surrogate light chain VpreB is one of the components of the pre-B-cell receptor complex. #Expressed in cytoplasm of pro-B cells and on the surface of pre-B cells.	16-18/					+#							22q11.22	**CD179a**
CD179b	λ5, 14.1	B	CD179a, μ heavy chain	λ5 is one of the components of the pre-B-cell receptor complex. #Expressed in cytoplasm of pro-B cells and on the surface of pre-B cells.	-/22					+#							22q11.23	**CD179b**
CD180	RP105/Bgp95	B	LPS, MD-1	May regulate the LPS signaling in B cells in concert with TLR4; ligation of CD180 induces proliferation of B cells and increases susceptibility to BCR induced cell death.	95-105/95-105		+	+			+						5q12	**CD180**
CD183	CXCR3	CK/CKR	IP-10, Mig, I-TAC	Involved with inflammation-associated effector T-cell chemotaxis.	40-41		+	+			+						8p12-p11.2, Xq13	**CD183**
CD184	CXCR4	CK/CKR	HIV-1	Homing receptor of hematopoietic progenitor cells; co-stimulation of B cells; induces apoptosis; involved with the entry of HIV-1.		+	+	+		+	+	+	+	−	+	+	2q21	**CD184**
CD195	CCR5	CK/CKR	HIV-1	Regulates lymphocyte chemotaxis activation and transendothelial migration during inflammation. Neutralizes HIV infection. #Expressed on immature dendritic cells.	37.0/40.6	+	−	+#	−		+	+	−	−	−			**CD195**
CDw197	CCR7, EBI1, BLR2	CK/CKR	SLC/6Ckine, ELC/MIP-3b	Lymphocytes and dendritic cell homing to lymphoid organs.	90	+	+	+	+		+	+	−	−			9p13	**CDw197**
CD200	OX2	Non-lineage	OX2R	Ig-SF, OX2 shares many biochemical similarities with Thy-1; may regulate myeloid cell activity.	40-45		+	+	−	+	−	−	−	−	+			**CD200**
CD201	EPCR	Endothelial cells	Protein C	Involved in protein C activation.	49/25										+		20q11.2	**CD201**
CD202b	TEK/Tie2	Endothelial cells	Angiopoietin-1,2,and4	Involved in vascular development.	140										+		9p21	**CD202b**
CD203c	PDNP3, B10, PDIβ, E-NPP3	Myeloid	Oligo-nucleotides	Multi-functional ectoenzyme involved in the clearance of extracellular nucleotides. #Expressed on basophils, mast cells and their precursors.	270/130,150					+#		+#					6q22	**CD203c**
CD204	MSR	Myeloid	LDL	Role in deposition of cholesterol through receptor mediated uptake of LDL; recognition and elimination of pathogenic microorganisms.	220						+							**CD204**
CD205	DEC-205	Dendritic cell	Unknown	Antigen-uptake receptor for mannosylated antigens; present on both CD11c+ blood dendritic cells and in lesser density on surface of T and B cells.	198	+	+	+		+	+							**CD205**
CD206	MMR	Dendritic cell	Sialodine sins and CD45	Mediates endocytosis of glycoconjugates with terminal mannose, fucose N-acetylglucosamine or glucose residues.	162-175			+		+	+						10p13	**CD206**

AV

CD	Gene Locus	Epithelial Cell	Endothelial Cell	Erythrocyte	Platelet	Granulocyte	Macrophage/Monocyte	Stem Cell/Precursor	NK Cell	Dendritic Cell	B Cell	T Cell	MW (kDa)	Description and Function	Ligand/receptor/substrate/associated molecule	HLDA Section	Alternative Name
CD207	2p13						+	+		+				Found on a subset of cultured blood CD11c+ DC and TGF beta differentiated MoDC. Provides new reagent for characterizing Langerhans histiocytosis. Endocytic receptor with functional lectin domain with mannose specificity.		Dendritic cell	Langerin
CD208	3q26.3-q27							+		+	–			Function unknown. Possible participation in peptide loading onto MHC class II.		Dendritic cell	DC-LAMP
CD209	19p13									+	–	–	44	Expressed on MoDC but not on blood DC even after activation; contributes to the initial adhesion interaction between MoDC and naïve T lymphocytes; regulation of T cell proliferation.		Dendritic cell	DC-SIGN
CDw210	11q23.3, 21q22.11					–	–			–	–	–	90	Receptors involved with cell signaling and immune regulation.	IL-10	CK/CKR	CK
CD212	19p13.1					–	–		+		–	⊕	~110	Tyrosine kinase membrane receptor for angiopoietin; involved in cell signaling and immune regulation.	IL-12	CK/CKR	CK
CD213a	x13		+			–	+		–		–	–		Receptors involved in cell signaling and immune regulation. CD213a1, CD213a2.	IL-13	CK/CKR	CK
CDw217	2p31			+		+	+	+			+	+		Involved in inflammation, osteogenesis, and granulopoiesis.	IL-17	CK/CKR	CK
CD220	19p13.3					–	+	+	–	–	+	+		Functions in the clearance of ligands rather then intracellular signaling.	Insulin	Non-lineage	Insulin R
CD221	15q25-26			+		+	+	+	+		+	+		Functions in the clearance of ligands rather then intracellular signaling.	Insulin	Non-lineage	IGF1 R
CD222				+		–	+	+	+		+	⊕	250	Plays role in the transport of newly synthesized acid hydrolases to lysomes.	Plasminogen, M6P & IGFII	Non-lineage	M6P/IGFII-R
CD223	12p13					–	–	+	⊕	–	+	+	70	Lymphocyte activation Gene-3, like CD4, interacts with MHC class II molecules.	MHC class II	Non-lineage	LAG-3
CD224						–	+	+	–		+	+	27-68	G-glutamyl transderase; ectoenzyme; maintains intracellular glutathione (GHS) concentrations and consequently a state of oxidative homeostasis within cellular microenvironments.	GSH	Non-lineage	GGT
CD225		–	+		+	–	+	+	+	+	+	+	17	Interferon-inducible protein may play role in controlling cell to cell interactions.	IFN-γ	Non-lineage	Leu13
CD226	18q22.3					–	–	+	+	–	+	⊕	65	Adhesion molecule; cytolytic function mediated by CTL and NK cells; platelet and T cell activation antigen 1.	LFA-1	T	DNAM-1, PTA1
CD227		+	+			–	⊕	+		+	+	–	300	Involved in cell surface protection and modulation of adhesion and cell migration.	CD54, CD169	Non-lineage	MUC1
CD228						–	–				–	–	97	GPI-anchored melanoma-associated protein.		Non-lineage	p97, gp95, MT
CD229	1q22			–		–	–		+	–	+	+	100	In activated T cells, the SAP protein binds to and regulates signal transduction events initiated through the engagement of SLAM, 2B4, CD84, and Ly-9.	SAP protein	Non-lineage	Ly9
CD230				–	–	–	+	+	+	+	+	+	33-37	Isoform PrPsc (pathological) is present in Transmissible Spongiform Encephalitis (TSE).		Non-lineage	Prion Protein (PrP)
CD231			+										30-45	Highly expressed on T-cell acute lymphoblastic leukemia; can be potentially useful as an anti-tumor agent.		Non-lineage	TALLA-1/A15, TALLA

AV

CD	Alternative name	Lineage	Ligand / Other names	Mol. wt (kDa)	Chromosome	Function
CD232	VESP-R	Non-lineage	CD108	200		Receptor for CD108 and semaphorin from virus; A39R (protein of semaphorin family) upregulates ICAM-1 and induces cytokine production.
CD233	Band 3/AE1	RBC		95-105	17q12-q21	Carrier of the Diego blood group system; maintains red cell morphology; Band 3 is essential for terminal erythroid differentiation.
CD234	DARC/Fy-glycoprotein	RBC	IL-8,MGSA, RANTES,MCP-1	35-43	1q22-23	Carrier of the Duffy blood group system; binds to a number of chemokines to modulate the intensity of inflammatory reactions.
CD235a	Glycophorin A	RBC			4q28-q31	Major membrane sialoglycoprotein of RBC membrane and carrier of blood group M and N specificities.
CD235ab	Glycophorin A & B	RBC			4q28-q31	Glycophorin B is the carrier of blood group S, s, and N specificities (for Glycophorin A see CD235a)
CD236	Glycophorin C & D	RBC		30-40	2q14-q21	One of the chored protein of red blood cell skeleton that maintains cell morphology; carrier of Gerbich blood group.
CD236R	Glycophorin C, GYPC	RBC		40	2q14-q21	Plays a role in the invasion and intra-erythrocytic development of P. falciparum.
CD238	Kell	RBC	Endothelin-3	93	7q33	Kell is classified as a member of the small neprilysin (M13) family of zinc metalloproteases, which include CD10. Kell antibodies inhibit erythropoeisis.
CD239	Lu/B-CAM	RBC	Laminin	78-85	19q13.2	Carrier of the Lutheran blood group; receptor for laminin; plays role in terminal erythroid differentiation; facilitates trafficking of more mature RBC.
CD240		RBC		30	1p34.3-p36.1	CD240 includes CD240CE (RhCE), CD240D (RhD), and CD240DCE (RhD/RhCE). Rh system is one of the most polymorphic in the blood group system comprising 45 different antigens; Rh antigen may promote export of ammonium.
CD241	RhAG/Rh50	RBC		50	6p11-p21.1	Promotes export of ammonium that accumulates within erythrocytes; promotes erythrocyte-mediated retention of ammonium from the plasma and its release to detoxifying organs.
CD242	ICAM-4/LW	RBC	LFA-1,Mac-1, VLA-4	37-43	19p13.3	Carrier of LW blood group system; involved in red cell senescence; interaction with VLA-4 may stabilize erythroblastic islands in normal BM.
CD243	MDR-1	Stem/Progenitor cells		180		p-glycoprotein, drug resistance pump.
CD244	2B4, P38, NAIL	NK	CD48	70/70	1q22	Engagement of 2B4 with its ligand, CD48, or with specific antibodies enhances NK cell cytokine production and cytolytic function. #Found only on basophils.
CD245	p220/240	T	lymphocyte receptor	220-250		Signal transduction and co-stimulation of T and NK cells; function is distinct from CD45 or CD148.
CD246	ALK	T	Tyrosine kinase R	200	2p23	Expressed in T-cell lymphoma subtype; suggested role in cellular proliferation, apoptosis and embryonic neural differentiation.
CD247	Zeta Chain	T			2p23	Essential signal sub-unit of activating receptor on T and NK cells.

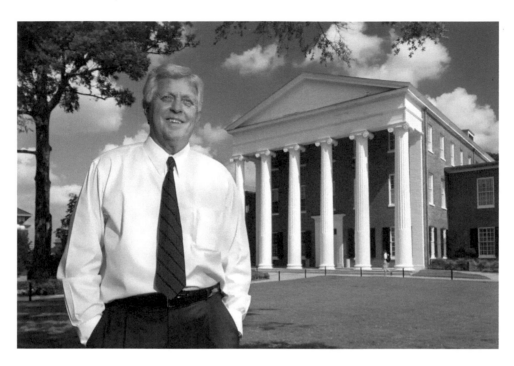

Dr. Robert C. Khayat
Chancellor, University Of Mississippi

In *Twelfth Night,* Shakespeare writes, "Be not afraid of greatness: Some are born great, some achieve greatness, and some have greatness thrust upon them." By popular consensus, Chancellor Khayat, the finest Ole Miss Chancellor since Frederick A.P. Barnard of the Civil War era, has achieved greatness by his indefatigable efforts to elevate the university's standing in the world, and had greatness thrust upon him by his eloquent responses to the obstacles of our troubled social past. He has faced every challenge with courage, conviction, and dignity to make Ole Miss respected for social justice, and academic and athletic excellence throughout America and the world.

Editorial Staff

Jeanann Lovell Suggs, M.D.–Ph.D. Candidate
Coordinating Editor

Julia C. Peteet
Copy Editor and Principal Transcriptionist

Joshua Ryan Goodin, B.S., B.S.N., R.N., H.T. (ASCP)
Contributing Editor

Will Singleterry, B.S.
Contributing Editor

Bradley J. Suggs, M.D.
Contributing Editor

G. Reid Bishop, B.S., Ph.D.
Assistant Professor of Chemistry, Mississippi College
Silicon Graphics Molecular Models
Illustrator

Rachel Webb, Ph.D.
Contributor

Taylor & Francis Editorial Staff

Barbara Ellen Norwitz
Executive Editor

Pat Roberson
Project Coordinator

Amy Rodriguez
Project Editor

Jonathan Pennell
Art Director

Scott Hayes
Prepress Manager

T - #0539 - 071024 - C818 - 279/216/36 - PB - 9780367452452 - Gloss Lamination